eat right. Academy of Nutrition and Dietetics

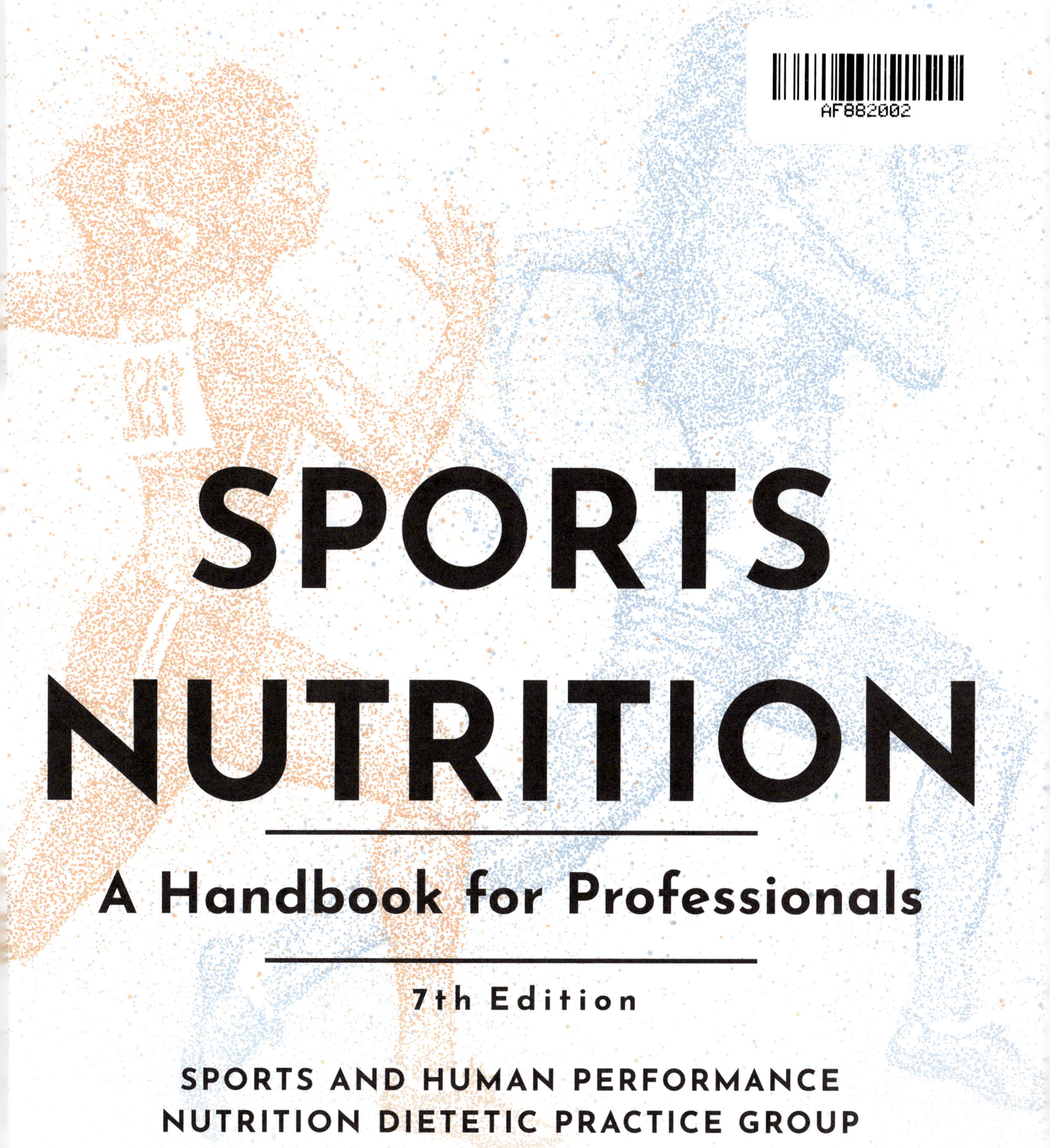

SPORTS NUTRITION

A Handbook for Professionals

7th Edition

SPORTS AND HUMAN PERFORMANCE NUTRITION DIETETIC PRACTICE GROUP

Melissa L. Brown, PhD, RD, CSSD, LD, Editor in Chief
Hope Barkoukis, PhD, RDN, LD, FAND, Assistant Editor

eat right. Academy of Nutrition and Dietetics

Sports Nutrition: A Handbook for Professionals, Seventh Edition

ISBN 978-0-88091-242-6 (print)
ISBN 978-0-88091-243-3 (eBook)
Catalog Number 411426 (print)
Catalog Number 411426e (eBook)

10 9 8 7 6 5 4 3 2 1
For more information on the Academy of Nutrition and Dietetics, visit www.eatright.org.

Library of Congress Cataloging-in-Publication Data
Names: Brown, Melissa L. (Dietitian) editor | Barkoukis, Hope editor | Academy of Nutrition and Dietetics. Sports and Human Performance Nutrition Dietetic Practice Group issuing body
Title: Sports nutrition : a handbook for professionals / Sports and Human Performance Nutrition Dietetic Practice Group ; Melissa L. Brown, PhD, RD, CSSD, LD, editor in chief ; Hope Barkoukis, PhD, RDN, LD, FAND, assistant editor.
Other titles: Sports nutrition (1986)
Description: 7th edition. | Chicago, IL : Academy of Nutrition and Dietetics, [2025] | Includes bibliographical references and index.
Identifiers: LCCN 2025023956 (print) | LCCN 2025023957 (ebook) | ISBN 9780880912426 paperback | ISBN 9780880912433 ebook
Subjects: LCSH: Athletes--Nutrition | Exercise--Physiological aspects
Classification: LCC TX361.A8 S66 2025 (print) | LCC TX361.A8 (ebook)
LC record available at https://lccn.loc.gov/2025023956
LC ebook record available at https://lccn.loc.gov/2025023957

"Success is no accident. It is hard work, perseverance, learning, studying, sacrifice, and most of all, love of what you are doing or learning to do."

—Pelé (Edson Arantes do Nascímento)
Brazilian professional soccer star
Recipient of the International Peace Award, 1978
Athlete of the Century, L'Equipe, 1980
Athlete of the Century, International Olympic Committee, 1980

Contents

Contributors

Elizabeth L. Abbey, PhD, RDN, CDN
Professor and Chair, Undergraduate Department of Health Sciences, Whitworth University
Spokane, WA

Roberta Anding, MS, RDN/LD, CSSD, CDCES, FAND
Director of Performance Nutrition,
Lecturer, Kinesiology Department
Rice University
Houston, TX

Hope Barkoukis, PhD, RDN, LD, FAND
Chair, Department of Nutrition, School of Medicine, Case Western Reserve University
Cleveland, OH

Nicholas Barringer, PhD, RDN, CSSD, CSCS
Program Director, Army-Baylor Master's Program in Nutrition, Department of Defense
San Antonio, TX

Katherine Beals, PhD, RD, FACSM, CSSD
Adjunct Instructor, Department of Kinesiology, Boise State University
Boise, ID

Melissa L. Brown, PhD, RD, CSSD, LD
Chair, Department of Nutrition and Public Health, University of Saint Joseph
West Hartford, CT

Nicholas A. Burd, PhD
Professor, University of Illinois Urbana-Champaign
Urbana, IL

Louise Burke, OAM, PhD, APD, FACSM
Chair of Sports Nutrition, Mary MacKillop Institute for Health Research, Australian Catholic University
Melbourne, Victoria, Australia

Ellen J. Coleman, MA, MPH, RD
Sports Dietitian
Riverside, CA

Max. T. Deutz, PhD, RD, CSSD
Sports Dietitian/Nutrition Professor,
Colorado State University
Fort Collins, CO

Karen Reznik Dolins, EdD, RDN, CSSD
Adjunct Associate Professor, Teachers College
Columbia University
New York, NY

Matthew Frakes, PhD, RD, LDN, CSCS, ISAK-2
Director of Performance Nutrition,
New York Football Giants
East Rutherford, NJ

Abby Gilman, PhD, RDN, LDN
Research Grants and Compliance Manager,
Bryn Mawr College
Bryn Mawr, PA

Kaneen Gomez-Hixson, MS, RDN, CSSD, CDN
Assistant Professor and Lead Sports Dietitian,
University of Saint Joseph
West Hartford, CT

Drew E. Gonzalez, PhD, SCCC, CISSN, CSCS,*D, TSAC-F,*D, EP-C
Assistant Professor, Department of Kinesiology
Director, Occupational, Performance, and Nutrition Lab, Sam Houston State University
Huntsville, TX

Carrie M. Hamady, EdD, MS, RD, LD, FAND
Chair, Department of Public and Allied Health,
Bowling Green State University
Bowling Green, OH

Charlotte Hayes, MMSc, MS, RDN, CSSD, CDCES, ACSM-CEP
Head of Diabetes, Wellness, and Education,
Team Novo Nordisk
Atlanta, GA

Isaac Hicks III, RDN, CSSD, LDN, CSCS
Director of Performance Nutrition,
Indiana University
Bloomington, IN

Sarah Johnson, MS
Doctoral student, Texas A&M University
College Station, TX

Jillian M. Joyce, PhD, RD
Associate Professor, Department of Nutritional Sciences, Oklahoma State University
Stillwater, OK

Douglas S. Kalman, PhD, RD, FACN, FISSN
Senior Vice President, Scientific and Regulatory Affairs, Natural Products Association
Faculty, College of Osteopathic Medicine, Nova Southeastern University
Davie, FL

Christine A. Karpinski, PhD, RD, CSSD, LDN
Professor and Chair, West Chester University
West Chester, PA

Jennifer Ketterly, MS, RD, CSSD, LDN
Associate Director Sports Performance, Duke Sports Science Institute;
Instructor, Duke University School of Medicine
Durham, NC

Richard B. Kreider, PhD, FACSM, FASEP, FISSN, FACN, FNAK
Professor and Director, Exercise & Sport Nutrition Lab, Department of Kinesiology & Sport Management, Texas A&M University
College Station, TX

Laura J. Kruskall, PhD, RDN, CSSD, LD, FACSM, FAND, ACSM EP-C
Nutrition Center Director, University of Nevada, Las Vegas
Las Vegas, NV

D. Enette Larson-Meyer, PhD, RD, CSSD, FACSM
Professor and Director of the Nutrition & Exercise Metabolism Lab, Department of Human Nutrition, Foods, and Exercise, Virginia Tech
Blacksburg, VA

Kayla Lawson, MS, RD, LDN
Director of Performance Nutrition, Olympic Sports, Louisiana State University
Baton Rouge, LA

Caroline Mandel, MS, RD, CSSD
Director of Performance Nutrition, University of Michigan Athletics
Ann Arbor, MI

Amy L. Morgan, PhD, FACSM
Professor, Bowling Green State University
Bowling Green, OH

Bob Murray, PhD, FACSM
Managing Principal, Sports Science Insights, LLC
Crystal Lake, IL

Kris Osterberg, PhD, RD, CSSD
Principal Scientist, Gatorade Sports Science Institute
Bradenton, FL

Eve Pearson, MBA, RDN
Registered Dietitian, Nutriworks, Inc.
Fort Worth, TX

Stuart Phillips, PhD, FACSM
Professor and Canada Research Chair, McMaster University
Hamilton, Ontario, Canada

Christine A. Rosenbloom, PhD, RDN, FAND
President, Chris Rosenbloom Food & Nutirtion Services, LLC
Professor Emerita, Georgia State University
Hartwell, GA

Christina Scribner, MS, RDN, CSSD, CEDS
Faculty, Arizona State University
Nutrition Consultant, Encompass Nutrition LLC
Littleton, CO

D. Travis Thomas, PhD, RDN, CSSD, LD, FAND
Associate Professor, University of Kentucky
Lexington, KY

Stella Lucia Volpe, PhD, RDN, ACSM-CEP, FACSM
Professor and Head, Department of Human Nutrition, Foods, and Exercise, Virginia Polytechnic Institute and State University
Blacksburg, VA

Reviewers

Elizabeth L. Abbey, PhD, RDN, CDN
Professor and Chair, Undergraduate Department of Health Sciences, Whitworth University
Spokane, WA

Roberta Anding, MS, RDN/LD, CSSD, CDCES, FAND
Director of Performance Nutrition, Lecturer, Kinesiology Department, Rice University
Houston, TX

Hope Barkoukis, PhD, RDN, LD, FAND
Chair, Department of Nutrition, School of Medicine, Case Western Reserve University
Cleveland, OH

Michelle Barrack, PhD, RD, CSSD, FACSM
Professor, Nutrition and Dietetics, California State University, Long Beach
Long Beach, CA

Julie Brake, MS, RDN, LD
Owner/Registered Dietitian, Positive Nutrition
Marietta, GA

Melissa L. Brown, PhD, RD, CSSD, LD
Chair, Department of Nutrition and Public Health, University of Saint Joseph
West Hartford, CT

Paige Crawford Blyth, MS, RD, CSSD
Team Dietitian, Los Angeles Chargers
Costa Mesa, CA
Owner/Sports Dietitian, Freestyle Nutrition Co, LLC
Scottsdale, AZ

Joanna Cummings, MS, RD-AP, CNSC, CSSD
Performance Dietitian, Owner, Altitude Sport & Performance Nutrition
Parker, CO

Karen Reznik Dolins, EdD, RDN, CSSD
Adjunct Associate Professor, Teachers College, Columbia University
New York, NY

Kaitlyn M. Eck, PhD, RDN
Assistant Professor, Thomas Jefferson University
Philadelphia, PA

Sotiria Everett, EdD, RD, CDN, CSSD
Clinical Assistant Professor, SUNY Stonybrook Medicine
Stony Brook, NY

Kimberly A. Feeney, PhD, RD, CSSD
Performance Dietitian, Department of Defense
Lillington, NC

Jennifer Fiske, MS, RDN, LD
Registered Dietitian Nutritionist
Lewisville, TX

Reyna Franco, MS, MBA, RDN, CSSD, FAND, DipACLM
Owner, Reyna Franco
New York, NY

Katie Frushour, MS, RD, CSSD
Performance Dietitian, Department of Defense
Albuquerque, NM

Karen Gibson, RDN, DCN, CSSD
Professor Emeritus, Viterbo University
La Crosse, WI

Kaneen Gomez-Hixson, MS, RDN, CSSD, CDN
Assistant Professor/Lead Sports Dietitian, University of Saint Joseph
West Hartford, CT

Drew E. Gonzalez, PhD, SCCC, CISSN, CSCS,*D, TSAC-F,*D, EP-C
Assistant Professor, Department of Kinesiology
Director, Occupational, Performance, and Nutrition Lab, Sam Houston State University
Huntsville, TX

Marilyn Gordon, EdD, RDN, CSSD, LDN, FAND
Assistant Professor, Department of Nutrition Dr. Kiran C. Patel College of Osteopathic Medicine, Nova Southeastern University, College of Osteopathic Medicine
Davie, FL

Satya S. Jonnalagadda, PhD, MBA, RDN
Vice President, Scientific and Clinical Affairs, Medifast Inc
Baltimore, MD

Douglas S. Kalman, PhD, RD, CCRC, FACN, FISSN
Clinical Associate Professor, Nutrition
Dr. Kiran C. Patel College of Osteopathic Medicine, Nova Southeastern University
Davie, FL

Tara LaRowe, PhD, RDN, CSSD
Assistant Teaching Professor, University of Wisconsin-Madison
Madison, WI

D. Enette Larson-Meyer, PhD, RD, CSSD, FACSM
Professor and Director of the Nutrition & Exercise Metabolism Lab, Department of Human Nutrition, Foods, and Exercise, Virginia Tech, Blacksburg, VA

Heidi Lynch, PhD, RDN
Professor, Point Loma Nazarene University
San Diego, CA

Allison Mankowski, MPH, RD, CSSD
Owner, Allison Mankowski Nutrition
Plymouth, MI

Anthony Paradis, MA, MS, RDN, CSSD, CSCS
Army Pregnancy & Postpartum Performance Training (P3T) Program Analyst, United States Army
Columbia, SC

Justin Robinson, MA, RD, CSSD, CSCS, TSAC-F, FAFS
Adjunct Faculty, Point Loma Nazarene University
San Diego, CA

Jesse Shaw, DO, USAW, CAQSM
Assistant Professor, Washington State University
Associate Professor Sports Medicine/Sports Performance, University of Western States
Team Physician, Washington State University
Team Physician, Team USA
Pullman, WA

Brett Singer, MS, RD, CSSD, LD
Sports Dietitian, Memorial Hermann Rockets Sports Medicine Institute
Houston, TX

Sherri Stastny, PhD, RD, CSSD, LRD
Professor, Health, Nutrition and Exercise Sciences, North Dakota State University
Fargo, ND

Elizabeth Stuart, MS, RD, CSSD, LD
Assistant Athletics Director of Performance Nutrition, University of Missouri Football
Columbia, MO

Cathy Tillery, MS, RDN, CSSD, LD
Director of Performance Nutrition, Assistant Professor, Life University
Marietta, GA

Mandy Tyler, MEd, RD, CSSD, LD, LAT
Sports Dietitian, Consultant, Private Practice
Bulverde, TX

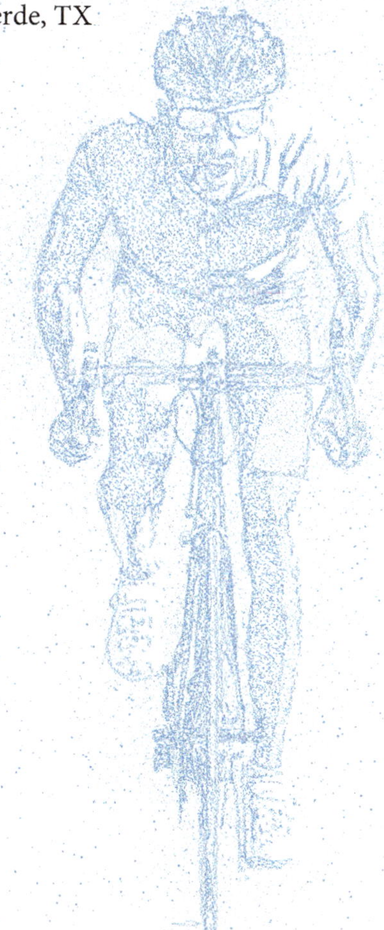

Foreword

As a sports nutrition veteran, I look back on my rookie years when we made do with the few resources we had available at the time. These limitations resulted in hours of research, conversations with others in the field to further our education, and the need to develop materials with clinical and relevant applications to sports nutrition. Nutrition operations management, budget creation, and supplement ordering were part of the "learn as you go" playbook. In addition, we learned to nurture collaborations with the sports medicine, training, strength and conditioning, and foodservice staff through open, constructive, and productive conversations.

As one of the few females in the field, it was quite daunting to learn how to be assertive, progressive, innovative, and creative as a department of 1 while aiming to be available and accessible to all athletes. Understanding the nuances, energy demands, and particulars of every sport, in addition to counseling on physique, physiology, performance, and practicality resulted in long days and significant challenges.

The seventh edition of *Sports Nutrition: A Handbook for Professionals* is the GPS to help both new and seasoned sports dietitians navigate the complexities of performance nutrition. The job demands a knowledge and mastery of exercise physiology, the energy demands of sports, fuel substrates, and hydration, and so we must have clinical competency in these areas. Additionally, the world of sport has expanded beyond collegiate and professional sports to include a need for our services in middle, club, and high school sports, and in working with masters athletes, the military, tactical first responders, and performance artists. All of this information is found within the pages of the book you are about to read.

Our audience pushes the boundaries in the quest to excel, therefore we must be able to respond with creative and compelling solutions. The abundance of misinformation and disinformation concerning body composition and weight management can detract from athlete performance and health. As sports dietitians we need to be able to help our athletes create plans that are attainable, sustainable, and maintainable.

Sports Nutrition: A Handbook for Professionals needs to be part of every sports dietitian's fuel kit. The information gleaned from this book will help our individual athletes, teams, and support staff strategize, optimize, and realize their goals. Being proficient and clinically competent not only enhances our scope of practice but leverages the role of the sports dietitian as an integral part of the performance team.

Leslie Bonci, MPH, RDN, CSSD, LDN, FAND
Owner, Active Eating Advice by Leslie Bonci, Inc.
Cofounder, Performance365
Former NFL sports dietitian (Kansas City Chiefs, Pittsburgh Steelers)
Former MLB sports dietitian (Pittsburgh Pirates, Cincinnati Reds, Milwaukee Brewers, Toronto Blue Jays, Washington Nationals)
Former NHL sports dietitian (Pittsburgh Penguins)
Former Olympic sports consultant
Former company nutritionist, Pittsburgh Ballet Theatre
Former chair, Sports, Cardiovascular, and Wellness Nutrition dietetic practice group

Acknowledgments

We would like to extend our appreciation to the authors and reviewers who contributed to the seventh edition of *Sports Nutrition* as well as the Academy Publications team for seeing this project through. We would like to specifically thank Stacey Zettle, MS, RDN, for her guidance, dedication, knowledge, and patience throughout this process and for keeping us on schedule. We would like to acknowledge those who came before us, for without them, there would be no seventh edition. Therefore, to the editors of the sixth edition, Dr Christine Karpinski and Dr Christine Rosenbloom, we thank you! You are both pillars in the sports nutrition field and role models to all. Lastly, we thank our families for their support and understanding through the long hours of work that have gone into this new edition.

Melissa L. Brown, PhD, RD, CSSD, LD
Hope Barkoukis, PhD, RDN, LD, FAND

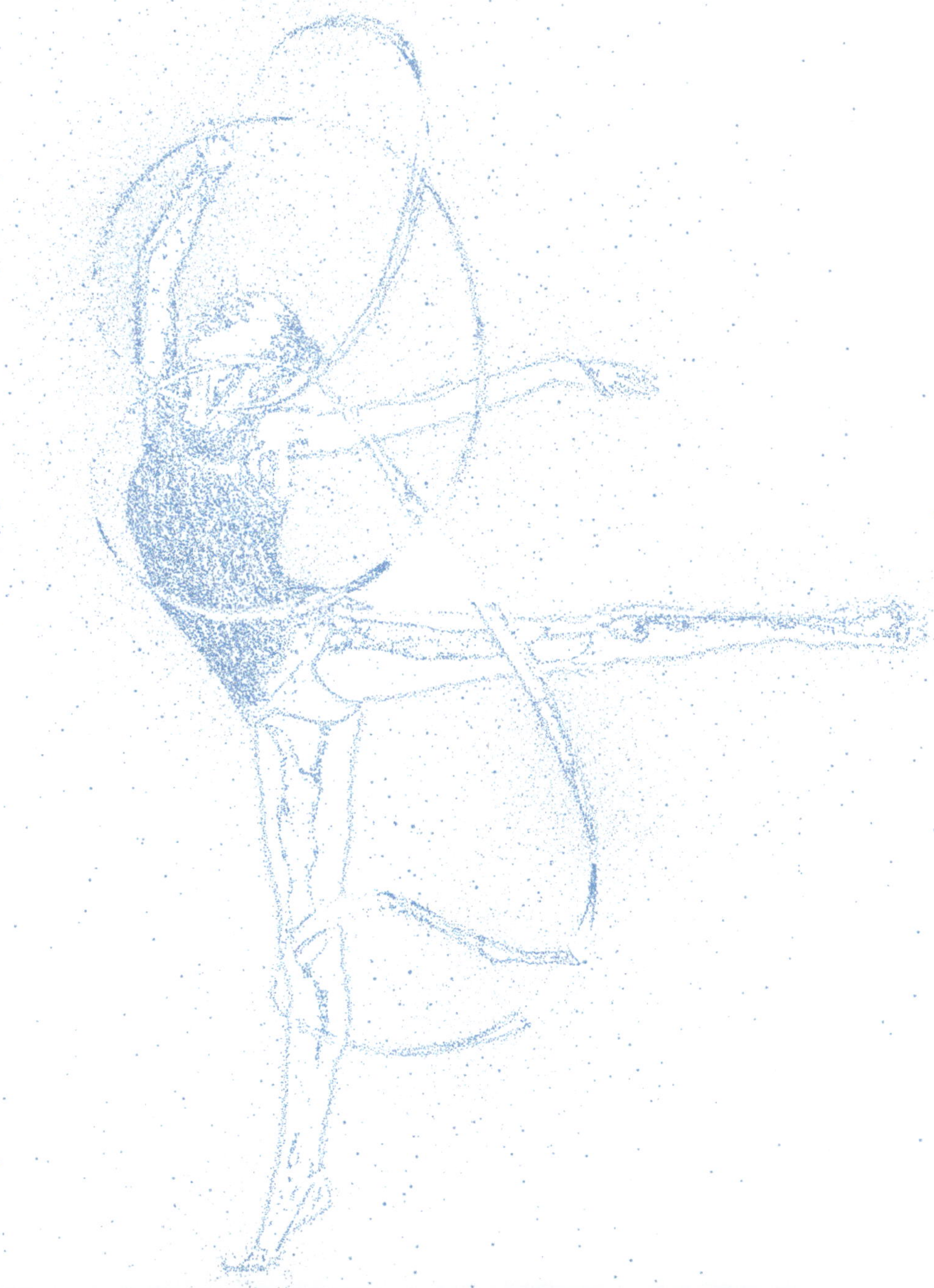

About the Editors

Melissa L. Brown, PhD, RD, CSSD, LD, has over 30 years of experience in the field of sports nutrition and is currently Chair of the Department of Nutrition and Public Health at the University of Saint Joseph in West Hartford, CT. Throughout her career, she has authored multiple peer-reviewed articles, contributed to several textbooks, given talks both nationally and internationally, and has been the recipient of many federally funded grants. In addition, Melissa has coauthored a series of CSSD exam prep materials through Pro-Style Nutrition Consulting, Inc.

Melissa has always been an athlete but did not become interested in sports nutrition until 1994 when she began her combined master's degree and dietetic internship at Rush University in Chicago. The mid-90s is often considered to be the start of sports nutrition and Melissa was incredibly fortunate to have been trained by some of the best in the field. Melissa has experience working with athletes at high school, collegiate, amateur adult, elite, and professional levels. She has also worked with teams and groups and has assisted with sports nutrition program development.

In addition to sports nutrition, Melissa also has decades of experience in the field of islet transplantation and diabetes research. To our knowledge, she is the only dietitian who has been trained to perform islet transplantations and maintains her islet and diabetes research laboratory to this day.

Hope Barkoukis, PhD, RDN, LD, FAND, is Chair of the Department of Nutrition in the School of Medicine at Case Western Reserve University, and the creator of/faculty lead for the Jack, Joseph, Morton Mandel Wellness & Preventive Care Pathway program for medical students. The Pathway introduces medical students to stress reduction techniques, social well-being habits, nutrition, exercise prescriptions, and culinary medicine. In 2018, the Pathway received the Alliance for a Healthier Generation's award for Innovation in Teaching future health care professionals.

Hope has advanced training in culinary arts and has presented countless culinary nutrition sessions for consumer and professional audiences. She has been coinvestigator on several National Institutes of Health research grants focused on dietary interventions and their impact on glucose metabolism, culinary medicine in medical education, and liver disease. Prior to assuming the role of Department Chair at Case Western Reserve Univeristy, Hope held various positions on the executive board of SCAN (Sports, Cardiovascular and Wellness Nutrition dietetic practice group) including Chair, and also had a private practice specializing in sports nutrition.

Overview of the 7th Edition

The much anticipated seventh edition of *Sports Nutrition: A Handbook for Professionals* builds upon the strong foundation set forth in previous editions. This new edition holds true to the need to provide fundamental sports nutrition information, clinical sports nutrition information, and practical applications of both. The seventh edition continues to offer cutting-edge research and evidence-based guidance for professionals working with athletes of all ages and levels.

This updated edition of *Sports Nutrition* is organized into 6 sections and is designed to be a complete reference manual for practicing professionals as well as a resource for undergraduate and graduate sports nutrition courses. We think that the changes made to this current edition will be of much benefit to the sports nutrition profession:

- We have enlisted 14 new authors for this edition. The manual is anchored by our esteemed returning authors who are a mix of board-certified specialist in sports dietetics (CSSD) RDNs, international sports RDNs, and our exercise physiologist colleagues.
- We have incorporated more practical information that you can implement into your daily practice. One way we accomplished this was by including learning objectives at the beginning of each chapter. These objectives then tie into the takeaway points provided at the end of the chapters.
- This edition includes updated references. If a related study was conducted since the last edition, you will most likely see it in the seventh edition.
- Brand-new chapters include Chapter 23, which provides an in-depth review of tactical performance nutrition; Chapter 25, which summarizes various dietary patterns important to athletes; and Chapter 26, which reviews fundamental knowledge related to sports nutrition operations and management.
- We have included guidelines from the most current position and practice papers.

Section 1 covers the foundation of sports nutrition. It begins with an overview of exercise physiology (Chapter 1), including a description of training principles and an important discussion about the scope of practice for sports RDNs. Chapters 2 through 6 utilize updated literature to provide practical advice on sports applications of dietary carbohydrates, protein, fat, vitamins, minerals, fluids, and electrolytes. Chapter 7 completes this section of the manual, focusing on the regulation of sports supplements and featuring the Australian Institute of Sport classification system.

Section 2 focuses on nutrition assessment and energy balance. Chapter 8 centers on assessment and how sports RDNs can incorporate the Nutrition Care Process, Standards of Practice, and Standards of Professional Performance into a sports nutrition practice. Chapter 9 was authored by a sports RDN and an exercise scientist, which helps to provide different approaches to the assessment of body size and composition. Both Chapters 10 (energy balance) and 11 (weight management) were written by 2 new authors, bringing a fresh perspective to these topics.

Section 3 puts these principles into practice. Chapters 12 through 19 provide practical applications of the sports nutrition basics discussed in Sections 1 and 2. We have kept the same population-specific topics included in the previous edition. It took the collaborative efforts of multiple experienced sports RDNs to complete this section, which offers you a plethora of information that you can incorporate into your practice.

Section 4 has been renamed "Activity-Specific Nutrition Guidelines" to include the exciting new chapter on tactical nutrition (Chapter 23) along with the traditional sport-specific recommendations. Chapters 20 and 21 feature updated research for sprint, power, and intermittent sports, and Chapter 22 reviews the research behind fueling endurance athletes.

Section 5 is brand new to this edition and is titled "Advancing the Future." It is led by Chapter 24, Emerging Opportunities in Sports Nutrition, which was first included in the sixth edition and explores a variety of nontraditional practice areas such as CrossFit, obstacle course races, motorsports, performance arts (eg, dancers, marching band), esports, and more. The *Sports Nutrition* textbook has always focused on being as inclusive as possible and now for the first time Chapter 24 also reviews the available evidence pertaining to transgender and gender nonconforming athletes. This chapter includes the current knowledge-base and best practices for providing evidence-based, compassionate care, recognizing that there is much that we still do not know and still have to learn about this understudied population. Section 5 also includes 2 brand new chapters. Chapter 25 introduces the term *dietary pattern* and discusses its role in health promotion and sports performance, along with a general overview of the core elements of the main US dietary patterns identified as "healthy" in the *Dietary Guidelines for Americans, 2020–2025*. The chapter also includes the metabolic impacts from each dietary pattern as they relate to athletes. Special attention is given to identifying the considerable gaps in knowledge regarding the prevalence of and adherence to the specific dietary patterns by athletes. Chapter 26 focuses on operations and management in sports nutrition. The information presented in the previous chapters collectively underscores the vital importance of performance nutrition for health and athletic performance. The RDN with advanced training in sports nutrition (often a CSSD) is the preferred provider of performance nutrition services.

Section 6 includes the At-A-Glance section, which has been expanded to include updated information on 24 sports. The book's appendixes include information on helpful sports nutrition–related position statements, position stands, consensus statements, and websites.

The role of the sports RDN has expanded tremendously over the years. Sports RDNs now play integral roles in operations, teams, and schools by focusing on individualized nutrition plans, evidence-based practice, advanced nutrition therapies, performance and recovery, cultural sensitivity, and program development. The sports RDN takes a holistic approach to athlete health and performance, reflecting the growing recognition of the critical role of nutrition in athletic success.

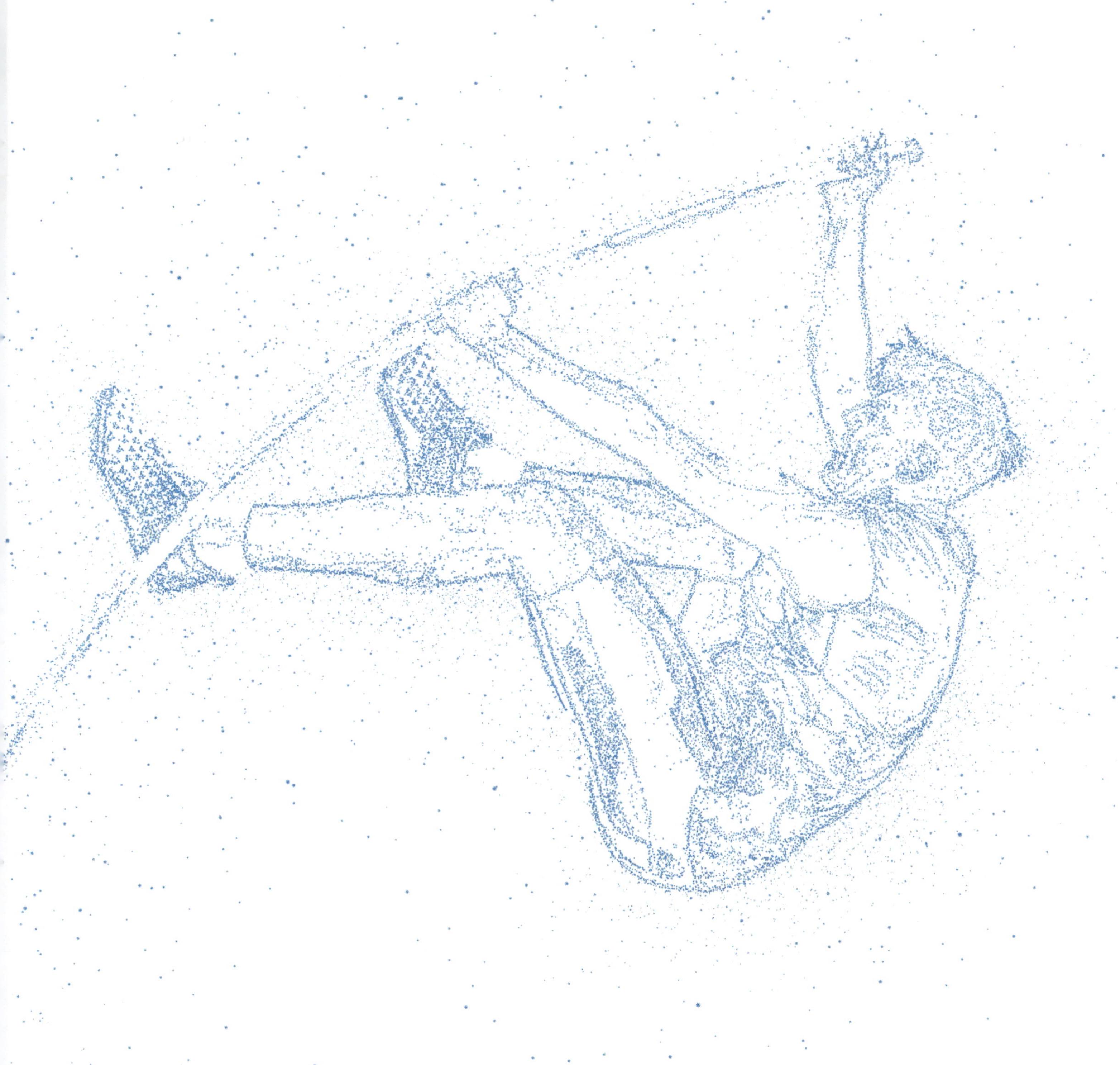

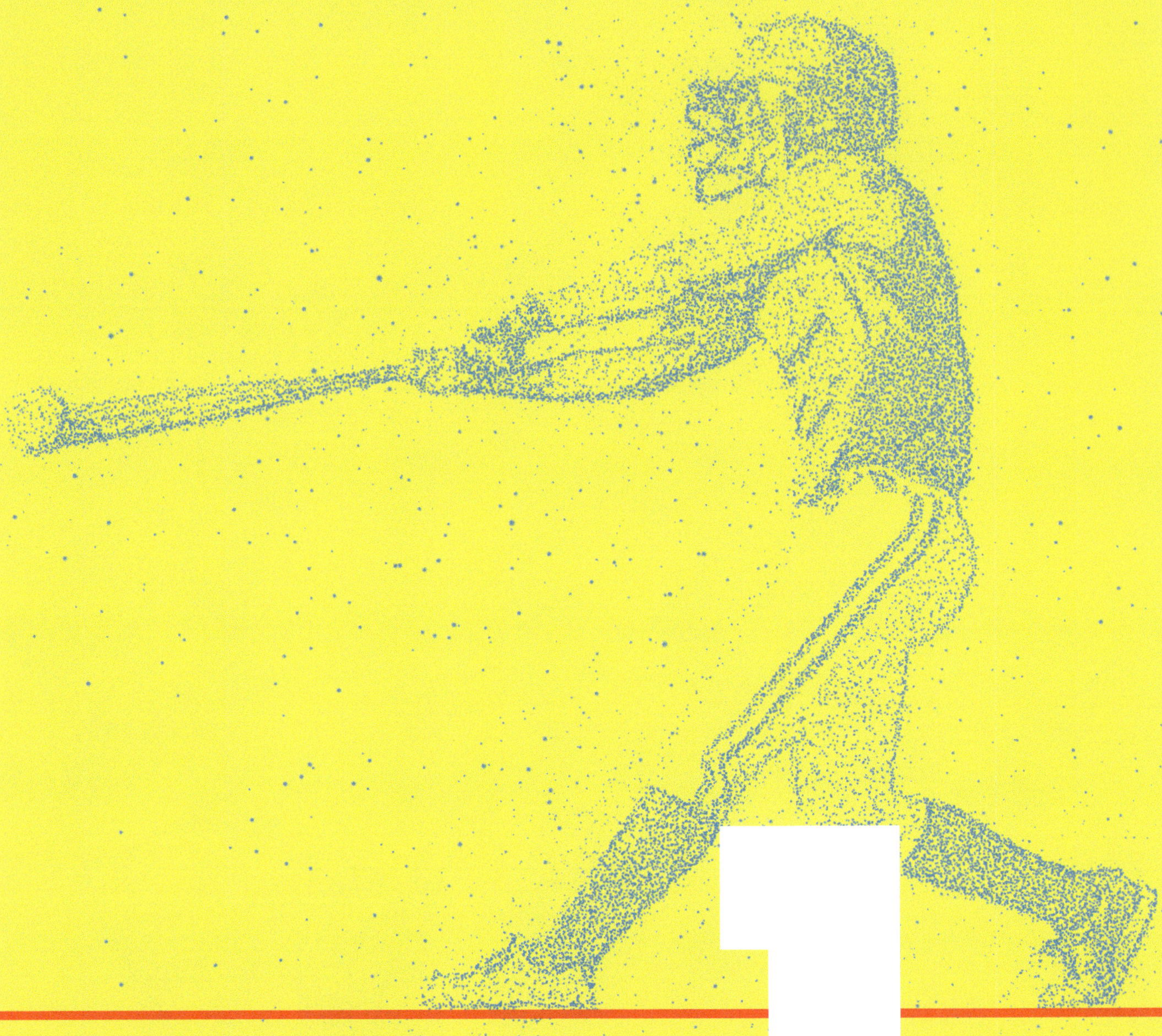

SECTION 1

SPORTS NUTRITION FOUNDATIONS

A thorough understanding of exercise physiology and the way nutrients support training and competition is essential for the registered dietitian nutritionist working with active people. The first section of *Sports Nutrition* seeks to enhance this understanding by examining the critical role of macronutrients and micronutrients in exercise performance.

The physiology of exercise includes more than just energy production. Athletic success depends on proper nutrition for growth and development and for effective immune system function, as discussed in Chapter 1. Our knowledge of the interrelated roles of dietary carbohydrate, protein, and fat has increased tremendously in the past 20 years, and this new information is incorporated into Chapters 2, 3, and 4. Micronutrients are covered in detail in Chapter 5, which presents the most current research on the effects of vitamin and mineral intake on sports performance. The most essential nutrient for athletes, water, is explained in both scientific and practical terms in Chapter 6, and further discusses fluid, electrolytes, and exercise. Finally, this section concludes with a comprehensive look at dietary supplements and sports foods that athletes use in the hope of improving performance in Chapter 7. Specifically, Chapter 7 discusses how the sports dietitian can critically evaluate dietary supplements and provide sound advice to athletes about using these supplements.

CHAPTER 1

Physiology of Exercise

Laura J. Kruskall, PhD, RDN, CSSD, LD, FACSM, FAND, ACSM EP-C

LEARNING OBJECTIVES

- Understand the basic principles of exercise physiology, the physiological responses to exercise, and adaptations to physical training.
- Identify the primary energy systems and substrates used to fuel the working muscle during physical activity.
- List the principles of exercise training.
- Utilize key concepts in the registered dietitian nutritionist scope of practice to discuss physical activity and exercise with clients.
- Explain the basic principles in the *Physical Activity Guidelines for Americans*, 2nd Edition.

INTRODUCTION

The human body is a dynamic organism composed of molecules, cells, tissues, whole organs, and systems working together to regulate the environment within itself—a process called *homeostasis*. Many factors can threaten the inner environment of the body; the body's response is always to attempt to maintain homeostasis. External extremes and challenges to the body include changes in temperature and altitude. Individuals can deliberately challenge the body by participating in physical activity and exercise. During physical activity and exercise, homeostasis in systems such as the cardiorespiratory system and musculoskeletal system is challenged, triggering a body response. With these challenges, the organ systems must coordinate and adjust to meet the increased energy and metabolic demands of the body.

Exercise physiology is the study of these adjustments. It also includes the responses to exercise that result from acute bouts of activity, as well as the chronic adaptations that occur from repeated exercise and long-term training.[1] This chapter provides a brief overview of the basics of the exercise physiology and includes a discussion of the role of the registered dietitian nutritionist (RDN)[2] or Board Certified Specialist in Sports Dietetics (CSSD)[3] and appropriate application to practice.

ACUTE RESPONSE TO EXERCISE

Even at rest, the body is in a constant state of flux—it remains metabolically active to maintain physiological function. This requires a continual supply of energy. During exercise, the energy demands of skeletal muscles greatly increase, and the respiratory and cardiovascular systems must work harder to allow for increased respiration and to supply blood to the working muscles with a concomitant reduction of blood flow to the gastrointestinal tract. This respiratory and cardiovascular response can continue for minutes to hours depending on the intensity of exercise and the physical training status of the individual. In some sports or events, the increased energy demand is relatively constant for an extended time (eg, a marathon). In others the energy demand is not constant and is often characterized by periods of high intensity followed by periods of active recovery or rest (eg, soccer, tennis). During both endurance and stop-and-go activities, the energy demand can increase by 2 to 20 times that at rest. Very high-intensity activities can exceed this range, though they can be sustained for only seconds to minutes. Ultimately, the body systems must work together to meet the increased energy demands.[1,4-7]

Skeletal Muscle and Exercise

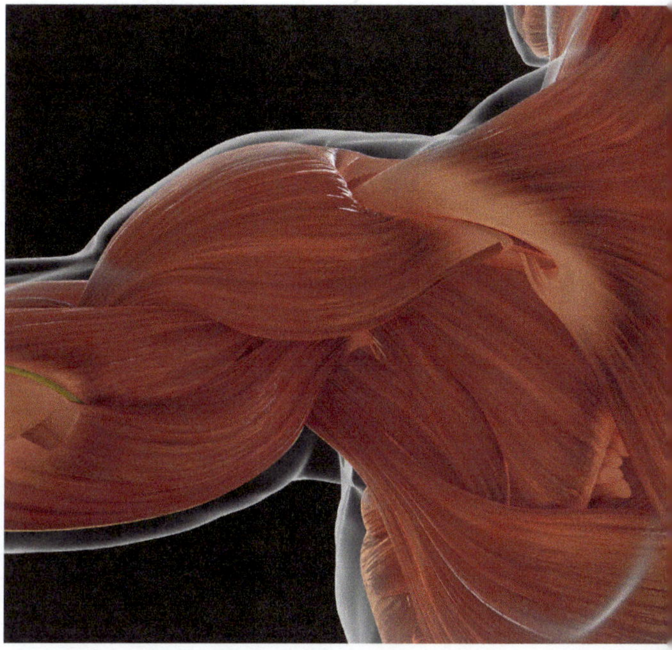

Skeletal muscles terminate where tendons attach to the skeleton. As these muscles contract and relax, they allow movement of the body. The human body has more than 600 skeletal muscles that allow for fine and gross movement. A muscle or muscle group (such as the biceps or quadriceps) is often thought of as a single unit. These units, however, are made of many complex components working together to complete a single contraction. A single nerve and the group of muscle fibers it innervates are referred to as a *motor unit*. *Muscle fiber* is the term used to describe a muscle cell. Each muscle fiber contains organelles, including mitochondria for aerobic energy production and hundreds to thousands of myofibrils. The functional units of a myofibril, *sarcomeres*, are responsible for the contractile properties of the muscle. Sarcomeres are composed of thin and thick filaments called *actin* and *myosin*, respectively. Activation of the motor unit causes these filaments to "slide" over one another, allowing the muscles to shorten, or contract. This slide, referred to as the *sliding filament theory*, is a process that requires energy. Not all available motor units are activated at once—only those needed to generate the appropriate force are used. The force and speed of movement needed determine the extent of the motor unit recruitment: the higher the force or speed of contraction required, the greater the number of individual muscle fibers that must be recruited for contraction. Muscle groups in opposition cannot contract at the same time—one contracts while the other relaxes or lengthens (eg, biceps and triceps). Nerve transmission is coordinated, so it is unlikely to stimulate the contraction of 2 antagonistic muscles at any time.[1,8-10]

Different types of muscle fibers contract at different speeds, producing varying amounts of force. *Type I fibers*, sometimes referred to as slow-twitch fibers, have a high level of aerobic endurance; they can use a continuous supply of energy from the aerobic metabolism of carbohydrate and fat. These fibers allow prolonged muscular contraction for long periods. They are primarily used during activities of daily living, such as walking, or during lower-intensity endurance events, such as bike riding or jogging. *Type II fibers*, sometimes referred to as fast-twitch fibers, have relatively poor endurance capacity and work better anaerobically. These are primarily used for activities such as a tennis serve or a weightlifting set. Although these fiber types can be further classified as type IIa, type IIx, and type IIc, experts are still researching the differences between the types.[1]

Most skeletal muscles consist of approximately 50% type I fibers and 50% type II fibers (25% type IIa fibers, 22%–24% type IIx, and 1%–3% type IIc). The precise percentages of fibers can vary greatly among individuals, and extreme variation in athletes from different sports is common. Type IIa fibers are recruited most frequently but are secondary to type I fibers. Type IIa fibers generate more force than type I fibers but fatigue more easily. Type IIa fibers also tend to be recruited during higher-intensity events of short duration, such as a half-mile run or a strength-training workout. Experts do not fully understand the importance of type IIx fibers. Research findings indicate that they are used in explosive activities such as a 50-meter dash or weightlifting. Type IIc fibers are recruited least frequently. Most muscle groups contain both type I and II fibers and recruit the appropriate type needed for an activity.[1,8-12]

There may be differences in skeletal muscle fiber types when athletes are compared to untrained individuals. Most studies show little to no difference in the proportion of type I muscle fibers between athletes and controls (although in contrast, some studies show large differences).[13-18] One study examining bodybuilders reported extremely high amounts of type IIx fibers,[13] yet other similar studies do not support this finding.[15,17,19] There do, however, appear to be proportional differences in type IIa and type IIx muscle fibers between strength and power athletes vs untrained control subjects. Some studies support the notion that strength and power athletes have a greater proportion of type IIa fibers and a smaller proportion of type IIx fibers, whereas other studies do not.[13-18] The majority of studies show a shift from type IIx to type IIa fibers with long-term resistance training.[14-19]

What is the relationship between fiber type and endurance performance success? Researchers believe that an increased number of type I fibers could benefit an athlete during long endurance activities and more type II fibers would benefit an athlete during high-intensity activities. Endurance athletes tend to possess a greater proportion of type I vs type II muscle fibers, but the difference does not appear to be caused by training. Furthermore, studies show that endurance athletes do not experience pronounced changes in their type IIa fiber profiles.[20-23] Studies examining the muscle fiber types in the gastrocnemius muscle in distance runners and sprinters support this hypothesis: endurance athletes have more type I fibers, and sprinters have more type II fibers. Health care practitioners and athletes should note that fiber type is just 1 piece of the puzzle. Other factors that affect performance include training, nutrition, and motivation.[1,8-10,24]

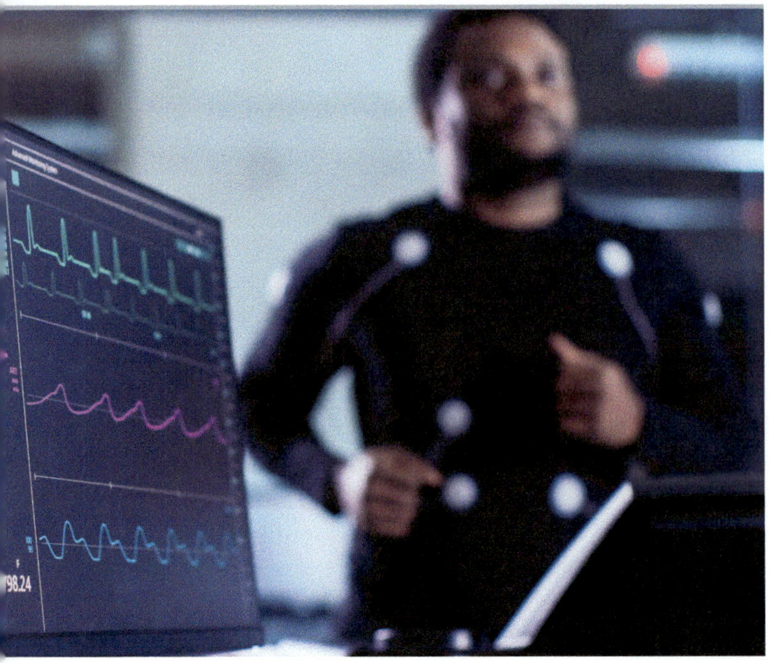

Cardiovascular and Respiratory Systems

The cardiovascular and respiratory systems work together to deliver oxygen and nutrients to working muscles and tissues and to remove metabolic waste products and carbon dioxide. Together, these systems are often referred to as the cardiorespiratory system, and this combined system consists of the heart, blood vessels, airways, and lungs. The cardiorespiratory system has many functions and supports all other physiological systems. Additional key functions include transporting compounds such as hormones, nutrients, oxygen, carbon dioxide, and waste such as urea; supporting thermoregulation and fluid balance; and maintaining acid-base balance.

Pulmonary ventilation describes breathing, or air moving in and out of the lungs. Ventilation happens in 2 phases: inspiration and expiration. *Inspiration* is an active process involving the activation of the diaphragm and external intercostal muscles, whereas *expiration* is usually a passive process as muscles relax and air is expelled from the lungs. Most of the oxygen in the blood is bound to hemoglobin and delivered to the working muscle. Once inside the muscle, oxygen is transported to the mitochondria by myoglobin and is then available for aerobic energy production in the muscle cells.[1]

The cardiac cycle occurs during each heartbeat and includes both electrical and mechanical events.[1] *Heart rate* describes the number of heartbeats, or the number of contractions of the ventricles (the lower chambers of the heart), per unit of time. Heart rate is usually measured and expressed as beats per minute (bpm). The normal heart rate range for untrained individuals is 60 to 100 bpm. *Tachycardia* refers to a heart rate that is faster than normal; *bradycardia* refers to a heart rate this is slower than normal. *Stroke volume* is the volume of blood pumped during 1 heartbeat. *Cardiac output* is the total volume of blood pumped from 1 heartbeat and is the product of heart rate multiplied by stroke volume. Resting cardiac output averages 5 L/min, but this number can vary with body size. Cardiac output increases with exercise and can range from less than 20 L/min in an untrained sedentary person to 40 L/min or more for individuals with elite endurance training. *Athlete heart* refers to anatomical alterations in which unique muscle thickness, electrical signals, and anatomical function develop as a result of physical training. This is usually seen in individuals who train at least 1 hour per day most days of the week.[1,25]

The volume of blood distributed throughout the body depends on the metabolic demands of the tissues, with the most active tissues receiving the greatest amount of blood. When the body is at rest, many organs require more blood than skeletal muscles. The muscle receives approximately 15% of the cardiac output at rest, but this can increase to as much as 80% during intense exercise to meet oxygen and nutrient demands of active muscle.[1,26]

Cardiovascular and Respiratory Responses to Acute Exercise

The initiation of exercise requires increased muscle oxygen and nutrient demand and the removal of more metabolic waste products. When exercise begins, pulmonary ventilation increases to meet the oxygen demand of the muscles. During lower-intensity activities, this demand can be met by simply moving more air in and out of the lungs. However, as exercise intensity increases, respiration rate also increases. During most common forms of endurance exercise, pulmonary ventilation typically does not reach maximum capacity and is not the limiting factor in performance; very high–intensity exercise may be the exception. During prolonged endurance exercise, respiratory muscles can withstand fatigue. However, there is a point at which athletes cannot take in a higher volume of air and the respiration rate cannot be any higher. At this point, athletes are at their aerobic capacity, and the energy required for continued activity must be supplied by anaerobic metabolism. The term used to describe this sequence is *maximal oxygen uptake*, also known as *VO_2 max*.

An athlete's VO_2 max is an important consideration for performance lasting more than a few minutes and can be measured in an exercise physiology laboratory. It is considered the best measurement of cardiovascular or aerobic fitness.[1,27-29] VO_2 max is usually expressed in units of milliliters per kilogram per minute ($mL \times kg^{-1} \times min^{-1}$). A sedentary individual may see a 10-fold increase in VO_2 max while exercising, whereas an endurance athlete may see a 23-fold increase. Studies show that a sedentary male has an average VO_2 max of 35 $mL \times kg^{-1} \times min^{-1}$, whereas a world-class male endurance athlete can have a VO_2 max as high as 80 $mL \times kg^{-1} \times min^{-1}$.[30,31]

Gas exchange in the lungs is not considered a limiting factor in endurance exercise performance. In endurance athletes, maximum cardiac output is closely related to VO_2 max and endurance performance. Heart rate increases linearly with exercise intensity and plateaus when maximum heart rate is achieved. Maximum heart rate (estimated as 220 – age in years) differs little between trained and untrained individuals, although the intensity level at which these individuals will reach their maximum heart rates will vary. For example, both a trained and an untrained person may have the same maximum heart rate of 170 bpm, but the trained person can work at a higher training workload before reaching that maximum heart rate.

Stroke volume is another key factor for determining cardiovascular endurance capacity. In an untrained person, stroke volume increases proportionally with exercise intensity but does not increase further once a person reaches 40% to 60% of their VO_2 max. In trained individuals, stroke volume can continue to increase past this threshold as exercise intensity increases. Because both heart rate and stroke volume increase with exercise, total increased cardiac output parallels the intensity of the exercise to meet the increased blood flow demands of the working muscle. Individuals do not usually exercise at maximum heart rate; instead, they perform submaximal exercise for an extended time. The point where the cardiovascular system is delivering the optimal amount of oxygen and nutrients to the muscle is called *steady-state heart rate*.[1,27,30-33]

FUEL FOR EXERCISE

The biologically usable form of energy in the human body is adenosine triphosphate (ATP). ATP is required for skeletal muscle contraction and relaxation. Skeletal muscles require increased energy during all movements, including intentional exercise. As exercise intensity or duration increases, the body may have difficulty keeping up with this increased energy demand, and a person will feel fatigue. If energy cannot be supplied to the muscles in a timely manner and in adequate amounts, movement will cease. Once energy from endogenous carbohydrate stores is exhausted, ATP production is limited by the availability of exogenous fuel from carbohydrates, fats, and proteins.[1,7,32]

Energy Substrates

Plants rely on photosynthesis to convert sunlight into chemical energy, and animals consume these plants. Human beings obtain energy by consuming plants and animals, thereby taking in energy nutrients. Energy nutrients consist of carbohydrate, fat, and protein. All cells in the body have the ability to break down these nutrients for energy, and each cell has a substrate preference in its resting state. The cells have metabolic pathways to process these energy substrates and generate ATP. For example, in muscle cells, ATP is hydrolyzed to release a phosphate group, adenosine diphosphate (ADP), and energy.[1,5-7]

The human body can acquire energy through the intake of foods and beverages (exogenous sources) or from the breakdown of substrates stored for later use (endogenous sources). Under normal circumstances, the primary nutrients for energy production come from carbohydrate and fat. Typically, protein contributes less than 5% to 10% of the body's energy needs because it is utilized for other important functions, such as acting as enzymes, hormones, and immune proteins and performing tissue maintenance, growth, and repair. The exception to this occurs during the later stages of prolonged endurance exercise when protein can contribute up to 15% of the energy needs if exogenous carbohydrate is not consumed and glycogen stores become depleted.

As previously noted, the primary nutrients for energy production come from carbohydrate and fat. The storage form of carbohydrate in human beings is glycogen, which consists of glucose and is found in both skeletal muscle and liver tissue. These organs can store a maximum capacity of glycogen. Liver tissue can store 75 to 110 g (300–440 kcal) of glycogen, whereas skeletal muscle can hold 300 to 400 g (1,200–1,600 kcal). Circulating glucose in the plasma provides only a small source of carbohydrate, approximately 5 g (20 kcal). Glycogen storage generally cannot be relied on as the only source of energy during exercise because the brain and central nervous system require glucose for energy and take priority. Fat is stored as triglycerides within adipose tissue and skeletal muscle. Unlike glycogen, adipose tissue triglyceride is limitless and can provide 70,000 kcal or more of energy.[1,5,34,35]

Energy Systems

ATP is stored in cells in very limited quantities, so the body must constantly generate ATP to meet the demands of cellular metabolism and muscle contraction during exercise. During rest, most of the cells and organs use a constant supply of ATP. With increased activity, the demand by skeletal muscle for ATP can increase greatly, depending on the intensity and duration of exercise. Each muscle contraction uses ATP, which is hydrolyzed to ADP and a single phosphate group. The ADP and phosphate group must then be rephosphorylized to ATP. There are 3 basic metabolic pathways to accomplish this: those that rely on the large amount of creatine found in muscle cells (phosphocreatine system), those that generate ATP without the use of oxygen (anaerobic), and those that require oxygen involvement (aerobic).[1,5,34,35]

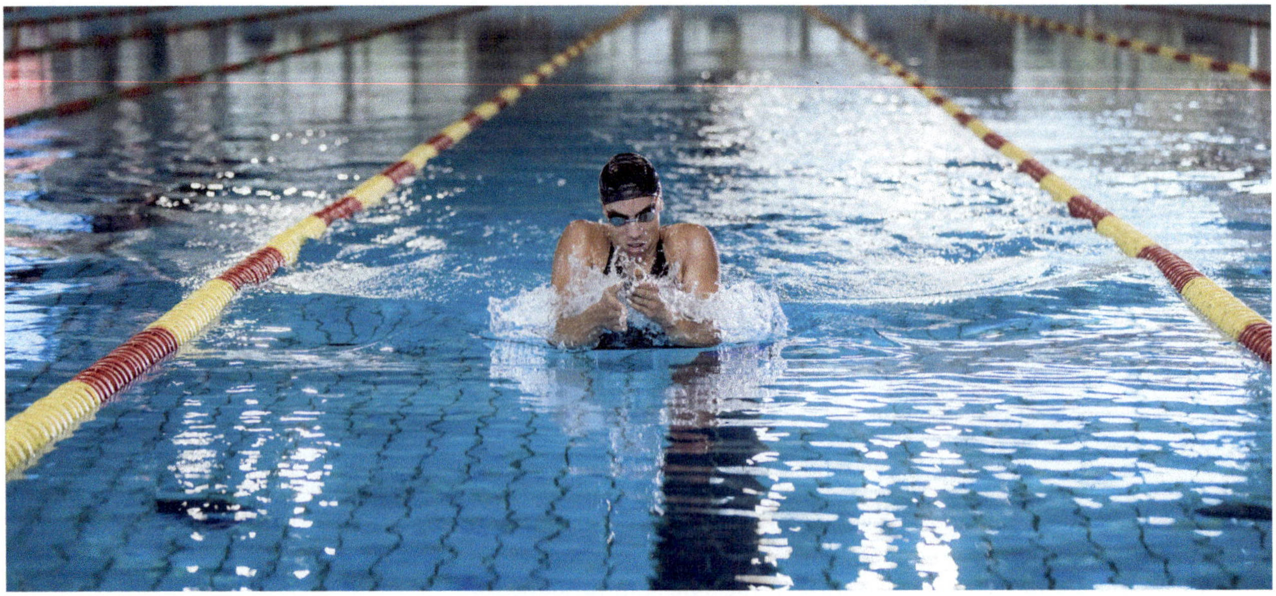

ADENOSINE TRIPHOSPHATE-PHOSPHOCREATINE SYSTEM

The adenosine triphosphate–phosphocreatine (ATP-PCr) system is the quickest way for the body to produce ATP. This anaerobic system is used during intensive, explosive movements, such as a tennis serve or a power lift. The ATP-PCr system generates ATP rapidly; however, it is very limited and only supplies ATP for up to 10 seconds. A key component in the ATP-PCr system is phosphocreatine (PCr), which is stored in skeletal muscle and consists of a molecule of creatine attached to a single molecule of phosphate. To generate ATP, a creatine kinase enzyme breaks the creatine and phosphate molecules apart, and the free phosphate then combines with ADP, forming new ATP. The ATP-PCr system is limited because the amount of PCr stored in the skeletal muscle is small. Once all PCr molecules have donated their phosphate groups to ADP, the system can no longer facilitate further ATP production until PCr is replenished. A combination of rest and dietary intake is the main way to replenish PCr.[1,5] Approximately 95% of the body's creatine is found in skeletal muscle and can easily be replenished by the diet. Athletes who include meat in their diet obtain plenty of creatine, but creatine can also be synthesized from the amino acids methionine, arginine, and glycine, which are obtained from other dietary sources.[1,5,34,35]

ANAEROBIC GLYCOLYSIS

The anaerobic glycolysis (AG) system oxidizes 1 glucose molecule (6 carbons) to form 2 pyruvic acid molecules (3 carbons each). Glucose can come from dietary intake (circulating blood glucose) or from glycogen stored in the muscles or liver. During AG, energy is generated in 2 ways. The first generates ATP directly from the breakdown of glucose to pyruvate. The second generates ATP through the oxidation of glucose, during which hydrogen molecules are removed from the carbon skeleton of glucose. Nicotinamide adenine dinucleotide (NAD) is a coenzyme that carries electrons and receives these hydrogen molecules to form NADH. NADH transports hydrogen to the electron transport chain (ETC) in the mitochondria where it undergoes oxidative phosphorylation so the body can generate ATP aerobically. Although this AG pathway does not produce large amounts of ATP, it does generate ATP fairly rapidly. AG and the ATP-PCr system are the predominant energy systems for the first few minutes of intense, continuous activity.[1,5,36] AG also provides energy during the first few moments of moderate, longer-duration activity as the aerobic system begins to generate ATP.[5,37,38]

AG is limited by the production and accumulation of lactate during high-intensity situations when the demand for ATP by skeletal muscle is high. Production of pyruvate from the AG process is not problematic when oxygen is present to be the final acceptor of these hydrogen molecules to form metabolic water. However, when oxygen is limited, such as during very high–intensity activity, the pyruvate is converted to lactic acid. Lactic acid is relatively unstable at normal body pH and loses a hydrogen ion or dissociates into lactate. As hydrogen molecules accumulate, the pH of the muscle cell drops, and glycolytic enzymatic activity is hampered, resulting in skeletal muscle fatigue. The body must slow down to recover before intense activity can continue. Lactate is constantly being produced, but it is easily cleared with time by several mechanisms, as follows[5,37,38]:

- Lactate is taken up and oxidized by the mitochondria in the same muscle cell. This occurs primarily in type I muscle fibers.
- Higher amounts of lactate are produced in type II muscle fibers and then transported to the type I fibers or to other cells in the body for oxidation.
- Lactate travels from the muscle to the liver, is converted to glucose via gluconeogenesis, and is sent back to the working muscle for fuel (the Cori cycle). Once lactate is cleared, activity can continue.

AEROBIC METABOLISM

Through aerobic metabolism, the body can break down carbohydrates, fats, and proteins with the involvement of oxygen through the Krebs cycle and the ETC. Unlike the ATP-PCr system and AG, aerobic metabolism can supply ATP on a fairly limitless basis as long as macronutrients and oxygen are available. Acetyl coenzyme A (CoA) is a metabolic intermediate of both glucose and fat oxidation and is ultimately oxidized through aerobic metabolism. Acetyl CoA combines with oxaloacetate to begin the Krebs cycle. Many hydrogen molecules produced during the Krebs cycle are shuttled by NAD and flavin adenine dinucleotide (FAD) to the ETC. As the hydrogen molecules are passed along the chain, ATP is generated. Oxygen, the final hydrogen acceptor, combines with these molecules to form water. The ETC is the most efficient way that the body produces ATP because there are no metabolic byproducts that lead to fatigue.[1,5,34]

CROSSOVER CONCEPT

All metabolic systems work concurrently. The relative contribution of each system depends on the physiological need for ATP. The oxidation of fatty acids produces more ATP per gram than that of carbohydrates, but at a lower rate and with a greater oxygen requirement. A 16-carbon fatty acid can produce 106 molecules of ATP, whereas oxidation of a 6-carbon glucose molecule nets approximately 32 molecules of ATP. More ATP can be produced from fatty acid because of its longer carbon chain, but ATP can only be generated from fat aerobically. A glucose molecule does not yield as much ATP, but it can be oxidized rapidly and without oxygen when necessary.[5,39]

During rest or low-intensity activity, ATP demand is low, and oxygen is plentiful. As a result, fat is the preferred fuel source during these times. With increased exercise intensity, skeletal muscle requires increased ATP, and oxygen delivery becomes more limited. In this scenario, the body relies more on carbohydrate than fat for fuel because glucose is oxidized more rapidly and is more oxygen efficient (more ATP is generated per oxygen molecule used). The point at which the body shifts from using predominantly fat to predominantly carbohydrate is known as the *crossover point*. Both carbohydrate and fat are always being used, but the ATP demand and oxygen availability determine which substrate and metabolic system is predominant in ATP generation.[1,34,36,39]

FATIGUE

Muscular fatigue refers to the impairment or inability of the muscle to produce force. At rest and during lower-intensity exercise, human beings are capable of producing enough ATP to fuel activity without muscular fatigue, as long as sufficient energy substrates (primarily carbohydrate and fat) are readily available in the body. At low exercise intensity, carbon-containing pyruvate is consistently oxidized to acetyl CoA. At the same time, hydrogen molecules are shuttled smoothly within cells to the ETC by the compounds NAD and FAD. At such low exercise intensities, ATP is readily produced in required amounts, and there are no metabolic byproducts that contribute to fatigue.[1,40-42]

Short-Term Fatigue

Short-term fatigue occurs when exercise intensity rises to levels that disturb the body's ability to derive energy from the primary exercise fuel substrates: carbohydrate and fat. Possible causes of short-term fatigue include the accumulation of metabolic products such as inorganic phosphate and lactate, the depletion of phosphocreatine, and changes in cellular calcium. However, the primary cause of short-term fatigue is the limited ability to inspire and transport oxygen to working muscles at a rate sufficient to keep up with increased ATP demand as exercise intensity rises. The process of short-term fatigue consists of the following steps[1,40-42]:

1) When oxygen levels at the working muscle are insufficient, hydrogen molecules that normally bind with oxygen to form water start to accumulate and eventually overwhelm the capacity for NAD and FAD to accept and transport all of the hydrogen molecules.
2) The normal metabolism of pyruvate to acetyl CoA diminishes, and instead pyruvate accepts these hydrogen molecules and forms lactic acid, which rapidly dissociates into lactate.
3) Lactate is formed faster than it can be cleared, and the acidic environment in the cell disrupts glycolytic enzymatic activity.
4) At this point, ATP production is hindered, and skeletal muscle contraction is impaired.
5) The only way to restore homeostasis is to reduce exercise intensity to enhance oxygen uptake and clear metabolic byproducts. Lactate is not just a waste product of metabolism; it is a fuel source for resting tissues and contracting cardiac and skeletal muscles. Endurance-trained individuals can

better utilize lactate for energy. Once the lactate is cleared (which is a rapid process), the fatigue dissipates, and the skeletal muscle can once again contract.

Long-Term Fatigue

Lactate accumulation is not significantly related to fatigue in prolonged endurance activities. Long-term or substrate fatigue, sometimes referred to as "hitting the wall" or "bonking," is thought to be a consequence of glycogen depletion. Because glycogen storage capacity is limited in skeletal muscles and liver tissue, depletion can occur fairly rapidly. Once glycogen stores are depleted, dietary carbohydrate absorption and gluconeogenesis cannot keep up with the ATP demand of the skeletal muscles, and movement must stop. The body cannot continue to perform until more carbohydrate (glucose) becomes available for ATP production. For endurance athletes, any strategy to maximize glycogen stores and provide a continuous supply of glucose during exercise will help delay the onset of substrate depletion.[1,40-42]

PRINCIPLES OF EXERCISE TRAINING

Exercise training refers to the body's response to physical activity repeated over time, resulting in positive physiological adaptations. Appropriate training coupled with proper fueling and adequate rest and recovery generally results in improved performance. Overtraining or undertraining will not result in a desirable effect. The principles of exercise training apply to the novice beginning an exercise program to improve health, as well as to the elite athlete wishing to compete. Appropriate exercise training depends on factors such as the individual's body composition, the specificity of training, the ability to incorporate progressive overload and periodization, and the avoidance of detraining.

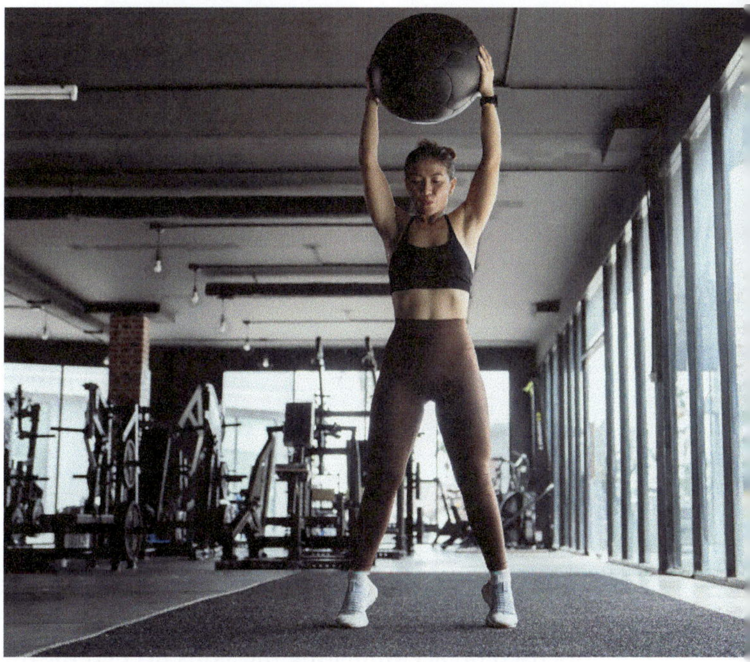

Individual Body Composition

An individual's body composition depends on both genetic and environmental factors. Although genetics creates a starting point and boundaries that determine fat patterning and muscularity, this does not mean that one's ultimate body shape and size are completely outside individual control. The ability to alter physique can be influenced to an extent with nutrition and training. It is, however, important to be realistic about genetic potential. People have different body shapes and can respond differently to the same training. For example, a very tall and lean person may never be able to achieve the physique of a professional bodybuilder through resistance training. On the other hand, a stout, muscular person may never be light or fast enough to compete as an elite marathon runner. Furthermore, some people are considered "higher responders" to training and seem to achieve desired results more easily than "lower responders." It is important for individuals to be realistic in terms of body type and athletic potential.[43,44]

Specificity of Training

Specificity dictates that physiological adaptations and performance enhancements are specific to the mode, intensity, and duration of the exercise training. A training regimen must induce a physical stress specific to the system needed for performance gains. For example, a distance runner must perform endurance activities of long enough duration to promote cellular training adaptations, such as increases in mitochondrial density. Anaerobic sprints or weightlifting promote increased muscle strength and hypertrophy, which are not beneficial to an endurance athlete. Similarly, cardiovascular training will not result in the increased muscular strength and hypertrophy desired for the high-intensity activity needed by athletes specializing in stop-and-go sports. The training program must mimic the desired activity.[1,45,46]

Progressive Overload

To see improvements, athletes need to overload the system being trained (eg, cardiovascular, muscular), resulting in continuous demands on that system. For example, if a person wants to gain strength, they may initially bench press 100 lb for 8 repetitions, and over time, they will be able to do 12 to 15 repetitions at that weight before reaching fatigue. As training continues, the athlete will need to add weight until again reaching fatigue at 8 repetitions. In addition to the weight and number of repetitions performed, muscles can reach fatigue in other ways. For example, one can increase the number of sets of the exercise, decrease the rest period between sets, or emphasize the eccentric contraction by decreasing the speed of the lowering motion. With endurance performance, the athlete must increase the total training volume with intensity, duration, or both, to see an improvement.[1,45,46]

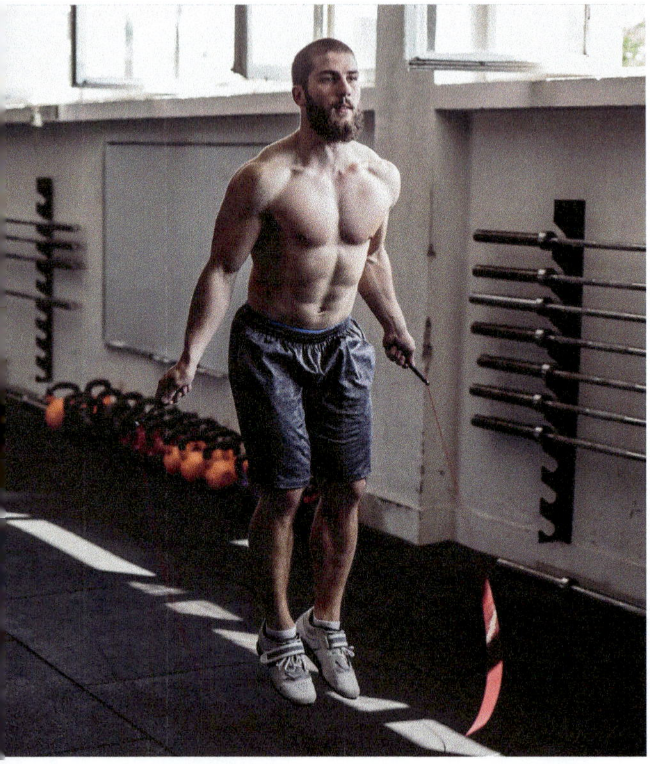

Periodization or Variation

The principle of periodization involves breaking exercise training for a particular sport or event into smaller periods based on desired outcomes. Proper periodization allows for the intensity of training to be adjusted as needed to produce the desired performance outcome while working in adequate rest and recovery to prevent overtraining. Traditional (linear) periodization typically occurs over a longer time frame, such as 1 to 4 years. Within that time, there are various cycles of months (macrocycles), weeks (mesocycles), days (microcycles), and individual training sessions. Appropriately planned periodization programming should consider the athlete's goals and the demands of their sport. Well-rounded athletes require many systems and skills that make use of a combination of aerobic, anaerobic, and strength training.

Block periodization is a newer area of training that incorporates training blocks that can be individualized based on the desired sport or event. These blocks can be specific and focus on a minimum number of performance outcomes. Training consists of performing a small number of blocks at 1 time (eg, 3 or 4) over the span of a few weeks. The sequence can be customized for the sport or event. In 1 example, top-performing canoe and kayak paddlers utilized block periodization. Block 1 focused on accumulating the skills needed for the sport, with general conditioning for aerobic endurance and muscular strength and endurance. Block 2 focused on specialized movements and proper technique, combining anaerobic and aerobic conditioning along with continued muscular strength and endurance. Block 3 emphasized modeling a specific race and obtaining optimal speed and recovery between sessions. This regimen resulted in outstanding performance outcomes.[1,45-47]

Detraining

Detraining is defined as a partial or full reduction in training-induced physiological adaptations as a result of inactivity or lower training load. As both resistance and aerobic training result in increased strength and cardiovascular endurance, stopping this training (detraining) results in the opposite. Continued training is necessary to prevent this detraining effect. Systematically increasing the physical demands on the body with training will be necessary for further improvements, whereas maintenance-level training regimens prevent physiological decline from the trained state. It appears that there is a larger substantial loss of cardiorespiratory endurance gains than loss of muscular endurance, strength, and power. Fortunately, 3 training sessions per week at approximately 70% VO_2 max can maintain cardiorespiratory fitness levels and provide adequate skeletal muscle stimulatory load to retain any gains made with strength training. Formal rehabilitation is recommended for the retention of skeletal muscle mass in an injured person.[1,45,46]

PHYSIOLOGICAL ADAPTATIONS TO ENDURANCE TRAINING

Cardiorespiratory fitness is the ability to perform prolonged endurance exercise using large muscle groups. VO_2 max is one of the best measures of cardiorespiratory endurance. As discussed previously, both the respiratory and cardiovascular systems play important roles in facilitating endurance activity in acute responses to exercise. Training has minimal effect on lung structure and function, but maximal effort does increase pulmonary ventilation, pulmonary diffusion, the distribution of arterial blood away from inactive tissue and toward active skeletal muscle, and the ability of the muscle to take up delivered oxygen.[1,29]

The cardiovascular system undergoes numerous adaptations to regular endurance training. All of these changes result in a greater delivery of oxygen and nutrients to the working skeletal muscle, including the following[1,29]:

- Increases in left ventricular internal space, wall thickness, and mass allow for a stronger contraction and ultimately greater stroke volume. Increased stroke volume in trained individuals is seen both at rest and during exercise.
- Resting heart rate decreases with endurance training; the rate can be 40 bpm or lower (compared with the 60 to 80 bpm rate of a typical sedentary person).
- Exercise heart rate is also lower at a given training load (eg, 60% VO_2 max) with endurance training, but maximum heart rate does not change markedly.
- Cardiac output does not change much during rest and submaximal exercise, but it does increase considerably during maximal effort and is an important contributor to the increased VO_2 max achieved with training.
- Resting blood pressure is reduced.
- Increased capillarization, blood volume, plasma volume, and red blood cell volume improve tissue perfusion and oxygen delivery.
- Increases occur in the percentage and cross-sectional area of type I muscle fibers (those primarily used in endurance activities).
- Increases occur in mitochondria, oxidative enzymes, and myoglobin content (more machinery for ATP production).

PHYSIOLOGICAL ADAPTATIONS TO RESISTANCE TRAINING

Individuals can undertake regular resistance training to improve muscular strength and power. *Strength* is the maximum force generated by the muscle, whereas *power* is a product of muscle force and velocity. Power is an indicator of the rate at which the work of the muscle is performed. Changes in strength and power require numerous adaptations in the neuromuscular system depending on the type of resistance training. The neuromuscular system is highly responsive to training, and improvements in strength and/or power can be seen within months. Skeletal muscle is very dynamic. Training can improve muscle size (hypertrophy) and strength, whereas disuse or immobility can result in decreased size (atrophy) and strength. The primary neuromuscular adaptations to regular resistance training include:

- improved neural adaptations (increased motor unit recruitment, decreased neurologic inhibition) with strength gains, with or without hypertrophy, especially in the early stages of training;
- strength gains related to muscle hypertrophy in later stages of training; and
- increased size of the individual skeletal muscle fibers and increased numbers of myofibrils and actin and myosin filaments from hypertrophy.

Genetic potential plays a large role in body type. Muscles can be trained to improve strength and size, but there is a limit beyond which further adaptation is not possible.[43,44]

OVERREACHING AND OVERTRAINING

It is clear that proper training and adequate recovery result in increased performance, but many athletes develop the belief that "more is better" and that there is no ceiling for performance enhancement. Excessive training usually results in a performance decrement, for which the athlete often compensates with even more effort. The different stages of training-induced fatigue and subsequent restoration are known as functional overreaching and nonfunctional overreaching, also referred to as overtraining syndrome.[48] The American College of Sports Medicine and the European College of Sports Science[49] issued a joint consensus statement on this topic. *Functional overreaching* refers to a short-term training-induced decrement in performance thought to be necessary for optimal physiological adaptations. *Nonfunctional overreaching* describes excessive training that results in short-term performance decrements that may take several weeks to months to reverse with proper training and rest. During this time, it is critical that the athlete take in adequate amounts of fluid to restore hydration, carbohydrate to replenish glycogen stores, and protein to optimize protein synthesis and healing.

The symptoms leading to performance decrements include overall fatigue, muscular fatigue, chronic muscle tenderness and soreness, lack of concentration, and disrupted eating habits or loss of interest in eating. Persistent training with lack of physiological and psychological recovery can result in long-term and potentially permanent incomplete recovery, referred to as overtraining syndrome (OTS). OTS is more serious because long-term decrements in performance can take months to recover from. OTS includes both physiological maladaptation and psychological dysfunction stemming from increased physical and psychological stress. Because of a lack of standardization and because symptoms vary from person to person, experts have not reached a consensus on diagnostic criteria for OTS. It is important for an athlete with suspected OTS to seek medical care to rule out other confounding diseases or conditions and to develop a sound recovery plan, which consists of deloaded activity, rest, and functional treatment based on symptoms. Box 1.1 provides a list of some symptoms of overtraining syndrome.[1,49,50]

BOX 1.1 Signs and Symptoms of Overtraining Syndrome[1,49,50]

Decline in performance despite continued training

Fatigue, with loss of skeletal muscle strength, endurance capacity, and overall coordination

Decrease in appetite

Weight or fat loss

Anxiousness, restlessness, and sleep disruption

Inability to concentrate, loss of motivation, and even depression

SCOPE OF PRACTICE FOR REGISTERED DIETITIAN NUTRITIONISTS

Scope of practice is an important issue for all health professionals.[51] States that license various health professions have a defined scope of practice for each profession.[52] For RDNs interested in sports dietetics, there is a natural desire to discuss exercise with patients and clients, regardless of whether the RDN has the appropriate educational training or certification to do so. Current nutrition and dietetics educational programs accredited by the Accreditation Council for Education in Nutrition and Dietetics do not require courses, certain knowledge, or competencies specific to exercise science.[53] As a result, many RDNs graduating from traditional nutrition and dietetics programs are not qualified to discuss detailed issues regarding fitness assessment and exercise prescription. RDNs seeking to obtain more knowledge and skill related to nutrition and physical activity, exercise performance, or both should review the *Revised 2021 Standards of Practice and Standards of Professional Performance for Registered Dietitian Nutritionists*

(Competent, Proficient, and Expert) in Sports and Human Performance Nutrition to see if this is an area of specialty in which to seek additional credentialing.[54]

It is critical for the practitioner to understand the laws of the state(s) where they practice.[52] The exercise profession relies largely on self-regulated certification. Many states regulate the profession of dietetics, yet most states (except Louisiana) do not regulate the practice of exercise professionals. If a state licenses any health profession, licensure supersedes any registration or certification.

Physical Activity Guidance

RDNs with an interest in sports dietetics should be comfortable discussing some aspects of exercise and physical activity with their patients and clients. At a minimum, they should be familiar with the current federal *Physical Activity Guidelines for Americans*[45,46] and the overall health benefits of exercise. In general, RDNs can assist medically cleared patients and clients with planning and implementing ways to increase their physical activity levels to match these guidelines. RDNs should use the patient's or client's current level of physical activity and stage of readiness to change as a basis for planning physical activity goals. It is critical for the RDN to fully assess their current knowledge and scope of practice in the area of exercise science. Most RDNs who specialize in sports dietetics should be able to discuss the health benefits of exercise and the principles of exercise training discussed earlier in this chapter. Conducting a fitness assessment and prescribing exercise require specialized knowledge and skills and, ideally, an appropriate certification, both of which can be obtained by RDNs. If a patient or client needs physical activity information, a fitness assessment, or an exercise prescription that is outside of the RDN's scope of practice, the RDN must then provide a referral to a qualified exercise professional.

Fitness Assessment and Exercise Prescription

A fitness assessment measures cardiorespiratory fitness, musculoskeletal strength and endurance, flexibility, balance, and body composition. This information is used to develop a detailed exercise plan, known as an *exercise prescription*, tailored to the individual's current fitness level and health goals. The exercise prescription should be created by a qualified exercise professional. Conducting fitness assessments and writing exercise prescriptions may be outside the scope of practice for some RDNs, depending on whether they hold additional training and certification.

The American College of Sports Medicine (ACSM) ProFinder (www.acsm.org/certification/about/profinder) and the US Registry of Exercise Professionals (USREPS, https://usreps.org) are reputable websites that list qualified exercise professionals.[55,56] ACSM has certified more than 34,000 health professionals worldwide. USREPS is a nationally recognized registry of exercise professionals and an advocate for the exercise professionals who hold accredited exercise certifications from the National Commission of Certifying Agencies (NCCA).[57]

Reputable Exercise and Fitness Certifications

Unlike in nutrition and dietetics, no single accrediting body for college-level programs in kinesiology or exercise science results in a nationally recognized credential in either specialty. Academic programs in these fields may voluntarily become accredited through the Commission on Accreditation of Allied Health Education Programs (CAAHEP)[58] with the goal of achieving some consistency among all exercise science programs. Many CAAHEP-accredited programs provide a track for students to prepare for and earn an exercise-based certification.

If an RDN is not qualified to conduct fitness assessments and provide exercise prescriptions, it is important that they have a network of qualified exercise professionals for patient or client referral, and this should be documented when using the Nutrition Care Process.[59] Both physicians and exercise professionals can be a valuable resource for patients and clients. Fellowship-trained or board-certified sports medicine physicians can guide the client and may have a network of qualified exercise professionals for collaboration. Numerous exercise-related certifications are available; therefore, it is important to research the qualifications for certification and the knowledge and skills assessed in the process. The NCCA[57] governs many of the exercise certifications. Several reputable organizations and their certifications are listed in Box 1.2 on page 14.[60-62]

BOX 1.2 Example Certifications for Exercise Professionals[a,60-62]

Certification	Qualifications	Purpose
American College of Sports Medicine (ACSM) (www. acsm.org)		
Certified Personal Trainer	At least 18 years of age High school diploma or the equivalent Adult CPR/AED certification Must also pass examination	Plan and implement exercise programs for healthy individuals
Certified Group Exercise Instructor	At least 18 years of age High school diploma or the equivalent Adult CPR/AED certification Must also pass examination	Supervise participants or lead instructional sessions for healthy individuals
Certified Exercise Physiologist	Minimum of a bachelor's degree in exercise science, exercise physiology, or kinesiology Adult CPR/AED certification Must also pass examination	Conduct fitness assessments, create exercise plans, conduct personal training for those with medically controlled diseases
Certified Clinical Exercise Physiologist	Master's degree in clinical exercise physiology or the equivalent and 600 hours of hands-on clinical experience **OR** Bachelor's degree in exercise science, exercise physiology, or the equivalent and 1,200 hours of hands-on clinical experience Basic Life Support or CPR for the Professional Rescuer certification	Conduct fitness assessments; create exercise plans; conduct personal training for those with medically controlled diseases and those with cardiovascular, pulmonary, and metabolic diseases

Certification	Qualifications	Purpose
Exercise is Medicine Credential	Minimum of a bachelor's degree in exercise science, exercise physiology, or kinesiology ACSM certification or other National Commission for Certifying Agencies (NCCA)-accredited or International Organization for Standardization/International Electrotechnical Commission 17024 fitness certification Must complete all modules of the Exercise is Medicine online course and pass all online exams with a score of 80% or higher	Help individuals with common chronic diseases lead healthier, more active lives Credential holders are also more likely to be seen as trusted referral resource by health care providers
Autism Exercise Specialist Certificate	Available to exercise professionals, physical education or adapted physical education teachers, physical therapists, recreational therapists, or special education professionals Must complete online course and pass virtual or in-person examination	Incorporate specialized strategies to implement individual or group exercise programs for those with autism in a gym, home, or classroom setting
ACSM in Collaboration with the American Cancer Society (ACS) (www.acsm.org)		
ACSM/ACS Certified Cancer Exercise Trainer	ACSM- or NCCA-accredited health or fitness certification Adult CPR/AED certification Bachelor's degree (in any field) with 500 hours of experience training older adults or individuals with chronic conditions **OR** 10,000 hours of experience training older adults or individuals with chronic conditions Must also pass examination	Work with clients who have been cleared by their physician for independent exercise and physical activity

Continued on next page

BOX 1.2 Example Certifications for Exercise Professionals[a,60-62] (CONTINUED)

Certification	Qualifications	Purpose
ACSM in collaboration with the National Center on Health, Physical Activity and Disability (NCHPAD) (www.acsm.org)		
ACSM/NCHPAD Certified Inclusive Fitness Trainer	Complete online preparation course and pass examination	Empower those who are challenged by physical, sensory, or cognitive disabilities to engage in physical activity
ACSM in Collaboration with the National Physical Activity Society (NPAS) (www.acsm.org)		
ACSM/NPAS Certified Physical Activity in Public Health Specialist	Bachelor's degree in a health-related field from a regionally accredited college or university **OR** Bachelor's degree in any subject with 1,200 hours of experience in settings promoting physical activity, healthy lifestyle management, or other health promotion Must also pass examination	Promote physical activity with a focus on the public health setting; develop key partnerships to establish legislation, policies, and programs that promote physical activity for people throughout the country
National Strength and Conditioning Association (NSCA) (www.nsca.org)		
Certified Strength and Conditioning Specialist (CSCS)	Minimum of a bachelor's degree or currently enrolled as a college senior Current CPR/AED certification Must pass an exam that tests knowledge, skills, and abilities in 2 areas of professional practice: scientific foundations and practical/applied	Apply scientific knowledge to train athletes for the primary goal of improving athletic performance; conduct sport-specific testing sessions, design and implement safe and effective strength-training and conditioning programs, and provide guidance regarding nutrition and injury prevention
NSCA-Certified Personal Trainer (CPT)	At least 18 years of age High school diploma or an equivalent Current CPR/AED certification Must pass an exam that tests knowledge, skills, and abilities in 4 domains: client consultation/fitness assessment, program planning, exercise techniques, and safety/emergency issues	Assess, motivate, educate and train clients regarding their personal health and fitness needs; design safe and effective exercise programs, provide guidance to help clients achieve their personal health and fitness goals, and respond appropriately in emergency situations

Certification	Qualifications	Purpose
Certified Special Population Specialist (CSPS)	Minimum of a bachelor's degree OR A license in 1 of a number of occupations Current CPR/AED certification Must pass an exam that tests knowledge, skills, and abilities in 4 domains: basic pathophysiology and science of health status, condition, disorder or disease; client consultation; program planning; and safety, emergency procedures, and legal issues	Assess, motivate, educate, and train special population clients of all ages regarding their health and fitness needs, preventively and in collaboration with health care professionals
American Council on Exercise (ACE) (www.acefitness.org)		
Personal Trainer Certification	At least 18 years of age High school diploma or the equivalent Adult CPR/AED certification Must also pass examination	May work as a virtual coach or online trainer, athletic coach, gym owner, self-employed corrective exercise and injury prevention specialist
Group Fitness Instructor Certification	At least 18 years of age High school diploma or the equivalent Adult CPR/AED certification Must also pass examination	Lead various fitness classes for healthy individuals
Medical Exercise Specialist Certification	At least 18 years of age Adult CPR/AED certification Bachelor's degree in exercise science or a related field Proof of 500 hours of work experience designing and implementing exercise programs for apparently healthy individuals and/or high-risk individuals	Work as part of a client's health care team, helping them prevent or effectively manage chronic disease

Continued on next page

BOX 1.2 Example Certifications for Exercise Professionals[a,60-62] (CONTINUED)

Certification	Qualifications	Purpose
American Council on Exercise (ACE) (www.acefitness.org) (continued)		
Health Coach Certification	At least 18 years of age Adult CPR/AED certification Must also submit proof of at least 1 of the following: • Current NCCA-accredited certification in fitness, nutrition, health care, wellness, human resources, or a related field • Associate's degree or higher from an accredited college or university in fitness, exercise science, nutrition, health care, wellness, or a related field • Minimum of 2 years of documented work experience in coaching, leading, designing, implementing, or facilitating 1 or more of the areas behavior or lifestyle change, exercise, wellness, nutrition, or physical activity • Completed health coach training and education program approved by the National Board for Health and Wellness Coaches (NBHWC)	Recognize unique dietary, emotional, and physical needs of individuals and help people reach their goals and implement lifestyle changes that improve their overall health and wellness with exercise, nutrition, and psychology; can work in a variety of settings from health clubs to corporations, virtual coaching to health care

[a] This is not an all-inclusive list. Please see the organization websites for updated information.

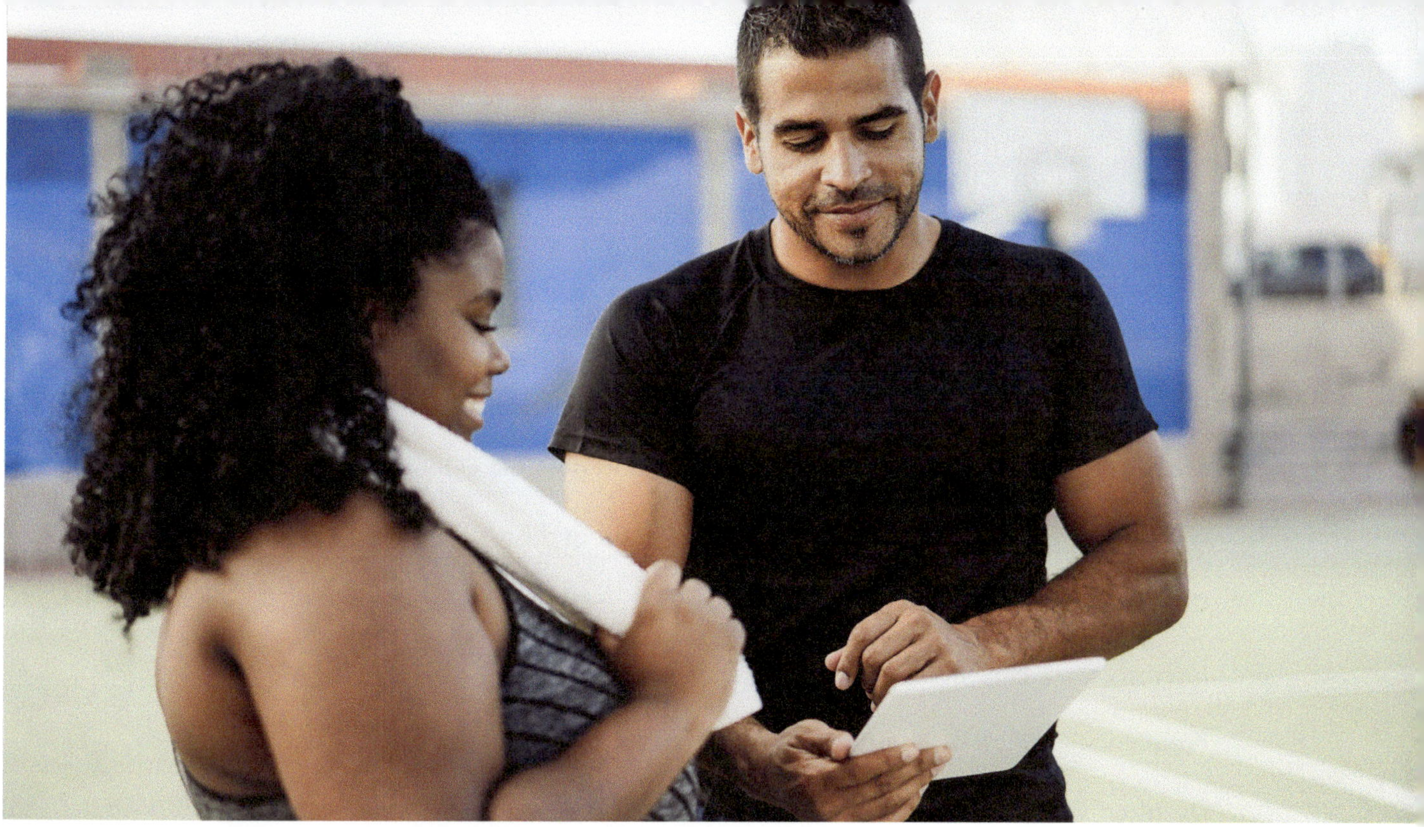

Physical Activity Guidance and the Nutrition Care Process

The Nutrition Care Process consists of nutrition assessment, diagnosis, intervention, monitoring, and evaluation.[63] These steps as they relate to physical activity guidance are detailed further below.

Assessment The RDN may assess an individual's readiness to change, weight and body composition, physical activity history, and current level of physical activity.

Diagnosis The RDN can document any problems and create a diagnosis (problem, etiology, signs and symptoms) statement. The diagnosis often references the individual's level of physical activity or inactivity, readiness to change, or something in the behavioral domain.

Intervention The RDN can choose to provide education if it is within their scope of practice, provide a referral to a qualified exercise professional, or do a combination of the 2. For most RDNs, education can include a discussion of topics such as the health benefits of exercise, the way to start an exercise program, and the key concepts presented in the *Physical Activity Guidelines for Americans*,[45,46] as well as providing additional resources (eg, handouts, names of community centers, list of professionals).

Monitoring and evaluation The RDN should include follow-up on the physical activity–related goals set for the patient or client.

For more information on how to discuss physical activity guidance using the Nutrition Care Process, refer to the Academy of Nutrition and Dietetics publication *A Physical Activity Toolkit for RDNs: Exercise is Medicine*.[64] This tool kit contains extensive links to usable resources and handouts on the topic of discussing physical activity with patients.

Physical Activity Guidelines for Americans

RDNs with an interest in sports dietetics should be familiar with the *Physical Activity Guidelines for Americans* and be comfortable discussing these guidelines with their patients or clients.[45,46] The guidelines can be downloaded free of charge at the Health.gov website (https://health.gov/our-work/nutrition-physical-activity/physical-activity-guidelines). In addition to the document itself, a ready-made PowerPoint presentation that covers key concepts in the guidelines is available. Box 1.3 on page 20 provides definitions of the levels, components, and intensity of physical activity found in the guidelines.

BOX 1.3 Definitions of Levels, Components, and Intensity of Physical Activity in the Physical Activity Guidelines for Americans[45,46]

Levels of physical activity	
Inactive	No activity beyond baseline (this is considered unhealthy)
Low	Beyond baseline but fewer than 150 min/wk (better for health than inactive)
Medium	150 to 300 min/wk (additional and possible extensive health benefits)
High	More than 300 min/wk (additional and possible extensive health benefits)
Components of physical activity	
Intensity	How hard a person works
Frequency	How often an activity is performed
Duration	How long an activity lasts in 1 session or how many repetitions are performed
Intensity of physical activity	
Light	1.1 to 2.9 METs[a] (1.1-2.9 times rest)
Moderate	3.0 to 5.9 METs
Vigorous	6.0 METs or higher

[a] MET = metabolic equivalent. 1 MET represents the work at rest and is equivalent to an oxygen consumption (VO_2) of 3.5 mL × kg^{-1} × min^{-1}.

Metabolic equivalents (METs) are another way of defining exercise intensity. MET is the ratio of the rate of energy expended during exercise to the rate of energy expended at rest. One MET is equivalent to an oxygen consumption (VO_2) of 3.5 mL × kg^{-1} × min^{-1}. Multiples of this value can be used to quantify energy expenditure, as discussed in detail in Chapter 10. One MET is the work at rest, whereas 5 METs equals 5 times the energy expenditure at rest. The *Physical Activity Guidelines* also use MET-minutes for guidance. MET-minutes consider both physical activity intensity and duration. For example, a 4-MET activity done for 30 minutes is equivalent to 120 MET-minutes, and an 8-MET activity done for 15 minutes is also equivalent to 120 MET-minutes. For health benefits, one can exercise at a lower intensity for longer periods of time or at a higher intensity for shorter periods of time. Practitioners should note that these physical activity guidelines are for general health and are not exercise training guidelines for optimal performance. The goal for health is to achieve a minimum of 500 to 1,000 MET-min/wk, with potential greater health benefits found at greater than 1,000 MET-min/wk. The relationship between intensity and METs is summarized as follows:

- Light intensity = 1.1 to 2.9 METs
- Moderate intensity = 3.0 to 5.9 METs
  - For example, walking at a rate of 3 mph requires 3.3 METs of energy expenditure.
- Vigorous intensity = 6.0 METs or greater
  - For example, running a 10-minute mile (6 mph) is a 10-MET activity.

Key guidelines for health from the *Physical Activity Guidelines for Americans* are summarized in Box 1.4.[45,46]

BOX 1.4 Summary of Key Guidelines for Health from the *Physical Activity Guidelines for Americans*[45,46]

It is important to get people to sit less and move more.

Physical activity reduces the risk of many adverse health outcomes.

Some physical activity is better than none.

Physical activity has immediate health benefits.

Consistently meeting the recommendations in these guidelines can lead to even more long-term health benefits.

There is new evidence for many additional health benefits related to physical and mental health.

Additional benefits occur with increases in intensity, frequency, and duration.

Both cardiorespiratory and resistance exercise are beneficial.

Health benefits occur at all ages.

Benefits far outweigh the possibility of adverse outcomes.

Substantial health benefits are seen with 150 min/wk of moderate-intensity physical activity or 75 min/wk of vigorous physical activity or a combination.

Additional health benefits are seen with 300 min/wk of moderate-intensity physical activity or 150 min/wk of vigorous physical activity or a combination.

Resistance training—moderate or high in intensity—involving all major muscle groups is recommended 2 d/wk or more.

For health, 2 minutes of moderate physical activity is equivalent to 1 minute of vigorous physical activity.

SUMMARY

Exercise physiology is the study of the body alterations and responses to acute and chronic exercise. Exercise disrupts homeostasis, resulting in increased energy needs to meet the metabolic demands of active muscles. The respiratory and cardiovascular systems work in a coordinated fashion to supply oxygen and nutrients to working muscles in an attempt to meet this demand. At lower moderate-intensity exercise, the body can use carbohydrate and fat in aerobic metabolism, meeting the energy demands with ease. As exercise intensity increases, the body's reliance on carbohydrate as a fuel source with some ATP being generated through anaerobic glycolysis increases. Short-term or metabolic fatigue is a result of reliance on anaerobic metabolism, whereas long-term or substrate fatigue is a result of glycogen depletion. Exercise training results in positive physiological adaptations that improve performance. Several principles of exercise training are key for determining the performance outcome.

RDNs should be comfortable discussing exercise with their patients or clients while staying within their scope of practice. The extent of this discussion will depend on individual comfort level and any additional education and certification. All RDNs should be able to discuss the health benefits of exercise and the general principles in the *Physical Activity Guidelines for Americans.* Beyond this, if the RDN cannot complete a fitness assessment and exercise prescription, then the RDN should provide a referral to a qualified exercise professional.

KEY TAKEAWAYS

An understanding of exercise physiology basics is necessary for all RDNs interested in sports nutrition in order to understand the sports nutrition-specific guidelines and their effects on performance.

Exercise results in increased skeletal muscle ATP demand, and the cardiovascular and respiratory systems work in a coordinated fashion to deliver oxygen and nutrients to the working skeletal muscle.

The key nutrients providing energy during exercise are carbohydrate and fat. Carbohydrate can provide ATP through both anaerobic and aerobic metabolism, but fat can only be fully oxidized aerobically.

At all times, the body is using a mixture of carbohydrate and fat. As exercise intensity increases, there is an increased reliance on carbohydrate for fuel (crossover concept). Carbohydrate is a more oxygen-efficient fuel and can produce ATP quickly.

Short-term or metabolic fatigue is a result of a reliance on anaerobic metabolism under high exercise intensities. Long-term or substrate fatigue is a result of glycogen depletion.

Sound training results in physiological adaptations that improve performance. There are several principles of training that should be considered.

RDNs should include physical activity in their use of the Nutrition Care Process.

All RDNs interested in sports nutrition should be comfortable discussing the health benefits of exercise and the key principles presented in the *Physical Activity Guidelines for Americans, 2020-2025*.

An RDN may or may not have the education and training to conduct fitness assessments and develop exercise prescriptions. If not, the RDN must provide a referral to a qualified exercise professional.

REFERENCES

1. Kenny WL, Wilmore JH, Costill DL. *Physiology of Sport and Exercise.* 8th ed.: Human Kinetics; 2022.
2. Academy of Nutrition and Dietetics. About RDNs and NDTRs. www.eatright.org. Accessed December 1, 2022. www.eatright.org/about-rdns-and-ndtrs
3. Sports and Human Performance Nutrition. Board Certified Specialist in Sports Dietetics (CSSD). Accessed December 1, 2022. www.shpndpg .org/shpn/professional-resources/cssd
4. Achten J, Gleeson M, Jeukendrup AE. Determination of the exercise intensity that elicits maximal fat oxidation. *Med Sci Sports Exerc.* 2002;34(1):92-97. doi:10.1097/00005768-200201000-00015
5. Brooks GA. Bioenergetics of exercising humans. *Compr Physiol.* 2012;2(1):537-562. doi:10.1002/cphy.c110007
6. Gollnick PD. Metabolism of substrates: energy substrate metabolism during exercise and as modified by training. *Fed Proc.* 1985;44(2):353-357.
7. Newsholme EA. The control of fuel utilization by muscle during exercise and starvation. *Diabetes.* 1979;28(suppl 1):1-7. doi:10.2337/diab.28.1.s1
8. Fry AC, Allemeier CA, Staron RS. Correlation between percentage fiber type area and myosin heavy chain content in human skeletal muscle. *Eur J Appl Physiol Occup Physiol.* 1994;68(3):246-251. doi:10.1007/BF00376773
9. Herzog W, Powers K, Johnston K, Duvall M. A new paradigm for muscle contraction. *Front Physiol.* 2015;6:174. doi:10.3389/fphys.2015.00174
10. Staron RS, Karapondo DL, Kraemer WJ, et al. Skeletal muscle adaptations during early phase of heavy-resistance training in men and women. *J Appl Physiol (1985).* 1994;76(3):1247-1255. doi:10.1152/jappl.1994.76.3.1247
11. Barnard RJ, Edgerton VR, Furukawa T, Peter JB. Histochemical, biochemical, and contractile properties of red, white, and intermediate fibers. *Am J Physiol.* 1971;220(2):410-414. doi:10.1152/ajplegacy.1971.220.2.410
12. Brooke MH, Kaiser KK. Muscle fiber types: how many and what kind? *Arch Neurol.* 1970;23(4):369-379. doi:10.1001/archneur.1970.00480280083010
13. D'Antona G, Lanfranconi F, Pellegrino MA, et al. Skeletal muscle hypertrophy and structure and function of skeletal muscle fibres in male body builders. *J Physiol.* 2006;570(Pt 3):611-627. doi:10.1113/jphysiol.2005.10164214
14. Fry AC, Schilling BK, Staron RS, Hagerman FC, Hikida RS, Thrush JT. Muscle fiber characteristics and performance correlates of male Olympic-style weightlifters. *J Strength Cond Res.* 2003;17(4):746-754. doi:10.1519/1533-4287(2003)017
15. Jürimäe J, Abernethy PJ, Quigley BM, Blake K, McEniery MT. Differences in muscle contractile characteristics among bodybuilders, endurance trainers and control subjects. *Eur J Appl Physiol Occup Physiol.* 1997;75(4):357-362. doi:10.1007/s004210050172
16. Kesidis N, Metaxas TI, Vrabas IS, et al. Myosin heavy chain isoform distribution in single fibres of bodybuilders. *Eur J Appl Physiol.* 2008;103(5):579-583. doi:10.1007/s00421-008-0751-5
17. Klitgaard H, Zhou M, Richter EA. Myosin heavy chain composition of single fibres from m. biceps brachii of male body builders. *Acta Physiol Scand.* 1990;140(2):175-180. doi:10.1111/j.1748-1716.1990.tb08989.x
18. Shoepe TC, Stelzer JE, Garner DP, Widrick JJ. Functional adaptability of muscle fibers to long-term resistance exercise. *Med Sci Sports Exerc.* 2003;35(6):944-951. doi:10.1249/01.mss.0000069756.17841.9e
19. MacDougall JD, Sale DG, Alway SE, Sutton JR. Muscle fiber number in biceps brachii in bodybuilders and control subjects. *J Appl Physiol Respir Environ Exerc Physiol.* 1984;57(5):1399-1403. doi:10.1152/jappl.1984.57.5.1399
20. Costill DL, Coyle EF, Fink WF, Lesmes GR, Witzmann FA. Adaptations in skeletal muscle following strength training. *J Appl Physiol Respir Environ Exerc Physiol.* 1979;46(1):96-99. doi:10.1152/jappl.1979.46.1.96
21. Gollnick PD, Armstrong RB, Saubert CW 4th, Piehl K, Saltin B. Enzyme activity and fiber composition in skeletal muscle of untrained and trained men. *J Appl Physiol.* 1972;33(3):312-319. doi:10.1152/jappl.1972.33.3.312
22. Harber MP, Gallagher PM, Creer AR, Minchev KM, Trappe SW. Single muscle fiber contractile properties during a competitive season in male runners. *Am J Physiol Regul Integr Comp Physiol.* 2004;287(5):R1124-R1131. doi:10.1152/ajpregu.00686.2003
23. Trappe S, Harber M, Creer A, et al. Single muscle fiber adaptations with marathon training. *J Appl Physiol (1985).* 2006;101(3):721-727. doi:10.1152/japplphysiol.01595.2005
24. Saltin B, Gollnick, PD. Skeletal muscle adaptability: significance for metabolism and performance. In: Peachey LD, ed. *Handbook of Physiology–Skeletal Muscle.* American Physiological Society; 1983:555-631.
25. Concu A, Marcello C. Stroke volume response to progressive exercise in athletes engaged in different types of training. *Eur J Appl Physiol Occup Physiol.* 1993;66(1):11-17. doi:10.1007/BF00863393
26. Casey DP, Joyner MJ. Local control of skeletal muscle blood flow during exercise: influence of available oxygen. *J Appl Physiol (1985).* 2011;111(6):1527-1538. doi:10.1152/japplphysiol.00895.2011
27. Bassett DR Jr, Howley ET. Limiting factors for maximum oxygen uptake and determinants of endurance performance. *Med Sci Sports Exerc.* 2000;32(1):70-84. doi:10.1097/00005768-200001000-00012
28. Howley ET, Bassett DR Jr, Welch HG. Criteria for maximal oxygen uptake: review and commentary. *Med Sci Sports Exerc.* 1995;27(9):1292-1301.
29. Taylor HL, Buskirk E, Henschel A. Maximal oxygen intake as an objective measure of cardio-respiratory performance. *J Appl Physiol.* 1955;8(1):73-80. doi:10.1152/jappl.1955.8.1.73
30. Foster C, Kuffel E, Bradley N, et al. VO2max during successive maximal efforts. *Eur J Appl Physiol.* 2007;102(1):67-72. doi:10.1007/s00421-007-0565-x

31. Stromme SB, Ingjer F, Meen HD. Assessment of maximal aerobic power in specifically trained athletes. *J Appl Physiol Respir Environ Exerc Physiol.* 1977;42(6):833-837. doi:10.1152/jappl.1977.42.6.833
32. Gollnick PD, Riedy M, Quintinskie JJ, Bertocci LA. Differences in metabolic potential of skeletal muscle fibres and their significance for metabolic control. *J Exp Biol.* 1985;115:191-199. doi:10.1242/jeb.115.1.191
33. Wilmore JH, Stanforth PR, Gagnon J, et al. Cardiac output and stroke volume changes with endurance training: the HERITAGE Family Study. *Med Sci Sports Exerc.* 2001;33(1):99-106. doi:10.1097/00005768-200101000-00016
34. Baar K. Nutrition and the adaptation to endurance training. *Sports Med.* 2014;44(suppl 1):S5-S12. doi:10.1007/s40279-014-0146-1
35. Bergström J, Hermansen L, Hultman E, Saltin B. Diet, muscle glycogen and physical performance. *Acta Physiol Scand.* 1967;71(2):140-150. doi:10.1111/j.1748-1716.1967.tb03720.x
36. Jeukendrup AE. Performance and endurance in sport: can it all be explained by metabolism and its manipulation? *Dialog Cardiovasc Med.* 2012;17(1):40-45.
37. Brooks GA. Lactate production under fully aerobic conditions: the lactate shuttle during rest and exercise. *Fed Proc.* 1986;45(13):2924-2929.
38. Stainsby WN, Brooks GA. Control of lactic acid metabolism in contracting muscles and during exercise. *Exerc Sport Sci Rev.* 1990;18:29-63.
39. Brooks GA, Mercier J. Balance of carbohydrate and lipid utilization during exercise: the "crossover" concept. *J Appl Physiol.* 1985;76(6):2253-2261. doi:10.1152/jappl.1994.76.6.2253
40. Allen DG, Lamb GD, Westerblad H. Skeletal muscle fatigue: cellular mechanisms. *Physiol Rev.* 2008;88(1):287-332. doi:10.1152/physrev.00015.2007
41. Enoka RM, Stuart DG. Neurobiology of muscle fatigue. *J Appl Physiol (1985).* 1992;72(5):1631-1648. doi:10.1152/jappl.1992.72.5.1631
42. Fitts RH. Cellular mechanisms of muscle fatigue. *Physiol Rev.* 1994;74(1):49-94. doi:10.1152/physrev.1994.74.1.49
43. Manore MM. Weight management in the performance athlete. *Nestle Nutr Inst Workshop Ser.* 2013;75:123-33. doi:10.1159/000345831
44. Manore MM. Weight management for athletes and active individuals: a brief review. *Sports Med.* 2015;45 (suppl 1):83-92. doi:10.1007/s40279-015-0401-0
45. US Department of Health and Human Services, Office of Disease Prevention and Health Promotion. Physical Activity Guidelines for Americans. Accessed December 1, 2022. https://health.gov/our-work/nutrition-physical-activity/physical-activity-guidelines
46. US Department of Health and Human Services, Office of Disease Prevention and Health Promotion. 2018 Physical Activity Guidelines for Americans Advisory Committee Scientific Report. February 2018. Accessed December 1, 2022. https://health.gov/paguidelines/second-edition/report
47. Issurin VB. New horizons for the methodology and physiology of training periodization. *Sports Med.* 2010;40(3):189-206. doi:10.2165/11319770-000000000-00000
48. Bellinger P. Functional overreaching in endurance athletes: a necessity or cause for concern? *Sports Med.* 2020;50(6):1059-1073. doi:10.1007/s40279-020-01269-w
49. Meeusen R, Duclos M, Foster C, et al. Prevention, diagnosis, and treatment of the overtraining syndrome: joint consensus statement of the European College of Sport Science and the American College of Sports Medicine. *Med Sci Sports Exerc.* 2013;45(1):186-205. doi:10.1249/MSS.0b013e318279a10a
50. Kreher JB, Schwartz JB. Overtraining syndrome: a practical guide. *Sports Health.* 2012;4(2):128-138. doi:10.1177/1941738111434406
51. Academy of Nutrition and Dietetics. Scope and Standards of Practice. Accessed December 1, 2022. www.eatrightpro.org/practice/dietetics-resources/scope-and-standards-of-practice
52. Academy of Nutrition and Dietetics. Licensure and Professional Regulation of Dietitians. Accessed December 1, 2022. www.eatrightpro.org/advocacy/licensure/professional-regulation-of-dietitians
53. Academy of Nutrition and Dietetics. Accreditation Council for Education in Nutrition and Dietetics. Accessed December 1, 2022. www.eatrightpro.org/acend
54. Daigle K, Subach R, Valliant M. Academy of Nutrition and Dietetics: Revised 2021 Standards of Practice and Standards of Professional Performance for Registered Dietitian Nutritionists (Competent, Proficient, and Expert) in Sports and Human Performance Nutrition. *J Acad Nutr Diet.* 2021;121(9):1813-1830.e55. doi:10.1016/j.jand.2021.04.018
55. American College of Sports Medicine. ACSM ProFinder. Accessed December 1, 2022. www.acsm.org/certification/about/profinder
56. US Registry of Exercise Professionals. Welcome to the United States Registry of Exercise Professionals. Accessed December 1, 2022. www.usreps.org/Pages/Default.aspx
57. Institute for Credentialing Excellence. NCCA Accreditation. Accessed December 1, 2022. www.credentialingexcellence.org/Accreditation/Earn-Accreditation/NCCA
58. Commission on Accreditation of Allied Health Education Programs. Accessed November 14, 2022. www.caahep.org
59. Academy of Nutrition and Dietetics. Nutrition Care Process. Accessed November 11, 2022. www.eatrightpro.org/research/projects-tools-and-initiatives/nutrition-care-process
60. American College of Sports Medicine. Accessed December 1, 2022. www.acsm.org
61. National Strength and Conditioning Association. Accessed December 1, 2022. www.nsca.com
62. American Council on Exercise. Accessed December 1, 2022. www.acefitness.org
63. Academy of Nutrition and Dietetics. Electronic Nutrition Care Process Terminology (eNCPT). Accessed November 21, 2022. www.ncpro.org
64. Academy of Nutrition and Dietetics. A Physical Activity Toolkit for RDNs: Exercise is Medicine. Accessed November 21, 2022. www.eatrightpro.org/practice/dietetics-resources/sports-nutrition-and-athletic-performance/a-physical-activity-toolkit-for-rdns-exercise-is-medicine

CHAPTER 2

Carbohydrate and Exercise

Ellen J. Coleman, MA, MPH, RD

LEARNING OBJECTIVES

- Describe nutritional strategies to enhance carbohydrate availability in athletes.
- Explain why the energy demands of exercise dictate that carbohydrate is the predominant fuel for exercise.
- Define the recommended daily carbohydrate intake based on the athlete's exercise intensity and duration.
- Define the recommended carbohydrate intake during exercise based on exercise intensity and duration.
- Define the recommended carbohydrate intake to promote recovery following glycogen-depleting exercise.
- Describe the potential benefits and risks of training with low carbohydrate availability.

INTRODUCTION

Adequate carbohydrate stores (in muscle and liver glycogen and blood glucose) are critical for optimum performance and training adaptations during both intermittent high-intensity work and prolonged endurance exercise. Experts can recommend nutritional strategies to enhance carbohydrate availability to match the fuel demands of key training sessions (those designed to mimic the physiological demands of competition), as well as competitive events.[1-3]

Consuming carbohydrate before exercise can help performance by topping off existing muscle and liver glycogen stores. Consuming carbohydrate during exercise can improve performance by maintaining blood glucose levels and carbohydrate oxidation, sparing muscle glycogen, or activating reward centers in the central nervous system. Ingesting carbohydrate after glycogen-depleting exercise facilitates rapid glycogen restoration, especially among athletes engaged in daily hard training, multiday endurance events, or tournaments.[1-3]

CARBOHYDRATE AVAILABILITY AND PERIODIZATION

Consuming adequate carbohydrate is necessary to replenish muscle and liver glycogen between key training sessions and competitive events and to help meet the energy requirements of the athlete's training program.[1-3] *Carbohydrate availability* is defined as the sum of the endogenous carbohydrate (eg, muscle and liver glycogen) and exogenous carbohydrate (eg, carbohydrate consumed before and/or during exercise) that is available to sustain the required exercise intensity and duration. A diet with high carbohydrate availability provides sufficient endogenous and/or exogenous carbohydrate to sustain the required exercise workload, whereas a diet with low carbohydrate availability does not. It is possible to have low carbohydrate availability (even if exercise is started with high muscle glycogen stores) if inadequate carbohydrate is consumed during exercise to sustain the desired workload. On the other hand, it is possible to start exercise with reduced muscle glycogen stores but have high carbohydrate availability if the carbohydrate consumed during exercise sustains the desired workload.[3,4] High carbohydrate availability can be achieved by consuming carbohydrate in the hours or days before exercise, ingesting carbohydrate during exercise, and consuming carbohydrate after exercise.[1-3,5-7]

Training with high carbohydrate availability supports the intensity and duration of key training sessions.[1,3,5-7] Undertaking key training sessions with high carbohydrate availability also allows the athlete to practice fueling strategies before and during competition and helps to train the gut by improving gastric emptying and intestinal absorption.[1,3,5,6,8] Training with high carbohydrate availability enhances the energy pathways of oxygen-independent glycolysis and carbohydrate oxidation.[3,9]

Athletes should "fuel for the work required" and adjust carbohydrate intake (periodization) according to the fuel demands of the specific training session or competitive event.[3,4] With carbohydrate periodization, the total daily carbohydrate intake and distribution can be altered day by day and meal by meal to manipulate carbohydrate availability.[1,3,5-8] Training with low carbohydrate availability during carefully selected exercise sessions *may* enhance training adaptations, as discussed later in this chapter.[1,3,4,7]

Energy Availability

Athletes should consume sufficient energy, as well as carbohydrate, to support the range of body functions needed for optimal health and performance. *Energy availability* is calculated as energy intake minus energy cost of exercise relative to fat-free mass. A value of 45 kcal per kilogram of fat-free mass per day equates energy balance in healthy adults.[1] Low energy availability may occur as a result of insufficient energy intake, high energy cost of exercise, or a combination of the 2.[1,10] Low energy availability may be associated with disordered eating, extremely rapid weight loss, or an unintentional failure to meet energy requirements during periods with frequent training sessions and heavy training loads. *Relative energy deficiency in sport* (REDs) is a group of physiological complications caused by low energy availability that includes, but is not limited to, impairments in metabolic rate, menstrual function, bone health, immunity, protein synthesis, and psychological and cardiovascular health. Potential performance effects of REDs include decreased endurance, increased injury risk, decreased training response, impaired judgment, depression, and reduced muscle strength.[1,10,11] More information on REDs can be found in Chapter 18.

CARBOHYDRATE USE DURING EXERCISE

The size of the body's endogenous carbohydrate stores is relatively limited and can be acutely altered by daily dietary intake and exercise.[1] Muscle glycogen represents the major source of carbohydrate in the body (300–400 g or 1,200–1,600 kcal), followed by liver glycogen (75–110 g or 300–440 kcal) and, lastly, blood glucose (5 g or 20 kcal). Untrained individuals have muscle glycogen stores of roughly 80 to 90 mmol per kilogram of wet muscle weight. Endurance athletes have muscle glycogen stores of 130 to 135 mmol per kilogram of wet muscle weight. Carbohydrate loading increases muscle glycogen stores to 210 to 230 mmol per kilogram of wet muscle weight.[5] Muscle glycogen is used most rapidly during early stages of exercise and is exponentially related to exercise intensity.[12]

The energy demands of exercise dictate that carbohydrate is the predominant fuel for exercise. Unlike fat (intramuscular lipid and adipose tissue triglycerides), carbohydrate can be used by both the glycolytic (anaerobic) and oxidative (aerobic) energy pathways.[1] Muscle glycogen and blood glucose provide about half of the energy for moderate-intensity exercise (65% of maximal oxygen uptake [VO_2 max]) and two-thirds of the energy for high-intensity exercise (85% of VO_2 max).[12] It is impossible to meet the adenosine triphosphate (ATP) requirements for high-intensity, high-power-output exercise when these carbohydrate fuels are depleted.[1,12] Carbohydrate also offers advantages over fat as a substrate because it provides approximately 5.5% more ATP per liter of oxygen consumed, thereby improving gross exercise efficiency.[1,3]

Liver glycogen stores maintain blood glucose levels both at rest and during exercise. At rest, the brain and central nervous system use most of the blood glucose, and muscle accounts for less than 20% of blood glucose utilization. However, during exercise, muscle glucose uptake can increase 30-fold, depending on exercise intensity and duration. Initially during exercise, the majority of hepatic glucose output comes from glycogenolysis; however, as exercise duration increases and liver glycogen decreases, the contribution of glucose from gluconeogenesis increases. Liver glycogen stores can be depleted by a 15-hour fast, decreasing from a typical level of 490 mmol on a mixed diet to 60 mmol on a low-carbohydrate diet. A high-carbohydrate diet can increase liver glycogen content to approximately 900 mmol.[12]

At the beginning of exercise, the hepatic glucose output matches the increased muscle glucose uptake, so blood glucose levels remain near resting levels. Although muscle glycogen is the primary source of carbohydrate during exercise intensities between 65% and 85% of VO_2 max, blood glucose becomes an increasingly important source of carbohydrate as muscle glycogen stores decrease. Hypoglycemia occurs when the hepatic glucose output can no longer keep up with muscle glucose uptake during prolonged exercise.[12]

DAILY CARBOHYDRATE RECOMMENDATIONS

Muscle glycogen depletion is associated with fatigue and reduced exercise intensity, whereas insufficient carbohydrate for the central nervous system impairs concentration, motor skills, and pacing and increases the perception of effort. Experts recommend promoting high carbohydrate availability to promote optimal performance in key training sessions and competitive events.[1-3]

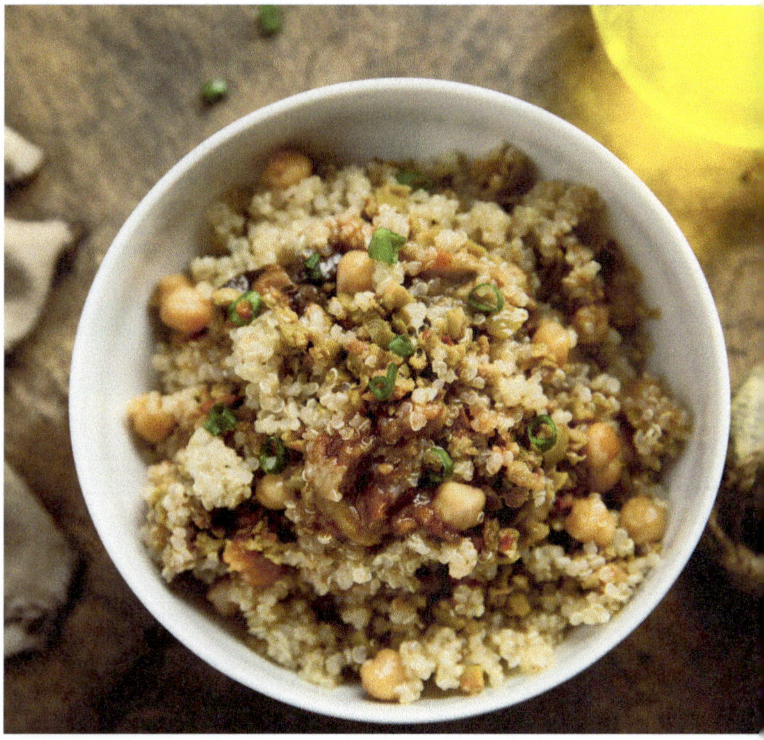

Manipulating nutrition and exercise before a key training session allows the athlete to start with glycogen stores that match the estimated fuel costs of the session. In the absence of muscle damage, muscle glycogen stores can be normalized with 24 hours of reduced training or rest and a carbohydrate intake of 7 to 10 g of carbohydrate per kilogram per day. These stores appear adequate for muscle fuel needs during 60 to 90 minutes of exercise.[1,5,13,14]

Targets for daily carbohydrate intake are based on the athlete's body weight (to account for the size of the athlete's muscle mass) and the athlete's training load. Recommendations for daily carbohydrate intake range from 3 to 12 g of carbohydrate per kilogram per day. Athletes with very light training programs (low-intensity exercise or skill-based exercise) should consume 3 to 5 g of carbohydrate per kilogram of body weight per day. These targets may also be suitable for athletes with a large body mass or athletes who need to reduce energy intake to lose weight. Athletes engaged in moderate-intensity training programs for 60 min/d should consume 5 to 7 g of carbohydrate per kilogram of body weight per day. Athletes participating in moderate- to high-intensity endurance exercise lasting for 1 to 3 hours should consume 6 to 10 g of carbohydrate per kilogram of body weight per day. Athletes undertaking moderate- to high-intensity endurance exercise for 4 to 5 h/d or more (eg, the Tour de France) should consume 8 to 12 g of carbohydrate per kilogram of body weight per day.[1] Recommended daily carbohydrate intake is summarized in Box 2.1 on page 28.[1,2]

These recommendations for carbohydrate intake are general and should be adjusted with consideration for the athlete's total energy needs, specific training needs, and feedback from their training performance.[1,2] Carbohydrate availability can be strategically periodized and adjusted around important training sessions

BOX 2.1 Recommended Daily Carbohydrate Intake for Athletes[a,1,2]

Type of activity	Recommended carbohydrate intake
Very light training program (low-intensity or skill-based exercise)	3 to 5 g per kilogram of body weight
Moderate-intensity training programs, 60 min/d	5 to 7 g per kilogram of body weight
Moderate- to high-intensity endurance exercise, 1 to 3 h/d	6 to 10 g per kilogram of body weight
Moderate- to high-intensity exercise, 4 to 5 h/d	8 to 12 g per kilogram of body weight

[a] Recommended daily carbohydrate intake ranges from 3 to 12 g per kilogram of body weight. Adjust with consideration for the athlete's total energy needs, specific training needs, and feedback from training performance. Carbohydrate intake should be spread over the day to promote fuel availability for key training sessions—before, during, and after exercise.

and competitions to enhance performance and promote recovery. An athlete's carbohydrate requirement may change based on alterations in daily, weekly, or seasonal exercise goals.[1-3]

Foods that provide approximately 25 g of carbohydrate per serving are listed in Box 2.2. These are typical serving sizes that can be useful when planning meals and snacks. Athletes who train heavily and have difficulty eating enough food to consume adequate carbohydrate and energy can use a high-carbohydrate liquid supplement. Most products contain glucose polymers (maltodextrins) or modified starches to reduce the solution's osmolality and potential for gastrointestinal distress.[5] Liquid meals (eg, Ensure and Boost) may also be beneficial during heavy training when energy requirements are extremely elevated.[1,5,13]

BOX 2.2 Carbohydrate-Rich Foods: 25-g Portions

Grains

- 2 slices whole-wheat bread
- ½ deli-style bagel
- 2-oz English muffin
- 1 cup oatmeal
- 1 cup ready-to-eat breakfast cereal
- 1 package snack-type cheese crackers (6 per package)
- 2 fig cookie bars
- ½ cup rice
- ½ cup cooked pasta
- 5 cups popcorn
- ½ large soft pretzel
- 17 mini pretzels
- 1 flour tortilla (12-in diameter)
- 1 oz tortilla chips and ¼ cup salsa

Dairy products and other beverages

- 2 cups milk (low-fat or nonfat)
- 1 cup low-fat chocolate milk
- 4.5-oz container fruit-flavored yogurt
- 6 oz plain yogurt
- 1 cup vanilla-flavored soy milk
- 1 package instant hot chocolate (made with water)

Beans and starchy vegetables

½ cup black beans
½ cup baked beans
1 cup green peas
½ cup corn
¾ cup kidney beans
½ cup lima beans
¾ cup mashed potatoes
½ medium baked potato with skin

Sports drinks, bars, and gels

2 cups sports drink (6%–8% carbohydrate-containing sports drink)
½ sports nutrition bar (25 g is average; individual brands may differ)
1 carbohydrate gel
½ bottle nutrition shake
½ bottle meal replacement shake

Mixed dishes

1 slice thin-crust pizza with meat or veggie toppings
½ slice thick-crust pizza with meat or veggie toppings
1 small bean and rice burrito
½ cup black beans and rice
1½ cups canned chicken noodle soup
¾ cup tomato soup
1 cup cooked ramen noodles
½ 6-in submarine sandwich
½ cup macaroni and cheese

Fruit and juice

2 cups fresh strawberries
1 large orange
¾ cup orange juice
½ cup cranberry-apple juice
1 medium apple

CARBOHYDRATE LOADING

Depletion of muscle glycogen is a well-recognized limitation to endurance performance lasting longer than 90 minutes. Carbohydrate loading (glycogen supercompensation) can increase muscle glycogen stores from resting levels of 100 to 120 mmol per kilogram of wet muscle weight to approximately 150 to 250 mmol per kilogram of wet muscle weight after carbohydrate loading. The regimen can postpone fatigue, extend the duration of steady-state exercise by about 20%, and improve endurance performance in which a set distance is covered as quickly as possible by about 2% to 3%.[5,15]

The classic regimen of carbohydrate loading involved a 3-day depletion phase (hard training and low carbohydrate intake) followed by a 3-day loading phase (tapered training and high carbohydrate intake) before the event.[5,14,15] Subsequent research established that high glycogen concentrations can be achieved without a depletion phase by tapering training for 3 days and consuming a high-carbohydrate diet of 10 g of carbohydrate per kilogram of body weight per day.[5,14,16] Current evidence indicates that muscle glycogen can be significantly increased from 90 to 180 mmol per kilogram of wet muscle weight with 24 hours of rest and a high-carbohydrate diet of 10 g of carbohydrate per kilogram per day.[5,14,17] Current guidelines for carbohydrate loading recommend that athletes taper or rest for 36 to 48 hours and consume 10 to 12 g of carbohydrate per kilogram of body weight per day.[1,2,5] These guidelines are summarized in Box 2.3 on page 30.[1,2,5]

An athlete may not be able to carbohydrate load within a short period of time.[5,18] McInerney et al[18] found that athletes could not supercompensate muscle glycogen levels after undertaking a second carbohydrate loading session (12 g of carbohydrate per kilogram of body weight per day) within 48 hours but that the athletes maintained their performance on the subsequent exercise test. Current evidence

BOX 2.3 Carbohydrate Loading Guidelines[1,2,5]

Day	Training	Carbohydrate
1	Taper/rest	10 to 12 g/kg/d
2	Taper/rest	10 to 12 g/kg/d
3	Competition	Follow carbohydrate guidelines for intake before competition, during competition, and after competition

indicates that 4 days of a high-carbohydrate diet (10 g of carbohydrate per kilogram of body weight per day) is sufficient to repeatedly supercompensate muscle glycogen following exhaustive exercise, and it also enhances work capacity.[5,19]

Most athletes need to eat frequently throughout the day to consume adequate carbohydrate and energy for glycogen supercompensation. The athlete may benefit from consuming low-fiber foods such as pasta, white rice, pancakes, cereal and fruit bars, sports nutrition bars and gels, yogurt, baked goods, and low-fat or nonfat sweets (eg, hard candy).[1,2,5,13] Carbohydrate-rich fluids, such as sports drinks, low-fat chocolate milk, liquid meals, liquid high-carbohydrate supplements, yogurt drinks, and fruit smoothies, help to augment carbohydrate and energy intake.[1,2,5] A low-fiber diet may reduce the risk of gut distress during an event and promote a small loss of weight to partially offset the additional weight gained from muscle glycogen supercompensation.[1,2,5,13] As with other nutrition strategies, athletes should first test their carbohydrate loading regimen prior to a key training session or a low-priority race.[5]

PREEXERCISE MEAL

Consuming carbohydrate-rich foods and fluids in the 4 hours before exercise helps to restore liver glycogen (especially for morning exercise when liver glycogen is depleted from an overnight fast), increase muscle glycogen stores (if they are not fully restored from the previous exercise session), and provide glucose for the central nervous system. The preexercise meal may also add to the performance benefits of consuming carbohydrate during endurance exercise.[5,20-22]

The preexercise meal should contain 1 to 4 g of carbohydrate per kilogram of body weight and be consumed 1 to 4 hours before exercise. The carbohydrate and energy content of the meal should be reduced the closer to exercise that the meal is consumed to avoid potential gastrointestinal distress when blood is diverted from the gut to the exercising muscles. For example, a carbohydrate feeding of 1 g per kilogram of body weight is appropriate 1 hour before exercise, whereas 4 g per kilogram of body weight can be consumed 4 hours before exercise.[1,2,20,23-25] The type, timing, and amount of carbohydrate in the preexercise meal should be individualized based on the athlete's specific event, gut comfort, and individual preferences.[1,2,5]

Athletes may also need to avoid foods high in fat, protein, and fiber to reduce the risk of gastrointestinal issues during exercise.[1,2,5,13] Liquid meals (eg, Ensure and Boost) are quickly digested and may be useful for athletes who are tense or anxious prior to competition. They produce a low stool residue and may help athletes "make weight" for their event.[1,13]

If the athlete is unable to eat breakfast before early morning exercise, consuming approximately 30 g of an easily digested carbohydrate-rich food or fluid (eg, banana, carbohydrate gel, or sports drink) 5 minutes before exercise may improve endurance performance.[26] Recommendations for carbohydrate intake before exercise are summarized in Box 2.4.

Glycemic Index of the Preexercise Meal

In theory, a low glycemic index preexercise meal promotes sustained carbohydrate availability during exercise and increases endurance. However, current evidence indicates that a low glycemic index preexercise meal does not significantly improve performance whether or not carbohydrate is consumed during

BOX 2.4 Recommended Carbohydrate Intake Before Exercise

The type, timing, and amount of carbohydrate consumed should be individualized.

Athletes should avoid foods high in fat, protein, and fiber to reduce the risk of gastrointestinal issues during exercise.

If an athlete is unable to eat breakfast, they can consume approximately 30 g of easily digested carbohydrate 5 minutes before exercise, which may improve performance.

Foods with a low glycemic index may be beneficial when carbohydrate cannot be consumed during exercise.

Timing before exercise	Recommended carbohydrate intake
1 hour	1 g per kilogram of body weight
2 hours	2 g per kilogram of body weight
3 hours	3 g per kilogram of body weight
4 hours	4 g per kilogram of body weight

exercise.[5,27] In addition, consuming carbohydrate during exercise negates the effects of the glycemic index of the preexercise meal on performance and metabolism.[5,22] Most athletes have opportunities to consume carbohydrate during competition. However, a low glycemic index preexercise meal may be useful prior to prolonged exercise when access to carbohydrate is logistically difficult (eg, trail runs, adventure races) or not well tolerated (eg, gastrointestinal distress).[5]

Carbohydrate in the Hour Before Exercise

Preexercise carbohydrate feedings generally improve performance. However, on rare occasions, an athlete may react negatively to carbohydrate feedings in the hour before exercise and experience symptoms of hypoglycemia and fatigue as a result of elevated blood insulin levels.[5,28] Experts do not fully understand the reason for this unusual reaction. In most cases, the decrease in blood glucose observed during the first 20 minutes of exercise is self-correcting and has no apparent effects on the athlete.

Preventive strategies for athletes who react negatively to carbohydrate feedings an hour before exercise include consuming carbohydrate a few minutes before exercise, waiting until exercising to consume carbohydrate, or consuming a low glycemic index preexercise meal to attenuate glucose and insulin responses.[2] The metabolic and performance effects of ingesting carbohydrate a few minutes before exercise are similar to those of consuming carbohydrate during exercise. The exercise-induced increase in the hormones epinephrine, norepinephrine, and growth hormone inhibit the release of insulin and thus counter insulin's effect in reducing blood glucose.[5,28]

CARBOHYDRATE INTAKE DURING EXERCISE

The literature has established that consuming carbohydrate during endurance exercise can increase exercise capacity and improve performance. For endurance exercise lasting longer than 2 hours, the effects are primarily metabolic: carbohydrate ingestion prevents hypoglycemia, maintains high rates of carbohydrate oxidation, and improves endurance. During prolonged exercise, blood glucose becomes an increasingly important fuel source as muscle glycogen stores decrease. Carbohydrate feedings both maintain blood glucose levels at a time when muscle glycogen stores are diminished and also reduce the reliance on gluconeogenesis. Thus, carbohydrate oxidation (and therefore ATP production) can continue at a high rate, and performance is enhanced.[6,29-31]

Carbohydrate feedings may also improve performance during high-intensity (>75% VO_2 max), relatively short-duration (approximately 1 hour) exercise. Because this type of activity is not limited by the availability of muscle glycogen or blood glucose, the underlying mechanism for performance appears to be tied to the central nervous system.[6,31-33]

When individuals rinse their mouths with a carbohydrate solution, the improvements in performance are very similar to those seen with carbohydrate ingestion. It is possible that carbohydrate receptors in the oral cavity signal the central nervous system to positively modify motor output, thereby improving performance. The precise receptors in the oral cavity have not yet been identified, and the exact roles of various brain areas are not clearly understood.[6,31-33] Current evidence suggests that using a carbohydrate mouth rinse or drinking a carbohydrate beverage during high-power exercise lasting 30 to 75 minutes improves performance by 2% to 3%. The benefits are more pronounced after an overnight fast, but they are evident even after a preexercise meal. Athletes who experience gastrointestinal distress from carbohydrate beverages may benefit from taking small sips of a carbohydrate drink or using a carbohydrate mouth rinse.[33]

Guidelines for Carbohydrate Intake During Exercise

There is no relationship between body weight and exogenous carbohydrate utilization during exercise; therefore, guidelines for intake during exercise are absolute and not based on body weight.[1,2,6,31] Recommendations depend on exercise duration, exercise intensity, and individual gut tolerance to intake, as well as the sport and its rules and regulations.

In general, carbohydrate intake should increase as the duration of exercise increases[1,2,6,31]:

- Carbohydrate consumption is not necessary during exercise lasting less than 45 minutes.
- During sustained high-intensity exercise lasting 45 to 75 minutes, the consumption of small amounts of carbohydrate or a carbohydrate mouth rinse may enhance performance.
- During endurance and intermittent, high-intensity exercise lasting 1 to 2.5 hours, athletes should consume 30 to 60 g of carbohydrate per hour.[1,2]
- During endurance and ultraendurance exercise lasting 2.5 hours or more, athletes should consume up to 90 g of carbohydrate per hour.[1,2]
- The ingestion of carbohydrate significantly improves performance in a dose-dependent manner, and the greatest benefit is observed with between 60 and 80 g of carbohydrate per hour.[34,35] Products providing multiple transportable carbohydrates (glucose-fructose mixtures, discussed further in the next section) help to achieve high rates of carbohydrate oxidation during prolonged exercise.[1,2,31]

Athletes who perform at lower absolute intensities will have lower carbohydrate oxidation rates and may need to adjust these recommendations downward.[31] Recommendations for carbohydrate intake during exercise are summarized in Box 2.5.

BOX 2.5 Recommended Carbohydrate Intake During Exercise

Type of activity	Recommended carbohydrate intake
Exercise lasting less than 45 minutes	Not necessary or practical
High-intensity exercise lasting 45 to 75 minutes	Small amounts of carbohydrate or carbohydrate mouth rinse
Endurance and intermittent, high-intensity exercise lasting 1 to 2.5 hour	30 to 60 g/h
Endurance and ultraendurance exercise lasting 2.5 hours or longer	Up to 90 g/h Multiple transportable carbohydrates (glucose-fructose mixtures) help achieve high rates of carbohydrate oxidation

A combination of foods and fluids can be used to meet carbohydrate goals during exercise. Athletes can consume sports products (eg, drinks, gels, chews, bars) and foods that are low in fat, protein, and fiber.[31,36-39] Although carbohydrate-rich foods are as effective as sports products, they may increase the risk of gastrointestinal distress in events exceeding 2 hours.[39] Fuel selection should be guided by personal preference and gut tolerance.[6,31,40] The carbohydrate content of selected foods are listed in Table 2.1.

TABLE 2.1 Carbohydrate Content of Selected Foods

Food	Portion	Carbohydrate content
Sports drink	1 qt (~1 L)	60 g
Sports nutrition bar	1 bar	47 g
Energy gel pack	2 gels	50 g
Caffeinated jelly beans	28 pieces	50 g
Energy chews	6 chews	50 g
Graham crackers	3 large	66 g
Fig bars	4 bars	42 g
Banana	1 whole	30 g

Carbohydrate intake must be balanced with hydration. Solid foods and highly concentrated carbohydrate solutions reduce the absorption of fluid. Using products with multiple transportable carbohydrates optimizes gastric emptying and intestinal absorption of carbohydrate.[31] Athletes should practice their nutrition strategies during training to "train the gut." Training with a high carbohydrate intake during exercise increases gastric emptying and intestinal absorption, thereby reducing the risk of gastrointestinal distress and enhancing performance.[6,31,40]

Multiple Transportable Carbohydrates

A high rate of intestinal carbohydrate absorption is necessary to increase exogenous carbohydrate oxidation. The maximum amount of glucose that can be absorbed during exercise is about 1 g/min (60 g/h) because the sodium-dependent glucose transporter 1 (SGLT1) becomes saturated. However, when glucose is combined with fructose (which uses glucose transporter type 5 [GLUT5]) the rate of carbohydrate oxidation exceeds 1 g/min. Consuming these multiple transportable carbohydrates (glucose-fructose mixtures) increases the rate of carbohydrate oxidation by up to 75%.[6,31,41]

Several studies have demonstrated that the increased exogenous carbohydrate oxidation rates observed with multiple transportable carbohydrates delay fatigue and improve performance. However, the performance benefits of multiple transportable carbohydrates are observed only during endurance exercise lasting 2.5 hours or longer and when carbohydrate is consumed at high rates (eg, 90 g/h). Multiple transportable carbohydrates provide the same performance benefits as other carbohydrate sources during shorter-duration exercise.[6,31,41]

Carbohydrate Intake During Intermittent Sports

Intermittent sports (eg, team sports) are characterized by intermittent bursts of high-intensity exercise and require intricate sport-specific skills and cognitive tasks over a prolonged period of time. This type of exercise can significantly reduce muscle glycogen stores and impair high-intensity performance; therefore, carbohydrate intake is crucial.[6,31,42]

Studies using intermittent running protocols to simulate soccer, rugby, field hockey, and basketball have consistently demonstrated that carbohydrate feedings delay fatigue and increase time to exhaustion.[6,31,42-47] The effects of carbohydrate intake on sprinting, jumping, skill, change-of-direction speed, and cognition (attention and response time) are mixed.[6,31,42] Researchers have found more benefits from carbohydrate ingestion in soccer than in other intermittent sports. This may be due to the endurance-based nature of soccer, the use of more rigorously validated soccer protocols, or the limited data available for other intermittent sports.[42]

Carbohydrate feedings may improve performance in intermittent, high-intensity sports by decreasing muscle glycogen utilization, increasing blood glucose, or both. The beneficial effects of carbohydrate ingestion may also be mediated by the central nervous system. Carbohydrate ingestion seems to have the greatest impact on performance in intermittent sports toward the end of the exercise, by which time the activity has caused extreme muscular fatigue and/or hypoglycemia.[6,31,42]

CARBOHYDRATE INTAKE POSTEXERCISE

The restoration of muscle and liver glycogen is essential for recovery between key training sessions or competitive events, particularly when the athlete works out multiple times per day and has limited time to recover before the next exercise session. The use of effective refueling strategies after strenuous exercise helps to promote optimal glycogen resynthesis.[1,2,7,48-50]

When strenuous workouts or competitions are less than 8 hours apart, the athlete should consume carbohydrate *as soon as possible* after the first exercise session to maximize the recovery time between sessions. For speedy refueling during the first 4 hours after glycogen-depleting exercise, the athlete should consume 1 to 1.2 g/kg of carbohydrate per kilogram of body weight each hour. Eating small amounts frequently (every 15–30 minutes) can help the athlete consume adequate carbohydrate.[1,2,7] During longer recovery periods (24 hours or more), timing of intake is not as critical, provided that the athlete consumes sufficient carbohydrate and energy. Adequate energy intake is necessary to optimize glycogen storage. Restrained eating practices interfere with meeting carbohydrate intake goals and glycogen restoration.[1,2,7]

The foods consumed during recovery meals and snacks should contribute to the athlete's overall nutrient intake. Nutrient-dense carbohydrate sources contain vitamins and minerals essential for performance and health.[1,2,7] There is no difference in muscle glycogen synthesis between liquid and solid carbohydrate sources.[51] However, an athlete may prefer fluids (fruit juices and smoothies, sports drinks, milkshakes, liquid high-carbohydrate supplements, and liquid meals) when feeling decreased appetite because of fatigue or dehydration.[7]

The highest rates of muscle glycogen repletion occur during the first hour after exercise for several reasons: the depletion of muscle glycogen activates glycogen synthase, exercise increases insulin sensitivity, and the muscle cell membrane is more permeable to glucose. Consuming carbohydrate immediately after exercise enhances these effects by increasing blood glucose and insulin concentrations.[7] Recommendations for postexercise carbohydrate intake are summarized in Box 2.6.

BOX 2.6 Recommended Carbohydrate Intake After Glycogen-Depleting Exercise

When exercise sessions are less than 8 hours apart, start consuming carbohydrate immediately after exercise to maximize recovery time.

Consume 1 to 1.2 g of carbohydrate per kilogram per hour for the first 4 hours after glycogen-depleting exercise.

Speedy refueling may be enhanced by consuming small amounts of carbohydrate more frequently (every 15-30 minutes) for up to 4 hours postexercise.

Adding 0.3 g of protein per kilogram of body weight (about 20 g) or more immediately after exercise stimulates muscle protein synthesis and repair and may enhance glycogen storage when carbohydrate intake is suboptimal (<1 g/kg).

Protein in Postexercise Feedings

When carbohydrate intake is suboptimal for refueling during the first 4 hours of recovery (<1 g per kilogram of body weight per hour), adding protein in the amount of at least 0.3 g per kilogram of body weight can enhance glycogen repletion. However, when carbohydrate intake is adequate (≥1.2 g per kilogram of body weight per hour), adding protein has no further effect on glycogen synthesis.[1,2,7,52-54]

Experts recommend consuming at least 0.3 g of protein per kilogram of body weight (about 20 g) immediately after exercise to stimulate muscle protein synthesis, inhibit protein breakdown, and enhance muscle protein accretion.[1,52,55,56] For example, athletes may consume 24 oz of fat-free milk (20 g of protein), 3 large eggs (21 g of protein), or 3 oz of lean red meat (21 g of protein) to reach this goal.

TRAINING WITH LOW CARBOHYDRATE AVAILABILITY

In addition to its role as a muscle substrate, muscle glycogen plays an important role in regulating the muscle's adaptation to training. Deliberately training with low carbohydrate availability activates acute cell signaling pathways that increase many of the characteristic skeletal muscle adaptations associated with endurance training, such as mitochondrial biogenesis, angiogenesis, and increased lipid oxidation.[1,3,4,7,57-59]

Impey et al[4] reported that periodically completing some endurance training sessions (eg, 30%–50%) with low carbohydrate availability augments cell signaling pathways (8 of 11 studies, or 73%) and oxidative skeletal muscle adaptations (7 of 9 studies, or 78%). However, despite improved metabolic adaptations associated with the periodization of low carbohydrate availability, only 4 of 11 studies (37%) demonstrated improvements in performance.

There are many ways to reduce carbohydrate availability for exercise: training after an overnight fast, training twice per day so that the second session is performed with reduced glycogen stores, restricting carbohydrate intake during exercise, or restricting carbohydrate intake after exercise. Athletes can also "sleep low" by training in the evening to deplete carbohydrate stores, going to sleep without refueling, and then training in the fasted state the next morning.[3,4,7,58,59]

A training with low carbohydrate availability must be carefully incorporated into the athlete's periodized training program. Prolonged training (>3–5 days) with low carbohydrate availability may limit the athlete's ability to perform high-intensity exercise and reduce the training stimulus. Chronic use of the regimen may also impair bone health, immunity, and endocrine function.[3,57-59] Although select workouts may be undertaken with low carbohydrate availability to promote skeletal muscle adaptations, the strategy is best suited for sessions in which exercise intensity and duration lend themselves to the approach. Athletes should commence high-intensity training sessions with high carbohydrate availability to practice pacing and fueling strategies for competition.[3,57-59]

The best way to periodize low-carbohydrate–availability training into an athlete's training program is still unclear. In addition, notwithstanding the evidence of improved metabolic adaptations, experts question whether this strategy enhances real-world measures of exercise performance.[3,57-60] As with all nutritional strategies, carbohydrate periodization should be done only in conjunction with appropriately qualified nutrition professionals.[3,7]

The ability to generate high-power outputs and high work rates is a critical component of a periodized training program. Furthermore, the strategic moves that occur during competition depend on the athlete's ability to work at high intensities, which are fueled by carbohydrate. Thus, a diet with high carbohydrate availability is recommended during periods of heavy training and when an athlete is preparing to peak for competition.[3,57-59]

SUMMARY

Carbohydrate is the predominant fuel for moderate- to high-intensity endurance exercise and intermittent high-intensity exercise. The depletion of endogenous carbohydrate stores is associated with reduced work rates, impaired skill and concentration, and increased perception of effort. Strategies that promote high carbohydrate availability are recommended to promote optimal performance in key training sessions and competitive events.

KEY TAKEAWAYS

Athletes should "fuel for the work required," whereby carbohydrate availability is adjusted and periodized according to the fuel demands of the specific training session or competitive event.

Athletes with very light training programs (low-intensity exercise or skill-based exercise) should consume 3 to 5 g of carbohydrate per kilogram of body weight per day. Athletes engaged in moderate-intensity training programs for 60 min/d should consume 5 to 7 g of carbohydrate per kilogram of body weight per day. During moderate- to high-intensity endurance exercise for 1 to 3 hours, athletes should consume 6 to 10 g of carbohydrate per kilogram of body weight per day. Athletes participating in moderate- to high-intensity endurance exercise for 4 to 5 h/d or more (eg, Tour de France) should consume 8 to 12 g of carbohydrate per kilogram of body weight per day.

Between 1 and 4 hours prior to endurance and intermittent, high-intensity exercise, athletes should consume 1 to 4 g of carbohydrate per kilogram of body weight to top off muscle and liver glycogen stores.

Consuming carbohydrate is not necessary during exercise lasting less than 45 minutes. During sustained high-intensity exercise lasting 45 to 75 minutes, the consumption of small amounts of carbohydrate or a carbohydrate mouth rinse may enhance performance. Athletes should consume 30 to 60 g of carbohydrate per hour during endurance and intermittent, high-intensity exercise lasting 1 to 2.5 hours. During endurance and ultraendurance exercise lasting 2.5 hours or more, athletes should consume up to 90 g of carbohydrate per hour.

When strenuous workouts or competitions are less than 8 hours apart, the athlete should consume carbohydrate as soon as possible after the first exercise session to maximize the effective recovery time between sessions. For speedy refueling after glycogen-depleting exercise, the athlete should consume 1 to 1.2 g of carbohydrate per kilogram per hour for the first 4 hours. Consuming carbohydrate at frequent intervals (every 15-30 minutes) for up to 4 hours can help the athlete consume adequate carbohydrate. During longer recovery periods (≥24 hours), the timing of carbohydrate intake does not matter, provided that the athlete consumes adequate carbohydrate and energy.

The consumption of at least 0.3 g of protein per kilogram of body weight (about 20 g) immediately after exercise is recommended to stimulate muscle protein synthesis, inhibit protein breakdown, and enhance muscle protein accretion. When carbohydrate intake is suboptimal for refueling during the first 4 hours of recovery (<1 g per kilogram of body weight per hour), the addition of at least 0.3 g of protein per kilogram of body weight can enhance glycogen repletion.

Chronic periods (>3–5 days) of training with low carbohydrate availability should be avoided because of the potential negative effects of low carbohydrate and energy availability on training quality, competitive performance, and health outcomes.

These are general recommendations and should be individualized with consideration of the athlete's total energy requirements, specific training needs, gut tolerance, and feedback from training and competition.

REFERENCES

1. Thomas DT, Erdman KA, Burke LM. Position of the Academy of Nutrition and Dietetics, Dietitians of Canada, and the American College of Sports Medicine: nutrition and athletic performance. *J Acad Nutr Diet.* 2016;116(3):501-528. doi:10.1016/j.jand.2015.12.006
2. Burke LM, Hawley JA, Wong S, Jeukendrup AE. Carbohydrates for training and competition. *J Sports Sci.* 2011;29(suppl 1):S17-S27. doi:10.1080/02640414.2011.585473
3. Stellingwerff T, Morton JP, Burke LM. A framework for periodized nutrition for athletics. *Int J Sport Nutr Exerc Metab.* 2019;29(2):141-151. doi:10.1123/ijsnem.2018-0305
4. Impey SG, Hearris MA, Hammond KM, et al. Fuel for the work required: A theoretical framework for carbohydrate periodization and the glycogen threshold hypothesis. *Sports Med.* 2018;48(5):1031-1048. doi:10.1007/s40279-018-0867-7
5. Burke LM, Hall R. Preparation for competition. In: Burke L, Deakin V, Minehan M, eds. *Clinical Sports Nutrition.* 6th ed. McGraw-Hill; 2021:313-334.
6. Jeukendrup AE, Carter J. Competition fluid and fuel. In: Burke L, Deakin V, Minehan M, eds. *Clinical Sports Nutrition.* 6th ed. McGraw-Hill; 2021:336-369.
7. Burke LM. Nutrition for recovery after training and competition. In: Burke L, Deakin V, Minehan M, eds. *Clinical Sports Nutrition.* 6th ed. McGraw-Hill; 2021:375-416.
8. Jeukendrup AE. Periodized nutrition for athletes. *Sports Med.* 2017;47(suppl 1):51-63. doi:10.1007/s40279-017-0694-2
9. Cox GR, Clark SA, Cox AJ, et al. Daily training with high carbohydrate availability increases exogenous carbohydrate oxidation during endurance cycling. *J Appl Physiol (1985).* 2010;109(1):126-134. doi:10.1152/japplphysiol.00950.2009
10. Mountjoy M, Sundgot-Borgen JK, Burke LM, et al. IOC consensus statement on relative energy deficiency in sport (RED-S): 2018 update. *Br J Sports Med.* 2018;52(11):687-697. doi:10.1136/bjsports-2018-099193
11. Melin AK, Heikura IA, Tenforde A, Mountjoy M. Energy availability in athletics: health, performance, and physique. *Int J Sport Nutr Exerc Metab.* 2019;29(2):152-164. doi:10.1123/ijsnem.2018-0201
12. Coyle EF. Substrate utilization during exercise in active people. *Am J Clin Nutr.* 1995;61(suppl 4):968S-979S. doi:10.1093/ajcn/61.4.968S
13. Burke LM, Jeukendrup AE, Jones AM, Mooses M. Contemporary nutrition strategies to optimize performance in distance runners and race walkers. *Int J Sport Nutr Exerc Metab.* 2019;29(2):117-129. doi:10.1123/ijsnem.2019-0004
14. Burke LM, van Loon LJC, Hawley JA. Postexercise muscle glycogen resynthesis in humans. *J Appl Physiol (1985).* 2017;122(5):1055-1067. doi:10.1152/japplphysiol.00860.2016
15. Hawley JA, Schabort EJ, Noakes TD, Dennis SC. Carbohydrate-loading and exercise performance. An update. *Sports Med.* 1997;24(2):73-81. doi:10.2165/00007256-199724020-00001
16. Sherman WM, Costill DL, Fink WJ, Miller JM. Effect of exercise-diet manipulation on muscle glycogen and its subsequent use during performance. *Int J Sport Med.* 1981;2(2):114-118. doi:10.1055/s-2008-1034594
17. Bussau VA., Fairchild TJ, Rao A, Steele P, Fournier PA. Carbohydrate loading in human muscle: an improved 1 day protocol. *Eur J Appl Physiol.* 2002;87(3):290-295. doi:10.1007/s00421-002-0621-5
18. McInerney P, Lessard SJ, Burke LM, et al. Failure to repeatedly supercompensate muscle glycogen stores in highly trained men. *Med Sci Sport Exerc.* 2005;37(3):404-411. doi:10.1249/01.mss.0000155699.51360.2f
19. Doering TM, Cox GR, Areta JL, Coffey VG. Repeated muscle glycogen supercompensation with four days' recovery between exhaustive exercise. *J Sci Med Sport.* 2019;22(8):907-911. doi:10.1016/j.jsams.2019.03.009
20. Wright DA, Sherman WM, Dernbach AR. Carbohydrate feedings before, during, or in combination improves cycling performance. *J Appl Physiol (1985).* 1991;71(3):1082-1088. doi:10.1152/jappl.1991.71.3.1082
21. Chryssanthopoulos C, Williams C. Pre-exercise carbohydrate meal and endurance running capacity when carbohydrates are ingested during exercise. *Int J Sports Med.* 1997;18(7):543-548. doi:10.1055/s-2007-972679
22. Burke LM, Claassen A, Hawley JA, Noakes TD. Carbohydrate intake during exercise minimizes effect of glycemic index of pre-exercise meal. *J Appl Physiol (1985).* 1998;85(6):2220-2226. doi:10.1152/jappl.1998.85.6.2220
23. Coyle EF, Coggan AR, Hemmert MK, Lowe RC, Walters TJ. Substrate usage during prolonged exercise following a preexercise meal. *J Appl Physiol (1985).* 1985;59(2):429-433. doi:10.1152/jappl.1985.59.2.429
24. Nuefer PD, Costill DL, Flynn MG, Kirwan JP, Mitchell JB, Houmard J. Improvements in exercise performance: effects of carbohydrate feedings and diet. *J Appl Physiol (1985).* 1987;62(3):983-988. doi:10.1152/jappl.1987.62.3.983
25. Sherman WM, Brodowicz G, Wright DA, Allen WK, Simonsen J, Dernbach A. Effects of 4 hour pre-exercise carbohydrate feedings on cycling performance. *Med Sci Sports Exerc.* 1989;21(5):598-604
26. Anantaraman R, Carimines AA, Gaesser GA, Weltman A. Effects of carbohydrate supplementation on performance during 1 hour of high-intensity exercise. *Int J Sport Med.* 1995;16(7):461-465. doi:10.1055/s-2007-973038
27. Burdon CA, Spronk I, Cheng HL, O'Connor HT. Effect of glycemic index of a pre-exercise meal on endurance exercise performance: a systematic review and meta-analysis. *Sports Med.* 2017;47(6):1087-1101. doi:10.1007/s40279-016-0632-8
28. Jeukendrup AE, Killer S. The myths surrounding pre-exercise carbohydrate feeding. *Ann Nutr Metab.* 2011;57(suppl 2):18-25. doi:10.1159/000322698
29. Coyle EF, Hagberg JM, Hurley BF, Martin WH, Ehsani AA, Holloszy JO. Carbohydrate feeding during prolonged strenuous exercise can delay fatigue. *J Appl Physiol Respir Environ Exerc Physiol.* 1983;55(Pt 1):230-235. doi:10.1152/jappl.1983.55.1.230

30. Coyle EF, Coggan AR, Hemmert WK, Ivy JL. Muscle glycogen utilization during prolonged strenuous exercise when fed carbohydrate. *J Appl Physiol (1985).* 1986;61(1):165-172. doi:10.1152/jappl.1986.61.1.165
31. Jeukendrup AE. A step towards personalized sports nutrition: carbohydrate intake during exercise. *Sports Med.* 2014;44 (suppl 1):S25-S33. doi:10.1007/s40279-017-0694-2
32. Jeukendrup AE, Chambers ES. Oral carbohydrate sensing and exercise performance. *Curr Opin Clin Nutr Metab Care.* 2010;13(4):447-451. doi:10.1097/MCO.0b013e328339de83
33. Jeukendrup AE. Oral carbohydrate rinse: placebo or beneficial? *Curr Sports Med Rep.* 2013;12(4):222-227. doi:10.1249/JSR.0b013e31829a6caa
34. Smith JW, Zachwieja JJ, Peronnet F, et al. Fuel selection and cycling endurance performance with ingestion of [13C]glucose: evidence for a carbohydrate dose response. *J Appl Physiol (1985).* 2010;108(6):1520-1529. doi:10.1152/japplphysiol.91394.2008
35. Smith JW, Pascoe DD, Passe DH, et al. Curvilinear dose-response relationship of carbohydrate (0-120 g·h−1) and performance. *Med Sci Sports Exerc.* 2013;45(2):336-341. doi:10.1249/MSS.0b013e31827205d1
36. Pfeiffer B, Stellingwerff T, Zaltas E, Jeukendrup AE. CHO oxidation from a CHO gel compared with a drink during exercise. *Med Sci Sports Exerc.* 2010;42(11):2038-2045. doi:10.1249/MSS.0b013e3181e0efe6
37. Pfeiffer B, Stellingwerff T, Zaltas E, Jeukendrup AE. Oxidation of solid versus liquid CHO sources during exercise. *Med Sci Sports Exerc.* 2010;42(11):2030-2037. doi:10.1249/MSS.0b013e3181e0efc9
38. Hearris MA, Pugh JN, Langan-Evans C, et al. 13C-glucose-fructose labeling reveals comparable exogenous CHO oxidation during exercise when consuming 120 g/h in fluid, gel, jelly chew, or coingestion. *J Appl Physiol (1985).* 2022;132(6):1394-1406. doi:10.1152/japplphysiol.00091.2022
39. Reynolds KM, Clifford T, Mears SA, James LJ. A food first approach to carbohydrate supplementation in endurance exercise: a systematic review. *Int J Sport Nutr Exerc Metab.* 2022;32(4):296-310. doi:10.1123/ijsnem.2021-0261
40. Jeukendrup AE. Training the gut for athletes. *Sports Med.* 2017;47 (suppl 1):101-110. doi:10.1007/s40279-017-0690-6
41. Jeukendrup AE. Carbohydrate and exercise performance: the role of multiple transportable carbohydrates. *Curr Opin Clin Nutr Metab Care.* 2010;13(4):452-457. doi:10.1097/MCO.0b013e328339de9f
42. Baker LB, Rollo I, Stein KW, Jeukendrup AE. Acute effects of carbohydrate supplementation on intermittent sports performance. *Nutrients.* 2015;7(7):5733-5763. doi:10.3390/nu7075249
43. Nicholas CW, Williams C, Lakomy HK, Phillips G, Nowitz A. Influence of ingesting a carbohydrate-electrolyte solution on endurance capacity during intermittent, high-intensity shuttle running. *J Sport Sci.* 1995;13(4):283-290. doi:10.1080/02640419508732241
44. Foskett A, Williams C, Boobis L, Tsintzas K. Carbohydrate availability and muscle energy metabolism during intermittent running. *Med Sci Sports Exerc.* 2008;40(1):96-103. doi:10.1249/mss.0b013e3181586b2c
45. Patterson SD, Gray SC. Carbohydrate-gel supplementation and endurance performance during intermittent high-intensity shuttle running. *Int J Sport Nutr Exerc Metab.* 2007;17(5):445-455. doi:10.1123/ijsnem.17.5.445
46. Welsh RS, Davis JM, Burke JR, Williams HG. Carbohydrates and physical/mental performance during intermittent exercise to fatigue. *Med Sci Sports Exerc.* 2002;34(4):723-731. doi:10.1097/00005768-200204000-00025
47. Rodriguez-Giustiniani P, Rollo I, Witard OC, Galloway SDR. Ingesting a 12% carbohydrate-electrolyte beverage before each half of a soccer match simulation facilitates retention of passing performance and improves high-intensity running capacity in academy players. *Int J Sport Nutr Exerc Metab.* 2019;29(4):397-405. doi:10.1123/ijsnem.2018-0214
48. Beelen M, Burke LM, Gibala MJ, van Loon L JC. Nutritional strategies to promote postexercise recovery. *Int J Sport Nutr Exerc Metab.* 2010;20(6):515-532. doi:10.1123/ijsnem.20.6.515
49. Ivy JL, Katz AL, Cutler CL, Sherman WM, Coyle EF. Muscle glycogen synthesis after exercise: effect of time of carbohydrate ingestion. *J Appl Physiol (1985).* 1988;6(4):1480-1485. doi:10.1152/jappl.1988.64.4.1480
50. Ivy JL, Lee MC, Broznick JT, Reed MJ. Muscle glycogen storage after different amounts of carbohydrate ingestion. *J Appl Physiol (1985).* 1988;65(5):2018-2023. doi:10.1152/jappl.1988.65.5.2018
51. Reed MJ, Broznick JT, Lee MC, Ivy JL. Muscle glycogen storage postexercise: effect of mode of carbohydrate administration. *J Appl Physiol (1985).* 1989;66(2):720-726. doi:10.1152/jappl.1989.66.2.720
52. Moore D, Burd N, Slater G. Protein needs for the athlete. In: Burke L, Deakin V, Minehan M eds. *Clinical Sports Nutrition.* 6th ed. McGraw-Hill; 2021:67-85.
53. Betts JA, Williams C. Short-term recovery from prolonged exercise: exploring the potential for protein ingestion to accentuate the benefits of carbohydrate supplements. *Sports Med.* 2010;40(11):941-959. doi:10.2165/11536900-000000000-00000
54. Alghannam AF, Gonzalez JT, Betts JA. Restoration of muscle glycogen and functional capacity: role of post-exercise carbohydrate and protein co-ingestion. *Nutrients.* 2018;10(2):253. doi:10.3390/nu10020253
55. Moore DR. Maximizing post-exercise anabolism: the case for relative protein intakes. *Front Nutr.* 2019;6:147. doi:10.3389/fnut.2019.00147
56. Burd NA, Beals JW, Martinez IG, Salvador AF, Skinner SK. Food-first approach to enhance the regulation of post-exercise skeletal muscle protein synthesis and remodeling. *Sports Med.* 2019;49(suppl 1):59-68. doi:10.1007/s40279-018-1009-y
57. Bartlett JD, Hawley JA, Morton JP. Carbohydrate availability and exercise training adaptation: too much of a good thing? *Eur J Sport Sci.* 2015;15(1):3-12. doi:10.1080/17461391.2014.920926
58. Gejl KD, Nybo L. Performance effects of periodized carbohydrate restriction in endurance trained athletes - a systematic review and meta-analysis. *J Int Soc Sports Nutr.* 2021;18(1):37. doi:10.1186/s12970-021-00435-3
59. Hearris MA, Hammond KM, Fell JM, Morton JP. Regulation of muscle glycogen metabolism during exercise: implications for endurance performance and training adaptations. *Nutrients.* 2018;10(3):298. doi:10.3390/nu10030298
60. Burke LM, Ross ML, Garvican-Lewis LA, et al. Low carbohydrate, high fat diet impairs exercise economy and negates the performance benefit from intensified training in elite race walkers. *J Physiol.* 2017;595(9):2785-2807. doi:10.1113/JP273230

CHAPTER 3

Protein and Exercise

Max T. Deutz, PhD, RD, CSSD; Nicholas A. Burd, PhD; and Stuart Phillips, PhD, FACSM

LEARNING OBJECTIVES

- Understand how protein pools control muscle turnover (ie, the combined result of muscle protein synthesis and breakdown).
- Examine the impact that exercise and various dietary intake habits have on muscle regulation.
- Review strategies to optimize anabolic responses through protein ingestion.
- Outline general protein intake recommendations for both endurance- and resistance-based athletes.

INTRODUCTION

Proteins are made up of 20 unique organic molecules called amino acids. These amino acids (commonly called building blocks) are strung together in varied sequences and lengths via peptide bonds to form unique strands that determine the ultimate shape and function of a protein. From contractile, structural, mitochondrial, and hematologic proteins to regulatory enzymes, the wide array of bodily roles that proteins play is critically important for all humans. However, for athletes, skeletal muscle proteins have elevated importance, as they directly influence performance in a myriad of ways. Consequently, the primary focus of this chapter is on the nutritional considerations that allow for the optimization of muscle protein repair and remodeling.

In the 1800s, scientists hypothesized that the energy supporting muscle contraction was derived from the "explosive breakdown of protein molecules."[1] Although our capability to correct such notions has improved in modern times, a burgeoning supplement industry coupled with advances in social media and gym culture have played a role in countering such advances. Few narratives have been as omnipresent in the perpetuation of spreading nutrition misinformation as those involving dietary protein (and associated specific amino acids). The emphasis placed on elevated protein intakes and the overall mystique surrounding dietary protein have produced erroneous ideologies such as "more protein equals more (muscle) gains." Given the difficulty in understanding the many nuances of more complex arguments (eg, quality comparisons between plant- and animal-based proteins), everyone from the general public to elite athletes has more questions than answers. This lack of clarity poses a risk to the general well-being and health of both groups, but for athletes, such misunderstanding can also hinder performance.

Studies on athletes have demonstrated that focusing too much on protein may limit intake of other important nutrients such as carbohydrates and fats.[2-6] Though essential, protein alone cannot meet the varying demands that an athlete faces. For example, despite the aforementioned theory that muscle contraction results from the explosive breakdown of protein, current scientists and sports dietitians generally regard protein intake to be inconsequential for inducing muscle contraction, given that amino acids provide only a minor portion of energy contribution (<10%) during prolonged dynamic exercise.[7,8] Indeed, the body prefers to use carbohydrate as its direct energy source despite the capacity of human skeletal muscle to oxidize at least 7 amino acids during exercise.[9] Whereas the oxidation of amino acids to provide fuel during exercise is trivial, the profound influence dietary protein has on muscle turnover (ie, muscle protein synthesis [MPS] and muscle protein breakdown [MPB]) cannot be understated. Moreover, when different types of exercise (eg, endurance or resistance training) are coupled with consumption of dietary protein (as well as carbohydrates and fats), unique phenotypical adaptations occur. Generally speaking, endurance exercise leads to an enhanced muscular oxidative capacity, whereas resistance exercise leads to increased muscular hypertrophy. Regardless of the mode of exercise, athletes seeking to maximize skeletal muscle adaptations induced by training stimuli must rely on dietary protein to facilitate the repair, remodeling, and accretion of muscle. Proper manipulation of such protein intake to optimize these recovery processes permits ongoing peak performance and the capability to function at a high level over one's life span.

This chapter serves as a practical reference tool for both athletes and those who directly (eg, sports dietitians) and indirectly (eg, scientists) assist in the fueling of athletes. It provides a general overview of muscle protein turnover in the context of both resistance and endurance exercise, as well as information on the timing, quality, and quantity of protein ingestion for athletes engaged in these types of exercise. In addition, the chapter ends by highlighting key takeaways that can help athletes and those supporting them have a better understanding of both the scientific concepts and practical implementation strategies for using this knowledge.

MUSCLE PROTEIN TURNOVER

MPS is stimulated following the consumption of dietary protein. After protein ingestion, the concentration of amino acids in the blood, and subsequently muscle, are elevated, which ultimately stimulates MPS.[10] The intracellular pool of free amino acids in muscles functions as a link between the blood and muscle proteins. Although the amino acid inputs contributing to this pool can come from plasma during feeding (or from breaking down muscle proteins during fasting), not all amino acids are used for building muscle proteins. Rather, certain nonessential amino acids are used for intermediary metabolism or oxidation through de novo synthesis. To summarize, amino acids broken down from protein assume 1 of 3 fates: (1) as substrates for the synthesis of muscle protein, (2) as support for vital bodily functions, or (3) as an alternative source of fuel (ie, branched-chain amino acids) or energy source intermediate. Figure 3.1 illustrates the interaction between dietary amino acids and protein pools in the body.

Protein turnover is a synchronous and continuous process that is highly dynamic. Proteins that function in a regulatory (eg, enzymes) or signaling (eg, hormones) manner may turn over in minutes or days. In contrast, proteins that function structurally (eg, collagen) or act as contractile proteins (eg, actin and myosin) turn over at a much lower rate (ie, days or weeks). Many different techniques exist to estimate protein metabolism in the body. For example, concentrations of urea (a major constituent of urine and the principal means for disposing of nitrogen derived from amino acid metabolism) can be acutely measured in urine and sweat. Despite being a practical option, however, values are strongly affected by recent protein intake and

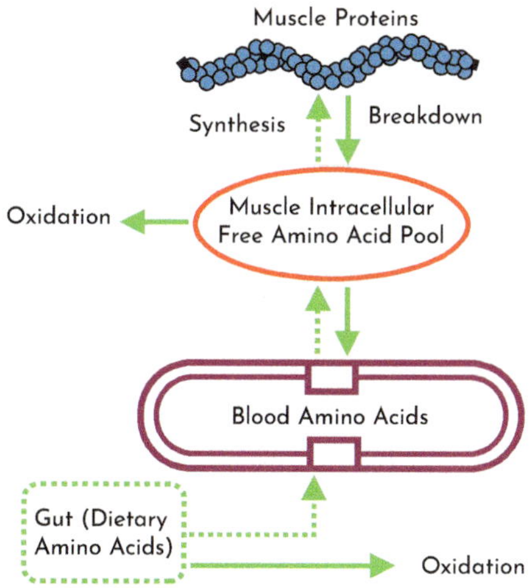

FIGURE 3.1 General overview of the fate of dietary amino acids and protein pools in the body *Muscle proteins* is a collective term referring to myofibrillar, sarcoplasmic, and mitochondrial proteins. These specific protein subfractions comprise approximately 60%, 30%, and 10%, respectively, of skeletal muscle. Solid arrows represent catabolic destinations. Dashed arrows represent anabolic destinations.

provide only approximate metabolism-related estimates. To provide long-term insight into how proteins are metabolized, researchers have traditionally employed nitrogen balance studies. In such studies, researchers carefully measure the intake of nitrogen and its excretion in urine, feces, and sweat for days to weeks at a time. Despite being the source from which most estimates of dietary protein intake have been derived, nitrogen balance studies are not exempt from shortcomings given that they are time-consuming, are highly dependent on subject compliance, and provide no direct insight into metabolic pathways.[2,11-13] To overcome this third limitation and gain more concrete and nuanced insights into protein flux within the body (to study either whole-body metabolism or specific amino acids), more demanding techniques (eg, use of stable isotopes and metabolic tracers) are often called upon to analyze muscle protein turnover.

Although advanced analyses of turnover are valuable in their own regard, fasted-state losses of muscle protein are generally offset by fed-state gains of muscle protein over the course of the day. Accordingly, the muscle net protein balance (NPB) equation (NPB = MPS – MPB) equilibrates, and skeletal muscle mass within the body remains essentially unchanged.[14] Pointed manipulation of NPB to achieve a goal such as muscle growth is possible with conscious effort. In addition to modifying dietary intake habits (discussed later in this chapter), the type of training an athlete undertakes plays a large role in determining how protein is turned over within the body.

Protein Turnover and Resistance Exercise

The fundamentally anabolic nature of resistance training means that it can have profound effects on muscle protein turnover. This relationship is not purely transient. In fact, following a single bout of resistance exercise in untrained individuals, NPB can be augmented for up to 48 hours.[15] Over time, the habitual application of such bouts of resistance exercise results in hypertrophic remodeling of muscle protein that is capable of inducing the accretion of myofibrillar protein (the predominant protein in skeletal muscle); increases in skeletal muscle fiber size; and ultimately, additional lean body mass (LBM).[15-17] Compared to those who are untrained, resistance-trained individuals exhibit elevated resting MPS and attenuated resting MPB.[18-21] As such, resistance-trained individuals are less responsive to dramatic NPB fluctuations in response to acute exercise. In other words, for trained individuals, both the acute amplitude (ie, 0–3 hours) and duration (16–48 hours) of MPS are not as large as those seen in untrained individuals.[22] In practical terms, these findings indicate that consistent training increases the need to focus on diverging exercise-based variables such as load, intensity, and type in order to maintain a relatively unique stimulus capable of inducing robust and prolonged MPS responses such as those seen in less-trained individuals.

Changes in dietary habits or patterns can be used to optimize muscle hypertrophy, strength, or oxidative capacity. Certain feeding patterns may be superior to others in terms of their ability to induce positive effects on skeletal muscle. To help offset natural MPB resulting from resistance training, it is especially important for athletes to consume the right quantity and quality of dietary protein to support augmentation of MPS. The consumption of essential amino acids (EAAs) is of particular importance, as they are the primary stimulators for MPS.[23] As such, the consumption of dietary protein (namely, EAAs) at a time close to training serves to be a practical way for athletes to optimize protein accretion and subsequent gains in muscle mass. Complementing this ingestion of protein at a time surrounding exercise (ie, periworkout) is the recommendation to also spread protein intake over the course of the day. Serum amino acid levels (in addition to MPS rates) transiently rise and stay elevated for a minimum of several hours following the ingestion of a meal containing protein.[24] Additional rationale behind this recommendation to separate protein feedings is further discussed in later sections of this chapter. To illustrate some of these concepts, NPB with and without resistance exercise is depicted in Figure 3.2.

Protein Turnover and Endurance Exercise

Even though the nature of aerobic exercise necessitates less focus on increasing total body muscle mass, enhancing protein turnover rates remains a fundamental part of optimizing how endurance athletes recover and adapt to training. Whereas carbohydrate- and fat-based fuels provide the majority of the energy required to support muscle contraction during sustained endurance exercise events, the oxidation of some classes of amino acids (eg, branched-chain amino acids) is capable of contributing up to 10% of total energy needs to support endurance exercise.[13] In addition to the intensity and duration of exercise being undertaken,

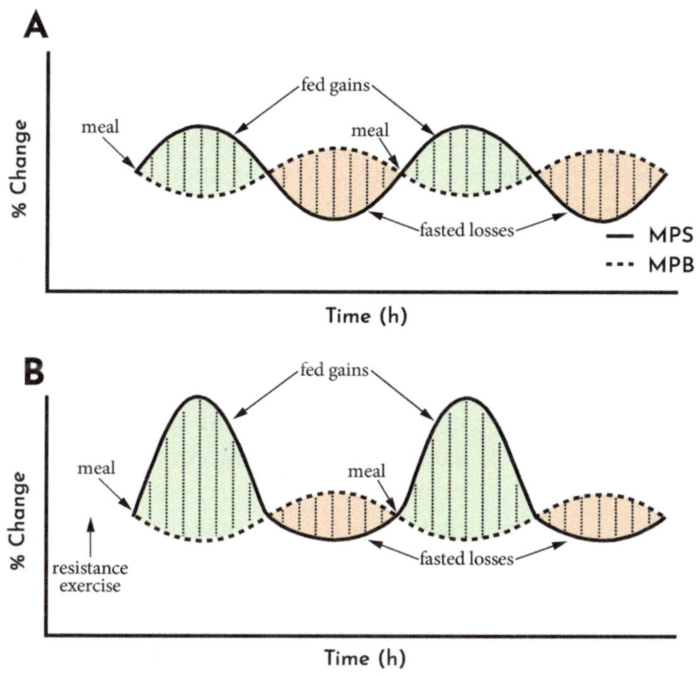

FIGURE 3.2 Daily muscle net protein balance with and without incorporation of resistance exercise (A) Changes in MPS and MPB in response to feeding. (B) Changes in MPS and MPB in response to feeding and resistance exercise. Chronic application of the stimuli shown in panel B results in muscular hypertrophy.
Abbreviations: MPB, muscle protein breakdown; MPS, muscle protein synthesis

several other factors, including sex, muscle glycogen availability, energy availability, and training status, all help determine the rate of oxidation for these amino acids.[7,25-29] Note that, in trained athletes, amino acid oxidation rates during aerobic exercise are often reduced due to a greater reliance on alternative fuels (ie, carbohydrate and fat) to provide the energy for muscle contraction.[29] However, regardless of training status, enhanced amino acid oxidation rates during aerobic exercise are thought to partially contribute to the overall elevated daily protein requirements of endurance athletes.[13,30]

The remodeling of muscle proteins during recovery from aerobic exercise is essential to replace damaged proteins and synthesize myofibrillar- and mitochondrial-related proteins and enzymes, in addition to angiogenic proteins. With prolonged aerobic training, this leads to an increased oxidative capacity of skeletal muscle. Research examining muscle protein turnover after acute aerobic exercise using stable isotope methodology suggests that aerobic exercise can induce increases in MPS, although the response is smaller in amplitude and duration than with resistance exercise.[15,19-21,31-34] The exercise intensity also directly influences the duration of the postexercise MPS response, with high-intensity exercise resulting in the MPS response being sustained longer than for low-intensity aerobic exercise.[35] This work supports the hypothesis that there is a relationship between the force placed on the muscle and the subsequent stimulation of MPS during postexercise recovery. In summary, whereas athletes focused on aerobic training are likely to be less focused on muscular hypertrophy than resistance athletes, optimizing protein turnover in their bodies is still an essential component to consider for proper recovery and adaptation.

TIMING OF DIETARY PROTEIN INTAKE

Historically, dietary protein recommendations for athletes focused on overall intake, de-emphasizing specified timing considerations. However, since the early 1990s, the narrative has shifted as a result of considerable research exploring the impact of adjusting the timing of protein ingestion to optimize recovery and performance. As highlighted in the preceding section, resistance- and endurance-based athletes have different training goals and adaptations; consequently, the timing of protein ingestion differs for the 2 groups.

Protein Timing for Resistance Exercise

The appropriate timing of resistance exercise and dietary protein intake can lead to substantial outcomes. Numerous studies have examined protein ingestion at various time points surrounding resistance exercise to determine the best time to deliver dietary amino acids to exercised muscle in pursuit of optimized anabolism.[14] However, regardless of the specific nutrition intervention used or the age-stratified population enlisted, research examining correlations between nutritional outcomes and resistance-exercise training is often difficult to reconcile because increases in muscle mass and strength are hallmark adaptations to such activity.[36-41]

PREEXERCISE FEEDING

Tipton et al[42] completed early work demonstrating that providing 6 g of EAAs (equivalent to approximately 15 g of high-quality protein in a food source such as eggs) and 35 g of sucrose before resistance exercise induced a 160% greater increase in muscle anabolism than consuming a similar drink after exercise. The researchers attributed this effect to the ability of the preexercise supplement to promote an exercise-induced hyperemia and an approximate fourfold increase in amino acid uptake by muscle.

Tipton and colleagues[43] subsequently studied the influence of intact proteins fed immediately before or after resistance exercise. Despite greater amino acid uptake in the group that received the preexercise feeding, the 2 eating patterns had similar anabolic responses. In this work, large individual differences were observed in the measured anabolic responses to the consumption of protein before and after resistance exercise. This finding coupled with the prior work led researchers to speculate that certain individuals may be more responsive to muscle anabolism induced by preexercise feeding.

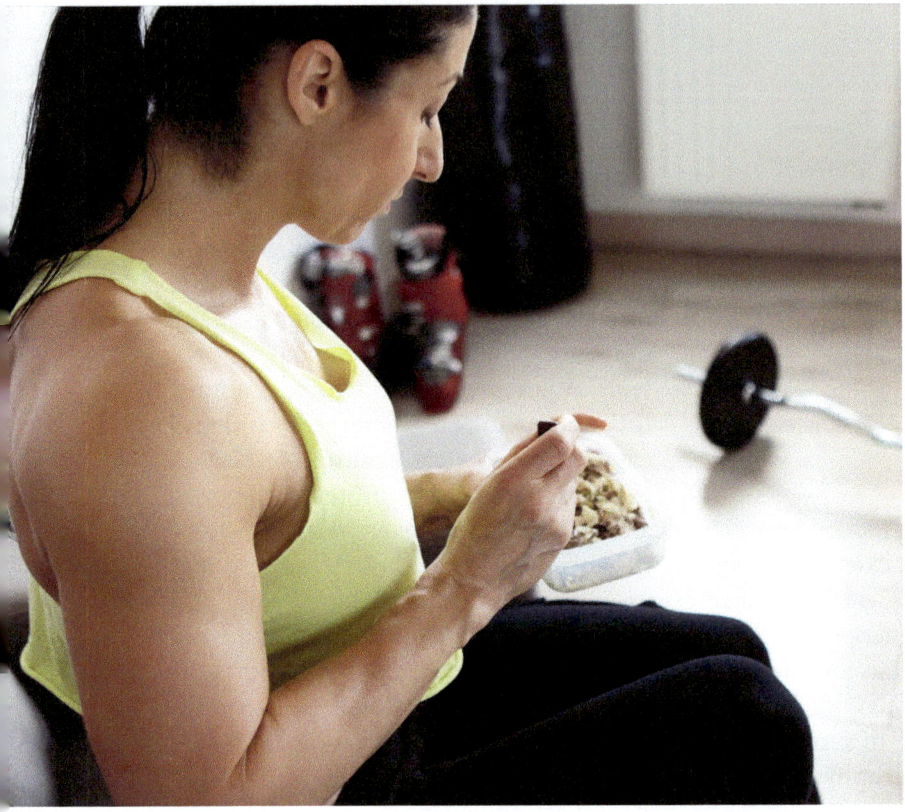

Later, Burk et al[44] attempted to delineate the importance of protein timing with resistance training by using a randomized within-subject crossover design. Young men in 1 group consumed a protein supplement (approximately 35 g of casein) twice daily, once in the morning and once in the evening (thus, the timing of protein intake was not immediately preworkout or postworkout). A second group consumed the same supplement twice daily, once in the morning and once immediately before a training session. Both groups were tasked with completing 8 weeks of resistance training. Although both groups demonstrated significant increases in strength markers, the first group (protein supplements taken in the morning and evening) demonstrated greater increases in fat-free mass than the second group (protein supplements taken in the morning and before exercise). In addition to demonstrating that more widely dispersed protein intake is perhaps more advantageous for resistance-trained athletes, these findings also appear to support the efficacy of presleep protein ingestion, discussed in a subsequent section.

Taken together, these results suggest that consumption of protein prior to exercise serves as a possible feeding opportunity to help meet overall daily needs but is not an obligatory time frame for athletes to augment MPS and obtain related benefits.

FEEDING DURING EXERCISE

A series of studies by Bird et al[45-47] were fundamental in assessing the acute impact of ingestion of protein (in addition to carbohydrate) during resistance exercise. These studies ranged from assessing hormonal and urinary protein breakdown measures to implementing a "triphasic" approach (providing protein before, during, and after exercise) and were able to demonstrate fairly successful outcomes (eg, reduced serum proteins indicative of muscle damage). However, a chronic study (12 weeks) completed by a similar group of authors was less noteworthy (eg, less of an increase in myofibrillar fiber size when carbohydrate was omitted from the protein and carbohydrate mixture).[48] These 4 studies were also accompanied by additional work completed by Beelen et al,[49] in which acutely fed participants were given carbohydrates and protein prior to, and during, a combined endurance and whole-body resistance exercise session.

Whereas sustained postworkout MPS stimulation was observed in the protein coingestion group, no further augmentation of net muscle protein accretion occurred during the subsequent overnight recovery period. Of note, the study by Beelen et al[49] employed an exercise protocol that also included endurance exercise (not just resistance exercise).

Athletes and trainers may well express concern about the physiological relevance of feeding protein during bouts of resistance exercise. Whereas endurance exercise requires constant adenosine triphosphate (ATP) utilization to fuel muscle that is perpetually working, the nature of resistance exercise is less constant. Research demonstrates that the energy-consuming process of MPS is not elevated during resistance exercise in the fasting state; this lack of enhanced regulation of MPS may be attributed to the activation of adenosine monophosphate protein kinase, the energy sensor in muscle cells.[34,50,51] Some individuals reason that the more promising results (such as those from Beelen et al[49]) of augmented in-exercise MPS rates may be considerably noteworthy for athletes who are completing extensive training bouts (ie, >2 hours) marked with particularly long rest periods. However, the practical notion remains that very little physiological value should be placed on such finite periods of relaxation considering that the majority of muscular protein remodeling still takes place in the hours and days following a training bout.[49] Future studies are warranted that focus exclusively on resistance exercise to determine if providing dose-appropriate protein during exercise is more advantageous than providing it before or after exercise. Until then, assuming that adequate quantities of protein are being consumed throughout the day (especially near at least 1 periworkout period), the choice to ingest protein throughout resistance training bouts will likely provide little added benefit regarding the ability to further induce muscle hypertrophy compared to ingestion at a more traditional time (ie, after training).

POSTEXERCISE FEEDING

Research demonstrating the notable synergy between resistance exercise and feeding has highlighted that such training works to prime the muscle to be more responsive to aminoacidemia (high concentrations of amino acids); consequently, this relationship renders the period following a workout as a theoretically sensible time to consume dietary protein when seeking to optimize hypertrophic responses.[14,52] Numerous studies have supported the concept that protein consumed following resistance training is capable of acute stimulation of MPS.[15,51,53-55] However, studies have reported widespread conflicting evidence regarding whether these benefits are truly due to both the protein and timing of consumption or are merely a byproduct of meeting bodily protein demands without respect to time frames.[56-59] As stated earlier, the fundamental anabolic nature of resistance training makes research findings difficult to extrapolate. In addition, marked differences in study designs (eg, participant training type and prior habits, diet history, and standardization) pose a challenge for practitioners trying to provide accurate recommendations about the *exact* timing of protein ingestion to best support MPS.[44,60,61]

Two classic studies have sought to examine the differences that emerge in protein turnover following different timings and patterns of protein ingestion. First, Moore et al[63] had participants consume 3 different variations of whey protein feeding schedules following a resistance-exercise bout. To provide each of the groups with a total dose of 80 g over 12 hours, the first group was given 40 g at intervals of 6 hours (2 total feedings), the second group was given 20 g at intervals of 3 hours (4 total feedings), and the third group was given 10 g at intervals of 1 hour (8 total feedings). The muscle-centric outcomes that were observed were strongest following the dosing scheme of 20 g every 3 hours.[62] Later, a group including many of the same researchers devised a similar study, this time again finding that 20 g of whey protein ingested every 3 hours following resistance exercise was optimal for enhancing MPS rates. Despite these rather clear findings, one should note that these studies were short-term and that 80 g of protein is likely inadequate to meet the augmented needs of many athletes. Nevertheless, such work provides support for the idea that NPB and MPS are influenced by both the timing and pattern of protein intake. More specifically, the 2 studies make a clear recommendation to athletes that moderate protein doses (ie, 20 g) dispersed over the course of the day (ie, 3–4 hours apart) promote favorable whole-body changes.[62,63]

In addition, the synergistic effect of exercise and feeding appears to persist well beyond the few hours following an acute bout of resistance exercise. Burd and colleagues[64] studied a group of young men who consumed 15 g of whey protein after a single bout of resistance exercise. Despite supporting the theory that MPS is elevated to the greatest extent shortly after resistance training, the results demonstrated that

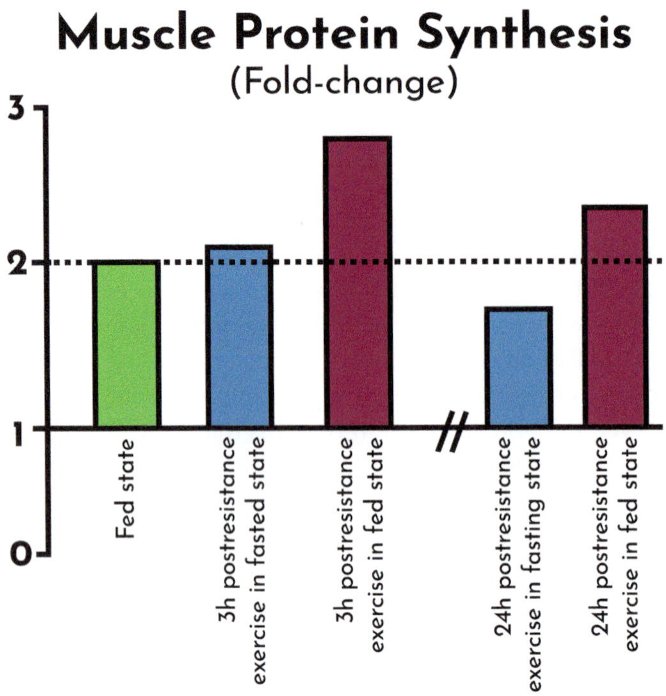

FIGURE 3.3 Fold-change from fasted-state resting conditions in muscle protein synthesis following feeding and resistance exercise Fold-change is a measure describing how much a quantity changes between an original measurement and a subsequent measurement; it is defined as the ratio of the second measurement to the original measurement. The anabolic sensitizing effect of resistance exercise is greatest during the immediate acute recovery period; however, this sensitizing effect is still conferred more than 1 day after exercise. The dashed line illustrates the sum of the fed response following exercise.

muscle remains more "anabolically sensitive" for up to 24 hours. Figure 3.3 illustrates these findings.

Researchers have not yet identified the exact underlying mechanisms behind this synergism of exercise and feeding, but the processes may involve anabolic signaling molecules that can potentiate, or "turn on," MPS and enhance sensitivity to feeding. Moreover, research demonstrates that resistance exercise and protein ingestion can upregulate skeletal muscle amino acid transporters, which, in turn, may assist in the transport of amino acids into the free amino acid pool.[65,66] Therefore, the resistance exercise–mediated increase in amino acid transport proteins in skeletal muscle tissue during late recovery after exercise may ultimately sensitize muscle to dietary protein–derived amino acids in a subsequent meal.[67] Note, however, that scientists still do not completely understand the role of increased expression of skeletal muscle amino acid transporter in modulating the postexercise or postprandial MPS response.

ADEQUATE PROTEIN INTAKE AT ANY TIME

Despite the information pointing to MPS-related benefits of consuming adequate protein following resistance training, further discussion of the notion of nonimmediate protein ingestion is warranted. A large 2013 meta-analysis examining the timing of protein ingestion for athletes supported the idea that, despite evidence of positive muscle-related outcomes when protein is ingested after resistance exercise, the exact timing of protein consumption is supplanted in importance by the strongest predictor of muscular hypertrophy: total daily protein intake.[57] In other words, even though the timing of protein intake appears to have some relevance, the factor that is of utmost importance when athletes are seeking to optimize training adaptations is the quantity of protein consumed, that is, satisfying the recommendations for daily protein intake. This stands somewhat in contrast to traditional mainstream focal points in which immediate and narrow (from 30 minutes to 1 hour) "windows of opportunity" are often viewed as compulsory feeding times for athletes to utilize. As seen in Figure 3.3, the anabolic sensitivity of muscle does not appear to necessitate such narrow preworkout or postworkout protein supplementation periods to induce MPS.[64]

Although research by Schoenfeld et al[68] considered periworkout time frames, the authors demonstrated that 10 weeks of supplementation with protein both preworkout and postworkout led to similar benefits in muscle mass and strength. Perhaps greater support for the theory of intake beyond periworkout periods can be found in a study by Hoffman et al,[61] in which collegiate football players completed 10 weeks of resistance training supplemented with protein either (1) immediately before and after their training or (2) in the morning and evening. Whereas both groups saw muscle-centric benefits, the variance in protein ingestion timing failed to produce any significant differences in strength, power, or body composition measures between groups. This research is an example of a more relaxed "big picture" approach in which athletes are not required to fixate on ingesting protein in tightly defined windows (but rather are tasked with focusing on overall daily needs). Nevertheless, studies have also indicated that protein intake close to exercise either helps or, at a minimum, has a neutral effect. In other words, consuming protein-containing foods, drinks, or supplements during a periworkout period provides another feeding opportunity with no notable downside. Furthermore, consumption at such times will still help athletes reach their adequate overall level of daily protein intake. This may be especially pertinent for athletes who have a hard time reaching their required intake because they must balance the need to accommodate scheduling demands with the requirement to consistently train at extremely high volumes and/or frequencies (eg, athletes attending school or working a full-time job while training). Nutrition practitioners should encourage athletes and those counseling them to view the periworkout "window of opportunity" as a valuable—but not essential—feeding occasion capable of helping the athlete meet total daily protein and caloric requirements.

INTERMITTENT FASTING

This relationship between postexercise protein requirements and the general recommendation to disperse protein intake over one's waking hours invites discussion of a popular dietary trend that has gained traction over recent years: intermittent fasting. (Approximately 40% of the roughly 800 registered research studies on intermittent fasting that occurred between 2010 and 2021 were conducted between 2020 and 2021.[69]) Intermittent fasting, a dietary tactic most commonly adopted to manage energy intake and encourage weight loss, can be broken into 3 subclasses: alternate-day fasting (alternating between ad libitum feeding and fasting days), whole-day fasting (fasting 1–2 d/wk paired with ad libitum feeding on the other days), and time-restricted eating (daily ad libitum feeding within a specific set of hours, usually 4–8 hours in duration, and fasting outside this time frame).[70] By nature, each subclass stands in contrast to evenly dispersed eating patterns. Many athletes may not set out to eat in such an intermittent pattern but could end up inadvertently adopting such habits. For example, 1 study examining the diets of college-level athletes found that the majority ate no breakfast and only 9% met their designated energy needs over the day.[71] Importantly, a high-protein breakfast helps shift an overnight negative NPB toward positive balance while also demonstrating the potential to improve aspects of weight management (improved satiety, reduced body fat gain, etc).[72] As Williamson and Moore[69] summarized in their 2021 perspective publication, "intermittent fasting likely represents a suboptimal dietary approach to remodel skeletal muscle, which could impact the ability to maintain or enhance muscle mass and quality, especially during periods of reduced energy availability."

PROTEIN INTAKE BEFORE SLEEP

The previously discussed work by Beelen et al[49] was an important foundational piece that prompted further work to assess the ability of ingesting protein before sleep to optimize MPS during overnight recovery. After this study, Res and colleagues[73] were among the first to demonstrate that protein consumed before sleep (40 g) was efficiently digested and absorbed into circulation. These augmented MPS responses observed during the overnight recovery period were seen despite participants receiving a full day of standardized nutritional intake, including immediate postexercise nutrition (20 g of protein, 60 g of carbohydrate) following an evening resistance-exercise bout.

In addition to these more acute studies, research examining longer intervention periods (ie, several weeks) has also been completed. For example, Snijders et al[74] enlisted men completing 12 weeks of resistance training to consume either 27.5 g of protein (plus 15 g of carbohydrate) or a noncaloric placebo each night. The authors found that those consuming the protein had greater improvements in both muscle mass and strength following the intervention. The individuals in the protein group did, however, consume far more daily protein (1.9 vs 1.3 g of protein per kilogram of body weight per day). These findings prompted Antonio et al[75] to carry out another study in an effort to determine whether the disparity between overall intake levels may have influenced the outcomes. This secondary study was conducted during 8 weeks of resistance training and, in addition to enlisting male participants, also included females. To better equate the overall daily protein intake between groups, those not consuming protein within 90 minutes of sleep were supplemented with an equal dose (54 g) of protein at a time in the morning (before 12 PM). When the groups were compared, no significant differences in either body composition or performance measures emerged, even though those who supplemented in the evening added almost 1 kg (0.4 vs 1.2 kg) more lean mass compared with the cohort supplementing in the morning. These studies and other works are supported by notable reviews that have provided additional evidence for the idea that consuming protein later in the evening (ie, before sleep) may improve body composition and performance through altered MPS, recovery, and metabolism.[76,77]

Despite the data provided by researchers to support the efficacy of consuming protein before sleep, much work remains to be done for athletes to buy into and take advantage of this "alternative feeding opportunity." For example, in a sizable survey of trained athletes,[79] the average intake of protein as part of an evening snack was a mere 7 g, an amount that is well below the larger doses (ie, 30–40 g) that have shown promising presleep benefits.[4,73,77,78] This is not the first study to indicate that athletes seeking to optimize training adaptations are taking in an insufficient amount of protein prior to sleep.[79] This lack of late-night protein ingestion has compounding implications considering research noting the lack of habitual breakfast intake among athletes.[71] One point of apprehension that may push athletes to avoid ingesting protein before bed is uncertainty about whether lipolysis or fat oxidation would be blunted by doing so. However, athletes can look to studies by Madzima et al[80] and Kinsey et al,[81] which demonstrated that such concerns are not valid. To properly inform athletes who might be considering eating more protein before bed, nutrition practitioners can point out that many of the aforementioned studies used casein, a slower-digesting protein, as their selected experimental protein source. (A variety of protein sources are discussed in the following sections.) Although experts are still forming concrete recommendations, the consumption of protein prior to sleep does appear to be an effective nutrient timing tactic to both modulate the adaptive response of skeletal muscle to exercise and also help increase the likelihood that both daily protein and energy needs are being met.[74]

Protein Timing for Endurance Exercise

Research investigating the effectiveness of protein consumed prior to endurance exercise is limited. Recent studies include the following:

- » A 2020 study investigated the effect of consuming either protein (dose of 0.5 g/kg LBM) or flavored water on trained cyclists before an endurance session. The protein intervention failed to increase MPS or NPB in exercising and nonexercising tissues, respectively. The researchers found that this lack of beneficial effects held true during and following exercise for both fasted and fed study subjects.[82]
- » A 2021 study revealed that cyclists training in a state of low carbohydrate availability while also consuming preexercise protein did not demonstrate altered fat oxidation or performance.[83]
- » A 2019 study found that, when insufficient carbohydrates were consumed before endurance exercise, athletes demonstrated increased requirements for dietary protein in general.[84]

Taken together, current research suggests that properly fueled athletes are unlikely to obtain direct MPS-related or performance benefits from consuming protein prior to normal endurance training.

During exercise, the expensive process of supporting muscle protein turnover generally comes secondary to supplying the constant high ATP requirements that working muscle demands.[85] Still, considerable research has been devoted to determining whether consuming protein during endurance exercise is an effective way to remodel muscle. Research in the early to mid-2000s by authors such as Ivy et al[86] and Saunders et al[87,88] suggested that feeding protein during endurance exercise may offer some additional performance benefits over the traditional tactic of feeding carbohydrates alone. However, in the years following this work, additional research emerged that led to concerns about the validity of this relationship.[89-93] For example, a well-designed, double-blind, repeated-measures, placebo-controlled, crossover study demonstrated that there was no additional time-to-exhaustion benefit from protein ingested with carbohydrate as opposed to carbohydrate alone.[89] Considering the overall body of evidence, Knuiman et al[94] concluded, in a perspective piece, that the need to include protein alongside carbohydrate to fuel normal endurance exercise is, like preexercise protein consumption, unlikely to further enhance performance and is thus not necessary, assuming that daily fueling requirements are being met.

Even though these recommendations fail to support mandating preexercise and intraexercise protein intake, the fundamental use of protein to replace exercise-induced amino acid oxidative losses and support positive NPB plus subsequent adaptations to aerobic exercise is worth mentioning. If athletes can tolerate coingestion of protein during (and perhaps prior to) training, there is certainly a potential for improved facilitation of protein toward muscle protein remodeling when exercise is stopped. Furthermore, the addition of protein (or other macronutrients) at such alternative times (ie, preexercise and intraexercise)

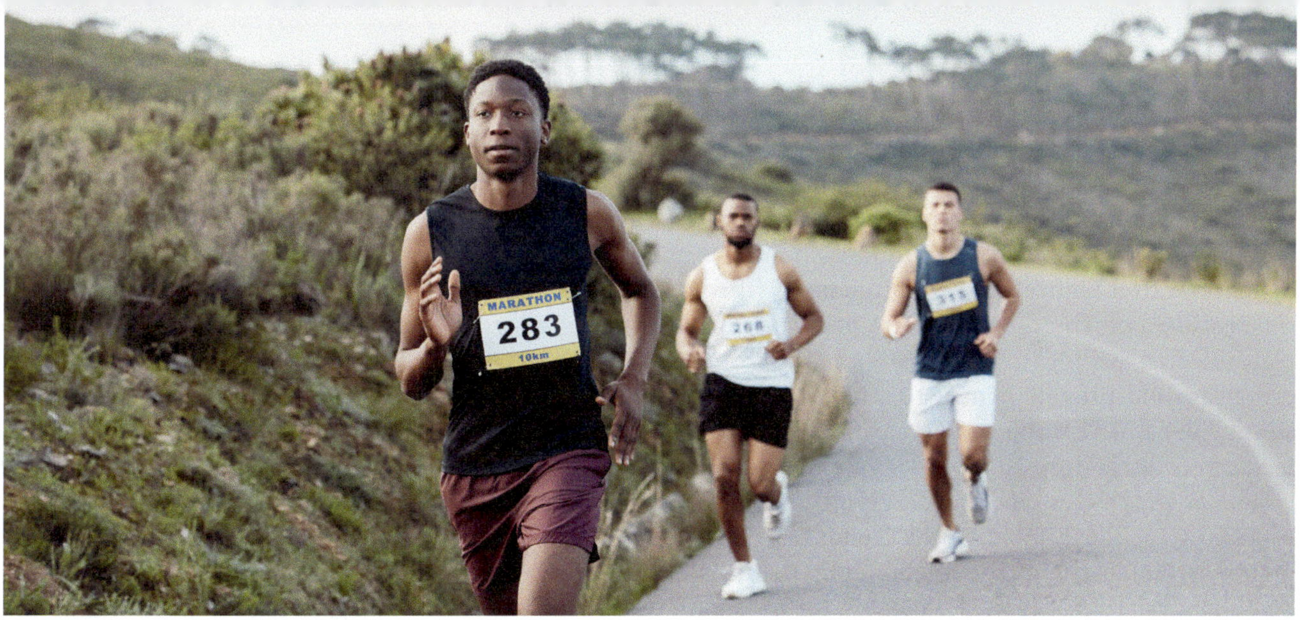

still stands as a useful way for an endurance athlete to meet their elevated daily protein requirements and, perhaps more importantly, total energy needs.

The most promising periworkout protein ingestion window for endurance athletes is also the most traditional: postexercise. Considering the glycolytic demands of aerobic exercise, many studies have sought to assess how protein may impact the ability to augment glycogen resynthesis.[95-98] Based on these studies, a 2021 meta-analysis maintained that, when adequate carbohydrate (ie, 1.2 g/kg/h) is being consumed following endurance training, the addition of protein likely provides no further benefit to glycogen recovery.[99] Beyond considerations of glycogen, several studies have established that acute aerobic exercise is capable of inducing increases in MPS.[15,19-21,31-34,100-103] A 2022 meta-analysis specifically emphasized that this notion should not be undervalued.[104] This statement can likely be attributed largely to the hallmark adaptations that occur following aerobic training, including increased capillarization, increased mitochondrial biogenesis, and increased abundance of glucose and fat transporters.[105-107] Each of these adaptations requires turning over of proteins and the net addition of new proteins; in other words, a positive NPB is needed to support optimal adaptation. Consequently, consuming protein following exercise serves as a very practical choice to increase the likelihood of optimizing these valuable adaptations while reducing the risk of being subject to added adverse side effects (eg, gastrointestinal discomfort) that often plague endurance athletes. Thus, without demanding specific adherence to this particular feeding window, it remains that protein consumed after exercise (endurance, resistance, or otherwise) can always be considered a suitable option for proper recovery nutrition.[28,108]

PROTEIN FOR ULTRAENDURANCE EXERCISE

Long in both distance and duration, ultraendurance activities are a unique form of exercise capable of inducing metabolic overload and/or mechanical strain, leading to significant muscle damage.[109-111] Following unusual bouts of exercise, an athlete's NPB may remain below normal levels for days.[2] Ultraendurance exercise entails unique fueling requirements, including adjusting protein intake. When compared to the traditional guidelines surrounding timing of protein intake for endurance athletes, recommendations for ultraendurance athletes are largely still being established.

In one of the foundational studies in this area of research, Koopman et al[112] sought to determine the response of whole-body protein turnover in triathletes, ultramarathon runners, cyclists, and others who exercise for more than 5 h/d. Participants were given either carbohydrate or carbohydrate plus protein before, during, and after exercise. The authors found that the athletes' protein balance remained negative when carbohydrates alone were ingested. More notably, when protein was ingested alongside carbohydrate, the researchers found that the whole-body NPB ratios were altered as increases in whole-body MPS and decreases in whole-body MPB occurred at rest, during prolonged moderate intensity exercise, and during recovery. However, standing in contrast to these results is another notable study in this area, which was conducted by Knechtle et al[113] in 2011. In this case, the researchers investigated the impact of acute supplementation with 52.5 g of amino acids before and during a 100-km ultramarathon. Although they anticipated a reduction in variables of skeletal muscle damage, decreases in muscle soreness, and improved performance, the authors found none of their hypothesized results.

Despite these equivocal and quite limited findings, providing periworkout protein to ultraendurance athletes seems like a sensible recommendation to make at the current time. Small boluses of protein taken in temporal proximity to long endurance bouts are not necessarily meant to provide a direct performance benefit or offset higher energy requirements (through direct oxidation), but rather are to try to optimize the processes of whole-body protein pool remodeling for longer-term benefit.[112,114] Nevertheless, it is still plausible that feeding such small amounts of protein (ie, 5–10 g) during each hour or so of ultraendurance exercise could provide benefit to athletes demanding so much of their bodies.[112] At the very least (assuming the athlete is able to tolerate in-exercise ingestion of protein without distress), such small frequent feedings could assist in dispersing protein appropriately (ie, ~20–30 g of protein every 3–4 hours) over the course of an athlete's day.[62,63] As a result, such athletes, who spend a large portion of their waking hours exercising, will also increase the likelihood that they are able to meet their markedly elevated energy demands, along with daily protein requirements. Meeting these amplified energy needs gives athletes the best chance of using ingested protein in the manner it is intended to be used (to optimize NPB) and reduce their risk of both injury and impaired performance.[114] With the exception of those who display adverse tolerability, there appears to be no reason to advise ultraendurance athletes to avoid consuming protein during periworkout phases, as failing to eat ensures that no benefits will be attained.

PROTEIN QUALITY

Amino acid composition and digestion rate kinetics are 2 vital variables that help determine the overall quality of a given dietary protein source.[115] In general, high-quality proteins have characteristics that optimize the magnitude and speed at which new proteins can be synthesized. Training adaptations such as muscle hypertrophy are often underpinned by net positive balances in protein, and protein quality is clearly important when seeking to augment such bodily turnover. Dietary protein is commonly separated into plant- and animal-based forms, and although there are considerable similarities between the two, they should not be considered equal. Inherently, animal-based proteins are understood to contain more robust concentrations of EAAs compared to plant-based proteins. When dietary protein sources are rich in these important amino acids and are rapidly digested, their associated protein quality score is raised, as is their capability to rapidly stimulate MPS following exercise.[116,117] One EAA that is especially notable to this critical concept is *leucine*.

Leucine as an Anabolic Trigger

As a foundational tenet of MPS stimulation, leucine targets a key signaling protein, the mammalian target of rapamycin complex 1 (mTORC1).[118] Leucine has an interesting relationship with insulin. Leucine is insulinogenic, but insulin is not particularly anabolic above levels already present in the fasting state (5 mcU/mL). Furthermore, the influence of leucine on MPB manifests at insulin levels of approximately 30 mcU/mL, a concentration that is commonly obtained after consuming a mixed meal.[119] When also considering the direct relationship between carbohydrate and insulin, researchers have notably demonstrated no further stimulation of MPS nor inhibition of MPB following ingestion of carbohydrate with protein compared to ingestion of protein alone. These findings were observed in both postexercise and resting states.[120] Although this might appear as an indictment suggesting that carbohydrates cannot be beneficial from the standpoint of muscle development, athletes should not dismiss the idea of consuming carbohydrate and protein together, as doing so confers other benefits such as muscle glycogen replenishment. Leucine may also serve as an anabolic mediator through its ability to increase the transport of other amino acids into muscle. In doing so, these amino acids can then accumulate in the muscle-free amino acid pool and be used for protein synthesis.[121] Moreover, research shows that the amino acid transporter that brings leucine into the muscle cell (L-type amino acid transporter 1 [LAT1]) may serve as an amino acid sensor to communicate with the protein synthetic machinery.[122] Thus, both supplements and foods rich in leucine tend to be considered anabolic and of high importance with respect to MPS and NPB.[58,123,124] Researchers generally suggest approximately 2 to 3 g of leucine as the dose that optimally "triggers" MPS.[124,125] Figure 3.4 illustrates this concept (ie, the "leucine trigger" hypothesis).

Even though leucine appears to be the primary stimulator of MPS (it can be metaphorically viewed as "the keys being used to turn on the car"), individuals must still consume other amino acids, especially EAAs, in adequate amounts. The fact that EAAs such as leucine are indispensable (ie, unable to be synthesized within the body) emphasizes their importance. However, the relative content of a specific amino acid in a given protein source diminishes as the total amount of protein consumed increases. In other words, one can compensate for foods with lower relative proportions of an EAA such as leucine through additional consumption.[126]

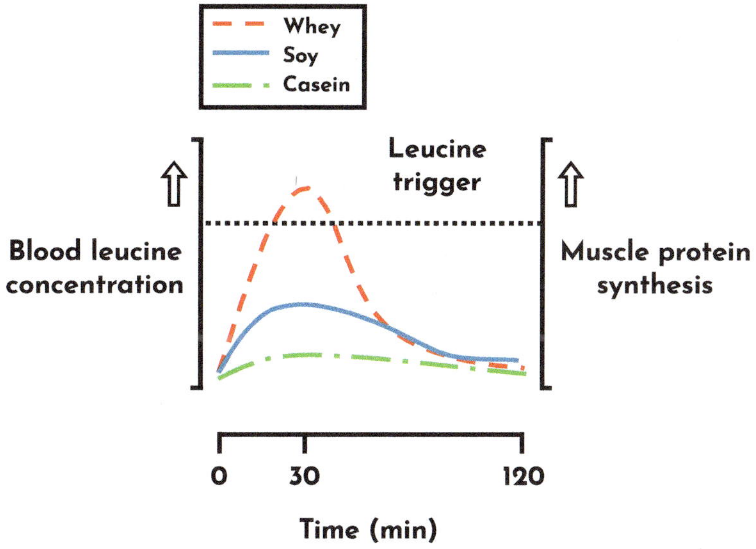

FIGURE 3.4 The leucine trigger hypothesis After consumption of whey protein (which is higher in leucine content than soy or casein), there is a rapid increase in plasma leucine concentration. This increase corresponds to the extent to which muscle protein synthesis is stimulated. The amount of leucine needed to achieve the "trigger" is understood to be approximately 2 to 3 g.

Finally, although supplemental protein options such as whey, casein, and soy can undoubtedly be practical options for athletes to use, high-quality whole-food proteins (chicken, beef, eggs, milk, salmon, soybeans, tofu, etc) should always be considered reliable options to build muscle protein and support overall health.

Comparative Analysis of Whey, Casein, and Soy

Whey, casein, and soy are the 3 primary types of isolated protein supplements that are typically studied in assessments of MPS and recovery.[116] For reference, milk is composed of approximately 20% whey protein and 80% casein protein. Whey digests quickly and is referred to as a "fast-digesting protein," whereas casein digests more slowly and is referred to as a "slow-digesting protein."[127] Soy has garnered considerable attention and use with more individuals seeking to consume plant-based proteins. Similarly to whey, soy is a more quickly digested protein source.

WHEY

Whey protein is the soluble fraction extracted from milk during cheese manufacturing and has become exceedingly popular among athletes as a dietary supplement. Whey protein powders are mainly available as a concentrate (generally >70% protein), isolate (generally >90% protein), or hydrolysate (protein content varies but is typically >80%); however, the protein content of these preparations can vary. In this chapter, the general term *whey protein* is used to describe all 3 forms.

Whey protein is considered a protein of exceptional quality because of its high protein digestibility–corrected amino acid score; its amino acid composition is close to, or in most cases exceeds, the digestibility of human body proteins. In addition to being a rapidly and easily digested protein source, whey protein contains very high concentrations of EAAs. Most notably, the total amino acid composition of whey protein has a surprisingly disproportionate amount of leucine (14%) relative to other high-quality protein sources. In comparison, milk and beef contain roughly 10% and 9% leucine, respectively, by total amino acid content.[128]

Considering the higher leucine content of whey and the ability of leucine to robustly stimulate mTORC1, researchers were able to demonstrate the effectiveness of whey in provoking significant rises (both at rest and following a single bout of resistance exercise) in both EAAs (ie, leucine) and MPS, notably in comparison to soy and casein.[116] Comparatively, whey contains approximately 3 g of leucine, casein contains approximately 2.5 g of leucine, and soy contains approximately 2 g of leucine per 30 g portion (ie, the general size of 1 scoop of protein powder). In an effort to confirm that leucine, and not another factor, was responsible for these findings, Reidy et al[129] demonstrated that a dairy-soy protein mixture was equally as effective at stimulating MPS as whey protein when the leucine contents were matched. Whey is a highly suitable protein option for athletes seeking to optimize MPS.

CASEIN

Casein, the acid-insoluble protein fraction of milk, is produced when milk is exposed to an acidic environment. Casein is less commonly used in sports drinks or bars because of solubility issues and production costs. Casein is commonly recommended for consumption in the late evening because it takes longer to digest.[127,130,131] As noted in the prior discussion on presleep protein, this slower, prolonged release of amino acids into the systemic circulation is hypothesized to promote a positive NPB during the overnight fast and recovery period and thus may result in a greater accretion of muscle proteins.

SOY

As a protein-rich legume, soy is the most commonly used and studied nonmeat protein source. When soy protein is extracted and used in isolated protein powders, it has a rate of digestion more closely resembling that of whey than casein.[132] However, the total amino acid content of soy protein includes a lower proportion of leucine than whey and casein. As a result, soy is thought to have a lower potential anabolic effect on skeletal muscle tissue.[133]

The superiority of higher-quality, animal-based proteins in inducing maximal responses after resistance exercise is not a novel phenomenon. Wilkinson et al[134] demonstrated that young men who consumed 500 mL of nonfat milk exhibited a greater anabolic response after an acute strength training bout than when they consumed an isonitrogenous, isoenergetic, and macronutrient-matched soy beverage. Another training study sought to build on these findings and had men consume various beverages over the course of 12 weeks. This longer study complemented the acute anabolic findings of Wilkinson et al and also found that nonfat milk led to greater total gains in LBM and significantly more loss of fat mass compared with soy- or carbohydrate-only products.[16] Shortly after, similar findings were also observed for females.[135] These results suggest that milk and its amino acid profile are favorable for inducing various important training adaptations compared to alternative plant-based options such as soy. As an additional aside on soy, males concerned about the potential impacts on androgenic hormones should know that chronic consumption of soy protein alongside resistance training was not found to significantly affect serum concentrations of sex hormones such as testosterone.[136]

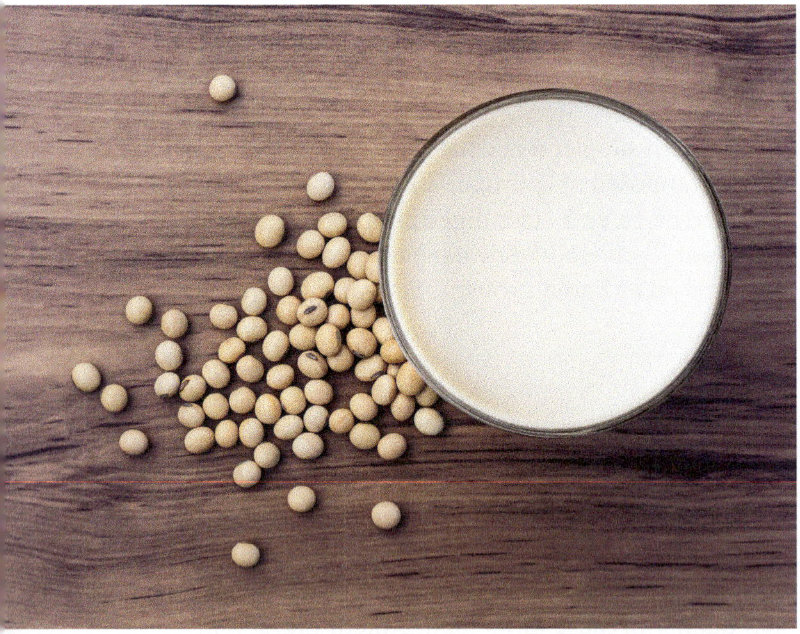

Plants make up a substantial portion of dietary intake for both carnivores and plant-based eaters.[4,133] Furthermore, well-trained athletes have reported that plants, and thus plant-based proteins, make up a substantial portion (approximately 40%) of their overall daily protein ingestion.[4] For those who are eating higher proportions of plant-based proteins (eg, vegetarians and vegans), the options of fortifying plant-based proteins with free amino acids or genetically manipulating or crossbreeding plants (such as high-quality maize protein) to improve the amino acid composition—leucine in particular—may serve as useful strategies to enhance muscle-centric adaptations. Other more practical options for athletes seeking to reduce their consumption of animal-based protein but still obtain such benefits also exist. For example, 1 study concluded that endurance athletes abstaining from meat consumption could simply seek out modest increases (approximately 10–20 g/d) of additional total protein intake to ensure that they are compensating for consuming only lower-quality proteins.[137] Alternatively, athletes might opt to use complementary food and supplement pairings to augment dietary protein quality.[138] For example, an athlete eating chickpeas might look to rice as a suitable pairing to meet EAA demands and presumably augment muscle repair and recovery. However, athletes and trainers should consider whether they have limited knowledge of the principles of nutrition and metabolism that would otherwise help them in making such pairings to meet their bodily demands (MPS-related and otherwise). In cases such as this or when other drastic dietary changes (eg, the decision to cut out large portions of one's typical diet such as animal-based proteins) are pursued, experts strongly recommend that athletes seek the assistance of a credentialed health care provider (such as a registered dietitian) to help ensure that they are taking the right steps for both their health and performance.

The Food Matrix

Most of the research regarding protein quality has involved the analysis of either (1) isolated amino acids (eg, leucine), (2) singular supplement sources (eg, whey protein), or (3) sole whole-food options (eg, milk). However, the reality is that the basis of human consumption consists of uniquely combined mixed meals, not isolated amino acids, singular supplement sources, or even individual whole-food options. As such, there is inherent value in promoting scientific research seeking to study the interplay between food sources. These relationships have been termed the *food matrix*, which is specifically defined by the US Department of Agriculture as "the nutrient and non-nutrient components of foods and their molecular relationships, ie, chemical bonds, to each other."[115,128,139-141]

Considering the complexity of whole foods, the fact that their unique amino acid profiles prompt distinctively dissimilar postmeal aminoacidemia responses compared to singular isolated protein fractions is not surprising.[142] For example, even though whole-food sources generally have lower total amounts of leucine and more prolonged release of amino acids into the circulation compared to options such as whey protein powder, the ingestion of various whole-food sources (eg, eggs, red meat, fish) has been found to exhibit the capability to induce robust posttraining MPS responses. Researchers such as Hodgkinson et al[143] have theorized that this capability of whole-food sources to overcome what appear to be inferior intrinsic MPS-inducing compositions (at least in terms of speed to induce) may be related to the interaction between nutrients (the food matrix) and alterations to food structure (ie, cooking).

Additional criteria aside from MPS should be considered when comparing the suitability of food sources to support training. For example, would the consumption of approximately 20 g of whey induce superior training adaptations compared to the consumption of 500 mL of milk? Although this specific comparison has never been investigated, an examination of the current literature suggests that gains in LBM and loss of fat mass would be relatively similar.[16,60,135,144-146] However, low-fat dairy seems to be exceptionally potent in decreasing fat mass, especially in young women who consume relatively low amounts of dairy.[135] This effect could potentially relate to the interplay between calcium and vitamin D and how it affects adipocyte metabolism and the inhibition of lipid accretion.[147,148] In addition, the consumption of protein in the form of nutrient-dense whole foods (milk, beef, chicken, seafood, etc) may offer additional benefits beyond simply stimulating the postprandial MPS response compared with the consumption of isolated protein sources that have lost many nutritional factors during processing. Thus, despite a keen interest in using protein blends (partly to reduce industrial manufacturing costs of single higher-quality protein sources) to augment the adaptive response of skeletal muscle, these simplified options will likely not offer any benefit beyond those that protein-dense foods are also able to provide (and they may, in fact, be inferior).[149] However, if used, the practice of blending different protein sources together (eg, adding whey protein along with pea protein) still appears to be a suitable option for increasing the likelihood of reaching one's anabolic potential.[133,149] From the perspective of the food matrix, the same logic could likely be applied to the benefits that nutrient-dense whole-food combinations can provide.

As athletes are often taught about the benefits of eating whole foods or making "performance plates," the fact that some of this initial work is pointing to whole foods as viable options for properly supporting athletic performance is promising. Nevertheless, this short discussion on the food matrix should not be mistaken as strict support for a "food-only" nutritional approach. Research-backed supplements such as isolated protein powders can certainly be seen as convenient complementary options to support healthy whole-food eating patterns for busy athletes with uniquely elevated needs. More research is warranted to truly elucidate how interactions within the food matrix may contribute to different metabolic responses.[124] Such possibilities should excite athletes, as this expansion of research on the intersection of whole foods with metabolic and training responses could lead to considerable practical implications in favor of simplifying their nutritional outlook.

PROTEIN QUANTITY

How much protein should an athlete consume to support training? The dose of protein required to optimize recovery from exercise is perhaps the best example of a classic sports nutrition debate that surfaces in groups ranging from sports scientists to everyday gym-goers. Detailed recommendations shared in this section address unique protein dosing recommendations for both resistance- and endurance-based athletes. Aging may alter the anabolic or aminoacidemia response to protein ingestion, and thus, older adults may require slightly more protein to meet their needs.[150-152] More information on this topic is provided in Chapter 14, Masters Athletes. With this in mind, the following section provides guidance largely intended for younger adult athletes without such augmented needs.

Quantity for Resistance Exercise

Resistance-trained athletes may assume that the more protein they eat, the more lean mass they will gain because amino acids in protein are the building blocks for muscle. Research suggests that this relationship only holds true to a certain extent.[153,154] Findings of a graded response relationship between protein dose and MPS stimulation showed that doubling a standard provision of 3 g of EAAs to 6 g of EAAs induced a similar twofold increase in MPS.[155] For reference, these doses of EAAs are approximately equivalent to 7.5 and 15 g, respectively, of a high-quality dietary protein. A related study demonstrated that experienced weight-trained men (weighing approximately 85 kg on average) who consumed varying doses of high-quality isolated egg protein alongside acute resistance exercise experienced the greatest degree of MPS stimulation at a dose of 20 g. Whereas that dose was notably superior to a 10-g dose, the authors found no further effect from doubling that 20-g dose to 40 g of protein.[153] Therefore, instead of doubling muscle size when twice as much protein is consumed, the additional amino acids end up being used alternatively for energy production or, at least in terms of MPS, being "wasted." Figure 3.5 illustrates this point.

Although this work was foundational in advancing the knowledge base regarding the amount of protein athletes should seek to consume, it is not without contest. A 2016 study by Macnaughton et al[156] did detect a statistically significant difference in MPS when greater amounts of protein (40 g vs 20 g) were consumed following resistance exercise. The finding that a larger protein dose further augmented MPS (approximately 20% here compared to 10% elsewhere) may be largely due to the type of exercise training that was completed by the study participants. Studies that indicated that 20 g of protein is sufficient to maximally stimulate MPS (eg, those by Moore et al[153] or Witard et al[154]) had participants complete more isolated muscle routines. Macnaughton et al[156] showed that a dose of 40 g could provide further MPS-related benefits to complete exercise

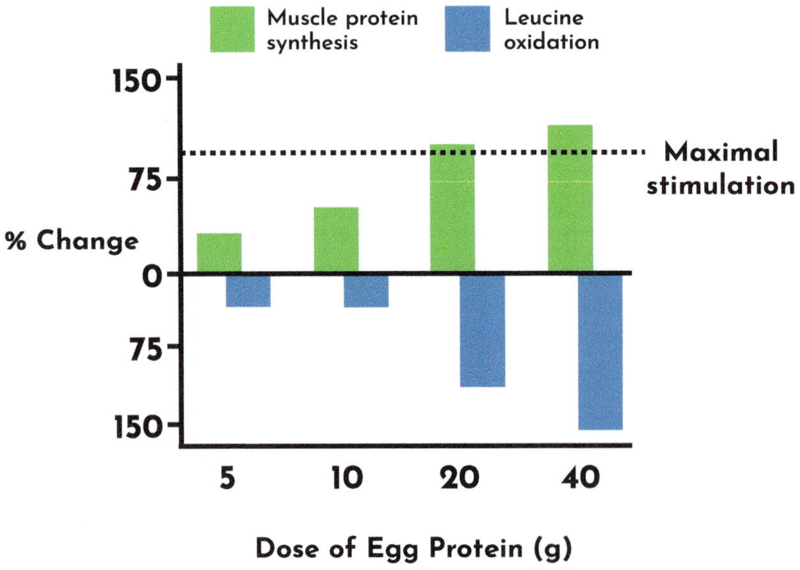

FIGURE 3.5 The relationship between protein dose and muscle protein synthesis The anabolic response to resistance exercise is maximized with 20 g of egg protein. No additional significant benefits are garnered from consuming 40 g of egg protein. Protein consumed in excess is either used for energy or "wasted" (excreted).

that was more taxing to their whole body. Because of the wide disparity between tested doses (ie, 20 g and 40 g), additional research is warranted to provide more clarity on a "middle ground" of protein intake between the 2 doses (eg, 30 g). Nevertheless, despite these findings making exact recommendations rather hard to provide, it is certainly not out of the question that athletes, especially those completing more robust whole-body exercise, might be able to further derive marginally greater (eg, 10%–20%) MPS-related benefits by increasing periworkout protein quantities above the commonly recommended dosage of 20 g to a level perhaps reaching 40 g.

Considering total protein intake levels over the entire day, a 2022 meta-analysis of 82 studies aimed to assess the dose-response relationship between protein intake and muscle strength (both with and without resistance training).[157] Not surprisingly, muscle strength was augmented only when resistance training was undertaken. More noteworthy is that a significant association was found between protein intake and muscle strength that demonstrated increases in strength for each 0.1 g of protein consumed per kilogram of body weight up to intake levels of 1.5 g/kg (daily). Beyond this level of intake, no further strength gains were achieved.[157] This finding from the meta-analysis complements that of a review by Morton et al[158] in which daily ingestion of protein at a level of 1.6 g per kilogram of body weight was deemed to be the limiting amount for muscle accretion under conditions of chronic resistance training. However, a study of resistance-trained athletes in a chronic energy deficit over a considerable amount of time found that higher intakes in the range from 2.4 g per kilogram of body weight up to exceptionally high levels of 3.0 g per kilogram of body weight may be warranted.[159] Work conducted in 2022 by Murphy and Koehler[160,161] expanded on these recommendations by concluding that lean mass accretion is impaired when an individual's total energy deficit exceeds 500 kcal/d. These unique guidelines may prove to be pivotal for weight-class athletes (eg, bodybuilders, wrestlers, mixed martial arts athletes) who must make significant alterations to their weight while still working to maintain optimal body composition measures. In these more extreme circumstances, it is imperative that athletes seeking to alter their body weight do so under detailed supervision from a group of health professionals.

How does body mass, or more appropriately LBM, factor into this recommendation? For example, do individuals with a greater degree of LBM (≥90 kg) require more protein than their smaller counterparts (≤50 kg)? Researchers have yet to systematically investigate this question. However, based on the notion that the amino acid concentrations in the blood after consumption of dietary protein are a primary factor in determining the increase in MPS after acute exercise (specifically, the leucine trigger hypothesis), it is reasonable to conclude that because larger individuals have a greater absolute volume of blood, these larger individuals would require more protein than their smaller counterparts.[162] Still, the theoretical "ceiling" recommendations for both smaller and larger individuals are most likely not so different (approximately ±5 g) that they would markedly alter the most widely recommended periworkout protein dose of 20 g.[153] Moore et al[152] provided insight into meal-based protein requirements for optimizing the postprandial MPS response relative to body weight. Their research indicated that a protein amount of about 0.24 g per kilogram of body weight (range: 0.18–0.30 g/kg) in a meal is sufficient to maximize postprandial MPS. However, these results were not obtained in the postexercise state. Nevertheless, the findings still provide reasonable estimates of the protein requirements of skeletal muscle tissue during recovery from resistance exercise.[152] Finally, even though Macnaughton et al[156] obtained statistically different results for MPS when 20 and 40 g of protein were ingested, the authors did not observe differential outcomes (in MPS) between individuals who had varying amounts of total LBM.

Whereas the general recommendations for protein intake do not fluctuate much based on body size, special considerations must be applied for individuals who have been consistently training for periods of 8 weeks or longer. If a sports dietitian were to base recommendations on the fact that resistance exercise increases protein synthesis, then they might plausibly assume that higher protein intakes are required to support this elevated level of synthesis.[14,163] Hartman et al[164] demonstrated that 12 weeks of resistance training actually decreased whole-body protein synthesis and breakdown, resulting in a greater NPB measured over the course of 24 hours compared with the untrained state. These findings imply a greater retention of dietary nitrogen (protein) after consistent resistance training than during the time before a person begins a training program. The findings can be considered consistent with the anabolic nature of resistance exercise in promoting muscle to hang on to more of its mass. Another group of researchers established that turnover of whole-body leucine decreased in both the fasting and fed states after 12 weeks of resistance training (with a concomitant increase in muscle fiber size).[165] This suggests that protein requirements are not elevated, at least in strength-trained individuals, to the level that some might expect.[166,167] The underlying mechanisms for the decreased protein requirements with training may be twofold: (1) resistance exercise in the fasted state increases NPB, suggesting a more efficient use of intracellular amino acids, and (2) aerobic exercise and resistance training preferentially stimulate specific muscle proteins.[15,19,20] This indicates that skeletal muscle can direct signals to turn on specific proteins in response to a specific exercise stimulus. Thus, repeated bouts of an anabolic stimulus on skeletal muscle may predispose muscle tissue to become a greater site of disposition of amino acids than would be the case in the absence of such training. In summary, research suggests that protein intake at a daily quantity of about 1.6 g per kilogram of body weight serves as a suitable general recommendation for which younger healthy adults completing resistance exercise can aim.[59,157]

Quantity for Endurance Exercise

As carbohydrates and fats are the primary fuel sources used during endurance exercise, protein consumption is often provided less attention by athletes looking to optimize their aerobic performance.[8,29,168] Yet, if dietary protein is not consumed in adequate quantities, MPB is the only alternative source to supply amino acids to the intracellular free amino acid pool to ultimately support protein synthesis (a counterproductive and undesirable outcome). Nitrogen balance studies analyzing nutrition practices in endurance athletes have shown that these athletes require protein intake at levels of approximately double the Recommended Dietary Allowance (RDA) of 0.8 g per kilogram of body weight per day.[169] Additionally, research has established that mitochondrial protein synthesis is stimulated after endurance exercise and that this protein fraction is responsive to protein feeding.[19,170] A 2020 study by Churchward-Venne et al[103] demonstrated that the postworkout ingestion of protein can maximize MPS among endurance-trained athletes and exhibited a dose-response element. In the study, consumption of 30 g and 45 g of protein elicited similar MPS results, 46% and 52%, respectively, above a nonprotein baseline. Compared to the similar but slightly lower amount (20 g) generally accepted as suitable for augmenting MPS following resistance exercise, this work indicates that equal or even larger amounts of protein are needed to help an athlete properly recover from endurance exercise. To support this work, future studies with similar experimental design are warranted. Ideally, such studies would incorporate plant-based protein sources in order to provide more nuanced, yet still highly practical, outcomes.

The daily quantity of protein that should be recommended to endurance athletes is largely variable and depends on factors such as an athlete's training status, training intensity, and workout duration. In addition, the heavy use of nitrogen balance studies to devise protein intake recommendations for endurance athletes also means that there is a lack of data coming from more robust study designs that directly measure MPS.[13,171-173] Endurance athletes are thus subject to a broader general range of theorized daily protein recommendations: from approximately 1.2 to 2.0 g per kilogram of body weight per day.[13,173-176] To help provide context for how variable endurance training (and associated needs) can be, consider the following 2 scenarios: (1) a recreational athlete training at a very moderate intensity (approximately 40% of VO_2 max) for approximately 1 h/d, 4 d/wk who would only expend approximately 2,000 kcal/wk more than their resting energy requirements and (2) an elite athlete training at intensities of 60% to 80% of VO_2 max for 8 to 40 h/wk who would expend approximately an additional 6,000 to 40,000 kcal/wk more than their resting energy requirements.[13] Whereas the first example would likely not require protein levels nearing the higher range of ~2.0 g per kilogram of body weight per day, the second example may require such amounts, especially if the athlete is unable to remain in overall energy balance. However, if advanced endurance athletes engaged in normal training are taking in the required number of calories needed to offset their large daily energy expenditure, they will likely have little issue consuming enough protein to ensure a state of nitrogen balance. For example, in work analyzing highly trained cyclists who engaged in long, exhaustive cycling (eg, Tour de France), only approximately 12% of their daily calories (6,000 kcal/d) came from protein, yet this still amounted to a total daily intake of protein of approximately 2.5 g per kilogram of body weight.[177,178] Considering that these athletes were found to require 1.5 to 1.8 g per kilogram of body weight to maintain nitrogen balance under such vigorous aerobic exercise conditions, this low percentage of overall intake coming from protein (12%) was still found to be sufficient to meet their needs.

Augmented protein requirements are recommended for endurance athletes in states of prolonged energy deficit. Researchers have demonstrated that individuals in a state of caloric deficit for 3 weeks yet still completing moderate bouts of endurance exercise were able to preserve their anabolic sensitivity to protein ingestions at doses of 1.6 and 2.4 g per kilogram of body weight. Even though all groups lost lean mass as a result of the intervention, those consuming protein at the RDA rate of 0.8 g per kilogram of body weight lost substantially more.[179] In addition, a diet containing 2.4 g of protein per kilogram of body weight was found to be more effective in optimizing body composition than a diet containing 1.2 g per kilogram of body weight when participants were completing both resistance and endurance exercise in a state of energy deprivation (approximately 40% below needs) for 4 weeks.[180] Such findings support the need for greater amounts of protein when endurance athletes are consuming insufficient amounts of energy over time; this recommendation is similar to that provided for resistance-trained athletes in similar energy-deprived states.[159] Beyond extreme situations, it is unlikely that endurance athletes need to be overly concerned with (1) the exact dose of protein they are consuming or, by extension, (2) the consumption of high-protein supplemental products, as long as they are meeting their augmented total body energy needs.

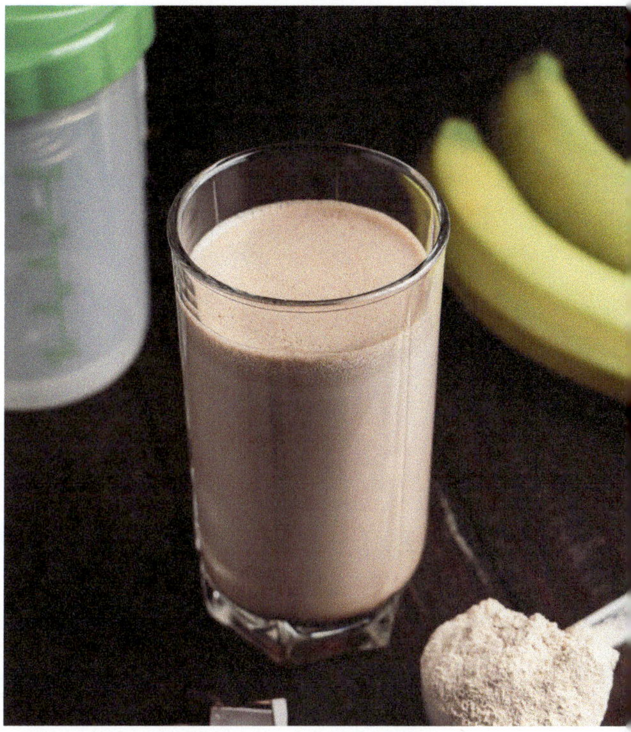

Concern for Excessive Protein Intake

Despite pervasive sentiments that high-protein diets pose substantial health risks (eg, danger to proper renal functioning), these concerns have been deemed unsubstantiated for otherwise healthy individuals.[181,182] For athletes, acute consumption of excessive protein also does not appear to have directly negative performance-related consequences. However, consumption of excessive protein (even short-term) is not recommended, as it could very likely come at the expense of the consumption of proper amounts of carbohydrate and fat. Thus, even though performance does not appear to be directly impacted by acutely high protein intakes, indirect consequences may produce such adverse performance (ie, inadequate carbohydrate intake leading to improperly fueled training sessions). Conversely, if an athlete consumes much higher than necessary quantities of protein while making sure they keep their carbohydrate and fat intake at appropriate levels, the ensuing caloric surplus could still indirectly lead to altered performance related to undesirable changes in body composition over time. Chronic overconsumption of protein appears to have more direct consequences, as perpetually elevated intake has been shown to increase amino acid oxidative capacities, leading to rather unfavorable adaptations that may artificially increase an athlete's general protein needs.[183] In other words, athletes eating excessive protein over time may raise their "baseline" and perpetually require such excessive doses to achieve their normally derived benefits. This information is particularly relevant considering that many athletes do appear to consume quantities of protein that may be closer to maximal than optimal (maximal not necessarily meaning excessive). In addition, eating excessive protein also decreases the importance of trying to optimize quality. This conversation is especially relevant when discussing how to meet nutritional needs with plant-based or animal-based nutrition regimes and underscores the importance of understanding EAA requirements when seeking to eat according to one's needs on a plant-based or plant-exclusive diet. Athletes are advised to follow, and not exceed, recommended protein intake ranges (discussed more in the next section).

GENERALIZED PROTEIN RECOMMENDATIONS

Even though adjustments in timing, quality, and quantity all likely influence the effectiveness of using dietary protein to augment MPS, strength, and training adaptations, such variables are still secondary to meeting the daily recommended protein intake levels suggested in this section.[158] Although guidelines for intake should always be individualized to the greatest extent possible, generalized recommendations are presented in Table 3.1 on page 58.[28,29,34,49,51,91,104,175,184]

TABLE 3.1 Daily Protein Recommendations for Endurance-Trained and Resistance-Trained Athletes[a,b,28,29,34,49,51,91,104,175,184]

Training type	Quantity of daily protein	Example of total daily protein intake
Endurance	~1.2-2.0 g/kg body mass	76-127 g for a 63.5-kg (140-lb) athlete
Resistance	~1.6-1.7 g/kg body mass	146-155 g for a 91-kg (200-lb) athlete

[a] Primary emphasis should be placed on the timing and distribution of dietary protein ingestion over the course of the day (eg, approximately 0.25 g of protein per kilogram of body mass per meal for 4 to 5 meals daily) to optimize the adaptive response of skeletal muscle in an athlete.
[b] The recommendations shown assume that daily energy needs are being met. In catabolic states in which energy intake is insufficient to meet energy demands, needs may be elevated (perhaps up to ~3.0 g/kg body mass).

TABLE 3.2 Protein Contents of Select Foods and Supplements[a,185]

Food or supplement	Amount (to provide 3 g of Leucine	Total protein content (g)	Energy content (kcal)
Whey protein isolate	25 g (1 scoop)	23	100
Poultry (lean and cooked)	4.75 oz	40	260
Beef (lean and uncooked)	5 oz	38	270
Salmon (cooked)	5.5 oz	36	280
Milk (skim)	30 oz (3.75 cups)	28	310
Tofu (firm and cooked)	14 oz (1.33 cups)	37	340
Eggs	5.5 large	34	390
Greek yogurt	19 oz (2.5 cups)	55	410
Milk (whole)	30 oz (3.75 cups)	28	540
Cheese (cheddar)	5 oz (1.25 cup)	35	570
Black beans (cooked)	15 oz (2.5 cups)	38	580
Peanuts	6 oz (1.25 cups)	44	970
Peanut butter	7 oz (3/4 cup)	42	1,170
Bread (multigrain)	20 slices	70	1,380
Rice (cooked)	60 oz (9 cups)	38	1,850

[a] Total protein content and caloric value relative to leucine amounts are also included. The foods in the table are listed in ascending order by energy content to simplify and showcase protein sources of higher biological value.

Table 3.1 shows that research indicates that both endurance- and resistance-trained athletes should consume protein well above the RDA value of 0.8 g per kilogram of body weight. Notably, it is important that athletes understand the content of protein, especially of the amino acid leucine, relative to total. Table 3.2 highlights the relationship between these quantities for various food and supplement sources.[185]

Given the elevated protein needs of athletes, determining how to appropriately distribute intake is an important consideration. For example, an athlete weighing 64 kg who is trying to meet protein needs determined to be approximately 100 g/d could set out to consume 20 g of protein at 5 different times during the day as a way to maximize MPS and avoid excess losses to oxidation.[153] Spreading protein intake out in such a way has been associated with augmented muscle mass (compared to skewed intake distributions) despite being accompanied by less conclusive evidence regarding a direct benefit to muscle strength.[63,186] Although, in theory, this tactic of eating consistent amounts of protein over the entire day does not sound overly daunting, athletes are commonly subject to demanding schedules that may not be conducive to such intake patterns. For example, a 2017 study looking at over 500 well-trained athletes found that dietary intake of protein was heavily skewed toward dinner (38% of total daily intake). This means that these athletes were more likely to have low protein intake (below 20 g) at breakfast (58%) and lunch (36%). These data points suggest a lack of optimal spacing of protein ingestion despite total daily intake patterns that habitually resulted in the consumption of more than 1.2 g per kilogram of body weight.[4] Because protein metabolism is altered for days, not just hours, after training, athletes should avoid differentiating their normal scheduled dietary plans too drastically when taking a day off.

Even if athletes are able to consume breakfast and/or approximately 5 meals per day, this is still no guarantee that the composition of such intake is dispersed in a way that properly promotes the plethora of various training adaptations that can accompany properly distributed protein intake. Consulting with a registered dietitian is a good way for athletes to become properly educated on the nuances related to appropriate protein distribution over the course of their day. Box 3.1 provides a single example of how such a dispersion varies from a more clustered daily intake of protein.[185]

BOX 3.1 Dispersed vs Clustered Intake of Sufficient Protein Over One Day[185]

Below are 2 different daily dietary plans for an 80-kg athlete consuming 3,000 kcal and 128 g of protein (1.6 g/kg body mass).

	Dispersed intake	Clustered intake
Breakfast	**27 g**	**10 g**
	3 hardboiled eggs (19 g)	2 pancakes (9 g)
	2 English muffins (8 g)	1/4 cup syrup (0 g)
	2 tbsp jam (0 g)	1 cup orange juice (1 g)
Morning snack	**16 g**	**2 g**
	5 oz Greek yogurt (15 g)	Granola bar, low protein (2 g)
	Banana (1 g)	
Lunch	**22 g**	**12 g**
	2 pitas (10 g)	2 pitas (10 g)
	1/3 cup hummus (6 g)	1/3 cup guacamole (1 g)
	1 cup chicken noodle soup (5 g)	1 cucumber (1 g)
	1 cucumber (1 g)	

Continued on next page

BOX 3.1 Dispersed vs Clustered Intake of Sufficient Protein Over One Day[185] (CONTINUED)

	Dispersed intake	Clustered intake
Periworkout snack	**20 g** 16 oz Gatorade (0 g) Protein bar (12 g) 1 cup chocolate milk (8 g)	**1 g** 16 oz Gatorade (0 g) 12 oz almond milk (1 g)
Dinner	**27 g** 3 oz pork loin (21 g) 1 cup rice (4 g) 1 cup broccoli (2 g)	**101 g** 12 oz pork loin (84 g) 2 cups rice (8 g) 1 cup broccoli (2 g) 1 slice cheese (7 g)
Pre-bed snack	**22 g** 2 pitas (10 g) 1/3 cup hummus (6 g) 1 cup chicken noodle soup (5 g) 1 cucumber (1 g)	

All decisions related to athletic fueling must be considered in the context of athlete tolerability. Although protein is likely not inducing as many adverse gastrointestinal-related issues as other nutrition tactics that can lead to concerns (eg, consuming too much fructose or high-fat food before exercise), some athletes may still struggle with tolerating it at certain times. Taking time to look at where possible benefits may be derived and using a trial-and-error approach during training should be cornerstones of any fueling strategy that athletes cultivate in preparation for fueling around their competitions. For example, if a resistance-based athlete struggling to meet daily needs sees that preexercise and postexercise protein ingestion are considered relatively equal in terms of potential benefits they provide for MPS, this individual may try to test their protein tolerability prior to a lifting session. If handled without issue, this athlete could then consider this period as another opportunity to provide additional protein and/or calories to a diet that may be lacking in quantity or proper timing.

Finally, as much of the research that makes up the current nutritional guidelines for athletes (protein and otherwise) was based on the study of adult males, there is a certain level of concern surrounding the capability to extrapolate research outcomes to their female counterparts, as there are distinct hormone-related differences. Research summarized in a 2022 article by Moore et al[187] suggested that it is premature to require a unique set of specified female guidelines for both carbohydrate and protein requirements if energy needs are being met. In addition to recommending more research in this area, the authors also suggested that female athletes should still consider their distinct personal symptoms (eg, hormonal cycle) to help develop an individualized approach to assist in meeting their specific training and competition goals. Therefore, taking only biological sex into consideration, research currently does not support the idea that female athletes have different protein needs than male athletes. Protein requirements for athletes with respect to age and pregnancy are discussed in Chapters 12 (Child and Adolescent Athletes), 14 (Masters Athletes), and 17 (Pregnant Athletes).

SUMMARY

Resistance and endurance exercise both stimulate MPS, but the significance of muscle accrual is directly related to the nature and stress of the stimulus, as noted by the diverse adaptations accompanying each type of work. Specifically, resistance exercise preferentially stimulates myofibrillar proteins to aid in force production, whereas endurance training typically stimulates the accretion of mitochondrial proteins to assist in sustained energy production during exercise. Ingesting dietary protein at a time near exercise is preferred, as it helps support a high rate of MPS and elicit an optimal adaptation to a chosen exercise stimulus. The quantity of protein required to achieve such benefits is generally lower than typically assumed, with a dose of 20 to 25 g being ideal for most circumstances and athletes. Food and supplements containing high-quality protein, such as lean meat, fish, eggs, milk, whey, casein, and soy, can positively influence the MPS response through differences in digestion and the subsequent rate at which amino acids appear in the blood. Incorporating food or supplements rich in leucine appears to be an important consideration when choosing which protein-containing foods to include in a balanced diet. Consuming approximately 2 to 3 g of leucine (the amount found in approximately 20–25 g of most high-quality protein-dense foods) should allow for this leucine threshold to be met. Consuming protein during the day in a dispersed rather than clustered fashion is recommended. Although supplements can help support an athlete in meeting their protein needs, they should be viewed as complementary to whole foods, especially considering the potential benefits of the food matrix effect. Finally, even though consuming ample high-quality dietary protein at a time that falls near exercise and spreading such intake over one's day should help elicit optimal adaptations, athletes should make achieving daily protein and energy requirements their principal nutrition goal. From this starting point of taking in the right amount of protein and total calories, athletes can use information from this chapter to help craft unique fueling programs that allow them to reach peak potential when the time for competition arrives.

KEY TAKEAWAYS

Muscle protein turnover can be assessed by using the NPB equation (NPB = MPS – MPB). Both feeding and training have marked effects on body proteins and thus can be employed to shift net protein balance to optimize both recovery and adaptation.

Consumption of a rapidly digesting protein rich in essential amino acids, especially leucine, is an effective way to induce enhanced acute protein synthesis. Although such proteins are readily available in supplements, proper plant- and animal-based whole-food options can also readily meet such demands.

Even though the recommended level of dietary protein intake for athletes is approximately twice what has been recommended for the general population (0.8 g per kilogram of body weight), most athletes are still consuming ample protein to support their unique training needs.

Endurance-based athletes should aim to consume between 1.2 and 2.0 g of protein per kilogram of body weight; strength- or resistance-based athletes should target levels of about 1.6 to 1.7 g of protein per kilogram of body weight. Chronic states of caloric insufficiency (≥500 kcal/d) may warrant higher recommended protein intakes (ie, values up to 3.0 g per kilogram of body weight).

Considering that the relationship between energy intake and protein intake is quite linear, excessive levels of protein intake (>2.0 g per kilogram of body weight) appear to pose no adverse risk to health but may impact performance negatively if protein is consumed at the expense of other macronutrients, namely, carbohydrates.

Although it is possible to do both, meeting overall daily protein needs should take priority over ingesting protein at a specified point in time within a determined "window of opportunity" (ie, immediately following a training session). Therefore, to meet daily demands and take advantage of the anabolic effect of exercise, athletes should aim to distribute their ingestion of dietary protein throughout the day (ie, by consuming approximately 0.25 g per kilogram of body weight at each meal over 4 to 5 meals daily), with one such eating bout surrounding their training session as appropriately tolerated. Additionally, special emphasis should be placed on breakfast and presleep time points considering (1) the natural decrease in muscle protein synthesis that accompanies sleep and (2) the propensity of athletes to skip such feeding opportunities.

REFERENCES

1. von Liebig J. Animal chemistry; or organic chemistry in its application to physiology and pathology. *Med Chir Rev.* 1842;37(74):337-371.
2. Phillips SM. Protein requirements and supplementation in strength sports. *Nutrition.* 2004;20(7-8):689-695. doi:10.1016/j.nut.2004.04.009
3. van Erp-Baart AM, Saris WH, Binkhorst RA, Vos JA, Elvers JW. Nationwide survey on nutritional habits in elite athletes. *Int J Sports Med.* 1989;10(suppl 1):S3-S10. doi:10.1055/s-2007-1024947
4. Gillen JB, Trommelen J, Wardenaar FC, et al. Dietary protein intake and distribution patterns of well-trained Dutch athletes. *Int J Sport Nutr Exerc Metab.* 2017;27(2):105-114. doi:10.1123/ijsnem.2016-0154
5. Wardenaar F, Brinkmans N, Ceelen I, et al. Macronutrient intakes in 553 Dutch elite and sub-elite endurance, team, and strength athletes: does intake differ between sport disciplines? *Nutrients.* 2017;9(2):119. doi:10.3390/nu9020119
6. Masson G, Lamarche B. Many non-elite multisport endurance athletes do not meet sports nutrition recommendations for carbohydrates. *Appl Physiol Nutr Metab.* 2016;41(7):728-734. doi:10.1139/apnm-2015-0599
7. Phillips SM, Atkinson SA, Tarnopolsky MA, MacDougall JD. Gender differences in leucine kinetics and nitrogen balance in endurance athletes. *J Appl Physiol (1985).* 1993;75(5):2134-2141. doi:10.1152/jappl.1993.75.5.2134
8. Tarnopolsky MA, Atkinson SA, Phillips SM, MacDougall JD. Carbohydrate loading and metabolism during exercise in men and women. *J Appl Physiol (1985).* 1995;78(4):1360-1368. doi:10.1152/jappl.1995.78.4.1360
9. Goldberg AL, Chang TW. Regulation and significance of amino acid metabolism in skeletal muscle. *Fed Proc.* 1978;37(9):2301-2307.
10. Rennie MJ, Edwards RHT, Halliday D, Matthews DE, Wolman SL, Millward DJ. Muscle protein synthesis measured by stable isotope techniques in man: the effects of feeding and fasting. *Clin Sci (Lond).* 1982;63(6):519-523. doi:10.1042/cs0630519
11. Phillips SM, Moore DR, Tang JE. A critical examination of dietary protein requirements, benefits, and excesses in athletes. *Int J Sport Nutr Exerc Metab.* 2007;17(suppl):S58-S76. doi:10.1123/ijsnem.17.s1.s58
12. Elango R, Humayun MA, Ball RO, Pencharz PB. Evidence that protein requirements have been significantly underestimated. *Curr Opin Clin Nutr Metab Care.* 2010;13(1):52-57. doi:10.1097/MCO.0b013e328332f9b7
13. Tarnopolsky MA. Protein requirements for endurance athletes. *Nutrition.* 2004;20(7-8):662-668. doi:10.1016/j.nut.2004.04.008
14. Burd NA, Tang JE, Moore DR, Phillips SM. Exercise training and protein metabolism: influences of contraction, protein intake, and sex-based differences. *J Appl Physiol (1985).* 2009;106(5):1692-1701. doi:10.1152/japplphysiol.91351.2008
15. Phillips SM, Tipton KD, Aarsland A, Wolf SE, Wolfe RR. Mixed muscle protein synthesis and breakdown after resistance exercise in humans. *Am J Physiol.* 1997;273(1):E99-E107. doi:10.1152/ajpendo.1997.273.1.E99
16. Hartman JW, Tang JE, Wilkinson SB, et al. Consumption of fat-free fluid milk after resistance exercise promotes greater lean mass accretion than does consumption of soy or carbohydrate in young, novice, male weightlifters. *Am J Clin Nutr.* 2007;86(2):373-381. doi:10.1093/ajcn/86.2.373
17. West DWD, Burd NA, Tang JE, et al. Elevations in ostensibly anabolic hormones with resistance exercise enhance neither training-induced muscle hypertrophy nor strength of the elbow flexors. *J Appl Physiol (1985).* 2010;108(1):60-67. doi:10.1152/japplphysiol.01147.2009
18. Kim PL, Staron RS, Phillips SM. Fasted-state skeletal muscle protein synthesis after resistance exercise is altered with training. *J Physiol.* 2005;568:283-290. doi:10.1113/jphysiol.2005.093708
19. Wilkinson SB, Phillips SM, Atherton PJ, et al. Differential effects of resistance and endurance exercise in the fed state on signalling molecule phosphorylation and protein synthesis in human muscle. *J Physiol.* 2008;586(15):3701-3717. doi:10.1113/jphysiol.2008.153916
20. Phillips SM, Parise G, Roy BD, Tipton KD, Wolfe RR, Tarnopolsky MA. Resistance-training-induced adaptations in skeletal muscle protein turnover in the fed state. *Can J Physiol Pharmacol.* 2002;80(11):1045-1053. doi:10.1139/y02-134
21. Phillips SM, Tipton KD, Ferrando AA, Wolfe RR. Resistance training reduces the acute exercise-induced increase in muscle protein turnover. *Am J Physiol.* 1999;276(1):E118-E124. doi:10.1152/ajpendo.1999.276.1.E118
22. Tang JE, Perco JG, Moore DR, Wilkinson SB, Phillips SM. Resistance training alters the response of fed state mixed muscle protein synthesis in young men. *Am J Physiol Regul Integr Comp Physiol.* 2008;294(1):R172-R178. doi:10.1152/ajpregu.00636.2007
23. Tipton KD. Nonessential amino acids are not necessary to stimulate net muscle protein synthesis in healthy volunteers. *J Nutr Biochem.* 1999;10(2):89-95. doi:10.1016/S0955-2863(98)00087-4
24. Phillips SM. A brief review of critical processes in exercise-induced muscular hypertrophy. *Sports Med.* 2014;44(suppl 1):S71-S77. doi:10.1007/s40279-014-0152-3
25. Lamont LS, McCullough AJ, Kalhan SC. Relationship between leucine oxidation and oxygen consumption during steady-state exercise. *Med Sci Sports Exerc.* 2001;33(2):237-241. doi:10.1097/00005768-200102000-00011
26. Haralambie G, Berg A. Serum urea and amino nitrogen changes with exercise duration. *Eur J Appl Physiol Occup Physiol.* 1976;36(1):39-48. doi:10.1007/BF00421632
27. Howarth KR, Phillips SM, MacDonald MJ, Richards D, Moreau NA, Gibala MJ. Effect of glycogen availability on human skeletal muscle protein turnover during exercise and recovery. *J Appl Physiol (1985).* 2010;109(2):431-438. doi:10.1152/japplphysiol.00108.2009
28. Moore DR. Nutrition to support recovery from endurance exercise: optimal carbohydrate and protein replacement. *Curr Sports Med Rep.* 2015;14(4):294-300. doi:10.1249/JSR.0000000000000180

29. McKenzie S, Phillips SM, Carter SL, Lowther S, Gibala MJ, Tarnopolsky MA. Endurance exercise training attenuates leucine oxidation and BCOAD activation during exercise in humans. *Am J Physiol Endocrinol Metab.* 2000;278(4):E580-E587. doi:10.1152/ajpendo.2000.278.4.E580
30. Moore DR, Camera DM, Areta JL, Hawley JA. Beyond muscle hypertrophy: why dietary protein is important for endurance athletes. *Appl Physiol Nutr Metab.* 2014;39(9):987-997. doi:10.1139/apnm-2013-0591
31. Carraro F, Stuart CA, Hartl WH, Rosenblatt J, Wolfe RR. Effect of exercise and recovery on muscle protein synthesis in human subjects. *Am J Physiol.* 1990;259(4):E470-E476. doi:10.1152/ajpendo.1990.259.4.E470
32. Harber MP, Konopka AR, Jemiolo B, Trappe SW, Trappe TA, Reidy PT. Muscle protein synthesis and gene expression during recovery from aerobic exercise in the fasted and fed states. *Am J Physiol Regul Integr Comp Physiol.* 2010;299(5):R1254-R1262. doi:10.1152/ajpregu.00348.2010
33. Miller BF, Olesen JL, Hansen M, et al. Coordinated collagen and muscle protein synthesis in human patella tendon and quadriceps muscle after exercise. *J Physiol.* 2005;567:1021-1033. doi:10.1113/jphysiol.2005.093690
34. Dreyer HC, Fujita S, Cadenas JG, Chinkes DL, Volpi E, Rasmussen BB. Resistance exercise increases AMPK activity and reduces 4E-BP1 phosphorylation and protein synthesis in human skeletal muscle. *J Physiol.* 2006;576:613-624. doi:10.1113/jphysiol.2006.113175
35. Di Donato DM, West DWD, Churchward-Venne TA, Breen L, Baker SK, Phillips SM. Influence of aerobic exercise intensity on myofibrillar and mitochondrial protein synthesis in young men during early and late postexercise recovery. *Am J Physiol Endocrinol Metab.* 2014;306(9):E1025-E1032. doi:10.1152/ajpendo.00487.2013
36. Frontera WR, Meredith CN, O'Reilly KP, Knuttgen HG, Evans WJ. Strength conditioning in older men: skeletal muscle hypertrophy and improved function. *J Appl Physiol (1985).* 1988;64(3):1038-1044. doi:10.1152/jappl.1988.64.3.1038
37. Trappe S, Williamson D, Godard M. Maintenance of whole muscle strength and size following resistance training in older men. *J Gerontol A Biol Sci Med Sci.* 2002;57(4):B138-B143. doi:10.1093/gerona/57.4.B138
38. Kosek DJ, Kim J-S, Petrella JK, Cross JM, Bamman MM. Efficacy of 3 days/wk resistance training on myofiber hypertrophy and myogenic mechanisms in young vs. older adults. *J Appl Physiol (1985).* 2006;101(2):531-544. doi:10.1152/japplphysiol.01474.2005
39. Fiatarone MA, Marks EC, Ryan ND, Meredith CN, Lipsitz LA, Evans WJ. High-intensity strength training in nonagenarians. Effects on skeletal muscle. *JAMA.* 1990;263(22):3029-3034.
40. Kalapotharakos VI, Michalopoulou M, Godolias G, Tokmakidis SP, Malliou PV, Gourgoulis V. The effects of high- and moderate-resistance training on muscle function in the elderly. *J Aging Phys Act.* 2004;12(2):131-143. doi:10.1123/japa.12.2.131
41. Slivka D, Raue U, Hollon C, Minchev K, Trappe S. Single muscle fiber adaptations to resistance training in old (>80 yr) men: evidence for limited skeletal muscle plasticity. *Am J Physiol Regul Integr Comp Physiol.* 2008;295(1):R273-R280. doi:10.1152/ajpregu.00093.2008
42. Tipton KD, Rasmussen BB, Miller SL, et al. Timing of amino acid-carbohydrate ingestion alters anabolic response of muscle to resistance exercise. *Am J Physiol Endocrinol Metab.* 2001;281(2):E197-E206. doi:10.1152/ajpendo.2001.281.2.E197
43. Tipton KD, Elliott TA, Cree MG, Aarsland AA, Sanford AP, Wolfe RR. Stimulation of net muscle protein synthesis by whey protein ingestion before and after exercise. *Am J Physiol Endocrinol Metab.* 2007;292(1):E71-E76. doi:10.1152/ajpendo.00166.2006
44. Burk A, Timpmann S, Medijainen L, Vähi M, Ööpik V. Time-divided ingestion pattern of casein-based protein supplement stimulates an increase in fat-free body mass during resistance training in young untrained men. *Nutr Res.* 2009;29(6):405-413. doi:10.1016/j.nutres.2009.03.008
45. Bird SP, Tarpenning KM, Marino FE. Effects of liquid carbohydrate/essential amino acid ingestion on acute hormonal response during a single bout of resistance exercise in untrained men. *Nutrition.* 2006;22(4):367-375. doi:10.1016/j.nut.2005.11.005
46. Bird SP, Tarpenning KM, Marino FE. Liquid carbohydrate/essential amino acid ingestion during a short-term bout of resistance exercise suppresses myofibrillar protein degradation. *Metabolism.* 2006;55(5):570-577. doi:10.1016/j.metabol.2005.11.011
47. Bird SP, Mabon T, Pryde M, Feebrey S, Cannon J. Triphasic multinutrient supplementation during acute resistance exercise improves session volume load and reduces muscle damage in strength-trained athletes. *Nutr Res.* 2013;33(5):376-387. doi:10.1016/j.nutres.2013.03.002
48. Bird SP, Tarpenning KM, Marino FE. Independent and combined effects of liquid carbohydrate/essential amino acid ingestion on hormonal and muscular adaptations following resistance training in untrained men. *Eur J Appl Physiol.* 2006;97(2):225-238. doi:10.1007/s00421-005-0127-z
49. Beelen M, Tieland M, Gijsen AP, et al. Coingestion of carbohydrate and protein hydrolysate stimulates muscle protein synthesis during exercise in young men, with no further increase during subsequent overnight recovery. *J Nutr.* 2008;138(11):2198-2204. doi:10.3945/jn.108.092924
50. Durham WJ, Casperson SL, Dillon EL, et al. Age-related anabolic resistance after endurance-type exercise in healthy humans. *FASEB J.* 2010;24(10):4117-4127. doi:10.1096/fj.09-150177
51. Rasmussen BB, Tipton KD, Miller SL, Wolf SE, Wolfe RR. An oral essential amino acid-carbohydrate supplement enhances muscle protein anabolism after resistance exercise. *J Appl Physiol (1985).* 2000;88(2):386-392. doi:10.1152/jappl.2000.88.2.386
52. Kumar V, Selby A, Rankin D, et al. Age-related differences in the dose-response relationship of muscle protein synthesis to resistance exercise in young and old men. *J Physiol.* 2009;587:211-217. doi:10.1113/jphysiol.2008.164483
53. Tipton KD, Ferrando AA, Phillips SM, Doyle D, Wolfe RR. Postexercise net protein synthesis in human muscle from orally administered amino acids. *Am J Physiol.* 1999;276(4):E628-E634. doi:10.1152/ajpendo.1999.276.4.E628

54. Tipton KD, Elliott TA, Cree MG, Wolf SE, Sanford AP, Wolfe RR. Ingestion of casein and whey proteins result in muscle anabolism after resistance exercise. *Med Sci Sports Exerc.* 2004;36(12):2073-2081. doi:10.1249/01.mss.0000147582.99810.c5
55. Biolo G, Maggi SP, Williams BD, Tipton KD, Wolfe RR. Increased rates of muscle protein turnover and amino acid transport after resistance exercise in humans. *Am J Physiol.* 1995;268(3):E514-E520. doi:10.1152/ajpendo.1995.268.3.E514
56. Cermak NM, Res PT, de Groot LC, Saris WH, van Loon LJ. Protein supplementation augments the adaptive response of skeletal muscle to resistance-type exercise training: a meta-analysis. *Am J Clin Nutr.* 2012;96(6):1454-1464. doi:10.3945/ajcn.112.037556
57. Schoenfeld BJ, Aragon AA, Krieger JW. The effect of protein timing on muscle strength and hypertrophy: a meta-analysis. *J Int Soc Sports Nutr.* 2013;10(1):53. doi:10.1186/1550-2783-10-53
58. Stokes T, Hector AJ, Morton RW, McGlory C, Phillips SM. Recent perspectives regarding the role of dietary protein for the promotion of muscle hypertrophy with resistance exercise training. *Nutrients.* 2018;10(2):180. doi:10.3390/nu10020180
59. Nunes EA, Colenso-Semple L, McKellar SR, et al. Systematic review and meta-analysis of protein intake to support muscle mass and function in healthy adults. *J Cachexia Sarcopenia Muscle.* 2022;13(2):795-810. doi:10.1002/jcsm.12922
60. Cribb PJ, Hayes A. Effects of supplement timing and resistance exercise on skeletal muscle hypertrophy. *Med Sci Sports Exerc.* 2006;38(11):1918-1925. doi:10.1249/01.mss.0000233790.08788.3e
61. Hoffman JR, Ratamess NA, Tranchina CP, Rashti SL, Kang J, Faigenbaum AD. Effect of protein-supplement timing on strength, power, and body-composition changes in resistance-trained men. *Int J Sport Nutr Exerc Metab.* 2009;19(2):172-185. doi:10.1123/ijsnem.19.2.172
62. Moore DR, Areta J, Coffey VG, et al. Daytime pattern of post-exercise protein intake affects whole-body protein turnover in resistance-trained males. *Nutr Metab (Lond).* 2012;9(1):91. doi:10.1186/1743-7075-9-91
63. Areta JL, Burke LM, Ross ML, et al. Timing and distribution of protein ingestion during prolonged recovery from resistance exercise alters myofibrillar protein synthesis. *J Physiol.* 2013;591:2319-2331. doi:10.1113/jphysiol.2012.244897
64. Burd NA, West DWD, Moore DR, et al. Enhanced amino acid sensitivity of myofibrillar protein synthesis persists for up to 24 h after resistance exercise in young men. *J Nutr.* 2011;141(4):568-573. doi:10.3945/jn.110.135038
65. Drummond MJ, Fry CS, Glynn EL, et al. Skeletal muscle amino acid transporter expression is increased in young and older adults following resistance exercise. *J Appl Physiol (1985).* 2011;111(1):135-142. doi:10.1152/japplphysiol.01408.2010
66. Drummond MJ, Glynn EL, Fry CS, Timmerman KL, Volpi E, Rasmussen BB. An increase in essential amino acid availability upregulates amino acid transporter expression in human skeletal muscle. *Am J Physiol Endocrinol Metab.* 2010;298(5):E1011-E1018. doi:10.1152/ajpendo.00690.2009
67. Dickinson JM, Gundermann DM, Walker DK, et al. Leucine-enriched amino acid ingestion after resistance exercise prolongs myofibrillar protein synthesis and amino acid transporter expression in older men. *J Nutr.* 2014;144(11):1694-1702. doi:10.3945/jn.114.198671
68. Schoenfeld BJ, Aragon A, Wilborn C, Urbina SL, Hayward SE, Krieger J. Pre- versus post-exercise protein intake has similar effects on muscular adaptations. *PeerJ.* 2017;5:e2825. doi:10.7717/peerj.2825
69. Williamson E, Moore DR. A muscle-centric perspective on intermittent fasting: a suboptimal dietary strategy for supporting muscle protein remodeling and muscle mass? *Front Nutr.* 2021;8:640621. doi:10.3389/fnut.2021.640621
70. Tinsley GM, La Bounty PM. Effects of intermittent fasting on body composition and clinical health markers in humans. *Nutr Rev.* 2015;73(10):661-674. doi:10.1093/nutrit/nuv041
71. Shriver LH, Betts NM, Wollenberg G. Dietary intakes and eating habits of college athletes: are female college athletes following the current sports nutrition standards? *J Am Coll Health.* 2013;61(1):10-16. doi:10.1080/07448481.2012.747526
72. Leidy HJ, Hoertel HA, Douglas SM, Higgins KA, Shafer RS. A high-protein breakfast prevents body fat gain, through reductions in daily intake and hunger, in "breakfast skipping" adolescents. *Obesity (Silver Spring).* 2015;23(9):1761-1764. doi:10.1002/oby.21185
73. Res PT, Groen B, Pennings B, et al. Protein ingestion before sleep improves postexercise overnight recovery. *Med Sci Sports Exerc.* 2012;44(8):1560-1569. doi:10.1249/MSS.0b013e31824cc363
74. Snijders T, Res PT, Smeets JS, et al. Protein ingestion before sleep increases muscle mass and strength gains during prolonged resistance-type exercise training in healthy young men. *J Nutr.* 2015;145(6):1178-1184. doi:10.3945/jn.114.208371
75. Antonio J, Ellerbroek A, Peacock C, Silver T. Casein protein supplementation in trained men and women: morning versus evening. *Int J Exerc Sci.* 2017;10(3):479-486.
76. Kinsey A, Ormsbee M. The health impact of nighttime eating: old and new perspectives. *Nutrients.* 2015;7(4):2648-2662. doi:10.3390/nu7042648
77. Snijders T, Trommelen J, Kouw IWK, Holwerda AM, Verdijk LB, van Loon LJC. The impact of pre-sleep protein ingestion on the skeletal muscle adaptive response to exercise in humans: an update. *Front Nutr.* 2019;6:17. doi:10.3389/fnut.2019.00017
78. Groen BBL, Res PT, Pennings B, et al. Intragastric protein administration stimulates overnight muscle protein synthesis in elderly men. *Am J Physiol Endocrinol Metab.* 2012;302(1):E52-E60. doi:10.1152/ajpendo.00321.2011
79. Erdman KA, Tunnicliffe J, Lun VM, Reimer RA. Eating patterns and composition of meals and snacks in elite Canadian athletes. *Int J Sport Nutr Exerc Metab.* 2013;23(3):210-219. doi:10.1123/ijsnem.23.3.210
80. Madzima TA, Panton LB, Fretti SK, Kinsey AW, Ormsbee MJ. Night-time consumption of protein or carbohydrate results in increased morning resting energy expenditure in active college-aged men. *Br J Nutr.* 2014;111(1):71-77. doi:10.1017/S000711451300192X
81. Kinsey A, Cappadona S, Panton L, et al. The effect of casein protein prior to sleep on fat metabolism in obese men. *Nutrients.* 2016;8(8):452. doi:10.3390/nu8080452

82. Larsen MS, Holm L, Svart MV, et al. Effects of protein intake prior to carbohydrate-restricted endurance exercise: a randomized crossover trial. *J Int Soc Sports Nutr.* 2020;17(1):7. doi:10.1186/s12970-020-0338-z

83. Rothschild JA, Kilding AE, Broome SC, Stewart T, Cronin JB, Plews DJ. Pre-exercise carbohydrate or protein ingestion influences substrate oxidation but not performance or hunger compared with cycling in the fasted state. *Nutrients.* 2021;13(4):1291. doi:10.3390/nu13041291

84. Gillen JB, West DWD, Williamson EP, Fung HJW, Moore DR. Low-carbohydrate training increases protein requirements of endurance athletes. *Med Sci Sports Exerc.* 2019;51(11):2294-2301. doi:10.1249/MSS.0000000000002036

85. Rose AJ, Richter EA. Regulatory mechanisms of skeletal muscle protein turnover during exercise. *J Appl Physiol (1985).* 2009;106(5):1702-1711. doi:10.1152/japplphysiol.91375.2008

86. Ivy JL, Res PT, Sprague RC, Widzer MO. Effect of a carbohydrate-protein supplement on endurance performance during exercise of varying intensity. *Int J Sport Nutr Exerc Metab.* 2003;13(3):382-395. doi:10.1123/ijsnem.13.3.382

87. Saunders MJ, Kane MD, Todd MK. Effects of a carbohydrate-protein beverage on cycling endurance and muscle damage. *Med Sci Sports Exerc.* 2004;36(7):1233-1238. doi:10.1249/01.MSS.0000132377.66177.9F

88. Saunders MJ, Luden ND, Herrick JE. Consumption of an oral carbohydrate-protein gel improves cycling endurance and prevents postexercise muscle damage. *J Strength Cond Res.* 2007;21(3):678-684. doi:10.1519/R-20506.1

89. van Essen M, Gibala MJ. Failure of protein to improve time trial performance when added to a sports drink. *Med Sci Sports Exerc.* 2006;38(8):1476-1483. doi:10.1249/01.mss.0000228958.82968.0 a

90. Jeukendrup AE, Tipton KD, Gibala MJ, Saunders MJ. Protein plus carbohydrate does not enhance 60-km time-trial performance. *Int J Sport Nutr Exerc Metab.* 2009;19(4):335-339. doi:10.1123/ijsnem.19.4.335

91. Breen L, Tipton KD, Jeukendrup AE. No effect of carbohydrate-protein on cycling performance and indices of recovery. *Med Sci Sports Exerc.* 2010;42(6):1140-1148. doi:10.1249/MSS.0b013e3181c91f1a

92. Beelen M, Zorenc A, Pennings B, Senden JM, Kuipers H, van Loon LJC. Impact of protein coingestion on muscle protein synthesis during continuous endurance type exercise. *Am J Physiol Endocrinol Metab.* 2011;300(6):E945-E954. doi:10.1152/ajpendo.00446.2010

93. Hulston CJ, Wolsk E, Grøndahl TS, Yfanti C, Van Hall G. Protein intake does not increase vastus lateralis muscle protein synthesis during cycling. *Med Sci Sports Exerc.* 2011;43(9):1635-1642. doi:10.1249/MSS.0b013e31821661ab

94. Knuiman P, Hopman MTE, Verbruggen C, Mensink M. Protein and the adaptive response with endurance training: wishful thinking or a competitive edge? *Front Physiol.* 2018;9:598. doi:10.3389/fphys.2018.00598

95. Ivy JL, Goforth HW, Damon BM, McCauley TR, Parsons EC, Price TB. Early postexercise muscle glycogen recovery is enhanced with a carbohydrate-protein supplement. *J Appl Physiol (1985).* 2002;93(4):1337-1344. doi:10.1152/japplphysiol.00394.2002

96. Berardi JM, Price TB, Noreen EE, Lemon PWR. Postexercise muscle glycogen recovery enhanced with a carbohydrate-protein supplement. *Med Sci Sports Exerc.* 2006;38(6):1106-1113. doi:10.1249/01.mss.0000222826.49358.f3

97. Howarth KR, Moreau NA, Phillips SM, Gibala MJ. Coingestion of protein with carbohydrate during recovery from endurance exercise stimulates skeletal muscle protein synthesis in humans. *J Appl Physiol (1985).* 2009;106(4):1394-1402. doi:10.1152/japplphysiol.90333.2008

98. Jentjens R, Jeukendrup AE. Determinants of post-exercise glycogen synthesis during short-term recovery. *Sports Med.* 2003;33(2):117-144. doi:10.2165/00007256-200333020-00004

99. Craven J, Desbrow B, Sabapathy S, Bellinger P, McCartney D, Irwin C. The effect of consuming carbohydrate with and without protein on the rate of muscle glycogen re-synthesis during short-term post-exercise recovery: a systematic review and meta-analysis. *Sports Med Open.* 2021;7(1):9. doi:10.1186/s40798-020-00297-0

100. Knuiman P, van Loon LJC, Wouters J, Hopman M, Mensink M. Protein supplementation elicits greater gains in maximal oxygen uptake capacity and stimulates lean mass accretion during prolonged endurance training: a double-blind randomized controlled trial. *Am J Clin Nutr.* 2019;110(2):508-518. doi:10.1093/ajcn/nqz093

101. Breen L, Philp A, Witard OC, et al. The influence of carbohydrate-protein co-ingestion following endurance exercise on myofibrillar and mitochondrial protein synthesis. *J Physiol.* 2011;589:4011-4025. doi:10.1113/jphysiol.2011.211888

102. Lunn WR, Pasiakos SM, Colletto MR, et al. Chocolate milk and endurance exercise recovery: protein balance, glycogen, and performance. *Med Sci Sports Exerc.* 2012;44(4):682-691. doi:10.1249/MSS.0b013e3182364162

103. Churchward-Venne TA, Pinckaers PJM, Smeets JSJ, et al. Dose-response effects of dietary protein on muscle protein synthesis during recovery from endurance exercise in young men: a double-blind randomized trial. *Am J Clin Nutr.* 2020;112(2):303-317. doi:10.1093/ajcn/nqaa073

104. Bagheri R, Robinson I, Moradi S, et al. Muscle protein synthesis responses following aerobic-based exercise or high-intensity interval training with or without protein ingestion: a systematic review. *Sports Med.* 2022;52(11):2713-2732. doi:10.1007/s40279-022-01707-x

105. Holloszy JO, Coyle EF. Adaptations of skeletal muscle to endurance exercise and their metabolic consequences. *J Appl Physiol Respir Environ Exerc Physiol.* 1984;56(4):831-838. doi:10.1152/jappl.1984.56.4.831

106. Hood DA. Invited Review: Contractile activity-induced mitochondrial biogenesis in skeletal muscle. *J Appl Physiol (1985).* 2001;90(3):1137-1157. doi:10.1152/jappl.2001.90.3.1137

107. Hood DA, Takahashi M, Connor MK, Freyssenet D. Assembly of the cellular powerhouse: current issues in muscle mitochondrial biogenesis. *Exerc Sport Sci Rev.* 2000;28(2):68-73.

108. Phillips SM, van Loon LJC. Dietary protein for athletes: from requirements to optimum adaptation. *J Sports Sci.* 2011;29(suppl 1):S29-S38. doi:10.1080/02640414.2011.619204

109. Eston RG, Mickleborough J, Baltzopoulos V. Eccentric activation and muscle damage: biomechanical and physiological considerations during downhill running. *Br J Sports Med.* 1995;29(2):89-94. doi:10.1136/bjsm.29.2.89

110. Shin KA, Park KD, Ahn J, Park Y, Kim YJ. Comparison of changes in biochemical markers for skeletal muscles, hepatic metabolism, and renal function after three types of long-distance running. *Medicine (Baltimore).* 2016;95(20):e3657. doi:10.1097/MD.0000000000003657

111. Fallon KE, Sivyer G, Sivyer K, Dare A. The biochemistry of runners in a 1600 km ultramarathon. *Br J Sports Med.* 1999;33(4):264-269. doi:10.1136/bjsm.33.4.264

112. Koopman R, Pannemans DLE, Jeukendrup AE, et al. Combined ingestion of protein and carbohydrate improves protein balance during ultra-endurance exercise. *Am J Physiol Endocrinol Metab.* 2004;287(4):E712-E720. doi:10.1152/ajpendo.00543.2003

113. Knechtle B, Knechtle P, Mrazek C, et al. No effect of short-term amino acid supplementation on variables related to skeletal muscle damage in 100 km ultra-runners - a randomized controlled trial. *J Int Soc Sports Nutr.* 2011;8(1):6. doi:10.1186/1550-2783-8-6

114. Rodriguez NR, Vislocky LM, Gaine PC. Dietary protein, endurance exercise, and human skeletal-muscle protein turnover. *Curr Opin Clin Nutr Metab Care.* 2007;10(1):40-45. doi:10.1097/MCO.0b013e3280115e3b

115. Burd NA, Beals JW, Martinez IG, Salvador AF, Skinner SK. Food-first approach to enhance the regulation of post-exercise skeletal muscle protein synthesis and remodeling. *Sports Med.* 2019;49(suppl 1):59-68. doi:10.1007/s40279-018-1009-y

116. Tang JE, Moore DR, Kujbida GW, Tarnopolsky MA, Phillips SM. Ingestion of whey hydrolysate, casein, or soy protein isolate: effects on mixed muscle protein synthesis at rest and following resistance exercise in young men. *J Appl Physiol (1985).* 2009;107(3):987-992. doi:10.1152/japplphysiol.00076.2009

117. West DW, Burd NA, Coffey VG, et al. Rapid aminoacidemia enhances myofibrillar protein synthesis and anabolic intramuscular signaling responses after resistance exercise. *Am J Clin Nutr.* 2011;94(3):795-803. doi:10.3945/ajcn.111.013722

118. Phillips SM. The impact of protein quality on the promotion of resistance exercise-induced changes in muscle mass. *Nutr Metab (Lond).* 2016;13(1):64. doi:10.1186/s12986-016-0124-8

119. Greenhaff PL, Karagounis LG, Peirce N, et al. Disassociation between the effects of amino acids and insulin on signaling, ubiquitin ligases, and protein turnover in human muscle. *Am J Physiol Endocrinol Metab.* 2008;295(3):E595-E604. doi:10.1152/ajpendo.90411.2008

120. Staples AW, Burd NA, West DWD, et al. Carbohydrate does not augment exercise-induced protein accretion versus protein alone. *Med Sci Sports Exerc.* 2011;43(7):1154-1161. doi:10.1249/MSS.0b013e31820751cb

121. Hagenfeldt L, Eriksson S, Wahren J. Influence of leucine on arterial concentrations and regional exchange of amino acids in healthy subjects. *Clin Sci (Lond).* 1980;59(3):173-181. doi:10.1042/cs0590173

122. Hundal HS, Taylor PM. Amino acid transceptors: gate keepers of nutrient exchange and regulators of nutrient signaling. *Am J Physiol Endocrinol Metab.* 2009;296(4):E603-E613. doi:10.1152/ajpendo.91002.2008

123. Bohé J, Low A, Wolfe RR, Rennie MJ. Human muscle protein synthesis is modulated by extracellular, not intramuscular amino acid availability: a dose-response study. *J Physiol.* 2003;552:315-324. doi:10.1113/jphysiol.2003.050674

124. Zaromskyte G, Prokopidis K, Ioannidis T, Tipton KD, Witard OC. Evaluating the leucine trigger hypothesis to explain the post-prandial regulation of muscle protein synthesis in young and older adults: a systematic review. *Front Nutr.* 2021;8:685165. doi:10.3389/fnut.2021.685165

125. Kramer IF, Verdijk LB, Hamer HM, et al. Both basal and post-prandial muscle protein synthesis rates, following the ingestion of a leucine-enriched whey protein supplement, are not impaired in sarcopenic older males. *Clin Nutr.* 2017;36(5):1440-1449. doi:10.1016/j.clnu.2016.09.023

126. Joy JM, Lowery RP, Wilson JM, et al. The effects of 8 weeks of whey or rice protein supplementation on body composition and exercise performance. *Nutr J.* 2013;12(1):86. doi:10.1186/1475-2891-12-86

127. Boirie Y, Dangin M, Gachon P, Vasson MP, Maubois JL, Beaufrère B. Slow and fast dietary proteins differently modulate postprandial protein accretion. *Proc Natl Acad Sci U S A.* 1997;94(26):14930-14935. doi:10.1073/pnas.94.26.14930

128. Burd NA, Gorissen SH, van Vliet S, Snijders T, van Loon LJ. Differences in postprandial protein handling after beef compared with milk ingestion during postexercise recovery: a randomized controlled trial. *Am J Clin Nutr.* 2015;102(4):828-836. doi:10.3945/ajcn.114.103184

129. Reidy PT, Walker DK, Dickinson JM, et al. Protein blend ingestion following resistance exercise promotes human muscle protein synthesis. *J Nutr.* 2013;143(4):410-416. doi:10.3945/jn.112.168021

130. Pennings B, Boirie Y, Senden JM, Gijsen AP, Kuipers H, van Loon LJ. Whey protein stimulates postprandial muscle protein accretion more effectively than do casein and casein hydrolysate in older men. *Am J Clin Nutr.* 2011;93(5):997-1005. doi:10.3945/ajcn.110.008102

131. Paul GL. The rationale for consuming protein blends in sports nutrition. *J Am Coll Nutr.* 2009;28(suppl 4):464S-472S. doi:10.1080/07315724.2009.10718113

132. Bos C, Metges CC, Gaudichon C, et al. Postprandial kinetics of dietary amino acids are the main determinant of their metabolism after soy or milk protein ingestion in humans. *J Nutr.* 2003;133(5):1308-1315. doi:10.1093/jn/133.5.1308

133. van Vliet S, Burd NA, van Loon LJ. The skeletal muscle anabolic response to plant- versus animal-based protein consumption. *J Nutr.* 2015;145(9):1981-1991. doi:10.3945/jn.114.204305

134. Wilkinson SB, Tarnopolsky MA, MacDonald MJ, MacDonald JR, Armstrong D, Phillips SM. Consumption of fluid skim milk promotes greater muscle protein accretion after resistance exercise than does consumption of an isonitrogenous and isoenergetic soy-protein beverage. *Am J Clin Nutr.* 2007;85(4):1031-1040. doi:10.1093/ajcn/85.4.1031

135. Josse AR, Tang JE, Tarnopolsky MA, Phillips SM. Body composition and strength changes in women with milk and resistance exercise. *Med Sci Sports Exerc.* 2010;42(6):1122-1130. doi:10.1249/MSS.0b013e3181c854f6
136. Kalman D, Feldman S, Martinez M, Krieger DR, Tallon MJ. Effect of protein source and resistance training on body composition and sex hormones. *J Int Soc Sports Nutr.* 2007;4(1):4. doi:10.1186/1550-2783-4-4
137. Ciuris C, Lynch HM, Wharton C, Johnston CS. A comparison of dietary protein digestibility, based on DIAAS scoring, in vegetarian and non-vegetarian athletes. *Nutrients.* 2019;11(12):3016. doi:10.3390/nu11123016
138. Rafii M, Pencharz PB, Ball RO, Tomlinson C, Elango R, Courtney-Martin G. Bioavailable methionine assessed using the indicator amino acid oxidation method is greater when cooked chickpeas and steamed rice are combined in healthy young men. *J Nutr.* 2020;150(7):1834-1844. doi:10.1093/jn/nxaa086
139. US Department of Agriculture. Food matrix. National Agricultural Library (NAL) Agricultural Thesaurus website. Accessed September 14, 2023. https://lod.nal.usda.gov/nalt/17238
140. van Vliet S, Shy EL, Abou Sawan S, et al. Consumption of whole eggs promotes greater stimulation of postexercise muscle protein synthesis than consumption of isonitrogenous amounts of egg whites in young men. *Am J Clin Nutr.* 2017;106(6):1401-1412. doi:10.3945/ajcn.117.159855
141. Abou Sawan S, van Vliet S, West DWD, et al. Whole egg, but not egg white, ingestion induces mTOR colocalization with the lysosome after resistance exercise. *Am J Physiol Cell Physiol.* 2018;315(4):C537-C543. doi:10.1152/ajpcell.00225.2018
142. Burke LM, Winter JA, Cameron-Smith D, Enslen M, Farnfield M, Decombaz J. Effect of intake of different dietary protein sources on plasma amino acid profiles at rest and after exercise. *Int J Sport Nutr Exerc Metab.* 2012;22(6):452-462. doi:10.1123/ijsnem.22.6.452
143. Hodgkinson SM, Montoya CA, Scholten PT, Rutherfurd SM, Moughan PJ. Cooking conditions affect the true ileal digestible amino acid content and digestible indispensable amino acid score (DIAAS) of bovine meat as determined in pigs. *J Nutr.* 2018;148(10):1564-1569. doi:10.1093/jn/nxy153
144. Rankin JW, Goldman LP, Puglisi MJ, Nickols-Richardson SM, Earthman CP, Gwazdauskas FC. Effect of post-exercise supplement consumption on adaptations to resistance training. *J Am Coll Nutr.* 2004;23(4):322-330. doi:10.1080/07315724.2004.10719375
145. Cribb PJ, Williams AD, Carey MF, Hayes A. The effect of whey isolate and resistance training on strength, body composition, and plasma glutamine. *Int J Sport Nutr Exerc Metab.* 2006;16(5):494-509. doi:10.1123/ijsnem.16.5.494
146. Cribb PJ, Williams AD, Stathis CG, Carey MF, Hayes A. Effects of whey isolate, creatine, and resistance training on muscle hypertrophy. *Med Sci Sports Exerc.* 2007;39(2):298-307. doi:10.1249/01.mss.0000247002.32589.ef
147. Teegarden D. The influence of dairy product consumption on body composition. *J Nutr.* 2005;135(12):2749-2752. doi:10.1093/jn/135.12.2749
148. Zemel MB. Role of calcium and dairy products in energy partitioning and weight management. *Am J Clin Nutr.* 2004;79(5):907S-912S. doi:10.1093/ajcn/79.5.907 S
149. Reidy PT, Walker DK, Dickinson JM, et al. Soy-dairy protein blend and whey protein ingestion after resistance exercise increases amino acid transport and transporter expression in human skeletal muscle. *J Appl Physiol (1985).* 2014;116(11):1353-1364. doi:10.1152/japplphysiol.01093.2013
150. Yang Y, Breen L, Burd NA, et al. Resistance exercise enhances myofibrillar protein synthesis with graded intakes of whey protein in older men. *Br J Nutr.* 2012;108(10):1780-1788. doi:10.1017/S0007114511007422
151. Katsanos CS, Kobayashi H, Sheffield-Moore M, Aarsland A, Wolfe RR. A high proportion of leucine is required for optimal stimulation of the rate of muscle protein synthesis by essential amino acids in the elderly. *Am J Physiol Endocrinol Metab.* 2006;291(2):E381-E387. doi:10.1152/ajpendo.00488.2005
152. Moore DR, Churchward-Venne TA, Witard O, et al. Protein ingestion to stimulate myofibrillar protein synthesis requires greater relative protein intakes in healthy older versus younger men. *J Gerontol A Biol Sci Med Sci.* 2015;70(1):57-62. doi:10.1093/gerona/glu103
153. Moore DR, Robinson MJ, Fry JL, et al. Ingested protein dose response of muscle and albumin protein synthesis after resistance exercise in young men. *Am J Clin Nutr.* 2009;89(1):161-168. doi:10.3945/ajcn.2008.26401
154. Witard OC, Jackman SR, Breen L, Smith K, Selby A, Tipton KD. Myofibrillar muscle protein synthesis rates subsequent to a meal in response to increasing doses of whey protein at rest and after resistance exercise. *Am J Clin Nutr.* 2014;99(1):86-95. doi:10.3945/ajcn.112.055517
155. Børsheim E, Tipton KD, Wolf SE, Wolfe RR. Essential amino acids and muscle protein recovery from resistance exercise. *Am J Physiol Endocrinol Metab.* 2002;283(4):E648-E657. doi:10.1152/ajpendo.00466.2001
156. Macnaughton LS, Wardle SL, Witard OC, et al. The response of muscle protein synthesis following whole-body resistance exercise is greater following 40 g than 20 g of ingested whey protein. *Physiol Rep.* 2016;4(15):e12893. doi:10.14814/phy2.12893
157. Tagawa R, Watanabe D, Ito K, et al. Synergistic effect of increased total protein intake and strength training on muscle strength: a dose-response meta-analysis of randomized controlled trials. *Sports Med Open.* 2022;8(1):110. doi:10.1186/s40798-022-00508-w
158. Morton RW, Murphy KT, McKellar SR, et al. A systematic review, meta-analysis and meta-regression of the effect of protein supplementation on resistance training-induced gains in muscle mass and strength in healthy adults. *Br J Sports Med.* 2018;52(6):376-384. doi:10.1136/bjsports-2017-097608
159. Helms ER, Zinn C, Rowlands DS, Brown SR. A systematic review of dietary protein during caloric restriction in resistance trained lean athletes: a case for higher intakes. *Int J Sport Nutr Exerc Metab.* 2014;24(2):127-138. doi:10.1123/ijsnem.2013-0054
160. Murphy C, Koehler K. Caloric restriction induces anabolic resistance to resistance exercise. *Eur J Appl Physiol.* 2020;120(5):1155-1164. doi:10.1007/s00421-020-04354-0

161. Murphy C, Koehler K. Energy deficiency impairs resistance training gains in lean mass but not strength: a meta-analysis and meta-regression. *Scand J Med Sci Sports*. 2022;32(1):125-137. doi:10.1111/sms.14075

162. Mier CM, Domenick MA, Turner NS, Wilmore JH. Changes in stroke volume and maximal aerobic capacity with increased blood volume in men women. *J Appl Physiol (1985)*. 1996;80(4):1180-1186. doi:10.1152/jappl.1996.80.4.1180

163. Lemon PW, Tarnopolsky MA, MacDougall JD, Atkinson SA. Protein requirements and muscle mass/strength changes during intensive training in novice bodybuilders. *J Appl Physiol (1985)*. 1992;73(2):767-775. doi:10.1152/jappl.1992.73.2.767

164. Hartman JW, Moore DR, Phillips SM. Resistance training reduces whole-body protein turnover and improves net protein retention in untrained young males. *Appl Physiol Nutr Metab*. 2006;31(5):557-564. doi:10.1139/h06-031

165. Moore DR, Del Bel NC, Nizi KI, et al. Resistance training reduces fasted- and fed-state leucine turnover and increases dietary nitrogen retention in previously untrained young men. *J Nutr*. 2007;137(4):985-991. doi:10.1093/jn/137.4.985

166. Campbell WW, Crim MC, Young VR, Joseph LJ, Evans WJ. Effects of resistance training and dietary protein intake on protein metabolism in older adults. *Am J Physiol*. 1995;268(6):E1143-E1153. doi:10.1152/ajpendo.1995.268.6.E1143

167. Campbell WW, Trappe TA, Jozsi AC, Kruskall LJ, Wolfe RR, Evans WJ. Dietary protein adequacy and lower body versus whole body resistive training in older humans. *J Physiol*. 2002;542:631-642. doi:10.1113/jphysiol.2002.020685

168. Tarnopolsky LJ, MacDougall JD, Atkinson SA, Tarnopolsky MA, Sutton JR. Gender differences in substrate for endurance exercise. *J Appl Physiol (1985)*. 1990;68(1):302-308. doi:10.1152/jappl.1990.68.1.302

169. Rodriguez NR, DiMarco NM, Langley S. Special Communications: Position Stands: Nutrition and athletic performance [Retired Statement]. *Med Sci Sports Exerc*. 2009;41(3):709-731. doi:10.1249/MSS.0b013e31890eb86

170. Burd NA, Tardif N, Rooyackers O, van Loon LJC. Optimizing the measurement of mitochondrial protein synthesis in human skeletal muscle. *Appl Physiol Nutr Metab*. 2015;40(1):1-9. doi:10.1139/apnm-2014-0211

171. el-Khoury AE, Forslund A, Olsson R, et al. Moderate exercise at energy balance does not affect 24-h leucine oxidation or nitrogen retention in healthy men. *Am J Physiol*. 1997;273(2):E394-E407. doi:10.1152/ajpendo.1997.273.2.E394

172. Forslund AH, El-Khoury AE, Olsson RM, Sjödin AM, Hambraeus L, Young VR. Effect of protein intake and physical activity on 24-h pattern and rate of macronutrient utilization. *Am J. Physiol*. 1999;276(5):E964-E976. doi:10.1152/ajpendo.1999.276.5.E964

173. Houltham SD, Rowlands DS. A snapshot of nitrogen balance in endurance-trained women. *Appl Physiol Nutr Metab*. 2014;39(2):219-225. doi:10.1139/apnm-2013-0182

174. Bolster DR, Pikosky MA, Gaine PC, et al. Dietary protein intake impacts human skeletal muscle protein fractional synthetic rates after endurance exercise. *Am J Physiol*. 2005;289(4):E678-E683. doi:10.1152/ajpendo.00060.2005

175. Kato H, Suzuki K, Bannai M, Moore DR. Protein requirements are elevated in endurance athletes after exercise as determined by the indicator amino acid oxidation method. *PLoS One*. 2016;11(6):e0157406. doi:10.1371/journal.pone.0157406

176. Williamson E, Kato H, Volterman K, Suzuki K, Moore D. The effect of dietary protein on protein metabolism and performance in endurance-trained males. *Med Sci Sports Exerc*. 2019;51(2):352-360. doi:10.1249/MSS.0000000000001791

177. Brouns F, Saris WH, Stroecken J, et al. Eating, drinking, and cycling. a controlled Tour de France simulation study, part 1. *Int J Sports Med*. 1989;10(suppl 1):S32-S40. doi:10.1055/s-2007-1024952

178. Brouns F, Saris WH, Stroecken J, et al. Eating, drinking, and cycling. a controlled Tour de France simulation study, part 2. Effect of diet manipulation. *Int J Sports Med*. 1989;10(suppl 1):S41-S48. doi:10.1055/s-2007-1024953

179. Pasiakos SM, Cao JJ, Margolis LM, et al. Effects of high-protein diets on fat-free mass and muscle protein synthesis following weight loss: a randomized controlled trial. *FASEB J*. 2013;27(9):3837-3847. doi:10.1096/fj.13-230227

180. Longland TM, Oikawa SY, Mitchell CJ, Devries MC, Phillips SM. Higher compared with lower dietary protein during an energy deficit combined with intense exercise promotes greater lean mass gain and fat mass loss: a randomized trial. *Am J Clin Nutr*. 2016;103(3):738-746. doi:10.3945/ajcn.115.119339

181. Martin WF, Armstrong LE, Rodriguez NR. Dietary protein intake and renal function. *Nutr Metab (Lond)*. 2005;2(1):25. doi:10.1186/1743-7075-2-25

182. Tipton KD. Efficacy and consequences of very-high-protein diets for athletes and exercisers. *Proc Nutr Soc*. 2011;70(2):205-214. doi:10.1017/S0029665111000024

183. Tinline-Goodfellow CT, West DWD, Malowany JM, Gillen JB, Moore DR. An acute reduction in habitual protein intake attenuates post exercise anabolism and may bias oxidation-derived protein requirements in resistance trained men. *Front Nutr*. 2020;7:55. doi:10.3389/fnut.2020.00055

184. Tiller NB, Roberts JD, Beasley L, et al. International Society of Sports Nutrition Position Stand: Nutritional considerations for single-stage ultra-marathon training and racing. *J Int Soc Sports Nutr*. 2019;16(1):50. doi:10.1186/s12970-019-0312-9

185. US Department of Agriculture, Agricultural Research Service, Beltsville Human Nutrition Research Center. FoodData Central [Internet], 2019. Accessed September 14, 2023. fdc.nal.usda.gov

186. Jespersen SE, Agergaard J. Evenness of dietary protein distribution is associated with higher muscle mass but not muscle strength or protein turnover in healthy adults: a systematic review. *Eur J Nutr*. 2021;60(6):3185-3202. doi:10.1007/s00394-021-02487-2

187. Moore DR, Sygo J, Morton JP. Fuelling the female athlete: carbohydrate and protein recommendations. *Eur J Sport Sci*. 2022;22(5):684-696. doi:10.1080/17461391.2021.1922508

CHAPTER 4

Dietary Fat and Exercise

D. Travis Thomas, PhD, RDN, CSSD, LD, FAND

LEARNING OBJECTIVES

- Describe the physical structures of different dietary fats.
- Distinguish among different dietary fat intake patterns and current public health recommendations.
- Discuss the influence of exercise and training on lipid metabolism.
- Summarize the expected metabolic adaptations to a high-fat diet.
- Provide recommendations and practical advice to help athletes choose dietary fat for daily training and competition.

INTRODUCTION

Fat, also known as lipid, is an important fuel source for athletes. It constitutes a broad range of molecules that play vital roles in multiple physiological functions. Indeed, the intricacies surrounding recommendations for fat intake seem to be overshadowed by interest in carbohydrate and protein needs to support, sustain, and improve athletic performance. However, given the critical role of dietary fat in both energy metabolism and many other physiological functions, athletes should view fat as a necessary component of the diet—an essential dietary macronutrient that can affect overall wellness and performance during exercise and sport. Dietary fat, dietary carbohydrate, and endogenous fat stores all have the capacity to influence fat metabolism. They work separately and in concert to regulate substrate utilization and availability during exercise and at rest. Many details of how fatty acids serve as energy sources and how exercise intensity affects fatty acid metabolism during exercise and in postexercise recovery are well established in the scientific literature. Researchers show continued interest in looking into the metabolic adaptations that may occur in response to a high-fat diet and the ways in which these changes may translate into improved training capacity and athletic performance.[1] This chapter provides a brief overview of lipids and reviews current evidence to help practitioners understand dietary strategies involving fat manipulation that may influence athletic performance and health.

PHYSICAL STRUCTURE AND FOOD SOURCES OF DIETARY FAT

Among the multiple varieties of lipids in the food supply, triglycerides, also known as triacylglycerols, make up more than 90% of the lipid consumed in the human diet.[2] Phospholipids and sterols are also classes of lipid found in food that exhibit essential functions in metabolism. Nonenergy-producing metabolic functions of phospholipids include imparting structure to cell membranes, emulsification, molecular signaling, and participating in biochemical reactions and pathways, such as hormone synthesis. Phospholipids are found in a wide range of foods and are characterized by a polar, hydrophilic head group with hydrophobic tails composed of 2 longer-chain fatty acids. Cholesterol is found only in foods of animal origin and is highest in animal-based diets, whereas phytosterols are found in plant materials and are therefore more abundant in plant-based diets. Generally, all cholesterol needs are met through endogenous synthesis; the body uses cholesterol as an essential component of cell membrane structure and many physiological pathways, including the biosynthesis of steroid hormones. Given their plant-based origins, dietary intake of phytosterols depends on diet composition and may impart some health benefits by reducing low-density lipoprotein cholesterol.[3] Athletes generally consume enough fat in their diets to receive adequate amounts of both phospholipids and sterols, or their bodies can synthesize these compounds. Because of the disproportionate number of triglycerides and various fatty acids that make up dietary triglycerides, these lipids are the focus of this chapter.

Triglycerides are composed of 3 fatty acid groups attached by ester bonds to a glycerol backbone (refer to Figure 4.1). These lipids serve as a substantial source of energy and contribute to the essential fatty acids that humans must consume to avoid a dietary deficiency. Many foods found in an athlete's diet are sources of dietary lipids, so it is important to carefully evaluate food labels and ingredient lists to understand and accurately assess the lipid composition of an athlete's diet.

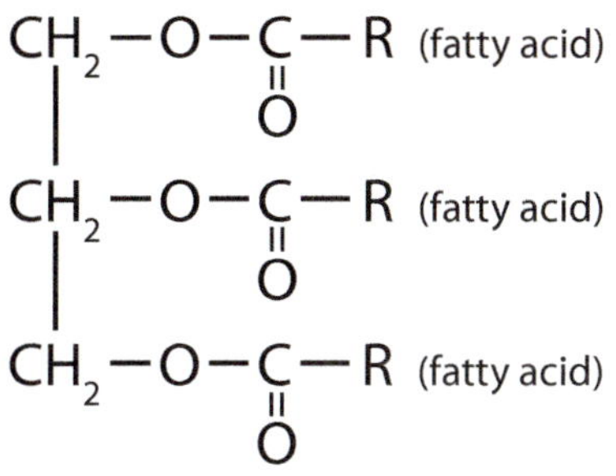

FIGURE 4.1 General structure of a triglyceride

All fatty acid molecules are described by their physical structure and characterized by the presence of a hydrocarbon chain linked to a carboxylic acid group. Fatty acids can be classified based on the length of the hydrocarbon chain or based on their degree of saturation with hydrogen atoms. Fatty acids with 1 to 3 carbon atoms in the chain are referred to as volatile fatty acids, whereas short-chain fatty acids have 4 to 6 carbons. Fatty acids can also be composed of 6 to 12 carbons (medium-chain fatty acids), 14 to 22 carbons (long-chain fatty acids), and more than 22 carbons (very-long-chain fatty acids). Small amounts of short- and medium-chain fatty acids are obtained as naturally occurring components of foods, such as dairy products and coconut oil. Most dietary fatty acids are 16 to 18 carbons in length.

A fatty acid that is saturated contains the maximal amount of hydrogen atoms possible and is thus "saturated" with hydrogens, whereas unsaturated fatty acids have 1 or more double bonds that displace hydrogen atoms. Unsaturated fatty acids are broadly characterized by the number of double bonds (unsaturated carbons) within each molecule. Fatty acids with 1 double bond are monounsaturated fatty acids (MUFAs), and those with multiple double bonds are polyunsaturated fatty acids (PUFAs). Unsaturated fatty acids are further classified by the position of the first double bond within the hydrocarbon chain in relation to the omega (terminal) carbon, as well as the *cis* or *trans* configurations of the double bonds (refer to Figure 4.2 on page 72).

For example, α-linolenic acid can be referred to as all-*cis* 18:3 or omega-3. This chapter will use omega-3, but in some of the literature, omega-3 takes the form Ω-3 or n-3, used to represent the same information, where the number 3 refers to the position of the first double bond in relation to the omega carbon. Most dietary sources of unsaturated fatty acids are found in *cis* conformation, with a smaller amount having a *trans* conformation (refer to Figure 4.2D). *Trans* fatty acids have 1 or more double bonds in the *trans* configuration and were previously found in vegetable oils used to produce shortening and margarine. These *trans* bonds, resulting from a chemical hydrogenation process, changed the chemical and metabolic nature of these lipids and were highly associated with an increased risk of cardiovascular disease. Manufactured hydrogenated oils were a major source of *trans* fat in processed foods prior to 2018. As of 2015, *trans* fats were no longer recognized as safe by the US Food and Drug Administration and are no longer allowed in the United States food supply.[4] Whereas manufactured *trans* fats have been eliminated, a very small amount of naturally occurring *trans* fats exist in milk, butter, and beef fat.

The *Dietary Guidelines for Americans, 2020–2025,* recommends keeping *trans* fat and dietary cholesterol intake as low as possible and limiting saturated fat intake to less than 10% of fat calories consumed.[5] This is a prudent recommendation for all athletes and an important consideration when evaluating the relationship between popular low-carbohydrate, high-fat diets and cardiovascular risk factors.[6,7] Foods that are rich sources of various types of fatty acids are presented in Box 4.1.

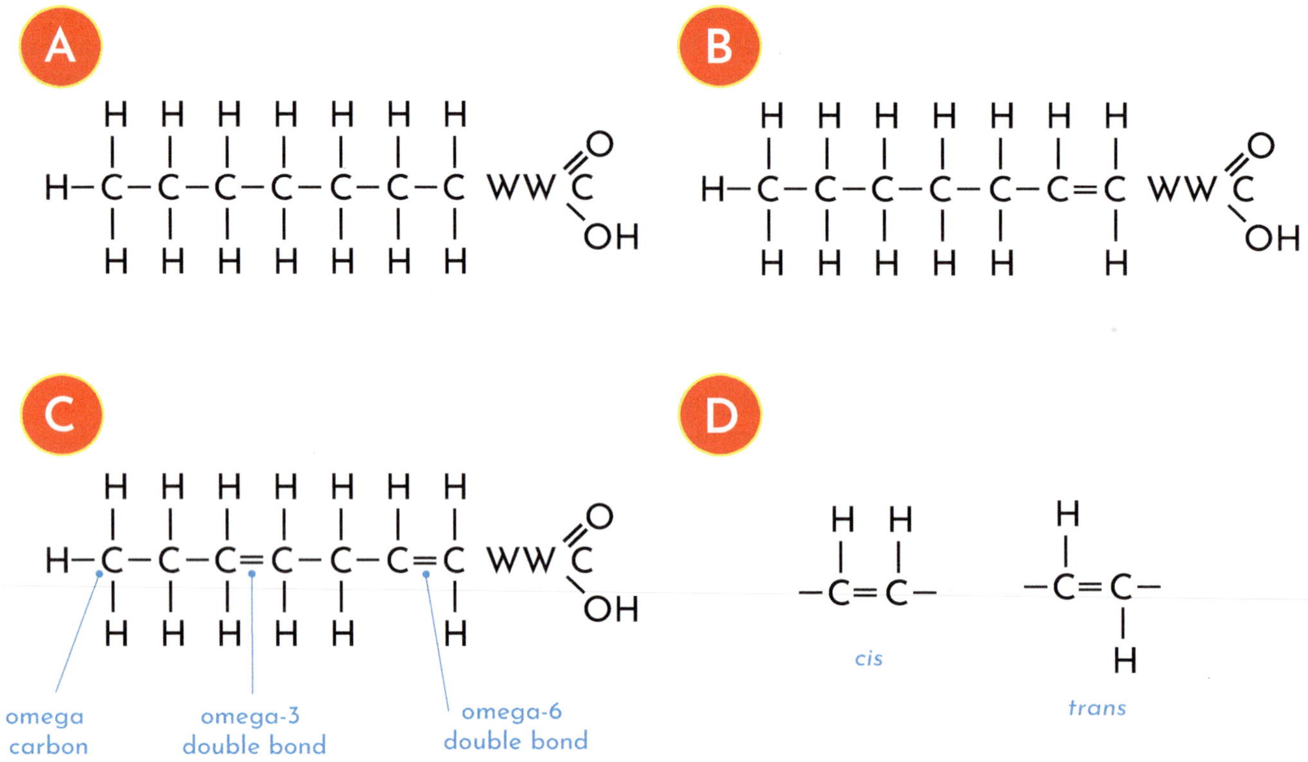

FIGURE 4.2 Structures of various types of fatty acids[a]
A = saturated fatty acid; B = monounsaturated fatty acid; C = polyunsaturated (omega 3) fatty acid; D = *cis* and *trans* double bonds
[a] WW represents variable carbon chain length.

Various foods contain different types of fatty acids, which should be balanced by consuming a complete, well-chosen diet. Foods that are rich sources of saturated fatty acids include many animal foods, cocoa butter, and tropical plant oils (eg, coconut oil, palm oil, and palm kernel oil). Plant foods such as canola oil, olives and olive oil, and avocados are good sources of MUFAs, whereas most other plant foods (eg, soy, corn, nuts, and seeds) and fish tend to be rich in PUFAs. Dietary sources of omega-3 PUFAs include certain fatty fish, such as salmon and lake trout, as well as walnuts, canola oil, and flaxseed, whereas omega-6 fatty acids are found in relatively high levels in most, but not all, other plant foods.

Examples of PUFAs include the essential fatty acids linoleic acid and α-linolenic acid. Although these are the only fatty acids required in the diet, a healthy diet includes a variety of longer, more unsaturated fatty acids. For example, eicosapentaenoic acid (EPA) and docosahexaenoic acid (DHA), both of which are abundant in fatty fish, can help meet omega-3 fatty acid requirements. This serves as one example of why the types of fatty acids that make up the triglycerides within a food or diet are often as important as the total fat content.

The simple variations in fatty acid structure described previously can produce profoundly different metabolic effects that may directly influence chronic health and disease risk while indirectly influencing athletic performance. Long-term health implications are associated with both the amount and composition of the lipids consumed in the diet. Significant interest in performance and health outcomes associated with dietary fat continues to spark new research questions and debate. Some of the controversy is due to inconsistencies associated with public health messages surrounding fat intake guidelines and the latest fad diets that catch the eye of the public. Any confusion experienced by athletes and practitioners is likely exacerbated by the emergence of studies investigating the effects of a high-fat diet on athletic performance. This often leads to scenarios in which the wellness and athletic performance messages regarding proper fat

BOX 4.1 Select Dietary Sources of Various Fatty Acids

Type of fat	Food sources	
Polyunsaturated (omega-6) fatty acids	Corn oil Cottonseed oil Pumpkin seeds Safflower oil	Sesame seeds Soybean oil Walnuts
Polyunsaturated (omega-3) fatty acids	Anchovies Catfish Flaxseed, flax oil Herring High omega-3 eggs Lake trout	Mackerel Salmon Sardines Shrimp Tuna
Monounsaturated (omega-9) fatty acids	Avocados Canola oil Cashews Peanut butter	Peanut oil Peanuts Olive oil Olives
Saturated fatty acids	Bacon Butter Cheese Cheesecake Cream Cream cheese Coconut Coconut oil	Half-and-half Beef Ice cream Palm kernel oil Poultry skin Pork and beef ribs Sausage

DIETARY FAT INTAKE PATTERNS AND CURRENT PUBLIC HEALTH RECOMMENDATIONS

Dietary Fat Intake Patterns of Athletes

Data describing the macronutrient composition of the athlete's diet, including fat intake patterns, continue to emerge for various groups of athletes. In many cases, athletes report consuming a quantity of fat that consistently falls within the range of 20% to 35% of total energy but is highly variable within this range. This range is consistent with the acceptable macronutrient distribution range (AMDR) established for adults by the Institute of Medicine.[5] Several studies have documented fat intake in a wide variety of athletes, ranging from 23% of energy intake in Ethiopian distance runners to 33% in European rugby players.[8,9] In some cases, the variability of fat intake has extended above or below the AMDR. Total fat consumption has been reported as high as 36% in Spanish volleyball players and at more than 50% in ultraendurance athletes in Antarctica.[10,11] Conversely, some athletes have reported fat intakes well below the AMDR.[12-14] At various phases of the training cycle, some athletes may choose to restrict their fat intake in an effort to lose body weight or improve characteristics of their physique (ie, body size, shape, growth, and composition). This restriction is often well below the AMDR minimum of 20% of total energy intake from fat.

Although there is limited evidence to support or refute the claim that acute consumption of 20% or less of energy intake from fat affects athletic performance, research widely supports the notion that chronic and extreme restriction of dietary fat contributes to a decrease in diet quality. This type of restriction can also make it difficult for the athlete to consume adequate quantities and varieties of food to meet overall health and performance goals. For example, a study of endurance athletes found that fat intake was the major distinguishing factor between healthy female runners and those with menstrual dysfunction.[15] As a result of this study, researchers recommended that endurance athletes consume no less than 1 g of fat per kilogram of body weight per day. Although this specific recommendation is likely prudent and easy for practitioners to remember, strong evidence to support this guideline is lacking. Most importantly, athletes should be discouraged from avoiding fat and implementing chronic extreme fat restriction. When acute fat restriction is practiced—as is common for athletes trying to make weight—it should be limited to very short-term scenarios. Fat restriction is widely considered acceptable in making-weight sports for the 2 to 3 days leading up to competition weigh-ins. Acute fat restriction may also be beneficial just before or after a sporting event or training session or during carbohydrate loading, when fueling (carbohydrate), repair (protein), or gastrointestinal comfort have priority. It is important to note that the requirements associated with extreme fat restriction will likely reduce the athlete's intake of a variety of nutrients and food components. Chronic fat restriction may also specifically limit the intake of key fat-related nutrients, such as fat-soluble vitamins, essential fatty acids (especially omega-3 fatty acids), and fat-soluble phytonutrients. These nutrients are of value to the overall health of an athlete, and lack of these nutrients may lead to acute or chronic decrements in athletic performance.

Some athletes may be interested in following extremely high-fat diets based on claims that this practice can promote beneficial metabolic adaptations to support or improve athletic performance. Several human studies have investigated this approach and have broadened scientific understanding of the concept.[16-22] Although it is clear that metabolic adaptations do occur in response to high-fat feeding, claims that extremely high-fat, carbohydrate-restricted diets provide a benefit to the performance of *competitive* athletes are not supported by the scientific community. Current literature describing metabolic adaptations that occur in athletes on high-fat diets is outlined later in the chapter. However, given the variability in fat intake among athletes, the many different athlete types and training demands, and the differences in fat utilization by fast- and slow-twitch muscles, it is not easy to recommend a universal level for fat consumption that may significantly influence athletic performance. Further adding to the complexity of the conversation are the ways in which fat intake influences chronic health and disease and the emerging evidence describing genetic differences in fat utilization.[23]

Public Health Recommendations Regarding Fat Intake

The AMDR provides a good starting point for evaluating and recommending dietary fat intake for athletes. Total fat intake recommendations are often fine-tuned after other macronutrient demands are determined based on training macrocycles and microcycles and day-to-day training periodization. Consuming 20% to 35% of total energy from fat as part of a well-chosen diet will allow athletes to meet their needs for essential fatty acids without increasing their risk for coronary heart disease. These intake recommendations are also aligned with the American College of Cardiology (ACC) and American Heart Association (AHA) recommendations for total fat intake. These guidelines suggest that the overall dietary pattern is more important than individual foods and call for a diet that emphasizes incorporating plant-based foods low in saturated fat.[24] ACC/AHA guidelines support a Mediterranean diet pattern that provides dietary fat primarily from fatty fish, avocados, nuts, and olive and canola oils. These guidelines indicate that the type of dietary fat is much more important than the quantity in relation to heart health.[5] Given the elevated energy needs of most athletes, a well-chosen diet that includes dietary fat from many heart-healthy food sources aligned with the AMDR is likely to meet essential fatty acid needs without added risk for heart disease. When making recommendations for athletes, consider the following factors:

- » total fat intake demands for the training and competition stages of the training cycle
- » the importance of promoting gastrointestinal tolerance
- » whether added fat intake is displacing other essential macronutrients
- » whether recommendations align with public health guidelines.

Recommendations for athletes regarding fat composition can and should be centered on supporting both long-term cardiovascular health and athletic performance. Science in these areas continues to evolve, providing the basis for the types of dietary lipids athletes should strive to consume regularly during training and competition. The 2021 report by the ACC/AHA task force provides guidelines for lipid intake based on a large expert panel's comprehensive review of the literature.[24] Although the report centers on reducing risk factors for individuals at the highest risk for having a cardiovascular event, it also suggests that there is moderate to strong evidence that everyone would benefit from an energy intake that is relatively lower in saturated fatty acids than other dietary fatty acids. To be clear, this message is not to completely avoid saturated fat but to limit intake to align with the current AHA guidelines, which recommend less than 10% of total daily calories from saturated fat. Despite these guidelines, not all recommendations from the scientific literature or those expressed by the media are consistent with ACC/AHA guidelines. For example, the Dietary Guidelines Advisory Committee (DGAC) issued a report in 2010 that addressed many questions consumers and professionals commonly have regarding dietary fat intake.[25] The report recommended a universal de-emphasis on the classification of saturated fat as a nutrient of concern because the effect of saturated fat intake on disease end points is unclear.

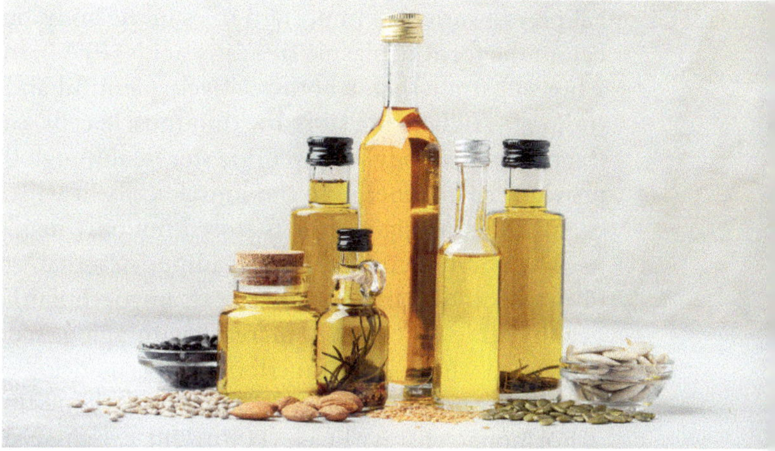

What is often lost in discussions surrounding saturated fat intake is the long-held consistent organizational messages on recommended dietary fat intake patterns. All evidence-based organizations appear to agree that there should be a greater emphasis on consuming a larger proportion of MUFAs and PUFAs relative to saturated fat intake. This recommendation may be particularly helpful in supporting cardiovascular health when these fatty acids replace a portion of energy intake from refined carbohydrates and sugar. Most dietary fats should come from monounsaturated or polyunsaturated food sources as part of a diet emphasizing vegetables, fruits, whole grains, low-fat dairy, and seafood, with lower consumption of red meat and processed meat. The AHA continues to recommend eating 1 to 2 seafood meals per week to reduce the risk of several negative cardiovascular outcomes, particularly when this seafood containing high levels of omega-3 fatty acids replaces less healthy foods.[26,27]

Current recommendations for dietary fat intake, on which most organizations seem to agree, support both cardiovascular health and athletic performance. Although the DGAC suggested that the most effective recommendation for reducing cardiovascular disease is to reduce carbohydrate intake and replace it with PUFAs, many athletes may experience performance decrements when following such a strategy. Therefore, the literature cautions against any casual recommendation for an athlete to reduce carbohydrate intake in favor of lipid intake. If a reduction in carbohydrate intake is indicated, many athletes would simply benefit from reducing their intake of sugar-sweetened beverages (eg, soft drinks) and other confections in favor of carbohydrate-containing foods that are nutrient dense and higher in naturally occurring fiber. Independent of carbohydrate considerations, there are many opportunities for sports dietitians to impact and influence the fat composition of an athlete's diet. By increasing the proportion of MUFAs and omega-3 PUFAs consumed, athletes may benefit from the metabolic advantages of reduced inflammation and the maintenance of proper vascular function, which may indirectly support athletic performance.

The *Dietary Guidelines for Americans, 2020–2025,* provides additional guidance to further refine the practical recommendations regarding health messages associated with dietary fat intake. In general, the *Dietary Guidelines* recommend that the consumption of *trans* fat, saturated fat, and dietary cholesterol be as low as possible without compromising the nutritional adequacy of the diet.[5] It is prudent for athletes to limit these sources of fat while concomitantly modifying their diet to include more nutrient-dense versions of foods within each food group. The newest version of the *Dietary Guidelines* has not changed much from the preceding version regarding saturated fat intake. The guidelines state that intake of saturated fats should be limited to less than 10% of calories per day, while keeping total dietary fats within the age-appropriate AMDR.

Sports dietitians should consider the athlete's sport, goals for physique, and risk factors for chronic disease before recommending total and specific dietary fat intake levels. Practitioners should also stay abreast of emerging science investigating the role of fat adaptation in athletic performance with special attention to protocol details such as scientific design, subject characteristics, and diet and exercise interventions. Such attention to detail is imperative for promoting the critical evaluation of evidence and clarifying the applicability of the research findings to the athlete or athletic groups to whom sports dietitians are assigned.

INFLUENCE OF EXERCISE AND TRAINING ON LIPID METABOLISM

Fat plays a variety of important roles in the body, but the key function for the athlete is energy production. Fat, in the form of plasma free fatty acids (FFAs), muscle lipid, and stored lipid in adipose tissue, provides a fuel substrate that is both relatively plentiful and readily available to the muscle to support endurance training. Triglyceride stored within muscle cells, called intramyocellular lipid (IMCL), represents a small fraction of the body's triglyceride stores, although this amount increases with aerobic training. IMCLs can provide critical energy to the muscle cells in which they are stored, particularly during long endurance events. Muscle triglyceride is stored not only inside muscle cells in lipid droplets but also within muscle tissues as an accumulation of adipocytes that appear as fatty streaks between muscle fibers, called intramyocellular triglyceride or extramyocellular lipid (EMCL). EMCL stores are typically low in young, healthy athletes, but they increase with aging, sedentary behavior or muscular injury and are inversely associated with muscle functional performance.[28]

Adipose tissue triglycerides are exported into the circulation as protein-bound fatty acids by the action of hormone-sensitive lipase (HSL). HSL activity is stimulated by rising concentrations of epinephrine, norepinephrine, glucagon, adrenocorticotropic hormone, thyroxine, and growth hormones during exercise. These fatty acids can be taken up by muscle cells, where they are subsequently catabolized, which allows them to contribute to energy demands by providing adenosine triphosphate (ATP) for muscle movement. Fatty acids that enter muscle cells are linked to coenzyme A (CoA) by fatty acyl-CoA synthetase. These fatty acids must first be translocated to the mitochondrion by means of carnitine and the enzymes carnitine-acylcarnitine translocase, carnitine palmitoyltransferase I, and carnitine palmitoyltransferase II. These molecules work in concert to transfer the fatty acids across mitochondrial membranes and to re-esterify them to CoA. Within the mitochondria, β-oxidation results in 1 molecule of acyl-CoA, 1 reduced flavin adenine dinucleotide, and 1 reduced nicotinamide adenine dinucleotide for every 2 carbons cleaved from the fatty acid. These molecules can then undergo further mitochondrial oxidation via oxidative phosphorylation to regenerate ATP from adenosine diphosphate.

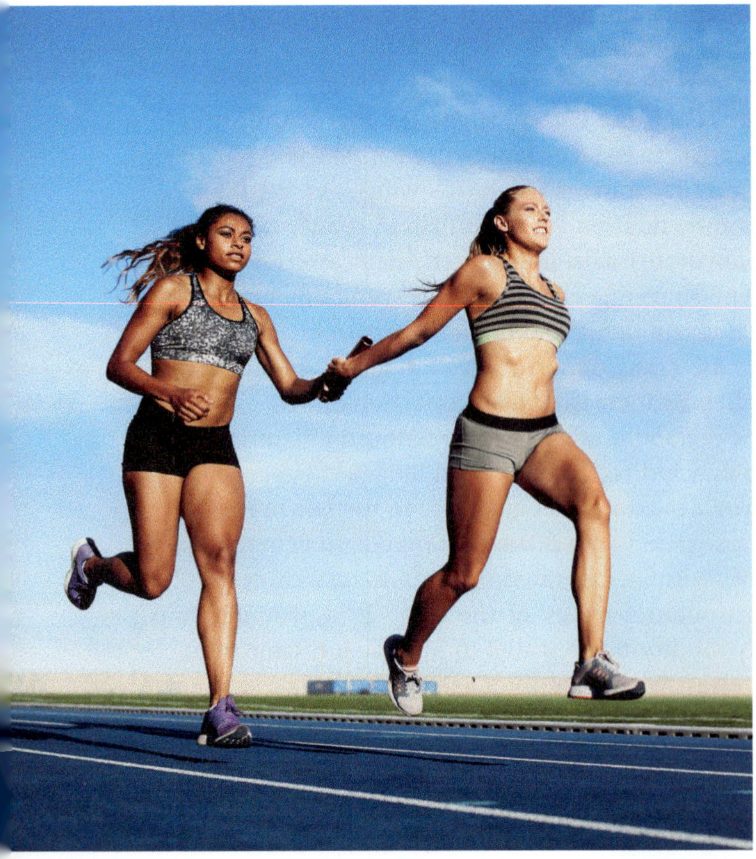

Factors Affecting Fat Metabolism During Exercise

The relative proportions of macromolecule energy sources (eg, carbohydrate, fat) oxidized during exercise are influenced by many variables. Regarding lipid, most of the relative contribution to energy turnover varies as a function of exercise intensity and duration. The contributions of different body stores of fat to energy turnover are influenced by many of the same factors that influence the proportion of substrate oxidation. Training, a function of exercise frequency, also influences fat metabolism principally by promoting metabolic adaptations that facilitate lipid delivery and lipid oxidation in working muscle. Although the effects of exercise intensity, duration, and training are the primary factors in determining the proportion and source of lipid utilized and total exercise energy expenditure, the contributions of the various lipid sources in the body to fat oxidation also depend on an individual's sex and dietary intake before and during exercise.

Lipid Sources and Integration With Macronutrient Metabolism During Exercise

Fatty acids represent a major fuel for muscle contractions and the major type of lipids used for energy during exercise. These fatty acids come principally from adipose tissue, muscle lipid depots EMCL and IMCL, and lipoproteins. Whereas albumin-bound fatty acids contribute more to fatty acid oxidation, very low-density lipoprotein triglycerides can contribute up to 10% of total energy expenditure during prolonged exercise of moderate intensity.[29] Regarding muscle lipid depots at lower exercise intensity, IMCL generally contributes only a minor portion of energy expended compared with fatty acids obtained from the plasma. IMCLs, found in lipid droplets, are generally located next to the mitochondria. The overall amount of IMCL within muscle tissue varies based on individual differences in fiber-type content, diet, and training. In addition, females typically have more IMCL than males relative to aerobic capacity, fitness level, and training history. Each of these factors is known to dictate the relative contribution of IMCL to energy turnover. Moreover, Roepstorff et al[30] found that females tend to have higher fatty acid oxidation rates during moderate-intensity prolonged endurance events, likely because of the presence of more type I muscle fibers and higher capillary density. Type I muscle fibers, which are more oxidative than type II fibers, also contain more IMCL. IMCL fatty acids are liberated from their triglyceride bond through sequential lipase hydrolyzation involving adipose tissue triglyceride lipase, HSL, and monoglyceride lipase. Endurance training increases IMCL concentration and adipose triglyceride lipase in athletes, suggesting improved lipolysis efficiency in response to training. The relative energy contribution of IMCL increases as exercise intensity increases.[31,32] The contribution of IMCL to energy turnover decreases, however, with extended endurance events, such as those that occur at consistent intensities, resulting in an increase in FFA concentration.[33]

The contribution of different stored fat sources to energy turnover is influenced by both the duration and intensity of the exercise bout, with plasma FFAs contributing a higher percentage of fat utilization and the relative utilization of muscle lipid decreasing as the duration progresses.[32] During prolonged endurance exercise in trained individuals, the carbohydrate-to-fat oxidation ratio is relatively stable, with carbohydrate contributing to a higher oxidation rate, particularly in exercise events lasting between 60 and 90 minutes. In general, regarding exercise duration, the oxidation of fatty acids is substantially higher than that of carbohydrate only in endurance events lasting more than 90 minutes. However, it should be noted that dietary intake both before and during exercise can have a significant effect on these observations, as can intensity of exercise and fitness of the individual.

During light to moderate exercise intensities and long-duration exercise, fatty acids are a major fuel for muscle contraction. This occurs as oxygen becomes more available to the working muscle, allowing the body to rely more on the aerobic (oxidative) pathways and less of the anaerobic (phosphagen and glycolytic) pathways. The crossover shift toward greater carbohydrate oxidation at increasing intensity is a limitation in fatty acid utilization in high-intensity sports and activities. The limitation is partially explained by the inverse relationship between the lactate concentration and the rate of lipolysis. Lipolysis is also limited by inadequate blood perfusion of adipose tissue and the sympathetic response to high-intensity exercise.[34] Aside from limitations with lipolysis, other explanations include the inability of mitochondria to completely oxidize fat under conditions of limited oxygen availability occurring at exercise intensities of more than 85% of VO_2 peak. Despite limited changes in plasma FFA availability, a decrease in total fatty acid oxidation during high-intensity exercise (72% of VO_2 peak) compared with that at moderate intensities (44% to 55% of VO_2 peak) suggests that reduced fatty acid oxidation cannot be fully explained by a decreased delivery of fatty acid to an exercising muscle.[35] As exercise intensity increases, there is a progressive increase in the respiratory exchange ratio (RER), indicating a shift to greater carbohydrate oxidation. However, even with greater carbohydrate oxidation, fatty acid oxidation remains elevated for several hours after exercise. The maximum lipid contribution as an energy source is reached at approximately 60% to 65% of VO_2 max, with the contribution from carbohydrate oxidation maintained at about 50% of the energy expenditure of exercise. Fatty acid transport across the sarcolemma of the muscle does not appear to be a limiting factor for fatty acid oxidation at high intensity; instead, research continues to point toward traditionally defined mitochondrial regulatory steps involving the inhibition of carnitine and carnitine palmitoyltransferase I.[32,35,36]

METABOLIC ADAPTATIONS TO A HIGH-FAT DIET

In trained athletes, additional exercise-induced adaptations do not appear to significantly increase fat oxidation rates, but rates can be increased further by dietary strategies, such as fasting, acute preexercise intake of fat, and chronic exposure to low-carbohydrate, high-fat (LCHF) diets.[37] Significant interest in the implications of high-fat feeding in promoting metabolic adaptation that may support or improve athletic performance has emerged over the past few decades, partially fueled by the knowledge that limited endogenous carbohydrate stores often limit endurance performance. Most endurance events (>90 minutes) and ultraendurance events (>4–5 hours) are completed between 65% and 85% of VO_2 max, at which approximately 50% of the athlete's energy is acquired from muscle glycogen. Because a well-trained human can store only approximately 350 to 500 g (1,400–2,000 kcal) of glycogen in liver and muscle tissues, glycogen availability is often a limiting factor in performance duration and intensity. However, even a very lean athlete (eg, a 70-kg cisgender male with 6% body fat) holds more than 4 kg of body fat, equivalent to more than 35,000 kcal. To extend performance, athletes and sports nutrition practitioners have attempted to implement dietary strategies to shift substrate utilization during exercise to favor fat utilization and carbohydrate sparing. Because fatty acids are digested slowly, acute dietary interventions to increase FFA availability and oxidation are not practical. Therefore, if availability and oxidation of FFAs is to be increased during exercise, a multiday strategy to significantly increase fat intake is usually implemented.

The science investigating fat adaptation began in the early 1980s as an attempt to reduce athletes' reliance on exogenous carbohydrate during endurance events. An early study examining a ketogenic diet for weight loss in overweight and obese individuals recognized a drop in RER at VO_2 max from 0.76 at baseline to 0.66 after 5 weeks of a ketogenic diet (<10 g of carbohydrate per day). This was accompanied by a decrease in resting muscle glycogen from 1.53 to 1.04 mg/100 g (on a wet weight basis) and complete sparing of muscle glycogen during an uphill treadmill walk to exhaustion.[38] A second study by the same group built on this finding and identified a 30% decrease in glucose oxidation at rest during consumption of a ketogenic diet.[39] However, participants noted a 30% increase in mean serum cholesterol despite a 28 mg/dL drop in mean serum triglyceride. Further examination of a ketogenic diet in endurance-trained individuals showed a drop in RER from 0.83 to 0.72 after 5 weeks of ketogenic adaptation. Further, ketosis-adapted athletes were shown to exhibit fat oxidation rates almost 50% higher (90 vs 60 g/h) during exercise than those eating a traditional diet.[40] These early studies showed potential metabolic advantages for athletes consuming a ketogenic diet and spurred several decades of research examining the metabolic and athletic adaptations to a high-fat diet. Recent strategies have diverged from this extreme carbohydrate restriction in hopes of better maintaining glycogen stores as well as high-intensity capability.

Practitioners and athletes continue to show interest in the use of protocols for short-term or long-term adherence to LCHF diets that increase the ability of fat to support the fuel needs of exercise.[18] Fat-adaptation interventions have sparked the interest of endurance athletes and generally include consuming an LCHF diet for at least 5 to 14 days while maintaining normal training. Protocols have been implemented both with and without carbohydrate restoration coupled with a training taper leading up to competition.[21] Whereas early efforts to identify a fat-adaptive diet strategy focused on ketogenic diets, more recent efforts have attempted less-restrictive approaches that maintain muscle glycogen for high-intensity training and competition. Historical dietary models that combined a period of fat adaptation with the subsequent restoration of endogenous and exogenous carbohydrate availability for a simulated endurance task failed to find benefits to overall endurance performance despite robust increases in fat utilization during exercise. In addition, these models also resulted in impaired performance during higher-intensity tasks within the protocol.[41-43] This was later explained further by evidence of a downregulation of carbohydrate metabolism even when glycogen was available.[44] A seminal 2015 review article described the effects of LCHF diets on performance and noted that, despite widespread anecdotal support and a surge in popularity on social media and in non–peer-reviewed sources, research failed to show an improvement in performance from LCHF diets.[18] A more recent review noted that low-carbohydrate diets may allow ultraendurance athletes (>4 hours) to increase their ability to oxidize fat to support exercise at intensities up to approximately 75% to 80% of VO_2 peak. However, enthusiasm for this conclusion was limited because most ultramarathon runners already exhibit a high capacity for fat oxidation, regardless of their dietary interventions.[45] Furthermore, the authors concluded that any increase in fat utilization across a wide range of exercise intensities comes with the cost of a greater oxygen demand during exercise and a downregulation of carbohydrate oxidation pathways. These findings may be considered maladaptations in endurance events requiring segments of higher exercise intensities (>80%–85% of VO_2 peak) and therefore limiting the utility of an LCHF diet.[45]

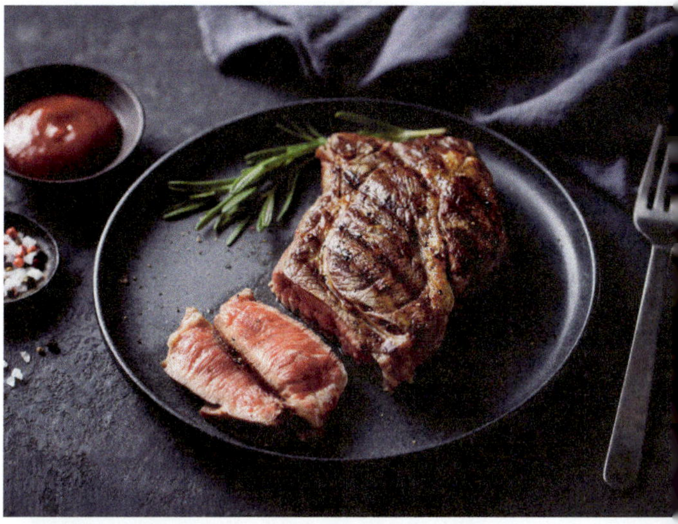

Ketogenic Diets

A very low-carbohydrate, high-fat diet has the potential to induce ketosis. A diet containing less than 10 g of carbohydrate per day can increase blood concentration of β-hydroxybutyrate from 0.06 mmol/L to approximately 2.5 mmol/L and raise total ketone body concentrations by more than a factor of 30 after only 1 week of diet exposure.[38] Such a diet has the theoretical potential to negate the need for exogenous macronutrients during extreme endurance events.[20] However, the first study that aimed to evaluate the effect of a ketogenic, LCHF diet on well-trained athletes concluded that chronic adaptation to a diet providing more than 80% of its energy from fat was, at best, able to maintain endurance capacity at only a moderate working intensity and sacrificed the ability and desire to exercise at higher workloads.[40]

One study reported weight loss and an increase in VO_2 max and lactic threshold (VO_2 LT) in well-trained, off-road cyclists after 4 weeks of a ketogenic diet consisting of 70% fat and 15% carbohydrate.[46] However, ketone bodies exhibited only a moderate increase (eg, the β-hydroxybutyrate concentration increased from 0.04 to 0.15 mmol/L) compared to other studies, and maximal power output was decreased following the ketogenic protocol, despite maintenance of absolute VO_2.[38,40] A 2020 study reproduced and confirmed that exercise economy and performance are impaired in race walkers on a ketogenic LCHF diet.[16] Whereas twice as much fat oxidation was observed in the LCHF group compared to high-carbohydrate and periodized carbohydrate groups, LCHF individuals experienced a higher rating of perceived exertion during the trial and a higher absolute oxygen cost of exercise. This reduction in exercise economy was observed when fat oxidation increased. The authors concluded that the increase in fat oxidation associated with keto-adaptation increases the oxygen cost of movement at any given speed and reduces the speed or power achieved at any given percentage of maximal aerobic capacity. In summary, the current literature on LCHF and ketogenic LCHF diets in endurance athletes points toward high carbohydrate availability being necessary to optimize performance in endurance exercise. There is no evidence of performance benefits associated with exposure to a ketogenic or nonketogenic LCHF diet—whether through adaptation or through a period of training under an LCHF diet before returning to high carbohydrate availability.

Other work in the area of LCHF sports nutrition has examined the impact of such diets on power athletes. One study examining gymnasts on a ketogenic LCHF diet (22 g of carbohydrate per day, 54% of calories from fat) found no change in performance markers such as pull-ups, push-ups, and triceps dips. However, the authors did observe a significant reduction in body weight from a loss of both fat and lean mass during the intervention.[47] Similar results were found by Sawyer et al[48] in both trained men and trained women. The researchers observed a decrease in body weight but no change in handgrip dynamometry, vertical jump, 1-repetition maximum bench press or back squat, maximum-repetition bench press, or 30-second Wingate anaerobic cycling test after 7 days of a diet with 53% of calories from fat. To date, some research has been published describing performance outcomes in power athletes. However, decreased high-intensity performance in endurance athletes suggests that no ergogenic effect would be seen in power athletes. More research must be conducted before sports nutrition practitioners can make informed recommendations encouraging high-fat diets to these athletes. Furthermore, there are research gaps in evaluating these diets in females. The limited data described previously suggest that performance in power athletes is either reduced or maintained as a result of following an LCHF ketogenic diet.

Training With Low Carbohydrate Availability

The implementation of a high-fat diet is as much of a low-carbohydrate challenge as it is a high-fat challenge. Although "training low" (ie, training with low carbohydrate availability) does not explicitly refer to the practice of training while on a high-fat diet, these practices frequently overlap, particularly if the athlete is in energy balance. The restriction of exogenous carbohydrate availability while exercising in a fasted state promotes an extended signaling response, albeit less robustly than when an athlete exercises with low endogenous carbohydrate stores.[49] These strategies enhance the cellular outcomes of endurance training, such as increased maximal mitochondrial enzyme activities or mitochondrial content and increased rates of lipid oxidation, with the augmentation of responses likely explained by enhanced activation of key cell-signaling kinases (eg, adenosine 5'-monophosphate–activated protein kinase [AMPK], p38 class of mitogen-activated protein kinases [p38 MAPK]), transcription factors (eg, p53, peroxisome proliferator-activated receptor delta [PPARδ]), and transcriptional coactivators (eg, peroxisome proliferator-activated receptor gamma coactivator 1-alpha [PGC-1α]).[49] Deliberate integration of such training-low exercise and dietary strategies within a periodized training program has become a recognized part of sports nutrition practice, despite its potential for misuse.[49,50]

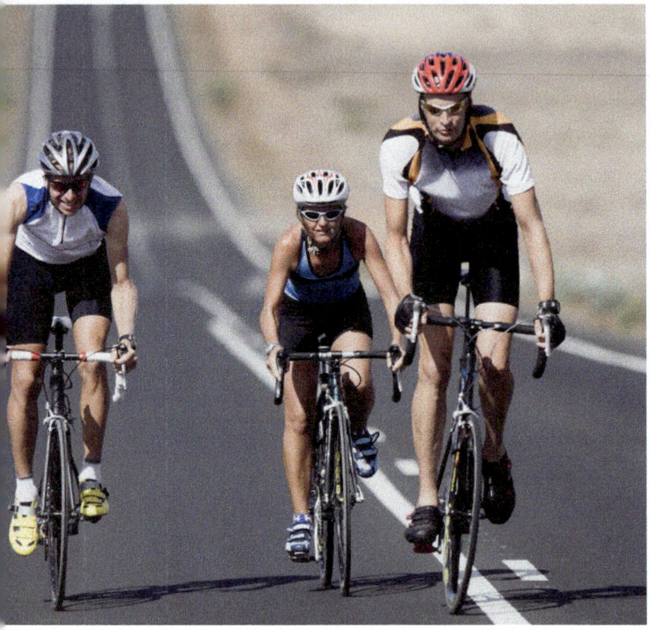

Exercising in a postabsorptive phase attempts to simulate a metabolic effect similar to that of a high-fat diet while allowing for moderate carbohydrate intake. Shimada et al[51] found that well-trained endurance athletes exhibited a metabolic shift away from glycogen oxidation when exercising before breakfast. During a before-breakfast 60-minute cycle ergometer training session at 50% of VO_2 max, athletes exhibited a lower RER (0.89 vs 0.94), increased 24-hour fat oxidation, and decreased 24-hour glycogen oxidation compared with the same workout performed in the afternoon. However, their study did not examine changes in performance. There is evidence that long-duration, low-intensity training in a fasted state increases mitochondrial biogenesis, and some researchers suggest that this pattern of training may improve performance.[52] A modified version of this strategy used a high-fat pretraining meal (as opposed to a high-carbohydrate meal) and found similar results. The data showed that a high-fat meal consumed 90 minutes before a 185-minute cycling workout reaching 82% peak power produced a lower RER than a high-carbohydrate meal given at the same time. However, despite substantial effects on plasma hormone concentrations and fuel utilization, there were no observed effects on performance.[53]

A variation on the training-low strategy is to complete 2 training sessions in 1 day with an LCHF diet and to include a carbohydrate restoration meal after the second training session. This strategy attempts to deplete muscle glycogen in the morning, creating an environment in which athletes rely more heavily on fat oxidation for the second workout. One study divided well-trained cyclists into 2 groups completing the same workouts on a different schedule. One group trained twice every other day (aerobic in the morning, high intensity in the afternoon) with a high-fat meal between the workouts. The other group completed an aerobic training session on 1 day and a high-intensity session on the next day with a regular diet. The cyclists who completed 2 training sessions every other day oxidized more fat and increased their β-hydroxyacyl-CoA dehydrogenase protein content relative to that of the athletes who completed the same training regimen on separate days. Both groups showed performance improvements over the 3-week study, and researchers observed no difference in performance improvements between the 2 groups.[54]

Dietary Periodization and Carbohydrate Restoration

The metabolic perturbations favoring the oxidation of fat persist even in the face of restored endogenous carbohydrate and increased exogenous carbohydrate availability.[21] Thus, to maximize possible fat-adaptation benefits from a high-fat diet without sacrificing endogenous carbohydrate stores, some researchers have proposed a method of diet periodization in which a high-fat diet (approximately 70% of energy from fat, 15% of energy from carbohydrate) is consumed for 5 to 14 days and then replaced with a traditional carbohydrate-loading diet directly before an event. This model replenishes glycogen stores at the time of competition in combination with increased rates of fat oxidation, albeit lower rates than are observed without carbohydrate replenishment. One of the original studies investigating diet periodization showed a successful increase of fat oxidation accompanied by a decrease in glucose oxidation and a decrease in RER after 5 days of a high-fat diet with 1 day of carbohydrate restoration in well-trained cyclists. However, performance improvements in an approximately 30-minute cycling time trial after 120 minutes of riding at 70% of VO_2 max were not significant.[55]

A variety of studies examining this dietary strategy have produced similar results. A 5-day high-fat diet followed by 1 day of rest and a high-carbohydrate diet resulted in lowered RER and carbohydrate oxidation during both a 2-hour steady-state workout and the following time trial but did not have significant effects on time trial performance.[56] Havemann et al[43] showed that a 7-day high-fat diet followed by 1 day of carbohydrate restoration increased fat oxidation and maintained endurance performance during a 100-km cycling time trial but compromised performance during intermediary sprints. The authors also noted the possibility of increased sympathetic activation or altered contractile function. The same study showed that metabolic adaptation to a high-fat diet can be observed in the form of decreased RER at rest and during exercise in as little as 3 days.

Whereas most studies have shown no statistically significant increases in performance with high-fat diets, several have demonstrated modest improvements. One of the strongest studies supporting dietary periodization for endurance athletes compared the effects of 3 diet conditions on cycling performance: 14 days of a high-carbohydrate diet, 14 days of a high-fat diet, and 11.5 days of a high-fat diet followed by 2.5 days of carbohydrate loading. The results indicated that the 11.5 days of high-fat diet plus 2.5 days of carbohydrate loading resulted in a nonsignificant 3% to 4% improvement in race time in a 100-km time trial.[57] The high-fat diet and the high-fat diet followed by carbohydrate loading attenuated an observed end-of-race power decline (last 5 km) seen under the high-carbohydrate conditions. Furthermore, power output during the last 5 km of this time trial was 1.3 times greater after the high-fat diet plus carbohydrate loading than after the high-carbohydrate diet. Another study showed a 4% improvement in a 20-km time trial preceded by a 150-minute preload at 70% of VO_2 max following a 10-day nonketogenic, high-fat diet with 3 days of carbohydrate loading.[58]

Potential Mechanisms of Fat Adaptation With Carbohydrate Restoration

Yeo et al[22] investigated mechanisms of fat adaptation with carbohydrate restoration. The authors studied a 5-day fat adaptation followed by 1 day of carbohydrate restoration with a 1-hour cycling workout at 70% of VO_2 peak. The results revealed higher AMPK-α1 and AMPK-α2 activity, lower RER and glycogen utilization, and increased resting muscle triglyceride stores and fat oxidation; however, the study did not examine performance. Bigrigg et al[59] observed a reduction in pyruvate dehydrogenase activity following 6 days of a high-fat protocol. Although this study did not measure performance, these findings provide some mechanistic insight for the reduction in glucose utilization observed in other trials. However, these effects were rapidly reversed after the reintroduction of carbohydrates. More research is needed to determine the significance of changes in pyruvate dehydrogenase and pyruvate dehydrogenase kinases in athletes with varying metabolic demands, including those needing to train or compete at high intensity with a greater reliance on anaerobic metabolism. Multiple studies have shown increases in fat oxidation and decreases in RER in response to both chronic and acute high-fat feeding compared with high-carbohydrate diets.[20,60] This is possibly in response to increased mitochondrial biogenesis activated through PGC-1α signaling.[52,61]

Another mechanism through which high-fat diets may alter performance is through increased muscle triglyceride stores. Increased storage of lipids in immediate proximity to mitochondria in the muscle increases their availability during exercise and may decrease muscles' demand on glycogen for energy production. A high-fat diet in combination with endurance training has been shown to increase intramyocellular triglyceride by 50% in type I muscle fibers and by 75% in type IIa muscle fibers over 6 weeks.[62] Other research has shown a 75% preexercise increase in total muscle triacylglycerol after 5 days of fat adaptation and 1 day of carbohydrate loading.

Summary of High-Fat Diet Literature and Need for Future Research

There seems to be very little contention that high-fat diets increase the amount of fat burned during exercise, but it remains unclear how this strategy directly affects athletic performance. This form of dietary periodization increases the rate of whole-body and muscle fat oxidation while attenuating the rate of muscle glycogenolysis during submaximal exercise. Sports dietitians should note that dietary periodization strategies such as this represent a low-carbohydrate challenge as well as a high-fat challenge because muscle glycogen is reduced during the adaptation phase. Furthermore, simply increasing fat oxidation does not increase performance and cannot be assumed to improve long-term metabolic health, as has been suggested in some studies. These concerns may be even more pronounced in recreational athletes who may misunderstand their carbohydrate needs and associated claims about the potential benefits of fat adaptation. Much of the controversy surrounding whether fat adaptation is a potentially helpful strategy for athletes is due to a long list of inconsistencies between study designs and outcomes. For example, research questions surrounding this topic have often been studied in cisgender males, ranging from recreationally active individuals to well-trained cyclists and ultraendurance athletes. Protocols have ranged from 1 day to several days, and the high-fat experimental groups have all experienced various degrees of carbohydrate restriction ranging from mild to ketogenic. Furthermore, some of the metabolic changes that have been reported use different methods for assigning high-fat treatment, many times using calorie percentages instead of dosing fat by body weight (g/kg). The discrepancies in research designs and the lack of chronic studies make it difficult to translate the results into conclusions about long-term effects on athletic performance and health.

Before recommending a fat-adaptation diet to athletes, sports dietitians should consider several factors. Most importantly, there is no consensus on the performance benefits of a high-fat adaptation diet. There has been speculation that some athletes respond better than others to fat-adaption diets in terms of tolerance, mood profile, and performance. However, these diets are associated with higher rated perceived exertion, especially for higher-intensity workouts, and athletes using these diets often need more encouragement to train.[63] Despite renewed attention and popular interest in this practice, recent reviews have concluded that there is no evidence to support widespread performance benefits.[20] This lack of evidence extends to the preparation of competitive athletes even in the face of metabolic adaptations to increase the mobilization, transport, and oxidation of fat as an exercise substrate.[41] Although there has been historical[39] and revived interest in chronic adaptation to LCHF diets, present evidence suggests that enhanced rates of fat oxidation can only match the exercise capacity and performance achieved by diets or strategies promoting high carbohydrate availability at moderate intensities.[20,40] However, the performance of exercise at the higher intensities representative of or important for competitive outcomes in most sporting activities seems to be impaired.[43,64]

Further research is warranted, in view of both the current discussions and the failure of recent studies to include an adequate reference diet that includes contemporary periodized dietary approaches.[20,41] Although specific scenarios may exist in which high-fat diets offer some benefits or at least are not disadvantageous to performance, in general, such diets appear to reduce rather than enhance metabolic flexibility by reducing carbohydrate availability and the capacity to use carbohydrate effectively as an exercise substrate. Therefore, competitive athletes would be unwise to sacrifice their ability to undertake high-quality training or high-intensity efforts during competition that could determine the competitive outcome.[41] Even when working at the highest intensities that can be supported by oxidative phosphorylation, carbohydrate offers advantages over fat as a substrate because it provides a greater yield of ATP per volume of oxygen that can be delivered to the mitochondria,[37] thus improving gross exercise efficiency.[65]

Fat is a key energy provider, and restriction may lead to low energy availability, resulting in unwanted loss of muscle mass; menstrual dysfunction and hormonal disturbances; suboptimal bone density; increased risk of fatigue, injury, and illness; impaired adaptation; and a prolonged recovery process. Adequate energy availability is needed to optimize protein metabolism. When energy availability is reduced (eg, to reduce body weight or fat), performance can suffer.[66]

PRACTICAL ADVICE: DAILY FAT INTAKE

An athlete's daily fat intake should help meet the energy demands of a periodized nutrition program to support proper training and competition. The percentage of energy consumed daily from fat will fluctuate based on changing energy needs, with specific target amounts generally determined after carbohydrate and protein goals are established. Once a general gram-per-day amount is determined, athletes should modify their planned intake to incorporate more MUFA and PUFA food sources and devise a plan for consuming a dietary source of omega-3 fatty acids several days per week. Sports dietitians should consider the ratio of omega-6 to omega-3 fats when counseling athletes about diet planning because this may have a greater impact on fatty acid nutrition than a relatively small dose of an omega-3 fatty acid supplement. With the exception of omega-3 fatty acids, lipid-based dietary supplements have shown limited efficacy as ergogenic aids and should only be used with caution. If athletes remain interested in these types of dietary supplements, the sports dietitian can assist them in undertaking a cost-benefit analysis of the use of such products and remind them that the greatest value will be observed only when added to a well-chosen eating plan. Research summaries on some popular lipid-based supplements are provided in Box 4.2.[67-80]

BOX 4.2 Functions, Efficacies, and Concerns About Common Lipid-Based Dietary Supplements[67-80]

Supplement	Claims	Efficacy and concerns
Conjugated linoleic acid (CLA)[67-71]	May alter blood lipids May support immune function Helps to reduce body fat, change body composition, and improve athletic performance	Has not been shown to enhance aerobic exercise performance Body composition and effects on immunity are equivocal Appears to improve high-density lipoprotein cholesterol (HDL-C) while increasing other lipoprotein concentrations May cause negative gastrointestinal (GI) side effects Evidence of effectiveness as a weight-loss aid is mixed in human studies
L-Carnitine[72-76]	Decreases heart rate Improves exercise performance Promotes recovery after exercise Increases loss of body fat	Does not affect whole-body fat utilization during short-duration exercise Performance outcomes are equivocal Safe at recommended doses of 2 to 4 g/d but not effective for improving performance
Medium-chain triglyceride (MCT) oil[77-80]	Can prolong performance and spare glycogen stores	MCT oils are ineffective in improving exercise performance in humans May cause GI distress in doses associated with performance enhancement Limited application to most sports Food sources may support healthy changes in body composition over other dietary lipids during a weight-loss program

Fat intake should be limited for 1 or 2 hours before exercise or competition to prevent gastrointestinal distress. Athletes often benefit from liquid meal supplements, especially if they suffer from preevent anxiety or an uncertain preevent timetable, thus favoring a more quickly digested option. The amount of fat recommended in a meal or snack 3 to 4 hours before the event is variable and depends on individual tolerance. A prudent goal for meals 3 to 4 hours prior to training or competition would be to consume less than 30% of calories from fat to promote gastric emptying at a rate unlikely to impede performance. Above all, athletes should choose a strategy that suits their situation and their past experiences and can be fine-tuned with further experimentation.[81,82] Generally, foods that are low in fat, low in fiber, and low to moderate in protein are preferred for a preevent menu because they are less prone to cause gastrointestinal problems, including flatulence, bloating, nausea, vomiting, intestinal cramps, and diarrhea.[83]

Omega-3 Fatty Acid Dietary Supplementation

Omega-3 fatty acids are required for structural integrity and fluidity of membrane lipids, for the synthesis of eicosanoids, and as substrates for metabolic products needed for structural and functional roles within many body systems.[84] Because of these essential roles, athletes who chronically restrict their fat intake to below the AMDR minimum of 20% of energy intake or who do not regularly consume sources of α-linolenic acid and EPA/DHA may benefit from taking an omega-3 fatty acid supplement. Furthermore, omega-3 fatty acid supplements may be useful in the prevention or treatment of nutrient deficiency in some athlete scenarios. For example, depending on the extent of dietary limitations, omega-3 fatty acid intake for vegetarians may be a concern that warrants supplementation.

Ideally, athletes considering purchasing and taking an omega-3 dietary supplement should do so under the supervision of an appropriate medical or nutrition expert. This is a prudent recommendation considering that routine high-dose omega-3 supplementation may not be scientifically justified based on the desired sports nutrition outcome of interest. Moreover, some studies have indicated that large doses of omega-3 supplements have increased oxidative stress markers after exercise and that some athletes who take high doses chronically may be at greater risk for immunosuppression and prolonged bleed times.[85-87] Despite these documented concerns, athletes who frequently restrict their energy intake may receive benefits from increasing omega-3 intake through diet or supplementation. Daily intake of up to 3 g of EPA/DHA from diet or supplements is considered safe and may help facilitate training and diet-induced performance improvements.

EPA and DHA are the most popular and most biologically active fatty acids found in omega-3 fish oil supplements and are responsible for many bioactive end products, such as anti-inflammatory resolvins and the antiarrhythmic, vasodilation, and platelet-inhibitor effects of the prostaglandin H_3 (PGH_3) family of molecules. EPA and DHA are also incorporated into cell membranes and function to make membranes more elastic, more flexible, and less prone to damage.[88] In addition, EPA and DHA supplementation is very effective at decreasing serum triglycerides.[89]

Specific to the realm of sports nutrition, most research on omega-3 supplementation has centered on outcomes related directly to sports performance, muscle soreness, sports-related concussions, and musculoskeletal injury risk and recovery. Athletes who take supplemental omega-3 fatty acids should know that these fatty acids have many diverse and important physiological roles, but the commonly discussed anti-inflammatory properties of these lipids have not been shown to directly enhance performance. Therefore, fish oil supplements should not be viewed as ergogenic aids.[88-92] Although there is some evidence that omega-3 supplementation may improve endurance capacity by reducing the oxygen cost of exercise,[93] their primary benefit may be to indirectly support athletic performance by supporting healthy physiological function and adaptations to exercise.

Several studies have examined the impact of varying doses of omega-3 supplements on muscle damage and hypertrophy.[94-96] Although there may be some utility for these supplements to promote recovery from muscle-damaging eccentric exercise,[79] studies that specifically examined muscle damage and functional changes, soreness, and recovery after resistance exercise and routine training activities have been inconclusive. Any hypertrophic effect appears to be equivocal when controlling for the independent hypertrophic effects of resistance training or when consuming postexercise protein in recommended amounts. To date, research does not support the claim that omega-3 supplementation facilitates muscle growth during resistance training or preserves muscle mass following injury in athletic populations.[93] Furthermore, because of inconclusive data, there is no scientific consensus on recommending a specific amount or duration of omega-3 supplementation for these outcomes.[87]

The role of omega-3 supplementation in preventing and treating negative neurological outcomes associated with sports-related concussions continues to garner substantial scientific attention. A 2021 multisite nonrandomized trial examined 2 football teams whose players received daily supplemental omega-3 fatty acids (2,000 mg of DHA, 560 mg of EPA, 320 mg of docosapentaenoic acid [DPA]).[97] The authors reported a reduction in serum neurofilament light (a biomarker of axonal injury associated with repetitive head impact exposure) following a 3-month supplementation protocol spanning preseason and in-season play. Although these findings complement animal data that show an attenuation in structural damage and cognitive decline and suggest neuroprotective potential,[94] the results are preliminary, and many new research questions exist. More clinical trials are underway to inform sports nutrition practice in the future.

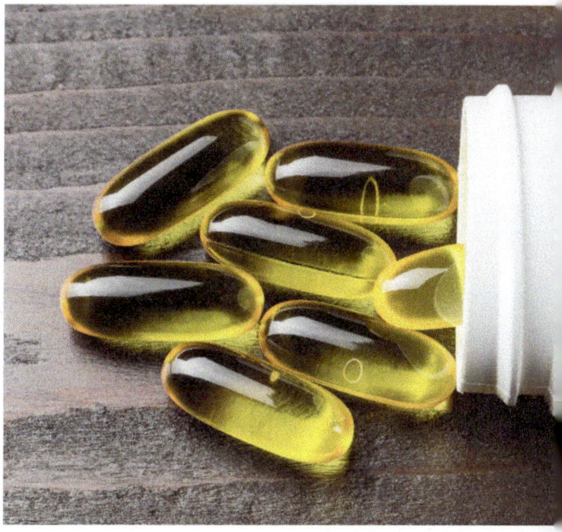

The most intriguing research outcomes related to omega-3 supplementation may be in the prevention and treatment of musculoskeletal injuries. Whereas the prophylactic use of these supplements for injury prevention is currently considered speculative, postinjury supplementation has been shown to improve muscle function and reduce inflammation when provided at a dose of approximately 3,500 mg of EPA and 900 mg of DHA.[98] This dose is higher than what is often recommended in uninjured athletes, permits a detectable increase in muscle omega-3 PUFA lipid composition, reduces the magnitude of a prolonged inflammatory response, and may aid in cell membrane production and regeneration.[94,99]

In the selection of an omega-3 supplement, it is important to note that 18:3 (omega-3, from plant sources) undergo limited conversion to EPA/DHA because of their entry point in the fatty acid conversion pathway, which requires competition with omega-6 fatty acids for the delta-6 desaturase enzyme.[100,101] Although EPA and DHA can be derived from algae, such preparations usually have a low concentration compared with EPA/DHA derived from fish.[102] It is important for sports nutrition practitioners to monitor the omega-3 supplemental intake of their athletes, as such supplementation may be done unnecessarily without appropriate supervision or monitoring.

SUMMARY

Dietary fat is essential for promoting both the health and performance of athletes. Although no athlete's diet should be devoid of fat, there are certain scenarios and acute time frames when recommending fat restriction as a temporary strategy is necessary. When acute fat restriction is practiced for making competition weight, it should be limited to very short-term scenarios. Other examples in which acute fat restriction may be beneficial are when considerations of preferred macronutrients or gastrointestinal comfort have priority, such as immediately before a sporting event or training session or during carbohydrate loading. Athletes who choose to excessively restrict their fat intake to lose body weight or improve physique should be cautioned that they may not be able to meet energy needs.

In most athletes, fat intakes associated with eating styles that accommodate public health recommendations typically range from 20% to 35% of total energy intake. Consuming less than 20% of energy intake from fat does not benefit performance, and extreme restriction of fat intake may limit the food range needed to meet overall health and performance goals. Claims that extremely high-fat (more than 35%), carbohydrate-restricted diets provide a benefit to the performance of competitive athletes are also not supported by the current research.

The choice of what fats to include in the diet should be based on taste preference while incorporating a wide range of foods consistent with the *Dietary Guidelines for Americans, 2020–2025*. Many athletes would benefit from consuming more plant-based fatty acids and fewer foods containing significant sources of animal fat. Dietary sources of omega-3 PUFAs include fish, walnuts, canola oil, and flaxseed, whereas omega-6 fatty acids are found in relatively high levels in most, but not all, other plant foods.

KEY TAKEAWAYS

Different lipids can produce profoundly different metabolic effects; therefore, it is very important for nutrition practitioners to understand the differences among sources of dietary fat and make clear, evidence-based recommendations for both athletic performance and general wellness.

A well-chosen diet with balanced fatty acid intake includes a larger proportion of MUFAs and PUFAs relative to saturated fat as part of a mixed diet that emphasizes vegetables, fruits, whole grains, low-fat dairy, and seafood, with lower consumption of red and processed meats.

As exercise duration increases and intensity decreases, endogenous fat stores contribute a greater percentage of total energy sources relative to carbohydrate and amino acids.

Fat intake patterns may fluctuate daily to help the athlete meet the energy demands of a periodized nutrition program and support proper training and competition.

In very short-term scenarios (up to 72 hours), fat restriction may be effective for acute weight reduction for weigh-ins or when preferred macronutrients or gastrointestinal comfort have priority.

Adequate fat consumption is crucial to health, and chronic fat restriction may contribute to low energy availability that can result in both decreased performance and serious long-term health concerns.

Although metabolic adaptations do occur in response to high-fat feeding, claims that high-fat, carbohydrate-restricted diets improve performance in competitive athletes are not supported by the current literature.

REFERENCES

1. Thomas DT, Erdman KA, Burke LM. American College of Sports Medicine joint position statement: Nutrition and athletic performance. *Med Sci Sports Exerc.* 2016;48(3):543-568. doi:10.1249/mss.0000000000000852
2. Jones PJH, Kubow S. Lipids, sterols and their metabolites. In: Shils ME, Shike M, Ross AC, Caballero B, Cousins RJ, eds. *Modern Nutrition in Health and Disease.* 10th ed. Lippincott Williams & Wilkins; 2006:65-87.
3. Bard JM, Paillard F, Lecerf JM. Effect of phytosterols/stanols on LDL concentration and other surrogate markers of cardiovascular risk. *Diabetes Metab.* 2015;41(1):69-75. doi:10.1016/j.diabet.2014.11.006
4. Final determination regarding partially hydrogenated oils. Fed Regist. 2015;80(116):34650-34670. Accessed September 1, 2023. www.federalregister.gov/documents/2015/06/17/2015-14883/final-determination-regarding-partially-hydrogenated-oils
5. US Department of Agriculture and US Department of Health and Human Services. *Dietary Guidelines for Americans, 2020-2025.* 9th ed. December 2020. Accessed September 1, 2023. www.dietaryguidelines.gov/sites/default/files/2021-03/Dietary_Guidelines_for_Americans-2020-2025.pdf
6. Kosinski C, Jornayvaz FR. Effects of ketogenic diets on cardiovascular risk factors: evidence from animal and human studies. *Nutrients.* 2017;9(5):517. doi:10.3390/nu9050517
7. Buren J, Ericsson M, Teixeira Damasceno NR, Sjödin A. A ketogenic low-carbohydrate high-fat diet increases LDL cholesterol in healthy, young, normal-weight women: a randomized controlled feeding trial. *Nutrients.* 2021;13(3):814. doi:10.3390/nu13030814
8. Beis LY, Willkomm L, Ross R, et al. Food and macronutrient intake of elite Ethiopian distance runners. *J Int Soc Sports Nutr.* 2011;8:7. doi:10.1186/1550-2783-8-7
9. Bradley WJ, Cavanagh B, Douglas W, et al. Energy intake and expenditure assessed 'in-season' in an elite European rugby union squad. *Eur J Sport Sci.* 2015;15(6):469-479. doi:10.1080/17461391.2015.1042528
10. Mielgo-Ayuso J, Zourdos MC, Calleja-Gonzalez J, Urdampilleta A, Ostojic SM. Dietary intake habits and controlled training on body composition and strength in elite female volleyball players during the season. *Appl Physiol Nutr Metab.* 2015;40(8):827-834. doi:10.1139/apnm-2015-0100
11. Paulin S, Roberts J, Roberts M, Davis I. A case study evaluation of competitors undertaking an antarctic ultra-endurance event: nutrition, hydration and body composition variables. *Extrem Physiol Med.* 2015;4:3. doi:10.1186/s13728-015-0022-0
12. Kopp-Woodroffe SA, Manore MM, Dueck CA, Skinner JS, Matt KS. Energy and nutrient status of amenorrheic athletes participating in a diet and exercise training intervention program. *Int J Sport Nutr.* 1999;9(1):70-88. doi:10.1123/ijsn.9.1.70
13. Waly MI, Kilani HA, Al-Busafi MS. Nutritional practices of athletes in Oman: a descriptive study. *Oman Med J.* 2013;28(5):360-364. doi:10.5001/omj.2013.103
14. Wright HH, Garthe I. Weight-category sports. In: Maughan LJ, ed. *The Encyclopaedia of Sports Medicine: An IOC Medical Commission Publication.* John Wiley & Sons Ltd; 2013:639-650.
15. Tomten S, Høstmark A. Energy balance in weight stable athletes with and without menstrual disorders. *Scand J Med Sci Sports.* 2006;16(2):127-133. doi:10.1111/j.1600-0838.2005.00451.x
16. Burke L, Sharma A, Keikura I, et al. Crisis of confidence averted: Impairment of exercise economy and performance in elite race walkers by ketogenic low carbohydrate, high fat (LCHF) diet is reproducible. *PLoS One.* 2020;15(6):e0234027. doi:10.1371/journal.pone.0234027
17. Burke LM. Fueling strategies to optimize performance: training high or training low? *Scand J Med Sci Sports.* 2010;20(suppl 2):48-58. doi:10.1111/j.1600-0838.2010.01185.x
18. Burke LM. Re-examining high-fat diets for sports performance: did we call the 'nail in the coffin' too soon? *Sports Med.* 2015;45(suppl 1):S33-S49. doi:10.1007/s40279-015-0393-9
19. Noakes T, Volek JS, Phinney SD. Low-carbohydrate diets for athletes: what evidence? *Br J Sports Med.* 2014;48(14):1077-1078. doi:10.1136/bjsports-2014-093824
20. Volek JS, Noakes T, Phinney SD. Rethinking fat as a fuel for endurance exercise. *Eur J Sport Sci.* 2015;15(1):13-20. doi:10.1080/17461391.2014.959564
21. Yeo WK, Carey AL, Burke L, Spriet LL, Hawley JA. Fat adaptation in well-trained athletes: effects on cell metabolism. *Appl Physiol Nutr Metab.* 2011;36(1):12-22. doi:10.1139/h10-089
22. Yeo WK, Lessard SJ, Chen Z-P, et al. Fat adaptation followed by carbohydrate restoration increases AMPK activity in skeletal muscle from trained humans. *J Appl Physiol (1985).* 2008;105(5):1519-1526. doi:10.1152/japplphysiol.90540.2008
23. Fumagalli M, Moltke I, Grarup N, et al. Greenlandic Inuit show genetic signatures of diet and climate adaptation. *Science.* 2015;349(6254):1343-1347. doi:10.1126/science.aab2319
24. Lichtenstein AH, Appel L, Vadiveloo M, et al. 2021 Dietary Guidance To Improve Cardiovascular Health: A Scientific Statement from the American Heart Association. *Circulation.* 2021;144(23):e472-e487. doi:10.1161/CIR.0000000000001031
25. Dietary Guidelines Advisory Committee. Report of the Dietary Guidelines Advisory Committee on the Dietary Guidelines for Americans, 2010, to the Secretary of Agriculture and the Secretary of Health and Human Services. US:Agricultural Research Service, Department of Agriculture: May 2010.

26. Arnett D, Blumenthal R, Albert M, et al. ACC/AHA Guideline on the Primary Prevention of Cardiovascular Disease: Executive Summary: A Report of the American College of Cardiology/American Heart Association Task Force on Clinical Practice Guidelines. *Circulation.* 2019;140(11):e563-e595. doi:10.1161/CIR.0000000000000678
27. Rimm EB, Appel LJ, Chiuve SE, et al. Seafood long-chain n-3 polyunsaturated fatty acids and cardiovascular disease: a science advisory from the American Heart Association. *Circulation.* 2018;138(1):e35-e47. doi:10.1161/CIR.0000000000000574
28. Manini TM, Clark BC, Nalls MA, Goodpaster BH, Ploutz-Snyder LL, Harris TB. Reduced physical activity increases intermuscular adipose tissue in healthy young adults. *Am J Clin Nutr.* 2007;85(2):377-384. doi:10.1093/ajcn/85.2.377
29. Enevoldsen LH, Simonsen L, Bulow J. Postprandial triacylglycerol uptake in the legs is increased during exercise and post-exercise recovery. *J Physiol.* 2005;568(Pt 3):941-950. doi:10.1113/jphysiol.2005.091975
30. Roepstorff C, Thiele M, Hillig T, et al. Higher skeletal muscle α2AMPK activation and lower energy charge and fat oxidation in men than in women during submaximal exercise. *J Physiol.* 2006;574(Pt 1):125-138. doi:10.1113/jphysiol.2006.108720
31. Alsted TJ, Nybo L, Schweiger M, et al. Adipose triglyceride lipase in human skeletal muscle is upregulated by exercise training. *Am J Physiol Endocrinol Metab.* 2009;296(3):E445-E453. doi:10.1152/ajpendo.90912.2008
32. Romijn JA, Coyle EF, Sidossis LS, et al. Regulation of endogenous fat and carbohydrate metabolism in relation to exercise intensity and duration. *Am J Physiol.* 1993;265(3 Pt 1):E380-E391. doi:10.1152/ajpendo.1993.265.3.E380
33. Watt MJ, Heigenhauser GJF, Spriet LL. Effects of dynamic exercise intensity on the activation of hormone-sensitive lipase in human skeletal muscle. *J Physiol.* 2003;547(Pt 1):301-308. doi:10.1113/jphysiol.2002.034595
34. Frayn KN. Fat as a fuel: emerging understanding of the adipose tissue-skeletal muscle axis. *Acta Physiol (Oxf).* 2010;199(4):509-518. doi:10.1111/j.1748-1716.2010.02128.x
35. van Loon LJ, Greenhaff PL, Constantin-Teodosiu D, Saris WH, Wagenmakers AJ. The effects of increasing exercise intensity on muscle fuel utilisation in humans. *J Physiol.* 2001;536(Pt 1):295-304. doi:10.1111/j.1469-7793.2001.00295.x
36. Kiens B, Jeppesen J. Fat metabolism during and after exercise. In: Maughan RJ, ed. *The Encyclopaedia of Sports Medicine: An IOC Medical Commission Publication.* John Wiley & Sons Ltd; 2013:156-165.
37. Spriet LL. New insights into the interaction of carbohydrate and fat metabolism during exercise. *Sports Med.* 2014;44(suppl 1):S87-S96. doi:10.1007/s40279-014-0154-1
38. Phinney SD, Horton ES, Sims EA, Hanson JS, Danforth E Jr., LaGrange BM. Capacity for moderate exercise in obese subjects after adaptation to a hypocaloric, ketogenic diet. *J Clin Invest.* 1980;66(5):1152-1161. doi:10.1172/jci109945
39. Phinney SD, Bistrian BR, Wolfe RR, Blackburn GL. The human metabolic response to chronic ketosis without caloric restriction: physical and biochemical adaptation. *Metabolism.* 1983;32(8):757-768. doi:10.1016/0026-0495(83)90105-1
40. Phinney SD, Bistrian BR, Evans WJ, Gervino E, Blackburn GL. The human metabolic response to chronic ketosis without caloric restriction: preservation of submaximal exercise capability with reduced carbohydrate oxidation. *Metabolism.* 1983;32(8):769-776. doi:10.1016/0026-0495(83)90106-3
41. Burke LM, Kiens B. "Fat adaptation" for athletic performance: the nail in the coffin? *J Appl Physiol (1985).* 2006;100(1):7-8. doi:10.1152/japplphysiol.01238.2005
42. Havemann L. *Nutritional Strategies for Endurance and Ultra-Endurance Cycling [dissertation]*: Department of Human Biology, University of Cape Town; 2008.
43. Havemann L, West SJ, Goedecke JH, et al. Fat adaptation followed by carbohydrate loading compromises high-intensity sprint performance. *J Appl Physiol (1985).* 2006;100(1):194-202. doi:10.1152/japplphysiol.00813.2005
44. Stellingwerff T, Spriet LL, Watt MJ, et al. Decreased PDH activation and glycogenolysis during exercise following fat adaptation with carbohydrate restoration. *Am J Physiol Endocrinol Metab.* 2006;290(2):E380-E388. doi:10.1152/ajpendo.00268.2005
45. Burke LM, Castell LM, Casa DJ, et al. International Association of Athletics Federations Consensus Statement 2019: Nutrition for Athletics. *Int J Sport Nutr Exerc Metab.* 2019;29(2):73-84. doi:10.1123/ijsnem.2019-0065
46. Zajac A, Poprzecki S, Maszczyk A, Czuba M, Michalczyk M, Zydek G. The effects of a ketogenic diet on exercise metabolism and physical performance in off-road cyclists. *Nutrients.* 2014;6(7):2493-2508. doi:10.3390/nu6072493
47. Paoli A, Grimaldi K, D'Agostino D, et al. Ketogenic diet does not affect strength performance in elite artistic gymnasts. *J Int Soc Sports Nutr.* 2012;9(1):34. doi:10.1186/1550-2783-9-34
48. Sawyer JC, Wood RJ, Davidson PW, et al. Effects of a short-term carbohydrate-restricted diet on strength and power performance. *J Strength Cond Res.* 2013;27(8):2255-2262. doi:10.1519/JSC.0b013e31827da314
49. Bartlett JD, Hawley JA, Morton JP. Carbohydrate availability and exercise training adaptation: too much of a good thing? *Eur J Sport Sci.* 2015;15(1):3-12. doi:10.1080/17461391.2014.920926
50. Stellingwerff T. Contemporary nutrition approaches to optimize elite marathon performance. *Int J Sports Physiol Perform.* 2013;8(5):573-578. doi:10.1123/ijspp.8.5.573
51. Shimada K, Yamamoto Y, Iwayama K, et al. Effects of post-absorptive and postprandial exercise on 24 h fat oxidation. *Metabolism.* 2013;62(6):793-800. doi:10.1016/j.metabol.2012.12.008
52. Baar K. Nutrition and the adaptation to endurance training. *Sports Med.* 2014;44(suppl 1):S5-S12. doi:10.1007/s40279-014-0146-1

53. Rowlands DS, Hopkins WG. Effect of high-fat, high-carbohydrate, and high-protein meals on metabolism and performance during endurance cycling. *Int J Sport Nutr Exerc Metab.* 2002;12(3):318-335. doi:10.1123/ijsnem.12.3.318
54. Hulston CJ, Venables MC, Mann CH, et al. Training with low muscle glycogen enhances fat metabolism in well-trained cyclists. *Med Sci Sports Exerc.* 2010;42(11):2046-2055. doi:10.1249/MSS.0b013e3181dd5070
55. Burke LM, Angus DJ, Cox GR, et al. Effect of fat adaptation and carbohydrate restoration on metabolism and performance during prolonged cycling. *J Appl Physiol (1985).* 2000;89(6):2413-2421. doi:10.1152/jappl.2000.89.6.2413
56. Burke LM, Hawley JA, Angus DJ, et al. Adaptations to short-term high-fat diet persist during exercise despite high carbohydrate availability. *Med Sci Sports Exerc.* 2002;34(1):83-91. doi:10.1097/00005768-200201000-00014
57. Rowlands DS, Hopkins WG. Effects of high-fat and high-carbohydrate diets on metabolism and performance in cycling. *Metabolism.* 2002;51(6):678-690. doi:10.1053/meta.2002.32723
58. Lambert EV, Goedecke JH, Zyle C, et al. High-fat diet versus habitual diet prior to carbohydrate loading: effects of exercise metabolism and cycling performance. *Int J Sport Nutr Exerc Metab.* 2001;11(2):209-225. doi:10.1123/ijsnem.11.2.209
59. Bigrigg JK, Heigenhauser GJF, Inglis JG, LeBlanc PJ, Peters SJ. Carbohydrate refeeding after a high-fat diet rapidly reverses the adaptive increase in human skeletal muscle PDH kinase activity. *Am J Physiol Regul Integr Comp Physiol.* 2009;297(3):R885-R891. doi:10.1152/ajpregu.90604.2008
60. Shaw DM, Merien F, Braakhuis A, Maunder ED, Dulson DK. Effect of a ketogenic diet on submaximal exercise capacity and efficiency in runners. *Med Sci Sports Exerc.* 2019;51(10):2135-2146. doi:10.1249/MSS.0000000000002008
61. Margolis LM, Pasiakos SM. Optimizing intramuscular adaptations to aerobic exercise: effects of carbohydrate restriction and protein supplementation on mitochondrial biogenesis. *Adv Nutr.* 2013;4(6):657-664. doi:10.3945/an.113.004572
62. Van Proeyen K, Szlufcik K, Nielens H, et al. High-fat diet overrules the effects of training on fiber-specific intramyocellular lipid utilization during exercise. *J Appl Physiol (1985).* 2011;111(1):108-116. doi:10.1152/japplphysiol.01459.2010
63. Hawley JA. Fat adaptation science: low-carbohydrate, high-fat diets to alter fuel utilization and promote training adaptation. *Nestle Nutr Inst Workshop Ser.* 2011;69:59-71; discussion 71-57. doi:10.1159/000329283
64. Burke LM, Sharma AP, Heikura IA, et al. Crisis of confidence averted: impairment of exercise economy and performance in elite race walkers by ketogenic low carbohydrate, high fat (LCHF) diet is reproducible. *PLoS One.* 2020;15(6):e0234027. doi:10.1371/journal.pone.0234027
65. Cole M, Coleman D, Hopker J, Wiles J. Improved gross efficiency during long duration submaximal cycling following a short-term high carbohydrate diet. *Int J Sports Med.* 2014;35(3):265-269. doi:10.1055/s-0033-1348254
66. Nindl BC, Friedl KE, Frykman PN, Marchitelli LJ, Shippee RL, Patton JF. Physical performance and metabolic recovery among lean, healthy men following a prolonged energy deficit. *Int J Sports Med.* 1997;18(5):317-324. doi:10.1055/s-2007-972640
67. Jenkins ND, Buckner SL, Baker RB, et al. Effects of 6 weeks of aerobic exercise combined with conjugated linoleic acid on the physical working capacity at fatigue threshold. *J Strength Cond Res.* 2014;28(8):2127-2135. doi:10.1519/JSC.0000000000000513
68. Liang CW, Cheng HY, Lee YH, Liou TH, Liao CD, Huang SW. Effects of conjugated linoleic acid and exercise on body composition and obesity: a systematic review and meta-analysis. *Nutr Rev.* 2023;81(4):397-415. doi:10.1093/nutrit/nuac060
69. Onakpoya IJ, Posadzki PP, Watson LK, Davies LA, Ernst E. The efficacy of long-term conjugated linoleic acid (CLA) supplementation on body composition in overweight and obese individuals: a systematic review and meta-analysis of randomized clinical trials. *Eur J Nutr.* 2012;51(2):127-134. doi:10.1007/s00394-011-0253-9
70. Song HJ, Grant I, Rotondo D, et al. Effect of CLA supplementation on immune function in young healthy volunteers. *Eur J Clin Nutr.* 2005;59(4):508-517. doi:10.1038/sj.ejcn.1602102
71. Asbaghi O, Ashtary-Larky D, Naseri K, et al. The effects of CLA supplementation on lipid profile in adults: A systematic review and dose-response meta-analysis. *Front Nutr.* 2022;9:953012. doi:10.3389/fnut.2022.953012
72. Orer GE, Guzel NA. The effects of acute l-carnitine supplementation on endurance performance of athletes. *J Strength Cond Res.* 2014;28(2):514-519. doi:10.1519/JSC.0b013e3182a76790
73. Mielgo-Ayuso J, Pietrantonio L, Viribay A, Calleja-González J, González-Bernal J, Fernández-Lázaro D. Effect of acute and chronic oral l-carnitine supplementation on exercise performance based on the exercise intensity: A systematic review. *Nutrients.* 2021;3;13(12):4359. doi:10.3390/nu13124359
74. Kraemer WJ, Volek JS, Dunn-Lewis C. l-Carnitine supplementation: influence upon physiological function. *Curr Sports Med Rep.* 2008;7(4):218-223. doi:10.1249/JSR.0b013e318180735c
75. Broad EM, Maughan RJ, Galloway S DR. Effects of exercise intensity and altered substrate availability on cardiovascular and metabolic responses to exercise after oral carnitine supplementation in athletes. *Int J Sport Nutr Exerc Metab.* 2011;21(5):385-397. doi:10.1123/ijsnem.21.5.385
76. Colombani P, Wenk C, Kunz I, et al. Effects of l-carnitine supplementation on physical performance and energy metabolism of endurance-trained athletes: a double-blind crossover field study. *J Appl Physiol Occup Physiol.* 1996;73(5):434-439. doi:10.1007/BF00334420

77. Calbet JA, Mooren FC, Burke LM, Stear SJ, Castell LM. A-Z of nutritional supplements: dietary supplements, sports nutrition foods and ergogenic aids for health and performance: part 24. *Br J Sports Med.* 2011;45(12):1005-1007. doi:10.1136/bjsports-2011-090397
78. Clegg ME. Medium-chain triglycerides are advantageous in promoting weight loss although not beneficial to exercise performance. *Int J Food Sci Nutr.* 2010;61(7):653-679. doi:10.3109/09637481003702114
79. Dunford M, Coleman EJ. Ergogenic aids, dietary supplements, and exercise. In: Rosenbloom C, Coleman EJ, eds. *Sports Nutrition : A Practice Manual for Professionals.* 5th ed. Academy of Nutrition and Dietetics; 2012:128-161.
80. St-Onge MP, Bosarge A. Weight-loss diet that includes consumption of medium-chain triacylglycerol oil leads to a greater rate of weight and fat mass loss than does olive oil. *Am J Clin Nutr.* 2008;87(3):621-626. doi:10.1093/ajcn/87.3.621
81. Burke LM, Kiens B, Ivy JL. Carbohydrates and fat for training and recovery. *J Sports Sci.* 2004;22(1):15-30. doi:10.1080/0264041031000140527
82. Ormsbee MJ, Bach CW, Baur DA. Pre-exercise nutrition: the role of macronutrients, modified starches and supplements on metabolism and endurance performance. *Nutrients.* 2014;6(5):1782-1808. doi:10.3390/nu6051782
83. Rehrer NJ, van Kemenade M, Meester W, Brouns F, Saris WH. Gastrointestinal complaints in relation to dietary intake in triathletes. *Int J Sport Nutr.* 1992;2(1):48-59. doi:10.1123/ijsn.2.1.48
84. Kapoor B, Kapoor D, Guatam S, Singh R, Bhardwaj S. Dietary polyunsaturated fatty acids (PUFAs): uses and potential health benefits. *Curr Nutr Rep.* 2021;10(3):232-242. doi:10.1007/s13668-021-00363-3
85. Filaire E, Massart A, Portier H, et al. Effect of 6 weeks of n-3 fatty-acid supplementation on oxidative stress in judo athletes. *Int J Sport Nutr Exerc Metab.* 2010;20(6):496-506. doi:10.1123/ijsnem.20.6.496
86. McAnulty SR, Nieman DC, Fox-Rabinovich M, et al. Effect of n-3 fatty acids and antioxidants on oxidative stress after exercise. *Med Sci Sports Exerc.* 2010;42(9):1704-1711. doi:10.1249/MSS.0b013e3181d85bd1
87. Mickleborough TD. Omega-3 polyunsaturated fatty acids in physical performance optimization. *Int J Sport Nutr Exerc Metab.* 2013;23(1):83-96. doi:10.1123/ijsnem.23.1.83
88. Heaton LE, Davis JK, Rawson ES, et al. Selected in-season nutritional strategies to enhance recovery for team sport athletes: a practical overview. *Sports Med.* 2017;47(11):2201-2218. doi:10.1007/s40279-017-0759-2
89. Innes JK, Calder PC. The differential effects of eicosapentaenoic acid and docosahexaenoic acid on cardiometabolic risk factors: a systematic review. *Int J Mol Med.* 2018;19(2):532. doi:10.3390/ijms19020532
90. Bloomer RJ, Larson DE, Fisher-Wellman KH, Galpin AJ, Schilling BK. Effect of eicosapentaenoic and docosahexaenoic acid on resting and exercise-induced inflammatory and oxidative stress biomarkers: a randomized, placebo controlled, cross-over study. *Lipids Health Dis.* 2009;8:36. doi:10.1186/1476-511x-8-36
91. Buckley JD, Burgess S, Murphy KJ, Howe PRC. DHA-rich fish oil lowers heart rate during submaximal exercise in elite Australian Rules footballers. *J Sci Med Sport.* 2009;12(4):503-507. doi:10.1016/j.jsams.2008.01.011
92. Nieman DC, Henson DA, McAnulty SR, Jin F, Maxwell KR. n-3 polyunsaturated fatty acids do not alter immune and inflammation measures in endurance athletes. *Int J Sport Nutr Exerc Metab.* 2009;19(5):536-546. doi:10.1123/ijsnem.19.5.536
93. Philpott JD, Witard OC, Galloway SR. Applications of omega-3 polyunsaturated fatty acid supplementation for sport performance. *Res Sports Med.* 2019;27(2):219-237. doi:10.1080/15438627.2018.1550401
94. Maughan RJ, Burke L, Dvorak J, et al. IOC consensus statement: dietary supplements and the high-performance athlete. *Br J Sports Med.* 2018;52(7):439-455. doi:10.1136/bjsports-2018-099199
95. Rossato LT, Schoenfeld B, de Oliveira EP. Is there sufficient evidence to supplement omega-3 fatty acids to increase muscle mass and strength in young and older adults? *Clin Nutr.* 2020;39(1):23-32. doi:10.1016/j.clnu.2019.01.001
96. Visconti LM, Cotter JA, Schick EE, et al. Impact of varying doses of omega-3 supplementation on muscle damage and recovery after eccentric resistance exercise. *Metabol Open.* 2021;12:100133. doi:10.1016/j.metop.2021.100133
97. Heileson JL, Anzalone AJ, Carbuhn AF, et al. The effect of omega-3 fatty acids on a biomarker of head trauma in NCAA football athletes: a multi-site, non-randomized study. *J Int Soc Sports Nutr.* 2021;18(1):65. doi:10.1186/s12970-021-00461-1
98. Close GL, Sale C, Baar K, Bermon S. Nutrition for the prevention and treatment of injuries in track and field athletes. *Int J Sport Nutr Exerc Metab.* 2019;29(2):189-197. doi:10.1123/ijsnem.2018-0290
99. Smith-Ryan A, Hirsch KR, Saylor HE, Gould LM, Blue MNM. Nutritional considerations and strategies to facilitate injury recovery and rehabilitation. *J Athl Train.* 2020;55(9):918-930. doi:10.4085/1062-6050-550-19
100. Goyens PLL, Spilker ME, Zock PL, Katan MB, Mensink RP. Conversion of α-linolenic acid in humans is influenced by the absolute amounts of α-linolenic acid and linoleic acid in the diet and not by their ratio. *Am J Clin Nutr.* 2006;84(1):44-53. doi:10.1093/ajcn/84.1.44
101. Nakamura MT, Nara TY. Structure, function, and dietary regulation of Δ6, Δ5, and Δ9 desaturases. *Annu Rev Nutr.* 2004;24:345-376. doi:10.1146/annurev.nutr.24.121803.063211
102. Jump DB, Depner CM, Tripathy S. Omega-3 fatty acid supplementation and cardiovascular disease. *J Lipid Res.* 2012;53(12):2525-2545. doi:10.1194/jlr.R027904

CHAPTER 5

Vitamins, Minerals, and Exercise

Stella Lucia Volpe, PhD, RDN, ACSM-CEP, FACSM, and Abby Gilman, PhD, RDN, LDN

LEARNING OBJECTIVES

- Review the Dietary Reference Intakes for vitamins and minerals.
- Describe the roles of vitamins and minerals within the body.
- Explain the specific and general roles of vitamins and minerals in exercise.
- Identify vitamins and minerals that have performance-enhancing effects on exercise.

INTRODUCTION

Micronutrients (vitamins and minerals) differ from macronutrients in that they are required in much smaller quantities; however, the use of macronutrients for all physiological processes is facilitated by micronutrients.[1-3] Vitamins and minerals are necessary for numerous metabolic processes in the body, including protein synthesis, cellular energy metabolism and storage, glucose metabolism, and fat metabolism, all of which are important in exercise and physical activity.[2-7]

Scientists and practitioners often debate the micronutrient needs of individuals who are physically active and those who exercise. Some researchers and practitioners have shown that individuals who exercise require more vitamins and minerals than those who do not exercise; however, not all research supports an increased need. The intensity, duration, and frequency of activity, as well as an individual's overall energy and nutrient intake, affect micronutrient requirements.[7-9] This chapter reviews the vitamin and mineral needs of those who are physically active and those who exercise.

DIETARY REFERENCE INTAKES

The recommended intakes of all known vitamins and some essential minerals for healthy, moderately active people were updated beginning in 1997.[10-13] Although Dietary Reference Intakes (DRIs) were updated for calcium and vitamin D in 2011, values for other vitamins and minerals have not been as recently updated.[14-17] Several related terms fall under the umbrella of the DRIs and are defined as follows:

- Recommended Dietary Allowance (RDA) is the dietary intake level that is adequate for approximately 98% of healthy people.
- Adequate Intake (AI) is an estimated value used when an RDA cannot be determined.

- Estimated average requirement (EAR) is used to approximate the nutrient needs of half of the healthy people in a group, from which an RDA is then established.[10]
- Tolerable Upper Intake Level (UL) is the highest amount of a nutrient that most people can consume without adverse effects.[11]

DRI tables have been published online by the National Academies of Sciences, Engineering, and Medicine (National Academies) (www.nationalacademies.org/hmd/Activities/Nutrition/SummaryDRIs/DRI-Tables.aspx).

In general, if the energy intakes of physically active individuals are adequate, their vitamin and mineral needs will typically be met; thus, the DRIs should be appropriate for their micronutrient needs. Some athletes may have increased requirements because of excessive losses of nutrients in sweat and urine, and these athletes may need supplementation. Because many physically active people choose to supplement with vitamins and minerals, practitioners may use ULs to give guidelines to those who take supplements to prevent adverse reactions from excess consumption.

The research on micronutrients for athletes has limitations. Many of the studies on micronutrients were conducted prior to 2000, calling into question their relevance today. Contradictory findings in the literature also make it difficult for practitioners to give definitive advice to athletes. Research limitations include small sample sizes, mostly cisgender male participants, differences in type of exercise performed or level of training and fitness, lack of strong longitudinal data, differences in assessment methodology or study design, and various types and amounts of supplements researched. In an effort to keep this chapter relevant, studies published prior to 2000 were not included unless they were considered seminal or no other studies have been published on that micronutrient.

VITAMINS AND MINERALS OF CONCERN DURING TRAINING

Exercise can affect vitamin and mineral requirements because of increased physiological demands and the stress of exercise. In addition, there may be increased losses of certain micronutrients (eg, sodium through sweat) and decreased absorption due to diminished gastrointestinal tract function during exercise. The level of alteration depends on the volume of training and competition. Studies have reported that 30% to 50% of athletes, in particular endurance athletes, experience some type of gastrointestinal upset. In addition, those who train more often and more intensely seem to report gastrointestinal upset the most. Nonetheless, little research has been conducted to identify long-term effects of gastrointestinal problems with exercise and micronutrient deficiency.[18]

The following sections review specific vitamins and minerals as they relate to energy metabolism, antioxidant function, bone health, red blood cell function, and immune health. The discussion of each micronutrient includes a review of background information, function, effects of exercise (if known), intake in athletes (if known), and intake recommendations. The information is summarized in Tables 5.1 through 5.4.

Energy Metabolism

Energy metabolism is the process of generating energy in the form of adenosine triphosphate (ATP) from nutrients. Energy metabolism is vital to life and is especially necessary during exercise. Interconnected pathways continuously produce energy with or without the presence of oxygen. Whereas macronutrients are metabolized to produce energy, micronutrients play a crucial supporting role in metabolic processes. This section focuses on the primary vitamins and minerals involved in energy metabolism as coenzymes and cofactors.

THIAMIN

Thiamin, also known as vitamin B1, is a water-soluble vitamin. In the body, 80% of thiamin is in the form of thiamin pyrophosphate (also known as thiamin diphosphate). Thiamin participates in several energy-producing reactions as part of thiamin pyrophosphate, including glycolysis, the Krebs cycle (citric acid cycle), branched-chain amino acid (BCAA) catabolism, and the pentose phosphate pathway. For example, thiamin is required to convert pyruvate to acetyl coenzyme A (CoA) during carbohydrate metabolism. Acetyl CoA is an important intermediate in fat, carbohydrate, and protein metabolism.[19] Thiamin also assists in the conversion of α-ketoglutarate into succinyl-CoA in the Krebs cycle, as well as in the decarboxylation of BCAAs, which increases with physical activity.[20,21] These conversions are all essential for the metabolism of glucose, BCAAs, fatty acids, and exercise performance. Health and performance may be impaired if these conversions do not occur.[2]

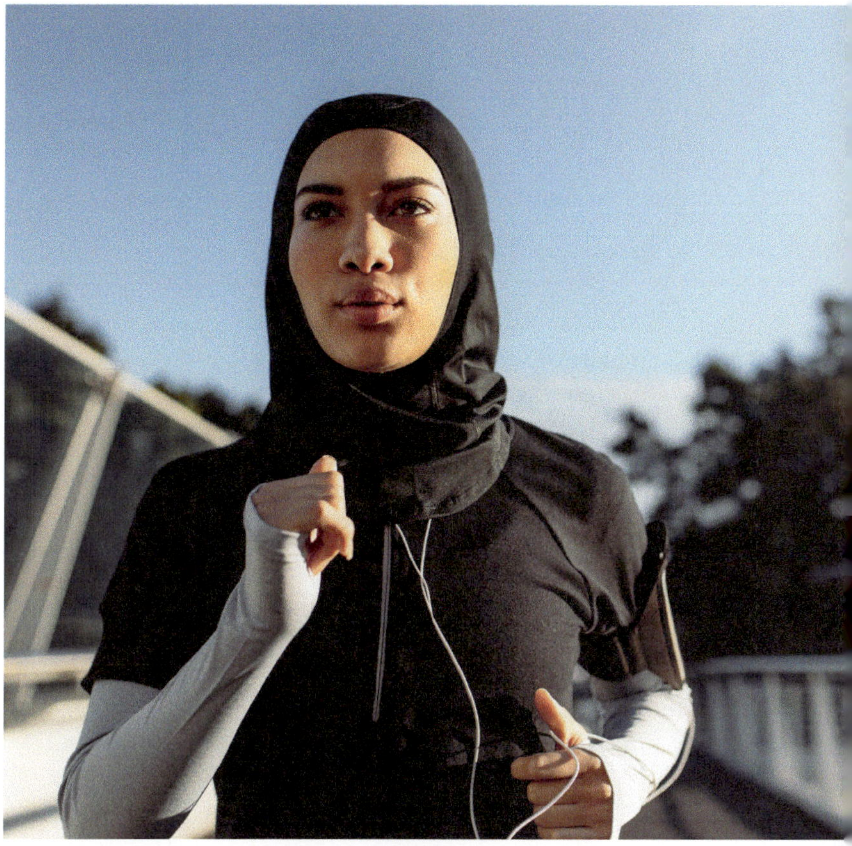

Researchers have not determined whether exercise results in an increase in thiamin excretion. Kim et al[22] showed that regular, moderate exercise training in rats elicited an increased urinary excretion of thiamin. However, this excretion was not significantly different ($P < .05$) from that of nonexercise-trained rats.

Although research on the effects of exercise on thiamin is limited, especially in human trials, Sato et al[23] conducted a cross-sectional study to evaluate the effect of high-intensity swim training on blood thiamin concentrations in 13 female and 6 male collegiate swimmers. The swimmers were assessed during a preparation period and an intensive training period. Whereas anthropometric variables and dietary intake did not change during the training period, energy expenditure increased significantly. In addition, blood thiamin concentrations decreased sharply during the intensive training period compared with the preparation period (38 ± 10 ng/mL vs 31 ± 5 ng/mL for females, $P = .004$; 41 ± 6 ng/mL vs 36 ± 3 ng/mL for males, $P = .048$). Although these results suggest that high-intensity training decreases blood thiamin concentrations, more research is required to determine whether thiamin requirements are greater in people who exercise.

Nichols et al[24] reported the thiamin intake of 105 female and 93 male collegiate and masters athletes. The researchers reported an average thiamin intake of 1.88 ± 0.50 mg/d (collegiate athletes) and 1.95 ± 0.40 mg/d (masters athletes), which is above the RDA of 1.0 and 1.2 mg/d for females and males, respectively, 14 years of age and older.[14]

Thiamin requirements may parallel the intensity, duration, and frequency of exercise, but because so little research has been conducted on thiamin and exercise, practitioners should not recommend thiamin intakes greater than the DRI for physically active people unless a thiamin deficiency has been determined. Dietary sources of thiamin are listed in Table 5.1 on page 94.

RIBOFLAVIN

Riboflavin, also known as vitamin B2, is a water-soluble vitamin involved in several key metabolic reactions that are important during exercise: glycolysis, the Krebs cycle, and the electron transport chain. Riboflavin is the precursor in the synthesis of the flavin coenzymes flavin mononucleotide and flavin adenine dinucleotide, which assist in oxidation-reduction reactions by acting as 1- and 2-electron transfers.[19]

Research has shown that initiating an exercise program may alter an individual's riboflavin status; however, it is unclear whether the effect is transient or long term.[19] Sato et al[23] reported no significant change in blood riboflavin concentrations in female and male collegiate swimmers during the offseason period compared with the intensive training period. This could indicate that, unlike thiamin, riboflavin is less susceptible to changes in exercise habits or that riboflavin status is unaltered entirely by exercise.

TABLE 5.1 Water-Soluble Vitamin Needs for Athletes and Respective Food Sources

Vitamin	Effect of exercise on requirements[a]	Recommended intake for athletes[b]	Food sources	Comments
Vitamin B6	Exercise does not cause transient changes in vitamin B6 status	RDA; supplementation may be necessary in the case of preexisting deficiencies	Liver, chicken, bananas, potatoes, spinach	
Vitamin B12	Exercise does not seem to increase vitamin B12 needs	RDA	Fish, milk and milk products, eggs, meat, poultry, fortified breakfast cereals	Vegan athletes will likely need to supplement to ensure adequate intake
Folate	Exercise does not seem to increase folate needs	RDA	Leafy greens (eg, spinach, turnip greens), dry beans, peas, fortified cereals, grain products, strawberries	
Thiamin	Exercise does not seem to increase thiamin needs	RDA; supplementation may be necessary in the case of preexisting deficiencies	Wheat germ, brewer's yeast, oysters, beef liver, peanuts, green peas, raisins, collard greens	Ergogenic effects are equivocal
Riboflavin	Exercise does not seem to increase riboflavin needs	RDA	Organ meats, milk, cheese, oily fish, eggs, dark green leafy vegetables	
Niacin	Exercise does not seem to increase niacin needs	RDA	Beef, pork, chicken, wheat flour, eggs, milk	Does not seem to have ergogenic effects
Pantothenic acid	Not enough information	AI	Eggs, sunflower seeds, mushrooms, peanuts, brewer's yeast, yogurt, broccoli, whole-grain cereals, meat	
Choline	Exercise does not seem to increase choline needs	AI	Liver, egg yolks, peanuts, cauliflower, soybeans, grape juice, cabbage	Does not seem to have ergogenic effects
Vitamin C	Increased vitamin C intakes may prevent infections of the upper respiratory tract	At least the DRI; ultraendurance athletes need more than the DRI, but less than the UL	Brussels sprouts, broccoli, chili peppers, bell peppers, kiwi, oranges, papaya, guava	Strong antioxidant properties reported for endurance and ultraendurance athletes

Abbreviations: AI, Adequate Intake; DRI, Dietary Reference Intake; RDA, Recommended Dietary Allowance; UL, Tolerable Upper Intake Level

[a] Unless noted otherwise, statements regarding the lack of an impact of exercise on specific nutrient needs rely solely on the limited data available at the time of publication.

[b] Summary tables are available online at the National Library of Medicine website (www.ncbi.nlm.nih.gov/books/NBK56068/table/summarytables.t2/?report=objectnly).

This research indicates that people who are physically active and consume adequate amounts of dietary riboflavin may not be at risk for depletion and may not require intakes higher than the RDA.

Hoffman et al[25] conducted a double-blind, placebo-controlled trial to evaluate whether riboflavin could decrease muscle soreness during and after a 161-km ultramarathon. The 32 runners were randomly assigned to receive either 100 mg riboflavin (18 runners) or placebo (95 mg maltodextrin and 5 mg 10% beta carotene) (14 runners) before the race and at 90 km during the race. Participants provided muscle pain and soreness ratings before, during, and immediately after the race and for the 10 subsequent days. Participants also completed 400-m runs at high intensity 3, 5, and 10 days after the race. The researchers reported that muscle pain and soreness ratings were significantly lower ($P = .043$) for the riboflavin-supplemented group during and after the race. In addition, those in the riboflavin group had significantly faster ($P < .05$) 400-m run times compared to the placebo group on days 3 and 5. Although this study was conducted on a small sample size, this research shows some promise for riboflavin as a potential ergogenic (performance-enhancing) aid. Nonetheless, more research is required before definitive conclusions can be made.

Nichols et al[24] reported the riboflavin intake of 105 female and 93 male collegiate and masters athletes. They found an average riboflavin intake of 1.98 ± 0.50 mg/d (collegiate athletes) and 2.06 ± 0.41 mg/d (masters athletes), which is greater than the RDAs of 1.0 and 1.3 mg/d for females and males, respectively, 14 years of age and older.[14] Deficiencies in riboflavin are uncommon in Western countries because it is found in a wide variety of foods; however, athletes who restrict their food intake for weight loss may be at greater risk for riboflavin deficiency. Dietary sources of riboflavin are listed in Table 5.1.

VITAMIN B6

The 3 major forms of vitamin B6 are pyridoxine, pyridoxal, and pyridoxamine. The active coenzyme forms of vitamin B6 are pyridoxal 5'-phosphate and pyridoxamine 5'-phosphate. Vitamin B6 is involved in approximately 100 metabolic reactions, including those involving gluconeogenesis, niacin synthesis, and lipid metabolism.[19] Pyridoxal 5'-phosphate is a required coenzyme of glycogen phosphorylase, the enzyme needed for glycogen metabolism.

Zhang et al[26] conducted a cross-sectional study to evaluate nutrient intake with various types of exercise in 217 women and 210 men, 21 to 35 years of age. Participants engaged in various types of exercise (endurance exercise, resistance training, walking, various sports). Exercise was self-reported, and 24-hour dietary intake was evaluated by telephone interviews. The researchers reported that resistance exercise was significantly and positively associated with intakes of vitamins B2, B3, B5, B6, and B12. In addition, only vitamin B6 intake was positively associated with time spent in aerobic exercise.[26] This research in physically active young adults indicates the need to ensure that they consume a varied diet and, in particular, be made aware of the importance of obtaining the appropriate amount of B vitamins. Endurance exercisers should be especially aware of their B6 intake.

The effects of maximal-effort exercise on vitamin B6 concentrations are unknown. Researchers found that vitamin B6 supplementation in conjunction with a maltodextrin supplement in elite mountain biking athletes during maximal-effort cycling significantly increased concentrations of available blood glucose compared with the results for the control group. Nonetheless, there was no significant difference in performance between the maltodextrin-supplemented group compared with the maltodextrin plus vitamin B6–supplemented group, suggesting that the maltodextrin provided the increased blood glucose concentrations.[27] Although supplementation with vitamin B6 has not been found to enhance glucose availability, it has been shown that poor vitamin B6 status can impair exercise performance.[28] Manore[29] reported that vitamin B6 plays a key role in producing energy during exercise, and therefore, those with an inadequate intake of vitamin B6 have a decreased ability to perform physical activity optimally. Considering the limited amount of research that has been conducted, it seems that individuals who exercise do not have increased needs for vitamin B6. However, Manore reported that work capacity improves as vitamin B6 status improves, whereas deficiencies of vitamin B6 negatively affect aerobic capacity. Therefore, if deficiencies exist, it may be necessary to supplement with vitamin B6 at the level of the DRI. It is worth noting that assessing vitamin B6 status is complicated. Ueland et al[30] stated that "[v]itamin B6 status is best assessed by using a combination of biomarkers because of the influence of potential confounders, such as inflammation, alkaline phosphatase activity, low serum albumin, renal function, and inorganic phosphate." Dietary sources of vitamin B6 are listed in Table 5.1.

NIACIN

Niacin, also known as vitamin B3, represents a family of molecules that includes nicotinic acid and nicotinamide. The coenzyme forms of niacin are nicotinamide adenine dinucleotide and nicotinamide adenine dinucleotide phosphate. Both are involved in glycolysis, the pentose phosphate pathway, the Krebs cycle, lipid synthesis, and the electron transport chain. Pharmacologic doses of nicotinic acid may also augment the use of carbohydrate as a substrate during exercise by decreasing the availability of free fatty acids. However, little research has been conducted on pharmacological doses (500–2,000 mg) of nicotinic acid with exercise. Trost et al[31] reported a reduction in free fatty acid concentrations in 5 male cyclists who cycled at 65% of their maximal oxygen consumption (VO_2 max) compared to a control trial. The cyclists were provided 500 mg of nicotinic acid prior to exercise and consumed 100 mg doses at 15, 30, and 45 minutes during exercise, as well as 30 minutes during recovery. These researchers noted that the free fatty acid blockade from nicotinic acid significantly reduced excess postexercise oxygen consumption. The researchers noted that their results emphasize the need for "increased free fatty acid metabolism during exercise and recovery."

Despite this strong connection to exercise metabolism, no solid data presently support increased niacin supplementation for individuals who exercise. Furthermore, pharmacologic doses of niacin can result in a "niacin flush," in which blood vessel dilation causes reddening of the face and extreme itching.[32] Athletes may take high doses of niacin thinking "more is better." However, taking too much niacin, as with taking too much of any vitamin or mineral, can be detrimental to both health and exercise performance.

Although niacin has not been shown to elicit ergogenic effects on exercise performance, Schaefer et al[33] evaluated whether supplementing mice who had the heart-muscle adenine nucleotide translocator isoform 1 (ANT1) mutation with nicotinamide riboside (a derivative of niacin) would improve exercise intolerance and muscle weakness (due to a mitochondrial disorder) associated with this mutation. They reported that nicotinamide riboside supplementation reduced exercise intolerance associated with the ANT1 mutation. Although this research was conducted in mice, it could indicate a therapeutic effect of niacin for those with mitochondrial disorders.

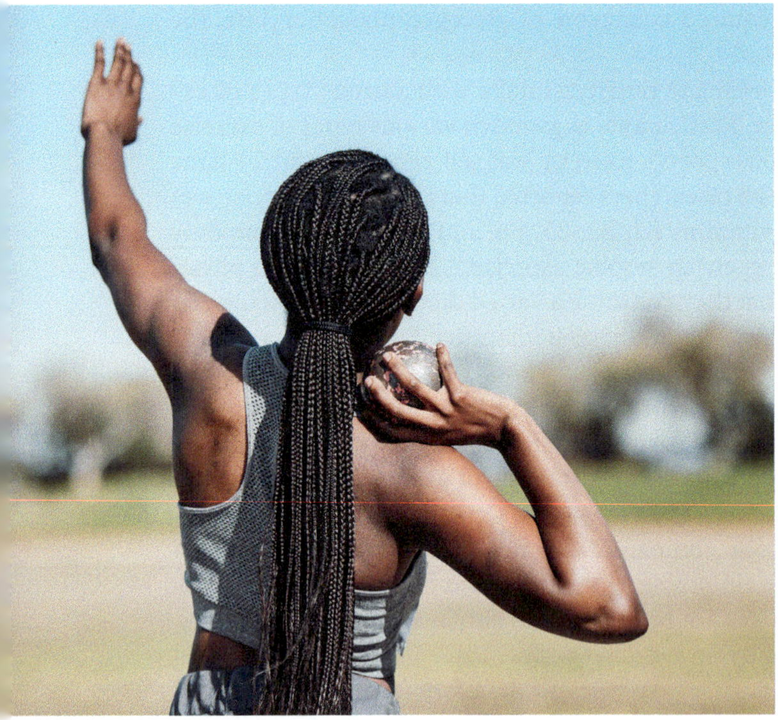

Nichols et al[25] reported the niacin intake of 105 female and 93 male collegiate and masters athletes. The researchers reported average niacin intake of 21.49 ± 5.13 mg/d (collegiate athletes) and 22.64 ± 4.19 mg/d (masters athletes), which is higher than the RDAs of 14 and 16 mg/d for females and males, respectively, 14 years of age and older.[14]

More research is needed to determine how niacin affects the depletion of glycogen stores and, therefore, its potential to indirectly affect performance.[1-6] It is important for people who exercise to obtain the DRI for niacin to ensure adequate intake and prevent alterations in fuel utilization, but they should not exceed the UL. Dietary sources of niacin are listed in Table 5.1 on page 94.

PANTOTHENIC ACID

Pantothenic acid, a water-soluble vitamin whose biologically active forms are CoA and acyl carrier protein, is involved in acyl group transfers, such as the acylation of amino acids.[14,34] Pantothenic acid coenzymes are also involved in lipid synthesis and metabolism, as well as the oxidation of pyruvate and α-ketoglutarate. Acetyl CoA is an important intermediate in fat, carbohydrate, and protein metabolism.[19]

Researchers have demonstrated that supplementation of D-pantothenic acid and L-cysteine does not affect fuel selection in the muscle or work output.[34] In 2021, Whitfield et al[35] evaluated whether daily supplementation of 6 g of pantothenic acid (vs a placebo) would increase muscle CoA concentrations, and thus exercise performance, in 14 trained male cyclists. The participants had to cycle incremental time to exhaustion, cycling at baseline and after 4, 8, and 16 weeks. Muscle biopsies were taken before and after each cycling exercise. The researchers did not find any change in muscle CoA concentrations or exercise performance as a result of pantothenic acid supplementation. Because little research has been conducted with pantothenic acid and exercise, it would be appropriate to suggest that athletes consume the AI for pantothenic acid. Dietary sources for pantothenic acid are listed in Table 5.1 on page 94.

CHOLINE AND BETAINE

Choline is an essential nutrient found in some foods, but it can also be provided as a supplement. Choline delivers methyl groups for several metabolic pathways in the body and is also required to synthesize phosphatidylcholine and sphingomyelin, 2 key phospholipids necessary for the integrity of cell membranes. Furthermore, choline is required for the synthesis of acetylcholine, a neurotransmitter needed for memory, mood, and muscle control. Choline is also required for muscle contraction.[14,36-39]

Blood choline concentrations have been reported to decrease after exercise, which may lead to a decrease in exercise performance. Warber et al[40] conducted a double-blind, crossover study to evaluate whether there is a relationship between plasma choline concentrations and exercise performance. Fourteen participants were given either a beverage containing 8.425 g of choline citrate or a placebo before and at 2 hours of a 4-hour treadmill exercise, in which they carried a 34.1-kg load at a treadmill speed of 5.6 km/h at 3% grade. After the treadmill test, the participants performed a run to exhaustion and squats. The researchers reported that plasma choline concentrations increased by 128% after the run to exhaustion only with the choline supplementation; no changes occurred with the placebo beverage. Despite the 128% increase in plasma choline concentrations, there were no changes in exercise performance with the choline supplementation.

Betaine, a metabolic derivative of choline widely found in many plant foods, acts similarly to choline (donating a methyl group in the same metabolic pathways), thus reducing the amount of choline required. Betaine supplementation may work as an ergogenic aid in improving power output.[41-43] Lee et al[42] conducted a randomized, double-blind, crossover study to determine whether betaine supplementation (1.25 g of betaine in a 300-mL sports drink) increased strength and power performance. Significant increases ($P < .05$) in force and power production were observed in the upper but not the lower body. Whereas Lee et al[42] found significant changes in force and power production in the upper body, Hoffman et al[43] reported that the effects of betaine supplementation (1.25 g of betaine mixed in a 240-mL sports drink) were more evident in the vertical jump than in the bench press throw. Although the research designs and measures varied, these studies provide a foundation for future research on betaine supplementation in athletes.

Soleimani et al[44] evaluated the interactive effects of dietary choline, betaine, and physical activity on creatine kinase, glycemic and metabolic markers, and body composition in 120 individuals, 18 to 35 years of age. They reported that increased dietary choline and betaine intakes were significantly related to increased ($P < .05$) waist-to-hip ratio, fat-free mass, and bone mass. They also reported that increased dietary betaine intake was related to decreased total cholesterol ($P = .032$) and increased high-density lipoprotein cholesterol (HDL-C) concentrations ($P = .049$). In addition, the researchers also reported that the interaction of dietary choline with physical activity was significantly related to improved insulin resistance ($P < .05$), whereas the interaction of betaine intake with physical activity increased HDL-C concentrations ($P = .049$). The combination of choline and betaine intake were found to interact with physical activity and lower fasting blood glucose concentrations.[44] The researchers demonstrated an interaction among choline, betaine, and physical activity that can lead to many improved metabolic outcomes. Because this was a cross-sectional study and no cause-and-effect conclusions can be made, more prospective research needs to be conducted to more definitely evaluate the effects of choline and betaine on metabolic outcomes.

Antioxidants and Oxidative Damage

Antioxidants are compounds that help counteract the damaging effects of free radicals in the body. Biological free radicals, most importantly reactive oxygen species and reactive nitrogen species, are compounds that contain 1 or more unpaired electrons that can react with various organic substrates, leading to tissue damage and contributing to chronic disease. Free radicals are endogenously produced through oxidation reactions such as energy metabolism; however, they are also created through exogenous sources, such as excess intake of micronutrients (eg, vitamins C and A) and exercise. Exercise type, mode, duration, and intensity all affect the amount of free radicals produced. When free-radical production overwhelms antioxidant availability, the resultant oxidation may decrease physical performance and health. It is important to note, however, that regular exercise and conditioning may lead to responses that adapt to the increased oxidative stress and prevent associated damage.[48-53] It is also important to note that many in vivo experiments use fruit and vegetable extracts to elucidate the effects of individual antioxidants. This can be misleading, because it may be the *combination* of various micronutrients and phytochemicals that contribute to the desired outcomes. Researchers often use combinations of vitamin and mineral supplements in their research; therefore, practitioners must use caution not to attribute individual outcomes to 1 antioxidant or micronutrient.[41,46]

VITAMIN C

Vitamin C, also referred to as ascorbic acid, ascorbate, or ascorbate monoanion, is a water-soluble vitamin involved in maintaining collagen synthesis, oxidizing fatty acids, and forming neurotransmitters. It is also an antioxidant.[15] Vitamin C protects against oxidative stress in endurance and ultraendurance athletes, especially in preventing upper respiratory tract infections.[54,55] Although aerobic exercise increases oxidative stress, it also increases enzymatic and nonenzymatic antioxidants as an adaptation to training.[48-53] Vitamin C concentrations in the blood can be increased for up to 24 hours after exercise, but they may decrease to below preexercise concentrations in the days following prolonged exercise. These changes might be a result of the increased oxidative stress that occurs with exercise. At present, there are few data to definitively establish whether regular exercise increases the metabolism of vitamin C. Thus, practitioners should exercise caution when plasma vitamin C concentrations are used as assessment parameters in research studies because they may not be truly reflective of status.[54,55] This phenomenon is fairly common for all antioxidants; therefore, researchers must be cognizant of their measurement techniques and timing.

Robson et al[56] reported significantly greater neutrophil oxidative activity following exercise after 7 days of supplementing athletes with an antioxidant combination of 900 mg of vitamin C, 18 mg of beta carotene, and 90 mg of vitamin E. Because the researchers also supplemented with beta carotene and vitamin E, a definitive effect of vitamin C cannot be determined.

Conversely, Gomez-Cabrera et al[57] reported that vitamin C supplementation delayed the positive changes associated with exercise in healthy sedentary men. They found that VO_2 max increased significantly (P = .019) after 8 weeks of training in both vitamin C–supplemented (1,000 mg/d) and nonsupplemented men. None of the expected changes associated with exercise, such as increased production of endogenous antioxidant enzymes, increased skeletal muscle protein concentrations, and increased protein concentration (indicative of mitochondrial adaptations) were seen in the supplemented men. These researchers presented conflicting evidence regarding the use of vitamin C in athletes.

Gabrial et al[58] evaluated the effects of supplementation with 500 mg of vitamin C compared to a placebo in 20 recreationally active male adolescents (who exercised 2–3 days per week) on muscle damage, oxidative stress, and inflammatory markers. After 90 days of supplementation, the individuals who supplemented with vitamin C had significantly lower (P < .05) concentrations of creatine kinase (muscle damage marker), lactate dehydrogenase (muscle damage marker), malondialdehyde (lipid peroxidation marker), and C-reactive protein (inflammatory marker) compared to the placebo group. Despite these positive results, evidence for vitamin C supplementation to support performance is still equivocal. Thus, athletes should not consume vitamin C beyond the DRI. Vitamin C also plays a role in the immune system and is discussed again in that respect later in this chapter. Dietary sources of vitamin C are listed in Table 5.1 on page 94.

VITAMIN E

Vitamin E refers to a family of 8 related fat-soluble compounds consisting of 4 tocopherols and 4 tocotrienols. Like vitamin C, vitamin E is well known for its antioxidant function in preventing free-radical damage to cell membranes. Vitamin E also plays a role in immune function.[15] Researchers have reported that vitamin E intakes were lower than intakes of other antioxidants in female figure skaters and heptathletes, as well as female and male rowers.[59,60]

Because athletes have reported low dietary intakes of vitamin E, supplementation may be beneficial in reducing exercise-induced oxidative stress.[28,59,60] Garelnabi et al[61] determined how vitamin E supplementation affects VO_2 max, oxidative stress, and lipid profile during short-duration, moderate-intensity activity. They randomly assigned 455 healthy participants into 2 groups: those receiving a placebo and those supplemented with 80 IU of vitamin E. The participants engaged in moderate aerobic exercise for at least 30 minutes per day, 3 times per week for 8 weeks. The researchers determined that myeloperoxidase (MPO), a protein released after oxidation of low-density lipoprotein cholesterol, increased in both the supplemented and placebo groups following the exercise regimen. MPO concentrations generally drop to clinically normal concentrations over time after oxidative stress; however, the vitamin E–supplemented participants had MPO concentrations that remained high after the 8-week intervention.

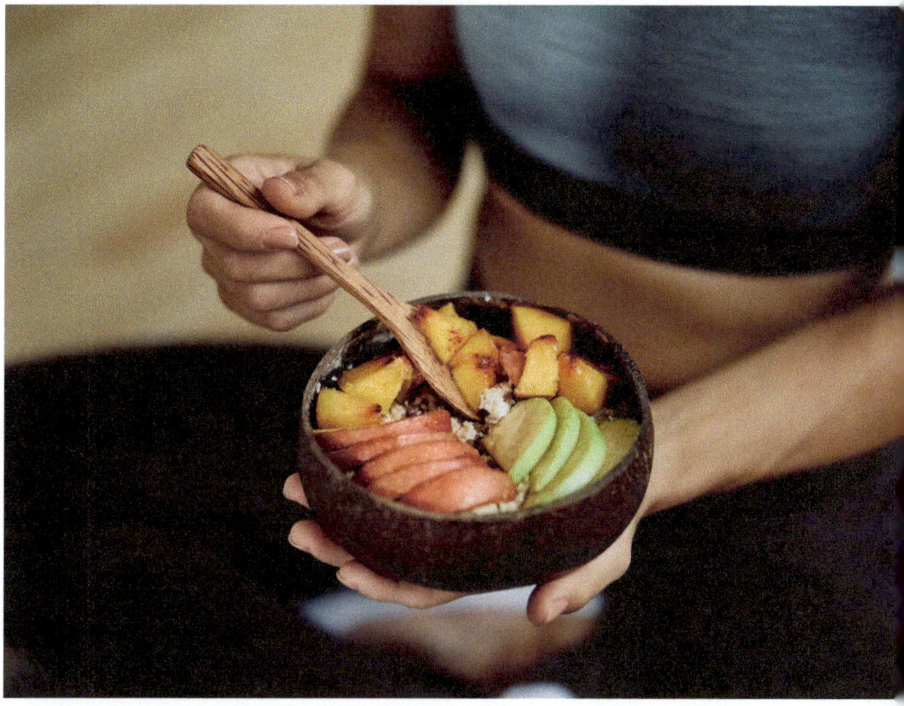

Antioxidant combination therapies are frequently tested to assess their additive effects. Bryant et al[62] examined different doses and combinations of antioxidant supplements in 7 trained male cyclists (approximately 22 years of age) who participated in 4 separate supplementation phases. They ingested 2 capsules per day containing the following treatments: placebo (placebo plus placebo), vitamin C (1 g/d plus placebo), vitamins C and E (vitamin C at 1 g/d plus vitamin E at 200 IU/kg of body weight), and vitamin E (400 IU/kg of body weight plus placebo). The researchers found that vitamin E alone was more effective at reducing the concentration of malondialdehyde, a marker of oxidative damage, than the other treatments.

In 2023, Sarkar et al[63] evaluated the effects of 8 weeks of supplementation with vitamins C and E on changes in lipid profile and hematological variables after high-intensity interval training (HIIT) in 49 Indian male football (soccer) players and 57 field hockey players, 15 to 16 years of age. They randomly assigned the 106 players into 5 groups: control (no exercise plus placebo), HIIT (placebo), HIIT plus 1,000 mg of vitamin C per day, HIIT plus 400 IU of vitamin E per day, and HIIT plus vitamins C and E. Supervised HIIT was conducted 3 times per week. The researchers found that supplementation with vitamins C and E, both individually and in combination, resulted in an improved lipid profile, decreased hemolysis, and improved inflammatory blood markers. However, vitamins C and E did not provide improved aerobic capacity in this group of male adolescent athletes. Despite their positive results, Sarkar et al stated that athletes should consider supplementation with vitamins C and E only if they have a deficiency or severe oxidative stress.

The effects of vitamin E supplementation on resistance training performance are still unknown. Avery et al[64] assessed the effects of vitamin E at a dose of 1,200 IU/d in comparison with a placebo on the recovery responses to repeated bouts of resistance training. No significant differences were found in muscle soreness, exercise performance, or plasma malondialdehyde concentrations between the group taking the vitamin E supplement and the placebo group.

Stepanyan et al[65] reported that vitamin E supplementation did not provide significant protection against lipid peroxidation or muscle damage from exercise. They stated that "[t]he complex antioxidant nature of tocopherols and low accumulation rates in muscle tissues could underlie an absence of protective effects." Long-term research is needed to assess the effects of vitamin E supplementation on oxidative stress from exercise. Dietary sources of vitamin E are listed in Table 5.2 on page 100.

TABLE 5.2 Fat-Soluble Vitamin Needs for Athletes and Respective Food Sources

Vitamin	Effect of exercise on requirements[a]	Recommended intake for athletes[b]	Food sources	Comments
Vitamin A	Exercise may increase vitamin A needs; results equivocal	RDA	Carrots, broccoli, tomatoes	Although vitamin A can be an antioxidant, intakes greater than the DRI may result in adverse effects in athletes
Vitamin D	Exercise does not seem to increase vitamin D needs	RDA; higher intakes may be needed in the winter if living in northern states (to prevent bone loss)	Oily fish; liver; eggs; fortified foods such as margarine, breakfast cereals, bread, milk, and powdered milk	
Vitamin E	Exercise may increase vitamin E needs	RDA	Plant oils (eg, soybean, corn, olive oils), nuts, seeds, wheat germ	Strong antioxidant effects in endurance athletes and older athletes
Vitamin K	Exercise does not seem to increase vitamin K needs	AI	Leafy green vegetables (eg, spinach, turnip greens), cabbage, green tea, alfalfa, oats, cauliflower	Increased intakes may be needed for bone formation

Abbreviations: AI, Adequate Intake; DRI, Dietary Reference Intake; RDA, Recommended Dietary Allowance

[a] Unless noted otherwise, statements regarding the lack of impact of exercise on specific nutrient needs rely solely on the limited data available at the time of publication.

[b] Summary tables are available online at the National Library of Medicine website (www.ncbi.nlm.nih.gov/books/NBK56068/table/summarytables.t2/?report=objectnly).

VITAMIN A

Vitamin A, which comprises a subset of retinoids, is a fat-soluble vitamin best known for the role it plays in vision. Other important functions of vitamin A include its roles in cellular differentiation, reproduction, gestation, fetal development, and bone formation; it also serves as an antioxidant (as beta carotene, a vitamin A precursor). Plants can synthesize carotenoids, which can serve as precursors of vitamin A; however, humans and other animals convert carotenoids into retinol or acquire preformed vitamin A from animal foods or supplements.[66] Assessments of vitamin A intake in individuals who are physically active have shown varied results, likely because the sources of vitamin A (plant vs animal) were not specified.[28,66]

Vitamin A antioxidant status may alleviate the oxidative load associated with endurance training. Braakhuis et al[60] analyzed how the intake of antioxidants, including that of vitamin A, and training status affect total antioxidant capacity (TAC) in competitive rowers. TAC measures how well a biological sample (or food product) can reduce an oxidant and is measured in units of the number of moles of radicals neutralized per gram of tested sample. The researchers found that blood TAC was correlated with total dietary antioxidant intake (correlation factor, $r = 0.29$; 90% ± 0.27% confidence limit). A negative association was also observed between the degree of training and TAC. This association was also reported between vitamin A intake and TAC, but to a much lesser extent. These results indicate that, although dietary intake of vitamin A is correlated with the TAC of an individual, exercise training has a stronger influence on increasing the TAC.[60]

Aguiló et al[67] reported decreased blood concentrations of beta carotene in well-trained professional cyclists after a 170-km endurance cycling bout, but this effect was not found in amateur cyclists. Nonetheless, daily vitamin A (as beta carotene) supplementation (50,000 IU) for 60 days (in combination with supplementation with 1,000 mg vitamin C and 200 mg vitamin E) was shown to be effective in decreasing the oxidative response after a 45-minute bout of cycling at 70% of VO_2 max in untrained, healthy people. As with other studies in which researchers combined antioxidants, it is difficult to determine whether any 1 vitamin had a greater effect than another. In general, athletes are encouraged to consume fruits and vegetables containing beta carotene; however, supplementation is not recommended.

Nichols et al[24] reported the vitamin A intake of 105 female and 93 male collegiate and masters athletes. The researchers reported average daily vitamin A intake of 859.3 ± 130.37 mcg retinol activity equivalents (RAE) (collegiate athletes) and 992.14 ± 106.88 mcg RAE (masters athletes), which is greater than the RDAs of 700 and 900 mcg RAE/d for females and males, respectively, 14 years of age and older.[16]

Because vitamin A is a fat-soluble vitamin that is stored in the body, athletes should not exceed the UL. Furthermore, athletes should be aware that, of all the fat-soluble vitamins, vitamin A is the most toxic. Table 5.2 on page 100 lists some dietary sources of vitamin A. Vitamin A is further discussed later in this chapter in terms of its relationship to bone health.

SELENIUM

Selenium is a trace mineral well known for its role as an antioxidant in the body (eg, as a component of the metalloenzyme glutathione peroxidase). Selenium is a crucial constituent of selenoproteins, which also play significant roles in antioxidant defense.[68] Selenium also functions to maintain normal thyroid hormone metabolism.[4-7] Limited data are available about whether people who exercise require more selenium than those who are sedentary.

Researchers have reported that supplementation with 150 mcg of selenium, combined with 2,000 IU of retinol, 120 mg of ascorbic acid, and 30 IU of α-tocopherol, increased total plasma antioxidant status after exercise.[68] However, as stated previously, when micronutrients are combined for supplementation, it is difficult to delineate the effects of 1 single micronutrient.

Fernandez-Lazaro et al[68] conducted a systematic review of the effect of selenium supplementation on athletic performance and various biomarkers in physically active populations. They found that selenium supplementation at levels of 180 or 240 mcg/d (as selenomethionine) or 200 mcg/d (as sodium selenite) significantly decreased lipid peroxide concentrations and increased glutathione peroxidase concentrations in plasma, erythrocyte, and muscle. They reported that selenium supplementation did not have significant effects on athletic performance, testosterone concentrations, or muscle damage markers (creatine kinase).

Because few data are available and excess selenium is toxic, individuals who exercise should consume no more than the DRI for selenium and should never exceed the UL. The selenium content of food can vary greatly with the soil content. Good sources of selenium are listed in Table 5.3 on page 102.

SULFUR

Sulfur is a mineral present in the body in a nonionic form and is a constituent of some vitamins (eg, thiamin and biotin), some amino acids (eg, methionine and cysteine), and some proteins. Sulfur also helps maintain the acid-base balance in the blood. If protein needs are met, sulfur is not required in the diet because it is present in protein foods.[4-8]

Sulfur is part of several proteins; therefore, the small body of research examining its effects on exercise performance is limited to sulfur-containing amino acids. Research has established that dietary sulfur-containing amino acids affect glutathione synthesis; however, their acute effects under conditions of oxidative stress, such as exercise, are not known. Aoi et al[69] investigated the effects of oral glutathione supplementation on muscle metabolism and fatigue in mice and humans. They reported that all mice (both those supplemented with glutathione and the control group) had significantly reduced interstitial pH levels in muscle following exercise ($P < .001$). However, the mice supplemented with glutathione had significantly higher serum pH levels ($P < .05$) than those in the control group, demonstrating an

TABLE 5.3 Trace Mineral Needs for Athletes and Respective Food Sources

Mineral	Effect of exercise on requirements[a]	Recommended intake for athletes[b]	Food sources	Comments
Copper	Exercise does not seem to increase copper needs	RDA	Red meat, fish, soy products, mushrooms, sweet potatoes	
Fluoride	Exercise does not seem to increase fluoride needs	AI	Fluoridated water, fish, tea	
Iodide	Exercise does not seem to increase iodide needs	RDA	Eggs, milk, strawberries, mozzarella cheese, cantaloupe	
Iron	Exercise may increase iron requirements	RDA; may need more in the case of preexisting iron depletion or iron deficiency anemia	Clams, red meat, oysters, egg yolks, salmon, tofu, raisins, whole grains, legumes, leafy greens	May have an ergogenic effect in the case of iron depletion or iron deficiency anemia; may impact thyroid hormone function in the case of iron deficiency
Manganese	Exercise does not seem to increase manganese needs	RDA	Liver, kidneys, wheat germ, legumes, nuts, black tea	
Selenium	Despite antioxidant properties, exercise does not seem to increase selenium needs	RDA	Fish, meat, poultry, cereal, grains, mushrooms, asparagus, Brazil nuts	
Zinc	Exercise does not seem to increase zinc needs; however, transient losses are often observed	RDA	Oysters, red meat, poultry, fish, wheat germ, fortified cereals, legumes	May have ergogenic effects, but not definitive; may impact thyroid hormone function if zinc deficient

Abbreviations: AI, Adequate Intake; RDA, Recommended Dietary Allowance

[a] Unless noted otherwise, statements regarding the lack of impact of exercise on specific nutrient needs rely solely on the limited data available at the time of publication.

[b] Summary tables are available online at the National Library of Medicine website (www.ncbi.nlm.nih.gov/books/NBK545442/table/appJ_tab3/?report=objectonly).

improved pH-buffering system in the muscle, which may lead to improved performance. These results were also replicated in human participants. After glutathione supplementation, participants who performed an exercise bout exhibited a decrease in intermuscular pH following exercise. This was shown by increased blood lactate concentrations following exercise. The participants who were supplemented reported significantly improved ratings of perceived exertion ($P < .05$), a psychological parameter of fatigue, compared with the placebo group. Additional research is needed to validate these results before recommendations may be warranted.

Kovacs et al[70] evaluated the blood sulfur concentrations in 26 Brazilian amateur male runners, 18 to 36 years of age, compared to an age-matched control group. The blood sulfur concentrations were 44% higher in athletes compared to the control group, likely due to the runners consuming high amounts of sulfated amino acids in their diets. Athletes should be cautioned not to consume sulfated amino acids and other foods high in sulfur in excess, because doing so could result in toxicity.

Those who consume appropriate amounts of complete protein in their diet will most probably be consuming adequate amounts of sulfur. Vegans can combine grains and legumes to obtain all of the essential amino acids. Refer to Table 5.4 on pages 104 and 105 for dietary sources of sulfur.

MANGANESE

Manganese is a trace mineral and an essential cofactor for many enzymes in the body. Manganese plays an essential role as an antioxidant as part of superoxide dismutase.[2] Data do not show that people who exercise require more manganese in their diet nor that manganese contributes as an ergogenic aid. However, Maynar et al[71] reported that moderate- and high-intensity exercise significantly decreased erythrocyte manganese concentrations in 24 moderately trained athletes and 22 professional cyclists who were about 23 years of age. The researchers stated that monitoring erythrocyte concentrations of manganese (and other minerals) in athletes would be prudent. Nonetheless, because of a lack of current research and an unknown risk of toxicity, athletes should not increase manganese consumption. Dietary sources of manganese are listed in Table 5.3 on page 102.

Bone Health and Development in Athletes

Bone health is critical for the health and physical performance of athletes. Bone is capable of being resorbed and remodeled in response to hormonal and mechanical changes. Weight-bearing exercise and hormonal activity determine the quantity and location of resorption and reformation. Certain minerals and vitamins are crucial for bone health and development.

CALCIUM

Calcium is the fifth most common element in the human body.[10] Ninety-nine percent of calcium exists in bones and teeth, and the remaining 1% is distributed in extracellular fluids, intracellular structures, cell membranes, and various soft tissues.[1-3,10,28] The major functions of calcium in the body include bone metabolism, blood coagulation, neuromuscular excitability, cellular adhesiveness, transmission of nerve impulses, maintenance and functionality of cell membranes, and activation of enzymatic reactions and hormonal secretions.[28]

Calcium Homeostasis Serum calcium concentrations are tightly controlled within a range of 8.8 to 10.0 mg/dL (2.2 to 2.5 mmol/L) by the calcitotropic hormones parathyroid hormone (PTH), vitamin D, and calcitonin.[1-3,10,28] When serum calcium concentrations decrease below 8.8 mg/dL, PTH responds by increasing the synthesis of calcitriol (the most active form of vitamin D) in the kidneys.[28] Calcitriol responds by increasing calcium reabsorption in the kidneys, increasing calcium absorption in the intestines, and increasing osteoclastic activity in the bone (releasing calcium from the bone into circulation and decreasing bone mineral density). When serum calcium concentrations are greater than 10 mg/dL, the hormone calcitonin responds by increasing renal excretion of calcium, decreasing calcium absorption in the intestines, and increasing osteoblastic activity by placing more calcium into the bone.[10,28]

TABLE 5.4 Major Mineral Needs for Athletes and Respective Food Sources

Mineral	Effect of exercise on requirements[a]	Recommended intake for athletes[b]	Food sources	Comments
Calcium	Individuals who consistently exercise in the heat may have greater calcium needs	RDA; those who exercise in the heat should consume more than the DRI but less than the UL	Milk, cheese, yogurt, tofu processed with calcium, kale, almonds, collard greens, spinach, canned salmon with bones, bok choy, soy milk fortified with calcium	Higher calcium intakes may also be related to fat loss; important for athletes in sports with weight categories or aesthetic sports (eg, wrestling, gymnastics, lightweight rowers, jockeys)
Chloride	Exercise typically results in increased chloride needs, especially for those who exercise in the heat	AI	Foods with high sodium; also found in salt substitutes with potassium chloride	
Magnesium	Exercise does not seem to increase magnesium needs; however, those exercising in hot environments may require more magnesium	AI	Peanuts, tofu, broccoli, spinach, Swiss chard, tomato paste, nuts, seeds, pulses, legumes, whole grains	No ergogenic effects established
Phosphorus	Exercise does not seem to increase phosphorus needs	RDA	Oranges, bananas, tomatoes, sardines, flounder, salmon, potatoes, beans, blackstrap molasses, milk	No ergogenic effects observed at this time
Potassium	Exercise does not seem to increase potassium needs; however, individuals with a high sweat rate may require more potassium	RDA	Oranges, bananas, tomatoes, sardines, flounder, salmon, potatoes, beans, blackstrap molasses, milk	No ergogenic effects observed at this time

Mineral	Effect of exercise on requirements[a]	Recommended intake for athletes[b]	Food sources	Comments
Sodium	Exercise typically results in increased sodium needs, especially for those who exercise in the heat and who sweat a lot of salt	AI	Bread, milk, beets, celery, carrots, spinach, chard, lean meats	
Sulfur	Exercise does not seem to increase sulfur needs	RDA; vegans need to ensure that they consume adequate sulfur	Garlic, legumes, nuts, seeds, red meat, eggs, asparagus	

Abbreviations: AI, Adequate Intake; DRI, Dietary Reference Intake; RDA, Recommended Dietary Allowance; UL, Tolerable Upper Intake Level.

[a] Unless noted otherwise, statements regarding the lack of impact of exercise on specific nutrient needs rely solely on the limited data available at the time of publication.

[b] Summary tables are available online at the National Library of Medicine website (www.ncbi.nlm.nih.gov/books/NBK545442/table/appJ_tab3/?report=objectonly)

Average Calcium Intakes Although serum calcium concentrations are easy to identify, precise levels of calcium intake are more difficult to determine. Serum calcium concentrations do not accurately correlate with calcium intake, primarily because of poor precision in dietary records and varying amounts of calcium in foods. Both teenage and adult females tend to consume less calcium than teenage and adult males.[2,6,72] Female athletes older than 50 years of age consume approximately 79% of the recommended intake.[73,74]

Although calcium's relationship to bone has been well documented, Zamboni et al[75] assessed self-reported calcium intake and bone mineral density among mountain bike cyclists (n = 30), road cyclists (n = 39), and controls (n = 27). They reported that calcium intake was not related to bone mineral density; however, this was a cross-sectional study, and thus, only a relationship was reported.

Physically active individuals should strive to consume at least the DRI for calcium. Barry et al[76] sought to disrupt the exercise-induced calcium homeostasis through calcium supplementation in 20 healthy adult male endurance-trained cyclists and triathletes. Participants consumed either a calcium-fortified sports drink (100 mg/L) or placebo. The researchers measured exercise-induced increases in PTH, a response to calcium loss. The athletes who consumed the calcium-supplemented drink before exercise had attenuated concentrations of PTH relative to those who consumed the placebo ($P = +.04$); however, this change was not observed when calcium was supplemented during or after exercise.

More recently, Lundy et al[77] conducted a study in 16 elite Australian male rowers in a randomized crossover design, 1 week apart, where the rowers consumed either 1,000 mg of calcium prior to the row or less than 10 mg of calcium (control) prior to each exercise session. During each session, the athletes rowed on a rowing ergometer for 90 minutes, with a 150-minute rest, before a second 90-minute row. They reported that consumption of calcium-rich foods prior to exercise significantly decreased bone turnover markers ($P < .0001$). The researchers stated that "[s]uch practical strategies may be integrated into the athlete's overall sports nutrition plan, with the potential to safeguard long-term bone health and reduce the risk of bone stress injuries."

Barry et al[76] and Lundy et al[77] have shown the importance of preexercise calcium consumption for bone health. Thus, strong consideration should be given to encouraging athletes to consume foods that are higher in calcium preexercise.

Calcium and Body Weight Calcium has been studied for its possible effects on decreasing body weight.[78,79] This could be of significant value, especially for athletes in sports in which body weight is a concern (eg, wrestlers, jockeys, gymnasts, figure skaters, lightweight rowers). Results from numerous research studies on calcium and weight loss have been equivocal. Some of the first studies on calcium and weight loss were conducted in animals. Since then, others have reported that increased calcium intake is associated with weight loss and increased fat oxidation in humans as well.[78-85] In a cross-sectional study, Huang et al[81] reported that dietary calcium intake, but not elemental calcium from supplements, had beneficial effects for maintaining body composition and abdominal obesity. Others have reported similar results for calcium intake and decreases in body weight in adults. For example, Skinner et al[82] reported that higher calcium intakes correlated with a lower percentage body fat in healthy White women and men 18 to 28 years of age. Zhu et al[83] reported that 12 weeks of daily supplementation with 600 mg of elemental calcium and 125 IU of vitamin D resulted in a significantly greater reduction in fat mass compared to placebo ($P = .02$). Although there were no significant differences in body weight between the supplemental and placebo groups, the calcium plus vitamin D group had significantly lower visceral fat mass compared to the placebo group ($P < .05$).[83]

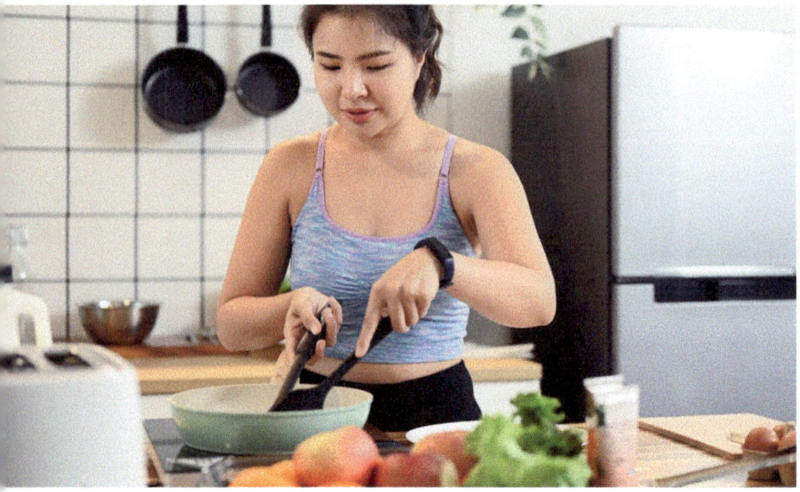

These results indicate a positive relationship between calcium intake and improved body composition; however, many researchers have failed to confirm this relationship.[86-89] For example, Palacios et al[86] conducted a 21-week randomized trial in 30 Puerto Rican adults (21–50 years of age) who were obese to determine the connection between dairy calcium intake/calcium supplementation and changes in body composition. The participants were randomized into 3 groups receiving 1 of the following interventions: high dietary dairy intake (about 1,300 mg of calcium per day) through the consumption of 4 servings of dairy products per day in place of other food groups, high elemental calcium (about 1,300 mg of calcium per day) from a combination of dietary dairy intake (about 700 mg of calcium per day) and a daily calcium carbonate supplement (600 mg), or a control group instructed to consume their usual diet. All participants were instructed to consume an isoenergetic diet throughout the intervention to prevent restricted energy intake from influencing changes in body composition. Although calcium intake increased throughout the trial in the 2 intervention groups, the researchers found no significant differences among the groups in body weight ($P = .77$), BMI ($P = .71$), total lean body mass ($P = .85$), or total body fat mass ($P = .71$), indicating that the type of calcium consumed (elemental supplement or dietary) does not significantly affect weight and body composition outcomes.[86]

Sources of Calcium The type of calcium consumed may not influence body weight and composition; however, the source of the dietary calcium consumed does affect bioavailability. Dairy sources and green vegetables with low amounts of oxalic acid (eg, bok choy, broccoli, cabbage, kale, and turnip greens) have the highest bioavailable form of calcium (about 30% absorption of calcium or higher). Vegetables with high amounts of oxalic acid (eg, spinach, collard greens, sweet potatoes, rhubarb, and beans) have only about 5% absorption of calcium. However, consuming a wide variety of foods will likely result in few or no nutritional concerns.[10,90]

If an individual is not consuming enough dietary calcium, experts recommend supplementation with calcium citrate or calcium carbonate because of the increased bioavailability of these supplements. Calcium supplements are best absorbed when taken in doses of 500 mg or less and when taken with meals. Thus, if a person requires 1,000 mg of calcium per day in the form of supplements, taking 500 mg in the morning and 500 mg in the evening would enhance absorption. Calcium supplements should be taken with vitamin D (contained within the supplement or separately) because adequate vitamin D status ensures maximal calcium absorption.[91,92]

Although a conclusive recommendation regarding calcium intake to maintain body composition has not been determined through research, it would be prudent to encourage athletes to consume the DRI for calcium through food to maintain bone health and integrity. Factors affecting calcium absorption are discussed later in this chapter. Various sources of calcium are listed in Table 5.4 on pages 104 and 105.

VITAMIN D

Vitamin D is considered both a hormone or secosteroid and a fat-soluble vitamin. Its well-established roles in maintaining calcium homeostasis and in bone remodeling are discussed later in this chapter.

Vitamin D Synthesis The best form of vitamin D is obtained from sunlight by which 7-dehydrocholesterol is converted into previtamin D3 in the skin. Conversion of vitamin D to its more active forms begins in the liver, where 25-α-hydroxylase adds a hydroxyl (OH) group to the 25th position on vitamin D to form 25-hydroxyvitamin D or calcidiol. The second hydroxylation of vitamin D occurs in the kidney, where 1-α-hydroxylase adds another hydroxyl group to the first position of calcidiol to form 1,25-dihydroxyvitamin D3, also known as calcitriol, the most active form of vitamin D. Although calcitriol is the most active form of vitamin D, concentrations of calcidiol are used to measure vitamin D status because it has a longer half-life than calcitriol. In addition, calcidiol better reflects vitamin D from dietary intake and supplements, as well as vitamin D synthesized in the body.[7,10,93]

Vitamin D Status It is important to note that researchers and clinicians do not all agree on the cutoff points for vitamin D sufficiency and insufficiency. According to the Endocrine Society's clinical guidelines, calcidiol concentrations of at least 30 ng/mL (≥75 nmol/L) are defined as sufficient. In addition, calcidiol concentrations of 21 to 29 ng/mL (52.5–72.5 nmol/L) are considered insufficient, and concentrations of 20 ng/mL or less (≤50 nmol/L) are considered deficient.[92] The Food and Nutrition Board of the Institute of Medicine (now the National Academy of Medicine)[10] assessed that calcidiol concentrations of less than 12 ng/mL (<30 nmol/L) are associated with rickets (in infants and children) and osteomalacia (in adults). Calcidiol concentrations ranging from 12 to less than 20 ng/mL (from 30 to <50 nmol/L) are "generally considered inadequate for bone and overall health in healthy individuals." Calcidiol concentrations of 20 ng/mL or higher (≥50 nmol/L) are considered "adequate for bone and overall health in healthy individuals," whereas concentrations higher than 50 ng/mL (>125 nmol/L) would be considered toxic. Thus, when reviewing the literature on vitamin D, it is important for practitioners to be aware that different cutoff values are used to assess deficiency. This makes it difficult to definitively ascertain the true prevalence of vitamin D deficiency in athletes and nonathletes around the world.

Vitamin D deficiency is fairly widespread, and certain people may be at higher risk for developing deficiencies. For example, individuals 65 years of age and older are at high risk for developing vitamin D deficiency, possibly because of low sunlight exposure from decreased time outdoors, decreased ability of older skin to synthesize vitamin D, or lower intake of dietary vitamin D.[94] In addition, those who live at or north of 42° latitude (eg, the northern United States and Canada) may require more vitamin D during the winter months to prevent increases in PTH secretion and decreased bone mineral density.[95] Kroll et al[96] used laboratory results (from the Quest Diagnostic database) to retrospectively determine the weekly mean concentrations of calcidiol and PTH of nearly 3.8 million adults from 20 to 99 years of age. The researchers reported variations in vitamin D status for women and men that changed seasonally; the highest vitamin D concentrations were reported in September and the lowest in March. The researchers also reported vitamin D deficiencies, even in those taking vitamin D supplements.

Close et al[97] evaluated the serum vitamin D concentration of 61 athletes based in the United Kingdom who did not supplement with vitamin D and compared them with the results for 30 age-matched healthy controls. The researchers reported that 62% of the athletes and 73% of the healthy controls had serum calcidiol concentrations of less than 50 nmoL/L (<20 ng/mL). These data further support the idea that living in northern latitudes (53° latitude in the northern United Kingdom) resulted in low calcidiol concentrations. The high percentage of participants, athletes and nonathletes alike, with low vitamin D concentrations echoes the overall low vitamin D status that Kroll et al[96] found in the general population.

Although vitamin D deficiencies tend to be higher in individuals with overweight or obesity, 56% of athletes are deficient in vitamin D,[98] which is much higher than the rate of deficiency in the general population

(24% to 40%, age-matched to athletes).[99] Decreased calcidiol concentrations are usually a result of decreased intake of vitamin D and/or low exposure to sunlight[100]; however, both seem unlikely among athletes. Researchers have reported a high percentage of athletes are vitamin D deficient, even among those who train outdoors at latitudes providing appropriate sun exposure for vitamin D conversion on the skin.[101-103]

Other factors likely play a role in vitamin D deficiency among athletes. Ip et al[104] stated there are important clinical considerations for assessing why athletes may be deficient in vitamin D:

- female athletes with oligomenorrhea or amenorrhea, coupled with low energy availability, and/or on oral contraceptives[105,106];
- athletes in jumping sports with a history of stress fractures (require more vitamin D and may have a low storage of vitamin D in the body)[107,108];
- athletes who train and compete indoors and who may also have weight restrictions[109]; and
- collegiate athletes who may have busy schedules and, thus, may not consume adequate vitamin D from the diet.[110]
- Erkal et al[111] stated that, although most athletes with vitamin D deficiency might not have symptoms, it is important that the health care professionals involved with their care clue into such general symptoms as muscle weakness, persistent musculoskeletal pain, and general fatigue. de la Puente Yague et al[93] stressed the importance of ensuring that athletes maintain sufficient concentrations of vitamin D (calcidiol) because of its role in immune function, musculoskeletal health, and injury prevention; however, they did not recommend unnecessary vitamin D supplementation if athletes' calcidiol status was sufficient.

Vitamin D Supplementation Leventis and Kiely[112] also investigated the difference between intramuscular vitamin D2 injections (300,000 IU) compared with oral vitamin D3 supplementation (300,000 IU) in 69 participants with insufficient vitamin D (calcidiol concentration <40 nmol/L [16 ng/mL]). The researchers determined that an oral vitamin D3 supplement significantly increased calcidiol concentrations at 6 and 12 weeks ($P<.0001$ and $P<.0001$, respectively) compared with baseline. In contrast, participants who were given vitamin D2 supplements by injection had modest but not significant increases in calcidiol.

Lehmann et al[113] studied the difference between daily supplementation with 50 mcg of oral vitamin D2 and D3 in healthy participants compared with a placebo. Their results were similar to those of Leventis and Kiely.[112] Lehmann et al[113] found that total serum calcidiol concentrations remained significantly higher ($P<.001$) in participants supplemented with vitamin D3 after 4 and 8 weeks of supplementation compared with participants receiving vitamin D2 or placebo.

Research has shown that vitamin D is necessary for optimal bone growth. Vitamin D deficiency may increase the risk of autoimmune diseases and nonskeletal chronic diseases, and it can affect muscle function and inflammation.[114] Some studies have suggested that exercise performance may be influenced by vitamin D status because of the wide functionality of vitamin D in the body; a key symptom of vitamin D deficiency is muscle weakness. Forney et al[115] investigated the relationship between calcidiol and fitness levels in 40 physically active college students (20 women and 20 men). Serum vitamin D concentrations were designated as low or high, that is, below or above the adequate serum concentration of 35 ng/mL (87.5 nmol/L). The researchers did not find a significant difference in aerobic capacity (measured by VO_2 max) based on vitamin D status in female participants. They did, however, report a significantly higher VO_2 max ($P<.01$) in men in the high vitamin D group compared with those in the low vitamin D group. Nonetheless, this difference was not seen when measuring anaerobic power output ($P=.34$). These results indicate that male participants with high vitamin D concentrations may have improved aerobic capacity compared with men with lower vitamin D concentrations. Incidentally, the researchers also reported that 20 of the 39 participants (1 female participant was not included in data analyses) presented with low concentrations of serum vitamin D.[115]

Carswell et al[116] conducted a 12-week randomized, placebo-controlled trial to determine the effects of obtaining sufficient vitamin D status (serum calcidiol concentrations of ≥50 nmol/L [20 ng/mL]) in 137 men, 22 years of age. The participants received either a placebo, simulated sunlight (3 times per week for 4 weeks, and then once per week for 8 weeks), or oral vitamin D3 (1,000 IU/d for 4 weeks, followed by 400 IU/d for 8 weeks). The researchers reported that both the simulated sunlight and the oral vitamin D3 supplementation were equally as effective in attaining serum calcitriol sufficiency in 97% of the participants. Nonetheless, the increased vitamin D status did not lead to improved exercise performance.

Sources of Vitamin D Sources of naturally occurring foods containing vitamin D are limited. The best dietary sources include fatty fish and fortified foods, such as milk, breakfast cereal, and orange juice. With the addition of fortified foods, it is possible to achieve adequate vitamin D intake from food alone (refer to Table 5.2 on page 100 for more foods rich in vitamin D). Furthermore, exposing the arms, legs, and either the chest or back to 15 minutes of sunlight per day for light-skinned persons or 30 minutes per day for dark-skinned persons will result in sufficient amounts of vitamin D.[91,92] However, confinement to indoors, geographic location, or use of sunscreen may make it difficult for some to acquire the necessary sunlight exposure on the skin to ensure vitamin D conversion. Because of the ubiquitous nature of vitamin D deficiency, athletes should aim to consume foods rich in vitamin D and obtain the appropriate amount of sun exposure. If a vitamin D deficiency is found, then taking a vitamin D3 supplement would be warranted because it is well documented that vitamin D3 has higher bioavailability than vitamin D2.[112,113]

PHOSPHORUS

Phosphorus is the second most abundant mineral in the body; approximately 85% of total body phosphorus is found in bone, mainly as hydroxyapatite crystals. Phosphate is important for bone mineralization in animals and humans. Even in the presence of high amounts of calcitriol in the blood, hypophosphatemia can disrupt the negative feedback loops regulating blood phosphate concentrations and result in bone matrix breakdown, which may lead to rickets in children and osteoporosis in adults. Although phosphorus is required for bone growth, excessive amounts may actually harm the skeleton, especially when accompanied by a low calcium intake.[19,117] Excessive phosphorus intakes have been negatively correlated with bone mineral density in the radius.[118]

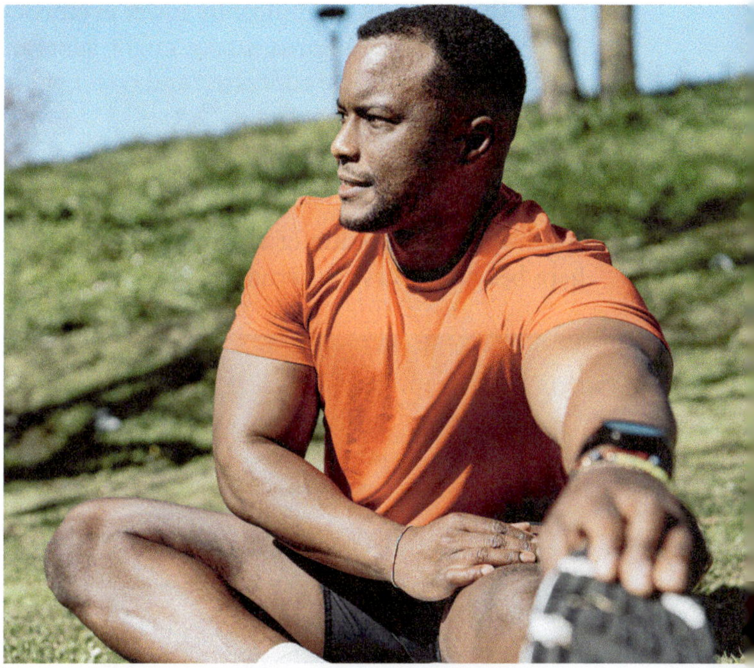

High phosphorus intakes reduce serum calcium concentrations, especially when calcium intake is low, because phosphorus carries calcium with it into soft tissues. The resulting hypocalcemia activates PTH secretion, which results in increased bone loss (resorption) to maintain serum calcium homeostasis. High phosphorus intakes can also decrease active vitamin D production, further reducing calcium absorption and producing secondary hyperparathyroidism.[118,119] Because of its ubiquitous nature, phosphorus intakes are usually higher than the recommended intakes.[117]

Because most people consume enough phosphorus in their diets, overconsumption is typically more concerning than underconsumption. Soft drinks contain high amounts of phosphate. This is especially concerning for children and teenagers because soft drinks often replace milk in their diets. Researchers have reported that the greater the consumption of carbonated beverages, especially cola beverages, the greater the risk of fracture.[120,121] This association was strongest in adult and young females. In addition, the intake of phosphorus-containing food additives (often used as a preservative and flavor enhancer) may lead to hyperphosphatemia and disrupt bone mineral density.[122]

High phosphorus intake may also indirectly lead to decreased physical activity. Peri-Okonny et al[123] evaluated serum inorganic phosphate concentrations, physical activity levels (by means of actigraphs), and left ventricular function (using magnetic resonance imaging) in 1,603 participants from phase 2 of the Dallas Heart Study. They reported that higher serum inorganic phosphate concentrations were significantly related ($P = .01$) to decreased moderate to vigorous physical activity levels and increased time in sedentary behavior ($P = .004$). The researchers did not find any significant relationship between serum inorganic phosphate concentrations and left ventricular function. They stated that dietary phosphorus intake could be a modifiable risk factor to increase physical activity.

Phosphate loading is another way many people, especially competitive athletes, consume excessive amounts of phosphorus. Phosphate loading is thought to decrease the buildup of hydrogen ions that increase during exercise and negatively affect energy production. Although research on phosphate loading as an ergogenic aid has shown equivocal results, Bremner et al[124] reported a 30% increase in plasma inorganic phosphate concentrations along with a 25% increase in erythrocyte 2,3-bisphosphoglycerate concentrations after 7 days of phosphate loading in healthy people. The researchers concluded that phosphate loading increased plasma and erythrocyte phosphate pools but that the increase in erythrocyte 2,3-bisphosphoglycerate was probably a result of the increase in cell inorganic phosphate. They did not assess the effect of phosphate loading on exercise performance. Brewer et al,[125] however, assessed the effects of sodium phosphate supplementation on short-duration (<15 minutes), high-intensity exercise performance. Competitive male cyclists were randomized into a sodium phosphate group and a placebo group and evaluated 1 and 8 days after supplementation. The researchers found no significant differences in time to completion of exercise, mean power output, or VO_2 max.[125] The long-term negative consequences of phosphate loading on bone mineral density have not been documented and should be considered before an athlete adopts this practice. Furthermore, research in this area is limited, and thus, the risk-to-benefit ratio of phosphate loading has not been established.

Conversely, Mariño et al[126] investigated the effects of exercise on erythrocyte phosphorus concentrations. They reported significantly lower erythrocyte concentrations in 46 male athletes, about 23 years of age. Although phosphorus intake might generally be above recommendations, loss of phosphorus with exercise should also be addressed and could affect performance. Table 5.4 on pages 104 and 105 lists some food sources of phosphorus.

VITAMIN A

An in-depth discussion of vitamin A was provided earlier in this chapter; however, it is mentioned again here because excessive serum vitamin A concentrations may be detrimental to bone health. Note that it is often difficult to accurately assess vitamin A status in research participants. Barker and Blumsohn[127] reviewed the methods employed in several animal and human studies of vitamin A status, along with the study results. Although they discussed several findings in their extensive review (including correlations between serum vitamin A concentrations and increased rate of bone resorption, ossification of cartilage, hypercalcemia, extraosseous calcification, suppressed PTH concentrations, and fractures), they also found the quality of the reviewed work to be inadequate. This review emphasized that the current state of research into the interaction between vitamin A and bone health is limited due to inaccurate assessments of vitamin A intake and varying definitions of intake thresholds. Although the current research is limited, it underscores the fact that vitamin A intakes of more than the UL can have detrimental effects on the body.

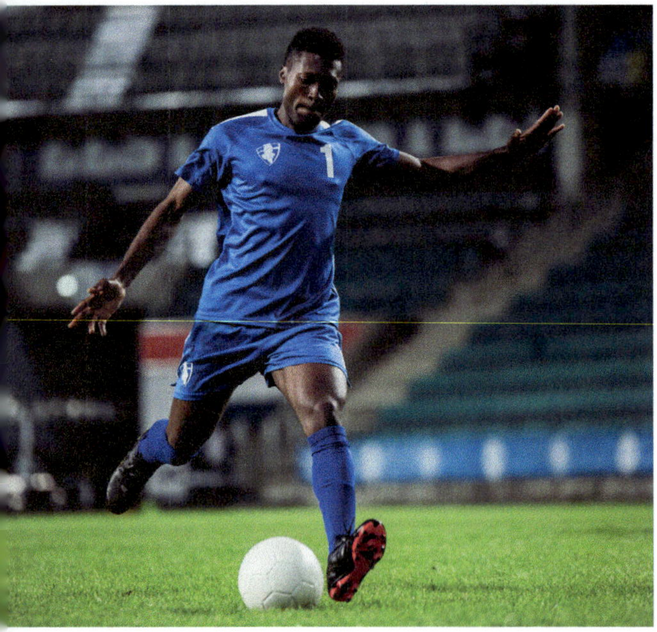

In a 2021 review on vitamin A and bone health, Yee et al[128] reported negative effects on cortical bone with high intakes of retinol in animals. They also reported that vitamin A intake and impaired bone mineral density were greater in those individuals who were obese and/or vitamin D–deficient. However, the researchers stated that provitamin A and vitamin A are likely bone-protecting compounds because of their role in osteogenesis and in the inhibition of osteoclast differentiation and development.

Red Blood Cell Function

The primary function of erythrocytes (red blood cells) is to deliver oxygen through the blood to the cells of the body. Because athletes have increased oxygen demands, the proper formation and function of red blood cells is critical for health and performance.

VITAMIN B12 AND FOLATE

Vitamin B12 (cyanocobalamin) and folate (folic acid) are both necessary for DNA synthesis[19] and are interrelated in their respective syntheses and metabolism reactions. Both vitamins are required for normal erythrocyte synthesis; creation of normal red blood cells is the function through which these 2 vitamins may affect exercise.[129] There is no evidence, however, to suggest that exercise increases the need for either of these vitamins. Lukaski[1] stated that, although the data assessing blood biochemical measures of folate status in physically active people are limited, physical performance did not improve in athletes who were folate deficient and received folate supplementation. A clinically normal blood concentration of vitamin B12 is between 200 and 900 pg/mL.[130] Normal blood concentrations of folate range from 2.7 to 17.0 ng/mL.[131] However, inadequate intakes of both vitamins can lead to megaloblastic anemia.[1,14]

Although injections of vitamin B12 are used clinically for persons diagnosed with megaloblastic anemia, oral supplementation is sufficient if frank anemia has not been diagnosed. A multivitamin and mineral supplement that includes 500 to 1,000 mg of vitamin C may decrease vitamin B12 bioavailability from food and may lead to vitamin B12 deficiency.[132] Vitamin B12 deficiency can be masked by high folate intakes; thus, if vitamin B12 deficiency is suspected, dietary intake will need to be assessed, especially if biochemical tests are negative for vitamin B12 deficiency. These nutrients are important for athletes who follow a vegan diet and are discussed later in this chapter.

Athletes who consume adequate amounts of vitamin B12 and folate in their diets are unlikely to be at risk for vitamin B12 or folate deficiencies. Nonetheless, a deficiency in vitamin B12 or folate can lead to increased serum homocysteine concentrations, a risk factor for cardiovascular disease. Normal blood homocysteine concentrations range between 4 and 15 mcmol/L, with optimal concentrations below 10 to 12 mcmol/L.[133] The risk of hyperhomocysteinemia (>15 mcmol/L) demonstrates that individuals who exercise need to be concerned not only about nutrition and performance but also about overall health.

To understand the effects of exercise intensity on homocysteine concentrations, Iglesias-Gutiérrez et al[134] studied changes in serum homocysteine concentrations in 8 sedentary males during and after low- and high-intensity interval exercises. Their findings indicated that high-intensity exercise raises serum homocysteine concentrations more quickly than lower-intensity exercise. Incidentally, the researchers also reported that serum concentrations of vitamin B12, folate, and vitamin B6 all significantly increased ($P < .05$) after both high- and low-intensity exercise.

König et al[135] also sought to identify changes in blood homocysteine concentrations in response to exercise. Their findings reiterated that serum homocysteine concentrations increase in response to exercise; however, they found that the timing of the alteration in concentration was not well defined.

Herrmann et al[136] had previously explored the relationship of exercise to homocysteine concentrations, and contrary to the findings of König et al,[135] they found that serum homocysteine concentrations increased during, not after, the bout of exercise. However, both groups of researchers agreed that homocysteine concentrations remained elevated following exercise cessation and continued to remain above normal throughout the 5-day recovery training period. They also found that serum vitamin B12 concentrations were unchanged during training but decreased during the recovery phase, indicating that serum vitamin B12 concentrations decreased postexercise. In contrast, the serum folate concentrations decreased during training but returned to normal by the end of the recovery period.[135,136]

Similarly, Kim et al[137] evaluated how regular exercise affected the plasma B12 and folate concentrations in 50 rats who were divided into either a nonexercise group (n = 25) or an exercise training group (n = 25). The exercise group ran on a treadmill for 30 min/d, 5 d/wk, for 5 weeks. After that, the exercise group was separated into 4 groups: 1 nonexercise group and 3 exercise groups with varying exercise durations (30 minutes, 1 hour, and 2 hours). The researchers reported that regular exercise significantly increased plasma vitamin B12 concentrations while significantly decreasing plasma folate concentrations ($P < .05$) compared to those of the nonexercising group. However, no differences were observed among the 3 durations of exercise.

Because vitamin B12 and folate are metabolically interrelated, changes in one but not the other at different times during exercise and recovery may indicate an adaptive response by each to protect the other. It is important for those who exercise to consume adequate amounts of vitamin B12 and folate despite evidence that supplementation may improve performance only if a nutritional deficit is present.[1] Dietary sources of vitamin B12 and folate are listed in Table 5.1 on page 94.

IRON

Iron plays a vital role in oxygen delivery and is paramount to overall exercise performance; yet iron-deficiency anemia affects 30% of the world's population (children and adults are both affected).[138-140] About 15% to 35% of female athletes have been diagnosed with iron deficiency anemia, and 5% to 11% of male athletes have been similarly diagnosed.[141] Athletes at highest risk for iron deficiency anemia include female endurance athletes, athletes who follow a vegetarian diet, and any athlete who practices weight restriction.[142] For athletes in particular, iron deficiency anemia may negatively affect exercise performance. Iron deficiency anemia negatively affects the oxidative production of ATP in skeletal muscle. It is therefore understandable that iron deficiency anemia has been shown to decrease overall aerobic capacity and, thus, overall athletic performance.[141-146]

Iron Supplementation For individuals with iron deficiency depletion or anemia, iron supplementation is the most prudent way to increase iron stores and prevent adverse physiological effects.[147] Ferrous sulfate or gluconate are the least expensive and most widely used forms of iron supplementation[146,147]; however, ferrous chelate and polysaccharide have been shown to be more bioavailable.[148] For adults diagnosed with iron deficiency anemia, a daily dose of 100 to 150 mg of elemental iron taken between meals is recommended.[147] However, Rosenzweig and Volpe[149] reported that daily intake of 23 mg of elemental iron, as ferrous fumarate, clinically corrected iron deficiency anemia in the 2 female athletes in their 4-month case study, demonstrating that lower amounts of iron can also be sufficient to reverse iron deficiency anemia. In 2023, Csulak et al[150] provided 65 male basketball players (15.8 ± 1.7 years of age) who had been diagnosed with iron deficiency with 100 mg of elemental iron or a placebo for 3 months. They reported that 3 months of iron supplementation increased serum ferritin concentrations compared to the placebo; however, sports performance was not improved.

Supplementation is also warranted for athletes with iron depletion (low serum ferritin concentrations) without iron deficiency anemia to prevent full-blown iron deficiency anemia from developing. DellaValle and Haas[151] assessed the effects of iron supplementation on 4-km run performance, VO_2 peak, energy expenditure, lactate response, and iron stores (serum ferritin concentrations) in 40 female rowers (about 19 years of age). Their goal was to show a relationship between iron depletion without anemia and physical performance. In this double-blind, placebo-controlled study, rowers received either a ferrous sulfate supplement (100 mg/d) or a placebo for 6 weeks. At baseline, rower characteristics did not differ; however, after supplementation, iron-supplemented rowers had a delayed lactate response during the first half of exercise ($P = .05$) and increased energy expenditure after 6 weeks of training ($P = .03$) compared with the rowers who received the placebo. These results suggest that because iron depletion may impair aerobic exercise performance and possibly diminish the effects of exercise, nutrition and dietetics practitioners need to understand the importance of treating iron depletion in addition to iron deficiency anemia in athletes. For adults with stage 1 iron deficiency (serum ferritin concentrations of <20 ng/mL), a daily dose of 25 to 65 mg of elemental iron taken between meals is recommended; 65 to 130 mg of elemental iron is recommended for stage 2 iron deficiency.

Factors Affecting Iron Absorption Several factors inhibit or enhance iron absorption. Factors that inhibit iron absorption include phytates and oxalates, tannins in tea and coffee, adequate iron stores, excessive intake of other minerals (eg, zinc, calcium, and manganese), reduced gastric acid production, and certain antacids. Factors that enhance iron absorption include heme iron; meat protein factor; ascorbic acid; low iron stores; normal gastric acid secretion; and a high demand for red blood cells, such as occurs with blood loss, exercise training (especially at altitude), and pregnancy.[1-8] Consuming foods or beverages that contain vitamin C with meals and consuming tea or coffee at least 1 hour before or after a meal rather than with a meal will enhance absorption of dietary iron. Table 5.3 on page 102 lists some examples of dietary sources of iron.

McCormick et al[152] compared the effects of 8 weeks of daily or alternate-day oral iron supplementation on iron status in 22 female and 9 male endurance-trained runners who had serum ferritin concentrations of less than 50 mcg/L. They reported that serum ferritin concentrations significantly increased in both groups ($P < .001$). They also reported less gastrointestinal upset in the individuals who took iron on alternate days. McCormick et al's research indicates that alternate-day iron supplementation could be considered for individuals who have gastrointestinal upset. To further enhance iron absorption, one should consume foods or meals high in iron (especially those high in heme iron) or iron supplements separated in time from intense workouts, so that absorption is not affected by the inflammatory response of exercise.[153]

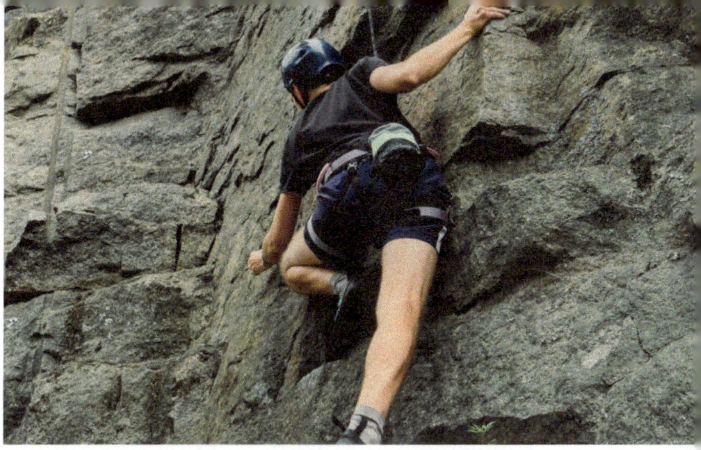

Sim et al[141] discussed other factors that may lead to altered iron metabolism in athletes. Hepcidin, a liver-derived iron regulatory hormone, is increased during exercise, thereby leading to a decrease in the amount of iron available during exercise.[141,154] A single bout of moderate to vigorous endurance exercise (about 60% to 90% of VO_2 peak) increased serum hepcidin concentrations between 0 and 6 hours postexercise, with a peak at 3 hours. The degree of the response of hepcidin was found to depend on ferritin and interleukin-6 concentrations prior to exercise.[154]

Bacchetta et al[155] reported that increased hepcidin concentrations and vitamin D deficiency are related to iron deficiency anemia. They reported that with a 1-dose supplementation of 100,000 IU of vitamin D, serum calcidiol concentrations significantly increased ($P < .001$), which resulted in a 34% reduction ($P < .05$) in hepcidin concentrations within 24 hours of the vitamin D supplementation.

The Immune System

The extreme physiological stress athletes impose on their bodies is associated with immunosuppression and increased risk of infection. Intense exercise exposes the body to stress-induced hormones, such as cortisol, and increased levels of oxidative stress. Elements of the immune system appear to be temporarily depressed following bouts of exercise, leading to susceptibility to infection.[156,157] Certain vitamins and minerals may alleviate the stress to the immune system associated with exercise.

Walsh[158] has proposed a new paradigm for exercise immunology. According to this paradigm, *resistance* is "the strength of immune weaponry" and *tolerance* is "the ability to endure microbes and dampen defense activity." Resistance, Walsh states, is not actually suppressed in athletes who train intensely, which is why nutritional supplements for "immunity" do not usually help athletes. However, Walsh also states that with nutritional supplements such as vitamins C and D that focus on tolerance might decrease the burden of infection in athletes.

VITAMIN C

Vitamin C is a well-known antioxidant discussed earlier in this chapter. Some people supplement vitamin C in very high doses (≥1,000 mg/d) because they believe that it can prevent or reduce the severity and duration of common colds; however, research on high doses of vitamin C and the common cold has been equivocal. Most of the existing data from supplementation and dietary studies do not support the concept that athletes require an increased amount of vitamin C for a variety of reasons. Hemilä and Chalker[159] conducted meta-analyses to assess the risk and duration of the common cold in placebo-controlled trials. One criterion of the studies they selected was that the researchers administered vitamin C to their participants in doses of at least 2 g/d. They determined that, among the general population, high-dose vitamin C supplementation does not reduce the occurrence of the common cold, but it does reduce the length of cold symptoms. In addition, the researchers determined that athletes (n = 598) undergoing short periods of extreme physical stress (marathon runners and skiers) in 5 separate studies presented with nearly half the risk of developing the common cold compared with the general population, indicating that exercise itself, although a stressor, can be protective in developing the common cold.

Athletes and individuals who are sedentary generally do not require different amounts of vitamin C. Some researchers have reported similar vitamin C intake between athletes and sedentary control participants. Note that plasma vitamin C concentrations are an indicator of recent dietary intake of vitamin C, whereas leukocyte vitamin C concentrations are an indicator of tissue stores.[160]

In addition, no difference has been reported between athletes and nonathletes in the excretion of ascorbic acid in urine, which is an assessment of the utilization of vitamin C within the body. However, people who consistently exercise may require at least 100 mg of vitamin C per day, which can be easily obtained from food, to maintain normal vitamin C status and protect the body from oxidative damage caused by exercise. Athletes competing in ultraendurance events may require up to 500 mg or more of vitamin C per day,[51,54] likely obtained from foods and supplements combined. Nonetheless, athletes should not exceed the UL for vitamin C (2,000 mg/d in adults, 19 years of age and older). Braakhuis[161] reported that vitamin C supplementation at levels of 1 g/d diminished athletic performance, potentially by decreasing mitochondrial biogenesis. Braakhuis suggested that athletes obtain their vitamin C from fruits and vegetables, which can reduce oxidative stress and provide additional health benefits. Dietary sources of vitamin C are listed in Table 5.1 on page 94.

VITAMIN D

Vitamin D also plays a role in immune function. Dubnov-Raz et al[162] evaluated whether 12 weeks of daily supplementation with 2,000 IU of vitamin D3 compared to a placebo would reduce the risk of upper respiratory tract infections in 55 competitive adolescent swimmers in Israel who were characterized as having vitamin D deficiency. The researchers reported that vitamin D supplementation did not decrease upper respiratory tract infections; however, the larger decreases in serum calcidiol concentrations seen in the placebo group led to significantly longer durations and greater severities for their upper respiratory tract infections.

In 2021, Harrison et al[163] determined the effects of simulated sunlight and oral vitamin D3 (1,000 IU/d for 4 weeks and then 400 IU/d) compared to a placebo for 8 weeks on upper respiratory tract infections in 250 men in military training who had vitamin D deficiency. The researchers reported that the simulated sunlight and vitamin D supplementation both were equally as effective in achieving vitamin D sufficiency (in 95% of the participants). Compared to the placebo, both types of vitamin D supplementation significantly reduced the severity of upper respiratory tract infection symptoms by 15% and decreased the number of days with an upper respiratory tract infection by 36% ($P < .05$).

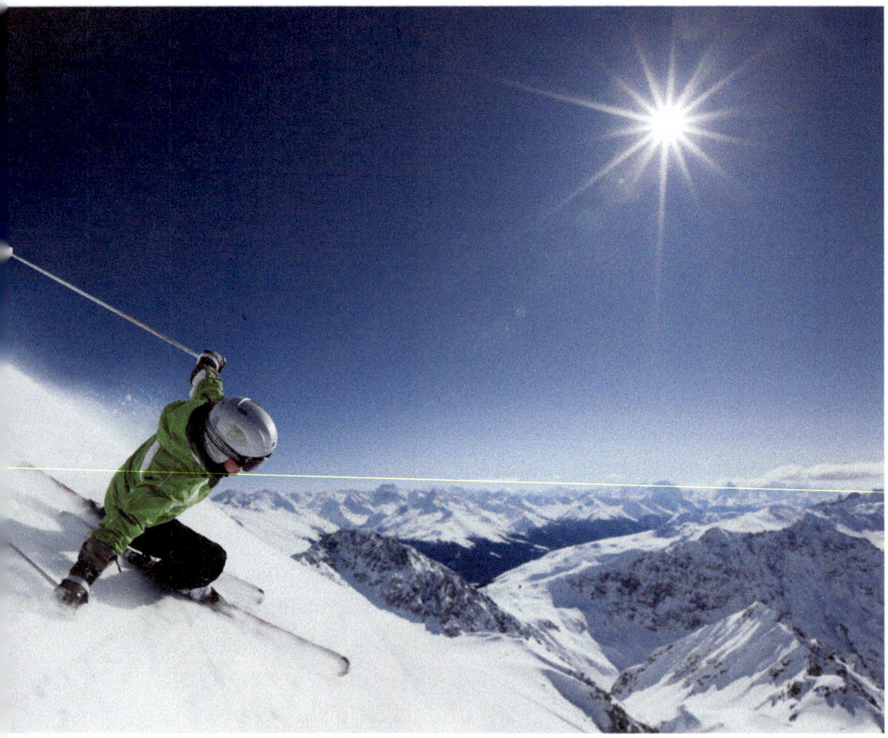

Jung et al[164] evaluated the effects of 4 weeks of vitamin D3 supplementation (5,000 IU/d) (n = 13) compared to a placebo (n = 12) in 25 male tae kwon do athletes, 19 to 22 years of age, who had vitamin D deficiency. They reported a significant increase in serum calcidiol concentrations ($P < .001$) compared to the placebo group. The increased calcidiol concentrations was significantly and inversely related to upper respiratory tract infections. Vitamin D3 supplementation may be effective in reducing upper respiratory tract infections in tae kwon do athletes during winter training.

It appears that vitamin D3 supplementation can significantly reduce upper respiratory tract infections in physically active individuals with vitamin D deficiency. Note that the doses varied among the trials, so dosing should be considered if supplementation is warranted.

ZINC

Zinc exists in all organs, tissues, fluids, and secretions. Approximately 60% of total body zinc is present in muscle, 29% in bone, and roughly 1% each in the gastrointestinal tract, skin, kidneys, brain, lungs, and prostate.[165]

Zinc Absorption Zinc is primarily absorbed in the jejunum of the small intestine. Most zinc is absorbed by a carrier-mediated system; however, some zinc can be absorbed by diffusion. Zinc absorption involves metallothionein (a small, cysteine-rich protein), which regulates zinc homeostasis within the intestinal mucosa. When the intestinal mucosa senses that there is enough zinc present, the synthesis and secretion of metallothionein are increased. Metallothionein releases zinc into the plasma if needed, or it releases zinc into the zinc pool within the mucosa if not needed in the plasma.[16]

Zinc absorption is enhanced when there is an increased need for zinc, with increased animal protein intake, and with increased vitamin D intake. In addition, amino acids (eg, histidine and methionine) and organic acids (eg, citrate) positively affect zinc absorption. Inhibitors of zinc absorption include fiber, phytates, oxalates, cadmium, and high intakes of iron.[166]

Zinc plays a role in more than 300 metabolic reactions in the body. Alkaline phosphatase, carbonic anhydrase, and copper-zinc superoxide dismutase are just a few of the zinc metalloenzymes.[16] Low zinc status can lead to poor growth, poor wound healing, and impaired immune function,[165] which can be detrimental to exercise and overall health.

One of the most discussed topics regarding zinc is the common cold. Are zinc lozenges effective in preventing the common cold? Hemilä[167] conducted a systematic review to determine whether zinc lozenges can prevent the common cold. Thirteen placebo-controlled trials in which zinc lozenges were used to alleviate the common cold were included, with the following results:

- In 5 trials, the researchers used zinc doses of less than 75 mg/d, and no effects of zinc on the common cold were reported.
- In 3 studies, the researchers used zinc acetate in doses greater than 75 mg/d, resulting in a 42% decrease in the length of colds.
- In 5 trials, the researchers had participants take zinc salts, not including zinc acetate, in doses greater than 75 mg/d, leading to a 20% decrease in the length of colds.

These results demonstrate strong evidence that ingesting zinc lozenges at more than 75 mg/d when experiencing cold symptoms can decrease the duration of colds.

Many athletes, like many people in the United States, do not consume the recommended amount of zinc, regardless of whether they are in or out of training season.[168-170] In a crossover study, Volpe et al[171] used stable isotopes of zinc to evaluate the effects of acute exhaustive exercise compared with rest on short-term zinc kinetics in 12 healthy, sedentary males, 25 to 35 years of age. They reported a significant decrease ($P < .05$) in plasma zinc concentrations after exercise. From the stable isotope data, they reported a shift of plasma zinc into the liver and interstitial fluid after exercise, likely demonstrating the acute stress response of exhaustive exercise. It is not clear whether these changes in zinc are transient or continue after exercise.

Maxwell and Volpe[172] evaluated the effects of zinc supplementation (as zinc gluconate) at a dose of 26.4 mg/d on thyroid hormone function in 2 physically active college women who were zinc deficient (case study). After 4 months of supplementation, the zinc deficiency was clinically corrected in both participants. In addition, zinc supplementation improved the participants' thyroid hormone concentrations. More research is required to assess athletes' zinc status, but it would be prudent for athletes to consume the DRI for zinc. Refer to Table 5.3 on page 102 for dietary sources of zinc.

RISK FACTORS AFFECTING VITAMIN AND MINERAL NEEDS

Training in Heat and Humidity

Athletes who exercise in excessive heat and humidity face challenges in replenishing fluid and electrolytes lost through sweat. The loss of electrolytes (sodium, potassium, calcium, and magnesium) is extensively covered in Chapter 6. Table 5.4 on pages 104 and 105 lists some food sources of these nutrients.

Training at Altitude

Training at altitude (7,000 to 8,000 feet above sea level), where oxygen concentrations are considerably lower than at atmospheric pressure, allows an athlete to increase their red blood cell volume and, in turn, oxygen delivery to their muscles. Such blood alterations allow for increased aerobic activity and improved performance.[173,174] Certain vitamins and minerals are crucial in the adaptations associated with altitude training.[175]

Iron is a crucial mineral for altitude acclimation. Many athletes follow the "live high, train low"[173] protocol to increase hemoglobin mass and, in turn, increase oxygen delivery to improve athletic performance. Govus et al[176] assessed hematologic data of 178 endurance athletes who were exposed to high-altitude training and discovered that daily oral ferrous sulfate supplements containing 210 mg of elemental iron slowed the decrease of serum ferritin concentrations that occurs after exposure to altitude compared with athletes who did not receive iron supplements. Thus, athletes who may be new to training or competing at high altitude should consider iron supplementation, especially if they have low serum ferritin concentrations when they begin training. Nonetheless, once an athlete becomes acclimatized to the altitude, iron supplementation will not be necessary.

Stellingwerff[175] emphasized the significant role that iron plays at altitude. The low-oxygen environment increases erythropoiesis, leading to increased hemoglobin levels, which are dependent on how much iron is available. Iron supplementation during altitude training appears to be more important than iron stores prior to altitude training.[177,178] In addition, it is important to monitor iron status during altitude training.[175]

Exposure to altitude also increases the production of reactive oxygen species and decreases plasma antioxidant concentrations. Pialoux et al[179] reported that antioxidant status remained low following simulated altitude training.

Nutritional Needs for Female Athletes

Female athletes require a complete and healthy diet to support their needs and recover from the physical stress of exercise. It is vital for female athletes to achieve proper nutrition as inadequate nutrition may lead to specific nutrient deficiencies.[180-182]

IRON

Some researchers have reported that as many as 60% of female athletes may have some degree of iron depletion. This is especially common in female athletes who participate in endurance sports.[141-143] Female athletes typically do not consume adequate amounts of dietary iron as a result of restricted energy consumption and a reduction in the heme iron content of the diet. These dietary patterns, paired with additional losses in the body (eg, sweat, menstruation, intravascular hemolysis, foot strike hemolysis in runners), may contribute to suboptimal iron content in the body.[142,144,145]

CALCIUM AND VITAMIN D

Calcium and vitamin D are important nutrients for developing and maintaining bone health. For female athletes, it is especially important to consume adequate amounts of calcium and vitamin D, because deficiencies are common. Median calcium intakes of female athletes in the United States are below recommended amounts,[72] and approximately one-third of female athletes are deficient in vitamin D.[93] All athletes, and especially female athletes, should be encouraged to consume adequate amounts of calcium and vitamin D in their diet to maintain healthy bones. Female athletes with low energy availability should have their calcium and vitamin D statuses assessed and addressed.[182]

VITAMIN K

Vitamin K is a fat-soluble vitamin that consists of the following 3 related substances:

- Phylloquinone, also known as phytonadione (vitamin K1), is found in plants.
- Menaquinone (vitamin K2) is produced by bacteria in the intestines, which supply an undetermined amount of the daily requirement of vitamin K.
- Menadione (vitamin K3) is the synthetic form of vitamin K.

All vitamin K variants are fat soluble and stable to heat. Alkalis, strong acids, radiation, and oxidizing agents can destroy vitamin K. It is absorbed from the upper small intestine with the help of bile or bile salts and pancreatic juices and then carried to the liver for the synthesis of prothrombin, a key blood-clotting factor.[16]

Much of the vitamin K research in athletes has focused on the interaction of vitamin K with estrogen and bone metabolism. Female athletes, especially those with abnormal menstrual cycles and those who are postmenopausal, are particularly vulnerable to bone metabolism disorders due to decreased circulating estrogen.[183] Braam et al[184] studied the effects of estrogen and vitamin K supplementation on bone loss in female endurance athletes. Based on their menstrual cycle status, 115 participants were assigned to 1 of 3 groups: (1) athletes with amenorrhea (no menstrual cycles per year) or oligomenorrhea (few menstrual cycles per year), (2) athletes with eumenorrhea (normal menstruation), and (3) athletes who used oral contraceptives (estrogen supplemented). The participants in each group were then randomized for treatment with either 10 mg of vitamin K1 per day or a placebo. All 3 groups and subgroups showed significant decreases in femoral neck bone mineral density after 2 years of supplementation or placebo. Athletes who were amenorrheic or oligomenorrheic had the most bone loss compared with those who were eumenorrheic and those who supplemented with estrogen. The researchers found that neither estrogen nor vitamin K supplementation helped decrease the rate of bone mineral density decline over the 2-year period in any of the groups. These results are concerning considering the rate of bone mineral density loss in all participants. Although vitamin K supplementation was not shown to prevent or reverse the loss of bone mineral density, it is important for athletes to consume adequate amounts of vitamin K in their diets.

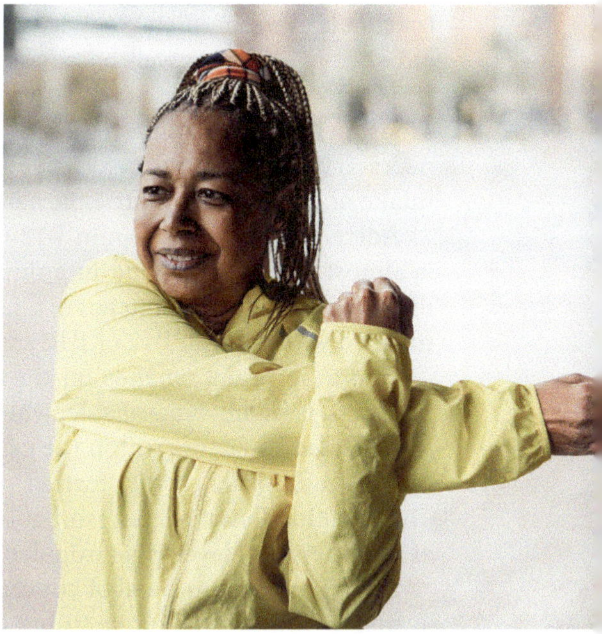

Volpe et al[185] conducted a double-blind, placebo-controlled, randomized trial to evaluate the effects of 6 months of vitamin K supplementation on bone mineral density and biomarkers of bone in 14 premenopausal and perimenopausal women, 25 to 50 years of age. Eight women were randomly assigned to receive 600 mcg of vitamin K per day as phylloquinone (vitamin K1), and 6 women were randomly assigned into the control group (placebo tablets). Although there were some positive changes in bone mineral density and biomarkers in both groups, the researchers reported no effects of 6 months of vitamin K1 supplementation on regional bone mineral density in their group of premenopausal and perimenopausal women. Perhaps they would have found significant changes in bone mineral density and biomarkers of bone if they had a larger sample size.

An average diet usually provides at least 75 to 150 mcg of total vitamin K per day (the suggested minimum intake); although 300 to 750 mcg/d may be optimal. Absorption of vitamin K ranges from 20% to 60% of total intake.[186] Vitamin K deficiency is more common than previously thought. Western diets high in sugar and processed foods, intake of vitamins A and E higher than the ULs, and use of antibiotics are all factors that may contribute to a decrease in intestinal bacterial function, resulting in a decrease in the production and/or metabolism of vitamins K1 and K2.[16,186] Dietary sources of vitamin K are listed in Table 5.2 on page 100.

VITAMINS AND MINERALS OF CONCERN DUE TO DIETARY INTAKE PATTERNS

Athletes who restrict certain foods or food groups may be at higher risk for deficiencies than those who eat a wide variety of foods. This section reviews specific dietary patterns and how they may affect athletes.

Vegetarian, Vegan, and Plant-Based Diets

According to the Academy of Nutrition and Dietetics, "appropriately planned vegetarian, including vegan, diets are healthful, nutritionally adequate and may provide health benefits for the prevention and treatment of certain diseases."[187] However, because of the increased demand placed on athletes, athletes who consume predominantly plant-based diets may be at higher risk for certain nutrient deficiencies. Nonetheless, individuals choose to consume vegetarian, vegan, and plant-based diets for many reasons, including concern for animals and the environment, religious practices and beliefs, and/or health benefits, all which need to be respected by health care professionals. Moreover, even though plant-based diets (particularly vegan diets) may lead to deficiencies in some nutrients, these diets can offer performance-enhancing benefits as well, because of their high carbohydrate, antioxidant, and phytochemical levels.[187,188] It is important that these diets be well-planned to ensure that they maximize the benefits of the variety of foods included. Although vegetarian, vegan, and plant-based diets provide high amounts of antioxidants necessary to attenuate the oxidative stress of exercise, avoidance of meat and poultry can lead to decreased intake of certain micronutrients, namely vitamin B12, iron, and zinc.[187,189]

Adequate intake of vitamin B12 is of special concern in athletes who are vegan because vitamin B12 is almost exclusively found in animal products.[14] Vegetarians who consume dairy products or eggs are likely to have adequate intakes of vitamin B12, but athletes who are vegan should regularly consume foods fortified with vitamin B12 or B12 supplements.[189]

Iron absorption depends on the type of iron consumed from the diet. Heme iron, found in animal products, is highly bioavailable, whereas nonheme iron, found in plant foods, is less bioavailable because it is affected by factors within the gastric lumen. In addition, some plant foods contain inhibitors, such as phytates and oxalates, that further restrict the bioavailability of all iron types, especially nonheme iron. The combination of a less absorbable iron and the inhibitors found in plants puts vegetarians and vegans at higher risk of developing iron depletion or iron deficiency anemia.[16]

Zinc is another mineral of concern to individuals following a vegetarian or vegan diet. Zinc is highly available from animal products but is not readily absorbed from plant foods, especially foods containing phytates, which inhibit zinc absorption. Vegans should consider including high-zinc foods in their diet, such as pumpkin and hemp seeds (each of which contains 5 of mg zinc per half-cup), or supplementing with zinc.[187-189] Additional information on vegetarian, vegan, and plant-based diets can be found in Chapter 16.

High- and Low-Carbohydrate Diets

There appears to be a strong correlation between high carbohydrate intake, physical activity, and thiamin requirements.[14] This may be a concern for individuals who exercise because a high-carbohydrate diet is recommended for athletes; however, there is no clear evidence indicating that people who exercise require more thiamin in their diets than those who are sedentary. Nonetheless, it is prudent to recommend that people who exercise obtain at least the DRI for thiamin to prevent depletion. Additionally, high carbohydrate intakes paired with low protein and fat intakes have been found to lead to suboptimal zinc intakes in 90% of all athletes.[168]

Low-carbohydrate diets may lead to nutrient deficiencies. Zhang et al[190] compared macronutrient and micronutrient intakes across several traditional diets (Chinese, Mediterranean/Italian, Japanese, and American). The researchers used dietary data derived from the China National Nutrition and Health Monitoring Survey (2010 to 2012) to compare nutrient intakes to those from other countries. Dietary data from other countries were obtained from the third National Food Consumption Survey in Italy, the National Health and Nutrition Survey in Japan, and the National Health and Nutrition Examination Survey (NHANES 2009 to 2010) in the United States. The Chinese data were collected from 3 consecutive 24-hour dietary recalls of 2,659 Chinese participants (1,385 females, 1,274 males) aged 2 to 89 years in the Zhejiang province. The researchers found that Chinese persons consuming diets with the lowest percentages of energy from carbohydrates consumed significantly lower ($P < .04$) amounts of vitamins B1, B2, A, and C than those who consumed the other diets studied. Although Zhang et al did not conduct this study in athletes, the findings suggest that low-carbohydrate diets can lead to nutrient deficiencies, which can ultimately affect athletic performance and overall health. Refer to Chapter 2 for more information on carbohydrates and exercise.

Energy-Restricted Diets

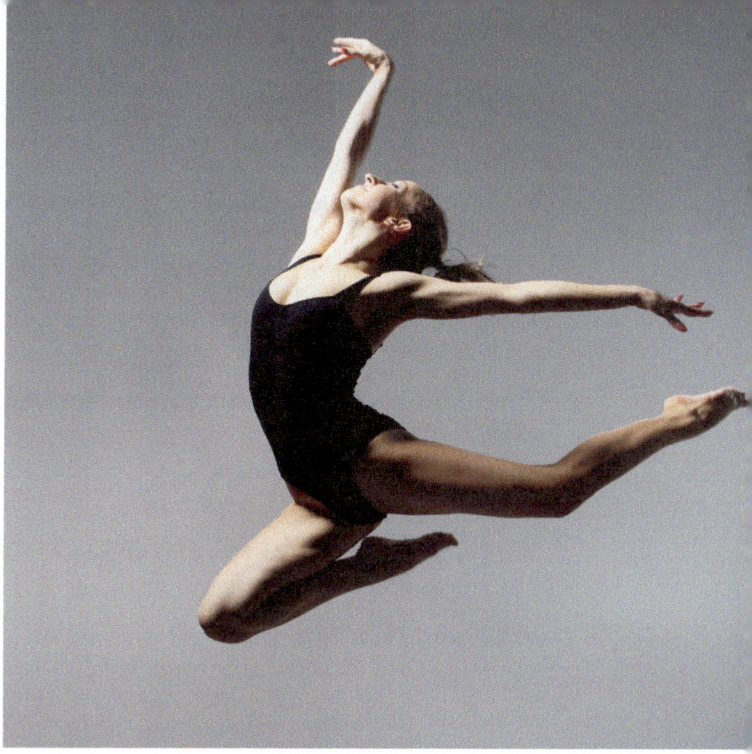

Athletes may consume an energy-restricted diet for many reasons. Elite athletes may have an idealized perception of a particular body type for their specific sport, may believe perceived energy restriction has performance benefits, and may feel social and cultural pressures toward thinness or a certain body shape.[191] Energy restriction is a common, albeit unhealthy, practice among athletes, especially those in weight-dependent sports, such as wrestling, gymnastics, jockeying, and rowing. Hinton et al[192] assessed the dietary intakes and behaviors of female and male collegiate athletes (N = 345) at National Collegiate Athletic Association Division I universities. The researchers reported that, on average, the athletes consumed only 15% of the recommended carbohydrates and 26% of the recommended protein. They also noted that more than half of the female athletes (62%) reported a desire to lose at least 5lb. This desire was associated with decreased energy and macronutrient consumption, but surprisingly, their micronutrient intakes were within the recommended ranges.

The desire to lose weight or exhibit an idealized body type drives many athletes to restrict food intake. El Ghoch et al[193] examined how restrictive eating disorder behaviors affected athletic performance. Although athletes who lost weight from restricted eating behaviors demonstrated improved physical performance initially, long-term effects of glycogen depletion, increased muscular pain, dehydration, and loss of lean body mass were all detriments of energy restriction. Additionally, low energy availability can significantly compromise immune function.[194] Although restrictive diets are common among athletes, the long-term detriments can compromise overall performance, and athletes should be taught proper dietary intake to optimize performance and overall long-term health. Refer to Chapters 10 and 11 for more information on energy balance and weight management.

SUMMARY

Active individuals must pay special attention to their micronutrient needs. Athletes and health care practitioners should consider the following factors when assessing micronutrient needs for physically active people: frequency, intensity, duration, and type(s) of physical activity; environment (hot or cold) in which exercise is performed; sex; and dietary intakes and food preferences. It is particularly important to evaluate usual dietary intakes of calcium and iron in female athletes.

Proper assessment will help practitioners counsel those who are physically active to consume adequate amounts of micronutrients for optimal health and performance. Athletes should be encouraged to consume adequate total energy. If they do so, they will typically consume adequate vitamins and minerals as well. Encouraging those who exercise to consume a varied diet rich in fruits, vegetables, and grains, with the proper amount of total energy from macronutrients (carbohydrate, fat, and protein), will also help to ensure that they obtain adequate amounts of vitamins and minerals needed for overall health and optimal performance. Individuals who exercise and consume a vegan diet should consider appropriate supplementation of micronutrients.

Box 5.1 on page 120 lists some helpful vitamin and mineral resources for practitioners.

BOX 5.1 Online Resources for Vitamins and Minerals

Food and Nutrition Board of the National Academies of Sciences, Engineering, and Medicine

- www.nationalacademies.org/fnb/food-and-nutrition-board

Institute for the Advancement of Food and Nutrition Sciences

- www.iafns.org

Food and Nutrition Board of the National Academies of Sciences, Engineering, and Medicine

Dietary Reference Intakes

- www.nationalacademies.org/our-work/summary-report-of-the-dietary-reference-intakes

National Institutes of Health, Office of Dietary Supplements

- https://ods.od.nih.gov

Food and Nutrition Information Center

- www.nal.usda.gov/programs/fnic

Nutrition.gov

- http://nutrition.gov

Vitamin D Council

- www.vitamindcouncil.org

Linus Pauling Institute

- https://lpi.oregonstate.edu/mic

KEY TAKEAWAYS

Overall, the vitamin and mineral needs of people who exercise or are physically active are similar to the requirements for all healthy people.

If dietary intakes are adequate (ie, meet 70% or more of the DRI for nutrients), supplementation is unnecessary.

Sweat losses may require some people to consume higher amounts of certain micronutrients, quantities that can be obtained with a varied diet of properly selected foods.

Supplementation may be necessary when intake is inadequate or when there is a deficiency in status. Care must be taken so that individuals do not exceed the UL, which could impair both exercise performance and health.

There are specific intricacies among all vitamins and minerals, especially with respect to athletes and exercise, between females and males, and among individuals. It is important to be aware of the special needs of each individual athlete, depending on sport, sex, and any condition they might have.

REFERENCES

1. Lukaski HC. Vitamin and mineral status: effects on physical performance. *Nutrition.* 2004;20(7-8):632-644. doi:10.1016/j.nut.2004.04.001
2. Volpe SL. Micronutrient requirements for athletes. *Clin Sports Med.* 2007;26(1):119-130. doi:10.1016/j.csm.2006.11.009
3. Volpe SL. Minerals as ergogenic aids. *Curr Sports Med Reports.* 2008;7(4):224-229. doi:10.1249/JSR.0b013e31817ed0e2
4. Ggazzawi HA, Hussain, MA, Raziq KM, et al. Exploring the relationship between micronutrients and athletic performance: a comprehensive scientific systematic review of the literature in sports medicine. *Sports (Basel).* 2023;11(6):109. doi:10.3390/sports11060109
5. Beck KL, von Hurst PR, O'Brien WJ, Badenhorst CE. Micronutrients and athletic performance: a review. *Food Chem Toxicol.* 2021;158:112618. doi:10.1016/j.fct.2021.112618
6. Peeling P, Sim M, McKay AKA. Considerations for the consumption of vitamin and mineral supplements in athlete populations. *Sports Med.* 2023;53(suppl 1):15-24. doi:10.1007/s40279-023-01875-4
7. Byrd-Bredbenner C, Moe G, Beshgetoor D, Berning J. *Wardlaw's Perspectives in Nutrition.* 9th ed. McGraw-Hill; 2013.
8. Burke L, Deakin V. *Clinical Sports Nutrition.* 4th ed. McGraw-Hill; 2009.
9. Kimura N, Fukuwatari T, Sasaki R, Hayakawa F, Shibata K. Vitamin intake in Japanese women college students. *J Nutr Sci Vitaminol (Tokyo).* 2003;49(3):149-155. doi:10.3177/jnsv.49.149
10. Committee to Review Dietary Reference Intakes for Vitamin D and Calcium, Food and Nutrition Board, Institute of Medicine. Ross AC, Taylor CL, Yaktine AL, Del Valle HB, eds. *Dietary Reference Intakes for Calcium and Vitamin D.* National Academies Press; 2011.
11. Barr SI. Introduction to Dietary Reference Intakes. *Appl Physiol Nutr Metab.* 2006;31(1):61-65. doi:10.1139/h05-019
12. Collins AC, Ward KD, Mirza B, Slawson DL, McClanahan BS, Vukadinovich C. Comparison of nutritional intake in US adolescent swimmers and non-athletes. *Health (Irvine Calif).* 2012;4(10):873-880. doi:10.4236/health.2012.410133
13. Vaz M, Paulin M, Unni US, et al. Micronutrient supplementation improves physical performance measures in Asian Indian school-age children. *J Nutr.* 2011;141(11):2017-2023. doi:10.3945/jn.110.135012
14. Standing Committee on the Scientific Evaluation of Dietary Reference Intakes and Its Panel on Folate, Other B Vitamins, and Choline, Food and Nutrition Board, Institute of Medicine. *Dietary Reference Intakes for Thiamin, Riboflavin, Niacin, Vitamin B6, Folate, Vitamin B12, Pantothenic Acid, Biotin, and Choline.* National Academies Press; 1998.
15. Panel on Dietary Antioxidants and Related Compounds, Food and Nutrition Board, Institute of Medicine. *Dietary Reference Intakes for Vitamin C, Vitamin E, Selenium, and Carotenoids.* National Academies Press; 2000.
16. Panel on Micronutrients, Food and Nutrition Board, Institute of Medicine. *Dietary Reference Intakes for Vitamin A, Vitamin K, Arsenic, Boron, Chromium, Copper, Iodine, Iron, Manganese, Molybdenum, Nickel, Silicon, Vanadium, and Zinc.* National Academies Press; 2001.
17. Panel on Dietary Reference Intakes for Electrolytes and Water, Standing Committee on the Scientific Evaluation of Dietary Reference Intakes, Food and Nutrition Board, Institute of Medicine. *Dietary Reference Intakes for Water, Potassium, Sodium, Chloride, and Sulfate.* National Academies Press; 2005.
18. Prado de Oliveira E, Burini RC, Jeukendrup A. Gastrointestinal complaints during exercise: prevalence, etiology, and nutritional recommendations. *Sports Med.* 2014;44(suppl 1):S79-S85. doi:10.1007/s40279-014-0153-2
19. Erdman JW Jr, Macdonald IA, Zeisel SH. *Present Knowledge in Nutrition.* 10th ed. Wiley-Blackwell; 2012.
20. Woolf K, Manore MM. B-vitamins and exercise: does exercise alter requirements? *Int J Sport Nutr Exerc Metab.* 2006;16(5):453-484. doi:10.1123/ijsnem.16.5.453
21. National Institutes of Health, Office of Dietary Supplements. Thiamin: Fact Sheet for Health Professionals. Updated February 9, 2023. Accessed July 27, 2023. https://ods.od.nih.gov/factsheets/Thiamin-HealthProfessional
22. Kim Y-N, Choi JY, Cho Y-O. Regular moderate exercise training can alter the urinary excretion of thiamin and riboflavin. *Nutr Res Pract.* 2015;9(1):43-48. doi:10.4162/nrp.2015.9.1.43
23. Sato A, Shimoyama Y, Ishikawa T, Murayama N. Dietary thiamin and riboflavin intake and blood thiamin and riboflavin concentrations in college swimmers undergoing intensive training. *Int J Sport Nutr Exerc Metab.* 2011;21(3):195-204. doi:10.1123/ijsnem.21.3.195
24. Nichols QZ, Ramadoss R, Stanzione JR, Volpe SL. Micronutrient supplement intakes among collegiate and masters athletes: a cross-sectional study. *Front Sports Act Living.* 2023;5:854442. doi:10.3389/fspor.2023.854442
25. Hoffman MD, Valentino TR, Stuempfle KJ, Hassid BV. A placebo-controlled trial of riboflavin for enhancement of ultramarathon recovery. *Sports Med Open.* 2017;3(1):14. doi:10.1186/s40798-017-0081-4
26. Zhang J, Chen J, Sui X, Drenowatz C, Wang Q. Association between different types of exercise and intake of nutrients including carbohydrate, fat, protein, and B vitamins in young adults. *Nutrients.* 2023;15(4):806. doi:10.3390/nu15040806
27. Bronkhorst I, Da Silva LA, Freitas L, Martins M, Martins H, Malfatti C. Vitamin B6 and maltodextrin sports drink modify glucose levels of elite mountain biking athletes. *J Exerc Physiol Online.* 2014;17(4):113-121.

28. Wolinsky I, Driskell JA, eds. *Sports Nutrition: Energy Metabolism and Exercise*. 2nd ed. Nutrition in Exercise and Sport Series. CRC Press; 2007.
29. Manore MM. Effect of physical activity on thiamine, riboflavin, and vitamin B-6 requirements. *Am J Clin Nutr*. 2000;72(2 suppl:598S-606S. doi:10.1093/ajcn/72.2.598S
30. Ueland PM, Ulvik A, Rios-Avila L, Midttun O, Gregory, JF. Direct and functional biomarkers of vitamin B6 status. *Annu Rev Nutr*. 2015;35:33-70. doi:10.1146/annurev-nutr-071714-034330
31. Trost S, Wilcox, A, Gillis, D. The effect of substrate utilization, manipulated by nicotinic acid, on excess postexercise oxygen consumption. *Int J Sports Med*. 1997;18(2):83-88. doi:10.1055/s-2007-972600
32. Kamanna VS, Ganji SH, Kashyap ML. The mechanism and mitigation of niacin-induced flushing. *Int J Clin Pract*. 2009;63(9):1369-1377. doi:10.1111/j.1742-1241.2009.02099.x
33. Schaefer PM, Huang J, Butic A, et al. Nicotinamide riboside alleviates exercise intolerance in ANT1-deficient mice. *Mol Metab*. 2022;64:101560. doi:10.1016/j.molmet.2022.101560
34. Wall BT, Stephens FB, Marimuthu K, Constantin-Teodosiu D, Macdonald IA, Greenhaff PL. Acute pantothenic acid and cysteine supplementation does not affect muscle coenzyme A content, fuel selection, or exercise performance in healthy humans. *J Appl Physiol (1985)*. 2012;112(2):272-278. doi:10.1152/japplphysiol.00807.2011
35. Whitfield J, Harris RC, Broad EM, et al. Chronic pantothenic acid supplementation does not affect muscle coenzyme A content or cycling performance. *Appl Physiol Nutr Metab*. 2021;46(3):280-283. doi:10.1139/apnm-2020-0692
36. National Institutes of Health, Office of Dietary Supplements. Choline: Fact Sheet for Health Professionals. Updated June 2, 2022. Accessed July 27, 2023. https://ods.od.nih.gov/factsheets/Choline-HealthProfessional/#en1
37. Zeisel SH. Choline. In: Coates PM, Betz JM, Blackman MR, et al. eds. *Encyclopedia of Dietary Supplements*. 2nd ed. Informa Healthcare; 2010:136-143.
38. Ross AC, Cabalero B, Cousins RJ, Tucker KL, Ziegler TR. *Modern Nutrition in Health and Disease*. 11th ed. Wolters Kluwer Health/Lippincott Williams & Wilkins; 2014.
39. Penry JT, Manore MM. Choline: an important micronutrient for maximal endurance-exercise performance? *Int J Sport Nutr Exerc Metab*. 2008;18(2):191-203. doi:10.1123/ijsnem.18.2.191
40. Warber JP, Patton JF, Tharion WJ, et al. The effects of choline supplementation on physical performance. *Int J Sport Nutr Exerc Metab*. 2000;10(2):170-181. doi:10.1123/ijsnem.10.2.170
41. Dunford M, Doyle JA. *Nutrition for Sport and Exercise*. 3rd ed. Aspen Publishing; 2012.
42. Lee EC, Maresh CM, Kraemer WJ, et al. Ergogenic effects of betaine supplementation on strength and power performance. *J Int Soc Sports Nutr*. 2010;7:27. doi:10.1186/1550-2783-7-27
43. Hoffman JR, Ratamess NA, Kang J, Rashti SL, Faigenbaum AD. Effect of betaine supplementation on power performance and fatigue. *J Int Soc Sports Nutr*. 2009;6:7. doi:10.1186/1550-2783-6-7
44. Soleimani E, Ardekani AM, Fayyazishishavan E, Farhangi MA. The interactive relationship of dietary choline and betaine with physical activity on circulating creatine kinase (CK), metabolic and glycemic markers, and anthropometric characteristics in physically active young individuals. *BMC Endocr Disord*. 2023;23(1):158. doi:10.1186/s12902-023-01413-3
45. McCarthy CG, Farney TM, Canale RE, Dessoulavy ME, Bloomer RJ. High-fat feeding, but not strenuous exercise, increases blood oxidative stress in trained men. *Appl Physiol Nutr Metab*. 2013;38(1):33-41. doi:10.1139/apnm-2012-0222
46. Sies H, Stahl W, Sevanian A. Nutritional, dietary and postprandial oxidative stress. *J Nutr*. 2005;135(5):969-972. doi:10.1093/jn/135.5.969
47. Fisher-Wellman K, Bloomer RJ. Acute exercise and oxidative stress: a 30-year history. *Dyn Med*. 2009;8:1. doi:10.1186/1476-5918-8-1
48. Bloomer RJ. Effect of exercise on oxidative stress biomarkers. *Adv Clin Chem*. 2008;46:1-50. doi:10.1016/s0065-2423(08)00401-0
49. Djordjevic DZ, Cubrilo DG, Barudzic NS, et al. Comparison of blood pro/antioxidant levels before and after acute exercise in athletes and non-athletes. *Gen Physiol Biophys*. 2012;31(2):211-219. doi:10.4149/gpb_2012_025
50. Ferreira LF, Reid MB. Muscle-derived ROS and thiol regulation in muscle fatigue. *J Appl Phys (1985)*. 2008;104(3):853-860. doi:10.1152/japplphysiol.00953.2007
51. Slattery K, Bentley D, Coutts AJ. The role of oxidative, inflammatory and neuroendocrinological systems during exercise stress in athletes: implications of antioxidant supplementation on physiological adaptation during intensified physical training. *Sports Med*. 2015;45(4):453-471. doi:10.1007/s40279-014-0282-7
52. Vassilakopoulos T, Karatza MH, Katsaounou P, Kollintza A, Zakynthinos S, Roussos C. Antioxidants attenuate the plasma cytokine response to exercise in humans. *J Appl Physiol*. 2003;94:1025-1032. doi:10.1152/japplphysiol.00735.200
53. Margaritis I, Palazzetti S, Rousseau AS, Richard MJ, Favier A. Antioxidant supplementation and tapering exercise improve exercise-induced antioxidant response. *J Am Coll Nutr*. 2003;22(2):147-156. doi:10.1080/07315724.2003.10719288
54. Peake JM. Vitamin C: effects of exercise and requirements with training. *Int J Sport Nutr Exerc Metab*. 2003;13(2):125-151. doi:10.1123/ijsnem.13.2.125
55. Rogers DR, Lawlor DJ, Moeller JL. Vitamin C supplementation and athletic performance: a review. *Curr Sports Med Rep*. 2023;22(7):255-259. doi:10.1249/JSR.0000000000001083
56. Robson PJ, Bouic PJ, Myburgh KH. Antioxidant supplementation enhances neutrophil oxidative burst in trained runners following prolonged exercise. *Int J Sport Nutr Exerc Metab*. 2003;13(3):369-381. doi:10.1123/ijsnem.13.3.369

57. Gomez-Cabrera M-C, Domenech E, Romagnoli M, et al. Oral administration of vitamin C decreases muscle mitochondrial biogenesis and hampers training-induced adaptations in endurance performance. *Am J Clin Nutr*. 2008:87(1):142-149. doi:10.1093/ajcn/87.1.142

58. Gabrial SGN, Shakib M-CR, Gabrial GN. Protective role of vitamin C intake on muscle damage in male adolescents performing strenuous physical activity. *Open Access Maced J Med Sci*. 2018;6(9):1594-1598. doi:10.3889/oamjms.2018.337

59. Mullins VA, Houtkooper LB, Howell WH, Going SB, Brown CH. Nutritional status of US elite female heptathletes during training. *Int J Sport Nutr Exerc Metab*. 2001;11(3):299-314. doi:10.1123/ijsnem.11.3.299

60. Braakhuis AJ, Hopkins WG, Lowe TE. Effect of dietary antioxidants, training, and performance correlates on antioxidant status in competitive rowers. *Int J Sports Physiol Perform*. 2013;8(5):565-572. doi:10.1123/ijspp.8.5.565

61. Garelnabi M, Veledar E, White-Welkley J, et al. Vitamin E differentially affects short term exercise induced changes in oxidative stress, lipids, and inflammatory markers. *Nutr Metab Cardiovasc Dis*. 2012;22(10):907-913. doi:10.1016/j.numecd.2011.03.002

62. Bryant RJ, Ryder J, Martino P, Kim J, Craig BW. Effects of vitamin E and C supplementation either alone or in combination on exercise-induced lipid peroxidation in trained cyclists. *J Strength Cond Res*. 2003;17(4):792-800. doi:10.1519/1533-4287(2003)017<0792:eoveac>2.0.co;2

63. Sarkar S, Dey SK, Datta G, Bandyopadhyay A. Vitamin C and E supplementation and high intensity interval training induced changes in lipid profile and haematological variables of young males. *Sports Med Health Sci*. 2023;5(2):137-145. doi:10.1016/j.smhs.2023.03.006

64. Avery NG, Kaiser JL, Sharman MJ, et al. Effects of vitamin E supplementation on recovery from repeated bouts of resistance exercise. *J Strength Cond Res*. 2003;17(4):801-809. doi:10.1519/1533-4287(2003)017<0801:eoveso>2.0.co;2

65. Stepanyan V, Crowe M, Haleagrahara N, Bowden B. Effects of vitamin E supplementation on exercise-induced oxidative stress: a meta-analysis. *Appl Physiol Nutr Metab*. 2014;39(9):1029-1037. doi:10.1139/apnm-2013-0566

66. Young AJ, Lowe GM. Antioxidant and prooxidant properties of carotenoids. *Arch Biochem Biophys*. 2001;385(1):20-27. doi:10.1006/abbi.2000.2149

67. Aguiló A, Tauler P, Pilar Guix M, et al. Effect of exercise intensity and training on antioxidants and cholesterol profile in cyclists. *J Nutr Biochem*. 2003;14(6):319-325. doi:10.1016/s0955-2863(03)00052-4

68. Fernandez-Lazaro D, Fernandez-Lazaro CI, Mielgo-Ayuso J, Navascués LJ, Córdova Martínez A, Seco-Calvo J. The role of selenium mineral trace element in exercise: antioxidant defense system, muscle performance, hormone response, and athletic performance. A systematic review. *Nutrients*. 2020;12(6):1790. doi:10.3390/nu12061790

69. Aoi W, Ogaya Y, Takami M, et al. Glutathione supplementation suppresses muscle fatigue induced by prolonged exercise via improved aerobic metabolism. *J Int Soc Sports Nutr*. 2015;12:7. doi:10.1186/s12970-015-0067-x

70. Kovacs L, Zamboni C, Lourenço T, Macedo D. Sulfur status in long distance runners. *J Phys Conf Ser*. 2015;630:012009. doi:10.1088/1742-6596/630/1/012009

71. Maynar M, Grijota FJ, Siguier-Coll J, et al. Erythrocyte concentrations of chromium, copper, manganese, molybdenum, selenium and zinc in subjects with different physical training levels. *J Int Soc Sports Nutr*. 2020;17(1)35. doi:10.1186/s12970-020-00367-4

72. Mehlenbeck RS, Ward KD, Klesges RC, Vukadinovich CM. A pilot intervention to increase calcium intake in female collegiate athletes. *Int J Sport Nutr Exerc Metab*. 2004;14(1):18-29. doi:10.1123/ijsnem.14.1.18

73. Deldicque L, Francaux M. Recommendations for healthy nutrition in female endurance runners: an update. *Front Nutr*. 2015;2:17. doi:10.3389/fnut.2015.00017

74. Beshgetoor D, Nichols JF. Dietary intake and supplement use in female master cyclists and runners. *Int J Sport Nutr Exerc Metab*. 2003;13(2):166-172. doi:10.1123/ijsnem.13.2.166

75. Zamboni F, Ferrari P, Cazzoletti L, et al. Bone mineral density in mountain, road cyclists and untrained controls: exercise, diet and hormones. *Res Q Exerc Sport*. 2024;95(2):423-430. doi:10.1080/02701367.2023.2242417

76. Barry DW, Hansen KC, Van Pelt RE, Witten M, Wolfe P, Kohrt WM. Acute calcium ingestion attenuates exercise-induced disruption of calcium homeostasis. *Med Sci Sports Exerc*. 2011;43(4):617-623. doi:10.1249/MSS.0b013e3181f79fa8

77. Lundy B, McKay AKA, Fensham NC, et al. The impact of acute calcium intake on bone turnover markers during a training day in elite male rowers. *Med Sci Sports Exerc*. 2023;55(1):55-65. doi:10.1249/MSS.0000000000003022

78. Moyad MA. The potential benefits of dietary and/or supplemental calcium and vitamin D. *Urol Oncol*. 2003;21(5):384-391. doi:10.1016/s1078-1439(03)00108-x

79. Zemel MB, Shi H, Greer B, Dirienzo D, Zemel PC. Regulation of adiposity by dietary calcium. *FASEB J*. 2000;14(9):1132-1138. doi:10.1096/fasebj.14.9.1132

80. Melanson EL, Sharp TA, Schneider J, Donahoo WT, Grunwald GK, Hill JO. Relation between calcium intake and fat oxidation in adult humans. *Int J Obes Relat Metab Disord*. 2003;27(2):196-203. doi:10.1038/sj.ijo.802202

81. Huang L, Xue J, He Y, et al. Dietary calcium but not elemental calcium from supplements is associated with body composition and obesity in Chinese women. *PLoS One*. 2011;6(12):e277703. doi:10.1371/journal.pone.0027703

82. Skinner ML, Randall Simpson JA, Buchholz AC. Dietary and total calcium intakes are associated with lower percentage total body and truncal fat in healthy adults. *J Am Coll Nutr*. 2011;30(6):484-490. doi:10.1080/07315724.2011.10719994

83. Zhu W, Cai D, Wang Y, et al. Calcium plus vitamin D3 supplementation facilitated Fat loss in overweight and obese college students with very-low calcium consumption: a randomized controlled trial. *Nutr J*. 2013;12:8. doi:10.1186/1475-2891-12-8
84. Samadi M, Sadrzadeh-Yeganeh H, Azadbakht L, Feizi A, Jafarian K, Sotoudeh G. Dietary calcium intake and risk of obesity in school girls aged 8-10 years. *J Res Med Sci*. 2012;17(12):1102-1107. doi:10.1681/ASN.2013040355
85. Shapses SA, Heshka S, Heymsfield SB. Effect of calcium supplementation on weight and fat loss in women. *J Clin Endocrinol Metab*. 2004;89(2):632-637. doi:10.1210/jc.2002-021136
86. Palacios C, Bertrán JJ, Rios RE, Soltero S. No effects of low and high consumption of dairy products and calcium supplements on body composition and serum lipids in Puerto Rican obese adults. *Nutrition*. 2011;27(5):520-525. doi:10.1016/j.nut.2010.02.011
87. Lorenzen JK, Mølgaard C, Michaelsen KF, Astrup A. Calcium supplementation for 1 y does not reduce body weight or fat mass in young girls. *Am J Clin Nutr*. 2006;83(1):18-23. doi:10.1093/ajcn/83.1.18
88. Murakami K, Okubo H, Sasaki S. No relation between intakes of calcium and dairy products and body mass index in Japanese women aged 18 to 20 y. *Nutrition*. 2006;22(5):490-495. doi:10.1016/j.nut.2005.12.003
89. Gunther CW, Legowski PA, Lyle RM, et al. Dairy products do not lead to alterations in body weight or fat mass in young women in a 1-y intervention. *Am J Clin Nutr*. 2005;81(4):751-756. doi:10.1093/ajcn/81.4.754
90. Weaver CM, Heaney RP. Calcium. In: Ross AC, Caballero B, Cousins RJ, Tucker KL, Ziegler TR, eds. *Modern Nutrition in Health and Disease*. 11th ed. Lippincott Williams & Wilkins; 2014:133-149.
91. Hossein-Nezhad A, Holick MF. Vitamin D for health: a global perspective. *Mayo Clin Proc*. 2013;88(7):720-755. doi:10.1016/j.mayocp.2013.05.011
92. Holick MF, Binkley NC, Bischoff-Ferrari HA, et al. Evaluation, treatment, and prevention of vitamin D deficiency: an Endocrine Society clinical practice guideline. *J Clin Endocrinol Metab*. 2011;96(7):1911-1930. doi:10.1210/jc.2011-0385
93. de la Puente Yague M, Collado Yurrita L, Ciudad Cabanas MJ, Cuadrado Cenzual MA. Role of vitamin D in athletes and their performance: current concepts and new trends. *Nutrients*. 2020:12:579. doi:10.3390/nu12020579
94. Wicherts IS, van Schoor NM, Boeke JP, V et al. Vitamin D status predicts physical performance and its decline in older persons. *J Endocrinol Metab*. 2007;92(6):2058-2065. doi:10.1210/jc.2006-1525
95. Cashman KD, Hill TR, Lucey AJ, et al. Estimation of the dietary requirement for vitamin D in healthy adults. *Am J Clin Nutr*. 2008;88(6):1535-1542. doi:10.3945/ajcn.2008.26594
96. Kroll MH, Bi C, Garber CC, et al. Temporal relationship between vitamin D status and parathyroid hormone in the United States. *PLoS One*. 2015;10(3):e0118108. doi:10.1371/journal.pone.0118108
97. Close GL, Russell J, Cobley JN. Assessment of vitamin D concentration in non-supplemented professional athletes and healthy adults during the winter months in the UK: implications for skeletal muscle function. *J Sports Sci*. 2013;31(4):344-353. doi:10.1080/02640414.2012.733822
98. Farrokhyar F, Tabasinejad R, Dao D, et al. Prevalence of vitamin D inadequacy in athletes: a systematic-review and meta-analysis. *Sports Med*. 2015;45(3):365-378. doi:10.1007/s40279-014-0267-6
99. Amrein K, Scherkl M, Hoffmann M, et al. Vitamin D deficiency 2.0: an update on the current status worldwide. *Eur J Clin Nutr*. 2020;74(11):1498-1513. doi:10.1038/s41430-020-0558-y
100. Bikle DD. Vitamin D metabolism, mechanism of action, and clinical applications. *Chem Biol*. 2014;21(3):319-329. doi:10.1016/j.chembiol.2013.12.016
101. Allison RJ, Close GL, Farooq A, et al. Severely vitamin D-deficient athletes present smaller hearts than sufficient athletes. *Eur J Preventive Cardiol*. 2015;22(4):535-542. doi:10.1177/2047487313518473
102. Galan F, Ribas J, Sánchez-Martinez PM, Calero T, Sánchez AB, Muñoz A. Serum 25-hydroxyvitamin D in early autumn to ensure vitamin D sufficiency in midwinter in professional football players. *Clin Nutr*. 2012;31(1):132-136. doi:10.1016/j.clnu.2011.07.008
103. Hamilton B, Grantham J, Racinais S, Chalabi H. Vitamin D deficiency is endemic in Middle Eastern sportsmen. *Publ Health Nutr*. 2010;13(10):1528-1534. doi:10.1017/S136898000999320X
104. Ip TS-T, Fu S-C, Ong MT-Y, Yung PS-H. Vitamin D deficiency in athletes: laboratory, clinical and field integration. *Asia Pac J Sports Med Arthrosc Rehabil Technol*. 2022;29:22-29. doi:10.1016/j.asmart.2022.06.001
105. Moss SL, Randell RK, Burgess D, et al. Assessment of energy availability and associated risk factors in professional female soccer players. *Eur J Sport Sci*. 2021;21(6):861-870. doi:10.1080/17461391.2020.1788647
106. Sheridan HC, Parker LJF, Hammond KM. Dietary supplements for consideration in elite female footballers. *Eur J Sport Sci*. 2022;22(5):733-744. doi:10.1080/17461391.2021.1988149
107. Williams K, Askew C, Mazoue C, et al. Vitamin D3 supplementation and stress fractures in high-risk collegiate athletes - a pilot study. *Orthop Res Rev*. 2020;12:9-17. doi:10.2147/ORR.S233387
108. Knechtle B, Jastrzebski Z, Hill L, Nikolaidis PT. Vitamin D and stress fractures in sport: preventive and therapeutic measures–a narrative review. *Medicina*. 2021;57(3):223. doi:10.3390/medicina57030223
109. Larson-Meyer DE, Willis KS. Vitamin D and athletes. *Curr Sports Med Rep*. 2010;9(4):220e226. doi:10.1249/JSR.0b013e3181e7dd45
110. Brooks MA, Parks RB, Sanfilippo JL, Binkley NC, Stiffler MR. Assessment of dietary vitamin D intake and compliance with recommended vitamin D supplementation in Division I collegiate athletes. *Athl Train Sports Health Care*. 2015;7(5):204-213. doi:10.3928/19425864-20150831-06

111. Erkal MZ, Wilde J, Bilgin Y, et al. High prevalence of vitamin D deficiency, secondary hyperparathyroidism and generalized bone pain in Turkish immigrants in Germany: identification of risk factors. *Osteoporos Int.* 2006;17(8):1133-1140. doi:10.1007/s00198-006-0069-2
112. Leventis P, Kiely DW. The tolerability and biochemical effects of high-dose bolus vitamin D2 and D3 supplementation in patients with vitamin D insufficiency. *Scand J Rheumatol.* 2009;38(2):149-153. doi:10.1080/03009740802419081
113. Lehmann U, Hirche F, Stangl GI, Hinz K, Westphal S, Dierkes J. Bioavailability of D2 and D3 in healthy volunteers, a randomized placebo-controlled trial. *J Clin Endocrinol Metab.* 2013;98(11):4339-4345. doi:10.1210/jc.2012-4287
114. Willis KS, Peterson NJ, Larson-Meyer DE. Should we be concerned about the vitamin D status of athletes? *Int J Sport Nutr Exerc Metab.* 2008;18(2):204-224. doi:10.1123/ijsnem.18.2.204
115. Forney LA, Earnest CP, Henagan TM, Johnson LE, Castleberry TJ, Stewart LK. Vitamin D status, body composition, and fitness measures in college-aged students. *J Strength Cond Res.* 2014;28(3):814-824. doi:10.1519/JSC.0b013e3182a35ed0
116. Carswell AT, Oliver SJ, Wentz LM, et al. Influence of vitamin D supplementation by sunlight or oral D3 on exercise performance. *Med Sci Sports Exerc.* 2018;50(12):2555-2564. doi:10.1249/MSS.0000000000001721
117. Standing Committee on the Scientific Evaluation of Dietary Reference Intakes, Food and Nutrition Board, Institute of Medicine. *Dietary Reference Intakes for Calcium, Phosphorus, Magnesium, Vitamin D, and Fluoride.* National Academies Press; 1997.
118. Moe SM. Disorders involving calcium, phosphorus, and magnesium. *Prim Care.* 2008;35(2):215-237. doi:10.1016/j.pop.2008.01.007
119. Penido MG, Alon US. Phosphate homeostasis and its role in bone health. *Pediatr Nephrol.* 2012;27(11):2039-2048. doi:10.1007/s00467-012-2175-z
120. Wyshak G. Teenaged girls, carbonated beverage consumption, and bone fractures. *Arch Pediatr Adolesc Med.* 2000;154(6):610-613. doi:10.1001/archpedi.154.6.610
121. Tucker KL, Morita K, Qiao N, Hannan MT, Cupples LA, Kiel DP. Colas, but not other carbonated beverages, are associated with low bone mineral density in older women: the Framingham Osteoporosis Study. *Am J Clin Nutr.* 2006;84(4):936-942. doi:10.1093/ajcn/84.4.936
122. Gutiérrez OM, Luzuriaga-McPherson A, Lin Y, Gilbert LC, Ha S-W, Beck GR Jr. Impact of phosphorus-based food additives on bone and mineral metabolism. *J Clin Endocrinol Metab.* 2015;100(11):4264-4271. doi:10.1210/jc.2015-2279
123. Peri-Okonny P, Baskin KK, Iwamoto G. High-phosphate diet induces exercise intolerance and impairs fatty acid metabolism in mice. *Circulation.* 2019;139(11):1422-1434. doi:10.1161/CIRCULATIONAHA.118.037550
124. Bremner K, Bubb WA, Kemp GJ, Trenell MI, Thompson CH. The effect of phosphate loading on erythrocyte 2,3-bisphosphoglycerate levels. *Clin Chim Acta.* 2002;323(1-2):111-114. doi:10.1016/s0009-8981(02)00165-1
125. Brewer CP, Dawson B, Wallman KE, Guelfi KJ. Effect of sodium phosphate supplementation on cycling time trial performance and VO_2 1 and 8 days post loading. *J Sports Sci Med.* 2014;13(3):529-534.
126. Mariño MM, Grijota FJ, Bartolomé I, Siquier-Coll J, Román VT, Muñoz D. Influence of physical training on erythrocyte concentrations of iron, phosphorus and magnesium. *J Int Soc Sports Nutr.* 2020;17(1):8. doi:10.1186/s12970-020-0339-y
127. Barker ME, Blumsohn A. Is vitamin A consumption a risk factor for osteoporotic fracture? *Proc Nutr Soc.* 2003;62(4):845-850. doi:10.1079/PNS2003306
128. Yee MMF, Chin K-Y, Ima-Nirwana S, Wong SK. Vitamin A and bone health: a review on current evidence. *Molecules.* 2021;26(6):1757. doi:10.3390/molecules26061757
129. Koury MJ, Ponka P. New insights into erythropoiesis: the roles of folate, vitamin B12, and iron. *Ann Rev Nutr.* 2004:24:105-131. doi:10.1146/annurev.nutr.24.012003.132306
130. National Institutes of Health, Office of Dietary Supplements. Vitamin B12: Fact Sheet for Health Professionals. Updated December 22, 2022. Accessed August 30, 2023. https://ods.od.nih.gov/factsheets/VitaminB12-HealthProfessional/#h7
131. National Institutes of Health, Office of Dietary Supplements. Folate: Fact Sheet for Health Professionals. Updated November 30, 2022. Accessed August 30, 2023. https://ods.od.nih.gov/factsheets/Folate-HealthProfessional
132. Mayo Clinic Staff. Vitamin B-12. Updated August 10, 2023. Accessed August 30, 2023. www.mayoclinic.org/drugs-supplements-vitamin-b12/art-20363663#:~:text= Taking%20vitamin%20B%2D12%20with,a%20vitamin%20B%2D12%20supplement
133. Veeranna V, Zalawadiya SK, Niraj A, et al. Homocysteine and reclassification of cardiovascular disease risk. *J Am Coll Cardiol.* 2011;58(10):1025-1033. doi:10.1016/j.jacc.2011.05.028
134. Iglesias-Gutiérrez E, Egan B, Díaz-Martinez AE, et al. Transient increase in homocysteine but not hyperhomocysteinemia during acute exercise at different intensities in sedentary individuals. *PLoS One.* 2012;7(12):e51185. doi:10.1371/journal.pone.0051185
135. König D, Bissé E, Deibert P, Müller H-M, Wieland H, Berg A. Influence of training volume and acute physical exercise on the homocysteine levels in endurance-trained men: interactions with plasma folate and vitamin B12. *Ann Nutr Metab.* 2003;47(3-4):114-118. doi:10.1159/000070032
136. Herrmann M, Wilkinson J, Schorr H, et al. Comparison of the influence of volume-oriented training and high-intensity interval training on serum homocysteine and its cofactors in young, healthy swimmers. *Clin Chem Lab Med.* 2003;41911:1525-1531. doi:10.1515/CCLM.2003.234

137. Kim Y-N, Hwang JH, Cho Y-O. The effects of exercise training and acute exercise duration on plasma folate and vitamin B12. *Nutr Res Pract.* 2016;10(2):161-166. doi:10.4162/nrp.2016.10.2.161
138. World Health Organization. Haemoglobin concentrations for the diagnosis of anaemia and assessment of severity. Report WHO/NMH/NHD/MNM/11.1. *Vitamin and Mineral Nutrition Information System.* 2011. Accessed August 30, 2023. www.who.int/vmnis/indicators/haemoglobin.pdf
139. Bathla S, Arora S. Prevalence and approaches to manage iron deficiency anemia (IDA). *Crit Rev Food Sci Nutr.* 2022;62(32):8815-8828. doi:10.1080/10408398.2021.1935442
140. Kumar A, Sharma E, Marley A, Samaan MA, Brookes MJ. Iron deficiency anaemia: pathophysiology, assessment, practical management. *BMJ Open Gastroenterol.* 2022;9(1):e000759. doi:10.1136/bmjgast-2021-000759
141. Sim M, Garvican-Lewis LA, Cox GR, et al. Iron considerations for the athlete: a narrative review. *Eur J Appl Physiol.* 2019;119:1463-1478. doi:10.1007/s00421-019-04157-y
142. Hinton PS. Iron and the endurance athlete. *Appl Physiol Nutr Metab.* 2014;39(9):1012-1018. doi:10.1139/apnm-2014-0147
143. Haymes EM. Iron. In: Driskell JA, Wolinsky I, eds. *Sports Nutrition: Vitamins and Trace Elements.* 2nd ed. CRC/Taylor & Francis; 2006:203-216.
144. Woolf K, St Thomas M, Hahn N, Vaughan LA, Carlson AG, Hinton P. Iron status in highly active and sedentary young women. *Int J Sport Nutr Exerc Metab.* 2009;19(5):519-535. doi:10.1123/ijsnem.19.5.519
145. Di Santolo M, Stel G, Banfi G, Gonano F, Cauci S. Anemia and iron status in young fertile non-professional female athletes. *Eur J Appl Physiol.* 2008;102(6):703-709. doi:10.1007/s00421-007-0647-9
146. Hueglin S. A practical approach for developing an iron protocol for athletes. *SCAN's PULSE.* 2016;35(2):10-13.
147. Cook JD. Diagnosis and management of iron-deficiency anaemia. *Best Pract Res Clin Haematol.* 2005;18(2):319-332. doi:10.1016/j.beha.2004.08.022
148. Ashmead HD. The absorption and metabolism of iron amino acid chelate. *Arch Latinoam Nutr.* 2001;51(1 suppl 1):13-21.
149. Rosenzweig PH, Volpe SL. Effect of iron supplementation on thyroid hormone levels and resting metabolic rate in two college female athletes: a case study. *Int J Sports Nutr Exerc Metab.* 2000:10(4):434-443. doi:10.1123/ijsnem.10.4.434
150. Csulak E, Takács T, Babis B, et al. Iron deficiency in young basketball players: is a 100 μg/L ferritin cut-off appropriate for iron supplementation?: results of a randomized placebo-controlled study. *Clin Cardiol.* 2023;46(9):1116-1123. doi:10.1002/clc.24117
151. DellaValle DM, Haas JD. Iron supplementation improves energetic efficiency in iron-depleted female rowers. *Med Sci Sports Exerc.* 2014;46(6):1204-1215. doi:10.1249/MSS.0000000000000208
152. McCormick R, Dreyer A, Dawson B, et al. The effectiveness of daily and alternate day oral iron supplementation in athletes with suboptimal iron status (Part 2). *Int J Sport Nutr Exerc Metab.* 2020;30(3):191-196. doi:10.1123/ijsnem.2019-0310
153. Malcolm C. Nutrient timing guide to optimize iron absorption. CTS. Accessed July 27, 2023. https://trainright.com/nutrient-timing-guide-optimize-iron-absorption/#:~:text=Consume%20iron%20rich%20meals%2C%20especially,while%20body%20inflammation%20is%20lower
154. Dominguez R, Sánchez-Oliver AJ, Mata-Ordoñez F, et al. Effects of an acute exercise bout on serum hepcidin levels. *Nutrients.* 2018;10(2):209. doi:10.3390/nu10020209
155. Bacchetta J, Zaritsky JJ, Sea JL, et al. Suppression of iron-regulatory hepcidin by vitamin D. *J Am Soc Nephrol.* 2014;25(3):564-572. doi:10.1681/ASN.2013040355
156. Jin C-H, Paik I-Y, Kwak Y-S, Jee Y-S, Kim J-Y. Exhaustive submaximal endurance and resistance exercises induces immunosuppression via physical and oxidative stress. *J Exerc Rehabil.* 2014;11(4):198-203. doi:10.12965/jer.150221
157. Gleeson M, Nieman DC, Pedersen BK. Exercise, nutrition and immune function. *J Sports Sci.* 2004;22(1):115-125. doi:10.1080/0264041031000140590
158. Walsh NP. Nutrition and athlete immune health: new perspectives on an old paradigm. *Sports Med.* 2019;49(suppl 2):S153-S168. doi:10.1007/s40279-019-01160-3
159. Hemilä H, Chalker E. Vitamin C for preventing and treating the common cold. *Cochrane Database Syst Rev.* 2013;1:CD000980. doi:10.1002/14651858.CD000980.pub4
160. Mitmesser SH, Ye Q, Evans M, Combs M. Determination of plasma and leukocyte vitamin C concentrations in a randomized, double-blind, placebo-controlled trial with Ester-C®. *SpringerPlus.* 2016;25;5(1):1161. doi:10.1186/s40064-016-2605-7
161. Braakhuis AJ. Effect of vitamin C supplements on physical performance. *Curr Sports Med Rep.* 2012;11(4):180-184. doi:10.1249/JSR.0b013e31825e19cd
162. Dubnov-Raz G, Hemilä H, Cohen AH, Rinat B, Choleva L, Constantini NW. Vitamin D supplementation and upper respiratory tract infections in adolescent swimmers: a randomized controlled trial. *Pediatr Exerc Sci.* 2015;27(1):113-119. doi:10.1123/pes.2014-0030
163. Harrison SE, Oliver SJ, Kashi DS, et al. Influence of vitamin D supplementation by simulated sunlight or oral D3 on respiratory infection during military training. *Med. Sci. Sports Exerc.* 2021;53(7):1505-1516. doi:10.1249/MSS.0000000000002604
164. Jung HC, Seo M-W, Lee S, Kim SW, Song JK. Vitamin D3 supplementation reduces the symptoms of upper respiratory tract infection during winter training in vitamin D-insufficient taekwondo athletes: a randomized controlled trial. *Int J Environ Res Public Health.* 2018;15(9):2003. doi:10.3390/ijerph15092003
165. Cunnane SC. *Zinc: Clinical and Biochemical Significance.* CRC Press; 1988.
166. Lönnerdal B. Dietary factors influencing zinc absorption. *J Nutr.* 2000;130(5S suppl):1378S-1383S. doi:10.1093/jn/130.5.1378S

167. Hemilä H. Zinc lozenges and the common cold: a meta-analysis comparing zinc acetate and zinc gluconate, and the role of zinc dosage. *JRSM Open*. 2017;8(5):2054270417694291. doi:10.1177/2054270417694291

168. Micheletti A, Rossi R, Rufini S. Zinc status in athletes: relation to diet and exercise. *Sports Med.* 2001;31(8):577-582. doi:10.2165/00007256-200131080-00002

169. Nikić M, Pedišić Ž, Šatalić Z, Jackovljević S, Venus D. Adequacy of nutrient intakes in elite junior basketball players. *Int J Sports Nutr Exerc Metab.* 2014;24(5):516-523. doi:10.1123/ijsnem.2013-0186

170. Giolo De Carvahlo F, Rosa FT, Marques Miguel Suen V, Freitas EC, Padovan GJ, Marchini JS. Evidence of zinc deficiency in competitive swimmers. *Nutrition.* 2012;28(11-12):1127-1131. doi:10.1016/j.nut.2012.02.012

171. Volpe SL, Lowe NM, Woodhouse LR, King JC. Effect of maximal exercise on the short-term kinetics of zinc metabolism in sedentary men. *Br J Sports Med.* 2007;41(3):156-161. doi:10.1136/bjsm.2006.030346

172. Maxwell C, Volpe SL. Effect of zinc supplementation on thyroid hormone function. A case study of two college females. *Ann Nutr Metab.* 2007;51(2):188-194. doi:10.1159/000103324

173. Wehrlin JP, Zuest P, Hallén J, Marti B. Live high-train low for 24 days increases hemoglobin mass and red blood cell volume in elite endurance athletes. *J Appl Physiol (1985).* 2006;100(6):1938-1945. doi:10.1152/japplphysiol.01284.2005

174. Neya M, Enoki T, Ohiwa N, Kawahara T, Gore CJ. Increased hemoglobin mass and VO2max with 10 h nightly simulated altitude at 3000 m. *Int J Sports Physiol Perform.* 2014;8(4):366-372. doi:10.1123/ijspp.8.4.366

175. Stellingwerff T. Nutrition recommendations for altitude training. *Sports Sci Exch.* 2019;29(199):1-5. Accessed July 27, 2023. www.gssiweb.org/sports-science-exchange/article/nutrition-recommendations-for-altitude-training

176. Govus AD, Garvican-Lewis LA, Abbiss CR, Peeling P, Gore CJ. Pre-altitude serum ferritin levels and daily oral iron supplement dose mediate iron parameter and hemoglobin mass responses to altitude exposure. *PLoS One.* 2015;10(8):e0135120. doi:10.1371/journal.pone.0135120

177. Garvican-Lewis LA, Govus AD, Peeling P, Abbiss CR, Gore CJ. Iron supplementation and altitude: decision making using a regression tree. *J Sports Sci Med.* 2016;15:204-205.

178. Hall R, Peeling P, Nemeth E, Bergland D, McCluskey WTP, Stellingwerff T. Single versus split dose of iron optimizes hemoglobin mass gains at 2106 m altitude. *Med Sci Sports Exerc.* 2019;51:751-759. doi:10.1249/MSS.0000000000001847

179. Pialoux V, Mounier R, Rock E, et al. Effects of acute hypoxic exposure on prooxidant/antioxidant balance in elite endurance athletes. *Int J Sports Med.* 2009;30(2):87-93. doi:10.1055/s-0028-1103284

180. Cowell BS, Rosenbloom CA, Skinner R, Summers SH. Policies on screening female athletes for iron deficiency in NCAA Division I-A institutions. *Int J Sport Nutr Exerc Metab.* 2003;13(3):277-285. doi:10.1123/ijsnem.13.3.277

181. De Souza MJ, Nattiv A, Joy E, et al; Expert Panel. 2014 Female Athlete Triad Coalition Consensus Statement on Treatment and Return to Play of the Female Athlete Triad: 1st International Conference held in San Francisco, California, May 2012, and 2nd International Conference held in Indianapolis, Indiana, May 2013. *Br J Sports Med.* 2014;48(4):289. doi:10.1136/bjsports-2013-093218

182. Mountjoy M, Sundgot-Borgen J, Burke L, et al. The IOC consensus statement: Beyond the Female Athlete Triad—Relative Energy Deficiency in Sport (RED-S). *Br J Sports Med.* 2014;48(7):491-497. doi:10.1136/bjsports-2014-093502

183. Cheng C-H, Chen L-R, Chen K-H. Osteoporosis due to hormone imbalance: an overview of the effects of estrogen deficiency and glucocorticoid overuse on bone turnover. *Int J Mol Sci.* 2022;23(3):1376. doi:10.3390/ijms23031376

184. Braam LA, Knapen MH, Geusens P, Brouns F, Vermeer C. Factors affecting bone loss in female endurance athletes: a two-year follow-up study. *Am J Sports Med.* 2003;31(6):889-895. doi:10.1177/03635465030310062601

185. Volpe SL, Leung MM, Giordano H. Vitamin K supplementation does not significantly impact bone mineral density and biochemical markers of bone in pre- and perimenopausal women. *Nutr Res.* 2008;28(9):577-582. doi:10.1016/j.nutres.2008.06.006

186. Booth SL, Suttie JW. Dietary intake and adequacy of vitamin K. *J Nutr.* 1998;128(5):785-788. doi:10.1093/jn/128.5.785

187. Melina V, Craig W, Levin S. Position of the Academy of Nutrition and Dietetics: vegetarian diets. *J Acad Nutr Diet.* 2016:116(12):1970-1980. doi:10.1016/j.jand.2016.09.025

188. Shaw KA, Zello GA, Rodgers CD, Warkentin TD, Baerwald AR, Chilibeck PD. Benefits of a plant-based diet and considerations for the athlete. *Eur J Appl Physiol.* 2022;122(5):1163-1178. doi:10.1007/s00421-022-04902-w

189. Fuhrman J, Ferreri DM. Fueling the vegetarian (vegan) athlete. *Curr Sports Med Rep.* 2010;9(4):233-241. doi:10.1249/JSR.0b013e3181e93a6f

190. Zhang R, Wang Z, Fei Y, et al. The difference in nutrient intakes between Chinese and Mediterranean, Japanese and American diets. *Nutrition.* 2015;7(6):4661-4688. doi:10.3390/nu7064661

191. Sundgot-Borgen J, Torstveit MK. Aspects of disordered eating continuum in elite high-intensity sports. *Scand J Med Sci Sports.* 2010;20(suppl 2):112-121. doi:10.1111/j.1600-0838.2010.01190.x

192. Hinton PS, Sanford TC, Davidson MM, Yakushko OF, Beck NC. Nutrient intakes and dietary behaviors of male and female collegiate athletes. *Int J Sport Nutr Exerc Metab.* 2004;14(4):389-405. doi:10.1123/ijsnem.14.4.389

193. El Ghoch M, Soave F, Calugi S, Grave RD. Eating disorders, physical fitness and sport performance: a systematic review. *Nutrients.* 2013;5(12):5140-5160. doi:10.3390/nu5125140

194. Nazem TG, Ackerman KE. The female athlete triad. *Sports Health.* 2012;4(4):302-311. doi:10.1177/1941738112439685

CHAPTER 6

Fluid, Electrolytes, and Exercise

Bob Murray, PhD, FACSM, and Kris Osterberg, PhD, RD, CSSD

LEARNING OBJECTIVES

- Explain how disruptions in fluid and electrolyte balance affect key physiological functions that influence physical and mental performance.
- Describe the mechanisms by which the body regulates fluid and electrolyte balance.
- Develop a hydration plan that provides fluid and electrolyte recommendations before, during, and after exercise.
- Compare the ways in which environmental extremes such as heat, altitude, humidity, and cold impact fluid and electrolyte balance.

INTRODUCTION

In August 2021, a husband, wife, their 1-year-old daughter, and their dog were found dead on a hiking trail in northern California. When the family began their hike, the ambient temperature in the parking lot was 75 °F (~24 °C), but after 6 miles of hiking, the temperature had climbed to well over 100 °F (>38 °C). Without shade in which to rest and with no more than 85 oz (2.5 L) of fluid between them, all had died of hyperthermia complicated by dehydration.[1]

Such tragic events in sports, occupational, and military settings underscore the importance of staying well hydrated during physical activity to help delay the onset of fatigue as well as protect health and well-being by preventing the physiologically deleterious effects of dehydration. In fact, even a slight amount of dehydration (eg, 1% loss of body weight, which is 1.5 lb [0.7 kg] in a 150-lb [68-kg] individual) can adversely affect the body's ability to cope with physical activity, particularly when that activity occurs in a warm environment.[2,3] That is not to say that dehydration always impairs performance or negatively impacts health; there are many occasions when temporary mild dehydration has no deleterious consequences. However, during physical activity and heat exposure, it is always better to be euhydrated (normally hydrated) than hypohydrated (dehydrated), because euhydration helps sustain critical cardiovascular and thermoregulatory functions. The physiological consequences of dehydration during physical activity are comprehensively reviewed in the scientific literature.[4-7] However, when educating coaches and athletes, the emphasis is better placed on the physiological and performance benefits of hydration,[8-10] along with practical advice for keeping athletes well hydrated during training and competition.

Consuming adequate amounts of fluid and electrolytes before, during, and after physical activity protects physiological function, safeguards health, and improves performance. The information in this chapter is gleaned from decades of research on the physiological and performance-related responses to changes in hydration status. In addition, numerous position stands on the topic of hydration and exercise have been published by a variety of professional organizations,[11-21] and key points from those documents are included in this chapter.

For individuals who engage in vigorous physical activity or who spend considerable time in warm environments, daily water and electrolyte losses can be prodigious, increasing the prevalence and risks of dehydration. Even on days when no sweating occurs, it is not unusual for people to remain slightly dehydrated, a potential risk factor for the development of kidney stones and other ailments.[22] For those reasons, it is important for sports health professionals to have a fundamental understanding of daily fluid and electrolyte balance, beginning with the unique—some might say weird—characteristics of the simple water molecule.

THE UNIQUENESS OF WATER

To understand why the hydration status of the human body has such a great impact on virtually every physiological function, it is essential to first appreciate the fact that the simple water molecule is the most biologically active molecule in the body. No other nutrient is as acutely essential or is needed in as great an amount on a daily basis as water. Water is considered the universal solvent because it is capable of dissolving more substances than any other liquid. Water plays a central role in life, not just because it is a solvent but because it performs many other functions in roles such as solute, reactant, product, carrier, lubricant, shock absorber, coolant, catalyst, ionizing agent, messenger, and controller, as well as the primary volumetric constituent of most cells. It is this compendium of unique characteristics that makes water the most important molecule in biology.[23]

Despite this fact, water has been a somewhat neglected molecule in biology. Water molecules are rarely portrayed in structural drawings of other biological molecules; yet without water, those molecules could not function.[23] An important aspect of the utility of water is its small size: 1 L of water at room temperature contains nearly 1 septillion (10^{24}) molecules—in other words, a million, million, million, million molecules. The water molecule (H_2O) is smaller and lighter than molecules of gases such as oxygen (O_2) and carbon dioxide (CO_2). Most water on Earth is in liquid or solid (ice) form. Water molecules prefer to remain in liquid form largely because of the molecular structure of H_2O. Picture an individual water molecule as a plump sphere in which 1 portion bears a negative charge whereas the other portion is positively charged. That bipolar charge characteristic is what attracts 1 water molecule to the next, allowing water to exist on Earth mostly in liquid or solid form rather than as a gas. The bipolar charge also governs water's interactions with all other elements and compounds.

In cells, water molecules not only allow proteins to form three-dimensional shapes but are also indispensable for allowing proteins such as enzymes to perform their various functions.[23] For example, the enzymatic pathways within cells, along with water and mineral molecules, are organized into clusters associated with membranes and the cellular cytoskeleton. That arrangement allows metabolites to be channeled through these clusters (referred to as metabolons) rather than randomly circulating as free solutes in solution, which was the traditional vision of how the cytoplasm was organized.[24]

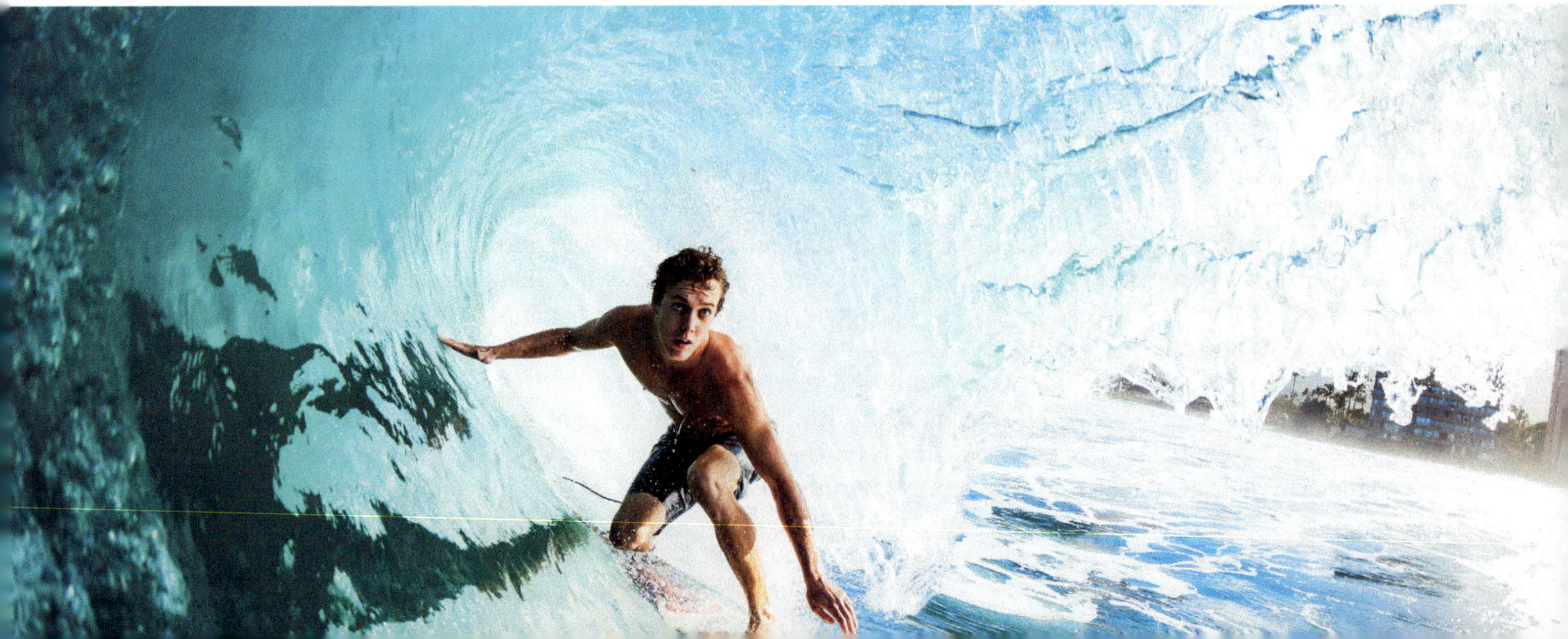

Other unique properties of water include its high heat capacity, high thermal conductivity, and high latent heat of evaporation, all of which help keep the body and its various parts (most of which have a high water content) from overheating during exercise and heat exposure. For example, the unique thermal characteristics of water prevent a runner's leg muscles from being destroyed by local overheating. Water allows the heat produced by muscles to be quickly transferred (with the help of circulating blood) away from active muscle. This heat is distributed throughout the body for eventual loss to the environment through the evaporation of sweat and through radiation, convection, and conduction to cooler surroundings.

DAILY FLUID AND ELECTROLYTE BALANCE

Control of Fluid Balance

Considering the crucial importance of water to every aspect of life, it should be no surprise that the human body contains intricate physiological systems responsible for maintaining water balance within a fairly narrow range. For example, when a person is at rest in thermoneutral conditions (environmental temperatures and activity levels in which the body can maintain a normal temperature), body fluid balance is maintained at ±0.2% of total body weight,[25,26] a very narrow tolerance befitting the critical importance of hydration status to physiological function, even under nonexercise conditions. The end result of this homeostatic control is that daily fluid intake usually matches or exceeds the volume of fluid lost in urine, feces, and sweat; through respiration; and through transcutaneous water loss. In other words, over 24 hours, individuals usually consume enough fluid from foods and beverages to replace fluid losses. However, there are many circumstances in which fluid intake lags behind fluid loss, resulting in dehydration.

Water mass (total body water) represents between 45% and 75% of body weight, a value that varies inversely with fat mass.[22] Regardless of the volume of total body water, maintenance of fluid balance in physically active people can be an ongoing challenge. Fluid is constantly lost from the body through the kidneys (urine), gastrointestinal tract (feces), respiratory tract (exhaled air that is saturated with water vapor), and skin, where the last 2 routes represent insensible water losses. Water and electrolytes are also periodically lost from eccrine sweat glands during exercise and heat exposure.[5,6,22] Eccrine sweat glands are responsible for secreting sweat onto the skin in response to physical activity and heat stress. Sweating is the most important thermoregulatory response in most circumstances because the evaporation of sweat from the skin removes heat from the body. (Apocrine sweat glands found in the armpits are not part of the thermoregulatory response.)

The total volume of fluid lost from the body on a daily basis is determined by a combination of factors, including environmental conditions; the size (and surface area) of the individual; the individual's metabolic rate, physical activity, and sweat loss; the composition of the diet; and the volume of excreted fluids. Insensible water loss via the skin is relatively constant (refer to Table 6.1 on page 132),[27] but water loss via the respiratory tract is affected by the ambient temperature, relative humidity, and ventilatory volume. Inhaled air is humidified during its passage through the respiratory tract, and as a result, exhaled air has a relative humidity of 100%. Inhaling warm, humid air reduces insensible water loss because the inhaled air already contains substantial water vapor. Athletes and workers (construction, agriculture, mining, etc) experience more insensible water losses via the respiratory tract because of the overall increase in breathing that accompanies physical activity. The air inhaled during cold-weather activity contains relatively little water vapor, so as it is warmed and humidified during its transit through the respiratory tract, additional water loss occurs. For this reason, during cold-weather activity, especially when conducted at altitude, transcutaneous and respiratory water loss can be quite high, at times exceeding 1 L/d.[22]

The composition of the diet can also influence daily water needs. In particular, consuming excess protein and sodium increases daily fluid requirements to meet the need for the increased urine volume required for sodium and urea excretion. For sedentary individuals consuming a high-protein diet (eg, >2.0 g per kilograms of body weight per day), the water required to excrete both urea nitrogen from protein (amino acid) degradation and excess sodium intake can represent a meaningful increase in daily water needs. However, for physically active people who already have an increased water requirement, the effect of protein and salt intake on overall water needs is usually quite small. For example, excreting the

TABLE 6.1 Typical Daily Fluid Losses in Milliliters for a 70-kg Athlete[a,27]

Water loss	Normal weather (68 °F/20 °C)	Warm weather (85 °F/29 °C)	Exercise in warm weather (85 °F/29 °C)
Skin	350	350	350
Respiratory tract	350	250	650
Urine	1,400	1,200	500
Feces	100	100	100
Sweat	100	1,400	5,000
TOTAL	**2,300**	**3,300**	**6,600**

[a] Daily fluid loss varies widely among athletes and can exceed 10 L/d under some circumstances.

urea produced from the degradation of 100 g of protein requires approximately 700 mL of water to be excreted from the body.[28] Healthy kidneys are well equipped to excrete excess dietary components, such as the urea from proteins and excess electrolytes from the diet. This is one reason why adequate daily fluid intake is important.

The volume of water produced during metabolism is also relatively small—approximately 130 mL/1,000 kcal in a mixed diet[22]—and is inconsequential for individuals consuming more than 2 L of fluid per day. To be more specific, the oxidation of carbohydrate, fat, and protein produces 15, 13, and 9 mL of water, respectively, per 100 kcal of oxidized substrate.[22]

Considering the multiple and constant avenues by which fluid is lost from the body, maintaining fluid balance requires the constant integration of input from osmoreceptors in the hypothalamus that gauge the osmolality of the blood and from baroreceptors that gauge the pressure within major vessels. Feedback from these receptors helps ensure that daily fluid intake matches or modestly exceeds fluid loss. In this regard, the combination of thirst-driven drinking that results from input from osmoreceptors and baroreceptors and spontaneous drinking is such that fluid balance is normally maintained in most individuals over the course of a day. Interestingly, thirst-driven fluid intake accounts for only a small percentage of daily fluid intake; most fluid is spontaneously consumed with meals or snacks during the day and not directly in response to feeling thirsty.[22]

When sweating occurs, body fluid balance is additionally regulated by mechanisms that reduce urinary water and sodium excretion and stimulate thirst. Sweat loss is accompanied by a decrease in plasma volume and an increase in plasma osmolality (because more water than salt is lost in sweat, the sodium and chloride concentrations in blood plasma increase, resulting in increased plasma osmolality). These changes are sensed by baroreceptors, which respond to a drop in blood volume, and hypothalamic osmoreceptors, which respond to an increase in plasma sodium concentration (ie, increased plasma osmolality). In response to dehydration, integrated input from baroreceptors and osmoreceptors results in an increase in the release of vasopressin (antidiuretic hormone) from the pituitary gland and in renin release from the kidneys (refer to Figure 6.1). These hormones, along with angiotensin II and aldosterone, which result from an increase in plasma renin activity, increase water and sodium retention by the kidneys and provoke an increase in thirst.[26] During the course of a day, ingesting adequate water and electrolytes in foods and beverages eventually restores plasma volume and osmolality to normal levels. Whenever too much fluid is ingested, the kidneys excrete the excess. However, for physically active people, body fluid balance is often compromised because the human thirst mechanism is an imprecise gauge of immediate fluid needs and because it is sometimes difficult to ingest enough fluid to offset the large volume of sweat lost during physical activity.[29]

Common terminology related to hydration is summarized in Box 6.1.[30]

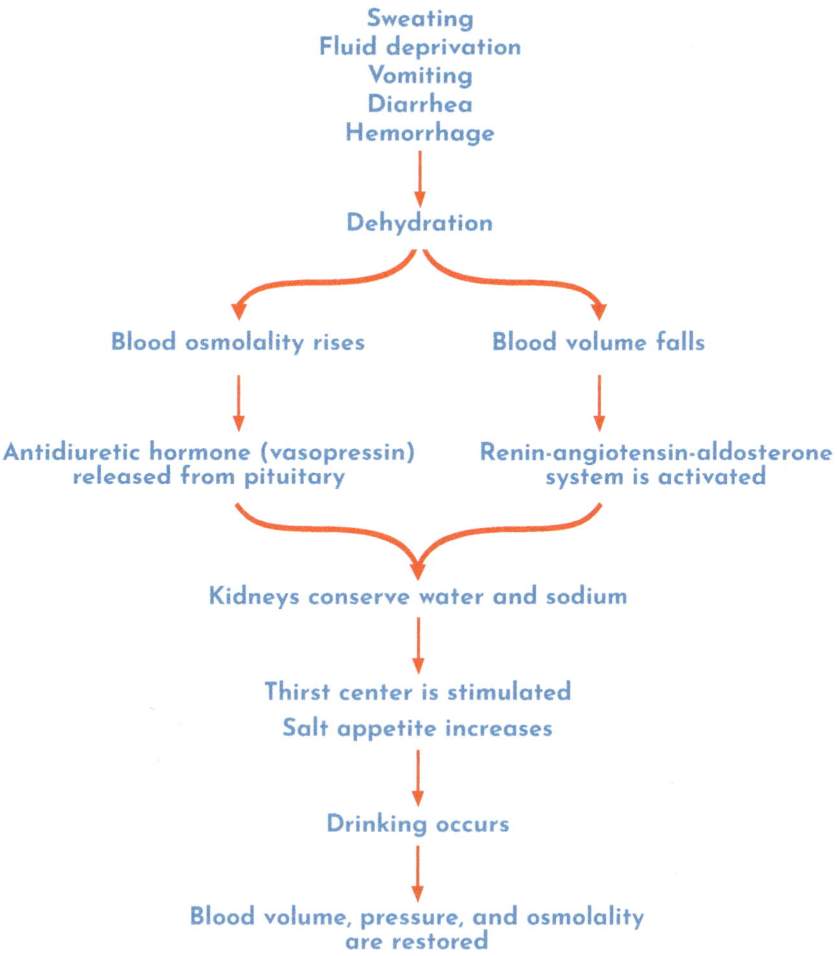

FIGURE 6.1 **Dehydration and thirst, simplified**

BOX 6.1 Hydration-Related Terms and Definitions[30]

Dehydration	Removal of water from the body or a fluid compartment *Example: Dehydration occurs whenever water is lost from the body.* Dehydration is often used interchangeably with hypohydration, although the 2 are not strictly synonymous.
Hypernatremia	Greater than normal blood sodium concentration *Example: As we sweat, more fluid than electrolytes is lost from the body, causing the blood to become hypernatremic.*
Hyponatremia	Lower than normal blood sodium concentration *Example: Consuming large volumes of water at rest or during exercise can cause a drop in blood sodium concentration, a dangerous condition known as hyponatremia.*

Continued on next page

BOX 6.1 Hydration-Related Terms and Definitions[30] (CONTINUED)

Euhydration	A state of water balance (that is more easily defined than measured) *Example: Euhydration is usually achieved by a combination of thirst-driven drinking and spontaneous drinking.*
Hyperhydration	A state of water excess *Example: Beverage consumption with meals typically results in a temporary state of hyperhydration.*
Hypohydration	A state of water deficit *Example: Dehydration produces a body water deficit known as hypohydration.* Synonymous with underhydration, subhydration, and hydration deficit
Hypovolemia	Reduced blood volume *Example: The hypovolemia caused by sweating is accompanied by an automatic increase in heart rate to help maintain cardiac output.*
Hypervolemia	Expanded blood volume *Example: Consuming fluids containing large amounts of glycerol results in hypervolemia as the glycerol molecules provide an osmotic impetus to retain water in the bloodstream.*
Hypertonic dehydration	Loss of predominantly water from the body *Example: Insufficient drinking and sweating both result in hypertonic dehydration because far more water than electrolytes is lost from the body.*
Isotonic dehydration	Loss of water and electrolytes from the body in a proportion similar to that found in the body *Example: Diarrhea and some diuretics produce isotonic dehydration, or a loss of water and electrolytes that leaves the water and electrolyte balance of blood unchanged.*
Hypotonic dehydration	Loss of water and large amounts of electrolytes *Example: Ironman triathletes and ultramarathon runners are at risk of hypotonic dehydration whenever large amounts of salt are lost in sweat and mostly plain water is consumed. In such cases, the athletes will be both dehydrated and possibly hyponatremic.*

Daily Fluid Needs

People are often confused by well-intended but errant hydration recommendations. One such recommendation is that everyone should consume eight 8-oz glasses of water per day to maintain proper hydration.[31] Although the genesis of this advice is a matter of debate, it is interesting that eight 8-oz servings amounts to 2 L (approximately 2 qt), the volume that has often been cited as the daily fluid requirement for sedentary adults.[27] In fact, there is no single fluid intake recommendation that will suffice for everyone because of the wide disparity in daily fluid needs created by differences in body size, body composition, physical activity, and environmental conditions.[22,32] For a small, sedentary older adult, 2 L per day might be too much fluid, but for a young, relatively large, and physically active individual, 2 L might represent the fluid loss during just 1 hour of physical activity. The 2004 Dietary Reference Intake (DRI) recommendations for water and electrolytes identify the adequate intake (AI) for water as 3.7 L/d for males (130 oz/d, or the equivalent of 16 cups of fluid per day) and 2.7 L/d for females (95 oz/d, or about 12 cups/d).[22] The AI is an estimate of the daily nutrient intake assumed to be adequate for most people. In other words, there is a low probability of inadequacy if sedentary individuals ingest between 2.7 and 3.7 L of fluid per day. The AI volumes are median values from the Third National Health and Nutrition Examination Survey, 1988–1994 (NHANES III), for adults ages 19 years and older; AI values for children and adolescents range from 1.3 to 3.3 L/d. In Europe, the recommended values for daily fluid intake are 2.5 L for males and 2.0 L for females.[33]

Suggesting AI for water intake in adult females is 12 cups of fluid per day does not mean that these individuals should literally drink at least 12 cups of water each day. Rather, it means that a total of 12 cups of fluid from all sources will meet the hydration needs of most adult females. This important distinction should be stressed when educating and counseling people about their hydration needs. Regardless of the extent of daily water needs, water can be supplied by a variety of foods and fluids such as fruits and vegetables, milk, soft drinks, fruit juices, sports drinks, coffee, tea, and soups. Approximately 80% of daily water needs are provided by fluids ingested during the day, and the remaining 20% comes from water found in food.[22] For example, bananas are roughly 75% water by weight; a chicken breast, 65%; and a hot dog, 50%. In brief, the prevailing scientific consensus is that sedentary individuals living in temperate environments can rely on the combination of thirst and spontaneous drinking to successfully maintain daily fluid balance, whereas physically active people and those living in warm environments often find it difficult to keep pace with their daily fluid needs.

Although accurately determining a minimum daily water need is difficult, such a minimum is likely to be no less than 1 L/d. This is because minimum urine flow is approximately 500 mL/d, transcutaneous water loss is approximately 400 mL/d, and respiratory loss is a minimum of 200 mL/d. This minimum value applies only to someone who is completely sedentary for the entire day in a thermoneutral environment (with no sweating). Current thinking is that the water requirement in most minimally active adults ranges between 3 and 4 L/d because of the transcutaneous, respiratory, and urinary water losses that accompany normal daily living.[34]

When individuals work, train, and compete in warm environments, their daily water needs can be considerably larger than those for sedentary individuals and might increase to more than 10 L/d.[35] For example, an athlete who trains 2 hours each day can easily lose an additional 3 to 4 L of body fluid, resulting in a daily fluid requirement in excess of 7 to 8 L. Some athletes and workers sweat for more than 2 hours each day, further increasing their fluid needs. Such losses can strain the capacity of the fluid regulatory system such that thirst becomes an inadequate stimulus for fluid intake and, coupled with limited opportunities for spontaneous drinking, persistent dehydration (hypohydration) can occur.

Acclimating to physical activity in warm or hot environments induces a number of physiological adaptations that affect hydration status. These adaptations include earlier onset of sweating, wider distribution of sweating, increased total sweat loss, lower sweat sodium concentration (but often increased total sodium loss due to increased sweat loss), increased hemoglobin mass, increased blood volume, lower resting heart rate, lower resting core temperature, slower rise in core temperature during exercise, increased VO_2 max, improved performance, increased total body water, and greater voluntary fluid intake.[36,37]

DRIs suggested by organizations in the United States indicate that daily fluid needs are lower in females, infants, children, adolescents, and older adult females compared with males over the age of 19 years.[22] Body size is one determinant of daily fluid needs, but the genetic predisposition to sweating, along with the fitness and environmental factors that influence sweating, combine to determine overall sweat loss and, thereby, daily hydration requirements. As previously noted, sweat loss can vary widely among people doing the same task, at the same intensity, in the same environment. Most athletes engaged in vigorous exercise will lose between 1 and 2 L of sweat per hour of exercise, and some people are capable of sweating more than 3 L/h.[5,7,21,35] In 1 study, Palmer and Spriet[38] reported an average sweat loss of 1.8 L/h in competitive ice hockey players during a training session. Three of the 44 players lost less than 1 L/h, whereas 12 players lost more than 2 L/h.

Control of Electrolyte Balance

The distribution of electrolytes across cell membranes must be tightly regulated to ensure proper function of cells throughout the body. Electrolytes such as sodium, potassium, chloride, magnesium, calcium, and bicarbonate play integral roles in the distribution and movement of water inside and outside cells, endocrine secretion, membrane permeability, acid-base buffering, and muscle contraction. In the case of cardiac muscle, for example, an electrolyte imbalance such as hyperkalemia can have fatal consequences if plasma potassium concentration increases just a few millimoles per liter. To maintain electrolyte balance, the kidneys have the capacity to increase or decrease the excretion of electrolytes into the urine. This is particularly true for sodium conservation (reabsorption) and secretion, which is controlled by the renin-angiotensin-aldosterone system in concert with antidiuretic hormone (vasopressin), essential responses in maintaining body fluid balance because of sodium's pivotal role in protecting the fluid volume of the extracellular space. In the case of other electrolytes, the sum of renal secretion and fecal excretion is roughly equal to intestinal absorption (also taking into consideration release or uptake from bone in the cases of calcium and phosphorus). The mechanisms of electrolyte reabsorption or secretion vary from electrolyte to electrolyte, with electrolyte loss influenced by the rate at which the kidneys filter blood (glomerular filtration rate) and the load of electrolytes presented to the kidneys. The kidney nephrons have different transporters (active and passive), channels, and pathways for different electrolytes, ensuring that electrolyte (and fluid) balance can constantly be maintained.

Although an appetite for sodium chloride does exist in humans,[34] there is no evidence to suggest that the intake of other minerals is governed similarly. In most individuals, when dietary energy intake is adequate, mineral intake is usually in excess of mineral needs, ensuring positive mineral balance. However, repeated days of profuse sweating can result in substantial electrolyte loss, especially of sodium and chloride, the 2 minerals found in greatest concentrations in sweat. Insufficient dietary mineral intake (particularly sodium intake) that cannot compensate for such large losses, can result in severe muscle cramping or hyponatremia.[39,40]

Daily Electrolyte Needs

Electrolytes are lost in urine, feces, and sweat. Some athletes, first responders, soldiers, and workers lose large volumes of sweat daily (eg, 4 to 10 L or more), and that loss is accompanied by a similarly large electrolyte loss. As shown in Table 6.2, the concentrations of potassium, magnesium, and calcium in sweat are low and relatively constant compared with the higher, more variable concentrations of sodium and chloride.[41] The fact that sodium concentration in sweat varies widely among individuals means that some athletes will be prone to large sodium losses, whereas others will not. A large salt loss in sweat is often characterized by dry, white residue on the skin and clothing after the sweat dries. An increased risk of heat-related problems, hyponatremia, and muscle cramps has been linked to large sodium chloride losses.[34,35,39,40]

FLUID AND ELECTROLYTE REPLACEMENT

Position Stands on Fluid and Electrolyte Replacement

Numerous position stands addressing fluid and electrolyte replacement before, during, and after physical activity have been published by professional organizations.[11-21] Box 6.2 summarizes the key recommendations from those publications.[12,14-16,18-21] Although the differences among the recommendations are relatively small, the recommendations do vary and have evolved over time. Nonetheless, the central intent of each position stand is to ensure that physically active individuals remain well hydrated. The common message among the position stands is that proper hydration practices reduce the risk of dehydration and heat illness, maintain cardiovascular and thermoregulatory function, and improve performance during vigorous physical activity.

TABLE 6.2 Mineral (Electrolyte) Losses in Sweat[41]

Mineral	Concentration in sweat, mmol/L (mg/L)	AI, mg/d	Possible AI lost in sweat, %AI/L
Sodium	20-80 (460-1,840)	1,300	35-140
Chloride	20-80 (710-2,840)	1,300	35-140
Potassium	4-8 (160-320)	4,700	3-8
Magnesium	0-1.5 (0-36)	240-420	0-15
Calcium	0-3 (0-120)	1,000-1,300	0-12

Abbreviation: AI, Adequate Intake

BOX 6.2 Recommendations for Fluid and Electrolyte Replacement When Exercising[12,14-16,18-21]

American College of Sports Medicine Position Stand: Exercise and Fluid Replacement (2007)[12]

Before exercise	Drink 5 to 7 mL per kilogram of body weight at least 4 hours before exercise. If needed, drink 3 to 5 mL per kilogram of body weight 2 hours before.
During exercise	Follow a customized fluid replacement program to prevent excessive dehydration (ie, >2% loss of body weight).
After exercise	Fully replace fluid and electrolyte deficits. For rapid rehydration, drink 1.5 L of fluid (with electrolytes) per kilogram of body weight lost.
Electrolyte replacement	Consume snacks and beverages with sodium to help stimulate thirst and retain fluids.

American College of Sports Medicine Roundtable on Hydration and Physical Activity: Consensus Statements (2005)[21]

Before exercise	No recommendation
During exercise	Replace but do not exceed sweat losses. Limit fluid deficits to less than 2% loss of body weight.
After exercise	Rehydration within 6 hours of exercise requires drinking 125% to 150% of body weight loss. Fluids should contain sodium. If 24 hours before next exercise, rely on normal food and fluid intake.
Electrolyte replacement	Rely on salty foods, fluids, and sports drinks.

Continued on next page

BOX 6.2 Recommendations for Fluid and Electrolyte Replacement When Exercising[12,14-16,18-21] (CONTINUED)

National Athletic Trainers Association Position Statement: Fluid Replacement for Athletes (2017)[14]

Before exercise	Begin an exercise bout euhydrated and be mindful of individual cues, such as thirst, body weight, urine color, and voiding frequency.
During exercise	Maintain hydration and do not allow more than a 2% loss of body mass.
After exercise	Up to 150% of the estimated fluid deficit should be consumed to effectively replace fluid losses after exercise over a short recovery period (<4 hours).
Electrolyte replacement	"Endurance athletes may be aided by fluids containing carbohydrates and electrolytes during extended training bouts and competitions. Individuals with much greater than average sweat sodium concentrations (>60 mEq/L) and high sweating rates (>2.5 L/h) may benefit from sodium supplementation in the fluids consumed during activity."

American Academy of Pediatrics: Climatic Heat Stress and the Exercising Child and Adolescent (2000)[15]

Before exercise	Before prolonged physical activity, the child should be well hydrated.
During exercise	Periodic drinking should be enforced, even if a child is not thirsty. Example: A child weighing 40 kg (88 lb) should drink 150 mL of water or a flavored, salted beverage every 20 minutes.
After exercise	No recommendation
Electrolyte replacement	Make water or a flavored, salted beverage available for active children.

Academy of Nutrition and Dietetics, Dietitians of Canada, and the American College of Sports Medicine: Nutrition and Athletic Performance (2016)[16]

Before exercise	To achieve euhydration, drink 5 to 10 mL per kilogram of body weight, 2 to 4 hours before exercise.
During exercise	Fluid intake depends on sweating rate, but a general guideline is 0.4 to 0.8 L/h.
After exercise	Drink 1.25 to 1.5 L of fluid for every 1 kg of body weight lost.
Electrolyte replacement	Ingest sodium during exercise when large sweat sodium losses occur.

Third International Exercise-Associated Hyponatremia Consensus Development Conference (2015)[18]

Before exercise	Do not overconsume fluids.
During exercise	Drink to thirst but have an idea of individual fluid needs.
After exercise	For those with asymptomatic hyponatremia, consume hypertonic saline solutions to reduce the risk of symptomatic hyponatremia.
Electrolyte replacement	Foods and beverages containing sodium should be available at marathon aid stations.

Inter-Association Task Force: Exertional Heat Illness Consensus Statement (2003)[19]

Before exercise	Athletes should begin exercise properly hydrated.
During exercise	Fluid intake should nearly approximate fluid losses. Individualized recommendations must be followed.
After exercise	No recommendation
Electrolyte replacement	Hydrating with a sports drink containing carbohydrates and electrolytes before and during exercise is optimal to replace losses and provide energy. Replacing lost sodium after exercise is best achieved by consuming food, in combination with a rehydration beverage.

USA Track & Field Advisory: Proper Hydration for Distance Running—Identifying Individual Fluid Needs (2003)[20]

Before exercise	Consume approximately 500 to 600 mL (17-20 oz) of water or sports drink 2 to 3 hours before exercise and 300 to 360 mL (10-12 oz) 0 to 10 minutes before exercise.
During exercise	During a race, drink no more than 1 cup (8-10 oz) every 15 to 20 minutes.
After exercise	Drink about 25% more than sweat loss to ensure optimal hydration 4 to 6 hours after the event.
Electrolyte replacement	Adding modest amounts of sodium (0.5-0.7 g/L) can offset sodium lost in sweat and may minimize medical events associated with electrolyte imbalances (eg, muscle cramps, hyponatremia).

Fluid and Electrolyte Replacement Before Exercise

How can athletes and others tell if they are well hydrated? This simple question continues to perplex scientists and clinicians because there is no single method that can accurately and reliably determine adequate hydration status. Measuring plasma osmolality is considered the gold standard for assessing hydration status and is commonly used in laboratory settings, but a blood sample and expensive equipment are required. The specific gravity of urine from the first void after rising in the morning can provide useful information about hydration status, but some equipment is needed, such as a refractometer or a hydrometer. The cost of such equipment is typically less than $200.

Noting the color and volume of urine is a practical way to help physically active individuals subjectively assess their hydration status. Darkly colored urine of relatively small volume is an indication of dehydration, a signal to ingest more fluid before activity. Monitoring urine output is a common recommendation in occupational settings, such as the mining industry where workers are constantly exposed to conditions of high heat and humidity. In addition to measuring body weight after waking, the use of some measure of urine concentration (specific gravity, osmolality, or color) may allow for the detection of dehydration.[14] (It should be noted that the intake of supplements of B vitamins, specifically riboflavin, can cause brightly colored urine, even when an individual is well hydrated.)

Achieving euhydration before physical activity helps optimize physiological and performance responses. For example, study subjects in a laboratory setting who ingested fluid in the hour before exercise exhibited lower core temperatures and heart rates during exercise than when no fluid is ingested.[3,5,7] Unfortunately, many athletes enter training sessions and competitive events already dehydrated. For example, Volpe et al[42] reported that more than 60% of the college athletes participating in their study (N = 174) had prepractice urine specific gravity measures indicative of hypohydration. Palmer and Spriet[38] noted similar findings in 50% of the ice hockey players they studied (N = 44), as did Chapelle et al[43] in a review of 24 studies on the preexercise hydration status (via urine specific gravity, osmolality, and color) of male and female professional and recreational soccer players, in which 37% to 63% of athletes were reported to be dehydrated prior to exercise.

Athletes who compete in a hypohydrated state are often at a competitive disadvantage.[7] For example, in a study by James et al,[44] study subjects completed 2 hours of intermittent cycle ergometer exercise in the heat (93 °F or 34 °C) before completing a 15-minute exhaustive performance effort. A unique aspect of this study was that the participants were blinded to the 2 treatments (euhydration and hypohydration of 2.4% of body weight) by allowing a portion of water intake to occur orally, while providing the remainder of the water through a nasogastric tube. In the hypohydration treatment, the tube was in place, but no water was introduced. The total work completed was 8% greater with euhydration, whereas the heart rate, rate of perceived exertion, core temperature, and thermal sensation were all lower. It is also well established that exercise in the heat exacerbates the performance-sapping effects of dehydration.[2,45]

When people live and are physically active in warm environments, voluntary fluid intake is often insufficient to meet fluid needs, as verified by a study conducted with soccer players in Puerto Rico. The athletes were studied during 2 weeks of training. When the players were allowed to drink fluids throughout the day as they wished (average intake equaled 2.7 L/d), their total body water at the end of 1 week was approximately 1.1 L less than when they were mandated to drink 4.6 L of fluid per day.[46] In other words, voluntary fluid consumption did not match fluid losses and caused the players to enter training and competition already dehydrated.

To help ensure adequate hydration prior to competition in the heat, some athletes have ingested glycerol solutions or used preexercise sodium loading in attempts to benefit from the cardiovascular and thermoregulatory advantages that might result from hyperhydration. Ingesting glycerol solutions before exercise does result in a reduction in urine production and in the temporary retention of fluid.[47] Glycerol-induced hyperhydration is accompanied by temporary weight gain proportional to the amount of water retained (usually approximately 0.5–1 kg). Fluid retention occurs because the presence of glycerol molecules (after they are absorbed and distributed throughout the body water, with the exception of the aqueous-humor and the cerebral-spinal fluid compartments) provokes a transient increase in plasma osmolality, prompting a temporary decrease in urine production. As glycerol molecules are removed from the body water in subsequent hours, plasma osmolality decreases, urine production increases, and excess water is excreted.

There are several reasons why hyperhydrating with glycerol could be problematic:

- In many sports, athletes pay a metabolic cost for carrying extra body weight.
- There is no compelling evidence that glycerol-induced hyperhydration results in a physiological benefit.[48]
- The side effects of ingesting glycerol can range from mild sensations of bloating and light-headedness to more severe symptoms of headaches, dizziness, and nausea.[47]
- Glycerol-induced hyperhydration can cause blood sodium levels to decrease,[49] potentially increasing the risk of hyponatremia.
- Glycerol used to be on the World Anti-Doping Agency list of prohibited substances out of concern that glycerol loading could be used to mask doping,[50] but it was removed in 2018 because research showed that even prolonged glycerol use did not influence the blood measures needed to mask doping.[51]

Fluid and Electrolyte Replacement During Exercise

Research has shown that an individual's cardiovascular, thermoregulatory, and performance responses are optimized by replacing sweat lost during exercise.[3,10,52,53] These and similar research findings are reflected in the various recommendations for fluid and electrolyte intake during exercise. For example, the American College of Sports Medicine recognizes the physiological and performance benefits of minimizing dehydration by simply recommending that "[i]ndividuals should develop customized fluid replacement programs that prevent excessive (>2% body weight reductions from baseline body weight) dehydration."[12] In some cases, minimizing dehydration during exercise may require little more than athletes drinking whenever they are thirsty[54]; in most cases, however, whenever performance is important, athletes are best advised to create a personal hydration plan to guide the frequency and volume of their fluid intake during exercise.

Developing a personal hydration plan requires that athletes periodically record body weights before and after activity. Using the simplest approach, weight loss indicates inadequate drinking, whereas weight gain indicates excessive drinking (refer to Figure 6.2).[55] Such basic feedback is often all athletes need to fine-tune their hydration practices. For athletes who continue to struggle with dehydration, calculations based on preexercise and postexercise body weights, fluid intake, and urine output can be used to prescribe the volume and frequency of fluid intake required to minimize dehydration. Such measurements should be made periodically throughout the season to reflect the change in sweating rate due to changes in environment, training intensity, fitness, and acclimation. To help assure a rapid gastric emptying rate and unimpeded delivery of fluid and electrolytes to the absorptive surface of the small intestine, athletes should begin activity with a comfortable volume of fluid already in the stomach and should take in additional fluid at 10- to 30-minute intervals (depending on sweating rate) to maintain gastric volume, an important driver of gastric emptying during exercise.[56]

A	Name	Shelby
B	Date	9/15
C	BW[a] Before Exercise, kg	61.7 kg
D	BW After Exercise, kg	60.3 kg
E	BW Lost, g (C – D) × 1,000	1,400 g
F	Drink Volume, mL	420 mL
G	Urine Volume,[b] mL	90 mL
H	Fluid Lost, mL (E + F – G)[c]	1,730 mL
I	Exercise Time, min	90 min
J	Sweating Rate, L/h (H/I × 60)	1.15 L (38 oz)

[a] BW , body weight
[b] Weight of urine, instead of volume, should be subtracted if urine was excreted before the postexercise body weight was measured.
[c] This approach assumes that 1 mL of sweat loss represents a 1-g loss of body weight.
Adapted with permission from reference 55: Murray R. Fluid replacement: the American College of Sports Medicine position stand. *Sports Sci Exch.* 1996;9(63):1-6.

FIGURE 6.2 Calculating sweating rates This table presents some simple steps for determining hourly sweating rate. In this example, Shelby should drink roughly 750 mL (25 oz) of fluid during each hour of activity to remain well hydrated.

Not surprisingly, most humans prefer—and drink more of—beverages that are flavored and sweetened.[57] This is an important consideration in preventing dehydration, because any step that can be taken to increase voluntary fluid intake will help reduce the risk of health issues associated with dehydration and heat stress. In addition to having palatable beverages available for athletes to drink, it is also important for athletes to periodically record body weights before and after vigorous physical activity as a way to assess the effectiveness of fluid intake and as a reminder of the importance of drinking adequate volumes of fluid during exercise.[55] Consuming sufficient fluid during exercise has well-established benefits that should be emphasized when nutrition practitioners speak to coaches and athletes about hydration strategies (see Table 6.3).[3,10,51,52]

TABLE 6.3 Beneficial Responses to Adequate Fluid Intake During Exercise[3,10,53,54]

Characteristic	Response
Heart rate	Lower
Stroke volume	Higher
Cardiac output	Higher
Skin blood flow	Higher
Core temperature	Lower
Perceived exertion	Lower
Performance	Better

CHANGES IN URINE VOLUME

During physical activity, urine production is reduced as the kidneys attempt to conserve water and sodium to offset losses due to sweating. When fluid intake is limited and dehydration occurs, the kidneys are capable of concentrating the urine to 4 to 5 times the concentration of blood. However, some renal fluid loss (approximately 500 mL/d) is obligatory for waste removal. Daily urine losses in some athletes and workers tend to be less than in sedentary individuals, a trend that is exacerbated by warm weather as the body strives to conserve fluid. However, most athletes consume large volumes of fluid during the day and, as a result, produce more urine than their sedentary counterparts. Reduced urine volume in physically active individuals usually indicates inadequate fluid intake. In general, urine volumes tend to be 800 to 1,500 mL/d in sedentary individuals and can easily exceed 4 L/d in physically active individuals who ingest large volumes of fluid to replace sweat losses. Measures of urine specific gravity (USG), urine osmolality, and urine color are commonly used to estimate hydration status at rest. For example, a USG value greater than 1.020 is indicative of hypohydration, as is a urine osmolality greater than 700 mOsm/kg.[58]

THE ROLE OF THIRST

Why can athletes, workers, and soldiers not simply rely on thirst to stay well hydrated? There are at least 3 reasons why thirst is an unreliable regulator of fluid needs during exercise. The first is behavioral: There are often many distractions during physical activity, so thirst signals can easily be missed or disregarded. The second reason is that fluid is often not readily available, so even if thirst is perceived, it might not be convenient to act on it. The third reason is rooted in the physiology of the thirst mechanism. Consider that the plasma osmolality of a well-hydrated (euhydrated) person is 285 mOsm/kg H_2O. The *thirst threshold* is the plasma osmolality above which thirst is triggered, and this is thought to be 293 mOsm/kg (this varies among individuals, but usually falls within the range from 290–295 mOsm/kg).[22] A simple calculation relying on total body water (TBW, in liters) illustrates the volume of fluid that must be lost from the body before thirst is stimulated: $V^{thirst} = TBW - [(TBW \times 285)/293]$. For example, consider a TBW value of 36 L: $36\ L - [(36\ L \times 285\ mOsm/kg) / 293\ mOsm/kg] \approx 1\ L$. Thus, if TBW is 36 L, then about 1 L of water must first be lost from the body for thirst to be initiated. This is the scientific rationale for the admonition that by the time thirst is perceived, some dehydration has already occurred.

One of many examples of the inadequacy of the human thirst mechanism during exercise can be found in the study by Passe et al.[59] Experienced runners participated in a 10-mile race conducted on a 400-meter track. The environmental conditions were moderate (69°F, 77% relative humidity) but sufficient for ample sweating to occur. Every 2 miles, the runners had the opportunity to grab a 24-oz sports bottle containing a commercial sports drink. They could drink from the bottle ad libitum; when they desired no more, the runners tossed the bottles onto the infield where the bottles were collected as part of a measurement system whereby drink volume for each runner was calculated. As in a road race, if the runners chose not to drink, they had to wait until the next 2-mile opportunity. After the race, each runner completed a questionnaire so that their impressions of the adequacy of their fluid intake could be recorded. On average, the runners replaced only 30% of their sweat loss (with a range from 5% to 67%), even though the conditions for fluid intake were purposefully optimized. Had thirst been an adequate stimulus for fluid intake, the runners—especially the ones who were most dehydrated—would have done a better job hydrating. The fact that they did not is evidence that other factors often conspire to produce the voluntary dehydration that is so often reported in the literature.[25,28,29] The postrun questionnaires revealed that the runners grossly underestimated the extent of their sweat loss despite accurately estimating their fluid intake. These results led the investigators to conclude that the inability to accurately estimate sweat loss contributed to the runners' inadequate fluid intake.[59] With this finding in mind, there are numerous steps athletes can take to help ensure that they consume enough fluid during exercise to minimize dehydration (refer to Box 6.3).

There are undoubtedly occasions when thirst can be an adequate gauge of fluid needs during physical activity.[60] For example, it is relatively easy to drink during long-duration, low-intensity activity, such as slow marathon runs lasting more than 4 hours, ultraendurance biking and running, hiking and backpacking, military marches, and similar activities. Under those circumstances, thirst may be an adequate stimulus for fluid intake in many people because there is ample opportunity to sense the presence of thirst and to drink accordingly. However, perceptions of thirst can also be inadequate in these circumstances, leading to dehydration and volume depletion in some participants and hyperhydration and hyponatremia in others.

BOX 6.3 Tips for Encouraging Drinking Before, During, and After Sweaty Physical Activity

Preparation

Know the warning signs of dehydration (thirst, unusual fatigue, light-headedness, headache, dark urine, dry mouth, infrequent urination, unusually rapid heartbeat).

Know where to find fluid (water fountains, stores, neighbors, etc).

Freeze fluid bottles overnight to allow the drink to stay cold longer during workouts.

Ideally, have a variety of beverage flavors to choose from.

Prehydrate to produce a light-colored urine and help ensure euhydration.

Training

When sweating is anticipated, start activity with a stomach comfortably full of fluid.

Practice drinking during training.

Bring fluids. Wear a bottle belt or fluid pack, and take along a cooler full of drinks.

Keep a comfortably full stomach during activity.

Train yourself to drink more during exercise.

One medium mouthful of fluid is about 1 oz.

Always carry money to buy drinks.

Periodically record your body weight before and after activity.

Complete rehydration requires full replacement of fluid and sodium losses.

After activity, drink 24 oz of fluid for every pound of weight lost during activity.

Continued on next page

BOX 6.3 *Tips for Encouraging Drinking Before, During, and After Sweaty Physical Activity* **(CONTINUED)**

Competition

Better hydration means better performance, so plan to drink during competition.

When sweating, drink early and often, but do not overdrink.

In distance running, stop to drink if that is what it takes to ensure adequate intake. Runners will more than make up the time by staying well hydrated.

During a road race, pinch the top of the drink cup to form a spout that will make drinking easier.

Carry fluid during a road race by folding the top of the cup over, keeping the fluid from spilling.

Put more fluid in the stomach than on the head. Pouring water over the head does nothing to maintain hydration, although it can reduce core temperature and improve thermal comfort.

If prone to dehydration, drink by schedule—not by thirst.

ELECTROLYTE REPLACEMENT

Electrolyte replacement during exercise—particularly sodium replacement—can help maintain blood volume and sustain the osmotic drive to drink and is therefore important during intense, prolonged exercise when sweat loss is high.[61] Large sweat and electrolyte losses commonly occur during 2-a-day practices, prolonged training sessions, and many types of competition. Sweat contains more sodium and chloride than other minerals, and although the sodium content of sweat is normally substantially less than the plasma value (plasma, 138–142 mmol/L; sweat, 20–80 mmol/L), large sweat losses can result in considerable salt loss (refer to Table 6.2). Chronic sodium deficits are uncommon among athletes and military personnel, in large part because a normal diet often provides more than enough salt to replace what is lost in sweat.[62]

However, persistent sodium losses can present short-term problems, as illustrated by Bergeron[63] in a case study of a nationally ranked tennis player who suffered from frequent muscle cramps. A high sweating rate (2.5 L/h) coupled with a higher-than-normal sweat sodium concentration (90 mmol/L) seemingly predisposed the player to severe muscle cramping. The cramps were eliminated when the player increased his daily dietary intake of sodium chloride from less than 10 g/d to between 15 and 20 g/d, relied on a sports drink during practices and games, and increased his daily fluid intake to ensure adequate hydration. A link between sweat sodium loss and cramping has also been reported in American football players,[64] although other research has questioned that conclusion.[65] Muscle cramping can be caused by many factors, but there is evidence that issues with sodium balance during exercise (eg, large sodium loss in sweat, decrease in blood sodium concentration) appear to be associated with the risk of cramping in some athletes.[64,66]

Some people mistakenly believe that potassium loss causes muscle cramps and suggest eating oranges and bananas to replace the potassium lost in sweat. However, potassium loss does not appear to be the culprit. Although potassium is lost in sweat (see Table 6.2),[67] the concentration of potassium in sweat (usually less than 10 mmol/L) is far less than that of sodium, which can be higher than 100 mmol/L in some people. In addition, the amount of potassium lost in a large volume of sweat represents only a small fraction of total body potassium content, whereas sweat sodium losses in a single 2-hour training session can approximate 20% of total body sodium content.

It is important to remember that ingesting sodium chloride in a beverage consumed during physical activity not only helps ensure adequate fluid intake but also stimulates more complete rehydration after activity.[68-70] These responses reflect the critical role that sodium plays in maintaining the osmotic drive to drink and in providing an osmotic stimulus to retain fluid in the extracellular space, including in the plasma and interstitial fluid compartments. The carbohydrate and electrolyte content of sports drinks can vary widely, so nutrition practitioners and coaches should read product nutrition labels carefully before recommending specific beverages or foods.

The sodium content of a fluid replacement beverage does not directly affect the rate of fluid absorption.[71] This is because the amount of sodium that can be included in a beverage is small compared to the amount of sodium that can move from the bloodstream into the intestine. Whenever fluid is ingested, sodium diffuses from plasma into the gut, driven by an osmotic gradient that strongly favors sodium influx. In brief, sodium chloride is an important constituent of a properly formulated sports drink because it improves beverage palatability, helps maintain the osmotic drive for drinking, reduces the amount of sodium that the blood has to supply to the intestine prior to fluid absorption, helps maintain plasma volume during exercise, and serves as the primary osmotic impetus for restoring extracellular fluid volume after exercise.[68-70]

A good example of the effect that beverage composition has on voluntary fluid intake is demonstrated by the work of Wilk and Bar-Or.[72] Preadolescent boys (aged 9–12 years) completed 3 hours of intermittent exercise in the heat, during which time they could drink 1 of 3 beverages ad libitum. The beverages tested included water, a sports drink, and a placebo (a flavored, artificially sweetened replica of the sports drink). The boys drank almost twice as much sports drink as they did water, whereas consumption of the placebo fell between these extremes. Flavoring and sweetness increased voluntary fluid intake (more intake with placebo vs water), and the presence of sodium chloride in the sports drink further increased consumption (the study subjects drank more sports drink than placebo).

These results are consistent with the physiology of the thirst mechanism. In humans, the sensation of thirst is a function of both changes in plasma sodium concentration (plasma osmolality) and changes in blood volume.[28,29,34] Drinking plain water removes the osmotic drive to drink (by quickly diluting the sodium concentration of the blood) and reduces the volume-dependent drive (by partially restoring blood volume), causing the premature satiation of thirst. Unfortunately, the resulting decrease in fluid intake occurs before adequate fluid has been ingested. As the Wilk and Bar-Or[72] research demonstrated, the osmotic drive for drinking can be maintained by the presence of low levels of sodium chloride in a beverage, resulting in greater fluid intake. This application of basic physiology is nothing new. For centuries, bartenders have known that salty foods and snacks help sustain beverage intake among their patrons.

ELECTROLYTE LOSS IN SWEAT

Considering that electrolytes play a critical role in fluid homeostasis at rest and during exercise, it is helpful to appreciate the extent of electrolyte loss in sweat. In addition to sodium, potassium, and chloride, human sweat contains small amounts of dozens of organic and inorganic substances, including amino acids; urea; lactic acid; and the minerals calcium, magnesium, and iron.[67] Even when sweat losses are large, it is unlikely that minerals such as magnesium, iron, and calcium will be lost in sufficient quantities in sweat to provoke a mineral imbalance in most people. However, for some individuals, such losses could constitute an additional dietary challenge, as might be the case with sweat calcium losses in physically active females (refer to Table 6.2). For example, a female athlete who loses 3 L of sweat in a day could lose 120 to 360 mg of calcium. Although this amount of calcium can be easily replaced by consuming a cup of milk, sweat calcium loss does increase the dietary calcium needs of active individuals.

For some individuals, the amount of sodium chloride lost in sweat is not trivial. Consider, for example, a football player who practices for 5 h/d, during which time he loses 8 L of sweat (average sweat loss of 1.6 L/h). If his sweat contains 50 mmol of sodium per liter, his total sodium loss will amount to 9,200 mg of sodium (23 g of NaCl). This sodium loss, which does not include the 50 to 200 mmol (1,150 to 4,600 mg) of sodium that is typically lost in urine, makes it apparent that physically active people often require a large salt intake to replace losses in sweat.

Advances in wearable technology now make it possible to monitor sweating responses, including the sodium content of sweat, via skin patches with Bluetooth connections to mobile phone apps and smartwatches.[73] This technology has the potential to benefit heavy, salty sweaters prone to dehydration, cramping, and hyponatremia by providing real-time feedback to encourage fluid and electrolyte intake during physical activity.

The 2004 DRI recommendations indicate that individuals should restrict their daily sodium intake to only 1.5 g/d (3.8 g of salt per day), with a Tolerable Upper Intake Level of 2.3 g of sodium per day (5.8 g of salt). The basis of this recommendation is that a reduction in dietary sodium intake can blunt the age-related increase in blood pressure. These stringent dietary recommendations are inadequate for athletes, fitness enthusiasts, and workers who lose considerably more salt in their sweat. However, this discrepancy is recognized in the DRI report: "This [recommendation] does not apply to highly active individuals . . . who lose large amounts of sweat on a daily basis."[22]

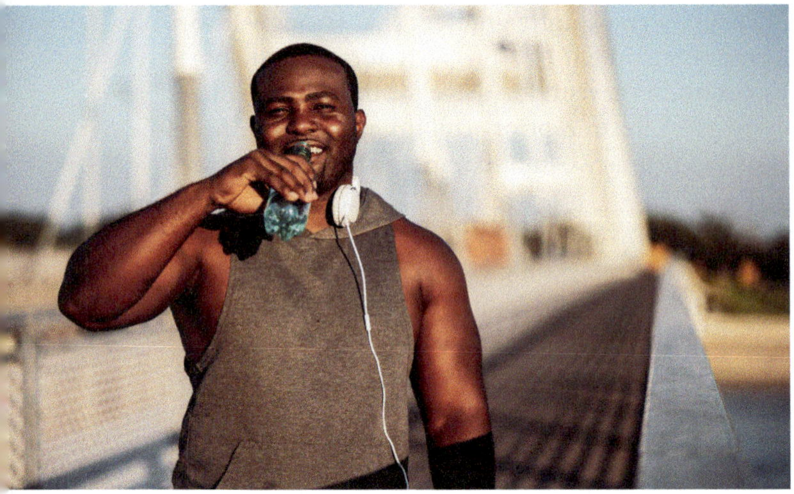

Athletes who incur large sodium and electrolyte losses can replace these nutrients through a variety of foods and fluids. During competition, oral rehydration solutions or powdered electrolyte supplements may be necessary for particularly heavy, salty sweaters. Higher-sodium meals should be stressed during periods of intense training (2-a-day practices, stage races) or hot, humid conditions in which cumulative sweat losses can be substantial. Foods such as soups or stir fries with soy or teriyaki sauces are healthy meal options that can help restore lost sodium. Simply keeping a saltshaker on the table can boost the sodium content of any meal (1 tsp = 2,300 mg). Providing athletes with salty snacks such as nuts, pretzels, or pita chips can also be helpful. Athletes should be educated regarding the importance of replacing sodium when sweat sodium losses are high. However, when losses are curtailed because of decreased activity or a change in the weather, sodium intake should also be reduced. Beyond sodium, diets rich in fruits, vegetables, whole grains, and low-fat dairy or plant-based alternatives will suffice to replace the other minerals such as potassium, magnesium, and calcium.

EXCESSIVE FLUID INTAKE

Some individuals may mistakenly interpret the current recommendations for fluid intake to mean that dehydration is to be avoided at all costs and that there is no such thing as drinking too much fluid during exercise—as well as throughout the rest of the day. This is certainly not true. Excessive fluid intake, even at rest, can result in life-threatening hyponatremia. Ingesting too much water, beer, or other low-sodium fluid can quickly dilute the plasma sodium concentration. When this occurs, the osmotic balance across the blood-brain barrier is disrupted, and water enters the brain, causing rapid swelling that can lead to seizures, coma, and even death.[74] In similar fashion, excessive drinking during prolonged exercise can also result in hyponatremia.[40,75] For that reason, physically active individuals should be counseled to limit their fluid intake to no more than is needed to minimize dehydration and to ingest sodium and other electrolytes in food or drink during prolonged exercise (>2 hours) (refer to Box 6.3 on page 144 and Box 6.5 on pages 152 and 153).[12,16,61]

Some sports scientists have argued that current hydration recommendations have increased deaths from hyponatremia and that hydration recommendations should be changed to encourage people to drink only when thirsty during exercise.[17,18] This argument defies logic, common sense, and the existing evidence. Symptomatic hyponatremia remains a rare disorder, which suggests that current hydration recommendations are not the cause of the problem. In addition, drinking to thirst—or what some perceive as thirst—obviously failed those who experienced exercise-associated hyponatremia. There is a large body of evidence demonstrating that those who drink enough fluid during exercise to minimize dehydration suffer no ill consequences and benefit from better cardiovascular and thermoregulatory function.[2-10,52,53]

DEHYDRATION AND PERFORMANCE

Does dehydration always impair performance? The simple answer is no. There are likely many circumstances when dehydration has minimal or no impact on performance. Of course, in science, simple answers rarely suffice, and in this case, the extent of dehydration, the environmental conditions, the individual's level of fitness and heat acclimation, and the intensity and duration of exercise combine to determine the impact of dehydration on exercise performance. In addition, some studies have reported no effect of dehydration on performance. However, the preponderance of evidence collected over many decades demonstrates that even low levels of dehydration (−1% of body weight) can negatively affect physiological and performance responses, including aerobic capacity, anaerobic power and capacity, muscle endurance, and strength.[2-10]

Because dehydration results in a loss of blood volume, numerous cardiovascular and thermoregulatory responses are adversely affected. The greater the level of dehydration and the hotter the environment, the greater the overall negative impact on physiological function.[10] For instance, Canadian researchers studied the effects of dehydration (−2% to −3% of body weight) during 2 hours of cycling at 65% of VO_2 peak and reported that carbohydrate oxidation, heart rate, core temperature, perceived exertion, and muscle glycogen use were all greater when the study subjects were allowed to dehydrate during exercise.[52,53]

Impaired physiological function often translates to impaired performance. Cross-country runners who were dehydrated by less than 1% of their body weight by overnight fluid restriction experienced a 3% reduction in 10-k running performance, even though heart rate and core temperature were not different between trials. The runners rated their perceived exertion as greater during dehydrated treatment, indicating that their effort felt more difficult even though they were running more slowly.[76]

Fluid and Electrolyte Replacement After Exercise

When hypohydration occurs after physical activity, it is often important to rehydrate quickly. An afternoon of working in the yard, 2-a-day football practices, a day-long sports tournament, and 8 hours of manual labor are all examples of activities in which rapid rehydration can be important. Full physical and mental recovery depends in part on adequate fluid and electrolyte intake after physical activity. Maughan et al[68] concluded that ingesting plain water is ineffective at restoring euhydration because water absorption causes plasma osmolality to decrease, suppressing thirst and increasing urine output. When sodium is provided in fluids or foods, the osmotic drive to drink is maintained, and urine production is decreased.[68-70]

In other words, plain water is a good thirst quencher but not an effective rehydrator. In short, consuming plain water turns off the thirst mechanism—by quickly lowering plasma osmolality and restoring some plasma volume—and turns on urine production. Only when water is ingested in combination with foods that contain sodium, chloride, and other minerals will sufficient water be consumed and retained to promote complete rehydration. Low-fat foods and beverages containing ample sodium include tomato juice, baked potato chips, pretzels, pickles, and crackers. These kinds of foods can be consumed as snacks on days when large sweat sodium losses are expected.

Maughan et al[68] also emphasized the importance of ingesting fluid in excess of the deficit in body weight to account for obligatory urine losses. In other words, the advice sometimes given to athletes—drink a pint (454 mL) of fluid for every pound (454 g) of body weight deficit—should be amended to drink *at least* a pint of fluid for every pound of body weight deficit. Ideally, fluids and foods consumed after exercise should contain sodium, chloride, and other minerals required for complete extracellular and intracellular rehydration. More precise recommendations for how much fluid athletes should ingest to ensure rapid and complete rehydration may evolve from future research; existing data indicate that ingesting 125% to 150% of weight loss is required to achieve normal hydration within 6 hours after exercise if only fluids are ingested.[69]

Finally, when *rapid* rehydration is the goal, consumption of alcoholic beverages is contraindicated because of alcohol's diuretic properties. Caffeine is, by comparison, a much milder diuretic and, in those who regularly ingest caffeine, might not be much of a diuretic at all with normal use (eg, <300 mg/d).[22,32] Outside of the exercise setting, beverages containing alcohol or caffeine are unlikely to compromise hydration status. The 2004 DRI recommendations conclude that, "[w]hile consumption of beverages containing caffeine and alcohol have been shown in some studies to have diuretic effects, available information indicates that this may be transient in nature, and that such beverages can contribute to total water intake and thus can be used in meeting recommendations for dietary intake of total water."[22] However, when rapid rehydration is required, athletes should rely on noncaffeinated and nonalcoholic beverages. Education efforts with athletes should reflect the reality that many individuals will choose to consume alcoholic and caffeinated beverages. For those who do drink coffee, colas, beer, and similar beverages, the best advice is to do so in moderation, avoiding such drinks in the first few hours after physical activity.

Fluid and Electrolyte Balance at Environmental Extremes

The environment has a major impact on fluid and electrolyte balance.[77,78] Exposure to extreme heat, high humidity, prolonged cold, water immersion, altitude, and reduced gravity increases the need for water and electrolytes to match the increased losses that occur in those circumstances. In extreme dry heat, combined water loss from sweating, respiration, and transcutaneous routes can increase water and salt needs to high levels, often exceeding 10 L and 20 g, respectively. Not surprisingly, a high proportion of children who live in hot and arid environments were found to be in a state of moderate to severe dehydration.[79] Although respiratory water loss is minimal during exposure to humid heat, sweating is profuse as the body struggles to lose heat through the evaporation of sweat from the skin. This can be particularly troublesome for unacclimated individuals exposed to high humidity; the inability of the sweat glands to respond maximally to environmental heat and humidity imposes a limit on both thermal comfort and the physiological capacity to sustain even mild exercise.[80]

During physical activity in cold environments, respiratory water loss increases because of the low humidity and increased ventilation rate, and it is also possible for sweating rates to exceed 1 L/h because of the warm, humid microenvironment created underneath clothing and equipment, such as during cross-country skiing and ice hockey. The risk of death due to periods of unusual heat and cold is greatest among sick, infirm, very young, and very old individuals. Interestingly, mortality rates are greater for unusual cold weather as opposed to hot weather.[80,81]

Being immersed in water increases urine production because the increase in plasma volume that accompanies immersion triggers high-pressure baroreceptors.[82] Athletes and health care practitioners should also note that competitive swimmers can sweat during tough workouts whenever their internal body temperature exceeds the sweat threshold, presenting another avenue for fluid loss.

Physical activity at altitude provokes the same responses as activity in the cold, with additional challenges to hydration posed by an altitude-induced reduction in food and fluid intake and increased urinary water and salt loss.[83] Astronauts who spend days in zero-gravity conditions lose considerable water and salt from the inevitable diuresis that occurs. All of these conditions promote fluid loss and increase the risk of dehydration.

Fluid and Electrolyte Balance With Gastrointestinal Disease

Diarrheal disease can cause rapid dehydration and has claimed the lives of millions of people worldwide. Each year in the United States, diarrheal illnesses in children result in roughly 3 million physician visits, 220,000 hospitalizations, and about 400 deaths.[84] The World Health Organization and various medical bodies recommend the use of oral rehydration solutions—simple concoctions of carbohydrates and electrolytes—to combat diarrheal fluid loss and save lives.[85] As is the case with sports drinks, a small amount of carbohydrate stimulates rapid water absorption in the small intestine, with sodium, chloride, and potassium replacing electrolytes lost in diarrhea and thereby helping sustain fluid and electrolyte balance. Oral rehydration is as effective as intravenous rehydration and is a home remedy that can be administered at a much lower cost and risk. Interestingly, fluid replacement during diarrheal disease does not reduce the duration of the disease; instead, fluid replacement saves lives by maintaining body fluid balance until the disease runs its course.[86]

HYDRATION Q&A

How Prevalent Is Dehydration Among Children?

Some research indicates that dehydration may be more prevalent in children than adults. For example, NHANES data found that more than half of the children examined were hypohydrated,[87] whereas about one-third of adults met the criteria.[88] Although this represents a cross-section of children in the United States, young athletes in particular should be encouraged to drink throughout the day. As is often the case with adults, children and adolescents are likely to be inadequately hydrated prior to training and competition.[89-91] Providing instruction and guidance can help them understand what beverages to drink and how much to drink, as well as how to monitor their own hydration status via urine color and volume. Drinking during training and competition should also be stressed, and providing easy opportunities to hydrate is imperative. In contrast to adults, when given access to palatable liquids during exercise, children and adolescents replace a greater percentage of their sweat losses compared to older athletes.[92] In addition to the research elucidating the negative effects of dehydration on physical performance in children,[93] several studies show cognitive improvements with water consumption.[94-96] Needless to say, the beneficial impact of hydration on memory and attention extends far beyond the court, field, or pitch. Box 6.4 lists tips for providing hydration education.

BOX 6.4 Tips for Hydration Education

Educate coaches, trainers, supervisors, parents, and athletes about the benefits of proper hydration.

Emphasize the positive aspects of staying well hydrated rather than the negative aspects of becoming dehydrated.

Create educational posters, flyers, brochures, and presentations for athletes, coaches, and parents.

Always have palatable fluids readily available.

Help athletes compare preexercise and postexercise weights and counsel them when needed on improving their hydration habits.

Establish individualized fluid replacement regimens that meet the unique needs of each athlete.

What Are the Current Recommendations Regarding Fluid Intake for Athletes?

Minimizing changes in body weight by drinking fluids sufficient to offset sweat losses is the goal for maintaining performance while safeguarding health. Current evidence indicates that a body weight deficit of 2% or more due to water loss negatively affects athletic performance, whereas overhydration can cause hyponatremia with potentially fatal consequences. Fluid intake recommendations from the American College of Sports Medicine provide hydration guidelines for fluid intake before, during, and after exercise,[12] as follows:

- Athletes should begin the exercise session well hydrated. Slowly drinking fluids that contain sodium or that are consumed with snacks that contain sodium allows for better fluid retention. Preexercise recommendations are to begin drinking 5 to 7 mL of fluid per kilogram of body weight 4 hours prior to allow sufficient time for fluids to be absorbed and urine production to return to normal. If urine is not being produced or is still dark in color 2 hours prior, an additional 3 to 5 mL/kg is recommended. However, if large volumes of clear urine are being produced, drinking more fluid is not necessary. Ideally, urine should be the color of light lemonade, and clear urine is a sign of overhydration.
- Fluid intake guidelines during exercise will vary widely based on individual sweating rates. Monitoring body weight changes during training will allow athletes and practitioners to design customized fluid replacement strategies with the goal of minimizing changes in body weight. Customizing a fluid intake strategy is important for both those who sweat heavily and those who sweat lightly. Individuals with low sweating rates and small body sizes who exercise over several hours (eg, marathon running) are at risk of developing hyponatremia, so a sound fluid replacement strategy is vital.
- Following exercise, fluid replacement should be 125% to 150% of body weight lost during exercise or 20 to 24 oz per pound of body weight lost. Again, consuming liquids with sodium or salty snacks helps retain fluid.

Figure 6.3 provides fluid and sodium replacement recommendations across a continuum of activities of varying intensities and durations.

Hydration Continuum

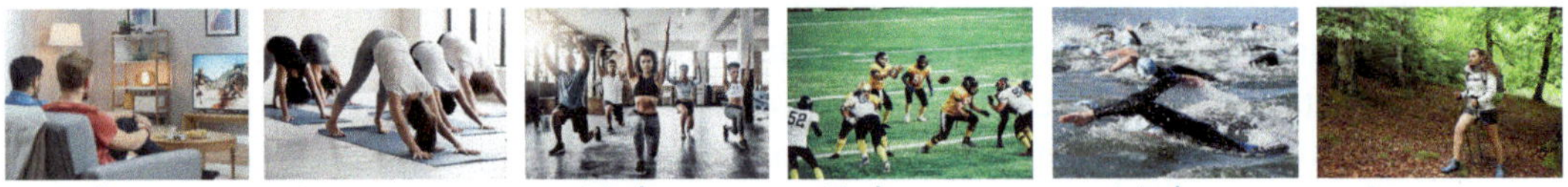

	Sedentary	Low-intensity	Moderate-intensity	High-intensity	Moderate-intensity	Low-intensity
	24 hours	Short-duration, 30 minutes	Moderate-duration, 60 minutes	Moderate-duration, 60-120 minutes	Long-duration, 2-8+ hours	Long-duration, 8+ hours
Typical sweat loss[a]	0 mL	0-0.5 L	0.5-1.5 L	1.0-3.0 L	1.0-16.0+ L	2.0-12.0+ L
Typical sodium loss[b]	1.5-3.0 g	0-0.5 g	0.5-1.5 g	1.0-3.0 g	1.0-16.0 g	2.0-12.0 g
Drink schedule	2.0-4.0 L/d	0-0.5 L	0.5-1.5 L	1.0-3.0 L	1.0-14.0 L	2.0-12.0 L
Beverage type	Water, coffee, tea, milk, fruit juice, soft drinks, soup	Nothing, water, fitness waters, sports drinks	Nothing, water, fitness waters, sports drink	Sports drinks, water	Sports drinks, water, extra sodium	Sports drinks, water, coffee, tea, milk, fruit juice, soft drinks, soup

[a] Typical sweating rates for most people under most conditions; some may sweat more.

[b] Assumes a loss of 1.0 g of sodium per liter of sweat (43 mmol of Na+/L).

Adapted with permission from www.sportsscienceinsights.com

FIGURE 6.3 **Hydration continuum with recommendations for fluid and sodium intake during various activities**

Can Dehydration Affect Driving Performance?

For race car drivers, any level of impairment that reduces vigilance, visual acuity, or reaction time not only diminishes performance but is dangerous. Maintaining hydration is crucial for success but also quite challenging. Reid and Lightfoot[97] provided an excellent review of the physiological stress of the driving athlete, but specific to hydration, the thermal load caused by the heat of the car, the safety suits, and helmets can result in sweat losses of about 1 L/h. Many motorsport races last 3 to 4 hours, resulting in cumulative sweat losses of 3% to 4% of body mass.[98] This level of dehydration negatively impacts both physical and cognitive performance.[99,100] Developing an effective hydration strategy for these athletes is essential for both health and safety.

For nonprofessional drivers, driving a car is likely the highest-risk activity that most of us do each day. The World Health Organization estimates 1.3 million people die and 20 to 50 million people are injured in road traffic accidents each year.[101] Although most drivers would likely not consider their hydration status to be an important aspect of safe driving, research has shown that mild hypohydration of just over 1% significantly increased driving errors in a simulated prolonged and monotonous driving task.[102] In fact, errors in judgment while driving have been correlated to a loss of vigilance behind the wheel.[103] Experts are uncertain whether the cause of the driving decrement is physiological or psychological, but the reduction in driving performance is similar to that of a blood alcohol content of 0.08% or driving while sleep deprived.[102] Although maintaining hydration on a long distance drive may result in more frequent stops, it is also likely the safer route.

When Is a Sports Drink Better Than Plain Water?

A properly formulated sports drink provides a convenient way to replace lost water and sodium while providing the muscles and brain with the carbohydrate needed to sustain the accelerated metabolism associated with exercise. Drinking water to replace sweat losses is often sufficient to prevent dehydration when exercise is short in duration (eg, <60 min), when exercise intensity is low, and when the environment is cool. Consuming carbohydrate during high-intensity, short-duration (<30 min) exercise generally does not impact performance. Likewise, low-intensity exercise (<50% of VO_2 max) that lasts less than 1 hour is not overly reliant on muscle glycogen for fuel. Sports drinks are beneficial to hydration and performance, however, when moderate- to high-intensity exercise lasts roughly an hour or when low- to moderate-intensity exercise lasts longer than 1 hour.

Carbohydrate metabolism is reviewed in detail in Chapter 2 but is discussed briefly here in the context of hydration and performance. Carbohydrate has been shown repeatedly to improve performance[16,35,104,105] through several mechanisms. First, a carbohydrate mouth rinse without ingestion improves high-intensity performance through the stimulation of oral receptors.[106,107] Second, carbohydrate consumed during exercise provides glucose to increase carbohydrate oxidation and possibly spare muscle and liver glycogen.[108,109] Finally, a sports drink that contains multiple transportable carbohydrates (eg, glucose, fructose, sucrose) stimulates fluid absorption, as the absorption of monosaccharides and sodium creates an osmotic gradient that speeds the movement of water molecules from the lumen of the small intestine into the bloodstream.[35,110-112] Sports drinks are formulated to contain no more than 6% to 7% carbohydrate (14–17 g/8 fl oz) to enable the fluid to quickly empty from the stomach and be absorbed into the body from the small intestine.[61,104,113] For trained endurance athletes who are accustomed to consuming carbohydrate during exercise, higher concentrations of carbohydrate may be well tolerated.[113]

Does Coconut Water Make a Good Hydration Beverage?

The nutritional composition of coconut water—fresh from a coconut—is such that it can be hydrating. Fresh, young coconuts have a higher water content than mature coconuts and a carbohydrate content of about 10 g/245 mL, or approximately 4% carbohydrate, including a blend of fructose, sucrose, and glucose. The same serving also provides about 400 mg of potassium, 65 mg of sodium, and 25 mg of vitamin C.[114] Coconut water has been used in tropical climates for generations as a treatment for diarrhea and dehydration. However, because sodium is the primary electrolyte driving rehydration, coconut water consumed during or after exercise for fluid replacement should be supplemented with a source of sodium to aid in fluid retention when sweat losses are substantial. In studies in which mild dehydration has been induced (~2% of body weight), rehydration with coconut water and sports drinks have produced similar degrees of fluid retention.[115] Coconut water also has a unique flavor profile that does not appeal to everyone, so those unaccustomed to drinking coconut water may curtail voluntary intake, causing inadequate fluid replacement.[116]

What Is the Relationship Between Hydration Status and the Risk of Disease?

Several health conditions have been associated with dehydration. Although all health conditions are multifactorial, with some having genetic causes, hydration may play a key role in their prevention, development, exacerbation, and treatment.

Urinary tract infections (UTIs) are common, particularly in females, with the lifetime risk being greater than 50%.[117] In a study of women who experienced recurrent UTIs, increasing water intake by 1.5 L/d significantly reduced the incidence of UTIs over the course of a year.[118]

Kidney stones caused by hyperoxaluria and the deposition or oxalate crystals in the kidney are usually genetic disorders of calcium oxalate metabolism. However, primary treatment, in addition to reducing oxalate intake and absorption, is high water intake to increase urine production to 2 to 3 L/d.[119]

Acute kidney injury (AKI) represents the rapid onset of kidney damage that can occur over a few hours or days. AKI is often seen in hospitalized patients who are being treated for other conditions; however, there is increasing recognition that the combination of mechanical load caused by work or exercise, a high heat index, and dehydration may contribute to AKI. Agricultural workers are at particular risk, and high urine specific gravity and heat index have been associated with an increased risk for the development of AKI.[120,121] In a study of ultramarathon runners, markers of transitional AKI (AKI that resolved within 24 h) were found in the majority of athletes; however, these markers were more closely associated with mechanical strain rather than dehydration or thermal stress.[122] Whereas the risk of AKI in athletes may be relatively low because of the short-term nature of racing or training, agricultural workers are at a greater risk of suffering chronic kidney disease resulting from months or years of laboring in the heat.[123]

Sickle cell trait (SCT) is caused by a single gene polymorphism resulting in a modification of normal hemoglobin that can damage deoxygenated red blood cells.[124] The damaged cells release adhesion molecules that can create a "logjam" that obstructs small blood vessels and impairs microcirculation.[125] Obstructed blood vessels cause complications including tissue ischemia, pain, organ failure, and possible death.[124] Experts estimate that 8% of the Black population in the United States have SCT,[126] and studies indicate that individuals with SCT have greater blood viscosity and red blood cell rigidity.[127] Dehydration also increases blood viscosity, and the combined effects of heat stress and dehydration may put athletes with SCT at greater risk of exercise-related sudden death. Athletes with SCT who are living or competing at altitude may also be at an increased risk because of greater insensible and evaporative water losses, as well as increased risk of hypoxia. Dehydration, hypoxemia, and a high blood lactate level resulting from reduced oxygen availability can all be precipitating factors in a sickle cell emergency.[128] In 2010, the National Collegiate Athletic Association required athletes to be screened for SCT and began educating athletes, coaches, and sports medicine professionals about the risks of SCT. The incidence of sudden death associated with SCT has significantly decreased since that time, although experts do know whether the decrease in death can be attributed to education or screening.[129] Nevertheless, awareness of the risk and vigilance in the care and treatment of these athletes are essential. Athletes with SCT are advised to acclimate to heat very slowly and to always be well hydrated.

Chronic dehydration may be associated with higher blood glucose concentrations, which may, over time, increase the risk of developing diabetes. Studies in the 1970s and 1980s linked blood concentrations of arginine vasopressin (AVP) with high blood glucose. AVP is synthesized and released from the hypothalamus in response to hypovolemia and hyperosmolarity of the blood. Its primary role is to act on the kidneys through the V2 receptor to conserve water, thereby increasing blood volume and reducing osmolarity. AVP, however, also has receptors (denoted V1aR and V2bR) in peripheral tissues and stimulates hepatic gluconeogenesis and glycogenolysis, in addition to triggering the release of glucagon and insulin from the pancreas.[130] Additionally, AVP is released as part of the stress response regulating the secretion of adrenocorticotropic hormone, which stimulates cortisol secretion and also stimulates hepatic glucose output.[131] Copeptin, a surrogate marker for AVP, has been associated with metabolic dysfunction in cross-sectional, population-based studies.[132]Although some studies have shown that higher self-reported water intake is associated with lower risk of hyperglycemia,[133,134] these results have not been consistent.[135] Whether AVP is the cause or the consequence of hyperglycemia has yet to be elucidated, and many questions remain, especially in relation to individuals who do not have diabetes. However, longitudinal studies are being conducted to determine if drinking water lowers the risk for developing insulin resistance and type 2 diabetes.

Box 6.5 summarizes the do's and dont's for appropriate hydration.

BOX 6.5 Hydration Do's and Dont's

Dehydration is the most common performance-sapping mistake, but it is also the most preventable. The following guidelines can help physically active people stay well hydrated.

Do	Don't
Do start exercise well hydrated. When heavy sweating is expected, drink 2 to 3 cups (475 to 700 mL; about 7 mL/kg of body weight [BW] or about 1 oz/10 lb of BW) of fluid 4 hours before exercise to allow excess fluid to be lost as urine. If urine output is still low 2 hours before exercise, drink 5 to 12 oz (150 to 355 mL; about 3 to 5 mL/kg of BW or about 0.6 oz/10 lb of BW). There is no benefit to hyperhydration, so do not drink excessively.	***Don't rely solely on water.*** If sweating lightly, water is an acceptable fluid replacement beverage. For heavier sweating (eg, >0.5 L/h), sports drinks help replace the electrolytes lost in sweat and supply performance-boosting carbohydrates to aid exercise performance. However, excessive drinking of any low-sodium beverage can lead to dangerous electrolyte disturbances (hyponatremia).

Do	Don't
Do monitor weight changes. The best way to determine if enough fluid is consumed during a workout is to determine how much weight has been lost. Minimal weight loss (eg, <2% of BW) means the athlete is well hydrated. Weight loss during an exercise session is water loss, not fat loss, and must be replaced.	**Don't overdrink.** Drinking large amounts of fluid is not only unnecessary but can be downright dangerous. A bloated stomach, puffy fingers and ankles, a bad headache, and confusion are warning signs of hyponatremia.
Do drink during exercise. When sweating, drink every 10 to 20 minutes during a workout. Those who sweat heavily can benefit from drinking more often (eg, every 10 min), whereas individuals who sweat lightly should drink less often (every 20 min or longer).	**Don't gain weight during exercise.** If an individual weighs more after exercise than before, too much fluid has been consumed. Cut back the next time so that no weight is gained.
Do ingest sodium during exercise. The best time to begin replacing the sodium lost in sweat is during exercise. This is one reason why a good sports drink is better than plain water. Sodium intake of 1 g/h is recommended during prolonged exercise where heavy sweat loss is expected.	**Don't restrict salt in your diet.** Ample salt (sodium chloride) in the diet is essential to replace the salt lost in sweat. Because athletes sweat a lot, their need for salt is often much more than that of nonathletes.
Do follow an individual plan. Everyone sweats differently, so every athlete should have a drinking plan tailored to their individual hydration needs.	**Don't use dehydration to lose weight.** Restricting fluid intake during exercise impairs performance and increases the risk of heat-related problems. Dehydration should be kept to a minimum by following an individualized fluid replacement plan.
Do drink plenty during meals. If unable to drink enough during exercise to keep from losing weight, be sure to drink enough before the next bout of exercise. Mealtime makes it easy to drink and to consume the sodium that comes along with food. When rapid rehydration is required, drink 50% more than the existing fluid deficit (eg, if a 2-lb [~1-kg] fluid deficit exists, drink 48 oz [1,500 mL] of fluid to catch up).	**Don't delay drinking during exercise.** Stick to a drinking schedule to avoid dehydration early in exercise. Once a person is dehydrated, it is next to impossible to catch up to what the body needs because dehydration actually slows the speed at which fluid exits the stomach.

Adapted with permission from reference 136: Murray R, Stofan J, Eichner ER. Hyponatremia and exercise. *Sports Sci Exch.* 2003;16:1-6.

SUMMARY

Water is constantly lost from the body, with each water-saturated breath; with the slow seeping of water through the skin; with the obligatory production of urine and feces; in substantial volumes in sweat; and when a person is ill, through emesis and diarrhea. Fortunately, the combination of thirst and spontaneous drinking is usually sufficient to match fluid intake to losses so that progressive, chronic dehydration is typically not an issue, even for older adults. However, for any individual who sweats profusely day after day, adequate water and salt replacement can pose a considerable challenge that can be met only by following practical yet scientifically founded recommendations for fluid and electrolyte intake.

The human body relies on an adequate volume of body water for all physiological and biochemical processes, so it should be no surprise that dehydration can adversely affect the health and performance of athletes and nonathletes. For that reason, it is essential that physically active people ingest ample fluids throughout the day to replace what is lost in sweat and urine. Two hours before a physical activity during which heavy sweating is expected, approximately 7 mL per kilogram of body weight (about 1 oz per 10 lb of body weight) of water or sports drink should be consumed. During exercise, the goal is to drink enough to minimize weight loss and dehydration. Those who sweat lightly require only modest volumes of fluid intake (<500 mL/h [<16 oz/h]), whereas those who sweat heavily may have to ingest in excess of 1.5 L/h (about 50 oz/h) to minimize dehydration. To fully restore hydration status after exercise, it is necessary to consume 125% to 150% of the existing fluid deficit. For example, if the fluid deficit after exercise is 2 lb (0.9 kg), 48 oz (1.4 L) of fluid should be consumed to ensure complete rehydration. For those who exercise only once per day, fluid deficits are usually corrected during the course of normal eating and drinking. Those who train or compete more than once a day, as well as those who sweat throughout the day (eg, workers and soldiers), should adopt a more aggressive fluid replacement plan, along with adequate salt intake, to avoid persistent dehydration.

KEY TAKEAWAYS

Water is essential for the body to function properly. Dehydration of just 1% to 2% of body weight can negatively impact performance, particularly in hot and humid climates.

Sodium is the primary electrolyte lost in sweat. Consuming sodium during and after exercise helps encourage drinking, maintain blood volume, reduce urine production, and stimulate more complete rehydration.

A practical way for athletes to monitor their hydration status is through the color and volume of their urine. A small volume of dark-colored urine likely indicates hypohydration and should signal greater fluid intake. Other approaches include assessing thirst, urine color, and body weight each morning; noticeable thirst, dark yellow urine, and loss of body weight signal dehydration and the need for increased fluid intake.

Diet generally has little impact on fluid requirements. However, high-protein and high-sodium diets may slightly increase fluid needs.

Daily fluid needs vary widely among and even within individuals depending on the intensity and duration of physical activity, environmental conditions, heat acclimation, and fitness.

Individual hydration plans can be established by periodically monitoring changes in body weight before and after exercise and encouraging athletes to consume enough fluid during activity to minimize postexercise weight loss.

REFERENCES

1. Vlamis, K. Heat and dehydration killed a family of 3 on a hike. A survival expert says such tragedies are more common than you think. *Business Insider*. October 28, 2021. Accessed November 12, 2022. www.insider.com/heat-dehydration-kill-family-hike-common-tragedy-survival-expert-2021-10
2. Cheuvront S, Carter R III, Castellani JW, Sawka MN. Hypohydration impairs endurance exercise performance in temperate but not cold air. *J Appl Physiol (1985)*. 2005;99(5):1972-1976. doi:10.1152/japplphysiol.00329.2005
3. Murray R. Hydration and physical performance. *J Am Coll Nutr*. 2007;26(5 suppl):542S-548S. doi:10.1080/07315724.2007.10719656
4. Murray R. Nutrition for the marathon and other endurance sports: environmental stress and dehydration. *Med Sci Sports Exerc*. 1992;24(9 suppl):S319-S323. PMID: 1406204
5. Sawka MN. Body fluid responses and dehydration during exercise and heat stress. In: Pandolf KB, Sawka MN, Gonzalez RR, eds. *Human Performance Physiology and Environmental Medicine at Terrestrial Extremes*. Benchmark Press; 1988:227-266.
6. Savoie FA, Kenefick RW, Ely BR, Cheuvront SN, Goulet ED. Effect of hypohydration on muscle endurance, strength, anaerobic power and capacity and vertical jumping ability: a meta-analysis. *Sports Med*. 2015;45(8):1207-1227. doi:10.1007/s40279-015-0349-0
7. Sawka MN. Physiological consequences of hypohydration: exercise performance and thermoregulation. *Med Sci Sports Exerc*. 1992;24(6):657-670. doi:10.1249/00005768-199206000-00008
8. Below PR, Mora-Rodríguez R, González-Alonso J, Coyle EF. Fluid and carbohydrate ingestion independently improve performance during 1 h of intense exercise. *Med Sci Sports Exerc*. 1995;27:200-210. PMID: 7723643
9. Coyle EF, Montain SJ. Benefits of fluid replacement with carbohydrate during exercise. *Med Sci Sports Exerc*. 1992;24(9 suppl):S324-S330. doi:10.1249/00005768-199209001-00004
10. Montain SJ, Coyle EF. The influence of graded dehydration on hyperthermia and cardiovascular drift during exercise. *J Appl Physiol (1985)*. 1992;73(4):1340-1350. doi:10.1152/jappl.1992.73.4.1340
11. American College of Sports Medicine position stand on the prevention of thermal injuries during distance running. *Med Sci Sports Exerc*. 1987;19(5):529-533. PMID: 3316906
12. American College of Sports Medicine; Sawka MN, Burke LM, Eichner ER, et al. American College of Sports Medicine position stand. Exercise and fluid replacement. *Med Sci Sports Exerc*. 2007;Feb;39(2):377-390. doi:10.1249/mss.0b013e31802ca597
13. Armstrong LE, Epstein Y, Greenleaf JE, et al. American College of Sports Medicine position stand on heat and cold illnesses during distance running. *Med Sci Sports Exerc*. 1996;28(12):i-x. PMID: 8970149
14. McDermott BP, Anderson SA, Armstrong LE, et al. National Athletic Trainers' Association Position Statement: fluid replacement for the physically active. *J Athl Train*. 2017;52(9):877-895. doi:10.4085/1062-6050-52.9.02
15. American Academy of Pediatrics, Committee on Sports Medicine and Fitness. Climatic heat stress and the exercising child and adolescent. *Pediatrics*. 2000;106(1 Pt 1):158-159. PMID: 7079049
16. Thomas DT, Erdman KA, Burke LM. Position of the Academy of Nutrition and Dietetics, Dietitians of Canada, and the American College of Sports Medicine: nutrition and athletic performance. *J Acad Nutr Diet*. 2016;116(3):501-528. doi:10.1016/j.jand.2015.12.006
17. Noakes T. Fluid replacement during marathon running. *Clin J Sports Med*. 2003;13(5):309-318. doi:10.1097/00042752-200309000-00007
18. Hew-Butler T, Rosner MH, Fowkes-Godek S, et al. Statement of the Third International Exercise-Associated Hyponatremia Consensus Development Conference, Carlsbad, California, 2015. *Br J Sports Med*. 2015; 25(4):303-320. doi:10.1136/bjsports-2015-095004
19. Inter-Association Task Force. Exertional heat illness consensus statement. *NATA News*. 2003;6:24-29.
20. Casa DJ. Proper hydration for distance running — identifying individual fluid needs. A USA Track and Field Advisory. April 2003. Accessed August 26, 2022. www.khsaa.org/sportsmedicine/heat/properhydrationfordistancerunning.pdf
21. Casa DJ, Clarkson PM, Roberts WO. American College of Sports Medicine Roundtable on Hydration and Physical Activity: consensus statements. *Curr Sports Med Rep*. 2005;4(3):115-127. doi:10.1097/01.csmr.0000306194.67241.76
22. Panel on Dietary Reference Intakes for Electrolytes and Water, Standing Committee on the Scientific Evaluation of Dietary Reference Intakes, Food and Nutrition Board, Institute of Medicine. *Dietary Reference Intakes for Water, Potassium, Sodium, Chloride, and Sulfate*. National Academies Press; 2005.
23. Ball P. Water as an active constituent in cell biology. *Chem Rev*. 2008;108(1):74-108. doi:10.1021/cr068037a
24. Shepherd VA. The cytomatrix as a cooperative system of macromolecular and water networks. *Curr Top Dev Biol*. 2006;75:171-223. doi:10.1016/S0070-2153(06)75006-2
25. Phillips PA, Rolls BJ, Ledingham ML, Morton JJ. Body fluid changes, thirst and drinking in man during free access to water. *Physiol Behav*. 1984;33(3):357-363. doi:10.1016/0031-9384(84)90154-9
26. Leib DE, Zimmerman CA, Knight ZA. Thirst. *Curr Biol*. 2016;26(24):R1260-R1265. doi:10.1016/j.cub.2016.11.019
27. Guyton AC, Hall JE. *Textbook of Medical Physiology*. 10th ed. WB Saunders Co; 2000.
28. Booth DA. Influences on human fluid consumption. In: Ramsay DJ, Booth DA, eds. *Thirst: Physiological and Psychological Aspects*. Springer-Verlag; 1991:53-76.

29. Greenleaf JE. Problem: thirst, drinking behavior, and involuntary dehydration. *Med Sci Sports Exerc*. 1992;24(6):645-656.
30. Lacey J, Corbett J, Forni L, et al. A multidisciplinary consensus on dehydration: definitions, diagnostic methods and clinical implications. *Ann Med*. 2019;51(3):232-251. doi:10.1080/07853890.2019.1628352
31. Valtin H. "Drink at least eight glasses of water a day?" Really? Is there scientific evidence for "8 × 8"? *Am J Physiol Regul Integr Comp Physiol*. 2002;283(5):993R-1004R. doi:10.1152/ajpregu.00365.2002
32. Grandjean AC, Reimers KJ, Buyckx ME. Hydration: issues for the 21st century. *Nutr Rev*. 2003;61(8):261-271. doi:10.1301/nr.2003.aug.261-271
33. EFSA Panel on Dietetic Products, Nutrition and Allergies. Scientific opinion on dietary reference values for water. *EFSA J*. 2010;8(3):1-48. doi:10.2903/j.efsa.2010.1459
34. Ladell WS. Water and salt (sodium chloride) intakes. In: Edholm O, Bacharach A, eds. *The Physiology of Human Survival*. Academic Press; 1965:235-299.
35. Baker LB, Jeukendrup AE. Optimal composition of fluid-replacement beverages. *Compr Physiol*. 2014;4(2):575-620. doi:10.1002/cphy.c130014
36. Lundby C, Hamarsland H, Hansen J, et al. Hematological, skeletal muscle fiber and exercise performance adaptations to heat training in elite female and male cyclists. *J Appl Physiol (1985)*. 2023;135(1):217-226. doi:10.1152/japplphysiol.00115.2023
37. Wenger CB. Human heat acclimation. In: Pandolf KB, Sawka MN, Gonzalez RR, eds. *Human Performance, Physiology, and Environment Medicine at Terrestrial Extremes*. Benchmark Press; 1988:153-197.
38. Palmer MS, Spriet LL. Sweat rate, salt loss, and fluid intake during an intense on-ice practice in elite Canadian male junior hockey players. *App Physiol Nutr Metab*. 2008;33(2):263-271. doi:10.1139/H08-011
39. Bergeron MF. Heat cramps: fluid and electrolyte challenges during tennis in the heat. *J Sci Med Sport*. 2003;6(1):19-27. doi:10.1016/s1440-2440(03)80005-1
40. Montain SJ, Sawka MN, Wenger CB. Hyponatremia associated with exercise: risk factors and pathogenesis. *Exerc Sports Sci Rev*. 2001;29(3):113-117. doi:10.1097/00003677-200107000-00005
41. Shirreffs SM, Maughan RJ. Whole body sweat collection in humans: an improved method with preliminary data on electrolyte content. *J Appl Physiol*. 1997;82(1):336-341.
42. Volpe SL, Poule KA, Bland EG. Estimation of prepractice hydration status of National Collegiate Athletic Association Division I athletes. *J Athl Train*. 2009;44(6):624-629. doi:10.4085/1062-6050-44.6.624
43. Chapelle L, Tassignon B, Rommers N, et al. Pre-exercise hypohydration prevalence in soccer players: a quantitative systematic review. *Eur J Sport Sci*. 2020;20(6):744-755. doi:10.1080/17461391.2019.1669716
44. James LJ, Moss J, Henry J, Papadopoulou C, Mears SA. Hypohydration impairs endurance performance: a blinded study. *Physiol Rep*. 2017;5(12):1-10. doi:10.14814/phy2.13315
45. González-Alonso J. New ideas about hydration and its impact on the athlete's brain, heart and muscles. *Sports Sci Exch*. 2019; 29(196):1-7.
46. Rico-Sanz J, Frontera WA, Rivera MA, Rivera-Brown A, Mole PA, Meredith CN. Effects of hyperhydration on total body water, temperature regulation and performance of elite young soccer players in a warm climate. *Int J Sports Med*. 1996;17(2):85-91. doi:10.1055/s-2007-972813
47. Riedesel ML, Allen DY, Peake GT, Al-Qattan K. Hyperhydration with glycerol solutions. *J Appl Physiol (1985)*. 1987;63(6):2262-2268. doi:10.1152/jappl.1987.63.6.2262
48. Latzka WA, Sawka MN, Montain SJ, et al. Hyperhydration: tolerance and cardiovascular effects during uncompensable exercise-heat stress. *J Appl Physiol (1985)*. 1998;84(6):1858-1864. doi:10.1152/jappl.1998.84.6.1858
49. Freund BJ, Montain SJ, Young AJ, et al. Glycerol hyperhydration: hormonal, renal, and vascular fluid responses. *J Appl Physiol (1985)*. 1995;79(6):2069-2077. doi:10.1152/jappl.1995.79.6.2069
50. World Anti-Doping Agency. *The World Anti-Doping Code: The 2015 Prohibited List International Standard*. Published September 20, 2014. Accessed October 4, 2023. www.wada-ama.org/sites/default/files/resources/files/wada-2015-prohibited-list-en.pdf
51. Polyviou TP, Easton C, Beis L, et al. Effects of glycerol and creatine hyperhydration on doping-relevant blood parameters. *Nutrients*. 2012;4(9):1171-1186. doi:10.3390/nu4091171
52. Logan-Sprenger HM, Heigenhauser GJ, Killian KJ, Spriet LL. Effects of dehydration during cycling on skeletal muscle metabolism in females. *Med Sci Sports Exerc*. 2012;44(10):1949-1957. doi:10.1249/MSS.0b013e31825abc7c
53. Logan-Sprenger HM, Heigenhauser GJ, Jones GL, Spriet LL. Increase in skeletal-muscle glycogenolysis and perceived exertion with progressive dehydration during cycling in hydrated men. *Int J Sport Nutr Exerc Metab*. 2013;23(3):220-229. doi:10.1123/ijsnem.23.3.220
54. Noakes TD. Hydration in the marathon: using thirst to gauge safe fluid replacement. *Sports Med*. 2007:37(4-5):463-466. doi:10.2165/00007256-200737040-00050
55. Murray R. Fluid replacement: the American College of Sports Medicine position stand. *Sports Sci Exch*. 1996;9:1-6.
56. Maughan RJ. Gastric emptying during exercise. *Sports Sci Exch*. 1993;6(5):1-6.
57. Hubbard RW, Szlyk PC, Armstrong LE. Influence of thirst and fluid palatability on fluid ingestion during exercise. In: Gisolfi CV, Lamb DR, eds. *Fluid Homeostasis During Exercise: Perspectives in Exercise Science and Sports Medicine; vol. 3*. Benchmark Press; 1990:39-96. Barley OR, Chapman DW, Abbiss CR. Reviewing the current methods of assessing hydration in athletes. *J Inter Soc Sports Nutr*. 2020;17(1):52. doi:10.1186/s12970-020-00381-6
58. Passe D, Horn M, Stofan J, Horswill C, Murray R. Voluntary dehydration in runners despite favorable conditions for fluid intake. *Int J Sports Nutr Exerc Metab*. 2007:17(3):284-295. doi:10.1123/ijsnem.17.3.284
59. Armstrong LE, Kavouras SA. Thirst and drinking paradigms: evolution from single factor effects to brainwide dynamic networks. *Nutrients*. 2019;11(12):2864. doi:10.3390/nu11122864

60. Horswill CA. Effective fluid replacement. *Int J Sport Nutr.* 1998;8(2):175-195. doi:10.1123/ijsn.8.2.175
61. Armstrong LE, Costill DL, Fink WJ. Changes in body water and electrolytes during heat acclimation: effects of dietary sodium. *Aviat Space Environ Med.* 1987;58(2):143-148.
62. Bergeron MF. Heat cramps during tennis: a case report. *Int J Sport Nutr.* 1996;6(1):62-68. doi:10.1123/ijsn.6.1.62
63. Stofan JR, Zachwieja JJ, Horswill CA, Murray R, Anderson SA, Eichner ER. Sweat and sodium losses in NCAA football players: a precursor to heat cramps? *Int J Sports Nutr Exerc Metab.* 2005;15(6):641-652. doi:10.1123/ijsnem.15.6.641
64. Miller KC, McDermott BP, Yeargin SW. Sweat characteristics of cramp-prone and cramp-resistant athletes. *Int J Sport Nutr Exerc Metab.* 2020;30(3):218–228. doi:10.1123/ijsnem.2019-0308
65. Murray B. How curiosity killed the cramp: emerging science on the cause and prevention of exercise-associated muscle cramps. *AMAA J.* 2016;(fall/winter):5-7.
66. Baker LB, Wolfe AS. Physiological mechanisms determining eccrine sweat composition. *Eur J Appl Physiol.* 2020;120(4):719-752. doi:10.1007/s00421-020-04323-7
67. Maughan RJ, Shirreffs SM, Leiper JB. Rehydration and recovery after exercise. *Sport Sci Exch.* 1996;9(62):1-5.
68. Shirreffs SM, Taylor AJ, Leiper JB, Maughan RJ. Post-exercise rehydration in man: effects of volume consumed and drink sodium content. *Med Sci Sports Exerc.* 1996;28(10):1260-1271. doi:10.1097/00005768-199610000-00009
69. González-Alonso J, Heaps CL, Coyle EF. Rehydration after exercise with common beverages and water. *Int J Sports Med.* 1992;13(5):399-406. doi:10.1055/s-2007-1021288
70. Gisolfi CV, Summers RW, Schedl HP, Bleiler TL. Effect of sodium concentration in a carbohydrate-electrolyte solution on intestinal absorption. *Med Sci Sports Exerc.* 1995;27(10):1414-1420.
71. Wilk B, Bar-Or O. Effect of drink flavor and NaCl on voluntary drinking and hydration in boys exercising in the heat. *J Appl Physiol (1985).* 1996;80(4):1112-1117. doi:10.1152/jappl.1996.80.4.1112
72. Uchida K, Ogawa Y, Kataoka Y, et al. New portable device for continuous measurement of sweat rate under heat stress during field tests. *J Appl Physiol (1985).* 2022;132(4):974-983. doi:10.1152/japplphysiol.00155.2021
73. Eichner ER. Six paths to hyponatremia. *Curr Sports Med Rep.* 2009;8(6):280-281. doi:10.1249/JSR.0b013e3181c1bb2c
74. Hew TD, Chorley JN, Cianca JC, Divine JG. The incidence, risk factors, and clinical manifestations of hyponatremia in marathon runners. *Clin J Sport Med.* 2003;13(1):41-47. doi:10.1097/00042752-200301000-00008
75. Davis BA, Thigpen LK, Hornsby JH, Green JM, Coates TE, O'Neal EK. Hydration kinetics and 10-km outdoor running performance following 75% and 150% between bout fluid replacement. *Eur J Sport Sci.* 2014;14(7):703-710. doi:10.1080/17461391.2014.894578
76. Piantodosi CA. *The Biology of Human Survival: Life and Death in Extreme Environments.* Oxford University Press; 2003.
77. Greenleaf JE. Environmental issues that influence intake of replacement beverages. In: Marriott BM, ed. *Fluid Replacement and Heat Stress.* National Academy Press; 1994:195-214.
78. Bar-David Y, Urkin J, Landau D, Bar-David Z, Pilpel D. Voluntary dehydration among elementary school children residing in a hot arid environment. *J Hum Nutr Diet.* 2009;22(5):455-460. doi:10.1111/j.1365-277X.2009.00960.x
79. Kenney WL, Havenith G, Jay O. Thermal physiology, more relevant than ever before. *J App Physiol.* 2022;133(3):676-678. doi:10.1152/japplphysiol.00464.2022
80. Berko J, Ingram DD, Saha S, Parker JD. Deaths attributed to heat, cold, and other weather events in the United States, 2006–2010. *National Health Statistics Report.* 2014;(76):1-15. www.cdc.gov/nchs/data/nhsr/nhsr076.pdf
81. Gasparrini A, Guo Y, Hashizume M, et al. Mortality risk attributable to high and low ambient temperature: a multicountry observational study. *Lancet.* 2014;386(9991):369-375. doi:10.1016/S0140-6736(14)62114-0
82. Hoyt RW, Honig A. Environmental influences on body fluid balance during exercise: altitude. In: Buskirk ER, Puhl SM. *Body Fluid Balance: Sport and Exercise.* CRC Press; 1996;183-196.
83. Diggins KC. Treatment of mild to moderate dehydration in children with oral rehydration therapy. *J Am Acad Nurse Pract.* 2008;20(8):402-406. doi:10.1111/j.1745-7599.2008.00338.x
84. WHO position paper on oral rehydration salts to reduce mortality from cholera. World Health Organization website. Published December 8, 2008. Accessed June 20, 2024. https://reliefweb.int/report/zimbabwe/who-position-paper-oral-rehydration-salts-reduce-mortality-cholera
85. Atia AN, Buchman AL. Oral rehydration solutions in non-cholera diarrhea: a review. *Am J Gastroenterol.* 2009;104(10):2596-2604. doi:10.1038/ajg.2009.329
86. Kenney EL, Long MW, Cradock AL, Gortmaker SL. Prevalence of inadequate hydration among US children and disparities by gender and race/ethnicity: National Health and Nutrition Examination Survey, 2009-2012. *Am J Public Health.* 2015;105(8):e113-e118. doi:10.2105/AJPH.2015.302572
87. Chang T, Ravi N, Plegue MA, Sonneville KR, Davis MM. Inadequate hydration, BMI, and obesity among US adults: NHANES 2009-2012. *Ann Fam Med.* 2016;14(4):320-324. doi:10.1370/afm.1951
88. Arnaoutis G, Kavouras SA, Angelopoulou A, et al. Fluid balance during training in elite young athletes of different sports. *J Strength Cond Res.* 2015;29(12):3447-3452. doi:10.1519/JSC.0000000000000400
89. Rivera-Brown AM, De Felix-Davila RA. Hydration status in adolescent judo athletes before and after training in the heat. *Int J Physiol Perform.* 2012;7(1):39-46. doi:10.1123/ijspp.7.1.39
90. Adams J, Kavouras SA, Robillard JI, et al. Fluid balance of adolescent swimmers during training. *J Strength Cond Res.* 2016;30(3):621-625. doi:10.1519/JSC.0000000000001132

91. Rowland T. Fluid replacement requirements for child athletes. *Sports Med.* 2011;41(4):279-288. doi:10.2165/11584320-000000000-00000
92. Kavouras SA, Arnaoutis G, Makrillos M, et al. Educational intervention on water intake improves hydration status and enhances exercise performance in athletic youth. *Scand J Med Sci Sports.* 2012;22(5):684-689. doi:10.1111/j.1600-0838.2011.01296.x
93. Fadda R, Rapinett G, Grathwol D, et al. Effects of drinking supplementary water at school on cognitive performance in children. *Appetite.* 2012;59(3):730-737. doi:10.1016/j.appet.2012.07.005
94. Perry CS 3rd, Rapinett G, Glaser NS, Ghetti S. Hydration status moderates the effects of drinking water on children's cognitive performance. *Appetite.* 2015;95:520-527. doi:10.1016/j.appet.2015.08.006
95. Edmonds CJ, Crosbie L, Fatima F, Hussain M, Jacob N, Gardner M. Dose-response effects of water supplementation on cognitive performance and mood in children and adults. *Appetite.* 2017;108:464-470. doi:10.1016/j.appet.2009.02.010
96. Reid MB, Lightfoot JT. The physiology of auto racing. *Med Sci Sports Exerc.* 2019;51(12):2548-2562. doi:10.1249/MSS.0000000000002070
97. Carlson LA, Lawrence MA, Kenefick RW. Hydration status and thermoregulation responses in drivers during competitive racing. *J Strength Cond Res.* 2018;32(7):2061-2065. doi:10.1519/JSC.0000000000002268
98. Sawka MN, Cheuvront SN, Kenefick RW. Hypohydration and human performance: Impact of environment and physiological mechanisms. *Sports Med.* 2015;45(suppl 1):S51-S60. doi:10.1007/s40279-015-0395.7
99. Lieberman HR. Hydration and cognition: A critical review and recommendations for future research. *J Am Coll Nutr.* 2007;26(suppl 5):555S-561S. doi:10.1111/j.1753-4887.2012.00524.x
100. Global Status Report on Road Safety 2018. World Health Organization; June 17, 2018. Accessed July 15, 2024. License: CC BY- NC-SA 3.0 IGO. www.who.int/publications/i/item/9789241565684
101. Watson P, Whale A, Mears SA, Reyner LA, Maughan RJ. Mild hypohydration increases the frequency of driver errors during a prolonged, monotonous driving task. *Physiol Behav.* 2015;147:313-318. doi:10.1016/j.physbeh.2015.04.028
102. Campagne A, Pabayle T, Muzet A. Correlation between driving errors and vigilance level: influence of driver's age. *Physiol. Behav.* 2004;80(4):515-524. doi:10.1016/j.physbeh.2003.10.004
103. Sawka MN, Francesconi RP, Young AJ, Pandolf KB. Influence of hydration level and body fluids on exercise performance in the heat. *JAMA.* 1984;252(9):1165-1169.
104. Casa DJ, Armstrong LE, Hillman SK, et al. National Athletic Trainers' Association Position Statement: Fluid replacement for athletes. *J Athl Train.* 2000;35(2):212-224.
105. Carter JM, Jeukendrup AE, Jones DA. The effect of carbohydrate mouth rinse on 1-h cycle time trial performance. *Med Sci Sports Exerc.* 2004;36(12):2107-2111. doi:10.1249/01.mss.0000147585.65709.6f
106. Rollo I, Williams C. Effect of mouth-rinsing carbohydrate solutions on endurance performance. *Sports Med.* 2011; 41(6):449-461. doi:10.2165/11588730-000000000-00000
107. Menzies, C Wood M, Thomas J, et al. Frequent carbohydrate ingestion reduces muscle glycogen depletion and postpones fatigue relative to a single bolus. *Int J Sport Nutr Exerc Metab.* 2020;30(3):203-209. doi:10.1123/ijsnem.2019-0291
108. Cermak NM, van Loon LJC. The use of carbohydrates during exercise as an ergogenic aid. *Sports Med.* 2013;43(11):1139-1155. doi:10.1007/s40279-013-0079-0
109. Gisolfi CV, Duchman SD. Guidelines for optimal replacement beverages for different athletic events. *Med Sci Sports Exerc.* 1992;24(6):679-687.
110. Coyle EF, Montain SJ. Carbohydrate and fluid ingestion during exercise: are there trade-offs? *Med Sci Sports Exerc.* 1992;24(6):671-678.
111. Ryan AJ, Lambert GP, Shi X, Chang RT, Summers RW, Gisolfi CV. Effect of hypohydration on gastric emptying and intestinal absorption during exercise. *J Appl Physiol (1985).* 1998;84(5):1581-1588. doi:10.1152/jappl.1998.84.5.1581
112. Hearris MA, Pugh JN, Langan-Evans, C, et al. ^{13}C-glucose-fructose labeling reveals comparable exogenous CHO oxidation during exercise when consuming 120 g/h in fluid, gel, jelly chew, or coingestion. *J Appl Physiol (1985).* 2022;132(6):1394-1406. doi:10.1152/japplphysiol.00091.2022
113. US Department of Agriculture, Agricultural Research Service, Beltsville Human Nutrition Research Center. FoodData Central[Internet], 2019. Accessed October 4, 2023. https://fdc.nal.usda.gov
114. Pérez-Idárraga A, Aragón-Vargas LF. Postexercise rehydration: potassium-rich drinks versus water and a sports drink. *Appl Physiol Nutr Metab.* 2014;30(10):1167-1174. doi:10.1139/apnm-2013-0434
115. Peart DJ, Hensby A, Shaw MP. Coconut water does not improve markers of hydration during sub-maximal exercise and performance in a subsequent time trial compared to water alone. *Int J Sport Nutr Exerc Metab.* 2017;27(3):279-284. doi:10.1123/ijsnem.2016.2016-0121
116. Foxman B, Barlow R, D'Arcy H, Gillespie B, Sobel JD. Urinary tract infection: self-reported incidence and associated costs. *Ann Epidemiol.* 2000;10(8):509-515. doi:10.1016/S1047-2797(00)00072-7
117. Hooton TM, Vecchio M, Iroz A, et al. Effect of increased daily water intake in premenopausal women with recurrent urinary tract infections. *JAMA Intern Med.* 2018;178(11):1509-1515. doi:10.1001/jamainternmed.2018.4204
118. Demoulin N, Aydin S, Gillion V, Morelle J, Jadoul M. Pathophysiology and management of hyperoxaluria and oxalate nephropathy: A review. *Am J Kidney Dis.* 2022;79(5):717-727. doi:10.1053/j.ajkd.2021.07.018
119. Mix J, Elon L, Vi Thein Mac V, et al. Hydration status, kidney function, and kidney injury in Florida agricultural workers. *J Occup Environ Med.* 2018;60(5):e253-e260. doi:10.1097/JOM.0000000000001261
120. Houser MC, Mac V, Smith DJ, et al. Inflammation-related factors identified as biomarkers of dehydration and subsequent acute kidney injury in agricultural workers. *Biol Res Nurs.* 2021;23(4):676-688. doi:10.1177/10998004211016070

121. Jouffroy R, Lebreton X, Mansencal N, Anglicheau D. Acute kidney injury during an ultra-distance race. *PLoS One*. 2019;14(9):e0222544. doi:10.1371/journal.pone.0222544

122. Clark WF, Sontrop JM, Huang SH, Moist L, Bouby N, Bankir L. Hydration and chronic kidney disease progression: A critical review of the evidence. *Am J Nephrol*. 2016;43(4):281-292. doi:10.1159/000445959

123. Piel FB, Steinberg MH, Rees DC. Sickle cell disease. *N Engl J Med*. 2017;376(16):1561-1573. doi:10.1056/NEJMa1510865

124. Eichner E. Sickle cell considerations in athletes. *Clin Sports Med*. 2011;30:537-549. doi:10.1016/j.csm.2011.03.004

125. Liem RI, Chan C, Vu TT, et al. Association among sickle cell trait, fitness, and cardiovascular risk factors in CARDIA. *Blood*. 2017;129(6):723-728. doi:10.1182/blood-2016-07-727719

126. Wang H, Martone M, Owens ME, et al. NCAA Division I American football players with sickle cell trait have altered hematological responses and hydration status. *Sci Rep*. 2021;11(1):1844. doi:10.1038/s41598-021-81473-4

127. Le Gallais D, Bile A, Mercier J, Paschel M, Tonellot JL, Dauverchain J. Exercise-induced death in sickle cell trait: role of aging, training, and deconditioning. *Med Sci Sports Exerc*. 1996;28(5):541-544. doi:10.1097/00005768-199605000-00001

128. Buchanan BK, Siebert DM, Zigman Suchsland ML, et al. Sudden death associated with sickle cell trait before and after mandatory screening. *Sports Health*. 2020;12(3):241-245. doi:10.1177/1941738120915690

129. Vanhaecke T, Perrier ET, Melander O. A journey through the early evidence linking hydration to metabolic health. *Ann Nutr Metab*. 2020;76(suppl 1):4-9. doi:10.1159/000515021

130. Perrier ET. Shifting focus: From hydration for performance to hydration for health. *Ann Nutr Metab*. 2017;70(suppl 1):4-12. doi:10.1159/000462996

131. Perrier ET, Armstrong LE, Bottin JH, et al. Hydration for health hypothesis: a narrative review of supporting evidence. *Eur J Nutr*. 2021;60(3):1167-1180. doi:10.1007/s00394-020-02296-z

132. Roussel R, Fezeu L, Bouby N, et al; DESIR Study Group. Low water intake and risk for new-onset hyperglycemia. *Diabetes Care*. 2011;34:2551-2554. doi:10.2337/dc11-0652

133. Carroll HA, Davis MG, Papadaki A. Higher plain water intake is associated with lower type 2 diabetes risk: A cross-sectional study in humans. *Nutr Res*. 2015;35(10):865-872. doi:10.1016/j.nutres.2015.06.015

134. Pan A, Malik VS, Schulze MB, Manson JE, Willett WC, Hu FB. Plain-water intake and risk of type 2 diabetes in young and middle-aged women. *Am J Clin Nutr*. 2012;95:1454-1460. doi:10.3945/ajcn.111.032698

135. Murray R, Stofan J, Eichner ER. Hyponatremia and exercise. *Sports Sci Exch*. 2003;16:1-6.

CHAPTER 7

Supplements and Sports Foods

Louise Burke, OAM, PhD, APD, FACSM

LEARNING OBJECTIVES

- Recognize that dietary supplements and sports foods do not have a single or universal set of characteristics but can be described by a range of features such as regulatory definitions, form, availability, mechanism of action, and robustness of supporting evidence for their use.
- Appreciate that products can be used by athletes to meet energy and macronutrient goals when it is inconvenient to consume everyday foods (eg, sports foods), prevent or treat clinical nutrient deficiencies (eg, micronutrient supplements), and directly or indirectly enhance sports performance (eg, dietary supplements targeting performance, recovery, health, or injury).
- Identify potential positive and negative outcomes associated with the use of sports foods and dietary supplements.
- Know how to be pragmatic in supporting athletes to make valuable use of evidence-based products by using research outputs and education resources to identify products that can make a valuable contribution to an athlete's nutrition plan, as well as third-party certification schemes to identify products with a reduced risk of health and doping concerns.

INTRODUCTION

Sports dietitians typically take a food-first approach to meeting sports nutrition goals. This is laudable because of the advantages of expense, safety, and the potential for whole foods and well-planned meals to achieve a wide range of nutritional goals and health benefits. However, to operate successfully, a sports dietitian should have an in-depth appreciation of the large range of dietary supplements and sports foods that are marketed to athletes and coaches. At one level, this knowledge is necessary because at least some of these products can confer benefits that may provide a small but critical part of an athlete's performance plan. On another level, expert knowledge about dietary supplements and sports foods is needed to gain the attention and respect of athletes and coaches because the marketing and allure around these products needs to be addressed with appropriate insight. The sheer number of dietary supplements and sports foods on the market makes it impossible to provide a summary of each. The aim of this chapter is to provide a framework to allow the sports dietitian to manage this challenging area of sports nutrition.

WHAT IS A SUPPLEMENT?

It is difficult to find a working definition that provides a simple but comprehensive summary of dietary supplements and sports foods. Supplements have been categorized according to a variety of characteristics including the mode of action and form or function of the active ingredients; supplements can also be categorized in terms of regulatory definitions. An overview of different perspectives is provided in Box 7.1, along with comments on how well the definition discriminates products based on safety and efficacy concerns.[1,2]

BOX 7.1 Frameworks for Defining Sports Supplements[1,2]

US Food and Drug Administration (FDA) definition[2]:

A product (other than tobacco) intended to supplement the diet that bears or contains 1 or more of the following dietary ingredients: a vitamin; a mineral; an herb or other botanical; an amino acid; a dietary substance for use by man to supplement the diet by increasing the total dietary intake; or a concentrate, metabolite, constituent, extract, or combination of any ingredient described previously.

Consumers often think that supplement safety and efficacy is guaranteed by FDA regulations. However, the FDA's role is typically reactive and begins after a product enters the marketplace. The FDA periodically inspects supplement manufacturing facilities and labeling information to verify that companies are meeting requirements. The FDA monitors adverse event reports as well as product complaints to evaluate the safety of products once they are on the market. It may work with companies that do not comply to recall products or enhance compliance.

Form

Pills Powders Drinks Bars Gels or confectionery	Historically, sports foods (bars, drinks, gels, etc) might have enjoyed a higher reputation for safety than pill-based supplements. This distinction has become blurred with the inclusion of new ingredients in many modern sports foods.

Availability

Prescription-only pharmacy Over-the-counter pharmacy Sports shops Health food shops Supermarkets Internet and mail order Multilevel marketing	The source of a sports food or supplement may provide some level of risk assessment regarding safety and efficacy, with products sold under some supervision (eg, pharmacies) being more reputable than products sold with less oversight (eg, internet sites). However, these distinctions have become more blurred with the exponential increase in online sales of supplements.

Function

Weight loss Weight gain Recovery illness prevention	Most supplements are marketed according to their (claimed) function. The efficacy of products cannot be judged from their claims because these products are not always regulated and regulations that do exist are not

Function *(continued)*	
Fuel support Preworkout activation Prevention or correction of nutrient deficiency	always enforced. In addition, many products are multi-ingredient and may not contain adequate doses of the evidence-based constituents.
Evidence base	
Well-supported benefits Equivocal support Minimal scientific support	Products fit in these categories on a dynamic basis because the evidence around products may evolve with new research findings. Moreover, the evidence base for a product is linked to a specific use, rather than universal application to all sports, all athletes, or all protocols of timing or size of dose. Although this classification system may help an athlete make some judgments about the potential use of a supplement product, it should not be the sole factor because other aspects of the product (eg, contamination risk, expense) should be included in decision making.

It is clear that none of these methods in isolation will assist an athlete in identifying products that could benefit their performance goals. Therefore, a composite of these categories was developed by the Australian Institute of Sport (AIS) Sports Supplement Program/Framework.[3] This system is covered in more detail later in this chapter.

SUPPLEMENT USE BY ATHLETES

Dietary supplements represent a multibillion-dollar industry, with increasing rates of use in the general population. For example in 2019, a survey by the Council for Responsible Nutrition (a body funded by the supplement industry) reported the highest prevalence of supplement use in the United States within its history.[4] The survey found that 77% of respondents (79% of females and 74% of males) reported using dietary supplements, with a 70% prevalence among young adults ages 18 to 34 years. Information about supplement use by athletes shows variable results; this can be partly explained by the use of protocols that are often neither standardized nor validated. Nevertheless, reviews and meta-analyses of surveys on supplement use with a range of athletic groups have found that, depending on the survey, the population, and the definition of a supplement, 40% to 100% of athletes are consumers of dietary supplements and sports foods.[5,6] Furthermore, there is evidence that supplement use among athletes starts at a younger age; is more prevalent than in the general community; and increases in conjunction with the athlete's age, training load, and sporting caliber.[5-7] In addition, evidence of different cultures of supplement use exists between the sexes, with several studies indicating that male athletes are more likely to use creatine and performance supplements, whereas female athletes are more likely to use vitamin supplements.[5,6] Although the reasons for these distinctions are likely to be multifactorial, some may reflect sex differences in body image. For example, Aguilar-Navarro et al[8] found that, whereas creatine use may be of interest to male athletes to support gains in muscle mass and strength, females may shun its potential benefits because of a fear of weight gain.

Pros of Supplement Use

CONVENIENCE IN MEETING NUTRIENT INTAKE GOALS

Some supplements and sports foods offer real benefits for athletic performance. The first such opportunity involves the use of sports foods to allow athletes to meet evidence-based sports nutrition guidelines and, as an indirect outcome, to support optimal health, recovery, and performance. Although sports foods technically meet the NOVA definition of ultraprocessed foods[9] in being hyperpalatable, packaged to have a long shelf life, and constituted from individual food ingredients, these features are often important in allowing athletes to achieve the intake of key nutrients on specific occasions. The most common scenarios of such use are preworkout, during exercise, and postexercise, when it may be impractical to consume whole foods to meet well-established nutrient targets. In such cases, the sports nutrition goals may be so well known that these uses of sports foods can be shown to enhance training outcomes or competition performance (for example, consuming carbohydrate during prolonged exercise activities[10] or protein after resistance-training sessions[11]).

Other aspects of the athlete's lifestyle, such as international travel or an "on-the-run" workday, are often associated with challenges to food availability. In such cases, multinutrient (eg, liquid meals) or key nutrient (eg, high quality protein) sports foods can offer value by being portable and nonperishable. The extreme energy demands of many athletes may make it impractical to consume and tolerate the gastrointestinal issues associated with intake of the required volume of everyday foods. Here, sports foods and liquids with a high energy density and low fiber content may facilitate the achievement of total energy demands.

Micronutrient supplements may also be important for some athletes to help correct or prevent deficiencies that might otherwise impair health or performance. Many athletes are at risk of suboptimal iron[12] and vitamin D status[13] and may benefit from supplementation. These supplements should be taken on the advice of an appropriate health professional and include appropriate assessment of nutrient status.[14] Sports foods that can be used to assist the athlete in meeting well-described demands for energy and macronutrients, as well as micronutrient supplements that can be used to prevent or reverse a nutrient deficiency, are listed in Group A of the AIS Sports Supplement Framework (Box 7.2).[3]

DIRECT PERFORMANCE ENHANCEMENT

Most of the interest in sports supplements is related to special food components that can directly enhance exercise capacity or performance, as well as others that can indirectly lead to better performance through support issues, such as adaptation, sleep, and illness and injury risk. Although these products are sometimes referred to as "ergogenic aids," this term will not be used in this chapter, because the description of ergogenic ("performance enhancing") can be applied to many resources and strategies used in sport. Although many single- and multi-ingredient products claim to provide measurable performance benefits, only a few of these claims can currently be considered evidence based by reputable authorities, such as the AIS Sports Supplement Framework[3] and the International Olympic Committee's Working Group on Supplements in High Performance Sport.[15] These products are summarized in Box 7.3 on page 168,[3,15-35] whereas others that offer reasonable evidence of indirect support are described elsewhere.[36] With regard to direct performance enhancement by caffeine, bicarbonate, nitrate/beetroot juice, β-alanine, creatine, and glycerol, there is evidence that each can enhance performance in specific types of sport, with a mean magnitude of benefit of about 1% to 3%.[16-31,37] Although such an improvement sounds small, these margins are similar to or larger than the intraindividual variability of performance in high-level competitors and likely to provide a worthwhile effect in real-world conditions.[38] The efficacy of these products is reliant on them being used according to an evidence-based protocol that is further personalized to the specific conditions of the event and the individual athlete. This includes considerations such as repeated use in multievent competitions, as well as coingestion with other supplements.[37] Practitioners and athletes can appreciate that some of these products can be used acutely to provide an immediate benefit to the sporting event (eg, caffeine or bicarbonate consumed before or during a race or game). Meanwhile, the protocols of use of other products within this group require a more chronic intake over days and weeks to achieve an increase in muscle stores before a targeted event (eg, creatine and β-alanine loading protocols). Finally, a direct performance enhancement also includes the concept of repeated use in training sessions to allow the athlete to train harder and with better quality (eg, creatine- or caffeine-supported training sessions).

SPORTS-SPECIFIC BENEFITS

In some cases, there may be specific benefits to consuming ingredients from a bespoke supplement or sports food rather than whole foods or conventional processed foods. Apart from the practical issues of easy storage, preparation, and ingestion, the supplement or sports food may be able to provide a known

BOX 7.2 The ABCD Categorization of Supplements and Sports Foods by the Australian Institute of Sport (AIS)[3]

Group A

Evidence level	Strong scientific evidence for use in specific situations in sport using evidence-based protocols
Use within supplement programs	Permitted for use by identified athletes according to best practice protocols

Sports foods

Specialized products used to provide a convenient source of nutrients when it is impractical to consume everyday foods

Examples	Sports drink Sports gel Sports confectionery Sports bar Electrolyte supplements	Isolated protein supplements Mixed macronutrient supplement (bar, powder, liquid meal)

Medical supplements

Supplements used to prevent or treat clinical issues including diagnosed nutrient deficiencies

Should be used within a larger plan under the expert guidance of a medical practitioner or accredited sports dietitian

Examples	Iron Calcium Vitamin D	Multivitamin Probiotics Zinc

Performance supplements

Supplements or ingredients that can support or enhance sports performance

Best used with an individualized and event-specific protocol, with the expert guidance of an accredited sports dietitian

Examples	Caffeine β-Alanine Sodium bicarbonate	Nitrate/beetroot juice Creatine monohydrate Glycerol

Group B

Evidence level	Emerging scientific support, deserving of further research
Use within supplement programs	Considered for use by identified individual athletes within research or clinical monitoring situations
Note	Some of the products currently listed in Group B have been included because of their historic interest to key stakeholders

Continued on next page

BOX 7.2 The ABCD Categorization of Supplements and Sports Foods by the Australian Institute of Sport (AIS)[3] (CONTINUED)

Food polyphenols

Food compounds that may have bioactivity including antioxidant and anti-inflammatory properties

May be consumed in food forms (whole or concentrate) or as isolated extracts

Examples	Fruit-derived polyphenols (eg, tart cherry, New Zealand blackcurrant, pomegranate)	

Antioxidants

Compounds often found in foods that protect against oxidative damage from free-radical chemicals

Examples	Vitamins C and E, astaxanthin	

Tastants

Food-derived compounds that interact with receptors in the mouth or gut to activate the central nervous system

Examples	Menthol	Quinine
	Pickle juice	

Other

Examples	Collagen supplement	Omega-3 fatty acids
	Curcumin	Carnitine
	Ketone supplements	N-Acetylcysteine

Group C

Evidence level	Scientific evidence not supportive of benefit among athletes or no research undertaken to guide an informed opinion
Use within supplement programs	Not advocated for use by athletes within supplement programs May be permitted for use by identified athletes when there is specific approval from, or reporting to, a sports supplement panel

Category A and B products used outside approved protocols

Examples	See list for Category A and B products

Named products

Specific supplements that were previously classified as Group B but whose use is less supported by the most recent research

Examples	Magnesium	Phosphate
	α-Lipoic acid	Prebiotics
	β-Hydroxy-β-methylbutyrate (HMB)	Vitamin E
	Branched-chain amino acids, leucine	L-Tyrosine

The rest

Ingredients or products not found in Groups A, B, or D probably deserve to be here

Group D[a]

Evidence level	Banned or at high risk of contamination with substances that could lead to a positive doping test[b]	
Use within supplement programs	Should not be used by athletes	
Stimulants		
Examples	Ephedrine Strychnine Sibutramine	Dimethylamylamine (DMAA) 1,3-dimethylbutylamine (DMBA) Other herbal stimulants
Prohormones and hormone boosters		
Examples	Dehydroepiandrosterone (DHEA) Androstenedione 19-Norandrostenione/ol	Other prohormones Tribulus terrestris and other testosterone boosters[c] Maca root powder[c]
Growth hormone releasers and "peptides"		
Examples	Growth hormone-releasing peptides 1 and 2 (GHRP-1 and GHRP-2) CJC-1293 and CJC-1295	
β-2 agonists		
Examples	Higenamine	
Selective androgen receptor modulators (SARMs)		
Examples	Andarine, ostarine, ligandrol	
Metabolic modulators		
Examples	GW1516 (Cardarine)	
Other		
Examples	Colostrum: not recommended by the World Anti-Doping Agency because of the inclusion of growth factors within its composition	

[a] Not a complete list.
[b] The World Anti-Doping Agency (WADA) list is updated on an annual basis and should be used as the first point of call for confirmation of the current list of banned substances and practices. Consult the WADA list for all examples (www.wada-ama.org).
[c] These products do not appear on the WADA list and are thus not specifically banned. However, they are often found in multi-ingredient products that contain banned ingredients or are at high risk of being contaminated. Therefore, they are not recommended for use.

BOX 7.3 Substances That Are Considered to Have a Robust Evidence Base of Direct Benefit to Sports Performance[3,15-35]

β-Alanine[22,23,33]

Increased intracellular buffering may be achieved by increases in muscle carnosine content via chronic supplementation with β-alanine. Carnosine may play other roles in the muscle.

Optimal supplementation protocol involves ingestion of about 3.2 to 6.4 g (~65 mg per kilogram of body weight) per day, consumed for a minimum of 2 to 4 weeks and up to 12 weeks, to enhance high-intensity exercise performance ranging from 30 seconds to 10 minutes in duration.

Split doses over the day or sustained-release preparations may reduce the common side effect of paresthesia (tingling).

Bicarbonate[20,21]

Bicarbonate is the main extracellular buffer, and an acute reduction in blood pH may increase the capacity to buffer the excess hydrogen produced by exercise that generates high rates of anaerobic glycolysis (eg, events lasting 2-10 minutes and perhaps intermittent team/racket sports).

Optimal protocol is 300 mg per kilogram of body weight taken in split doses over the 1.5 to 2.5 hours leading up to the event.

Gastrointestinal discomfort may be reduced by consuming the dose with large volumes of fluid and a carbohydrate-rich snack.

Caffeine[16-19,32]

The world's most widely used drug, caffeine is found in everyday beverages and specially formulated sports foods and supplements. The multifunctions include adenosine receptor antagonism, which reduces perception of effort, fatigue, and pain. Cafffeine is effective in sporting scenarios involving endurance, team/intermittent high intensity, sustained high intensity/power, and skill protocols.

Individualized protocols of use should be developed according to practical issues and personal experience of responsiveness. Evidence of individual responsiveness due to genotype is being explored.

Optimal dose appears to be 3 to 6 mg per kilogram of body weight and can be taken prior to and during the event, including just at the onset of fatigue.

Side effects can include insomnia and overarousal (jitters, anxiety, etc), as well as interference with sleep quality after the event. This effect may be important to consider in multiday sports.

Creatine monohydrate[27,29,34,35]

Creatine monohydrate is the most common product used to supplement dietary intake from meats and muscle sources and increase intramuscular creatine stores by close to 30%. Benefits are achieved by increasing the recovery of phosphocreatine stores during repeated high-intensity bouts of exercise; it may be used to directly enhance sports performance of this nature or to support the athlete to train harder. Although it is typically used by athletes with a resistance- or sprint-training background and may benefit performance in intermittent sports (eg, team games), this may also extend to endurance sports in which there are sequences of higher-intensity effort.

Creatine monohydrate may have other roles in the muscle, including direct effects to upregulate protein synthesis through changes in cellular osmolarity, as well as the potential to support brain function in scenarios of traumatic injury (eg, concussion) or fatigue (eg, sleep deprivation). Effects on bone health and other issues in aging populations (eg, masters athletes) are also being investigated.

Optimal protocol targeting muscle involves rapid loading of 4 doses of 5 g for 5 days or slower loading of 3 to 5 g/d for 1 month. Maintenance dose is 3 to 5 g/d.

In the case of increases in brain creatine stores, doses of up to 10 g/d may be needed.

Glycerol[30,31]

Glycerol, sold commercially as glycerin, is a naturally occurring metabolite, namely, the backbone of triglyceride (fat) molecules. When consumed orally, it is rapidly absorbed and distributed throughout the body's fluid compartments, until it is gradually excreted over the next 24 to 48 hours. The presence of glycerol exerts an osmotic effect that allows the body to temporarily retain extra fluid. This can allow an athlete to improve their hydration levels and promote better performance in hot environments. Hyperhydration strategies may be further enhanced when combined with sodium to add a separate osmotic effect.

Glycerol intake of 1 to 1.2 g per kilogram of body weight in conjunction with a moderate to large volume of fluid (25–30 mL per kilogram of body weight) results in a net retention of close to 600 mL of fluid above what can be achieved by water loading alone, increasing plasma volume by 5% to 15%.

Nitrate/beetroot juice[24-26]

Inorganic nitrate in beetroot, green leafy vegetables, and other ground vegetables works with the enterosalivary system to produce nitric oxide (NO) through an alternative and oxygen-independent pathway to arginine-based NO production. Nitrate is associated with improved exercise economy (reduction in oxygen cost of submaximal exercise) to improve endurance exercise performance and enhanced skeletal muscle contractile function to improve muscle power and sprint exercise performance. The effect of nitrate supplementation on longer events is inconsistent and may involve individual responsiveness, including observations that it seems less effective in elite and highly trained athletes.

Typical dose is about 8 mmol of nitrate taken 2 to 3 hours pre-event, especially with chronic intake for at least 3 days preevent.

and more suitable dose of the nutrient or compound compared to foods. For example, although β-alanine and creatine are both found in the food supply, it is difficult to consume adequate doses of these compounds from food sources such as meats.[1] Indeed, data derived from the 2017–2018 National Health and Nutrition Examination Survey (NHANES) reported that creatine-containing foods in the American diet (meat, fish, and poultry flesh, as well as foods derived from these) have a mean creatine content of 0.11 g/oz, with the mean daily intake across nearly 10,000 respondents being 1.38 g/d.[39] Furthermore, individuals following a vegetarian or vegan diet do not consume a dietary source of creatine, and such eating practices are associated with lower muscle creatine stores.[40] Similarly, beetroot juice concentrates and extracts have been manufactured to provide a known and less variable source of nitrate than what can be consumed from the intake of fruits and vegetables.[41] Although caffeine is consumed by most adults in everyday life, the caffeine content of common beverages is neither standardized nor identifiable by the consumer. For example, a study that purchased the same coffee beverage (an espresso) from 97 different retail outlets in the same city found a range in caffeine content from 25 to 214 mg per serving.[42] Such variation makes coffee unreliable as a performance aid because it could lead to either an ineffective dose or an excessive dose likely to cause side effects. Finally, some products may be manufactured with special features to enhance the bioavailability of their key ingredients. For example, carbohydrate supplements to be ingested during prolonged exercise activities may include specific formulas of glucose and fructose (ie, multiple transportable carbohydrates) to increase intestinal absorption,[43] as well as a hydrogel format that is claimed to increase gastric emptying.[44]

PLACEBO EFFECT

The placebo effect (a favorable outcome arising simply from an individual's belief that they have received a beneficial treatment or experience) may also contribute to the benefits associated with supplement use. Indeed, the mystique and glowing testimonials about a new product may confer positive expectations about the outcomes of its use. Although the placebo effect is often dismissed as not being a "real" consideration, there is evidence that it is a robust neurobiological phenomenon capable of delivering a worthwhile benefit to sports performance.[45,46] For example, in 1 study, performance in a 10-km cycling time trial was altered in a dose-response relationship according to participant beliefs about the amount of caffeine that they had consumed pretrial. Although no caffeine was consumed in any of the 3 experimental trials, when study subjects believed they had received a placebo treatment, their mean power output was *reduced* by 1.3% compared to baseline testing. Meanwhile, when they believed they had consumed caffeine doses of 4.5 and 9.0 mg/kg, mean power *increased* by 1.3% and 3.1% respectively.[47] Another study involving carbohydrate intake during a 40-km cycling time trial reported that participants performed best when they knew they were receiving the active treatment and worst when they were in doubt about what was consumed.[48]

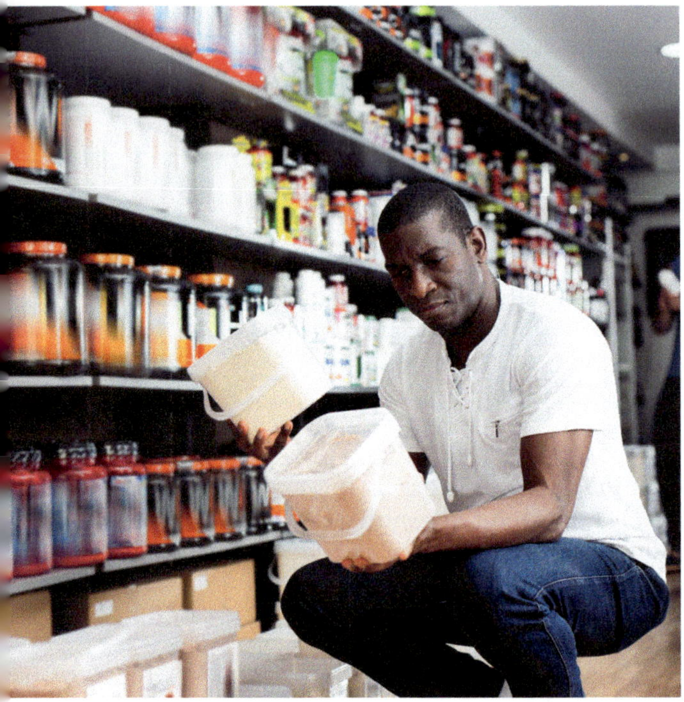

Additional well-controlled studies are needed to better describe the potential size and duration of the placebo effect and whether it applies equally to all athletes and across all types of performance. Although belief effects are sometimes employed as a justification for the use of any supplement (suggesting that, even if the product has no physiological benefit, the athlete may still benefit from a psychological boost), there is no guarantee that this will occur. It would be more valuable to apply the placebo effect to the use of evidence-based products, allowing athletes to be properly informed and confident about their use of such products to maximize both the physiologically and psychologically underpinned benefits.[45]

Cons of Supplement Use

EXPENSE

Sports foods and supplements are usually more expensive than the conventional food choices they replace. This may reflect the niche market, the price of the additional processing or packaging, the inclusion of novel or specialized ingredients, additional requirements such as third-party auditing, or simply what the market will pay for something that is perceived as valuable. Therefore, the use of supplements or sports foods may create an additional burden on an athlete's financial situation or displace expenditures on other items that might be of greater value. The cost of a product should be a deterrent when there is little scientific evidence to support a product's claims of benefits to athletic performance. However, even when benefits do exist, the athlete (or team) must acknowledge the expense and prioritize it appropriately within their resources. At times, a supplement or sports food may be deemed money well spent, particularly when the product provides the most practical and palatable way to achieve a nutrition goal or when the performance benefits have been well documented. On other occasions, the athlete may choose to limit the use of expensive products to the most important events or training periods. Lower-cost alternatives to some supplements and sports foods can be found for a budget-conscious athlete to use, particularly on less critical occasions. Education resources associated with the AIS Sports Supplement Framework provide suggestions for whole foods or conventional processed foods that can substitute for many of the evidence-based sports foods and supplements; for example, a fruit smoothie fortified with milk powder can replace a liquid meal product or bottled protein shake, and jelly candy can replace sports chews and gel products.[3]

HEALTH AND SAFETY RISKS

The use of supplements and sports foods carries a small but real risk of adverse effects related to the safety and composition of the product per se, as well as inappropriate practices around their use (eg, taking more than the recommended dose or taking several products at the same time). US Food and Drug Administration (FDA) regulations require supplements and sports foods to be manufactured in accordance with Good Manufacturing Practice standards. However, these products are considered low risk and allow only voluntary compliance to the appropriate code, with monitoring generally being targeted to scenarios in which noncompliance or safety issues have been identified postmarketing. The FDA's website-based database[49] reporting supplement recalls identifies cases of failure to gain a listing or registration, inclusion of undeclared ingredients on poison lists or prescription lists, presence of impurities (eg, lead, glass) or bacterial contamination, and failure to contain listed dosages of ingredients. Products or ingredients that have been removed from the market or reformulated with different ingredients because of serious health problems, include tryptophan supplements,[50] ephedra,[51] dimethylamylamine (DMAA),[52] hydroxycitric acid (*Garcinia cambogia*),[53] and the popular weight-loss supplements Hydroxycut and OxyElite Pro.[54] There are numerous reports of supplements containing irregular compositions. For example, in a pair of studies, DNA analysis of herbal supplements (eg, ginseng) identified that approximately 25% of products were adulterated or nonauthentic.[55,56] Even among products considered to be evidence based, there can be considerable variability in the dose of active ingredients. An analysis of 21 different beetroot juice products promoted for sports nutrition uses found a coefficient of variation of 30% in the nitrate content of different lots of the same product, an approximate 50-fold range in the nitrate content of different products, and clinically relevant doses provided in a single serving of only 2 products.[57] Another study of 134 protein powders found detectable levels of lead and other heavy metals in 70% of products, with vegetarian powders having higher levels than those derived from animals (eg, whey and egg) and organic products being more likely to be contaminated than nonorganic brands.[58]

Identifying the prevalence of adverse effects from supplement use is difficult, because most information comes from highlighted case reports, postmarketing surveillance by regulators, consumer complaints made to manufacturers, and hospital reports; these factors are likely to result in an underestimate of the true problems. In a study by the FDA Center for Food Safety and Applied Nutrition, data were captured from the FDA Adverse Event Reporting System[59] for the years 2004 to 2013, representing periods when notification by manufacturers of consumer complaints of adverse events was voluntary and then mandatory. The results showed a total of approximately 15,400 incidents of supplement-related adverse events over the decade, with greater numbers being reported during mandatory reporting periods and by female consumers. Among products used by individuals aged 20 to 35 years, most problems were associated with bodybuilding, weight-loss, and energy supplements such as energy drinks, "preworkout" products, and "fat-burner" products. Hospitalization was required in 25% of the reported events, and 2% of reports involved a death. In addition, such reports may fail to consider minor issues that may nevertheless interfere with an athlete's performance or training consistency.

ANTI-DOPING RULE VIOLATIONS

A number of ingredients found in supplements are included on anti-doping lists, the most well-known of which is the International Standard Prohibited List,[60] which forms part of the World Anti-Doping Code.[61] These substances belong to various categories of the Code, including anabolic agents, peptide hormones, β-agonists, hormone and metabolic modulators, and stimulants. Drug education programs highlight the need for athletes to read the labels of supplements and sports foods carefully to ensure that they do not contain such banned substances.[62] Although this is an athlete responsibility, in many cases, athletes do not consider it to be important because of the perception that supplements are "natural", or athletes are unable to recognize the different chemical and street names that can be used to describe various prohibited substances.

Most importantly, the inadvertent intake of banned substances from supplements can occur because of the presence of these substances as undeclared ingredients. This is typically a result of contamination or poor labeling within lax manufacturing processes, although there have been cases in which the deliberate inclusion of therapeutic doses of steroid compounds has been suspected in an effort by companies to gain "street popularity."[63,64] The first credible evidence of supplement contamination was reported in a 2004 study from a laboratory accredited by the International Olympic Committee (IOC).[65] Analysis of 634 supplements from 215 suppliers in 13 countries found that 94 (15% of the sample) contained banned hormones or prohormones (eg, testosterone, nandrolone) that were not stated on the product label. An additional 10% of samples provided technical difficulties in analysis such that the absence of hormones could not be guaranteed. Forty-nine of the supplements contained only 1 steroid, but 45 contained more than 1, with 8 products containing 5 or more different steroid products. Just over 20% of the products made by companies selling prohormones were positive for undeclared prohormones, but 10% of the products from companies that did not sell steroid-containing supplements were also positive. This suggests that contamination may occur from adulterated raw ingredients as well as from cross-contamination between different products in the same factory. Since this original report, evidence of poor product labeling, deliberate adulteration, and contamination have continued to emerge from independent studies[63,66] and from reports by commercial companies that undertake specific audits of supplement products.[67] In some cases, the data suggest that the risks of product contamination have reduced, whereas in others, there is evidence that there has merely been a change in the prohibited ingredients involved. Bodybuilding supplements promoting mass gain are the most likely to contain anabolic-androgenic substances, whereas products promoting weight loss or a boost in energy (such as preworkout supplements) are likely to contain banned stimulants. In any case, there is evidence that products from almost all categories of the World Anti-Doping Agency (WADA) Prohibited List have been found as undeclared ingredients in supplements.[68-73] Furthermore, a positive urinary test for many products or their metabolites can occur in the hours following intake of as little of 1 mcg of the substance, with risks being associated with the amount of the supplement consumed (eg, a 1-g tablet vs 30 g of powder) and the timing of intake in relation to the collection of the urine sample.[73]

Of course, there is no way to prove an athlete's claim that the presence of banned substances in their urine sample can be attributed to their unknowing ingestion of the product via a supplement.[73] Therefore, according to WADA's principle of strict liability, every athlete is responsible for the presence of a prohibited substance or its markers or metabolites in their biological samples, irrespective of whether the anti-doping rule violation (ADRV) was committed unintentionally or deliberately.[61] In various real-life cases, sanctions have varied from a suspended sentence to full imposition of a ban from participation in sport, with different outcomes occurring depending on the sporting authority or organizations involved, further referrals to courts of arbitration, and the detection of other mitigating circumstances. Regardless of the sanction, the athlete will carry an indelible reputation of having incurred an ADRV, with outcomes ranging from personal distress to loss of income. Therefore, the risk of an ADRV from supplement use is of major concern to sport.[73-75]

One way to reduce the risk of ingesting supplements containing banned substances is to make use of products that have been batch-tested by a third-party commercial certification protocol.[1] In the United States, LGC (Informed Sport, Informed Choice) and National Sanitation Foundation (NSF Certified for Sport) are well-recognized programs, and in other countries, similar services are provided by companies such as Human and Supplement Testing Australia (HASTA), Cologne List, and Banned Substances Control Group (BSCG). Third-party testing protocols currently offer services such as batch testing products for the presence of banned substances; undertaking audits of company adherence to Good Manufacturing Practice standards and origin of raw ingredients; and in some cases, testing for compliance to ingredient lists and absence of toxic elements. Such services are described within a consensus statement developed to identify essential features of such third-party testing schemes. Athletes should be encouraged to use only those products that have been certified by such programs, noting the batch and lot numbers of products that have been consumed in case problems later arise. Indeed, many sporting organizations such as the National Collegiate Athletic Association, National Basketball Association, Major League Baseball, and National Hockey League include this condition as a requirement. These schemes are not fool proof; testing occurs on random samples within batches rather than each individual bottle or item, and the product may not be tested for all substances that are banned. Importantly, athletes should be aware that such schemes do not provide endorsement from sporting agencies or WADA, nor are products included in such schemes guaranteed to be evidence based or able to meet their advertised claims.[76]

THE AUSTRALIAN INSTITUTE OF SPORT SPORTS SUPPLEMENT PROGRAM/FRAMEWORK

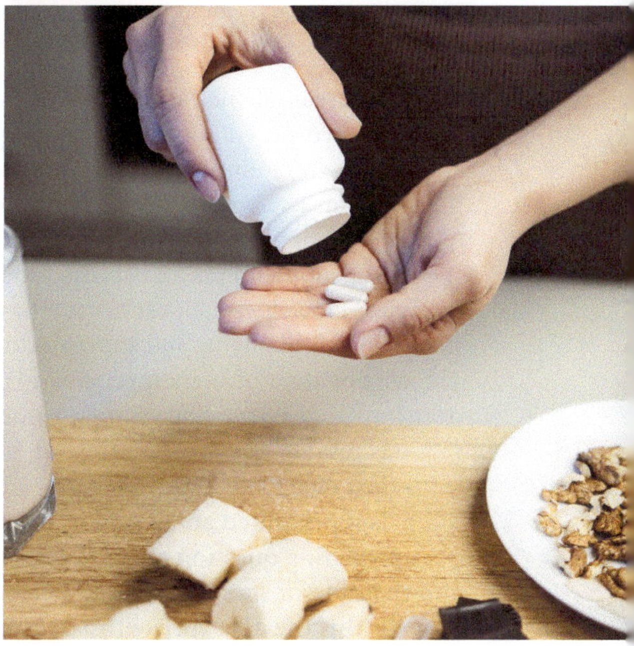

Many sporting organizations are interested in implementing policies or programs related to supplement use by the athletes within their care. The evolution of the AIS Sports Supplement Program/Framework provides a model for delivering best practices around supplements and sports foods to support their safe, effective, and permissible uses by athletes. The AIS Sports Supplement Program was developed in 2000 as a multidisciplinary approach to the use of supplements and sports foods within the AIS sports scholarship community. The activity was led by the AIS Department/Discipline of Sports Nutrition following an internal review of the culture, knowledge, and practices regarding supplements and sports foods within its populations of athletes and coaches. It identified that a number of factors had changed the landscape around supplement use by athletes, including increases in the number and marketing opportunities for products, research that confirmed the benefits of the use of some products according to clear protocols of use, and disengagement between athletes and coaches on one hand and sports science and medicine teams on the other because of the conservative attitude of the latter regarding supplement use. As a result, a multidisciplinary program involving supplement provision, education, research, and governance was implemented to meet the following key principles[1]:

- Athletes and coaches will collaborate effectively with sports scientist and medicine professionals and sports administrators when there is willingness to support a small but valuable role for the informed use of supplements and sports foods within a sports nutrition plan.
- Supplements and sports foods can be practically managed through the use of a classification hierarchy that divides products into groups based on the strength of the evidence base for their use, with an appreciation of the risk of an ADRV. In the case of the AIS Supplement Program, 4 groups were identified (A, B, C, D), with further stratification to identify strategies by which certain products could contribute to a sports nutrition plan. The placement of supplements and sports foods within these categories is a dynamic process that evolves with new knowledge and practice.

Note that these principles were considered novel and contradictory to the conventional advice of sporting authorities (eg, IOC) at the time of the program's inception, but they contributed to a later change in philosophy by major organizations to recognize the need to embrace judicious use of supplements by high-performance athletes.[15] The implementation of the Program from 2000 to 2012 led to a range of research outcomes,[77-83] as well as documentation of a reduced use of non-evidence-based supplements by stakeholder athletes.[84]

A reorganization of the Australian High Performance Sports System following the 2012 Olympic Games changed the role, responsibilities, and resources of its various sectors and organizations. In brief, gradual devolution of the AIS removed its direct responsibility for and involvement in the daily preparation of athletes. Meanwhile, it assumed a new leadership role, in conjunction with the state academies and institutes of sport (forming the National Institutes of Sport), to develop technical expertise and resources in the Australian High Performance Sports System. Such changes facilitated the evolution of the AIS Sports Supplement Program from an operational activity to a framework available to national sporting organizations and other agencies to support the development of bespoke sports supplement policies or programs according to specific needs. A Framework committee including various stakeholders, regular updates and reporting schedules, and the capacity to address new projects aims to further enhance best practices around supplement use within the Australian sports system. However, resources are made freely available to all athletes and international sporting agencies in the belief that a worldwide increase in supplement literacy is beneficial for all.[3] The current ABCD categorization of sports foods and supplements is provided in Box 7.2.

A PRAGMATIC APPROACH TO SUPPLEMENT USE

In many areas of life, a cautious or conservative approach to issues in which safety factors or health concerns are potentially involved is generally assumed. Therefore, it is understandable that sporting authorities, including national and international governing bodies, anti-doping agencies, and sports medicine and science authorities have traditionally taken the stance of advising athletes against the use of supplements. Because there is no practical way to completely remove the doping risk associated with the use of supplements and sports foods, it is likely that this will remain the official policy of anti-doping agencies. However, the past decade has seen a shift in the attitudes of other authorities to recognize that the use of supplements and sports foods is complex and warrants a more flexible and pragmatic approach. The cornerstone of such approaches is the use of decision trees that enable athletes to make considered decisions about a specific product before committing it to a specific use, including the following questions:

» Is it safe?

» Is it effective?

» Is it permitted and legal for use in its intended environment (eg, sporting code, military use)?

A preceding question related to the athlete is also suggested, particularly to account for junior athletes and their use of sports foods and performance supplements, namely

» Is this the appropriate time for me to consider using this product?

A decision tree related to the use of performance supplements (refer to Figure 7.1) was produced by the IOC Consensus on Supplements in High Performance Sport.[15] This diagram identifies scenarios in which the athlete is guided or required to seek professional assessment and advice, including a plan that is personalized for their intended use and a consideration of the evidence base for the product use. Of course, athletes must always abide by the supplement-related rules and programs of their specific sporting association or team and take notice of education resources produced for their specific environment, such as the Supplement Connect program of US Anti-Doping Agency.[62]

SUMMARY

Athletes and coaches are eager for sports foods and dietary supplements to be included within sports nutrition programs. This eagerness is partially vindicated by the potential valuable uses of some products to meet energy, macronutrient, and micronutrient needs that may go beyond the capacity of everyday food intake, as well as special compounds that may directly or indirectly enhance performance or its key determinants of recovery, adaptation, health, and injury risk. Although a range of potential concerns are associated with the use of supplements and sports foods, including expense, distraction, and health and safety concerns, there is opportunity for the sports nutrition practitioner to guide the athlete to make evidence-based, sports-specific, and personalized use of a small range of products. Resources from groups that are experts in sporting issues, such as the IOC and the AIS, as well as other well-credentialed groups and education hubs (refer to Box 7.4 on page 176), can aid the practitioner in working with athletes to develop such a plan. A decision tree approach can help the athlete work through key steps in deciding whether supplement use is appropriate and able to meet an acceptable risk–benefit outcome. The sourcing of products, particularly performance supplements, should make use of third-party auditing programs. Although such schemes cannot guarantee the identification of risk-free products, they raise awareness of the general issue and also support the availability of low-risk products. The various members of an athlete's support team and high-performance environment have clear roles to play in helping the athlete to make an informed decision about the use of supplements and sports foods and then act on it appropriately.

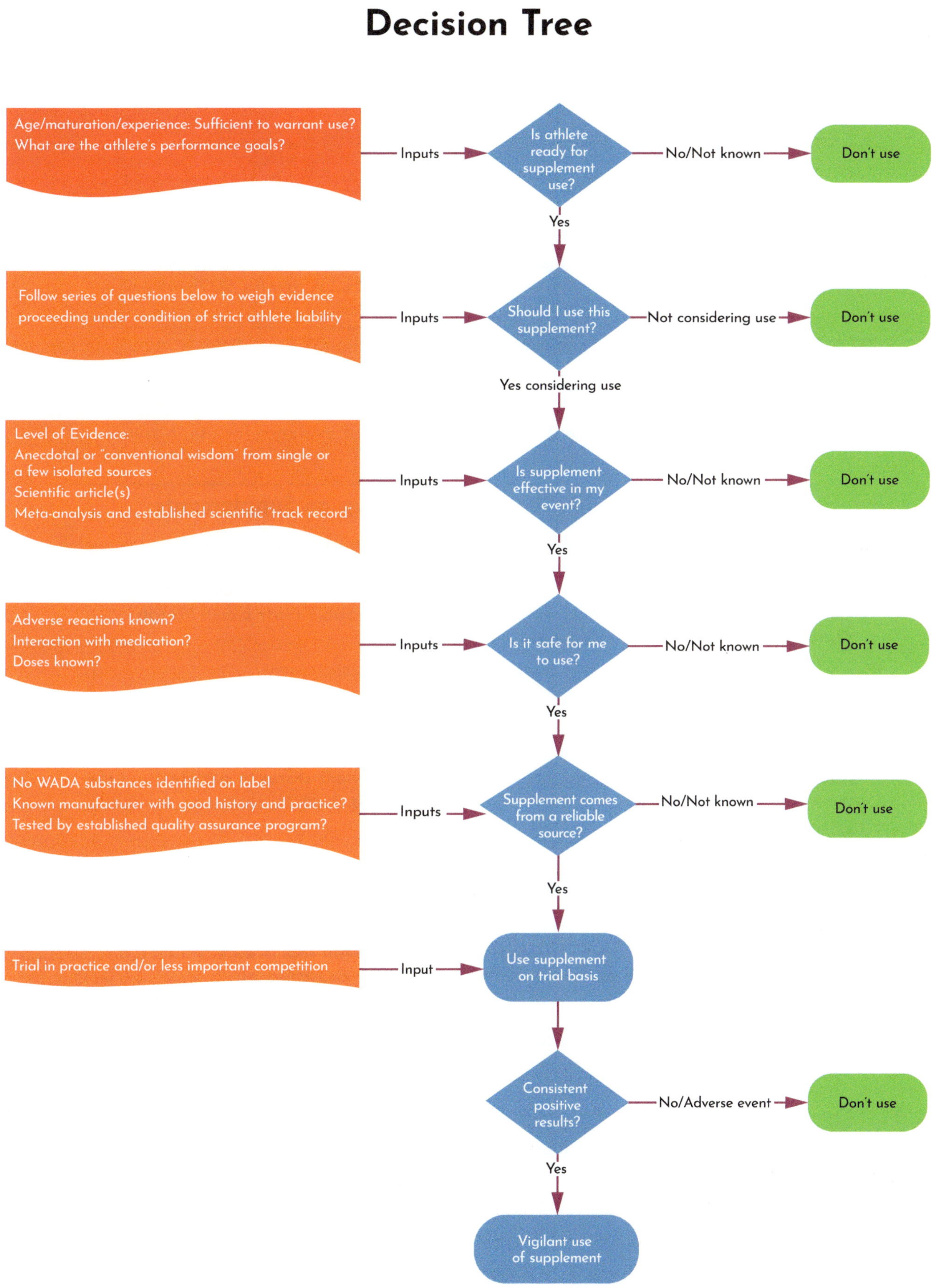

FIGURE 7.1 Decision tree for the use of performance supplements Reproduced with permission from reference 15: Maughan RJ, Burke LM, Dvorak J, et al. IOC Consensus Statement: Dietary Supplements and the High-Performance Athlete. *Int J Sport Nutr Exerc Metab.* 2018;28(2):104-1255. doi:10.1123/ijsnem.2018-0020
Abbreviation: WADA, World Anti Doping Agency

BOX 7.4 Additional Resources on Supplements

Australian Institute of Sport

www.ais.gov.au/nutrition/supplements

- Overview of program
- Fact sheets on Group A and B supplements

Burke LM, Slater GR. Supplements and sports foods in sport. In: Burke LM, Deakin V, Minehan M, eds. *Clinical Sports Nutrition*. 6th ed. McGraw-Hill Australia; 2021:445-477

US Office of Dietary Supplements

https://ods.od.nih.gov/factsheets/ExerciseAndAthleticPerformance-HealthProfessional

- Fact sheet on dietary supplements with various levels of evidence for use in sport

International Olympic Committee Working Group on Supplements

Consensus on use of supplements and sports foods in high-performance sport

- Maughan RJ, Burke LM, Dvorak J, et al. IOC Consensus Statement: Dietary Supplements and the High-Performance Athlete. *Int J Sport Nutr Exerc Metab*. 2018;28(2):104-125. doi:10.1123/ijsnem.2018-0020

Review papers providing evidence to support the consensus statement

- Garthe I, Maughan RJ. Athletes and supplements: prevalence and perspectives. *Int J Sport Nutr Exerc Metab*. 2018;28(2):126-138. doi:10.1123/ijsnem.2017-0429
- Larson-Meyer DE, Woolf K, Burke L. Assessment of nutrient status in athletes and the need for supplementation. *Int J Sport Nutr Exerc Metab*. 2018;28(2):139-158. doi:10.1123/ijsnem.2017-0338
- Burke LM, Peeling P. Methodologies for investigating performance changes with supplement use. *Int J Sport Nutr Exerc Metab*. 2018;28(2):159-169. doi:10.1123/ijsnem.2017-0325
- Hector AJ, Phillips SM. Protein recommendations for weight loss in elite athletes: a focus on body composition and performance. *Int J Sport Nutr Exerc Metab*. 2018;28(2):170-177. doi:10.1123/ijsnem.2017-0273
- Peeling P, Binnie MJ, Goods PSR, Sim M, Burke LM. Evidence-based supplements for the enhancement of athletic performance. *Int J Sport Nutr Exerc Metab*. 2018;28(2):178-187. doi:10.1123/ijsnem.2017-0343
- Rawson ES, Miles MP, Larson-Meyer DE. Dietary supplements for health, adaptation, and recovery in athletes. *Int J Sport Nutr Exerc Metab*. 2018;28(2):188-199. doi:10.1123/ijsnem.2017-0340
- Meeusen R, Decroix L. Nutritional supplements and the brain. *Int J Sport Nutr Exerc Metab*. 2018;28(2):200-211. doi:10.1123/ijsnem.2017-0314
- Maughan RJ, Shirreffs SM, Vernec A. Making decisions about supplement use. *Int J Sport Nutr Exerc Metab*. 2018;28(2):212-219. doi:10.1123/ijsnem.2018-0009

International Society of Sports Nutrition

Series of position stands on supplements and sports foods

- Wilson JM, Fitschen PJ, Campbell B, et al. International Society of Sports Nutrition position stand: beta-hydroxy-beta-methylbutyrate (HMB). *J Int Soc Sports Nutr.* 2013;10(1):6. doi:10.1186/1550-2783-10-6
- Trexler ET, Smith-Ryan AE, Stout JR, et al. International Society of Sports Nutrition position stand: beta-alanine. *J Int Soc Sports Nutr.* 2015;12:30. doi:10.1186/s12970-015-0090-y
- Kreider RB, Kalman DS, Antonio J, et al. International Society of Sports Nutrition position stand: safety and efficacy of creatine supplementation in exercise, sport, and medicine. *J Int Soc Sports* Nutr. 2017;14:18. doi:10.1186/s12970-017-0173-z
- Kerksick CM, Wilborn CD, Roberts MD, et al. ISSN exercise & sports nutrition review update: research & recommendations. *J Int Soc Sports Nutr.* 2018;15(1):38. doi:10.1186/s12970-018-0242-y
- Jäger R, Mohr AE, Carpenter KC, et al. International Society of Sports Nutrition position stand: probiotics. J *Int Soc Sports Nutr.* 2019;16(1):62. Published December 21, 2019. doi:10.1186/s12970-019-0329-0
- Guest NS, VanDusseldorp TA, Nelson MT, et al. International Society of Sports Nutrition position stand: caffeine and exercise performance. *J Int Soc Sports Nutr.* 2021;18(1):1. doi:10.1186/s12970-020-00383-4
- Grgic J, Pedisic Z, Saunders B, et al. International Society of Sports Nutrition position stand: sodium bicarbonate and exercise performance. *J Int Soc Sports Nutr.* 2021;18(1):61. doi:10.1186/s12970-021-00458-w
- Lowery LM, Anderson DE, Scanlon KF, et al. International Society of Sports Nutrition position stand: coffee and sports performance. *J Int Soc Sports Nutr.* 2023;20(1):2237952. doi:10.1080/15502783.2023.2237952
- Jagim AR, Harty PS, Tinsley GM, et al. International Society of Sports Nutrition position stand: energy drinks and energy shots. *J Int Soc Sports Nutr.* 2023;20(1):2171314. doi:10.1080/15502783.2023.2171314
- Ferrando AA, Wolfe RR, Hirsch KR, et al. International Society of Sports Nutrition position stand: Effects of essential amino acid supplementation on exercise and performance. *J Int Soc Sports Nutr.* 2023;20(1):2263409. doi:10.1080/15502783.2023.2263409

KEY TAKEAWAYS

The prior conservative approach of sporting organizations and sports nutrition experts regarding the use of sports foods and supplements contributed to a loss of their involvement in the expanding market and interests of athletes and coaches.

A more modern and pragmatic approach to sports foods and supplements involves recognition of both the risks and benefits of their use, providing for the development of an individualized plan for each athlete based on the needs of their event.

Evidence-based practices include the use of sports foods to meet energy and macronutrient targets, particularly around exercise or events; the use of micronutrient supplements to prevent or treat nutrient deficiencies; and the targeted use of dietary supplements containing compounds that enjoy robust support for their capacity to directly or indirectly enhance performance.

There is a valid role for the sports nutrition practitioner to help athletes to make sound decisions about the use of sports foods and dietary supplements and to source products with a low risk of negative effects including an anti-doping rule violation.

REFERENCES

1. Burke LM, Slater GR. Supplements and sports foods in sport. In: Burke LM, Deakin V, Minehan M, eds. *Clinical Sports Nutrition*. 6th ed. McGraw-Hill Australia; 2021:445-477.
2. Dietary Supplement Health and Education Act of 1994. 21 USC §321 (1994). Accessed July 15, 2024. www.congress.gov/bill/103rd-congress/senate-bill/784/text
3. AIS Sports Supplement Framework. Australian Institute of Sport. Accessed December 24, 2023. www.ais.gov.au/nutrition/supplements
4. Dietary supplement use reaches all time high. Council for Responsible Nutrition. September 30, 2019. Accessed December 24, 2023. www.crnusa.org/newsroom/dietary-supplement-use-reaches-all-time-high
5. Garthe I, Maughan RJ. Athletes and supplements: prevalence and perspectives. *Int J Sport Nutr Exerc Metab*. 2018;28(2):126-138. doi:10.1123/ijsnem.2017-0429
6. Knapik JJ, Steelman RA, Hoedebecke SS, Austin KG, Farina EK, Lieberman HR. Prevalence of dietary supplement use by athletes: systematic review and meta-analysis. *Sports Med.* 2016;46(1):103-123. doi:10.1007/s40279-015-0387-7
7. Sobal J, Marquart LF. Vitamin/mineral supplement use among athletes: a review of the literature. *Int J Sports Nutr.* 1994;4(4):320-334. doi:10.1123/ijsn.4.4.320
8. Aguilar-Navarro M, Baltazar-Martins G, Brito de Souza D, Muñoz-Guerra J, Del Mar Plata M, Del Coso J. Gender differences in prevalence and patterns of dietary supplement use in elite athletes. *Res Q Exerc Sport*. 2021;92(4):659-668. doi:10.1080/02701367.2020.1764469
9. Monteiro CA, Cannon G, Levy RB, et al. Ultra-processed foods: what they are and how to identify them. *Public Health Nutr*. 2019;22(5):936-941. doi:10.1017/S1368980018003762
10. Stellingwerff T, Cox GR. Systematic review: carbohydrate supplementation on exercise performance or capacity of varying durations. *Appl Physiol Nutr Metab*. 2014;39(9):998-1011. doi:10.1139/apnm-2014-0027
11. Cermak N, Res PT, de Groot LCPGM, Saris WHM, van Loon LJC. Protein supplementation augments the adaptive response of skeletal muscle to resistance-type exercise training: a meta-analysis. *Am J Clin Nutr.* 2012;96(6):1454-64. doi:10.3945/ajcn.112.037556
12. Sim M, Garvican-Lewis LA, Cox GR, et al. Iron considerations for the athlete: a narrative review. *Eur J Appl Physiol.* 2019;119(7):1463-1478. doi:10.1007/s00421-019-04157-y
13. Owens DJ, Allison R, Close GL. Vitamin D and the athlete: current perspectives and new challenges. *Sports Med.* 2018;48(suppl 1):3-16. doi:10.1007/s40279-017-0841-9
14. Larson-Meyer DE, Woolf K, Burke L. Assessment of nutrient status in athletes and the need for supplementation. *Int J Sport Nutr Exerc Metab*. 2018;28(2):139-158. doi:10.1123/ijsnem.2017-0338
15. Maughan RJ, Burke LM, Dvorak J, et al. IOC Consensus Statement: dietary supplements and the high-performance athlete. *Int J Sport Nutr Exerc Metab.* 2018;28(2):104-125. doi:10.1123/ijsnem.2018-0020
16. Burke LM. Caffeine and sports performance. *Appl Physiol Nutr Metab*. 2008;33(6):1319-1334. doi:10.1139/H08-130
17. Grgic J, Pickering C, Del Coso J, Schoenfeld BJ, Mikulic P. CYP1A2 genotype and acute ergogenic effects of caffeine intake on exercise performance: a systematic review. *Eur J Nutr* 2021;60(3):1181-1195. doi:10.1007/s00394-020-02427-6
18. Pickering C, Grgic J. A time and a place: a framework for caffeine periodization throughout the sporting year. *Nutrition*. 2020;82:111046. doi:10.1016/j.nut.2020.111046
19. Pickering C, Kiely J. What should we do about habitual caffeine use in athletes? *Sports Med.* 2019;49(6):833-842. doi:10.1007/s40279-018-0980-7
20. Grgic J, Pedisic Z, Saunders B, et al. International Society of Sports Nutrition position stand: sodium bicarbonate and exercise performance. *J Int Soc Sports Nutr.* 2021;18(1):61. doi:10.1186/s12970-021-00458-w
21. Burke LM, Pyne DB. Bicarbonate loading to enhance training and competitive performance. *Int J Sports Physiol Perform*. 2007;2(1):93-97. doi:10.1123/ijspp.2.1.93
22. Saunders B, Elliott-Sale K, Artioli GG, et al. β-Alanine supplementation to improve exercise capacity and performance: a systematic review and meta-analysis. *Br J Sports Med.* 2017;51(8):658-669. doi:10.1136/bjsports-2016-096396
23. Perim P, Marticorena FM, Ribeiro F, et al. Can the skeletal muscle carnosine response to beta-alanine supplementation be optimized? *Front Nutr*. 2019;6:135. doi:10.3389/fnut.2019.00135
24. Jones AM. Dietary nitrate supplementation and exercise performance. *Sports Med.* 2014;44(suppl 1):S35-S45. doi:10.1007/s40279-014-0149-y
25. Jones AM, Thompson C, Wylie LJ, Vanhatalo A. Dietary nitrate and physical performance. *Annu Rev Nutr* 2018;38:303-328. doi:10.1146/annurev-nutr-082117-051622
26. Shannon OM, Allen JD, Bescos R, et al. Dietary inorganic nitrate as an ergogenic aid: an expert consensus derived via the modified Delphi technique. *Sports Med.* 2022;52(10):2537-2558. doi:10.1007/s40279-022-01701-3
27. Kreider RB, Kalman DS, Antonio J, et al. International Society of Sports Nutrition position stand: safety and efficacy of creatine supplementation in exercise, sport, and medicine. *J Int Soc Sports Nutr.* 2017;14(1):18. doi:10.1186/s12970-017-0173-z
28. Roschel H, Gualano B, Ostojic SM, Rawson ES. Creatine supplementation and brain health. *Nutrients.* 2021;13(2):586. doi:10.3390/nu13020586
29. Forbes SC, Candow DG, Neto JHF, et al. Creatine supplementation and endurance performance: surges and sprints to win the race. *J Int Soc Sports Nutr.* 2023;20(1):2204071. doi:10.1080/15502783.2023.2204071

30. van Rosendal SP, Coombes JS. Glycerol use in hyperhydration and rehydration: scientific update. *Med Sport Sci.* 2012;59:104-112. doi:10.1159/000341959
31. Savoie FA, Asselin A, Goulet EDB. Comparison of sodium chloride tablets-induced, sodium chloride solution-induced, and glycerol-induced hyperhydration on fluid balance responses in healthy men. *J Strength Cond Res.* 2016;30(10):2880-2891. doi:10.1519/JSC.0000000000001371
32. Guest NS, VanDusseldorp TA, Nelson MT, et al. International Society of Sports Nutrition position stand: caffeine and exercise performance. *J Int Soc Sports Nutr.* 2021;18(1):1. doi:10.1186/s12970-020-00383-4
33. Trexler ET, Smith-Ryan AE, Stout JR, et al. International Society of Sports Nutrition position stand: beta-alanine. *J Int Soc Sports Nutr.* 2015;12:30. doi:10.1186/s12970-015-0090-y
34. Forbes SC, Cordingley DM, Cornish SM, et al. Effects of creatine supplementation on brain function and health. *Nutrients.* 2022;14(5):921. doi:10.3390/nu14050921
35. Forbes SC, Chilibeck PD, Candow DG. Creatine supplementation during resistance training does not lead to greater bone mineral density in older humans: a brief meta-analysis. *Front Nutr.* 2018;5:27. doi:10.3389/fnut.2018.00027
36. Rawson ES, Miles MP, Larson-Meyer DE. Dietary supplements for health, adaptation, and recovery in athletes. *Int J Sport Nutr Exerc Metab.* 2018;28(2):188-199. doi:10.1123/ijsnem.2017-0340
37. Burke LM. Practical issues in evidence-based use of performance supplements: supplement interactions, repeated use and individual responses. *Sports Med.* 2017;47(suppl 1):79-100. doi:10.1007/s40279-017-0687-1
38. Hopkins WG, Hawley JA, Burke LM. Design and analysis of research on sport performance enhancement. *Med Sci Sports Exerc.* 1999;31(3):472-485. doi:10.1097/00005768-199903000-00018
39. Ostojic SM. Dietary creatine intake in U.S. population: NHANES 2017-2018. *Nutrition.* 2021;87-88:111207. doi:10.1016/j.nut.2021.111207
40. Blancquaert L, Baguet A, Bex T, et al. Changing to a vegetarian diet reduces the body creatine pool in omnivorous women, but appears not to affect carnitine and carnosine homeostasis: a randomised trial. *Br J Nutr.* 2018;119(7):759-770. doi:10.1017/S000711451800017X
41. Jonvik KL, Nyakayiru J, van Dijk JW, Wardenaar FC, van Loon LJ, Verdijk LB. Habitual dietary nitrate intake in highly trained athletes. *Int J Sport Nutr Exerc Metab.* 2017;27(2):148-157. doi:10.1123/ijsnem.2016-0239
42. Desbrow B, Hughes R, Leveritt M, Scheelings P. An examination of consumer exposure to caffeine from retail coffee outlets. *Food Chem Toxicol.* 2007;45(9):1588-1592. doi:10.1016/j.fct.2007.02.020
43. Jeukendrup AE. Carbohydrate and exercise performance: the role of multiple transportable carbohydrates. *Curr Opin Clin Nutr Metab Care.* 2010;13(4):452-457. doi:10.1097/MCO.0b013e328339de9f
44. King AJ, Rowe JT, Burke LM. Carbohydrate hydrogel products do not improve performance or gastrointestinal distress during moderate-intensity endurance exercise. *Int J Sport Nutr Exerc Metab.* 2020;30(5):305-314. doi:10.1123/ijsnem.2020-0102
45. Hurst P, Schipof-Godart L, Szabo A, et al. The placebo and nocebo effect on sports performance: a systematic review. *Eur J Sport Sci.* 2020;20(3):279-292. doi:10.1080/17461391.2019.1655098
46. Raglin J, Szabo A, Lindheimer JB, Beedie C. Understanding placebo and nocebo effects in the context of sport: a psychological perspective. *Eur J Sport Sci.* 2020;20(3):293-301. doi:10.1080/17461391.2020.1727021
47. Beedie CJ, Stuart EM, Coleman DA, Foad AJ. Placebo effects of caffeine on cycling performance. *Med Sci Sports Exerc.* 2006;38(12):2159-2164. doi:10.1249/01.mss.0000233805.56315.a9
48. Clark VR, Hopkins WG, Hawley JA, Burke LM. Placebo effect of carbohydrate feedings during a 40-km cycling time trial. *Med Sci Sports Exerc.* 2000;32(9):1642-1647. doi:10.1097/00005768-200009000-00019
49. Recalls, outbreaks & emergencies. US Food and Drug Administration. January 25, 2022. Accessed December 24, 2023. www.fda.gov/food/recalls-outbreaks-emergencies
50. Kilbourne EM, Philen RM, Kamb ML, Falk H. Tryptophan produced by Showa Denko and epidemic eosinophilia-myalgia syndrome. *J Rheumatol Suppl.* 1996;46:81-91.
51. Phillips GC. Medicolegal issues and ergogenic aids: trade, tragedy, and public safety, the example of ephedra and the Dietary Supplement Health and Education Act. *Curr Sports Med Rep.* 2004;3(4):224-228. doi:10.1007/s11932-004-0020-2
52. Brown JA, Buckley NA. Toxicity from bodybuilding supplements and recreational use of products containing 1,3-dimethylamylamine. *Med J Aust.* 2013;198(8):414-415. doi:10.5694/mja12.11167
53. Crescioli G, Lombardi N, Bettiol A, et al. Acute liver injury following Garcinia cambogia weight-loss supplementation: case series and literature review. *Intern Emerg Med.* 2018;13(6):857-872. doi:10.1007/s11739-018-1880-4
54. Ronis MJJ, Pedersen KB, Watt J. Adverse effects of nutraceuticals and dietary supplements. *Annu Rev Pharmacol Toxicol.* 2018;58:583-601. doi:10.1146/annurev-pharmtox-010617-052844
55. Ichim MC. The DNA-based authentication of commercial herbal products reveals their globally widespread adulteration. *Front Pharmacol.* 2019;10:1227. doi:10.3389/fphar.2019.01227
56. Ichim MC, de Boer HJ. A review of authenticity and authentication of commercial ginseng herbal medicines and food supplements. *Front Pharmacol.* 2021;11:612071. doi:10.3389/fphar.2020.612071
57. Gallardo EJ, Coggan AR. What's in your beet juice? Nitrate and nitrite content of beet juice products marketed to athletes. *Int J Sport Nutr Exerc Metab.* 2019;29(4):345-349. doi:10.1123/ijsnem.2018-0223
58. Protein Powder White Paper. Clean Label Project. June 12, 2018. Accessed December 24, 2023. https://cleanlabelproject.org/protein-powder-white-paper/2018

59. Timbo BB, Chirtel SJ, Ihrie J, et al. Dietary supplement adverse event report data from the FDA Center for Food Safety and Applied Nutrition Adverse Event Reporting System (CAERS), 2004-2013. *Ann Pharmacother.* 2018;52(5):431-438. doi:10.1177/1060028017744316
60. The Prohibited List. World Anti-Doping Association. Accessed December 24, 2023. www.wada-ama.org/en/prohibited-list
61. The World Anti-Doping Code. World Anti-Doping Agency. Accessed December 24, 2023. www.wada-ama.org/en/what-we-do/world-anti-doping-code
62. Supplement Connect. US Anti-Doping Agency. Accessed December 24, 2023. www.usada.org/athletes/substances/supplement-connect
63. Geyer H, Parr MK, Koehler K, Mareck U, Schänzer W, Thevis M. Nutritional supplements cross-contaminated and faked with doping substances. *J Mass Spectrom.* 2008;43(7):892-902. doi:10.1002/jms.1452
64. Judkins C, Prock P. Supplements and inadvertent doping - how big is the risk to athletes. *Med Sport Sci.* 2012;59:143-152. doi:10.1159/000341970
65. Geyer H, Parr MK, Mareck U, Reinhart U, Schrader Y, Schänzer W. Analysis of non-hormonal nutritional supplements for anabolic-androgenic steroids - results of an international study. *Int J Sports Med.* 2004;25(2):124-129. doi:10.1055/s-2004-819955
66. Baume N, Mahler N, Kamber M, Mangin P, Saugy M. Research of stimulants and anabolic steroids in dietary supplements. *Scand J Med Sci Sports.* 2006;16(1):41-48. doi:10.1111/j.1600-0838.2005.00442.x
67. Judkins C, Hall D, Hoffman K. *Investigation Into Supplement Contamination Levels in the US Market.* HFL; 2007:1-11.
68. Mathews NM. Prohibited contaminants in dietary supplements. *Sports Health.* 2018;10(1):19-30. doi:10.1177/1941738117727736
69. Ayotte C, Lévesque JF, Cléroux M, Lajeunesse A, Goudreault D, Fakirian A. Sport nutritional supplements: quality and doping controls. *Can J Appl Physiol.* 2001;26(suppl):S120-S129. doi:10.1139/h2001-047
70. Catlin DH, Leder BZ, Ahrens B, et al. Trace contamination of over-the-counter androstenedione and positive urine test results for a nandrolone metabolite. *JAMA.* 2000;284(20):2618-2621. doi:10.1001/jama.284.20.2618
71. Green GA, Catlin DH, Starcevic B. Analysis of over-the-counter dietary supplements. *Clin J Sport Med.* 2001;11(4):254-259. doi:10.1097/00042752-200110000-00008
72. Kamber M, Baume N, Saugy M, Rivier L. Nutritional supplements as a source for positive doping cases? *Int J Sport Nutr Exerc Metab.* 2001;11(2):258-263. doi:10.1123/ijsnem.11.2.258
73. Walpurgis K, Thomas A, Geyer H, Mareck U, Thevis M. Dietary supplement and food contaminations and their implications for doping controls. *Foods.* 2020;9(8):1012. doi:10.3390/foods9081012
74. Abrahamson A. Olympic chance after 2-year ban. *Los Angeles Times.* October 9, 2005. Accessed December 24, 2023. www.latimes.com/archives/la-xpm-2005-oct-09-sp-oly9-story.html
75. Futterman M. Trials and tribulations of the angry swimmer. *Wall Street Journal.* Updated May 14, 2012. Accessed December 24, 2023. www.wsj.com/articles/SB10001424052702304203604577396561190319378
76. Eichner AK, Coyles J, Fedoruk M, et al. Essential features of third-party certification programs for dietary supplements: a consensus statement. *Curr Sports Med Rep.* 2019;18(5):178-182. doi:10.1249/JSR.0000000000000595
77. Hoon MW, Hopkins WG, Jones AM, et al. Nitrate supplementation and high-intensity performance in competitive cyclists. *Appl Physiol Nutr Metab.* 2014;39(9):1043-1049. doi:10.1139/apnm-2013-0574
78. Hoon MW, Johnson NA, Chapman PG, Burke LM. The effect of nitrate supplementation on exercise performance in healthy individuals: a systematic review and meta-analysis. *Int J Sport Nutr Exerc Metab.* 2013;23(5):522-532. doi:10.1123/ijsnem.23.5.522
79. Hoon MW, Jones AM, Johnson NA, et al. The effect of variable doses of inorganic nitrate-rich beetroot juice on simulated 2,000-m rowing performance in trained athletes. *Int J Sports Physiol Perform.* 2014;9(4):615-620. doi:10.1123/ijspp.2013-0207
80. Lane SC, Areta JL, Bird SR, et al. Caffeine ingestion and cycling power output in a low or normal muscle glycogen state. *Med Sci Sports Exerc.* 2013;45(8):1577-1584. doi:10.1249/MSS.0b013e31828af183
81. Lane SC, Bird SR, Burke LM, Hawley JA. Effect of a carbohydrate mouth rinse on simulated cycling time-trial performance commenced in a fed or fasted state. *Appl Physiol Nutr Metab.* 2013;38(2):134-139. doi:10.1139/apnm-2012-0300
82. Lane SC, Hawley JA, Desbrow B, et al. Single and combined effects of beetroot juice and caffeine supplementation on cycling time trial performance. *Appl Physiol Nutr Metab.* 2014;39(9):1050-1057. doi:10.1139/apnm-2013-0336
83. Chung W, Shaw G, Anderson ME, et al. Effect of 10 week beta-alanine supplementation on competition and training performance in elite swimmers. *Nutrients.* 2012;4(10):1441-1453. doi:10.3390/nu4101441
84. Shaw G, Slater G, Burke LM. Supplement use of elite Australian swimmers. *Int J Sport Nutr Exerc Metab.* 2016;26(3):249-258. doi:10.1123/ijsnem.2015-0182

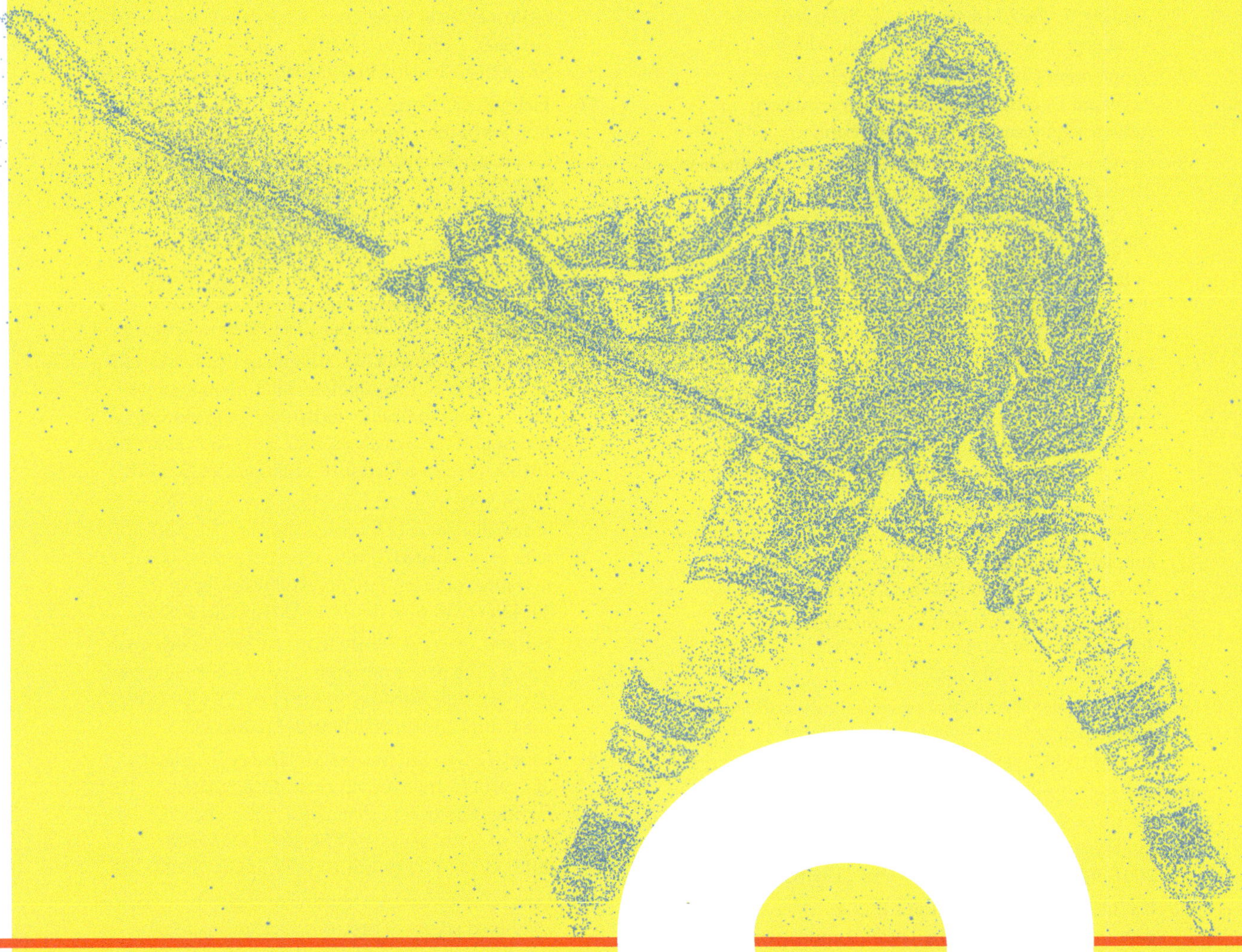

SECTION 2

SPORTS NUTRITION ASSESSMENT AND ENERGY BALANCE

Ask any sports dietitian and they will tell you that most athletes want to alter their body composition. Gaining or losing weight, increasing muscle mass, decreasing body fat, or a combination of such goals are top priorities for most competitive athletes. Chapter 8 provides an understanding of the nutrition assessment component of the Nutrition Care Process and Standards of Practice and Standards of Professional Performance, whereas Chapter 9 examines the various body composition measurement tools and summarizes the pros and cons of methods of measuring body composition to help the practitioner choose the appropriate technique. Chapter 10 presents a thorough explanation of energy balance, providing a foundational understanding of the factors that affect it. Finally, Chapter 11 provides the practitioner with an understanding of the research behind recommendations for weight management. These 4 chapters will answer many of the questions frequently asked by athletes and coaches.

CHAPTER 8

Nutrition Assessment

Karen Reznik Dolins, EdD, RDN, CSSD

LEARNING OBJECTIVES

- Identify the steps involved in performing a nutrition assessment of an athlete.
- Identify aspects of food- and nutrition-related history that are specific to athletes.
- Identify nutrients of particular concern to the active individual and the conditions under which a biochemical assessment might be warranted.
- Evaluate technological tools designed to aid in collecting data used to evaluate nutritional intake and exercise energy expenditure.
- Explain how to interpret data collected in the context of comparative standards used in sports nutrition.

INTRODUCTION

Nutrition assessment is the first step in the Nutrition Care Process, a systematic problem-solving method that registered dietitian nutritionists (RDNs) use to critically assess an individual's nutritional status, make decisions to address nutrition-related problems, and provide safe and effective quality nutrition care.[1] In the assessment step, data are collected, recorded, and interpreted. The Nutrition Care Process uses standardized language as described on the electronic Nutrition Care Process Terminology (eNCPT) website (www.ncpro.org).

Categories Included in Nutrition Assessment

The Revised 2021 Standards of Practice and Standards of Professional Performance for Registered Dietitian Nutritionists (Competent, Proficient, and Expert) in Sports and Human Performance Nutrition provides a detailed list of items that may be included in the nutrition assessment of the athlete.[2] Categories of nutrition assessment include the following:

- food- and nutrition-related history;
- anthropometric measurements;
- biochemical data, medical tests, and procedures;
- nutrition focused physical findings;
- client history; and
- comparative standards.

Much of the information required for the assessment can be obtained during a face-to-face interview with the athlete. Additional information may be obtained from the athlete's physician, certified athletic

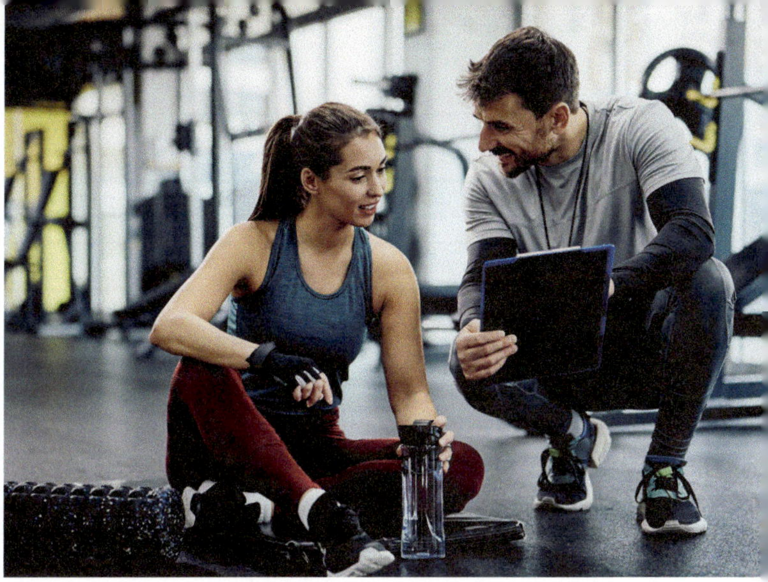

trainer, coach, psychologist, exercise physiologist, and family members. In the case of an athlete referred to the RDN by another professional, professional concerns will likely be communicated, and a referral form often provides initial information before the interview with the athlete. Current guidelines from the American College of Sports Medicine (ACSM) recommend a preexercise evaluation for physically inactive individuals with known cardiovascular, metabolic, or renal disease and for active individuals who develop symptoms of these diseases.[3] High school and collegiate athletes must also undergo a preseason medical examination. When available, results from these exams—which may include a medical history, physical examination, and laboratory data—will be included in the nutrition assessment. *ACSM's Guidelines for Exercise Testing and Prescription*[4] contains detailed information on the components of the preexercise evaluation and is an important resource for the sports nutrition professional.

An athlete may be referred to a sports RDN by a coach who is concerned about a lack of energy, drop in performance, or change in body weight. An athletic trainer may be concerned about injuries that have occurred, whereas a physician may have observed abnormal biochemical data with a possible nutrition etiology. An athlete who is self-referred is likely to be more highly motivated than an athlete who is referred by a concerned parent, coach, or member of the sports medicine team. The athlete's level of motivation and goals should be determined as part of the nutrition assessment.

In addition to understanding an athlete's goals and motivation, the sports RDN should assess their beliefs about and attitudes toward nutrition strategies. Athletes receive information from a variety of sources, not all of which are reliable, and the sports RDN should identify these sources to vet them. An athlete with firmly held but erroneous beliefs will likely need more counseling before they will adopt science-based recommendations. Behavior change theories provide a framework for describing behaviors and barriers to change. One of the most popular is the transtheoretical model, which finds that change occurs over time.[5]

The sports RDN must select the appropriate assessment tools, distinguish relevant and important data from irrelevant and unimportant data, and determine the need for additional information. As an example, Figure 8.1 on page 186 shows an assessment form used by the US Olympic Committee. Once all data are obtained, the data must be analyzed and interpreted, which requires identification of the appropriate standard for comparison. The most widely accepted standards in sports nutrition are the Joint Position Statement on Nutrition and Athletic Performance[6] and the International Olympic Committee (IOC) Consensus Statement on Sports Nutrition.[7] Once the nutrition assessment has been completed, the RDN can make a nutrition diagnosis and develop a plan for nutrition intervention. Continued monitoring and evaluation will determine whether revision of the assessment and updated recommendations are required.

The following sections provide the practitioner with an overview of the various components of the nutrition assessment as applied to the athlete. The sports RDN will need to use their judgment as to which components to include because a complete assessment is not always necessary or practical. For example, an athlete who is referred for low levels of vitamin D may not need an evaluation of body composition. The athlete's stated primary concern should be prioritized, but the RDN must be able to read between the lines to uncover other issues that may affect health and performance. For example, an athlete who requests guidance on recovery foods may reveal disordered eating ideations during the diet history.

ANTHROPOMETRIC MEASUREMENTS

Anthropometric measurements are used to estimate body composition. A 2-compartment model estimates the percentage of fat and fat-free mass. All methods of assessing body composition in live individuals involve indirect measurements and rely on prediction equations; therefore, all contain error and should not be thought of as precise measurements.

United States Olympic Committee		Sport Nutrition Assessment Form
Athlete Demographics	Sport:	Date:

Name:	DOB	Gender
Phone:	Email:	
Training location:	Coach:	
Purpose:		

Anthropometry

Date	WT	HT	Σ7-8 skinfol	%BF	Method	WT class	Comp WT	Problems and Solutions

Biochemistry (e.g., iron status, vit D status, Hb & Hct, other anemias, metabolic profile, lipids, hormones)

Hx

Date	Parameter	Comments	Treatment

Clinical (e.g., illness, injury, DE/ED, MD, bone, fatigue, GI, allergies, dehydration, sleep, overtraining, physical signs)

Hx

Date	Issue	Comments	Treatment

FIGURE 8.1 **US Olympic Committee sports nutrition assessment form** Reproduced with permission from the US Olympic & Paralympic Committee.

Clinical (e.g., Medications, Dietary/Sports Supplements)		
Date	Medication/Supplement & Dosage/Brand	Risks vs Benefits?

Dietary (e.g., usual intake, FFQ)			
Meal	Time	Food/Fluids	Intervention
Breakfast			
AM TR			
Lunch			
PM TR			
Dinner			
Snack			
Summary			

Food Frequency Questionnaire										
PRO	red meat	poultry	game	fish	soy	eggs	yogurt	milk	cheese	Risks?
CHO	pasta	rice	potatoes	cereals	breads	tortillas	grains	legumes	panc/waff	
F/V	fruit				vegetables					
FAT	nuts/seeds	butter	olive oil	other oils	dressings	mayo	mustard	olives	hummus	
FLUIDS	soda/diet	alcohol	coffee	tea	water					
SNACKS	cookies	ice cream	candy	crackers	chips					
#meals/d		#meals out/wk			#snacks/d			#meals cooked/wk		
Restaurants										

Environmental		PREP		PRE-COMP		COMP	OFF
Cycle	MON	TUE	WED	THU	FRI	SAT/SUN	Issues & Strategies: Training Nutrition
Intensity							
Intensity							
Intensity							

Peaking			
Date	COMPETITION	Location	Issues & Strategies: Competition Nutrition
Overall Summary			

Continued on next page

Summary and Follow Up Plan

USA

Nutrition Diagnosis (PES)

Goals & Intervention

Monitoring & Evaluation

Progress Notes

Date	
Date	
Date	
Date	
Date	
Date	
Date	

FIGURE 8.1 US Olympic Committee sports nutrition assessment form (continued) Reproduced with permission from the US Olympic & Paralympic Committee.

Some sports are associated with specific body types, although there is no consensus as to optimal body fat percentages for either health or physical performance.[4] Athletes participating in power sports may benefit from a specific power-to-weight ratio, whereas others, such as gymnasts and figure skaters, prefer minimal body fat. The purpose of collecting anthropometric data is to evaluate the body composition and growth of the athlete. Keep in mind that, because of genetic variation, no ideal body compositions have been identified for any specific sport.

BMI

The most basic and routine anthropometric measures are a person's height and weight. Height is measured using a stadiometer or measuring tape, and weight is measured using a balance or spring scale. The sports RDN should document if measuring equipment is unavailable and height and weight are reported by the individual rather than measured.

BMI is a metric that uses an individual's measured height and weight to estimate body fatness[2]:

$$\text{BMI} = \text{weight in kg} \div \text{height in m}^2$$

The National Heart, Lung, and Blood Institute (NHLBI) website provides a BMI calculator and discusses the strengths and limitations of using BMI as a screening or diagnostic tool.[8] The NHLBI's Expert Panel on the Identification, Evaluation, and Treatment of Overweight and Obesity in Adults defines a healthy weight as a BMI of 18.5 to 24.9, with values of 25.0 and greater indicating overweight or obesity.[9] BMI is not a useful tool for identifying overweight and obesity in athletes because it has been found to overestimate body fat in individuals who have a muscular build. The accuracy of BMI as an assessment of body fatness was assessed in collegiate athletes by comparing it with body fat percentage as measured using air displacement plethysmography in 226 collegiate athletes from a variety of sports.[10] Measurements were also taken from 213 nonathletes for comparison. Classifying overweight as a body fat percentage of greater than 20% in men and 33% in women, BMI resulted in a false positive for overweight for 67% of the male athletes compared with 25% of male nonathletes and for 31% of female athletes compared with 7% of female nonathletes. Another study of men and women ages 20 to 30 years also found that BMI had a limited ability to assess body fat.[11] Conversely, BMI may underestimate body fat in older individuals or others who have lost muscle mass. Although there is a positive relationship between percentage of body fat and BMI, the correlation is not perfect, and practitioners often find deviations.[12]

BMI classification differs for children and adolescents to account for continued growth. Although the same formula is used, the result is then plotted on BMI-for-age growth charts from the Centers for Disease Control and Prevention (CDC), and the results indicate a percentile for age.[13] The CDC defines respective BMI percentile categories in children and adolescents as follows[14]:

- Less than fifth percentile, underweight
- Fifth through 84th percentile, healthy weight
- 85th through 94th percentile, overweight
- 95th percentile and above, obesity
- 99th percentile and above, severe obesity

Waist Circumference

An adult athlete whose BMI classifies them as overweight or obese can be further evaluated by measuring the individual's waist circumference (WC). An android fat pattern, where fat is in the abdominal region, is associated with an increased risk of chronic diseases. Measurement of abdominal or visceral fat is also useful in determining whether BMI is accurately representing an estimate of body fat. The WC measurement should be taken horizontally at the height of the iliac crest using a cloth tape measure with a spring-loaded handle, which reduces skin compression and improves reliability of the measurement.[4] The NHLBI recommends a WC of 40 in (102 cm) or less for males and 35 in (88 cm) or less for females. Individuals whose WCs exceed these cutoffs and who have BMIs between 25 and 34.9 may have increased obesity-associated disease risks.[15]

Body Composition

Body composition can be further evaluated using a variety of methods. These other measurements are designed to assess body composition on the basis of a 2-compartment model (fat vs fat-free mass), a 3-compartment model (fat, fat-free mass, and bone mineral), or a 4-compartment model (fat, fat-free mass, bone mineral, and water). The most frequently used model is the 2-compartment model. Techniques for measuring body composition include the measurement of skinfold thickness, bioelectrical impedance analysis, dual-energy x-ray absorptiometry, underwater weighing, and air displacement plethysmography. Refer to Chapter 9 for further details on anthropometric measurements and body composition.

FOOD- AND NUTRITION-RELATED HISTORY

A complete history includes not only intake but also eating patterns, diet quality, and variety of foods consumed, as well as any consumption of alcohol, caffeine, and dietary supplements. Any previous modifications to the diet should be identified. One should also determine whether these modifications were prescribed by a physician, RDN, or other health professional or were self-selected without assessment of need. Any special dietary needs, including those related to food allergies or intolerances or medical conditions, must be clearly identified, along with any potential food-drug interactions.

Knowledge, beliefs, and attitudes toward food; eating behaviors; and environmental conditions affecting food choices are additional factors that must be included in the nutrition assessment. Medications must be identified so their potential interactions with or impact on food can be assessed.

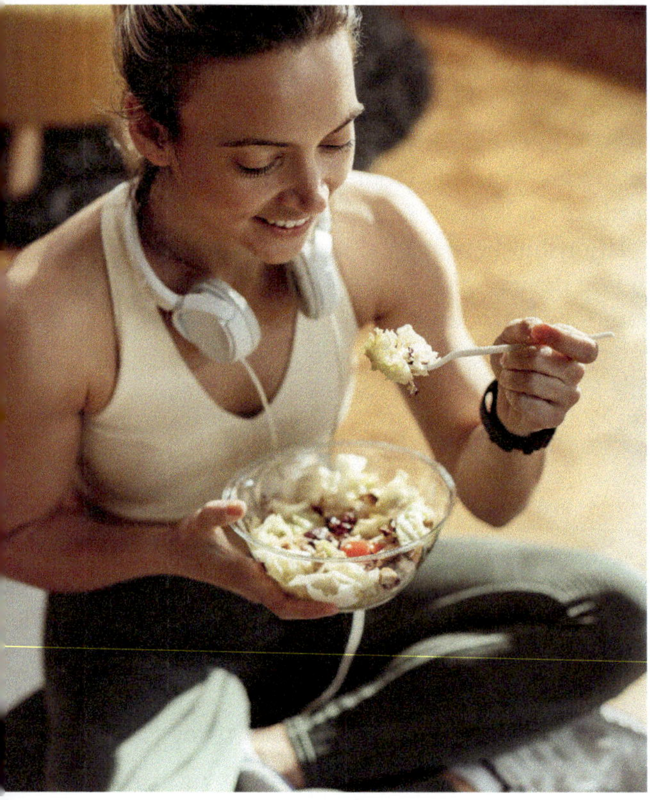

Diet and Weight History

The athlete should be asked about any previous dietary restrictions, the rationale behind them, and the outcome. An individual's weight history should also be obtained, and if available, current weight should be compared with previous weights. The individual should be asked whether weight is a concern and, if so, why. Is the concern performance-based or appearance-based? Does it arise from the athlete's own perceived need, or has it been communicated by a coach or other influential person? Has the athlete experienced recent or past weight changes? If so, additional questions about whether the weight change was intentional or unintentional are necessary, and the RDN should consider whether further investigation is warranted. Intentional weight change may occur during the offseason or in preparation for the competitive season. For example, an athlete may bulk up before the competitive season or gain weight as a result of glycogen loading. Conversely, an athlete who has reduced training during the offseason may observe an unintentional and undesirable weight gain. If this has occurred, the magnitude of weight change should be ascertained. Any history of extreme weight loss related to excessive physical activity or a history of large, repeated weight fluctuations should be identified. The weight history should include the individual's minimum and maximum weight (in adults) and the athlete's perception of their ideal weight. Athletes should be asked if they have difficulty maintaining their weight through the competitive season.

Assessment Tools

An accurate assessment of dietary intake is essential for the nutrition assessment. Data collected determine the adequacy of the diet relative to need and help diagnose any nutrition-related problems. Total intake of food, fluids, sports products, alcohol, and dietary supplements should be determined. In addition to general nutritional adequacy concerns, the sports RDN may need to assess nutrition patterns contributing to poor performance, slow recovery from training sessions, fatigue, increased incidence of injury, and difficulty maintaining an appropriate body weight.[16] It is essential to consider the timing of intake relative to training sessions or competitions and the specific demands of the exercise session.[17]

In the absence of instruments validated for the athletic population, those developed for the general population are typically used, including a 24-hour recall, a 3- to 7-day food record, and a food frequency questionnaire (FFQ). These may be modified to include foods and sports products typically used by the athlete.[18] Data may be collected retrospectively, as with 24-hour recalls and FFQs, or prospectively as with food records. Each method has its strengths and limitations. The clinician should be aware that research evaluating the validity of these methods in athletes is limited. Periodized exercise patterns, variations in day-to-day energy expenditure, and substantial energy requirements with frequent intake of food and beverages contribute to the challenge of accurately assessing nutrient intake in this population.[19]

24-HOUR RECALL

A 24-hour recall is typically conducted during the nutrition interview. The athlete is asked to describe all foods and beverages consumed the previous day or 24-hour period and to specify timing of meals and snacks. Although accuracy will be limited by the respondent's ability to accurately recall all items consumed, ability to estimate portion sizes, and knowledge of all ingredients used in preparation, this method is quick and easy and can provide a useful starting point for a conversation with the athlete about dietary patterns. The relationship between the interviewer and interviewee is key to enhancing the accuracy of information provided.[20] A rapport must be developed, and negative feedback and judgments on the part of the interviewer should be avoided so the athlete feels comfortable openly discussing food behaviors during the interview. A receptive interviewer will avoid obtaining a recall altered by the athlete's perception of what may or may not be acceptable. Gentle probing can help elicit additional information.

FOOD RECORD

Another commonly used dietary assessment method is a food record, which is generally gathered over a 3- to 7-day period. The individual is instructed in how to accurately complete the record and estimate portion sizes. The RDN reviews the records during the interview for the purpose of filling in missing information and clarifying portion sizes. Food models, measuring devices, or pictures can be used to help the athlete estimate portion sizes. Accuracy increases with the motivation of the individual, but staff might commonly observe underreporting.[21] It should be noted that individuals tend to alter their food choices when keeping logs.[16]

FOOD FREQUENCY QUESTIONNAIRES

FFQs are commonly used for assessing the intake of groups but can also be used to document and monitor intake in an individual. One benefit of this method is that it can evaluate intake over a longer time than a 24-hour recall or a 3- to 7-day food log, making it a more reliable tool for assessing the intake of specific nutrients. Heaney et al[18] modified an FFQ to include sports products and used this adapted FFQ to evaluate the dietary intake of elite female athletes from a variety of sports. Respondent cooperation was high, but the authors noted that this method has not been validated in athletes, results have not been compared with biological markers, and interpretation of results is difficult. Furthermore, athletes tend to change their diets according to training schedules. Because the FFQ provides a summary of foods and amounts consumed, these variations will not be evident, and content of specific meals and snacks cannot be assessed.

The inaccuracy of self-reported data limits the usefulness of these methods. Pooled data from 5 large validation studies of FFQs and 24-hour recalls that used doubly labeled water as a biological marker for energy intake and urinary nitrogen as a marker for protein intake found low correlation coefficients. Average correlation coefficients for the FFQ were 0.21 and 0.29 for energy and protein, respectively, and the correlation coefficients for a single 24-hour recall were 0.26 and 0.40 for energy and protein, respectively. This improved to 0.31 and 0.49 for the average of three 24-hour recalls. Researchers observed underreporting of 28% with an FFQ and 15% with a 24-hour recall; the underreporting was found to be related to BMI, education level, and age.[22]

Using a combination of methods will improve the accuracy of data collected. A diet history combines the 24-hour recall with an FFQ and can provide a more comprehensive assessment of the individual's nutrient intake.[16]

DIRECT OBSERVATION

In some instances, such as when a sports RDN works at a school or training camp, direct observation is an option for assessing food intake. Here the burden is placed on the RDN to accurately record all food and beverages consumed, rather than on the athlete to recall and record. Although this may be helpful in validating information obtained from other methodologies, observation is generally limited to specific meals and works best when the athlete is not aware that their behavior is being observed so that eating behavior is not altered.

TECHNOLOGY

Recently developed technology has been used to improve the accuracy of diet and exercise measurements.[23] Online food tracking apps on computers and smartphones linked to nutrient databases and used to analyze dietary intake have become widely popular.[23,24] These tools allow individuals to record food intake, from which a nutrient analysis can be derived. Many of these apps also include a physical activity component. A 2015 survey investigated the prevalence with which these products are being used by sports RDNs and perceptions of their usefulness in assessing and tracking dietary intake.[25] Although the response rate was a low 10.8%, approximately one-third of respondents reported using smartphone apps, with most finding them at least as useful as traditional assessment methods. Clinicians should be aware that there is a high burden for users to accurately input all food and beverages consumed, include all ingredients, and estimate portion sizes. As with other methods, self-reporting can affect accuracy. The quality of the database used may also limit the accuracy of the report. In 1 study, a comparison of nutrient analysis results from a 24-hour recall between 5 free popular apps and the Nutrition Data System for Research (developed by the Nutrition Coordinating Center at the University of Minnesota,) found significant differences, suggesting that these apps should be used with caution.[26]

The use of digital photography has also been explored as a means for enhancing the accuracy of dietary records.[27] Real-time data collection is preferable to methods that rely on memory. Image-based methods have the potential to reduce user burden and increase accuracy, but studies validating their use in the athletic population are limited.[28] This method may appeal to some who would prefer to snap a picture rather than keep a detailed food record, but ingredients used in preparation may not be apparent, and the respondent burden remains to ensure a complete record. The remote food photography method, often referred to as "snap-n-send," has been reported as a valid method for assessing energy intake in athletic populations.[29] Behavioral change strategies including coach support were found to improve motivation for complying with instructions.

The use of technology to assess dietary intake and exercise expenditure is rapidly expanding, and the potential exists for these tools to improve health outcomes. The RDN should use them with caution, as these technologies lack standardization and concerns remain regarding validation and privacy.[30]

Fluid and Electrolytes

Water intake must meet water loss, which is affected by body size and environmental conditions.[31] This requirement is met mostly by water in fluids and foods, with a small contribution coming from the oxidation of nutrients. The RDN should carefully evaluate the amount and type of fluid, along with electrolyte content. The RDN should be aware that some individuals may confuse energy drinks that contain caffeine and other stimulants for sports drinks. Caffeine-containing energy drinks often include a variety of other substances (eg, taurine, herbal extracts, vitamins, and more) and have become increasingly popular but may cause adverse effects.[32] An accurate assessment of intake will be best accomplished by asking the athlete to report all types of beverages consumed and to drink from measured containers rather than directly from water fountains or cups of unknown volume, which make quantification difficult. Refer to Chapter 6 for more information on fluids and electrolytes.

Dietary Supplements

The prevalence of dietary supplement use among athletes is high.[33] Athletes use dietary supplements to increase energy, build muscle, enhance athletic performance, aid in recovery, maintain health, and compensate for a poor diet.[34,35] Quality control for dietary supplements varies, and contamination with banned substances may occur.[36] All dietary supplements (along with dosing, frequency, and reason for use) should be identified during the nutrition assessment to determine appropriateness and potential risks. Refer to Chapter 7 for more information on supplements.

Environment and Access to Food

Where an individual eats, who purchases the food, how much access they have to food and to cooking facilities, and the people with whom the individual eats will all affect food choices and behaviors. Some barriers to healthy eating may include the following:

- A college athlete living in a dormitory room may be dependent on cafeteria food, which can vary widely in quality.
- Some schools are in areas where fast-food restaurants and delis are more accessible than grocery stores, leading the athlete to consume more highly processed foods and fewer fruits and vegetables.
- Team meals may be provided for athletes. Most often, coaching staff is responsible for ordering these meals, and the focus may be on cost rather than nutritional quality.
- Time constraints are often an issue for an athlete of any age because school or work responsibilities, in addition to training time, reduce the time available for food preparation and consumption.
- Athletes who travel may not have access to their customary foods while on the road.

The sports RDN can be instrumental in identifying foods that will be available and in creating performance-enhancing menu suggestions within those limitations. The athlete's food budget should be determined and used in planning. Identification of environmental obstacles to healthy eating will enable the sports RDN to help develop strategies to overcome such impediments.

Knowledge, Beliefs, and Attitudes

Athletes obtain nutrition information from a variety of sources, including team coaches, strength and conditioning coaches, certified athletic trainers, physicians, peers, parents, the media, and the internet. The reliability of this information is highly variable.[37-39] Athletes may enter the nutrition counseling session with a firm set of beliefs based on what they have read and heard. Certain practices may be part of the culture of the sport, as in the example of dehydration to "make weight" for weight-class sports. It may be helpful to identify sources of knowledge, beliefs, and attitudes so that science-based recommendations can be introduced in a nonjudgmental manner. The sports RDN should determine whether educational efforts also need to be directed toward key influencers such as parents and coaches.

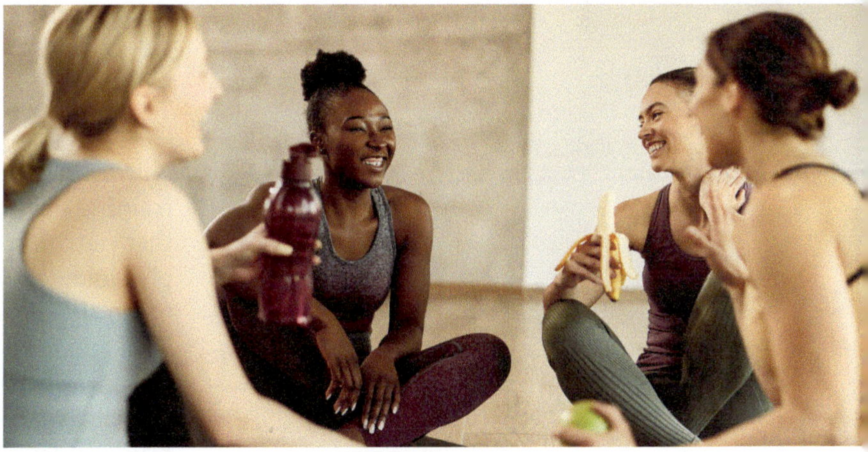

Sports RDNs develop nutrition strategies to enhance health, fitness, and optimal physical performance.[2] For such strategies to be effective, the recipient must be open to the guidance provided and willing to make behavioral changes. Nutrition education is more likely to be effective when based on research and theory. Integrative models of health behavior change have been developed.[40] The transtheoretical model of health behavior change is one such model that has been used to describe the progression of change over time as occurring through a series of stages: precontemplation, contemplation, preparation, action, maintenance, and termination.[5] Planned interventions, when appropriately designed according to stage, can help move people through the stages. This model has been applied to dietary changes and found to be useful for understanding the decision-making process and designing interventions to move the individual forward.[41] Advantages and disadvantages of making behavioral changes differ in the various stages, and evidence suggests a crossover effect—a point at which the advantages outweigh the disadvantages—occurs before the action stage where changes take hold. The University of California Los Angeles Center for Human Nutrition website provides a description of the 6 stages of this model of change, along with a discussion of techniques effective at each stage.[42] Research is still needed to evaluate the effectiveness of this approach in athletes.

Eating Behaviors

Certain behaviors related to food intake may affect an athlete's ability to achieve nutrition goals and, therefore, must be a part of the conversation. The athlete should be questioned about restrictive eating, rigidity or limited food preferences, and bingeing and purging, all of which may indicate disordered eating. Other behaviors of note include pace of eating, activities performed while eating that may distract and contribute to mindless eating, and emotional eating. Behaviors that interfere with goals will need to be addressed as a part of the nutrition intervention, and pathological eating behaviors will need to be addressed with a team approach including a psychologist and physician. Disordered eating is discussed in more detail in Chapter 18.

Challenges Specific to the Dietary Assessment of the Athlete

PERIODIZED TRAINING CYCLES

An athlete's training load, and therefore nutritional needs, will vary according to whether they are in preparation for the competitive season, in the competitive season, or transitioning out of the competitive season. A dietary assessment specific to the training cycle will most accurately meet the athlete's needs. A reassessment should be conducted each time the athlete enters a new period.[2]

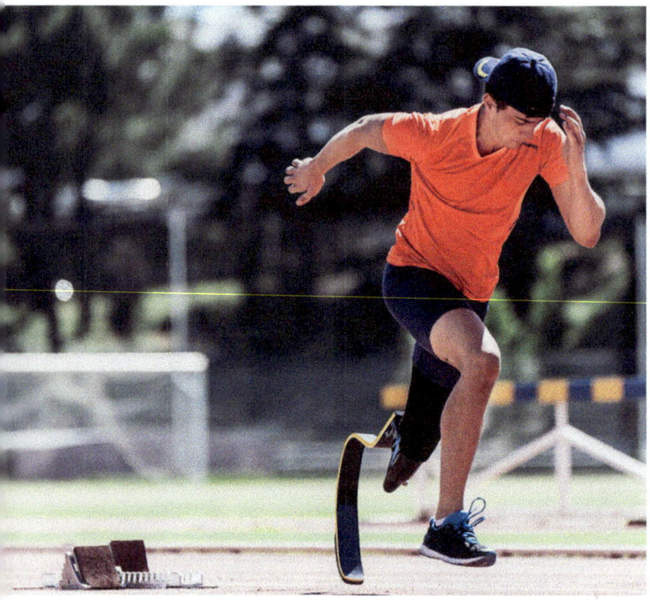

DIETARY MANIPULATION

An athlete may temporarily alter their diet in an attempt to improve performance, as in carbohydrate loading, or to change body composition before competition, as in weight-class sports. These periods of manipulation may last days or weeks and may not be indicative of the athlete's usual diet.

TRAINING DAYS VS COMPETITION DAYS

Nutritional needs and dietary intake typically vary between training days and competition days. Although it is essential that nutritional needs be met on training days to promote physiological adaptations and health, the goal on competition days may be more focused on providing foods and fluids that are well tolerated by the athlete. Foods and fluids for an athlete competing in tournaments must be appropriately spaced. Variability in nutritional needs between training days and competition days requires that intake on these days be assessed independently. Because dietary intake must be interpreted relative to the needs of the athlete, a training log should be collected in parallel with the food log.

SPORTS FOODS AND PRODUCTS

Athletes may consume sports drinks, protein shakes, gels, and other products not typically consumed by the general population. The specific products, the frequency at which they are used, and the timing of use should be ascertained. Product formulations may change over time. The RDN will find viewing product labels to be helpful.

PREEXERCISE AND POSTEXERCISE FUELING PATTERNS

Although distribution of energy and nutrients throughout the day is important for anyone, it is even more critical for athletes. Questions specific to foods and fluids consumed before exercise, during exercise, and after exercise are essential.[2]

Nutrient Analysis

Once all dietary information has been collected, the information can be entered into a nutrient analysis program. Programs vary in cost, ease of use, reports provided, and inclusion of items typically consumed by an athlete. Accurate entry is essential to prevent errors.

Nearly all nutrient analysis programs are based on information from the US Department of Agriculture Research Service's FoodData Central nutrient database (https://fdc.nal.usda.gov). Examples of free nutrition trackers include Cronometer (https://cronometer.com), LoseIt (www.loseit.com), and MyFitnessPal (www.myfitnesspal.com). Other websites, such as FitDay (www.fitday.com) and CalorieKing (www.calorieking.com), are useful for quickly looking up the nutrient content of foods but do not provide the high-quality analyses and reports that professional programs provide.[43] Some of the programs available for professional use include NutriBase Professional, Food Processor (ESHA Research), and Nutritionist Pro (Axxya Systems).

Assessment of Energy Requirements

An athlete's most basic need is for adequate energy intake to support normal body metabolism and physical activity including sport and exercise. Total daily energy expenditure is the sum of resting metabolic rate, thermic effect of food, and energy used in physical activity. Physical activity includes planned exercise, as well as the energy cost of normal daily activities and involuntary muscular activity such as fidgeting and shivering.[44]

Energy requirements can be directly measured by direct calorimetry, which measures heat production using a specialized chamber, or by using doubly labeled water (in which water labeled with stable isotopes of hydrogen and oxygen is ingested and subsequently collected when eliminated in the urine and breath).[45] In the latter case, energy expenditure is calculated by analyzing the isotope turnover rate. These methods provide greater accuracy than indirect methods, but they are costly and are generally reserved for research. Moreover, doubly labeled water provides a measure of energy expenditure as the individual goes about their normal activities, but it does not provide a measure of the energy use of each individual activity.

Indirect measures of energy include indirect calorimetry and movement monitors such as accelerometers and pedometers.[44] Indirect calorimetry uses the relationship between the volume of oxygen consumed (VO_2) and the respiratory quotient (RQ) to estimate energy expenditure. RQ describes the relationship between the volume of CO_2 produced (VCO_2) and the volume of O_2 consumed and is calculated as $RQ = VCO_2 \div VO_2$. RQ varies with the substrate used because the oxidations of carbohydrate, protein, and fat require different amounts of oxygen. Metabolic charts used to analyze inspired and expired gases are usually programmed with the Weir equation, which stipulates that the metabolic rate, or the kilocalories expended per minute, is equal to $[(1.1 \times RQ) + 3.9] \times VO_2$.[46] In this way, energy expenditure can be measured both at rest and during exercise. Handheld devices using the same principle to estimate resting energy expenditure have been developed and validated and may be useful in clinical practice.[47,48]

Prediction equations are used most commonly for estimating total daily energy expenditure in clinical practice, although most have been developed based on a sedentary population. A study that compared resting metabolic rate (RMR) measured in the laboratory for active men and women with those predicted by various equations found the Cunningham equation to be the most accurate, with the Harris-Benedict equation being the next best.[49] The Cunningham equation requires measurement of lean body mass. When this is not feasible, the Harris-Benedict equation offers a simple, though less accurate, alternative. Once the practitioner has determined RMR, they must add an appropriate activity factor and take into account the thermic effect of food.[50] Activity factors are a crude estimation of true amount of energy expended via physical activity. Refer to Chapter 10 for additional details on using energy prediction equations.

As noted earlier, reviewing an athlete's training log allows for a more accurate determination of energy and nutrient needs. Training protocols typically vary daily, and nutritional needs will vary accordingly. Some athletes require considerably more fuel on training days than competition days. A swimmer, for example, may expend 5,000 kcal in training daily, whereas their competition may involve a sprint with an energy cost of only several hundred kilocalories. Conversely, a competitive tennis athlete or triathlete needs to plan for adequate energy to delay fatigue in endurance events.

Energy availability refers to the energy left for body systems after exercise and is defined as the energy intake less the energy cost of exercise.[51] An assessment of energy availability will allow the practitioner to determine the adequacy of an athlete's caloric intake.

BIOCHEMICAL NUTRITION ASSESSMENT

Biochemical assessment involves the measurement of nutrient and metabolite levels in the blood and urine. A complete blood count, a comprehensive metabolic panel with a lipid profile, endocrine markers, and a urinary analysis are typically included as routine blood work in evaluating general health. Specific nutrients, such as vitamins, would be assessed only if a concern for deficiency or toxicity exists. Of particular concern in an athlete's assessment are the oxygen-carrying nutrients (iron, folic acid, and vitamin B12), the bone-building nutrients (vitamin D and calcium), and hormones. Because dehydration can alter the results of key tests, RDNs should assess hydration status at the time of testing (see the Fluids and Hydration section later in this chapter). The RDN should assess the adequacy of available laboratory work and make recommendations for additional evaluations when appropriate. Practitioners should note that some biochemical markers may be affected by mechanisms beyond dehydration (eg, exercise-induced inflammation, circadian rhythm) and that care should be taken when determining the timing of blood and urine samples.[52]

Protein

Both aerobic training and resistance training involve an upregulation of protein metabolism. Adequate dietary protein is essential for adaptations to occur. Protein status is evaluated in the laboratory using a variety of methods, including nitrogen balance, stable isotopes, and fractional synthetic rate (refer to Chapter 3). Key proteins, such as retinol-binding protein, prealbumin, and albumin, may be low in an athlete who is not consuming enough protein or calories.[52] Analysis of dietary intake and monitoring of body composition are useful in assessing adequacy of protein status.

Carbohydrate

Glucose metabolism is assessed by measuring fasting plasma glucose and HbA1c levels or by performing an oral glucose tolerance test. If an abnormal result is obtained in any of these measurements, additional tests would be warranted to rule out glucose intolerance, glucose sensitivity, and type 1 or type 2 diabetes.[53] The use of continuous glucose monitors by athletes to assess fluctuations in blood glucose and inform carbohydrate ingestion during and between exercise bouts is increasing in popularity; however, research is lacking showing correlation with this strategy and improvements in sports performance.[54]

Lipids

Lipids are generally assessed to rule out risk factors for cardiovascular disease. A basic lipid panel measures circulating levels of total cholesterol, high- and low-density lipoprotein cholesterol, and triglycerides in the serum.[55] Circulating levels of C-reactive protein and homocysteine levels may also be measured as additional risk factors for vascular disease.

Fluids and Hydration

Inadequate hydration can have a negative impact on aerobic exercise and can contribute to heat illness, making hydration status a critical component of an athlete's assessment. Various biomarkers can be used to assess hydration status, including plasma osmolality, urine osmolality, and urine specific gravity (USG).

The choice of biomarker will vary based on whether testing will be done by a laboratory or in the field and whether it will be done by a trained technician or an athlete or coach.[56]

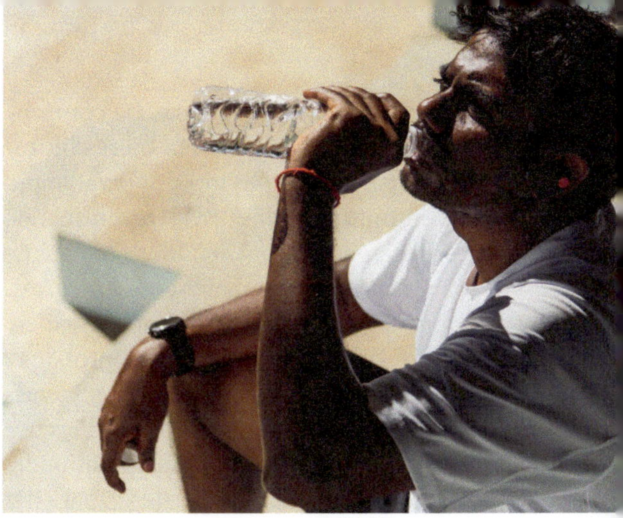

An athlete can assess their own fluid balance by monitoring daily morning weights after the first void and measuring urine concentration. Urine color and volume are simple, although subjective, ways of monitoring hydration. Darker urine indicates a greater degree of dehydration.[56] USG can be easily measured by placing a drop of urine in a refractometer or by using a reagent strip; however, this measure is prone to error, particularly during periods of fluctuating input and output of fluid.[57] When measured upon waking, a USG of 1.02 or less indicates euhydration, although diet, heavy exercise, and high lean body mass can alter these results.[56,58] Because of the limitations of any one simple assessment measure, a more accurate assessment of hydration status is provided by assessing weight, USG, and thirst concurrently.[58]

Exercise-associated hyponatremia, a potentially life-threatening condition, occurs when there is a relative excess of total body water, often as a result of excess fluid intake.[59] Diagnosis is based on a serum sodium concentration of less than 135 mEq/L accompanied by clinical symptoms, including an increase in body weight from baseline, nausea, vomiting, and altered mental status. A detailed discussion of this topic is found in Chapter 6.

Vitamin Status

Vitamin status is typically assumed based on the results of dietary intake. Athletes who consume adequate calories and eat a varied diet are unlikely to experience vitamin deficiencies. B vitamins play a vital role in the production of energy, and folate and vitamin B12 are required for the synthesis of red blood cells and the repair of damaged cells; it is possible that physical activity alters the need for these nutrients. A low red blood cell count coupled with an elevated mean corpuscular volume can indicate a deficiency of folate or vitamin B12. Although a vitamin deficiency is likely to impair athletic performance, deficiencies are rare in athletes.[60] A summary of biomarkers used for nutrition assessment of vitamins and other nutrients was published in 2018.[61]

VITAMIN D

Vitamin D has recently been identified as a nutrient of concern for athletes. In addition to its known effect on bone mineral density, vitamin D status has been associated with muscle strength.[62] Vitamin D status is known to vary with the season because the ultraviolet B rays in sunlight that trigger its activation are more plentiful in the spring and summer. Athletes who train indoors have been identified as a group at risk of inadequate vitamin D levels, as are those with dark skin, athletes who train with clothes providing little skin exposure, and athletes with higher levels of body fat.[63,64] Vitamin D status is determined by measuring the total serum concentration of 25-hydroxyvitamin D, although experts have suggested that the bioavailable 25-hydroxyvitamin D concentration may be a superior indicator.[65] According to current research, a level of at least 30 ng/mL is recommended to maintain skeletal health and muscle function (refer to Table 8.1 on page 198),[66] although an optimal level has yet to be identified.[67] Should a thorough assessment of vitamin status be required, refer to Chapter 10, Assessment of Vitamin Status, in *Nutritional Assessment of Athletes* by Driskell and Wolinsky.[68]

IRON

Iron deficiency may occur with or without anemia, and either can impair performance.[69] Stage 1 iron deficiency indicates inadequate stores of iron and is most commonly assessed by measuring serum ferritin levels. Suboptimal serum ferritin levels have been observed in significant numbers of elite athletes.[70] Note that ferritin is an acute-phase reactant and increases in response to both vigorous physical activity and inflammation, possibly resulting in a false-negative test result.[71] Although researchers have not reached a consensus regarding the ferritin cutoff point for a diagnosis of iron deficiency, many use a level of 12 mcg/mL.[72] However, exercise performance may be compromised before levels reach these clinical cutoffs. The US Olympic & Paralympic Committee (USOPC) recommends supplementation when levels fall below 35 mcg/mL for females and 4 mcg/mL for males.[73] Although not as widely used, soluble transferrin receptor may be preferable as a marker for identifying low iron stores in athletes because it does not respond to inflammation.[71]

Research has suggested that the iron-regulating hormone hepcidin may play a role in the development of iron deficiency in athletes. An inflammatory response may increase hepcidin levels for 3 to 6 hours postexercise, thereby decreasing iron absorption.[71]

TABLE 8.1 US Olympic Committee Protocol: Reference Ranges for Vitamin D

	ng/mL	nmol/mL
Vitamin D toxicity	75-150	188-375
Optimal status (bone and muscle)	40-70	100-175
Vitamin D sufficiency	>30	>75
Vitamin D insufficiency	21-29	52.5-72.5
Vitamin D deficiency	≤20	≤50

Republished with permission from reference 66: US Olympic & Paralympic Committee. Unpublished White Paper on Vitamin D and Athletes. 2020.

Iron is transported through the blood to the bone marrow by the protein transferrin. Transferrin is generally assessed by measuring total iron-binding capacity (TIBC). Transferrin saturation is then calculated by dividing serum iron by TIBC. Transferrin saturation of less than 16% is an indication of inadequate iron to support normal erythropoiesis.[74]

The hemoglobin and hematocrit concentrations are used to assess iron deficiency anemia. A decrease in these values will occur only during the late stages of iron deficiency, at which point performance will have clearly diminished because low levels of hemoglobin and hematocrit signify limited oxygen transport to working muscles.[71] Note that other nutrients involved in red blood cell production, such as folic acid, copper, and vitamin B12, also affect oxygen carrying ability and, therefore, performance.

Sports anemia may occur during the early phase of training, as increased blood volume dilutes hemoglobin, resulting in a reduction of its concentration. Yet, ferritin levels remain normal, indicating healthy iron stores, and performance is not affected. As training continues, increased erythropoiesis will lead to an increase in hemoglobin, and blood levels will normalize.

BOX 8.1 US Olympic Committee Protocol: Reference Ranges for Hematologic Iron Status Markers

Stage 1 iron depletion	Less than 35 mcg /L of ferritin Greater than 115 g/L hof emoglobin Greater than 16% transferrin saturation
Stage 2 iron deficient non-anemia	Less than 20 mcg/L of ferritin Greater than 115 g/L of hemoglobin Less than 16% transferrin saturation Total iron-binding capacity greater than 500 mcg/dL
Stage 3 iron deficiency anemia	Less than 12 mcg/L of ferritin Less than 115 g/L of hemoglobin Less than 16% transferrin saturation

Republished with permission from reference 73: US Olympic & Paralympic Committee. Unpublished White Paper on Iron Status in Athletes. 2020.

Vegetarian athletes and female athletes are at increased risk of iron depletion and deficiency. These athletes should pursue dietary strategies that will ensure the adequacy of their iron intake. Chapters 5 and 16 discuss this topic in detail.

Optimal iron levels for athletes may differ from clinical standards. Box 8.1 outlines recommended levels according to the USOPC protocol.[73] Because of the impact of hydration, exercise, and inflammation on markers of iron status, blood collection should occur in the morning before exercise and in a hydrated state.[71]

Organ Function

Biochemical tests are also used to measure organ function. Those most pertinent to nutrition assessment concern the organ systems involved in the digestion, absorption, metabolism, and excretion of nutrients and their end products. These include tests for malabsorption; screening for sickle cell trait or disease; studies of the endocrine system, including sex hormones; and bone mineral density testing.

NUTRITION FOCUSED PHYSICAL FINDINGS

Nutrition focused physical findings may be collected by a member of the health care team other than the sports RDN, such as the team physician or a certified athletic trainer. Findings pertinent to assessment of nutrition status include the following:

- clinical signs of fluid imbalance, such as skin turgor, fatigue, muscle cramps, dark urine, rapid weight change, constipation, and thirst,
- clinical signs of undernutrition or eating disorders, including muscle wasting, lanugo, hypothermia, dry or brittle hair and nails, bradycardia, tooth erosion, bony protrusions, parotid gland enlargement, and gastrointestinal distress;
- muscularity and subcutaneous fat distribution;
- oral health, including dentition and mouth sores; and
- clinical signs of digestive system impairment, such as bloating, cramping, and diarrhea.

CLIENT HISTORY

The client history includes current and past medical and social histories, including age; sport and position; number of years in the sport; current or past injuries; educational level; and preferred language, if pertinent. Any current or past medical conditions affecting the athlete or a family member that may impact nutrition should be noted. Socioeconomic factors and living situation can also be indicated.

COMPARATIVE STANDARDS

Once all data have been collected and analyzed, evidence-based standards on which the assessment will be based must be identified. The appropriate standard(s) will vary depending on age, health status, governing bodies, and goals of the athlete. For example, the *Dietary Guidelines for Americans, 2020–2025*, might be appropriate for addressing the dietary adequacy of an active individual whose goal is health and fitness, whereas a competitive athlete may benefit from use of the Nutrition and Athletic Performance joint position paper from the Academy of Nutrition and Dietetics, Dietitians of Canada, and ACSM or the IOC Consensus Statement on Sports Nutrition.[6,7] The ACSM has positions on a variety of issues relevant to nutrition assessment, including the female athlete triad, appropriate physical activity intervention strategies for weight loss and prevention of weight regain for adults, and exercise and fluid replacement.[56,75,76] The IOC consensus statement on relative energy deficiency in sport offers guidelines for education, detection, and treatment of this condition.[77] For school-aged athletes, the American Academy of Pediatrics offers a number of policy statements and other professional resources.[78] The National Athletic Trainers' Association and the National Strength and Conditioning Association have also published several position papers on subjects of interest to the RDN, including dietary supplements, weight management, and treatment of eating disorders in athletes.[79-81]

To tie the information presented in this chapter together, Box 8.2 on page 200 presents a case study of the nutrition assessment of a female marathon runner.[1,6,45,51,82]

BOX 8.2 Case Study: Female Marathoner[1,6,45,51,82]

Athlete description and goals

DW, a 22-year-old woman training for a marathon with a goal of completing it in under 4 hours

Anthropometrics

Height: 5'5"	Weight: 140 lb
BMI: 23.3	Waist circumference: 28"

Body composition as assessed with skinfold calipers: 25% body fat = 35 lb (16 kg) fat mass + 105 lb (48 kg) lean mass

Food- and nutrition-related history

Weight fluctuates between 135 and 140 lb. Athlete feels "lighter" at 135 lb. In the past, she has reduced her intake of breads and other grains to achieve weight loss.

A 24-hour recall and food frequency questionnaire were obtained.

- DW usually avoids food before her morning run, although she does drink a cup of coffee. She has a single-serve yogurt for breakfast once she gets to work, about 1.5 hours later. She alternates between a salad and a sandwich for lunch and will have a piece of fruit for an afternoon snack. If she is really hungry, she may eat 2 or 3 cookies or a small bag of chips. Dinner is variable. She may prepare chicken or fish and vegetables or pick up items such as a burrito bowl or 2 slices of pizza.
- She drinks a glass of wine an average of 3 nights per week, with 2 glasses on Saturday nights.
- On weekends, she will have half a bagel with butter and coffee before her long run and pancakes with butter and syrup after.
- DW drinks mostly water, although she does not drink during her runs.
- She takes a generic multivitamin and mineral supplement most days. She knows that carbohydrates are important for marathon running but also believes they lead to weight gain.

An analysis of DW's 24-hour recall indicates that she consumed 1,675 kcal, 100 g of protein, and 210 g of carbohydrate. Alcohol was not consumed on the day of the recall.

DW needs an estimated 1,740 kcal daily, with an additional 90 kcal for every mile she runs.[45,82] Her current training schedule ranges from 4 miles on short days to 11 miles on long days, requiring an additional 360 to 990 kcal, for a total energy expenditure of 2,100 to 2,730 kcal.

DW had an annual physical 1 month ago. Complete blood count, lipid profile, blood glucose, vitamin D, and electrolytes were all within normal limits.

DW presents as a well-nourished, fit individual. She has a normal menstrual cycle and does not report gastrointestinal or other medical issues. She reports infrequent urination and darker urine on days of long runs than on other days of the week.

Comparison with standards

Energy availability (EA)[51]

Energy intake (Ein) = 1,650 kcal

Energy expenditure of exercise (EEE) = 360 kcal

EA = Ein - EEE = 1,290 kcal

Recommended EA = 30 to 45 kcal/kg of fat-free mass = 30 × 48 kg = 1,440 kcal

Recommended carbohydrate intake = 6 to 7 g per kilogram of body weight = 384 to 448 g for current level of training.[6] This should increase to 7 to 8 g per kilogram of body weight as mileage increases.[6]

Recommended protein intake = 1.2 g per kilogram of body weight[6] = 77 g

Current carbohydrate intake: 210 g

Current protein intake: 100 g

Current fluid intake: Inadequate consumption before and during exercise

Current calcium intake: 600 mg (Dietary Reference Intake: 1,000 mg)

Current iron intake: 12 mg (Dietary Reference Intake: 18 mg)

Nutrition diagnoses[1]

- Inadequate energy availability
- Inadequate carbohydrate intake
- Excessive protein intake
- Inadequate fluid intake
- Inadequate calcium intake
- Inadequate iron intake

SUMMARY

Performing a nutrition assessment on an athlete requires knowledge and skill on the part of the sports RDN. Standards of practice for RDNs in sports nutrition and dietetics delineate the skills, training, and knowledge for the competent, proficient, and expert practitioner.[2] An expert level of competency may be required for more complex issues, such as the athlete with type 1 diabetes.

Appropriate use of assessment tools, effective interviewing methods, and clear organization of data collected contribute to the usefulness of the assessment.[2] The use of standard terminology enhances communication with other members of the team. All assessment data must be carefully recorded and dated, and results should be communicated in a timely fashion.

The experienced RDN will be able to differentiate between data that are pertinent to the situation and data that are not. For example, not all athletes will require anthropometric measurements beyond height and weight. In a healthy athlete, a complete biochemical workup may not be warranted. Conversely, the RDN may need to contact the physician or other provider to request additional tests if a specific concern arises. Athletes with an underlying health concern, such as type 1 or type 2 diabetes, celiac disease, hyperlipidemia, hypertension, or another disorder, will require more testing to determine appropriate dietary modifications. A complete discussion of medical nutrition assessment is beyond the scope of this chapter. Diabetes and exercise are thoroughly discussed in Chapter 19.

The sports RDN will benefit from understanding the logistics of an athlete's sport. It is important to understand the requirements of weight-class sports; periodized training protocols; and the strength, speed, and endurance needs of each athlete. After the RDN conducts a complete nutrition assessment of an athlete, the resulting nutrition diagnoses will provide the basis on which the intervention will be made. Periodic reassessment will determine whether alterations in the nutrition intervention are required.

KEY TAKEAWAYS

Categories included in the nutrition assessment are food- and nutrition-related history, anthropometric measurements, biochemical data, medical tests and procedures, nutrition focused physical findings, client history, and comparative standards.

A complete history includes not only intake but also eating patterns, diet quality, and variety of foods consumed, as well as any consumption of alcohol, caffeine, and dietary supplements.

In the absence of instruments validated for the athletic population, those developed for the general population are typically used, including a 24-hour recall, a 3- to 7-day food record, and a food frequency questionnaire.

Challenges specific to the assessment of the athlete include periodized training cycles; temporary manipulation of the diet; diets specific to training vs competition days; the use of dietary supplements, sports foods, and products; and the adequacy of preexercise and postexercise fueling.

Biochemical assessments of particular concern in the assessment an athlete are the oxygen-carrying nutrients (iron, folic acid, vitamin B12), bone-building nutrients (vitamin D and calcium), hormones, and markers of hydration status.

Collected data must be compared with evidence-based standards.

REFERENCES

1. Academy of Nutrition and Dietetics. Electronic Nutrition Care Process Terminology website. Accessed October 15, 2022. www.ncpro.org
2. Daigle K, Subach R, Valliant M. Academy of Nutrition and Dietetics: Revised 2021 Standards of Practice and Standards of Professional Performance for Registered Dietitian Nutritionists (Competent, Proficient, and Expert) in Sports and Human Performance Nutrition. *J Acad Nutr Diet.* 2021;121(9):1813-1830.e55. doi:10.1016/j.jand.2021.04.018
3. Riebe D, Franklin BA, Thompson PD, et al. Updating ACSM's recommendations for exercise preparticipation health screening. *Med Sci Sports Exerc.* 2015;47(11)2473-2479. doi:10.1249/MSS.0000000000000664
4. American College of Sports Medicine; Liguori G, Feito Y, Fountaine C, Roy BA, eds. *ACSM's Guidelines for Exercise Testing and Prescription;* 11th ed. Wolters Kluwer, 2022.
5. Prochaska J, Velicer W. The transtheoretical model of health behavior change. *Am J Health Promot.* 1997;12(1):38-48. doi:10.4278/0890-1171-12.1.38
6. Thomas DT, Erdman KA, Burke LM. Position of the Academy of Nutrition and Dietetics, Dietitians of Canada, and the American College of Sports Medicine: Nutrition and Athletic Performance. *J Acad Nutr Diet.* 2016;116(3):501-528. doi:10.1016/j.jand.2015.12.006
7. Maughan RJ, Shirreffs SM. IOC Consensus Conference on Nutrition in Sport, 25-27 October 2010, International Olympic Committee, Lausanne, Switzerland. *J Sports Sci.* 2011;29(suppl 1):S1. doi:10.1080/02640414.2011.619339
8. National Heart, Lung, and Blood Institute. Calculate Your Body Mass Index. Accessed November 6, 2022. www.nhlbi.nih.gov/health/educational/lose_wt/BMI/bmicalc.htm
9. Executive summary of the clinical guidelines on the identification, evaluation, and treatment of overweight and obesity in adults. *Arch Intern Med.* 1998;158(17):1855-1867. doi:10.1001/archinte.158.17.1855
10. Ode JJ, Pivarnik JM, Reeves MJ, Knous JL. Body mass index as a predictor of percent fat in college athletes and nonathletes. *Med Sci Sports Exerc.* 2007;39(3):403-409. doi:10.1249/01.mss.0000247008.19127.3e
11. Kruschitz R, Wallner-Liebmann SJ, Hamlin MJ, et al. Detecting body fat—a weighty problem BMI versus subcutaneous fat patterns in athletes and non-athletes. *PLoS One.* 2013;8(8):e72002. doi:10.1371/journal.pone.0072002.
12. Gallagher D, Heymsfield SB, Heo M, Jebb SA, Murgatroyd PR, Sakamoto Y. Healthy percentage body fat ranges: an approach for developing guidelines based on body mass index. *Am J Clin Nutr.* 2000;72(3):694-701. doi:10.1093/ajcn/72.3.694
13. Centers for Disease Control and Prevention. BMI percentile calculator for child and teen metric version. Accessed June 15, 2023. www.cdc.gov/healthyweight/bmi/calculator.html
14. Barlow SE; Expert Committee. Expert committee recommendations regarding the prevention, assessment, and treatment of child and adolescent overweight and obesity: summary report. *Pediatrics.* 2007;120(suppl 4):S164-S192. doi:10.1542/peds.2007-2329C
15. Flegal KM. Waist circumference of healthy men and women in the United States. *Int J Obes (Lond).* 2007;31(7):1134-1139. doi:10.1038/sj.ijo.0803566
16. Kerr D, Garcia CR, Boushey C. Nutritional assessment of athletes: clinical and research perspectives. In: Burke L, Deakin V, eds. *Clinical Sports Nutrition.* 6th ed. McGraw-Hill Education; 2021:26-47.
17. Kozior M, Jakeman PM, Norton C. Peri-training nutrition methods: advancements to dietary assessment in an athletic population. *Appl Physiol Nutr Metab.* 2020;45(5):564-568. doi:10.1139/apnm-2019-0622
18. Heaney S, O'Connor H, Gifford J, Naughton G. Comparison of strategies for assessing nutritional adequacy in elite female athletes' dietary intake. *Int J Sport Nutr Exerc Metab.* 2010;20(3):245-256. doi:10.1123/ijsnem.20.3.245
19. Capling L, Beck KL, Gifford JA, Slater G, Flood VM, O'Connor H. Validity of dietary assessment in athletes: a systematic review. *Nutrients.* 2017;9(12):1313. doi:10.3390/nu9121313
20. Moffatt RJ, Tomatis VB, Harris DA, Deetz AM. Estimation of food and nutrient intake of athletes. In: Driskell J, Wolinsky I, eds. *Nutritional Assessment of Athletes.* 2nd ed. CRC Press; 2010:3-50.
21. Koehler K, Braun H, De Marees M, et al. Parallel assessment of nutrition and activity in athletes: validation against doubly labelled water, 24-h urea excretion, and indirect calorimetry. *J Sports Sci.* 2010;28(13):1435-1449. doi:10.1080/02640414.2010.513482
22. Freedman LS, Commins JM, Moler JE, et al. Pooled results from 5 validation studies of dietary self-report instruments using recovery biomarkers for energy and protein intake. *Am J Epidemiol.* 2014;180(2):172-188. doi:10.1093/aje/kwu116
23. Rollo ME, Williams RL, Burrows T, Kirkpatrick SI, Bucher T, Collins CE. What are they really eating? A review on new approaches to dietary intake assessment and validation. *Curr Nutr Rep.* 2016;5(4), 307-314. doi:10.1007/s13668-016-0182-6
24. Ferrara G, Kim J, Lin S, Hua J, Seto E. A focused review of smartphone diet-tracking apps: usability, functionality, coherence with behavior change theory, and comparative validity of nutrient intake and energy estimates. *JMIR Mhealth Uhealth.* 2019;7(5):e9232. doi:10.2196/mhealth.9232
25. Jospe MR, Fairbairn KA, Green P, Perry TL. Diet app use by sports dietitians: a survey in five countries. *JMIR Mhealth Uhealth.* 2015;3(1):e7. doi:10.2196/mhealth.3345
26. Griffiths C, Harnack L, Pereira MA. Assessment of the accuracy of nutrient calculations of five popular nutrition tracking applications. *Public Health Nutr.* 2018;21(8):1495-1502. doi:10.1017/S1368980018000393

27. Ptomey LT, Willis EA, Honas JJ, et al. Validity of energy intake estimated by digital photography plus recall in overweight and obese young adults. *J Acad Nutr Diet.* 2015;115(9):1392-1399. doi:10.1016/j.jand.2015.05.006
28. Costello N, Deighton K, Dyson J, Mckenna J, Jones B. Snap-N-Send: A valid and reliable method for assessing the energy intake of elite adolescent athletes. *Eur J Sport Sci.* 2017;17(8):1044-1055. doi:10.1080/17461391.2017.1337815
29. Stables RG, Kasper AM, Sparks SA, Morton JP, Close GL. An assessment of the validity of the remote food photography method (termed Snap-N-Send) in experienced and inexperienced sport nutritionists. *Int J Sport Nutr Exerc Metab.* 2021;31(2):125-134. doi:10.1123/ijsnem.2020-0216
30. McClung HL, Raynor HA, Volpe SL, Dwyer JT, Papoutsakis C. A primer for the evaluation and integration of dietary intake and physical activity digital measurement tools into nutrition and dietetics practice. *J Acad Nutr Diet.* 2022;122(1):207-218. doi:10.1016/j.jand.2021.02.028
31. Maughan RJ. Water and electrolyte loss and replacement in training and competition. In: Maughan RJ, ed. *Sports Nutrition.* 2nd ed. John Wiley & Sons; 2013:174-184. *The Encyclopaedia of Sports Medicine: An IOC Medical Commission Publication.* Vol XIX.
32. Higgins JP, Babu K, Deuster PA, Shearer J. Energy drinks: a contemporary issues paper. *Curr Sports Med Rep.* 2018;17(2):65-72. doi:10.1249/JSR.0000000000000454
33. Daher J, Mallick M, El Khoury D. Prevalence of dietary supplement use among athletes worldwide: a scoping review. *Nutrients.* 2022;14(19):4109. doi:10.3390/nu14194109
34. Garthe I, Maughan RJ. Athletes and supplements: prevalence and perspectives. *Int J Sport Nutr Exerc Metab.* 2018;28(2):126-138. doi:10.1123/ijsnem.2017-0429
35. Wiens K, Erdman KA, Stadnyk M, Parnell JA. Dietary supplement usage, motivation, and education in young, Canadian athletes. *Int J Sport Nutr Exerc Metab.* 2014;24(6):613-622. doi:10.1123/ijsnem.2013-0087
36. Duiven E, van Loon LJC, Spruijt L, Koert W, de Hon OM. Undeclared doping substances are highly prevalent in commercial sports nutrition supplements. *J Sports Sci Med.* 2021;20(2):328-338. doi:10.52082/jssm.2021.328
37. Manore MM, Patton-Lopez MM, Meng Y, Wong SS. Sport nutrition knowledge, behaviors and beliefs of high school soccer players. *Nutrients.* 2017;9(4):350. doi:10.3390/nu9040350
38. Torres-McGehee TM, Pritchett KL, Zippel D, Minton DM, Cellamare A, Sibilia M. Sports nutrition knowledge among collegiate athletes, coaches, athletic trainers, and strength and conditioning specialists. *J Athl Train.* 2012;47(2):205-211. doi:10.4085/1062-6050-47.2.205
39. Werner EN, Guadagni AJ, Pivarnik JM. Assessment of nutrition knowledge in division I college athletes. *J Am Coll Health.* 2022;70(1):248-255. doi:10.1080/07448481.2020.1740234
40. Contento IR. Nutrition education: linking research, theory, and practice. *Asia Pac J Clin Nutr.* 2008;17(suppl 1):176-179.
41. Di Noia J, Prochaska JO. Dietary stages of change and decisional balance: a meta-analytic review. *Am J Health Behav.* 2010;34(5):618-632. doi:10.5993/AJHB.34.5.11
42. Prochaska and DiClemente's Stages of Change Model. UCLA Center for Human Nutrition website. Accessed November 15, 2022. www.cellinteractive.com/ucla/physcian_ed/stages_change.html
43. Aronson D. Ask the expert. Today's Dietitian. Accessed November 15, 2022. www.todaysdietitian.com/news/enews_0909_03.shtml
44. Manore, MM. Energy requirements and measurement of energy expenditure. In: Burke L, Deakin V, eds. *Clinical Sports Nutrition.* 6th ed. McGraw-Hill Education; 2021:86-105.
45. Ainsworth BE. How to assess the energy costs of exercise and sport. In: Maughan RJ, ed. *Sports Nutrition.* 2nd ed. John Wiley & Sons; 2013:61-71. *The Encyclopaedia of Sports Medicine*; vol XIX.
46. McArdle WD, Katch FI, Katch VL, eds. *Exercise Physiology: Nutrition, Energy, and Human Performance.* 8th ed. Wolters Kluwer Health/Lippincott Williams & Wilkins; 2015.
47. Metabolic Rate Test - Microlife MedGem and BodyGem Indirect Calorimeters. Microlife Medical Home Solutions, Inc. Accessed November 15, 2022. https://metabolicratetest.com/medgem-fda-approved-indirect-calorimeter
48. Zhao D, Xian X, Terrera M, et al. A pocket-sized metabolic analyzer for assessment of resting energy expenditure. *Clin Nutr.* 2014;33(2):341-347. doi:10.1016/j.clnu.2013.06.001
49. Thompson J, Manore MM. Predicted and measured resting metabolic rate of male and female endurance athletes. *J Am Diet Assoc.* 1996;96(1):30-34. doi:10.1016/S0002-8223(96)00010-7
50. Gerrior S, Juan W, Basiotis P. An easy approach to calculating estimated energy requirements. *Prev Chronic Dis.* 2006;3(4):A129.
51. Loucks AB, Kiens B, Wright HH. Energy availability in athletes. *J Sports Sci.* 2011;29(suppl 1):S7-S15. doi:10.1080/02640414.2011.588958
52. Larson-Meyer, DE. Nutrition assessment of the athlete. *Curr Sports Med Rep.* 2019;18(4):105-108. doi:10.1249/JSR.0000000000000586
53. Diabetes Tests & Diagnosis. National Institute of Diabetes and Digestive and Kidney. Accessed November 15, 2022. www.niddk.nih.gov/health-information/diabetes/overview/tests-diagnosis
54. Bowler AM, Whitfield J, Marshall L, Coffey VG, Burke LM, Cox GR. The use of continuous glucose monitors in sport: possible applications and considerations. *Int J Sport Nutr Exerc Metab.* 2022;33(2):121-132. doi:10.1123/ijsnem.2022-0139
55. Isselbacher EM, Preventza O, Black JH 3rd, et al; Peer Review Committee Members. 2022 ACC/AHA Guideline for the Diagnosis and Management of Aortic Disease: A Report of the American Heart Association/American College of Cardiology Joint Committee on Clinical Practice Guidelines. *Circulation.* 2022;146(24):e334-e482. doi:10.1161/CIR.0000000000001106

56. American College of Sports Medicine; Sawka MN, Burke LM, Eichner ER, Maughan RJ, Montain SJ, Stachenfeld NS. American College of Sports Medicine position stand. Exercise and fluid replacement. *Med Sci Sports Exerc.* 2007;39(2):377-390. doi:10.1249/mss.0b013e31802ca597
57. Cheuvront SN, Kenefick RW, Zambraski EJ. Spot urine concentrations should not be used for hydration assessment: a methodology review. *Int J Sport Nutr Exerc Metab.* 2014;25(3):293-297. doi:10.1123/ijsnem.2014-0138
58. Kenefick RW, Cheuvront SN. Hydration for recreational sport and physical activity. *Nutr Rev.* 2012;70(suppl 2):S137-S142. doi:10.1111/j.1753-4887.2012.00523.x
59. Hew-Butler T, Rosner MH, Fowkes-Godek S, et al. Statement of the Third International Exercise-Associated Hyponatremia Consensus Development Conference, Carlsbad, California, 2015. *Clin J Sport Med.* 2015;25(4):303-320. doi:10.1097/JSM.0000000000000221
60. Woolf K, Manore M. B-vitamins and exercise: does exercise alter requirements? *Int J Sport Nutr Exerc Metab.* 2006;16(5):453-484. doi:10.1123/ijsnem.16.5.453
61. Larson-Meyer DE, Woolf K, Burke L. Assessment of nutrient status in athletes and the need for supplementation. *Int J Sport Nutr Exerc Metab.* 2018;28(2):139-158. doi:10.1123/ijsnem.2017-0338
62. Grimaldi AS, Parker BA, Capizzi JA, et al. 25(OH) vitamin D is associated with greater muscle strength in healthy men and women. *Med Sci Sports Exerc.* 2013;45(1):157-162. doi:10.1249/MSS.0b013e31826c9a78
63. von Hurst PR, Beck KL. Vitamin D and skeletal muscle function in athletes. *Curr Opin Clin Nutr Metab Care.* 2014;17(6):539-545. doi:10.1097/MCO.0000000000000105
64. Wortsman J, Matsuoka LY, Chen TC, Lu Z, Holick MF. Decreased bioavailability of vitamin D in obesity. *Am J Clin Nutr.* 2000;72(3):690-693. doi:10.1093/ajcn/72.3.690
65. Rockwell MS, Kostelnik SB, McMillan RP, Lancaster M, Larson-Meyer DE, Hulver MW. An association between bioavailable 25-hydroxyvitamin D and bone mineral density in a diverse cohort of collegiate athletes. *Med Sci Sports Exerc.* 2022;54(3):371-376. doi:10.1249/MSS.0000000000002807
66. US Olympic & Paralympic Committee. Unpublished White Paper. *Vitamin D and Athletes.* 2020.
67. Owens DJ, Allison R, Close GL. Vitamin D and the athlete: current perspectives and new challenges. *Sports Med.* 2018;48(suppl 1):3-16. doi:10.1007/s40279-017-0841-9
68. Haub M, Loest H, Hubach K. Assessment of vitamin status of athletes. In: Driskell J, Wolinsky I, eds. *Nutritional Assessment of Athletes.* 2nd ed. CRC Press; 2010:289-310.
69. Pasricha S, Low M, Thompson J, Farrell A, De-Regil LM. Iron supplementation benefits physical performance in women of reproductive age: a systematic review and meta-analysis. *J Nutr.* 2014;144(6):906-914. doi:10.3945/jn.113.189589
70. Nabhan D, Bielko S, Sinex JA, et al. Serum ferritin distribution in elite athletes. *J Sci Med Sport.* 2020;23(6):554-558. doi:10.1016/j.jsams.2019.12.027
71. Sim M, Garvican-Lewis LA, Cox GR, et al. Iron considerations for the athlete: a narrative review. *Eur J Appl Physiol.* 2019;119(7):1463-1478. doi:10.1007/s00421-019-04157-y
72. Akabas SR, Dolins KR. Micronutrient requirements of physically active women: what can we learn from iron? *Am J Clin Nutr.* 2005;81(5):1246S-1251S. doi:10.1093/ajcn/81.5.1246
73. US Olympic & Paralympic Committee. Unpublished White Paper. *Iron Status in Athletes.* 2020.
74. Camaschella C. Iron-deficiency anemia. *N Engl J Med.* 2015;372(19):1832-1843. doi:10.1056/NEJMra1401038
75. Nattiv A, Loucks AB, Manore MM, Sanborn CF, Sundgot-Borgen J, Warren MP; American College of Sports Medicine. American College of Sports Medicine position stand. The female athlete triad. *Med Sci Sports Exerc.* 2007;39(10):1867-1882. doi:10.1249/mss.0b013e318149f111
76. Donnelly JE, Blair SN, Jakicic JM, Manore MM, Rankin JW, Smith BK; American College of Sports Medicine. American College of Sports Medicine position stand. Appropriate physical activity intervention strategies for weight loss and prevention of weight regain for adults. *Med Sci Sports Exerc.* 2009;41(2):459-471. doi:10.1249/MSS.0b013e3181949333
77. Mountjoy M, Sundgot-Borgen J, Burke L, et al. International Olympic Committee (IOC) Consensus Statement on Relative Energy Deficiency in Sport (RED-S): 2018 Update. *Int J Sport Nutr Exerc Metab.* 2018;28(4):316-331. doi:10.1123/ijsnem.2018-0136
78. American Academy of Pediatrics. Policy Collections. Accessed June 22, 2023. https://publications.aap.org/pediatrics/pages/policy
79. Turocy PS, DePalma BF, Horswill CA, et al; National Athletic Trainers' Association. National Athletic Trainers' Association position statement: safe weight loss and maintenance practices in sport and exercise. *J Athl Train.* 2011;46(3):322-336. doi:10.4085/1062-6050-46.3.322
80. Buell JL, Franks R, Ransone J, Powers ME, Laquale KM, Carlson-Phillips A; National Athletic Trainers' Association. National Athletic Trainers' Association position statement: evaluation of dietary supplements for performance nutrition. *J Athl Train.* 2013;48(1):124-136. doi:10.4085/1062-6050-48.1.16
81. Granger LR, Johnson CL, Malina RM, et al. National Athletic Trainers' Association position statement: preventing, detecting, and managing disordered eating in athletes. *J Athl Train.* 2008;43(1):80-108. doi:10.4085/1062-6050-43.1.80
82. Academy of Nutrition and Dietetics. Sports Nutrition Care Manual. Sports Nutrition Care Manual Calculators. Accessed October 4, 2023. www.nutritioncaremanual.org/calculators.cfm?ncm_category_id=10&ncm_heading

CHAPTER 9

Anthropometric Measurements and Body Composition

Carrie M. Hamady, EdD, MS, RD, LD, FAND, and Amy L. Morgan, PhD, FACSM

LEARNING OBJECTIVES

- Understand the uses and classifications of BMI.
- Define body composition and its use in the assessment of an athlete.
- State the differences, strengths, and weaknesses of specific body composition techniques.
- Interpret guidelines for the use and measurement of body composition in athletes of all abilities.
- Determine the appropriate timing and frequency of body composition measurements.
- Describe the overall limitations of measuring body composition in athletes.

INTRODUCTION

Anthropometric measurements, such as body weight, height, and waist circumference, along with body composition, are key components for assessing athletes. Monitoring changes in weight and height helps to evaluate the growth of a young athlete and can serve as a predictor of health and wellness in adulthood. Assessment of body composition can also be an indicator of energy balance, effects of training, and overall disease risk. The purpose of this chapter is to define body weight and body composition, review anthropometric measures that can be used as screening tools of health status, describe body composition measurement techniques, and illustrate how diet can assist an athlete in achieving body composition goals. For the purposes of this chapter, the standards discussed apply to sex assigned at birth. Research is emerging in some areas of practice regarding athletes who are transgender; however, the evidence available at this point is insufficient for general conclusions to be drawn. Future editions of this text will need to reevaluate and include the evidence as it emerges.

ANTHROPOMETRIC MEASUREMENTS

Weight, Height, and BMI

Weight and height are the most common anthropometric measurements taken during an assessment. To ensure accuracy, the athlete's weight should be taken with a calibrated scale and not as a self-reported measurement. Depending on the purpose of the visit (eg, weekly diet reviews, quarterly assessments, or seasonal physicals), weights should be taken on the same scale at every visit for consistency. The athlete's height should be taken without shoes on a stadiometer, which can be attached to the scale or affixed to the wall for reliability. For young athletes who are still growing, height should be measured at every visit to assess changes. A height can then be taken at the yearly physical once it has been determined that the athlete has achieved their adult height, the timing of which can vary from person to person.

Weight and height can be used to determine BMI. BMI is often thought of as a measure of body composition; however, it does not provide any values related to body fat or muscle content. BMI, described by the Centers for Disease Control and Prevention as a potential indicator of "high body fatness," is calculated as weight in kilograms divided by height in meters squared. Because there is no way to determine percent body fat from this method, BMI is a tool used to "screen for weight categories that may lead to health problems." The use of BMI is limited in athletes, primarily because high muscularity may lead to an elevated BMI without high body fatness. In many cases, athletes may be characterized as obese using standard ranges for BMI when, in fact, they are not overly fat. Thus, even though BMI is universally available and affordable and requires minimal time to assess, it is useful only as a screening tool and not as a measure of body composition. Table 9.1 lists BMI classifications for adults.[1]

TABLE 9.1 BMI Classifications[1]

Classification	Range
Underweight	<18.5
Healthy weight	18.5-24.9
Overweight	25.0-29.9
Obesity (class I)	30.0-34.9
Obesity (class II)	35.0-39.9
Extreme obesity (class III)	≥40.0

Waist Circumference

Waist circumference can be used to identify an individual's distribution of fat and is therefore a marker of disease risk. Individuals who carry excess fat in their abdominal region (ie, visceral fat) can experience metabolic changes leading to insulin resistance, hypercholesterolemia, hormonal imbalances, and hypertension. As a result, these individuals are at higher risk for many chronic diseases, such as cardiovascular disease, diabetes, stroke, and certain cancers.[2,3] According to the National Institutes of Health (NIH), a healthy waist circumference measurement is less than 35 in (88 cm) for females and less than 40 in (102 cm) for males.[4]

There are several methods for measuring waist circumference. As noted by the American College of Sports Medicine (ACSM), practitioners should be aware of how the measurement was taken to provide consistent evaluation of disease risk stratification over time.[5] For example, NIH guidelines indicate that the waist measurement be taken as follows[6]:

- Locate the upper hip bone and the top of the right iliac crest.
- Place a measuring tape in a horizontal place around the abdomen at the level of the iliac crest.
- Before reading the tape measure, ensure that the tape is snug, but does not compress the skin, and is parallel to the floor.
- Take the measurement at the end of a normal expiration.

Waist-to-Hip Ratio

Waist-to-hip ratio (WHR) is calculated by dividing an individual's waist circumference by their hip circumference (both in the same units, eg, inches). This measurement is a fast method to assess a person's overall health based on fat distribution.[7] This value is a measure not of body composition but rather of fat distribution and should be used only in adults and not in children. Studies in athletes indicate that WHR does not estimate overall adiposity and that there are sex differences in how WHR relates to body fat percentage.[8,9] There are also differences based on ethnicity. Although data are limited, populations of Asian descent may require alternative classifications. Table 9.2 on page 208 presents the World Health Organization (WHO) classifications of health risk based on WHR. Ensuring appropriate measurements is essential in determining an accurate ratio. Refer to the WHO guidelines for more detailed instructions on how to take these measurements.[10]

TABLE 9.2 Waist-to-Hip Ratio Health Risk Classifications[10]

Health risk	Men	Women
Low	<0.95	<0.80
Moderate	0.96-1.0	0.81-0.85
High	≥1.0	≥0.86

Waist-to-Height Ratio

Another indicator of adiposity is the waist-to-height ratio (WHtR), which is a predictor of risk for obesity-related cardiometabolic illnesses.[11] WHtR is calculated by dividing an individual's waist circumference by their height (both in the same units, eg, inches). A WHtR of 0.5 signifies risk, whereas 0.6 indicates substantial risk. These markers apply to all people, regardless of age, sex, and ethnicity.[12] As with other measurements, ensuring accuracy of the protocols used to measure waist size and height is essential for proper assessment and feedback over time. Evidence for a correlation between WHtR and lean body mass is limited; therefore, WHtR is best used as a screening tool for overweight, obesity, and distribution of adipose tissue.

BODY COMPOSITION

Definition of Body Composition

When people hear the term *body composition*, their immediate reaction is often to think about body fat and not about the other components that contribute to the overall makeup of the body (eg, muscle, water, bone, minerals). Body composition can be described in terms of a 2-compartment, 3-compartment, or 4-compartment model. For the purposes of this chapter, the 2-compartment model will be used. The 2-compartment model consists of (1) lean body mass (LBM), which includes muscle, bone, and organs, and (2) fat mass. Whereas fat-free mass (FFM) is described as all lipid-free components of the body (ie, water, muscle, bone, connective tissue, organs), LBM encompasses fat-free mass plus essential body fat.[13] Although not exactly synonymous, it is important to note that the descriptions *lean body mass* and *fat-free mass* are often used interchangeably. In the context of sport, body composition can contribute to performance, injury risk, and effective goal setting and intervention.

In the sport or athletic setting, the assessment of body composition is inclusive of bone, fat, and muscle, although there is often a focus on body weight or amount of fat. Although it may be important to measure body weight or fat to gauge or track the health of an athlete, there are many events in which individuals of various sizes and body compositions can be successful, such as baseball, softball, football, soccer, basketball, and tennis. For other events, body weight and composition may significantly affect an athlete's performance, perhaps because there are weight classes (eg, boxing, wrestling) or because the athlete needs to propel their body through space (eg, diving, gymnastics) in an efficient, athletic, and artistic manner. In any case, the sports dietitian must work with the athlete on an individual basis to develop and assess plans for maintaining a healthy level of body weight, fat mass, and LBM. Refer to Box 9.1 for a summary of reasons for measuring body composition in athletes.

BOX 9.1 Why Measure Body Composition in Athletes?

In the assessment of many sports medicine professionals, there are 3 reasons why one may choose to measure weight or body composition in athletes:

- to address concerns about the health of an athlete,
- to determine contributions to performance, and
- to best prepare an individual for a sport-specific performance.

These reasons are not independent, and in most cases, body composition is measured for some combination of these factors.

Body Composition to Gauge Health

Determining whether an individual has too much or too little body fat is important, as both situations are cause for concern for long-term health. Body fat is typically reported as a percentage of total body weight (percent body fat). The reference values for percent fat are determined in large part by sex, age, and activity level.[14] In general, males have lower body fat percentages than females, and body fat content tends to increase with age, particularly for those over the age of 40 years. As one might suspect, athletes and highly active individuals are leaner and have a lower fat percentages than those who are less active.

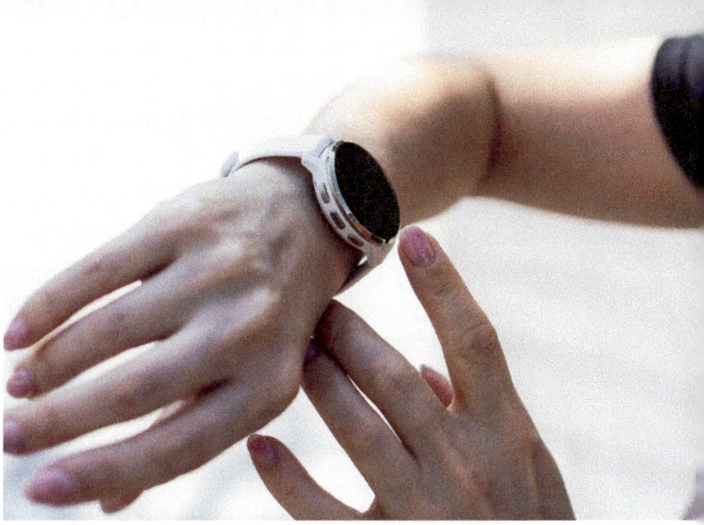

However, all individuals have a certain amount of body fat, known as *essential body fat*, that is imperative to overall health. Essential fat is found in vital organs, such as the heart, lungs, liver, spleen, kidneys, intestines, and muscles, as well as the central nervous system. In females, essential fat is also necessary to produce sex-specific hormones. Typically, females require about 10% to 13% essential fat and males require 2% to 5% essential fat.[15]

In general, high levels of fat are associated with a multitude of health concerns, including cardiovascular disease, type 2 diabetes, metabolic disease, and some cancers.[2,3] Other secondary issues such as joint problems (eg, osteoarthritis), limited functional movement, and compromised independence can result from long-term obesity.[16] Conversely, low levels of fat are also problematic, primarily in females. Females with too little fat may be at risk for reduced or no menstrual cycle, decreasing estrogen levels, and impaired bone development. These physiological changes can increase the risk of developing bone loss and osteoporosis later in life, despite participation in activities that are associated with bone health in other females of a similar age.[17-19] Changes in bone health and menstrual cycle can also be indicators for an assessment of relative energy deficiency in sport (REDs; see Chapter 10, Energy Balance, and Chapter 18, Disordered Eating in Athletes, for more information).

Body Composition as a Contributor to Performance

Perhaps one of the best uses of body composition measures in athletes is to assess muscle mass (ie, LBM), particularly over time. If an individual is underperforming, either in practice or in competition, low levels of LBM may be a contributing factor because the athlete does not have adequate muscle to perform at a level necessary to compete and/or has excess fat mass that is hindering performance. Refer to Chapter 11, Weight Management, for more information.

Lean body mass can also be assessed periodically to identify trends in body composition. For example, measuring body composition at preseason, midseason, and postseason will provide longitudinal evidence of gains or losses of muscle and fat across the season. If a coach has noted a drop in an athlete's performance, the change may be due to a loss of muscle. In this case, the athlete must work with strength and conditioning coaches, who can provide appropriate exercises to maintain muscle, and with a registered dietitian nutritionist (RDN), who can provide guidance on the most appropriate dietary intake, so the athlete can maintain performance and muscle mass across a season.

Body Composition to Best Prepare an Athlete for Performance

The assessment of body composition should not be a one-time measure during the season; it can be helpful for planning training regimens during the offseason as well. As discussed previously, an athlete should work with strength and conditioning coaches, along with an RDN, to develop a plan to regain any LBM lost during a season and to determine how to prevent such a loss from happening in the next season. Conversely, if an athlete gained weight or fat mass after the season, the athlete should work with the strength and conditioning staff and an RDN to achieve an optimal body composition before the next season. Trying to make significant changes to body composition during the season is not advised because of the potential for adverse effects on performance or endurance. The overall goal is to begin the preseason in peak condition to maximize the benefits of the training sessions. The Changing Body Composition section later in this chapter offers more details about this issue.

TECHNIQUES FOR ESTIMATING BODY COMPOSITION

A variety of methods can be used to estimate body composition. The techniques covered in this chapter include underwater weighing (UWW), dual-energy x-ray absorptiometry (DXA), air displacement plethysmography (ADP), bioelectrical impedance analysis (BIA), and skinfold thickness, as these are the most commonly used techniques. For each technique, a short description is provided, along with a discussion of the considerations for its use. For the purposes of this chapter, the techniques are divided into 2 categories: (1) traditional clinical techniques (ie, BIA and skinfolds) and (2) advanced techniques (ie, UWW, ADP, DXA). Newer methods include ultrasound and 3D body composition assessments; however, at present, these techniques are studied less and data are not readily available. For these reasons, they are not included in this chapter.

Until recently, all techniques for living humans were compared with UWW, also referred to as hydrodensitometry. Although UWW is often described as the gold standard and has traditionally been considered the criterion method, it is time intensive and less comfortable than numerous other techniques.[14] (For an excellent overview of body composition measurement techniques, see *ACSM's Resources for the Exercise Physiologist*[5] or *Advanced Fitness Assessment and Exercise Prescription*.[20]) In addition, UWW is mainly available within an exercise physiology laboratory and is thus less accessible than other methods. Newer techniques, such as DXA, are more precise and technologically advanced than UWW.[5] When determining which technique is best suited for a specific program or athlete population, factors to consider include cost, precision, comfort level, and time required per test (for both the athlete and the technician). Generally, skinfold thickness or ADP can provide relevant information while being cost-effective and efficient. Table 9.3 provides an outline of the techniques covered in this chapter.

TABLE 9.3 Factors to Consider When Choosing a Body Composition Technique

Method	Availability	Accuracy	Time		Cost
			Training[a]	Test	
Bioelectrical impedance analysis (BIA)	Limited	Moderate to high[b]	10-60 min, depending on device	1-3 min	Low to medium
Skinfold thickness	High	Moderate to high[b]	3-6 mo	~5 min	Low
Underwater weighing (UWW)	Limited	Historical gold standard	≥2 h	5-15 min	Medium
Air displacement plethysmography (ADP)	Limited	High	1-2 h through company	≤10 min	High
Dual-energy x-ray absorptiometry (DXA)	Limited	Modern standard	Formal certificate	≤15 min	High

[a] Training time for test administrator.
[b] Accuracy depends on external factors, such as participants following pretest precautions and availability of a trained technician.

Traditional Clinical Techniques

Two traditional clinical techniques have been identified: BIA and measures of skinfold thickness.

BIOELECTRICAL IMPEDANCE ANALYSIS

BIA involves the use of a device that allows a minimal, undetectable, electrical current to pass through the body. This device measures the resistance to the flow of the electrical current; in general, there is more resistance to flow in an individual with less water-containing tissue. As fat contains little water and muscle is well fortified with water, more resistance is indicative of an individual with a higher percent body fat, and less resistance is indicative of an individual with a higher percent LBM.

One of the benefits of BIA is that it is a rather quick measurement (1–3 minutes per person), so many athletes can be tested in a short time. It is also a fairly accurate measure of the fat percentage (ie, standard error of the estimate is between 2.7% and 6.3% compared with UWW) when high-quality equipment is used *and* when stringent pretest criteria are maintained (Box 9.2).[20] One additional benefit is that some research-grade devices can also provide segmental analysis. However, one should note that, in athletes, BIA tends to underestimate the fat percentage compared with UWW.[21]

BOX 9.2 Bioelectrical Impedance Analysis Pretest Criteria[20]

No food or drink within 4 hours

No moderate or vigorous exercise for 12 hours

No alcohol consumption for 48 hours

Maintenance of test position for a minimum of 5 minutes

The quality of BIA devices varies substantially; within reason, more expensive devices tend to be more accurate. The cost of BIA machines ranges from very inexpensive models that test using 2 points of contact (about $50 for a home model) to more costly, research-grade machines that can cost up to $18,000 and may not be locally available. These research-grade machines have up to 8 points of contact directly with the skin or through electrodes affixed to the skin. As stated previously, adherence to pretest criteria is critical for accuracy. Because results are determined by body water, testing in anything but a normally hydrated state (euhydration) will negatively affect the results.

SKINFOLD THICKNESS

The skinfold thickness measurement is used to estimate percent body fat. This measurement is readily available, fairly accurate, and low cost, and it requires only about 5 minutes per athlete. The following 3 factors can affect the accuracy of an estimate of percent fat by skinfold thickness:

- First, measurements need to be taken at the correct anatomical location. (Figures 9.1 through 9.7 on page 212 provide images of these measurements.) Each standardized site is clearly demarcated by bony landmarks.[14,22] Both the identification of these locations and the measurement of the skinfold thicknesses must be performed when the athlete is in the correct body position (ie, anatomical position without twisting or bending to make the site more available to the tester). Twisting and bending can affect the skin and thus the size of the subsequent fold.
- A second contributor to accuracy is equipment. A variety of calipers are available, but inexpensive ones with thin spring mechanisms may stretch or lose recoil over time, changing the force of the caliper on the skinfold. This may have an impact on the measured size of the folds over time. For high-quality fold measurements, either Lange or Harpenden calipers are recommended, as these tools provide a constant pressure of approximately 10 g/mm^2.
- Finally, skinfold thickness is most accurately measured when performed by a trained technician. Training includes learning from an expert and practicing until repeated measures at the same, properly identified site are consistent to within 1 to 3 mm. This is a learned skill.

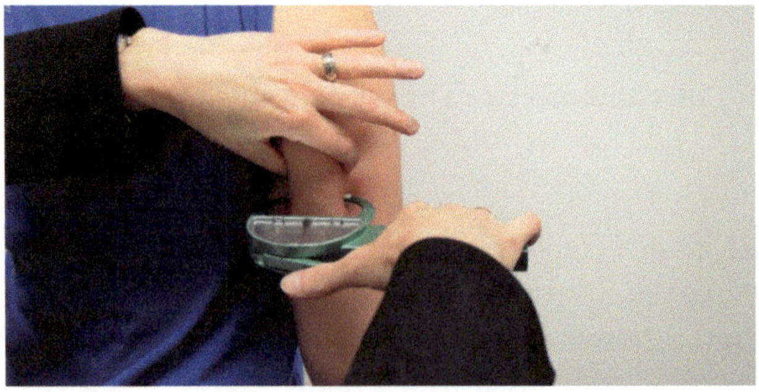

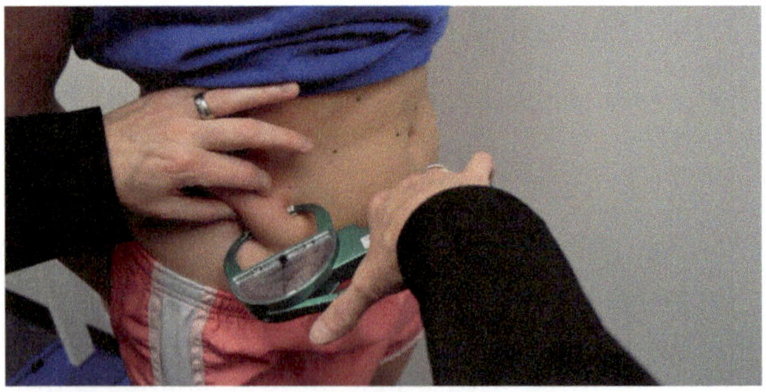

FIGURE 9.1 Demonstration of the triceps skinfold measurement A vertical pinch is made on the midline of the posterior (back) surface of the arm (over the triceps muscle), midway between the acromion process (bony tip of the shoulder) and olecranon process (approximately the elbow joint).

FIGURE 9.2 Demonstration of the iliac crest (suprailiac) skinfold measurement A diagonal pinch downward and medially (approximately 45°) is made immediately above the iliac crest on a vertical line from the front of the axilla (armpit).

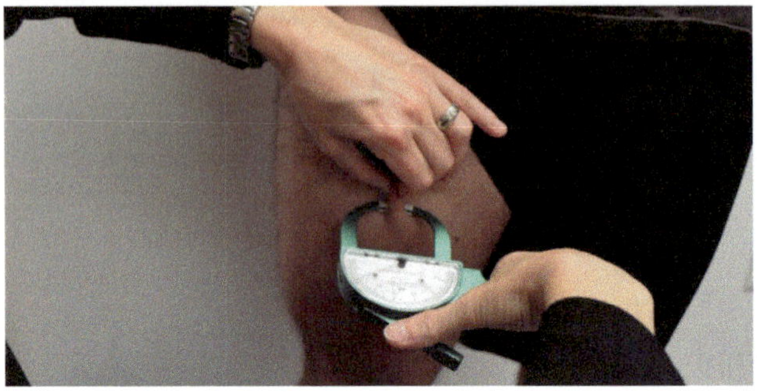

FIGURE 9.3 Demonstration of the thigh skinfold measurement A vertical pinch is made at the midpoint of the anterior (front) surface of the thigh, midway between the patella (kneecap) and the inguinal fold (crease at the top of the thigh).

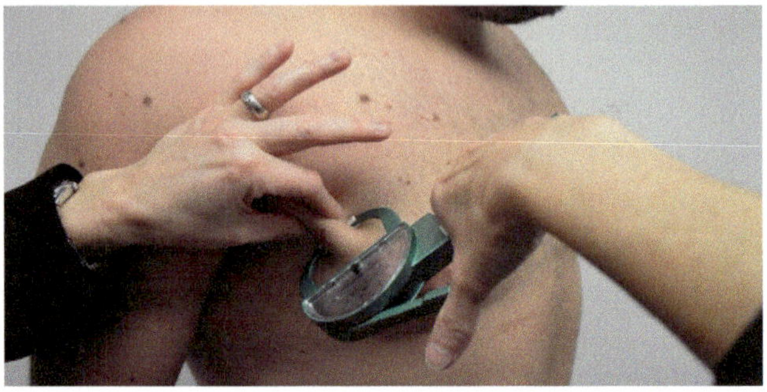

FIGURE 9.4 Demonstration of the (pectoral) chest skinfold measurement, usually only for males A diagonal pinch (about 45°) is taken on a line midway between the axilla and the nipple.

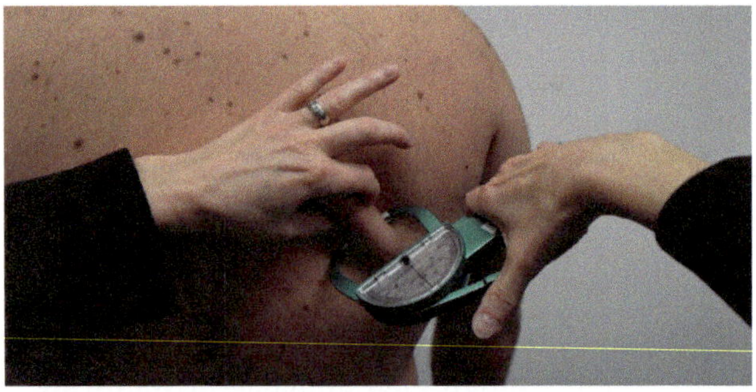

FIGURE 9.5 Demonstration of the subscapular skinfold measurement A diagonal pinch (at about 45°) is made following the natural fold of the skin 1 to 2 cm below the inferior angle of the scapula on a line running laterally (away from the body).

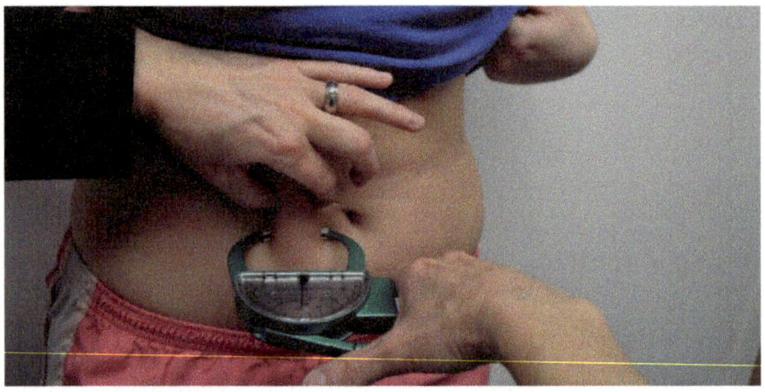

FIGURE 9.6 Demonstration of the abdominal skinfold measurement A vertical pinch is made 1 to 2 cm to the right of the umbilicus.

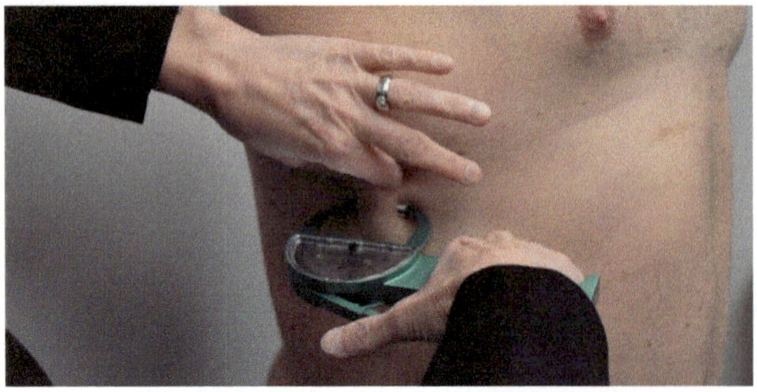

FIGURE 9.7 Demonstration of the midaxillary skinfold measurement With the athlete's arm held at chest height, a vertical pinch is made on a horizontal line extending from the bottom of the xiphoid process (breastbone) to the side of the torso until below the axilla (armpit).

When the aforementioned criteria are met and the proper equations (refer to Box 9.3[23-26]) are used for the specific population that is being tested, estimates of percent fat from skinfold thickness are within about 3.5% of UWW values.[23]

BOX 9.3 Skinfold Analysis Equations[24-26]

Generalized skinfold equations for 3 sites[24, 25]

Males (chest, abdomen, thigh)
Body density = 1.10938 – 0.0008267(sum of 3 skinfolds) + 0.0000016(sum of 3 skinfolds)^2 – 0.0002574(age)

Males (chest, triceps, subscapular)
Body density = 1.1125025 – 0.0013125(sum of 3 skinfolds) + 0.0000055(sum of 3 skinfolds)^2 – 0.0002574(age)

Females (triceps, suprailiac, thigh)
Body density = 1.0994921 – 0.0009929(sum of 3 skinfolds) + 0.0000023(sum of 3 skinfolds)^2 – 0.0001392(age)

Females (triceps, suprailiac, abdominal)
Body density = 1.089733 – 0.0009245(sum of 3 skinfolds) + 0.0000025(sum of 3 skinfolds)^2 – 0.0000979(age)

Calculation of fat percentage from body density[26]

Body fat (%) = (495/body density) – 450

As indicated earlier, the cost of skinfold thickness testing is fairly low. It includes the cost of calipers, which range from about $20 to $500, and any fees charged by the technician. The time per athlete depends mainly on the number of sites measured. For best results, 3 measurements should be taken at each site, and the median value should be used. Although measuring more sites results in higher accuracy, a reasonable trade-off may be available because measuring more sites takes more time and "good enough" values can usually be achieved with fewer sites. The number of sites should be determined by the purpose of the data. For health and across-season data, fewer sites (minimum of 3) can be used. If the data are to be used for research, more sites (eg, 5 to 7, depending on the equation) are appropriate.

In terms of availability, purchasing or gaining access to calipers is easy, whereas the availability of a trained technician may be more difficult. Because of the need to measure each site 3 times, the skinfold thickness method is a bit more time intensive than BIA, requiring about 5 minutes per athlete. However, skinfold thickness can be measured with limited pretest considerations, improving accessibility. Caution should be exercised if those being tested are sweaty or have used lotion at the test sites as the skin will be slippery and more difficult to pinch, reducing accuracy. Finally, keep in mind that if measurements will be repeated at the end of the season, athletes should report in the same state and measurements should be taken by the same trained technician as in previous sessions to ensure consistency.

Advanced Techniques

The 3 most common advanced methods of measuring body composition include UWW, ADP, and DXA. Although all 3 are considered highly accurate measures of body composition, they all also require specialized, costly equipment. Therefore, accessibility to such options is usually limited to hospitals or large universities that may have this equipment available, often through an exercise physiology laboratory. Because of equipment cost and the specialized nature of the tests, it is not unusual for charges to range from $20 to $200 per athlete depending on the technique used and the geographical area. Costs are typically higher for DXA testing. Refer to Box 9.4 for a breakdown of equipment and maintenance costs.

BOX 9.4 Equipment and Maintenance Costs for Advanced Body Composition Techniques

Underwater weighing

Initial cost	$2,000 to $15,000 Depends on the use of pool, newly built, or a commercially available tank
Estimated yearly costs	Minimal; water for filling, filters, and electrical costs for pump

Air displacement plethysmography (BOD POD)

Initial cost	$40,000 to $60,000 new Depends on testing options
Estimated yearly costs	$4,000 to $5,000 under a maintenance contract

Dual-energy x-ray absorptiometry

Initial cost	$90,000 to $200,000 Depends on model and options
Estimated yearly costs	$5,000 to $10,000 under a maintenance contract

Of these 3 techniques, ADP (measured with a device marketed under the brand name BOD POD) and DXA are the best options in terms of athlete comfort during the test. Generally, ADP and DXA can be completed in 10 minutes or less. The time required for UWW varies by individual; a minimum of 3 to 5 tests per session is required. The first time someone experiences UWW, there is a learning curve that may require extra time. Moreover, participant comfort plays a large role in how long each person will take. With repeated measures, time per test will diminish.

UNDERWATER WEIGHING

UWW has long been considered the gold standard in body composition assessment and has been used in exercise physiology laboratories for more than 50 years. This test requires an individual to be submerged underwater while suspended from a calibrated scale or load cell while expiring as much air as possible from the lungs. Weight in the water is measured after all of the air has been expired and the person is motionless.

Limits to this technique include the discomfort experienced upon maximal expiration; the difficulty testing those not comfortable in the water; and the challenges of accessibility for those who use wheelchairs, because ladders are often required to get in and out of the water. Because UWW is the method involved in much of the classic body composition research, many regression equations have been derived using this method as the standard.

AIR DISPLACEMENT PLETHYSMOGRAPHY

ADP requires an individual to sit in an egg-shaped chamber wearing tight-fitting clothing. This technique measures body volume by determining the amount of air displaced when the athlete is seated in the chamber. The commercial device most associated with this technique is the BOD POD.[27] According to the manufacturer, people who should not be tested in this device are individuals weighing more than

250 kg (550 lb) (equipment scale limit) and those with diagnosed claustrophobia. With some assistance, accessibility is available to those who use wheelchairs. Results from ADP are comparable to those from UWW in most populations (within 2% to 3%), although ADP has been shown to overestimate the fat percentage in some populations (eg, collegiate female athletes[28]) and to underestimate the fat percentage in others (eg, collegiate football players[29]). Practitioners should note that the equations programmed into the BOD POD software are for the general population and are not specific to athletes. Figures 9.8 and 9.9 show images of an individual in a BOD POD.

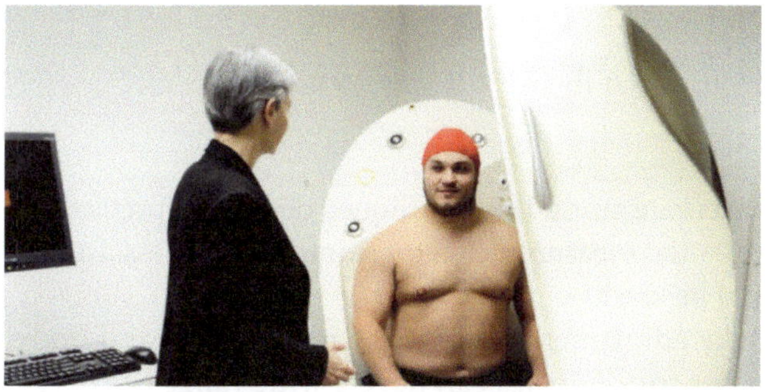

FIGURE 9.8 View of a participant seated in the BOD POD

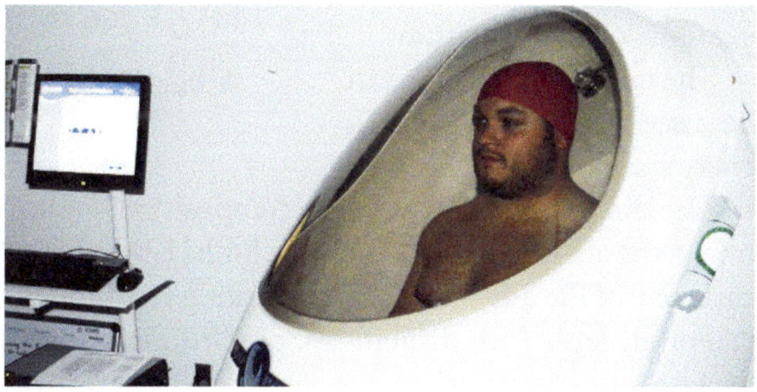

FIGURE 9.9 View of a participant being tested in the BOD POD

DUAL-ENERGY X-RAY ABSORPTIOMETRY

DXA is a tool that has been used mainly to determine bone density in medical or research settings. However, because this technology can measure the 3 compartments of bone, muscle, and fat, use of specialized software with DXA can also provide both muscle mass and body fat measurements. In addition, DXA allows for the determination of total body and regional (eg, trunk, limbs) values. Participant comfort is not a concern because athletes can be tested in any light clothing without zippers or jewelry. Note, however, that people who may be pregnant should not be tested using this technology. One challenge in testing athletes may be body size; extremely large or tall individuals may extend beyond the range of the scanner or may need to lie in a more cramped position, distorting regional measures. Whereas exposure to x-rays may be an initial concern, a whole-body DXA measurement is comparable to background radiation levels.[5] For athletes with spinal cord injuries, DXA is the most accurate tool because segmental or regional measurements can be made.

ATHLETES WITH DISABILITIES

As stated previously, DXA is the preferred method for assessing body composition in athletes with disabilities because it allows for segmental measurements.[30] (Note that some BIA analyzers can provide segmental analysis as well.) For example, if an athlete is paralyzed from the waist down, the athlete may have muscle atrophy in the lower half of the body, resulting in higher body fat in the lower half of the body compared to that in the upper half. Because only the upper torso is used for sport, determining the fat percentage for that section of the body is more important than obtaining the overall fat mass.

In addition, for athletes with amputations or spinal cord injuries, caloric intake recommendations may need to be adjusted as a result of changes in overall body mass and muscle mass. Athletes who have had an amputation will need to have their energy needs and weight goals adjusted according to which limb was removed. Table 9.4 provides more information on calculating

TABLE 9.4 Percent Weight by Body Part

Body part	Percent weight of body part
Arm	5.0%
Foot	1.5%
Portion of leg below the knee	5.9%
Portion of leg above the knee	8.1%
Whole leg	16.0%

ideal body weight (IBW) for individuals with missing limbs. To determine IBW, start with the Hamwi equation and then subtract the percentage of body weight that has been amputated.[31] Box 9.5 provides an example of this equation.

BOX 9.5 Sample Equation for Below-the-Knee Amputation

Example for a 5-ft 10-in male

Hamwi equation for ideal body weight (IBW) for males:
106 lb for 5 ft plus 6 lb for every inch thereafter

IBW = 166 lb × 5.9% (weight of amputated area) = 9.8 lb

Adjusted IBW = 166 lb – 9.8 lb = 156.2 lb ± 10%

The new adjusted IBW can be used when determining energy and weight goals for the athlete. Assessment of body composition should be accurate using the techniques described previously, unless the athlete does not have the limbs needed for the essential measurements for skinfold thickness. In that case, one of the advanced body fat testing techniques should be used.

For athletes with disabilities, practitioners should make adjustments for energy needs, IBW, and body fat testing as appropriate. For example, athletes with spinal cord injuries can have a wide range of energy needs (23–64 kcal/kg) depending on sex, sport, and initial level of training.[32] Studies have shown that in those with spinal cord injuries, 24-hour resting energy expenditure can be 75% of control values. This is related to muscle atrophy and a reduced sympathetic nervous system.[33] Therefore, indirect calorimetry is the preferred method for determining needs. If indirect calorimetry is not available, a thorough nutrition assessment including food records, weight records, and performance evaluations should be used to adjust total energy recommendations.

CHANGING BODY COMPOSITION

After analyzing the results of body composition testing, a nutrition practitioner may determine that the athlete should make changes in LBM, fat mass, or a combination of the two. If a change is desired, the athlete would benefit from the assistance of a strength and conditioning coach in addition to an RDN. In particular, diet alone cannot alter body composition—rather, a combination of exercise and diet is needed. This section reviews some practical nutritional implications for changing body composition, including the appropriate time for athletes to change body composition, how to monitor changes, potential effects on performance, and limitations in assessing body composition. Chapter 11 provides more information on diet strategies for weight loss or weight gain.

Goals for changing body composition should be established on an annual training cycle to promote realistic and timely approaches to changes in behavior or training schedules. Otherwise, some athletes may feel pressure to engage in unhealthy practices that could result in negative outcomes on performance and health. Some athletes, such as offensive and defensive linemen, shot putters, and powerlifters, may want to gain lean tissue in the offseason to start the season stronger than the year before. During this training period, the clinician should assess weight weekly to determine whether weight gain is occurring too rapidly or too slowly. Target weight gain should be 0.25 to 0.5 kg/wk to avoid negative side effects.[34] Rapid weight gain can cause adverse metabolic reactions, such as changes in hormone levels, increases in triglyceride production, and decreases in mitochondrial efficiency.[35] Adjustments in calorie levels should be based on the amount of weight gained until the final weight goal is achieved.

After determining body composition, some athletes may choose to focus on decreasing fat mass after their season is over while trying to either maintain or gain LBM. To achieve this goal, the athlete should work with an RDN to establish a calorie goal and macronutrient distribution tailored to individual needs based on training schedules and body weight or composition goals. To decrease fat mass, the diet will need to have a calorie deficit yet still provide adequate protein to promote the maintenance or growth of LBM during high-intensity training with a range of 1.6 to 2.4 g/kg/d.[36,37] This range is influenced by the amount of the calorie deficit, the intensity of the training, the quality of protein consumed, and the distribution of protein during the day. To minimize the use of protein for energy so that it will be available for synthesis, adequate calories—mainly in the form of carbohydrate—should be provided to meet caloric needs.[38] Weight loss should occur slowly. Athletes may be able to maintain FFM and performance at a greater level when weight loss is limited to less than 1% per week.[31] The goal is to establish the smallest deficit in calories that produces the desired results to avoid metabolic adaptations.[35] When weight loss occurs too quickly, the athlete loses more LBM and is at risk for negative effects once the weight-loss phase ends.[31,35] Some of these negative effects include rapid weight gain, increased hunger, and alterations to energy expenditure.

Practitioners should focus on both diet and exercise when the athlete desires to change fat mass and maintain or gain LBM over a period of more than 2 weeks. In fact, diet alone can lead to more loss of LBM when trying to lose weight.[39] Therefore, exercise—namely, resistance training—needs to accompany the changes in diet; aerobic exercise could potentially contribute to the loss of LBM.[40] It is the combination of exercise and proper nutrition that will bring the desired changes to body composition to achieve personal goals and maximize performance. Refer to Chapters 10 and 11 for more complete discussions of energy balance and weight management, respectively.

Timing of Body Composition Changes

Sports RDNs should also discuss the timing of weight-loss or weight-gain interventions with athletes. Experts do not recommend starting an aggressive plan to alter body composition during the active season. Instead, the athlete should address body composition goals in the offseason so they can begin preseason in peak condition. The macronutrient distribution recommended for changing body composition is often too low for carbohydrate intake to meet the needs for optimal performance.[39] Given that all athletes have different needs and training goals, there will be some exceptions to the rule. However, any attempt to lose weight or fat mass always involves the potential to lose LBM as well, which could negatively affect an athlete during the competitive season. In addition, nutritional barriers to the management of body composition may also exist, such as limited access to healthy foods, lack of time or skills for food preparation, lack of daily routine, and exposure to catering with "all you care to eat" portion sizes and energy-dense foods.[41] Therefore, the role of the clinician during the offseason is not only to help with body composition goals but also to help find creative and sustainable solutions to these barriers.

Frequency of Measurements, Measurement Error, and Reporting of Results

As a general rule, the minimum time between assessments of body composition should be 3 months. Changes in body composition are not usually measurable in shorter periods, largely because of the variability in measurements for most methods. For example, suppose the first time an athlete is assessed, their percent body fat measurement is 17%. If the assumption is that the measurement error is within 3%, the percent fat is actually 17% ±3% (ie, in the range between 14% and 20%). If a subsequent measure indicates a value of 15% and the same error is assumed, the individual's percent fat is then between 12% and 18%. In this example, the conclusion that a change in the individual's body composition has changed is not definitive because of the overlap in percent body fat from the 2 measurements. Therefore, measurements taken too frequently may give a false sense of change when it is possible that no relevant changes have occurred. When repeating measures for comparison purposes, best practice is to use the same technique each time (eg, if the first measurement used BIA, then BIA should be used each time thereafter), to minimize inflation of measurement errors.

Another concern regarding frequent assessments is the potential for negative alterations in dietary or activity behavior in response to findings. If the individual in the previous example is not made aware of the error inherent in the measurement, they may unnecessarily change behaviors to alter body composition, which could have negative long-term consequences. These examples highlight the caution that is necessary when interpreting and communicating results of body composition testing.

The preceding example highlights the importance of developing a plan for communicating body composition results. Sharing results with medical and/or sports medicine staff is appropriate. However, this information should be treated like other health information, and it should be shared only as it relates to the health and safety (mental and physical) of the athlete. Whether or not it is appropriate to share with each athlete is a decision to be made by the sports medicine personnel, taking into consideration factors such as risk to health, risk of negative behavior change, and level of athletic competition.

Practitoners should use caution when sharing body composition data with coaches, particularly if information related to the error of the method, appropriate ranges for health, and limitations of using body composition alone as a marker of performance have not been previously addressed. Coaches should be educated against using body composition (especially body fat) information as an independent variable that can or should be altered prior to an athlete receiving playing time.

Overall, each organization should come up with a protocol for both testing and reporting results. The protocol should be designed through conversations with representatives from the sports medicine staff, body composition experts, coaches, and athletes.

Girth Measurement

Although not an ideal tool for assessing body composition, many individuals rely on girth measures at certain sites as a short-term assessment (ie, usually in periods of less than 3 months) to determine whether an athlete is progressing in adding muscle or losing fat. There are several drawbacks to this approach. If an increase in girth size is noted at a specific site, this does not indicate whether the increase is due to an increase in muscle (a preferred improvement) or an increase in fat (not preferred). Conversely, a decrease in girth size at a specific site may indicate a loss from either muscle or fat. Because girth encompasses both components, there is no way to identify which interpretation is accurate. Coupling skinfold thickness with girth measurements does not solve this dilemma because appreciable changes in fat in less than 3 months cannot be measured accurately. This is an example of when reliance on other performance measures (eg, strength) is more appropriate for determining whether muscle quality has improved.

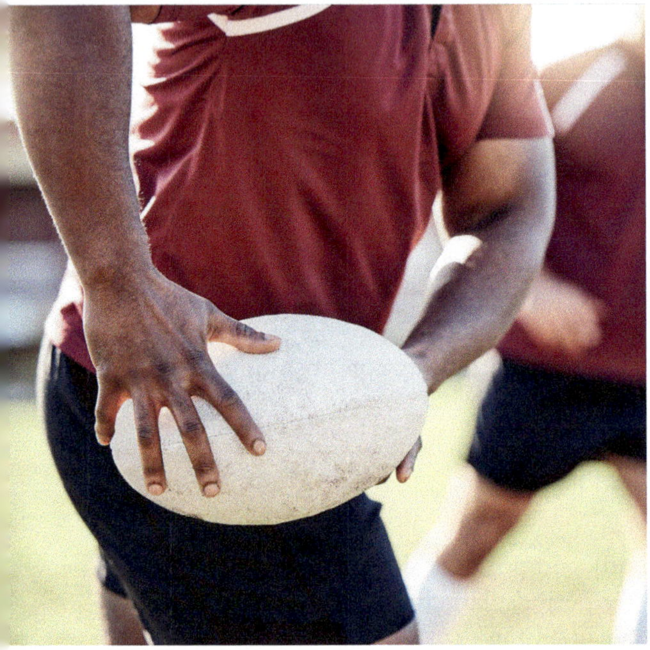

Limitations of Body Composition Data in Relation to Performance

Although body composition is a useful tool for the assessment of athletes, practitioners must exercise caution in the use and interpretation of these measures. There are many other variables that contribute much more significantly to athletic performance, such as muscular strength and endurance, cardiovascular endurance, and skill level within the sport. These variables can be improved and maximized through an appropriate training regimen. Daily performance (in training or competition) can be maximized through appropriate nutritional fueling and hydration status.

There are published values that represent common body composition ranges for a variety of sports.[42-45] What is clear from these numbers is that there is a large range between sexes and across sports. Note that these are averages, and they do not dictate guidelines that need to be enforced within a sport. Encouraging an athlete to meet a specific level of percent fat that is not realistic for the athlete's physiological makeup is counterproductive, particularly if performance has remained optimal.

The use of body composition is quite helpful for tracking both fat and muscle composition within an athlete and for identifying someone who may be at risk for health or performance concerns. Body composition measurements are best used to assist athletes in maximizing performance across a season.

ANTHROPOMETRIC SKILLS

Historically, instructional programs in dietetics have included very little, if any, hands-on anthropometric training. As a result, many current practicing RDNs lack these skills. More recently, many of these programs have created nutrition assessment courses that go beyond discussing anthropometrics to include hands-on training. Several options are available for RDNs who were never trained in measuring anthropometrics.

Many of the manufacturers of body composition equipment offer training with a representative. If an RDN works with a degreed exercise physiologist, the physiologist who has received training in anthropometrics may be able to train the RDN. Although nutrition and dietetics practitioners can also complete certification programs that include anthropometrics, such as those offered by the ACSM and the National Strength and Conditioning Association, these are often not skills-based assessments. Finally, the highly regarded International Society for the Advancement of Kinanthropometry trains and accredits people throughout the world in anthropometry. There are 4 levels of training, and they require reaccreditation every 4 years. (Visit the Society's website for more information: www.isak.global.)

SUMMARY

A variety of simple measurements can be used to screen for health status, along with body composition techniques that estimate levels of LBM and body fat. Professionals who work in sports nutrition or the sport performance field require proper training, not only in the techniques and measurements described in this chapter but also in the appropriate use of the information they provide. Body composition data should be assessed over time and can be part of the discussion involved in the evaluation of performance or in the planning of training regimens during the offseason. Each athlete should be evaluated based on their unique needs. Using these anthropometric data, RDNs and strength and conditioning professionals can work together with athletes to achieve their health and performance goals.

KEY TAKEAWAYS

Measures of percent fat in athletes should be used when there are concerns about health, performance, or injury, or to help determine levels of muscle or lean tissue.

Body composition measures provide a tool for tracking muscle and LBM across a season.

The technique selected for determining body composition should meet the needs of the situation while minimizing time and athlete discomfort.

RDNs and strength and conditioning professionals can work together to help athletes adjust LBM and percent fat, ideally during the offseason.

Other variables, such as muscular strength and endurance, cardiovascular endurance, and skill level within the sport, should be used in conjunction with body composition measures to assess an athlete's progression.

REFERENCES

1. Centers for Disease Control and Prevention. About adult BMI. Updated June 3, 2022. Accessed November 27, 2022. www.cdc.gov/healthyweight/assessing/bmi/index.html
2. Eckel RH. Obesity and heart disease: A statement for healthcare professionals from the Nutrition Committee, American Heart Association. *Circulation.* 1997;96(9):3248-3250. doi:10.1161/01.cir.96.9.3248
3. National Heart, Lung, and Blood Institute, National Institutes of Health. What is metabolic syndrome? Updated May 18, 2022. Accessed November 27, 2022. www.nhlbi.nih.gov/health/metabolic-syndrome
4. National Heart, Lung, and Blood Institute, National Institutes of Health. Overweight and obesity: causes and risk factors. Updated March 24, 2022. Accessed November 27, 2022. www.nhlbi.nih.gov/health/overweight-and-obesity/causes
5. Gibson AL, Chambliss H, Durstine JL, Jett DM, Ross LM, eds. *ACSM's Resources for the Exercise Physiologist: A Practical Guide for the Health Fitness Professional.* 3rd ed. Wolters Kluwer; 2022.
6. National Heart, Lung, and Blood Institute Obesity Education Initiative. The practical guide: identification, evaluation, and treatment of overweight and obesity in adults. Published October 2000. Accessed November 27, 2022. www.nhlbi.nih.gov/files/docs/guidelines/prctgd_c.pdf
7. Burgess L. Why is the hip-waist ratio important? *Medical News Today.* Updated September 17, 2017. Accessed November 27, 2022. www.medicalnewstoday.com/articles/319439#how-does-waist-to-hip-ratio-affect-health
8. Ashtary-Larky D, Vanani AN, Hosseini SA, Rafie R, Abbasnezhad A, Alipour M. Relationship between the body fat percentage and anthropometric measurements in athletes compared with non-athletes. *Zahedan J Res Med Sci.* 2018;20(2):e10422. doi:10.5812/zjrms.10422
9. Ramirez R, Gonzalez K. Body adiposity index in Colombian elite athletes: A comparison between the body mass index and other measures. *Rev Colomb Cardiol.* 2015;22(1):22-26. doi:10.1016/j.rccar.2014.10.008
10. Waist circumference and waist-hip ratio: Report of a WHO expert consultation. Geneva, 8-11 December 2008. Accessed November 27, 2022. https://apps.who.int/iris/bitstream/handle/10665/44583/9789241501491_eng.pdf;jsessionid=C7A8118F78F759B17FDA65CBE7E03779?sequence=1
11. Lee CM, Huxley RR, Wildman RP, Woodward M. Indices of abdominal obesity are better discriminators of cardiovascular risk factors than BMI: A meta-analysis. *J Clin Epidem.* 2008;61(7):646-653. doi:10.1016/j.jclinepi.2007.08.012
12. Swainson MG, Batterham AM, Tsakirides C, Rutherford ZH, Hind K. Prediction of whole-body fat percentage and visceral adipose tissue mass from five anthropometric variables. *PLoS One.* 2017;12(5):e0177175. doi:10.1371/journal.pone.0177175
13. McCardle WD, Katch FI, Katch VL. *Exercise Physiology: Nutrition, Energy and Human Performance.* 7th ed. Wolters Kluwer/Lippincott Williams & Wilkins; 2010.
14. American College of Sports Medicine; Liguori G, Feito Y, Fountaine C, Roy BA, eds. *ACSM's Guidelines for Exercise Testing and Prescription.* 11th ed. Wolters Kluwer; 2022.
15. American College of Sports Medicine. *ACSM's Health-Related Physical Fitness Assessment Manual.* 2nd ed. Wolters Kluwer/Lippincott Williams & Wilkins; 2008.
16. Marsh AP, Rejeski WJ, Espeland MA, et al. Muscle strength and BMI as predictors of major mobility disability in the Lifestyle Interventions and Independence for Elders pilot (LIFE-P). *J Gerontol A Biol Sci Med Sci.* 2011;66(12):1376-1383. doi:10.1093/gerona/glr158
17. Gordon CM, Nelson LM. Amenorrhea and bone health in adolescents and young women. *Curr Opin Obstet Gynecol.* 2003;15(5):377-384. doi:10.1097/00001703-200310000-00005
18. Nattiv A, Loucks AB, Manore MM, Sanborn CF, Sundgot-Borgen J, Warren MP; American College of Sports Medicine. American College of Sports Medicine Position Stand. The female athlete triad. *Med Sci Sports Exerc.* 2007;39(10):1867-1882. doi:10.1249/mss.0b013e318149f111
19. Maimoun L, Georgopoulos NA, Sultan C. Endocrine disorders in adolescent and young female athletes: Impact on growth, menstrual cycles and bone mass acquisition. *J Clin Endocrinol Metab.* 2014;99(11):4037-4050. doi:10.1210/jc.2013-3030
20. Gibson AL, Wagner DR, Heyward VH. *Advanced Fitness Assessment and Exercise Prescription.* 8th ed. Human Kinetics; 2019
21. Dixon CB, Deitrick RW, Pierce JR, Cutrufello PT, Drapeau LL. Evaluation of the BOD POD and leg-to-leg bioelectrical impedance analysis for estimating percent body fat in National Collegiate Athletic Association Division III collegiate wrestlers. *J Strength Cond Res.* 2005;19(1):85-91. doi:10.1519/14053.1
22. American College of Sports Medicine; Lohman TG, Milliken LA, eds. *ACSM's Body Composition Assessment.* Human Kinetics; 2020.
23. Heyward VH, Wagner DR. *Applied Body Composition Assessment.* 2nd ed. Human Kinetics; 2004.
24. Jackson AS, Pollock ML. Generalized equations for predicting body density of men. *Br J Nutr.* 1978:40(3):497-504. doi:10.1079/bjn19780152
25. Jackson AS, Pollock ML, Ward A. Generalized equations for predicting body density of women. *Med Sci Sports Exer.* 1980:12(3):175-182.
26. Siri WE. Body composition from fluid spaces and density: Analysis of methods. In: Brozek J, Henschel A, eds. *Techniques for Measuring Body Composition.* National Academy of Science; 1961:223-244.
27. COSMED - BOD POD GS-X - Gold Standard in Body Composition analysis. Accessed October 5,2023. www.cosmed.com/en/products/body-composition/bod-pod-gs-x

28. Vescovi JD, Hildebrandt L, Miller W, Hammer R, Spiller A. Evaluation of the BOD POD for estimating percent fat in female college athletes. *J Strength Cond Res.* 2002;16(4):599-605. doi:10.1007/s004210100459
29. Collins MA, Millard-Stafford ML, Sparling PB, et al. Evaluation of the BOD POD for assessing body fat in collegiate football players. *Med Sci Sports Exerc.* 1999;31(9):1350-1356. doi:10.1097/00005768-199909000-00019
30. Jones LM, Goulding A, Gerrard DF. DEXA: A practical and accurate tool to demonstrate total and regional bone loss, lean tissue loss, and fat mass gain in paraplegia. *Spinal Cord.* 1998;36(9):637-640. doi:10.1038/sj.sc.3100664
31. Garthe I, Raastad T, Refsnes PE, Koivisto A, Sundgot-Borgen J. Effect of two different weight-loss rates on body composition and strength and power-related performance in elite athletes. *Int J Sport Nutr Exerc Metab.* 2011;21(2);97-104. doi:10.1123/ijsnem.21.2.97
32. Figel K, Pritchett K, Pritchett R, Broad E. Energy and nutrient issues in athletes with spinal cord injury: are they at risk for low energy availability? *Nutrients.* 2018;10(8):1078. doi:10.3390/nu10081078
33. Price M. Energy expenditure and metabolism during exercise in persons with a spinal cord injury. *Sports Med.* 2010;40:681-696. doi:10.2165/11531960-000000000-00000
34. American College of Sports Medicine. American College of Sports Medicine position stand. Progression models in resistance training for healthy adults. *Med Sci Sports Exerc.* 2009;41(3):687-708. doi:10.1249/mss.0b013e3181915670
35. Trexler ET, Smith-Ryan AE, Norton LE. Metabolic adaptations to weight loss: implications for the athlete. *J Int Soc Sports Nutr.* 2014;11(1):7. doi:10.1186/1550-2783-11-7
36. Hector AJ, Phillips SM. Protein recommendations for weight loss in elite athletes: a focus on body composition and performance. *Int J Sport Nutr Exerc Metab.* 2018;28(2):170-177. doi:10.1123/ijsnem.2017-0273
37. Manore MM. Weight management for athletes and active individuals: a brief review. *Sports Med.* 2015;45(suppl 1):83-92. doi:10.1007/s40279-015-0401-0
38. Rodriguez NR, Vislocky LM, Gaine PC. Dietary protein, endurance exercise, and human skeletal-muscle protein turnover. *Curr Opin Clin Nutr Metab Care.* 2007;10(1):40-45. doi:10.1097/MCO.0b013e3280115e3b
39. Phillips S. Dietary protein for athletes: from requirements to metabolic advantage. *Appl Physiol Nutr Metab.* 2006;31(6):647-654. doi:10.1080/02640414.2011.619204
40. Phillips SM, Van Loon LJC. Dietary protein for athletes: From requirement to optimum adaptation. *J Sports Sci.* 2011;29(suppl 1):S29-S38. doi:10.1080/02640414.2011.619204
41. Thomas DT, Erdman KA, Burke LM. American College of Sports Medicine joint position statement. Nutrition and athletic performance. *Med Sci Sports Exerc.* 2016;48(3):543-568. doi:10.1249/MSS.0000000000000852
42. Jeukendrup A, Gleeson M. *Sport Nutrition.* 2nd ed. Human Kinetics; 2010
43. Bentzur KM, Kravitz L, Lockner DW. Evaluation of the BOD POD for estimating percent body fat in collegiate track and field female athletes: A comparison of four methods. *J Strength Cond Res.* 2008;22(6):1985-1991. doi:10.1519/JSC.0b013e318185f196
44. Glodt Baker AJ. *Evaluation of the Body Composition of Female Collegiate Athletes Using the BOD POD.* Master's thesis. University of Kentucky; 2012.
45. Ode JJ, Pivarnik JM, Reeves MJ, Knous JL. Body mass index as a predictor of percent body fat in college athletes and nonathletes. *Med Sci Sports Exerc.* 2007;39(3)403-409. doi:10.1249/01.mss.0000247008.19127.3e

CHAPTER 10

Energy Balance

Kaneen Gomez-Hixson, MS, RDN, CSSD, CDN

LEARNING OBJECTIVES

- Identify the key principles that underlie weight regulation from the perspective of bioenergetics.
- Explain the energy balance equation and the 4 specific principles important for understanding this equation.
- Describe the neuroendocrine regulation of energy balance.
- List the 4 components of total daily energy expenditure and identify the predictive equations and methods used to estimate resting metabolic rate.
- Recognize factors that affect energy expenditure and energy intake.
- Describe the complexities of the energy balance equation.

INTRODUCTION

Rapid increases in obesity throughout the United States and many other countries have spawned a weight-loss industry fraught with quick-fix approaches, diet gimmicks, misinformation, and confusion for the public. Athletes and other active individuals attempting to achieve a desired body weight and composition for reasons of health, metabolic fitness, and sports performance are not immune to marketing and uncertainty. A foundational understanding of the factors that affect energy balance will enable health practitioners to provide their clients with the most accurate scientific approaches possible and can help practitioners and clients sort through vast amounts of misinformation clamoring for their attention. Moreover, a greater understanding of what is involved in achieving energy balance will help health practitioners support their athletes' health and performance by helping them match their energy intake with their energy expenditure.

Energy balance is a function of energy input to the body (consumed as carbohydrates, proteins, fats, and alcohol) and the energy expenditure of the body at rest, during physical activity, and while processing ingested food. The magnitude and direction (positive or negative) of energy balance are reflected by changes in energy stores based on the equation

$$\Delta ES = EA - EEx$$

where ΔES is the change in bodily energy stores, EA is the energy ingested and available to the human body, and EEx is total body energy expenditure.[1] If food energy availability (input) and bodily energy expenditure (output) are equal, the energy stores in the body (glycogen, proteins, and fats) remain fairly constant over time, and the individual is said to be in energy balance or at zero energy balance.

A state of positive energy balance is characterized by greater energy input than expenditure, resulting in an increase in body energy stores. A state of negative energy balance is characterized by greater energy expenditure than energy intake, which causes a decrease in bodily energy stores. In this chapter, the fundamental principles of energy balance are examined, setting the stage for Chapter 11, which discusses dietary approaches to body weight regulation. The concepts presented in this chapter have relevance to competitive and recreational athletes attempting to alter body weight and composition and meet their fueling needs, as well as to nonathletes initiating diet and exercise changes. A central theme of the chapter is the dynamic nature of energy balance, wherein changes in energy intake can result in changes in energy expenditure and vice versa, which can have substantial effects on energy storage and body weight regulation and even on the health and athletic performance of athletes. Box 10.1 defines some of the terms that are used throughout this chapter.

BOX 10.1 Abbreviations Frequently Used in Energy Balance

ATP	adenosine triphosphate
BAT	brown adipose tissue
EA	energy available
EEx	total body energy expenditure
ΔES	change in bodily energy stores
ETS	electron transport system
ExEE	exercise energy expenditure
LEA	low energy availability
NAD	nicotinamide adenine dinucleotide
NEAT	nonexercise activity thermogenesis
PA	physical activity
PAEE	physical activity energy expenditure
PAL	physical activity level
RMR	resting metabolic rate
REDs	relative energy deficiency in sport
TCA cycle	tricarboxylic acid cycle (Krebs cycle)
TDEE	total daily energy expenditure
TEF	thermic effect of food

FOUNDATIONAL PRINCIPLES OF BIOENERGETICS

The key principles that underlie body weight regulation come from the field of bioenergetics. *Energy* is defined as the capacity to do work, and in the case of the human body, this work is a biological and physical function that includes a variety of cellular processes such as transport of ions against their concentration gradients, the synthesis of various compounds such as glycogen and proteins, and contraction of skeletal muscles for physical activity.

Figures 10.1 and 10.2 on page 224 provide schematic overviews of several fundamental aspects of energy metabolism in the human body. The energy available to athletes in food comes from macronutrients synthesized by plants and other animals (eg, proteins) and is used to synthesize the primary energy (the "currency") of the body: adenosine triphosphate (ATP). This energy contained in the chemical bonds of the ATP molecule is used for biological work. Upon hydrolysis of ATP to adenosine diphosphate (ADP) and inorganic phosphate (P_i), energy is released (exergonic process); this energy is used for vital cellular functions. The daily ATP requirement is met not by tapping into a large reservoir of stored ATP but primarily by rapidly resynthesizing ATP from ADP and P_i in the mitochondria.

If the ATP-resynthesizing processes were somehow impaired, the amount of stored, available ATP would be sufficient to provide only several seconds worth of energy to contracting skeletal muscle, thus highlighting the need for and ability of the body to recycle ADP into ATP.[2] This process of creating the high-energy phosphoanhydride bond of ATP from ADP and P_i is highly endergonic, with the necessary energy input coupled to the highly exergonic process of the oxidation of macronutrients, including carbohydrates, fatty acids, and deaminated amino acids. In oxidation reactions catalyzed by dehydrogenase enzymes, hydrogen atoms are removed from macronutrient intermediates by the coenzymes nicotinamide adenine dinucleotide (NAD^+) and flavin adenine dinucleotide (FAD), resulting in the reduction of these molecules to NADH and $FADH_2$, respectively. These reduced coenzymes, in turn, undergo oxidation in the electron transport system (ETS), where electrons are passed between conjugate redox pairs in the

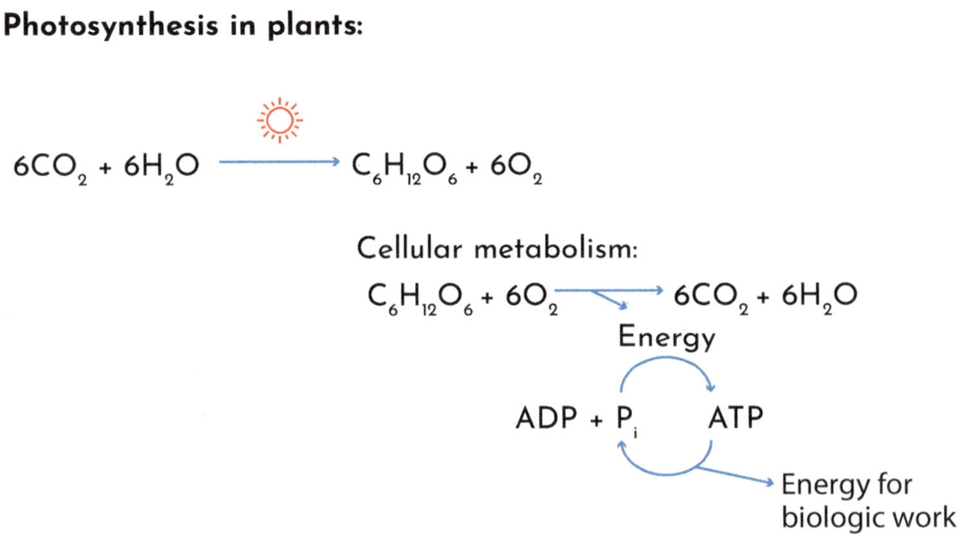

FIGURE 10.1 Plant photosynthesis and human glucose metabolism Synthesis of glucose in plants occurs in photosynthesis. Plants require radiant energy from the sun to synthesize glucose from carbon dioxide and water. After ingestion of glucose from plants, the human body uses the energy contained within the chemical bonds of glucose molecules to provide what is necessary to synthesize adenosine triphosphate (ATP) from adenosine diphosphate (ADP) and inorganic phosphate (Pi). ATP is the primary energy currency used by cells to perform biological work such as skeletal muscle contraction. The diagram shows how the exergonic process of glucose metabolism (oxidation) in cellular respiration provides the energy required for ATP synthesis. Lipids and proteins (amino acids) also undergo oxidation to provide the necessary energy for ATP synthesis.

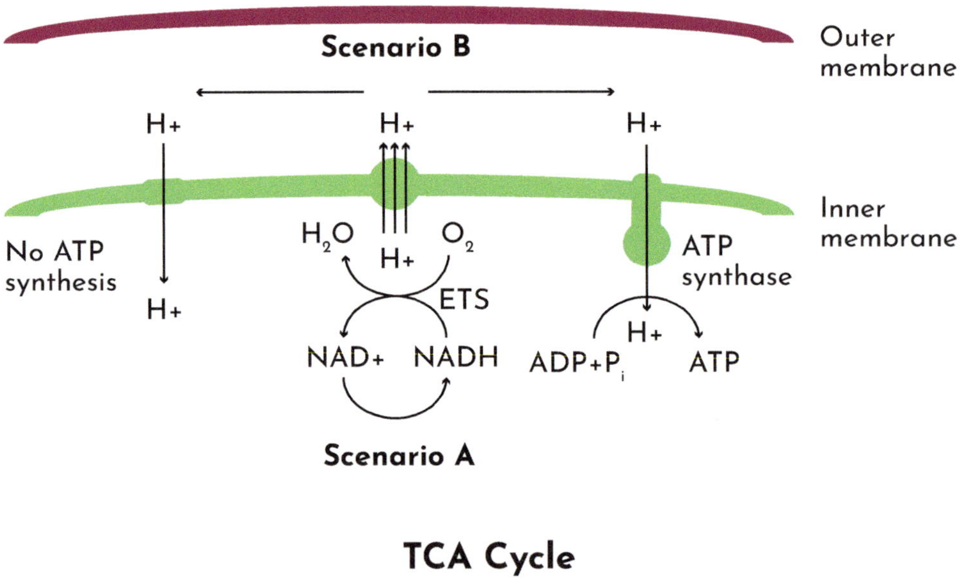

FIGURE 10.2 Simplified mitochondrial bioenergetics In the tricarboxylic acid cycle (TCA, also called the Krebs cycle), oxidation reactions catalyzed by dehydrogenase enzymes result in the removal of hydrogen atoms from substrates by the coenzymes nicotinamide adenine dinucleotide (NAD^+) and flavin adenine dinucleotide (FAD; not shown in diagram), resulting in the reduction of these molecules to NADH and $FADH_2$, respectively. These reduced coenzymes, in turn, undergo oxidation in the electron transport system (ETS); electrons are passed between conjugate redox pairs in the respiratory chain to ultimately reduce oxygen to form water. These oxidation/reduction reactions cause protons to move from the mitochondrial matrix across the inner mitochondrial membrane, resulting in the generation of a membrane potential and a pH gradient. As shown in scenario A, this energy is then used to drive the endergonic process of adenosine triphosphate (ATP) synthesis from adenosine diphosphate (ADP) and inorganic phosphate (Pi) as the hydrogen ions (protons) move back across the inner mitochondrial membrane by way of a specific conductance pathway associated with ATP synthase. If protons "leak" back into the matrix (inner portion of the mitochondrion) by conduction pathways not linked to ATP synthase shown by scenario B (eg, by uncoupling proteins found in highly thermogenic brown adipose tissue [BAT]), the coupling efficiency of oxidation and phosphorylation is reduced so that more heat is released and fewer ATP molecules are synthesized relative to the amount of oxygen consumed.

respiratory chain to ultimately reduce oxygen to form water. These oxidation/reduction reactions result in protons being pumped from the mitochondrial matrix across the inner mitochondrial membrane, resulting in the generation of a membrane potential and a pH gradient. This potential energy is then used to drive the endergonic process of ATP synthesis from ADP and P_i as the hydrogen ions (protons) move back across the inner mitochondrial membrane by way of a specific conductance pathway associated with ATP synthase.

In this way, oxidation reactions are coupled to the phosphorylation of ADP, hence the term *oxidative phosphorylation* used to describe the synthesis of ATP inside the mitochondria. Given the importance of oxygen as the final oxidizing agent in the electron transport chain and the liberation of carbon dioxide through the decarboxylation of macronutrient substrates, determining the rate of oxygen consumption and carbon dioxide production via indirect calorimetry provides an accurate measure of whole-body energy expenditure, except when substantial amounts of ATP are produced anaerobically. The latter process can occur when an individual's exercise intensity approaches their maximal capacity and the demand for ATP exceeds the capacity of skeletal muscle fibers to generate the ATP entirely by mitochondrial oxidative phosphorylation.

THE ENERGY BALANCE EQUATION: A SIMPLE CONCEPT WITH LAYERS OF COMPLEXITY

The first law of thermodynamics states that, in a closed system, energy is neither created nor destroyed, but it is transformed from one form to another. In humans, the energy balance equation is based on this law because the energy ingested (macronutrients) and the energy expended in carrying out the processes vital to life must both be taken into account. The energy balance equation dictates that energy available from foods and beverages in excess of expenditure—that is, a positive energy balance—will result in increased energy stores. Conversely, when energy expenditure is greater than the amount that is metabolically available from ingested food, negative energy balance will result in depletion of the body's energy stores.

Owing to episodic food intake via meals and snacks consumed during the day and episodic levels of daily physical activity and exercise, athletes are almost always in a state of acute energy imbalance. For example, during a meal, acute excess energy is available without a substantial increase in energy expenditure, making mealtimes a brief period characterized by an acute state of positive energy balance and storage of macronutrients. On the other hand, exercise during practice for a sport and other forms of physical activity during the day are characterized by an acute state of energy deficit as energy expenditure is substantially greater than energy intake. Thus, whereas energy intake and energy expenditure can be quantified for brief periods of time, the determination of chronic energy balance requires averaging acute energy balance over days, weeks, and months.[3]

During times of positive energy balance, adipocytes (fat cells) are the major storage depot for excess energy, with triacylglycerol molecules within adipocytes being the primary means of storing this energy. An excessive expansion of adipose tissue mass can jeopardize athletic performance and is associated with increased risk for a host of chronic inflammatory diseases such as type 2 diabetes and coronary heart disease.[4] The sequelae of excessive adiposity could lead one to assume that a lower fat mass means better health. However, adipose tissue plays an important functional role in ensuring that adequate energy is available during times of short-term (fasting) and long-term (hypocaloric diets) energy deprivation, as well as long-distance endurance exercise. Adipose tissue also has an important endocrine role, secreting regulatory signaling molecules such as leptin (discussed later in this chapter), which influences both energy intake and energy expenditure.[5] Thus, an excessively low degree of adiposity can detrimentally affect human health, and potentially performance, depending on the sport.

Despite the perceptions that some individuals are seemingly susceptible to weight gain and excessive fat storage, it is impossible to increase body energy stores without energy intake exceeding energy expenditure. One cannot overlook the first law of thermodynamics in an attempt to explain why some individuals are more prone to weight gain than others. An understanding of the various determinants of both sides of the balance—energy expenditure and intake—demonstrates the many nuances and complexities of this equation (refer to Figure 10.3 on page 226). Chapter 11 provides information regarding the achievement of weight management goals for sport-specific athletes.

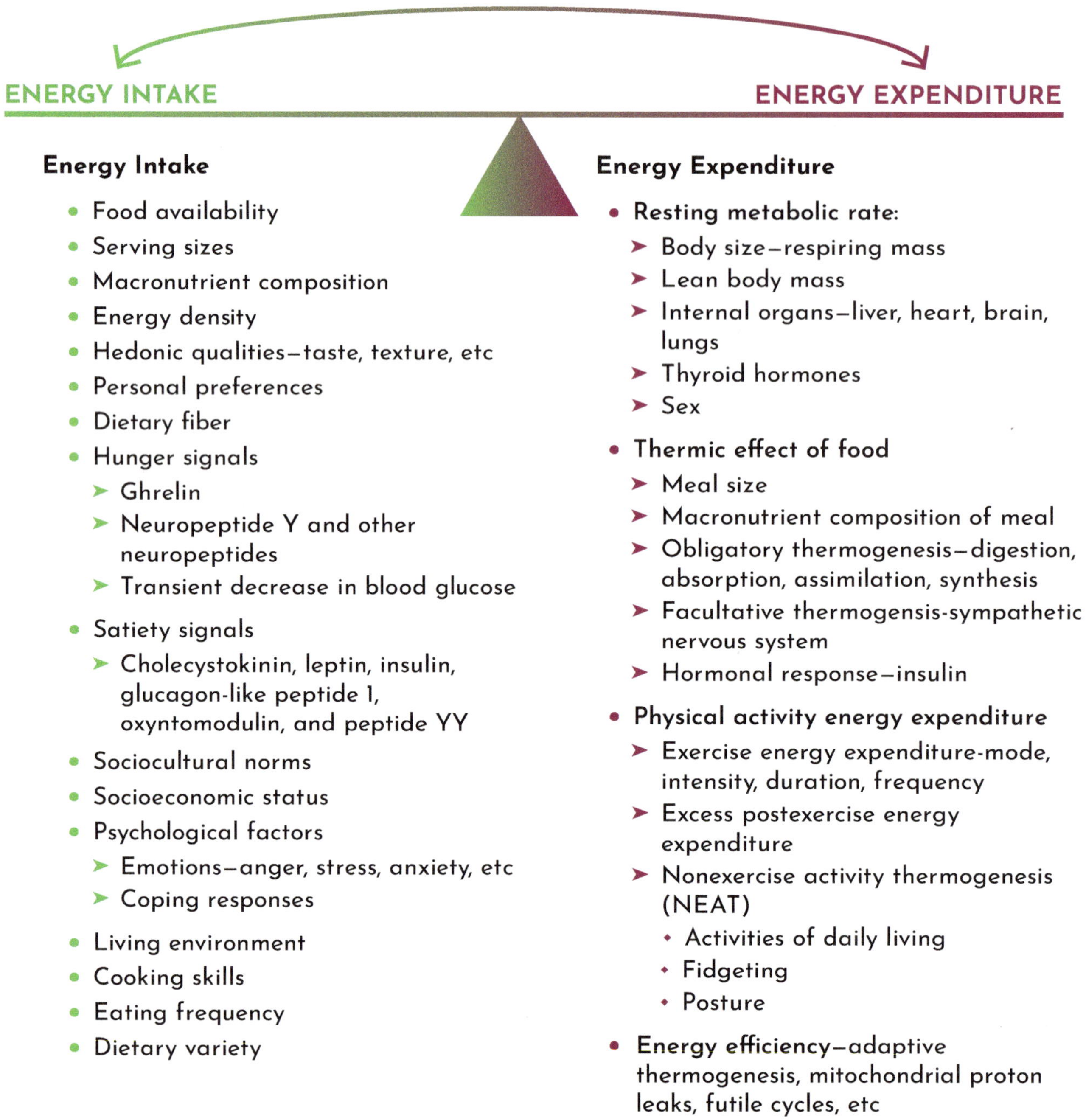

FIGURE 10.3 Dynamic energy balance The dynamic energy balance equation predicts that body energy stores are a function of energy intake and energy expenditure, both influenced by a multitude of factors. Sizable changes in energy intake usually bring about compensatory behavioral and metabolic changes in energy expenditure that defend the initial body weight. Conversely, sizable changes in energy expenditure may bring about changes in energy intake. These compensatory changes vary substantially between individuals and are related to neuroendocrine adjustments and cognitive factors.

Metabolic Efficiency

The second law of thermodynamics dictates that the cellular reactions that generate ATP are less than perfectly efficient—that is, at least a portion of energy released from oxidation of macronutrients will be lost as heat, rather than all of the available energy being conserved in the phosphoanhydride bonds of ATP molecules. Note that even under normal conditions, the cellular oxidation of glucose results in greater production of heat than energy conserved as ATP. Metabolic efficiency maximizes ATP production relative to heat loss, whereas metabolic inefficiency is characterized by increased heat production and lessened synthesis of ATP molecules relative to the potential energy in a macronutrient.[5]

The foundational principles of mitochondrial bioenergetics reveal that oxidation reactions in the mitochondria result in protons being pumped from the matrix, creating a proton gradient. If these protons "leak" back into the matrix by conduction pathways not linked to ATP synthase (eg, by uncoupling proteins found in highly thermogenic brown adipose tissue [BAT]), the coupling efficiency of oxidation and phosphorylation is reduced so that more heat is generated and fewer ATP molecules are synthesized relative to the amount of oxygen consumed. A person who produces more heat and less ATP per mole of substrate would thus be less energy efficient compared with an individual who produces more ATP relative to the amount of substrate oxidized. It follows, then, that energy inefficiency is characterized by an increased quantity of substrate required to synthesize a given amount of ATP, which, in turn, will require more oxygen consumption (reduction of oxygen to water) in the cellular mitochondria.

THE ROLE OF ADIPOSE TISSUE AND IRISIN

There is considerable interest in variable efficiency rates of cellular energy transduction, as they could theoretically help explain differences in individual susceptibility and resistance to obesity among humans living in the same obesogenic environment.[2] The commonly observed phenomenon that individuals subjected to the same magnitude of energy deficit or surplus do not lose or gain, respectively, the same amount of weight can be at least partially attributed to individual differences in energy efficiency in response to dieting or overeating.[6] Different types of fat cells can impact energy efficiency. There are 2 distinct types of adipose tissue: white and brown. White adipose tissue (WAT) is the primary site of energy storage and is responsible for the secretion of various hormones, including leptin. BAT is responsible for the dissipation of energy in the form of heat, by way of less efficient coupling of oxidation and phosphorylation. BAT was once thought to exist only in human infants; however, human adults also have variable amounts of brown fat depots.[7] Published observations of variations in the ability of brown fat to increase energy expenditure through the uncoupling of mitochondrial oxidation from ATP synthesis as well as observations that the amount of brown fat in adults is inversely correlated with BMI provide credible evidence for human differences in metabolic efficiency.[8] In addition, accumulating evidence indicates that white adipocytes can undergo some degree of "browning" (also referred to as "beiging"), resulting in beige-colored adipocytes with increased mitochondria that, upon stimulation, also exhibit greater uncoupled oxidative phosphorylation and thus more heat production.[9,10] Studies have encouraged interest in the possibility that exercise could cause the browning of WAT by way of a myokine called irisin, which may serve as an auspicious strategy for mitigating obesity and related metabolic disorders.[10]

Researchers first reported that the skeletal muscle of exercising mice secreted irisin, which stimulated mitochondrial biogenesis and the browning of white adipocytes. These changes were associated with increased energy expenditure and reduced energetic efficiency.[11] Animal studies have provided evidence to support the notion that irisin levels increase after exercise and may be metabolically beneficial; however, there is a scarcity of evidence supporting this notion in humans. Through the expression of the peroxisome proliferator-activated receptor γ (PPARγ) coactivator-1α (PGC-1α), the expression of fibronectin type III domain containing protein 5 (Fndc5) is triggered in skeletal muscle. Consequently, the cleavage of Fndc5 produces irisin, which is released into circulation and eventually reaches adipose tissue. At this time, researchers have not yet determined how long it takes until irisin levels rise with exercise or how long this up-regulation of irisin lasts, although different types of exercise do appear to have differing effects on the browning of WAT.[10] Furthermore, despite initial findings in animal studies that encouraged growing excitement about the role of exercise and WAT browning, recent research[12-15] in human study participants has tempered this excitement. Yet, certain methodological and sample selection concerns should be considered when evaluating the current evidence in this area. The following list includes an overview of emerging research involving human participants that has investigated the circulating levels of irisin and the activity of BAT after various types of exercise:

- In 1 study, investigators found that, although messenger RNA translated into the irisin protein increased in men following a 12-week endurance exercise training program, the circulating level of irisin was actually reduced after the 12 weeks of exercise, and there was little evidence for exercise-induced browning of WAT.[12]
- Similarly, in a cross-sectional comparison of endurance-trained athletes with lean sedentary counterparts, endurance training was actually associated with lower cold-stimulated BAT activity.[13]

- In a population-based sample of more than 700 men and women, circulating irisin concentrations were inversely associated with exercise capacity in men, although there was a trend toward a positive association of irisin with exercise capacity in women.[14]
- In another cross-sectional study, 86 adults were asked to perform 5 minutes of walking and running bouts at constant speeds of 4 and 8 km/h. Venous blood samples were obtained before and after the bout of exercise, and irisin concentrations were determined using an enzyme-linked immunosorbent assay (ELISA) protocol. No change in irisin concentration was observed after exercise among the majority of the participants, and the irisin concentration even decreased in 23% of the participants. However, the authors of this study did not describe the physical fitness status and habitual physical activity of the study participants, hindering the development of a better understanding of the effects of exercise on irisin levels among active individuals.[15] Moreover, the exercise protocol lasted only 5 minutes, which adds to the difficulty in understanding how such findings translate to various types of sport and durations of activity.

Overall, the findings from the current studies suggest that in humans, chronic exercise has little to no effect on circulating-irisin–induced beiging of WAT. However, research strongly suggests that some of the incongruities in study results stem from difficulties in accurately measuring the irisin peptide. For example, when Jedrychowski et al[16] used a better detection method, they measured an increase in irisin levels with aerobic exercise. If this controversy is adequately resolved by more accurate measurements of irisin and exercise is found to stimulate beiging of adipocytes via myokine, this would be yet another benefit of exercise to body weight regulation. More research is required to adequately determine the effects of exercise on irisin and beiging of white adipocytes. Furthermore, future studies should clearly identify the conditioning or physical fitness status of the human study participants involved, as well as their exercise intensity. These improvements in sample selection and description may help to improve the understanding of how the research findings translate to active individuals of different training statuses involved in various sports and other types of activity.

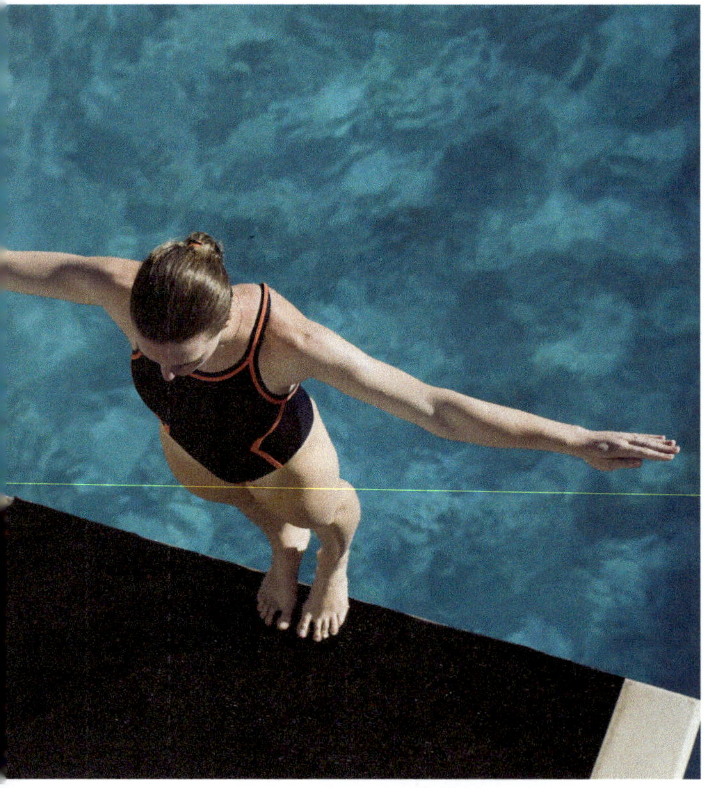

Important Energy Balance Concepts

Four specific principles are important for understanding the energy balance equation:

1) The laws of thermodynamics are inviolable.
2) The large variation in human responses to controlled diet and exercise changes likely results, at least in part, from differences in energetic efficiency that may be linked to genetic and epigenetic variation.[17]
3) Changes on 1 side of the energy balance equation will usually result in involuntary metabolic or behavioral changes on the other side as well.
4) Human responses to diet and exercise that seem contrary to our understanding of bioenergetics (eg, individuals losing far less weight than predicted based on their purported decreases in energy intake and increases in exercise) are not violations of the laws of thermodynamics.

Any apparent violations of the laws of thermodynamics are due, instead, to substantial limitations in our ability to accurately measure both energy intake and availability and total energy expenditure and its individual components, as well as our limited ability to measure changes in energetic efficiency in response to external perturbations, such as changes in diet and exercise.

NEUROENDOCRINE REGULATION OF ENERGY BALANCE

Both energy intake and expenditure can be modified by voluntary behavior. However, during the past several decades, considerable evidence has emerged showing that energy balance is regulated by a host of neuroendocrine factors. This notion has been summarized by Jeffrey Friedman, MD, PhD, an internationally recognized scientist known for his work in molecular genetics, energy regulation, and obesity. He wrote, "[the simplistic notion] that weight can be controlled by 'deciding' to eat less and exercise more is at odds with substantial scientific evidence illuminating a precise and powerful biologic system that maintains body weight within a relatively narrow range."[18] Although this view of the magnitude of genetic control over body weight is not shared by all scientists, it does highlight the fact that physiological regulatory controls of body weight do exist.

The hypothalamus, a portion of the central nervous system located just above the brainstem, integrates a host of signals from the liver, gut, and adipose tissue to regulate energy expenditure and the initiation, termination, and frequency of eating. The arcuate nucleus (ARC) is one of several important nuclei in the hypothalamus involved in the regulation of energy expenditure and intake. The ARC is composed of 2 neuronal populations with reciprocal functions. Neurons coexpressing neuropeptide Y (NPY) and agouti-related protein (AgRP) work in concert to increase food intake and decrease energy expenditure when stimulated.[19] Weight loss and the associated changes in various hormone concentrations activate these neurons to counter the weight loss by promoting positive energy balance and weight regain. Alternatively, the stimulation of neurons expressing proopiomelanocortin (POMC) induces decreases in food intake and increases in energy expenditure. These neurons are activated by homeostatic adjustments in response to weight gain to drive a negative energy balance and weight loss.[20]

Adiposity-Related Signals

Two circulating hormones have been identified as adiposity-related signals: insulin and leptin. As adiposity increases, so do circulating insulin and leptin concentrations.[21,22] Increases in insulin result from the well-characterized compensatory hyperinsulinemia in response to insulin resistance. Elevation of leptin occurs as a direct consequence of increased amounts of WAT, the primary site of leptin synthesis and secretion.[23] Effects on energy intake and expenditure are 2 of the many functions of these major adiposity-related signals, as shown in Figure 10.4 on page 230. These 2 hormones communicate to the brain the magnitude of the body's adiposity. Leptin receptors are located throughout the brain,[24] including both populations of ARC neurons. Binding to the leptin receptor in the ARC leads to a signaling cascade that ultimately inhibits NPY/AgRP neurons and excites POMC neurons to exert an antiadiposity effect.[25] In this way, increasing leptin concentrations due to increasing fat mass will promote weight loss. Similar to leptin, insulin interacts with the ARC of the hypothalamus to exert its anorexigenic (hunger-suppressing) effects. Insulin binds to the insulin receptor to inhibit NPY/AgRP neurons and reduce food intake.[26] As long as an individual does not develop insulin or leptin resistance, as their body weight fluctuates, changes in the circulating concentrations of leptin and insulin will activate and inhibit these neuronal circuits to return body weight to its preestablished level.

Powerful homeostatic regulation of food intake occurs such that severe energy restriction leading to weight loss typically results in a strong internal drive to eat, whereas an overabundance of food intake and weight gain is often followed by a reduction in food intake. These homeostatic compensatory responses, observed in both animals and humans, support the notion that body weight and composition are regulated within a typical range for a given individual. Many factors help determine this range, including genetic, environmental, and socioeconomic factors.[27] Substantial deviations from this range are met with metabolic and feeding changes that alter energy expenditure and intake in an effort to return one's body weight to its preestablished level, a concept that has been termed the *set-point theory*.[28] For example, as adipose tissue expands, adiposity-related signals, insulin and leptin, increase in circulation.[29-31] Through their effect on specific hypothalamic neurons, the signals stimulate increased energy expenditure and encourage a greater sense of satiety, leading to decreased food intake. Loss of body fat reduces these signals, leading to decreased energy expenditure and increased food intake.[30,31] This communication between adipose tissue and the brain suggests that the control of body weight extends beyond volitional behavior. The digestive tract also releases a number of peptides that interact with the hypothalamus to regulate short-term hunger and satiety. These will be briefly discussed in a later section of this chapter.

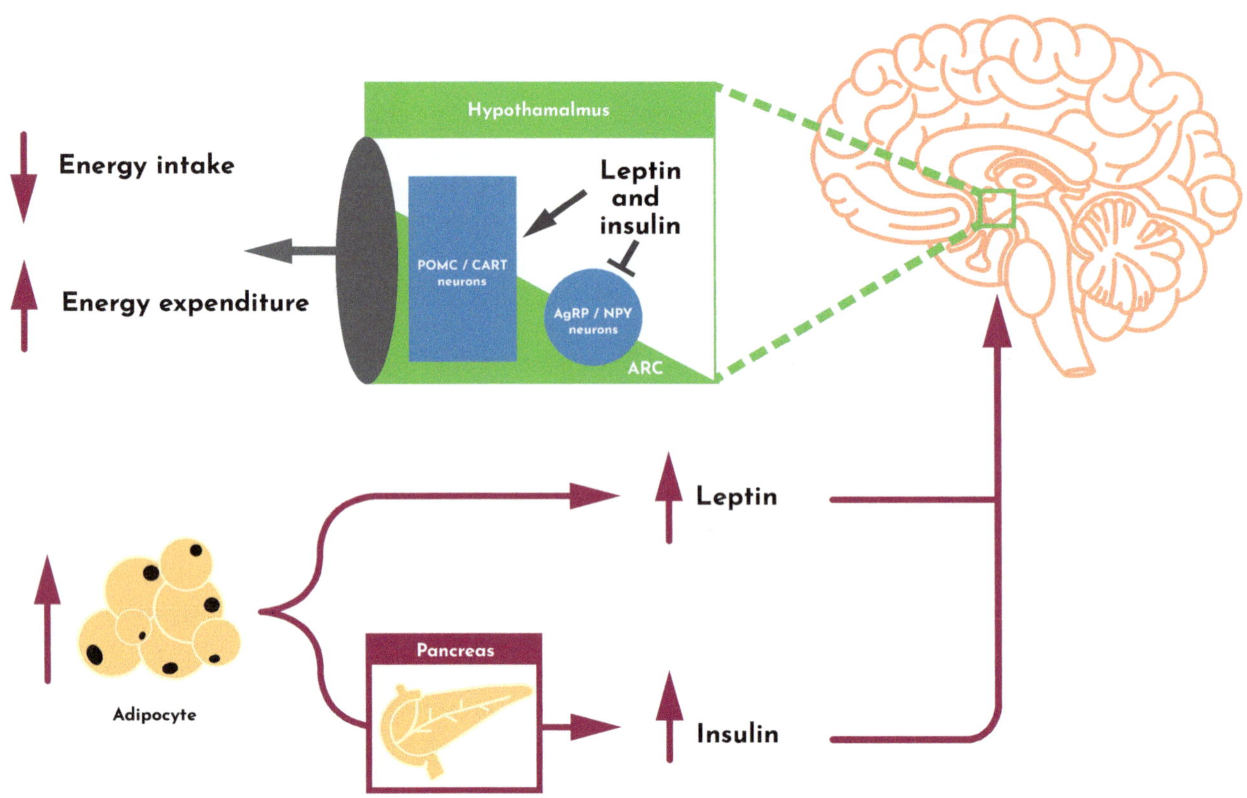

FIGURE 10.4 Effects of leptin and insulin on energy intake and expenditure Leptin and insulin are considered adiposity-related signals—that is, they alert the brain to the amount of body fat stores present. As body fat increases, the synthesis and release of leptin into circulation also increases. Insulin is secreted from the pancreas, not from adipocytes, but the amount circulating is proportional to the amount of body fat. Therefore, increased storage of fat is associated with increased blood concentrations of both leptin and insulin. These hormones travel to the brain where they bind to their respective receptors located on neurons throughout the hypothalamus, including specific neurons in the arcuate nucleus (ARC). They inhibit the expression of 2 orexigenic (hunger-stimulating) neuropeptides: agouti-related peptide (AgRP) and neuropeptide Y (NPY). These same hormones stimulate neurons that express the anorexigenic (hunger-suppressing) neuropeptides: proopiomelanocortin (POMC) and cocaine- and amphetamine-regulated transcript (CART). These latter neuropeptides also stimulate an increase in energy expenditure. Thus, as adipose tissue expands, the increased circulation of these hormones results in homeostatic adjustments to limit the expansion by decreasing energy intake and increasing energy expenditure.

The rapid increase in human obesity may seem to be at odds with set-point theory because it would appear that corrective internal actions must be lacking in a substantial portion of the population in the face of the current obesogenic environment. However, it is likely that the obesity-prone person regulates body weight, but at a higher set point than the obesity-resistant individual,[30] akin to an individual with hypertension regulating their blood pressure through endocrine and neural inputs but at a level that is higher than normal. Impairments in regulation may also occur such that the brain becomes resistant to peripheral signals such as leptin and insulin. The possibility also exists that most humans exhibit a stronger, more powerful defense against weight loss than against weight gain.[32] Regardless, it is evident that compensatory changes in energy intake occur in individuals who are obese and nonobese (including athletes) in response to energy excesses or deficiencies.[33,34] The magnitude of these compensatory responses is probably under both genetic control and environmental influences.

The dramatic increase in overweight and obesity during the past 30 to 40 years could primarily be due to environmental changes, given that any significant shifts in the human genetic constitution would not have occurred during such a brief time. Note, however, that in earlier periods, an underlying genetic predisposition toward obesity might have been masked by an environment in which hard manual labor and a lack of palatable food were the norms. However, such a genetic predisposition, coupled with the current obesogenic environment, could readily result in an obese phenotype today.[35] The individual contributions of genes and voluntary behavior in ultimately determining a person's body weight are unknown. The "either/or" debate (genetic/biological determinism vs voluntary choices) is not particularly helpful in dealing with individuals. What is important is to seek an understanding of the behavioral and metabolic features of the individual, with the aim of developing the most effective personalized approach to achieving a healthy and competitive body weight and composition.

ENERGY EXPENDITURE

Four components of total daily energy expenditure (TDEE) make up 1 side of the energy balance scale, namely, resting metabolic rate (RMR), the thermic effect of food (TEF), nonexercise activity thermogenesis (NEAT), and exercise energy expenditure (ExEE). Physical activity energy expenditure (PAEE) includes both NEAT and ExEE (refer to Figure 10.3). A brief discussion of each of the 4 components follows.

Resting Metabolic Rate

RMR is the energy expended by an individual for cellular processes necessary to maintain life while lying supine in a postabsorptive, awakened state.[36] For inactive individuals, the RMR accounts for approximately 70% to 75% of their daily energy expenditure.[37] For an athlete who engages in hours of exercise training each day, RMR may account for up to half of their total daily energy expenditure.[38] Many factors influence an individual's RMR, the most pronounced being body size (especially lean body mass), with a greater mass of respiring tissue accounting for greater energy expenditure. Among adults, RMR is generally lower in females than in males, mostly because of differences in lean body mass. Resting metabolism decreases with advancing age, primarily resulting from age-related declines in lean mass. RMR decreases by approximately 2% per decade in healthy adult females and by approximately 3% per decade in healthy adult males.[39] Although skeletal muscle accounts for a sizable portion of lean tissue, the internal organs, including the liver, heart, brain, kidneys, and lungs, together expend far more energy *at rest* than does skeletal muscle. Numerous hormones affect RMR as well, especially the thyroid hormone triiodothyronine. Individuals with a hypoactive thyroid gland have lower metabolic rates than their body size would predict, and they tend to readily gain weight and experience profound fatigue until the condition is corrected. On the other hand, a hyperactive thyroid gland leads to decreased energy efficiency characterized by an increased RMR and weight loss.

MEASUREMENT OF RESTING METABOLIC RATE

Typically, RMR is measured for 30 to 60 minutes in the early morning, approximately 10 to 12 hours after the previous evening's meal, while the individual being measured is lying quietly in a recumbent position in a thermoneutral environment.[36] Most often, RMR is determined by indirect calorimetry, a process involving the measurement of respiratory gases. Because oxygen (O_2) utilization in the mitochondria is directly tied to ATP synthesis and heat production, the measurement of oxygen consumption (and often carbon dioxide [CO_2] production as well) is used to accurately quantify energy expenditure. A ventilatory mask, mouthpiece, or canopy is used in conjunction with a metabolic cart equipped with a flow meter and CO_2 and O_2 analyzers. The energy equivalent per liter of O_2 ranges between 4.6 and 5.0 kcal, depending on the relative proportion of fats, carbohydrates, and deaminated amino acids oxidized. Based on the oxygen consumption per minute and the energy equivalent per liter of oxygen, energy expenditure per minute can be determined and can then be extrapolated to a 24-hour period. Some handheld measurement devices are also available to measure RMR. These devices are less expensive and can provide reasonably accurate measurements of RMR, but they are generally not capable of measuring the energy costs of exercise when a person's ventilation rates are much higher than they are during rest.[40]

An additional technique that can be used to measure energy expenditure is the doubly labeled water method.[41,42] The doubly labeled water method can be used in free-living individuals (that is, not subject to constraints), including during exercise or competition and under high-altitude conditions.[42] Although similar to indirect calorimetry, the doubly labeled water method does not account for oxygen consumption and is instead based on the difference between the turnover rates of the hydrogen and oxygen in body water as a function of carbon dioxide production.[43] More specifically, individuals receive a loading dose of the isotopes oxygen-18 (^{18}O) and deuterium (^{2}H), and the differential rates of elimination of these 2 isotopes in the urine allows for the calculation of carbon dioxide production.[41,42] Test participants experience minimal burden, illustrating the practicality of this method for use among active individuals. Moreover, this is an advantageous method for measuring energy expenditure during research studies with testing periods between 1 and 3 weeks.[42] However, cost is a major limitation of this method, and less expensive options are available for measuring energy expenditure.

ESTIMATION OF RESTING METABOLIC RATE BY PREDICTION EQUATIONS

Because indirect calorimetry and the doubly labeled water method are not accessible to all athletes, many RMR prediction equations have been developed. These typically include such variables as body size, age, and sex, with more sophisticated equations including some measures of lean and fat mass. Some commonly used equations are provided in Box 10.2,[44-50] which also highlights those found to be the most accurate in the athletic population. Unfortunately, the development of RMR equations for athletes has lagged behind the development of equations established for the general population. Moreover, the accuracy of the common equations may overestimate RMR values in obese individuals, owing to their lower lean-to-fat mass ratio, while these same equations may underestimate RMR values in athletes, who typically exhibit higher lean-to-fat mass ratios than characteristic of the general population. Given that the Cunningham equation for RMR estimation is based on fat-free mass, this equation would appear to work fairly well for athletes.[45]

BOX 10.2 Equations for Estimating Resting Metabolic Rate[44-50]

No single best equation exists for measuring resting metabolic rate (RMR) for all athletes because there is substantial diversity in body composition among athletes competing in different sports. If fat-free mass (FFM) can be accurately determined, the Cunningham equation often works well, but as the amount of body fat increases in athletes, its contribution to RMR will increase, which is not taken into account in this particular equation. For female athletes, the Owen equation is often used, as it was derived specifically from the study of elite female athletes. However, the number of female athletes studied to derive this equation was quite small (N = 8).

Harris-Benedict equation[44]

Highly accurate in the male athletic population

Males	RMR (kcal/d) = 66.4730 + 13.7516W + 5.0033H – 6.7750A
Females	RMR (kcal/d) = 665.0955 + 9.5634W + 1.8496H – 4.6756A where W = weight in kg, H = height in cm, and A = age in y

Cunningham equation[45]

Highly accurate in the athletic population

Males	RMR (kcal/d) = 370 + 21.6FFM
Females	RMR (kcal/d) = 370 + 21.6FFM where FFM = fat-free mass in kg

Owen equation[46,47]

Highly accurate in the female athletic population and in paralympic athletes

Males	RMR (kcal/d) = 879 + 10.2W
Females	RMR (kcal/d) = 795 + 7.18W
Female athletes	RMR (kcal/d) = 50.4 + 21.1W where W = weight in kg

Liu equation[48,49]

Highly accurate in the female athletic population

Males	RMR (kcal/d) = 13.88W + 4.16H - 3.43A - 112.40S + 54.34

Females	RMR (kcal/d) = 13.88W + 4.16H - 3.43A - 112.40S + 54.34
Female athletes	RMR (kcal/d) = 50.4 + 21.1W where W = weight in kg; H = height in cm; A = age in y; and S = sex, with male = 0 and female = 1

Mifflin-St. Jeor equation[50]

Highly accurate for all body sizes and types, including athletes who are obese and paralympic athletes

Males	RMR (kcal/d) = 10W + 6.25H - 5A + 5
Females	RMR (kcal/d) = 10W + 6.25H - 5A - 161 where W = weight in kg, H = height in cm, and A = age in y

EFFECT OF EXERCISE ON RESTING METABOLIC RATE

In a number of studies, endurance-trained athletes exhibited higher RMR values than nonathletes. However, this phenomenon does not seem to result from any adaptations to exercise training. It is more likely that the combination of high ExEE and high energy intake (high flux) in these athletes can temporarily, but not permanently, increase their RMR when measured the morning after exercise.[51] However, there is little evidence that the amount of physical activity for health maintenance and weight control used by recreational exercisers will produce any permanent increases in RMR, with the possible exception of such exercise in older individuals.[52]

Some fitness enthusiasts have promoted the idea that because regular weight lifting can increase skeletal muscle mass, such exercise will substantially increase RMR. Although this may be an attractive notion, a sizable increase in muscle mass is likely to occur only for the individual who becomes a serious weightlifter. The contribution of each pound of muscle mass to *resting* energy expenditure is far less than that of a similar mass of internal organs such as the liver and heart, so one would have to substantially increase muscle mass to increase RMR. Most people who lift weights for health rather than for bodybuilding or sports competition will not increase their muscle mass enough to produce more than a small increase in RMR. For the serious weight trainer, a single prolonged strenuous bout of weight lifting may increase RMR when measured the following morning.[53] Nevertheless, it is clear that for both athletes and nonathletes, young and old, the major impact of both endurance and resistance exercise on total daily energy expenditure occurs during the activity itself and not from any substantial increases in RMR.

Thermic Effect of Food

The *thermic effect of food* is defined as the increase in energy expenditure above RMR in response to ingestion of food. This increase in energy expenditure is attributable to obligatory components that include digestion, absorption, transport, and assimilation of the food consumed, as well as a facultative component. The latter is the portion of TEF resulting from the increase in sympathetic nervous system activity that accompanies food consumption.

MEASUREMENT OF THERMIC EFFECT OF FOOD

The TEF is usually measured in the same way as RMR, via indirect calorimetry. The athlete is provided with a meal of known macronutrient and calorie content, and technicians measure the increase in energy expenditure above RMR during the next 3 to 6 hours, with more accurate determinations made over at least 5 to 6 hours.[37] The average TEF for a mixed meal accounts for approximately 10% of energy ingested. The thermic effect of the individual macronutrients varies considerably, with fat having the lowest at approximately 3% of ingested fat calories, followed by carbohydrates at 5% to 10% of ingested carbohydrate energy, and proteins having the highest thermic effect at 20% to 30% of protein calories.[54]

Physical Activity Energy Expenditure

PAEE is the energy expenditure above resting values that results from skeletal muscle contraction, including the energy required for movement, balance, and maintenance of posture. This component can be further divided into ExEE and NEAT.

EXERCISE ENERGY EXPENDITURE

Exercise is defined as volitional movement done to improve or maintain 1 or more features of either health- or performance-related physical fitness.[55] Exercise is typically the most variable component of daily energy expenditure, and for the athlete attempting to modify body weight and composition, it is the component under the most volitional control. The energetic cost of daily exercise is based on the frequency, duration, intensity, and mode of exercise. On a given day, it can range from zero calories for someone who does not exercise to several thousand calories for an individual who participates in a long-distance endurance event, such as a marathon. Athletes who participate in regular strenuous and prolonged exercise training have very high TDEE values, which may require conscientious efforts to obtain adequate energy intake. For example, 1 study estimated the energy requirements in competitive cyclists to be approximately 4,300 kcal/d when they are in training and less than 2,400 kcal/d on very inactive days.[51]

The energy expended for a given exercise bout is usually determined by indirect calorimetry done in a laboratory and then extrapolated to a free-living situation with adjustments made for body size. A compendium of the energy expenditure values for many modes, durations, and intensities of exercise has been published by the American College of Sports Medicine. These values are useful in helping determine the contribution of PAEE to TDEE and energy balance.[56] Often the energetic cost of exercise is expressed in metabolic equivalents, or METs, which are multiples of RMR. For example, if an athlete expends 1.0 kcal/min at rest and has an ExEE of 13 kcal/min during a given training session, the athlete's exercise intensity is as follows:

$$13 \text{ kcal/min} \div 1.0 \text{ kcal/min} = 13 \text{ METs}$$

Energy expenditure is elevated for a period following exercise, with greater energy expenditure during this recovery period occurring for higher-intensity exercise. This phenomenon is a function of numerous factors, including elevated body temperature and elevated circulating catecholamines (epinephrine and norepinephrine). This excess postexercise energy expenditure should be considered part of the total ExEE.

NONEXERCISE ACTIVITY THERMOGENESIS

NEAT is the energy expenditure resulting from physical activity not considered exercise, such as activities of daily living and fidgeting. Maintaining body posture is also part of NEAT. This component of TDEE is difficult to measure and is often determined by default after measuring the other 3 components and subtracting them from TDEE or by using lightweight sensors to detect posture and motion. Primarily owing to the work of James Levine at the Mayo Clinic, NEAT is now widely recognized as an important and highly variable component of TDEE.[57,58] People who are obese spend more time sitting during the day than individuals who are not obese.[59] Sitting energy expenditure is lower than standing, as the latter requires muscle contractions necessary to maintain balance.[60] Therefore, altering daily activities, such as taking a flight of stairs instead of the elevator, can contribute to TDEE.

Determining Total Daily Energy Expenditure

Determining TDEE to identify a person's energy requirements, although difficult to do accurately, can be undertaken by a variety of methods. Whole-room calorimeters are used by some scientists but are not available for most people. Even when used by scientists, these instruments typically underestimate TDEE because ambulation is limited within the small chamber. The use of stable isotopes of hydrogen and oxygen (ie, doubly labeled water) provides accurate measures of TDEE in a free-living environment, but as previously mentioned, use of this approach is very expensive and impractical apart from access to a major research institution. The factorial method involves measuring individual components of TDEE and then summing these contributions to determine TDEE. However, this approach is very labor intensive and impractical.

Pedometers, accelerometers, and heart rate monitors can be useful in quantifying physical activity, especially when accompanied by activity diaries. Technological advances have made accelerometer-based activity monitors such as watches and fitness bands readily available to individuals. Although the features and capabilities of these devices vary, they all attempt to provide the user with information on their TDEE. These monitors estimate one's RMR using anthropometric data entered by the user—height, weight, sex, and age—and then base their TDEE on estimates of the calories expended above this RMR value. Some devices attempt to calculate calories for specific activities, whereas others use additional measurements, such as the temperature of the skin or barometric pressure, to more accurately consider intensity and activity. Initial research on the efficacy of some of these devices has shown promising results for increasing physical activity and weight loss.[61] When evaluated more directly and compared with research-grade instruments, these monitors have been found to exhibit strong validity for measuring step count but only moderate validity for measuring TDEE, with some devices differing in energy expenditure estimates by up to 900 kcal. Among different devices and activities, the validity of the monitors varied widely.[62,63] Additionally, wearable GPS tracking devices, such as GPS watches, are more frequently being used to quantify workload, describe intensity, and estimate energy expenditure. GPS is a satellite-based system that continuously monitors location and then computes caloric expenditure based on anthropometric data and distance traveled. When energy expenditure estimates from multiple GPS devices were compared against a validated accelerometer-based measure for participants walking at varying speeds, the GPS watches showed lower reliability than the accelerometer, especially at increased speeds. The researchers concluded that GPS watches may be limited in their ability to provide accurate values for energy expenditure; caution is advised when using these devices for such purposes.[64] Taken together, activity monitors may prove useful for keeping track of steps and physical activity, but they should be used reservedly when one is attempting to closely track energy expenditure, especially over a wide range of activities.

The conversion of data from steps walked, accelerometer counts, or changes in heart rate to precise energy expenditure values can be problematic. In light of these issues, TDEE is commonly estimated by multiplying either estimated or measured RMR by a specified physical activity level (PAL), which is a factor based on an estimated PAEE. For an inactive person, the estimates are likely to be more accurate, owing to a small contribution of physical activity to TDEE. However, for athletes, there is substantial room for error based on the significant contribution of ExEE to TDEE. The PAL values have been derived from a variety of methods, including the factorial approach and the use of doubly labeled water. Box 10.3 on page 236 provides the PAL values noted in the 2023 *Dietary Reference Intakes for Energy* based on a compilation of doubly labeled water values in free-living individuals.[38] The PALs range from 1.25 for an extremely inactive person with limited opportunity for ambulation to more than 2.5 for an athlete who spends hours per day in exercise training. For example, in the study mentioned earlier, competitive cyclists had resting metabolic rates of approximately 1,800 kcal/d and estimated TDEE values of 4,300 kcal/d, with a calculated PAL of 4,300 kcal/1,800 kcal or approximately 2.4. Interestingly, on inactive days, these same athletes exhibited TDEE reflective of a PAL of approximately 1.42.[51]

In 2023, the US and Canadian governments created an expert committee to update the estimated energy requirements based on age, sex, body size, body composition, PAL, and race/ethnicity for their populations. The expert committee created an approach to incorporate age dependency into PAL categories to develop new TDEE prediction equations, as evidence indicated that the PAL coefficients varied across age groups and could not be used for all life stages. These male- and female-specific equations are provided in Box 10.4. Box 10.5 provides a comparison of 2 estimations of an athlete's energy requirements, one using the Mifflin-St. Jeor formula and the other using the updated estimated energy requirement (EER) equations that the expert committee developed.[38] TDEE for this person varied by several hundred kilocalories, demonstrating the difficulty in accurately determining TDEE.

BOX 10.3 2023 Dietary Reference Intakes for Energy Based on Physical Activity Levels[38]

Physical Activity Level (PAL) category	Mean PAL value (range)	Example
Inactive	1.25 (1.1-1.39)	A person with an inactive occupation who spends their entire day sitting
Low Active	1.50 (1.40-1.59)	An office worker who sits most of the day other than the walking necessary to perform tasks of daily living
Active	1.75 (1.60-1.89)	An athlete who exercises approximately 1 h/d or a person with an active vocation equivalent to walking 6 to 8 mile/d
Very active	2.20 (1.90-2.50)	A competitive athlete engaging in several hours of vigorous exercise training each day

BOX 10.4 Estimated Energy Requirements for Adults (Age >19 y) Based on Predicted Total Daily Energy Expenditure[38]

Physical Activity Level (PAL) category	Estimated Energy Requirement (EER) equation[a] (kcal/d)
Males	
Inactive	EER = 753.07 - (10.83 × age) + (6.50 × height) + (14.10 × weight)
Low active	EER = 581.47 - (10.83 × age) + (8.30 × height) + (14.94 × weight)
Active	EER = 1,004.82 - (10.83 × age) + (6.52 × height) + (15.91 × weight)
Very active	EER = 517.88 - (10.83 × age) + (15.61 × height) + (19.11 × weight)
Females	
Inactive	EER = 584.90 - (7.01 × age) + (5.72 × height) + (11.71 × weight)
Low active	EER = 575.77 - (7.01 × age) + (6.60 × height) + (12.14 × weight)
Active	EER = 710.25 - (7.01 × age) + (6.54 × height) + (12.34 × weight)
Very active	EER = 511.83 - (7.01 × age) + (9.07 × height) + (12.56 × weight)

[a] In the equations, age is in years, height is in centimeters, and weight is in kilograms.

BOX 10.5 Sample Calculations of Total Daily Energy Expenditure

Athlete profile

A 30-year-old male endurance athlete (very active) is 1.75 m (5 ft 9 in) tall and weighs 73 kg (160.6 lb). The estimated physical activity level (PAL) for this athlete is 2.2. The estimated physical activity (PA) coefficient is 1.48.

Estimate using the Mifflin-St, Jeor equation and PAL

RMR in kcal/d = (10 × weight in kilograms) + (6.25 × height in centimeters) − (5 × age in years) + 5

RMR = (10 × 73) + (6.25 × 175) − (5 × 30) + 5 = 1,679 kcal/d

TDEE = RMR × PAL

TDEE = 1,679 × 2.2 = 3,694 kcal/d

Where RMR = resting metablic rate and TDEE = total daily energy expenditure.

Estimate using updated Estimated Energy Requirement (EER) equation

EER = 517.88 − (10.83 × age in years) + (15.61 × height in centimeters) + (19.11 × weight in kilograms)

EER = 517.88 − (10.83 × 30) + (15.61 × 175) + (19.11 × 73) = 4,317 kcal/d

ENERGY INTAKE

Many factors affect energy intake among active individuals, including the availability and palatability of food, macronutrient composition, social norms, peer pressure, economics, and psychological and emotional factors, to name a few (refer to Figure 10.3). Hall et al[65] have described *energy intake* as a function of the dynamic interplay between homeostatic feedback (hormonal signals from the periphery to the brain), hedonic feedback (stimulation of brain reward centers by foods and even food images), and cognitive feedback (self-regulation and feedback from the environment, including such things as measured body weight, social norms, etc). Although a thorough discussion of this dynamic interplay is beyond the scope of this chapter, some important aspects of neuroendocrine regulation are described later. Insulin and leptin are adiposity-related signals secreted from the periphery that have effects on food intake as mediated through the central nervous system. However, in humans, appetite and food intake are also regulated by a host of hunger and satiety signals originating from the gastrointestinal tract. Ghrelin, the only known orexigenic hormone, is produced primarily by the stomach.[66] This peptide is the endogenous ligand for the growth hormone secretagogue receptor type 1a, which is located throughout the body. Ghrelin binds to its receptor on vagal afferent neurons to mediate effects on appetite regulation.[67] These vagal afferents terminate on the nucleus tractus solitarius, which is connected to the ARC through noradrenergic neurons. Beyond the ARC, ghrelin has an additional effect in driving food intake through the stimulation of the reward centers of the brain. Fasting and weight loss lead to increases in circulating ghrelin concentrations to promote food intake. These concentrations drop rapidly upon meal ingestion, in proportion to the calorie content of the meal.[68]

Numerous peptide hormones released by the gastrointestinal tract are anorexigenic—that is, they decrease hunger and increase satiety. Cholecystokinin (CCK) is secreted by the intestines upon food ingestion. Its role in digestion includes stimulating enzyme release from the pancreas and bile ducts, slowing gastric emptying, and enhancing intestinal motility. CCK decreases hunger and increases satiety through its interactions with the vagus nerve.[69] Additionally, circulating CCK can cross the blood-brain barrier and directly affect the central nervous system. Weight loss decreases circulating CCK concentrations, a phenomenon shown to persist for at least 1 year and possibly much longer after initial weight loss.[2] Glucagon-like peptide 1 (GLP-1) is another anorexigenic hormone secreted by the gastrointestinal tract in response to food intake. Increases in the GLP-1 concentration stimulate the vagus nerve to decrease hunger and increase satiety. Peptide YY (PYY) is cosecreted with GLP-1, mediating its effects through binding to the Y family of G-protein–coupled receptors. PYY also acts to decrease hunger and increase satiety. Concentrations are lowest during fasting and peak about an hour after eating. Calorie content consumed and dietary composition of a meal will affect secretion of these gastrointestinal peptides.[70] These gut peptides, along with still other neuroendocrine signals not discussed in this chapter, coalesce to form the complicated web of signals that must be integrated to determine all aspects of food intake. Whereas the hypothalamus controls the homeostatic regulation of food intake, vast brain circuits beyond the hypothalamus are involved in the initiation and duration of food intake and in feeding behavior based on cognitive and hedonic feedback. When activated, these feedback pathways are capable of overriding the homeostatic control mechanisms designed to maintain energy balance.

The effects of exercise on the secretion of these neuroendocrine factors and the consequent manipulation of hunger and food intake are unclear. Studies have demonstrated how exercise can have a range of effects, including increasing, decreasing, and not affecting ratings of hunger, and these changes in hunger often fail to result in predictable changes in actual food intake.[71-76] The same ambiguous conclusions have been drawn in measurements of the effects of exercise on the concentrations of the hormones and peptides involved in regulating food intake.[76] The discrepancies in the results of these studies may be due to differences in exercise intensity, duration, and mode; participant characteristics such as sex, adiposity, and fitness level; whether the exercise was performed in a fed or fasted state; or even differences in the test meal composition and the amount of time during which intake was monitored after the exercise bout.

Effect of Dietary Composition on Energy Intake

Work by Stubbs et al[77] has demonstrated that habitual intake of high-fat, mixed meals promotes higher energy intake than lower-fat meals. Research has shown that participants are less likely to notice higher energy content in high-fat, mixed meals, a phenomenon termed *passive overconsumption*. Given the higher energy intake and the fact that of the 3 macronutrients, dietary fat is the weakest at promoting its own oxidation, one can envision why overfeeding and fat deposition can so readily occur when dietary composition is high in fat. Note, however, that individuals who consume high-fat, low-carbohydrate diets to lose weight may seem as though they are ingesting more than their usual intake of calories and still lose weight. In reality, such diets are typically hypocaloric because the reduction in carbohydrate calories is greater than the increase in fat and protein calories.

Measurement of Energy Intake

As for the measurement of energy expenditure, the accurate determination of one's energy intake is also fraught with difficulties. Self-reported energy intake can be derived from diet recalls, diet records, and food frequency questionnaires using computer software with the US Department of Agriculture database for the nutrient composition of foods. However, self-reported intake often substantially underestimates actual energy intake.[78-81] Inaccuracies in dietary self-reports severely limit their usefulness in an attempt to accurately quantify energy intake. Accurately measuring energy intake is difficult enough in itself, but energy intake is not always synonymous with metabolized energy in the form of macronutrients absorbed into circulation and available for energy use by cells in the body. The efficiency of absorption is not readily measured. It can be affected by a variety of factors, including the composition of microbiota in the gut. For a brief discussion of this topic, refer to Box 10.6.[82,83]

If an individual's body weight and body composition are stable, energy availability and energy expenditure will be similar over time. In a weight-stable individual, estimating energy expenditure by using an appropriate PAL or equation in Box 10.3 and then balancing the resulting value with caloric consumption is more likely to provide an accurate estimate of energy intake than self-reports of dietary intake. However, self-reported levels of physical activity used to establish an appropriate PAL (Box 10.3) or PA coefficient (Box 10.4) are often overestimated, and one must consider this possibility when there is a large mismatch between an individual's self-reported dietary intake and estimated energy requirements.[84]

BOX 10.6 Emerging Research on the Gut Microbiome of Athletes[82,83]

The human gut microbiome is fascinating, and recent gaps in knowledge regarding the interactions among diet, exercise, and the gut microbiota have been identified. Of particular interest is the impact of alterations in energy intake on the gut microbiome of athletes.

Energy deficiency can result in gastrointestinal distress in athletes, which may be related to negative changes in the gut microbiome (refer to Box 10.8 on page 244 to learn more about relative energy deficiency in sport). In extreme clinical cases of energy deficiency, patients with anorexia nervosa were found to have a decrease in the diversity of their gut microbiota, as well as a reduction in their concentration of short-chain fatty acids, which serve as an energy source in the gut.[82,83] These changes to the gut microbiome in individuals with anorexia nervosa were also found to be associated with poor bone health.[83]

Currently, no published studies have investigated the relationship between gastrointestinal distress, bone health, and changes to the gut microbiome in athletes with low energy availability. Future research should determine whether the clinical manifestations of low energy availability on the gastrointestinal tract and bone health are related to changes in the gut microbiome. Moreover, if the gut microbiome is found to be negatively impacted by low energy availability in athletes, these findings may help to establish microbiota-targeted nutritional guidelines to minimize negative symptoms related to gastrointestinal distress or bone-related injuries.

COMPLEXITIES OF THE ENERGY BALANCE EQUATION

An overly simplistic view of the energy balance equation may lead to projections or even promises of the magnitude of weight loss or weight gain an athlete should achieve based on certain changes in their diet or exercise. However, these projections often assume that all other factors that affect the energy balance equation remain the same. Such a static equation fails to account for homeostatic behavioral and metabolic adjustments in response to perturbations in energy intake and expenditure that render the static energy balance equation inadequate for accurately depicting the reality of the human experience. Less-than-predicted changes in body weight and composition can lead to discouragement and frustration in both athlete and counselor. Kevin Hall, PhD, at the National Institutes of Health, has written extensively about the dynamic aspects of energy balance, and the interested reader is referred to 1 of his reviews for further details.[85]

Dietary-Induced Changes in Energy Balance

In the same manner that acute and chronic exercise can influence energy balance by affecting TDEE and energy intake, so, too, can dietary changes affect energy balance, leading to increases or decreases in body energy stores.

ENERGY DEFICIT LEADING TO WEIGHT LOSS

Studies have shown that during the dynamic phase of weight loss (active weight loss), a hypocaloric diet results in a decrease in RMR and TDEE. Decreases in energy expenditure with active weight loss can be attributed to a loss of respiring body mass, as well as a decrease in energy expenditure per unit of body mass, the latter reflecting an increase in energy efficiency. However, controversy exists about whether this increased energy efficiency persists when the individual has maintained this lost weight for a considerable time. Increased energy efficiency that persists in the reduced-weight state could help explain the inability of so many individuals to maintain weight loss and the reported high levels of exercise and calorie-counting required of many individuals to maintain long-term weight loss.[86] A well-controlled inpatient study sheds some important light on this controversy. Investigators found that individuals who lost 10% or more of their body weight over a 5- to 8-week period had a reduction in TDEE greater than what could be explained by loss of body mass when measured within a few weeks of the weight loss. In the same study, another cohort of individuals who had maintained weight loss of 10% or more of their body weight for a minimum of 1 year was examined. The TDEE of this group was also significantly lower than predicted by their metabolic body size. The authors concluded that weight loss produces increased energy efficiency (lower energy requirements) that persists long term in individuals who are able to maintain the weight loss.[87] In an attempt to explain their findings, the same research group found in a separate study that weight loss was associated with an increased skeletal muscle work efficiency at very low exercise intensities (eg, pedaling a bicycle at 10–25 W of power).[88] As individuals lose weight, their TDEE decreases as a result of the loss of metabolically active tissue. However, TDEE actually decreases *beyond* what would be predicted by this loss in tissue, thus leading to a reduced caloric expenditure in the rested state and making sustained weight loss more difficult.

Given the aforementioned issues, the following scenario describes inappropriate use of the energy balance equation to determine the amount of weight to be lost by a dieting athlete. Suppose the health practitioner and athlete agree that a 17-lb weight loss would improve the athlete's sports performance. They set a goal of reducing the athlete's energy intake by 500 kcal/d, with specific daily food reductions identified after a comprehensive dietary assessment. Given that 1 lb of fat is equivalent to approximately 3,500 kcal, they might conclude that the dietary change would lead to a loss of 1 lb of fat per week (500 kcal/d × 7 days = 3,500 kcal), which, over a 4-month period (17 weeks), would result in a 17-lb decrease in body fat. However, the eventual weight loss is far less than predicted, and both athlete and practitioner are disappointed and frustrated. In reality, a static equation is not useful because changes in food intake can result in metabolic and behavioral changes in factors that influence energy expenditure. Owing to the hypocaloric state, RMR will decrease to an extent greater than can be explained by the loss of respiring tissue mass (ie, metabolic efficiency increases). Also, compared with the prediet state, the energy cost of any particular weight-bearing movement decreases as body mass is lost, and TEF is reduced as less food is consumed. Thus, an initial 500-kcal deficit shrinks over time with subsequent reduction in the velocity of weight loss. Additionally, not all weight loss is body fat (typically it is about 75% fat loss and 25% lean tissue loss), and the energy content of fat and lean tissue are not the same.[89] Given the dynamics induced by an energy deficit, the specific amount of weight lost in a given period is not readily predictable. Adding to this complexity are the difficulties in accurately reducing energy intake by 500 kcal/d, the possible changes in ExEE that can occur when dieting, and the considerable interindividual variation in changes in RMR and PAEE that can occur in response to a reduction in energy intake over a number of months.

Not only does diet-induced weight loss lead to decreases in energy expenditure as described previously, but it is also associated with increases in hunger and decreases in satiety. The term *energy gap* has been coined to identify the decrease in energy expenditure and increase in hunger that accompany diet-induced weight loss. Animal studies have shown that, despite many favorable changes in cardiometabolic features produced by weight loss, numerous metabolic changes almost inevitably lead the animal subjects to regain their lost weight.[90] This anabolic profile following weight loss in humans is characterized by reduced RMR; reduced TEF; increased metabolic efficiency; reduced circulating leptin and insulin; increased orexigenic peptides, such as ghrelin; and reduced anorexigenic peptides, such as PYY. These physiological changes result in an energy gap, in which the animal desires more calories than it requires. These metabolic changes induced by caloric restriction can readily alter the energy balance following weight loss and appear to be major contributors to the lack of successful long-term weight loss in many dieters. Registered dietitian nutritionists should be cognizant of the energy-gap phenomenon and seek ways to help their clients attenuate the decline in energy expenditure and the increase in hunger after weight loss. A high ExEE can help attenuate the drop in TDEE and allows for greater energy intake without resulting in a positive energy balance. Following diet-induced weight loss, individuals maintaining a relatively high TDEE through exercise with adequate calorie intake (a high-flux state) can attenuate the energy gap by increasing subjective feelings of fullness and increasing RMR compared with a sedentary low-flux state.[91]

ENERGY EXCESS LEADING TO WEIGHT GAIN

For the active individual attempting to gain weight (including athletes wanting to increase lean body mass), an increase in energy intake is crucial. However, increased energy consumption may be offset by compensatory changes in metabolism, such that TDEE will increase and thus attenuate increases in lean body mass. These compensatory changes in energy expenditure are highly variable, as are the magnitude of weight gain and increases in lean mass and body fat. For example, in several studies in which individuals were overfed an additional 1,000 kcal/d for several months, there were 3- to 5-fold differences in the magnitude of weight gain between the highest and lowest gainers.[92,93] In a study from the Mayo Clinic, a 10-fold difference was found in the amount of body fat deposition between the highest and lowest gainers, despite the same magnitude of overfeeding for all study participants (1,000 kcal in excess of maintenance requirements). Overfeeding increases RMR in most individuals beyond what would be expected by their changes in body size; that is, overfeeding results in decreased energy efficiency. Also, increases in TEF and the energy cost of movement contribute to an increase in TDEE. Adding to the complexity are the dramatic changes in NEAT that can occur in some individuals. In the Mayo Clinic study, an increase in NEAT was a much stronger predictor of attenuated weight gain than were increases in RMR and TEF.[92]

Exercise-Induced Changes in Energy Balance

Just as a change in energy intake can influence energy expenditure, an increase in PAEE can also influence energy intake. Although physical activity is the best means of increasing energy expenditure, the effects of exercise alone on weight loss are typically modest[94] unless substantial increases in ExEE occur without compensatory increases in energy intake.[95] The reasons why an exercise-only approach to weight loss produces such small losses of body weight for many individuals are discussed in Box 10.7.

BOX 10.7 Example of Limited Potential for Substantial Weight Loss From Exercise in a Previously Sedentary Person

Consider a sedentary male individual attempting to lose weight who decides to do so by starting an exercise program. He establishes a goal of walking for 40 minutes per day, 5 days per week. How much weight might this individual expect to lose over the course of several weeks and months if he tenaciously sticks to his new exercise regimen?

- Resting energy expenditure = 1.25 kcal/min = 1,800 kcal/d
- Sitting/standing energy expenditure = 1.5 kcal/min
- Exercise characteristics:
  - Duration: 40 min/exercise session
  - Frequency: 5 times/wk
  - Intensity: 5 metabolic equivalents = 6.25 kcal/min
- Gross daily energy cost of 40 minutes of exercise: 6.25 kcal/min × 40 min/d = 250 kcal/d
- Net energy cost of exercise per day: 250 kcal/d - (40 min/d × 1.5 kcal/min) = 190 kcal/d
- Net energy cost of exercise per week: 190 kcal/d × 5 d/wk = 950 kcal/wk

These data show that, whereas the gross energy cost of the walking exercise is 250 kcal for a 40-minute exercise session, the net energy cost is 60 kcal less, due to the fact that even if the person had not exercised, he would have expended at least 60 kcal while sitting or standing during those 40 minutes. Without any compensatory changes in dietary intake or other components of energy expenditure, the projected energy deficit over the course of a single month would be less than 4,000 kcal, equivalent to a monthly weight loss of slightly more than 1 lb, assuming no other metabolic or behavioral compensations, which is highly unlikely. This weight loss is far less than one might expect from a month-long diet. A head-to-head comparison of the amount of weight loss achieved by exercise only vs diet only is somewhat unfair, as the magnitude of energy deficit created by a hypocaloric diet is usually far greater than that created by starting an exercise program.

The magnitude of an exercise-induced energy deficit and weight loss can be affected by more than just the energy cost of the exercise, as compensatory changes in both NEAT and energy intake may occur. Just as with dieting and overfeeding, there is substantial individual variability in the amount of weight loss due to exercise. In an experimental investigation, people who were overweight or obese underwent prescribed and supervised exercise (500 kcal/session) for 5 days per week for 12 weeks. The average weight loss was 3.7 kg (8.1 lb), similar to that predicted using the static energy balance equation, suggesting no metabolic or compensatory changes. However, there was a very large variation in individual response, with 4 of the 30 study participants actually gaining weight. In the remaining 26 study participants, the weight loss ranged from 1 kg (2.2 lb) to 14.7 kg (32.3 lb). This occurred despite rigorous control and supervision of the exercise program so that all individuals were achieving the same energy cost of exercise. The major predictor of the magnitude of weight change was the change in energy intake that accompanied the exercise.[96] These findings suggest that, in response to initiating a sizable weekly energy expenditure in exercise, some individuals increase their energy intakes, whereas other individuals actually reduce them. Why there is a difference in response is not understood, but it is clear that there are very large differences in body weight and composition changes in response to the same amount of exercise.[97]

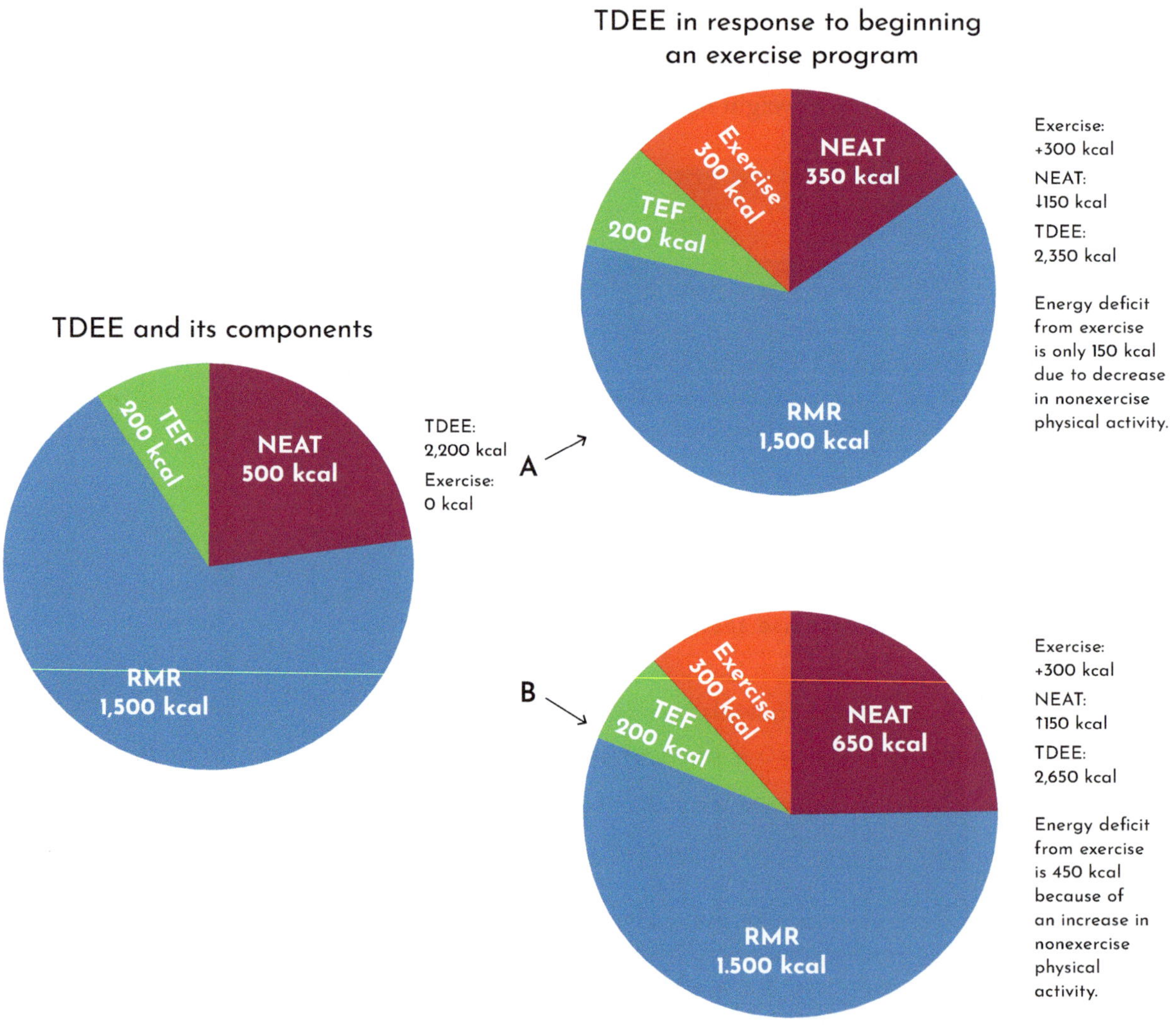

FIGURE 10.5 Illustration of change in energy balance in a sedentary person This figure illustrates 2 possible scenarios depicting the change in energy balance of a sedentary individual who begins an exercise program to create an energy deficit. Initially the person is in energy balance, with a total daily energy expenditure (TDEE) of 2,200 kcal (physical activity level [PAL] = 1.47), based on a resting metabolic rate (RMR) of 1,500 kcal, a thermic effect of food (TEF) of 200 kcal, and nonexercise activity thermogenesis (NEAT) of 500 kcal. The person begins an exercise program and adds a net 300 kcal to the energy expenditure side of the energy balance equation. However, in scenario A, the person compensates by reducing the activities of daily living, so the net change in energy expenditure is 150 kcal, not 300 kcal. In scenario B, in addition to the increase in exercise energy expenditure, the person actually increases NEAT by 150 kcal, and the net increase in TDEE is 450 kcal. Note that any change in energy intake as a result of a change in exercise must also be considered in an analysis of the overall impact on energy balance of beginning an exercise program.

It is also possible that in response to an increase in ExEE, compensatory decreases in NEAT could offset the impact on energy balance. For example, in 1 study, older adults who initiated an endurance exercise training program failed to significantly increase their TDEE, presumably because of a compensatory decline in NEAT during the nonexercise portion of the day.[98] Nevertheless, the reverse could be true in some individuals—that is, their NEAT may increase with improved physical fitness (Figure 10.5).

On the other end of the spectrum, a sudden cessation of ExEE can also have implications for body-weight regulation. This might occur, for example, when an athlete experiences a debilitating injury or when a collegiate athlete accustomed to a life of daily regimented physical activity graduates and no longer has the regular mandates of training and team practice. These scenarios exemplify a transition from a high-flux state—wherein a high TDEE must be matched with a high energy intake—to a low-flux state where energy intake must be substantially decreased to match the new state of low TDEE. Failure to lower energy intake in response to reduced energy expenditure, either mandated by injury or incurred by personal choice, will lead to a positive energy balance and an increase in adiposity. Unfortunately, owing to reduced exercise, atrophy of skeletal muscle often occurs as well.

Although little is known regarding the specific physiological phenomena occurring in the initial hours and days of reduced physical activity, these circumstances can result in substantial metabolic changes over time. One study found that with just 2 days of no exercise in endurance-trained individuals, insulin sensitivity dropped to those of sedentary levels.[99] In addition, increasing adiposity often accompanies retirement from sports participation. An estimated 30% of retired American football players have metabolic syndrome,[100] with a 60% prevalence in retired linemen specifically.[101] In another study, competitive cyclists exercised at a moderate-heavy intensity for 3 consecutive days and then abstained from exercise for the 2 subsequent days, while still maintaining a high energy intake. In just these 2 days, individuals displayed an RMR that was reduced from its value in a high-flux state and regained weight that had been lost in the previous 3 days of exercise.[51] Taken together, these data show potential implications for the effects of reductions in energy expenditure on body weight and markers for metabolic health and warrant modifications in intake during these periods. Though specific recommendations pertaining to alterations in total calories and macronutrient ratios are yet to be firmly established, changes in insulin sensitivity and resting metabolism lend support to the necessity of reevaluating nutrition strategies when transitioning out of a high-flux condition.

EFFECT OF ACUTE EXERCISE ON POSTEXERCISE ENERGY EXPENDITURE

Based on studies performed decades ago, many in the sports community held the common belief that upon completion of an exercise bout, individuals would continue to expend energy at an excess rate for a prolonged time, possibly up to 24 hours. Researchers believed that this excess postexercise energy expenditure provided a substantial contribution to TDEE in those who exercised. However, based on more carefully controlled studies, this is usually not the case. Although research has clearly shown that energy expenditure remains increased at higher-than-preexercise resting baseline levels immediately after exercise, the magnitude of this postexercise elevation of energy expenditure is almost always quite small unless the exercise bout is of high intensity and prolonged duration. Endurance exercise of the intensity and duration commonly put forth by recreational exercisers (for example, walking for 30 to 60 minutes or jogging at a pace of 8 to 10 minutes per mile for 30 minutes) typically results in a return to the baseline of energy expenditure well within the first hour of recovery.[102] The postexercise energy bonus for this type of exercise probably accounts for only about 10 to 30 additional kilocalories expended beyond the exercise bout itself.[103] Nevertheless, in athletes performing high-intensity, long-duration exercise, postexercise energy expenditure may remain elevated longer and could contribute a bit more to TDEE.[51,102] Endurance athletes who are in a state of high energy flux (high energy intake and expenditure) may have postexercise elevations that can be detected the morning after exercise,[51] but only the rare individual can regularly achieve this state of high flux. The average person who does considerably less strenuous exercise will likely experience little meaningful contribution of this postexercise bonus to their TDEE.

Several studies have suggested that vigorous weight-lifting exercise may increase energy expenditure to more than typical resting values for several hours and possibly even until the morning of the following day.[53,104] The possibility remains that, for both endurance and resistance exercise, the accumulation of even modest excess postexercise energy expenditure over the course of months and years can substantially impact energy expenditure. Yet, it is clear that the vast majority of energy expenditure occurs during the exercise itself rather than after.

EFFECT OF ACUTE EXERCISE ON ENERGY INTAKE

Numerous studies have examined the effects of acute and chronic exercise on energy intake. Many experimental studies have indicated that following acute strenuous exercise, increased energy intake during the next 24 hours does not completely compensate for the energy cost of the exercise.[96,105] Donnelly et al[106] conducted a systematic review of published studies and concluded that there is no consistent evidence that increased exercise affects energy intake or dietary macronutrient intake. These conclusions suggest that athletes who exhibit their desired body composition and increase exercise training to maximize performance may need to intentionally increase their energy intake accordingly. The consequences of energy imbalance in which energy expended through exercise exceeds energy intake, to the point that insufficient energy is left over to maintain normal physiologic function, is described in Box 10.8.[107-111]

BOX 10.8 Relative Energy Deficiency in Sport[107-111]

A perfect way to summarize the importance of energy balance is through the discussion of the impact of relative energy deficiency in sport (REDs) on athletes. The International Olympic Committee introduced the concept of REDs in 2014, and since then, emerging research has aimed to better understand the impact of REDs on the health and performance of various types of athletes. REDs is understood as a syndrome of impaired physiological function caused by energy deficiency relative to the balance between energy intake and energy expenditure. In REDs insufficient energy is left over after exercise to maintain the energy required for normal physiological function, which can inevitably lead to the impairment of several body systems, including, but not limited to, metabolic rate, menstrual function (in female athletes), bone health, and the immune system.[107,108] For example, energy deficiency has been found to have a dire impact on endocrine function, specifically leptin, triiodothyronine (T3), luteinizing hormone, follicle stimulating hormone, estradiol, testosterone, insulin-like growth factor 1 (IGF-1), and cortisol. Subsequently, reproductive function and bone health are negatively impacted, resulting in an increased risk of bone stress injury and musculoskeletal injury.[109]

Low energy availability (LEA) underpins the concept of REDs and occurs when an athlete's energy intake does not match their energy expenditure. Note that LEA also underpins the concepts of the female and male athlete triad, although these are viewed as separate, but equally meaningful, concepts to REDs.[110,111] The etiology of LEA may be due to a deficit of nutrition knowledge or to behaviors related to disordered eating or clinical eating disorders.[107,108]

Early identification of REDs is crucial to prevent significant harm to the athlete, such as injury or illness, and sports registered dietitian nutritionists are viewed as the key professionals in the identification of at-risk athletes and their care.

As previously discussed, many limitations exist regarding the collection of accurate energy intake and energy expenditure data. This serves as a major limitation of the accuracy of the results of energy availability equations, methodological approaches used in REDs research, and the attempt to develop evidence-based standards in the assessment of REDs in athletes.[108] Nonetheless, the issue of REDs is deserving of future research because of the deleterious effects this syndrome can have on the health, performance, and well-being of athletes. Refer to Chapter 18 for more information.

SUMMARY

Individual behavioral and metabolic characteristics affect acute and chronic energy balance and fundamentally explain the various body shapes and sizes present within the human population, including those of athletes. Energy balance is, in theory, a simple concept: if energy intake exceeds expenditure, the excess energy will be stored in the body, primarily as fat, unless concomitant exercise or physical maturation favors greater storage as lean body mass; if energy expenditure exceeds intake, body energy stores will be lost.

In reality, energy balance is best understood as a dynamic equation rather than a static one, wherein changes to one side of the scale can produce unintentional compensatory metabolic and behavioral changes in the other side of the scale. Because body weight is regulated by a host of neuroendocrine factors, because adaptive changes to energy intake and expenditure can modify energy balance and energy efficiency, and because there are considerable difficulties in accurately quantifying both intake and expenditure, the simplicity of this concept gives way to complexity. Even with intact regulatory systems, it seems that, in the face of our current obesogenic environment, the regulatory systems of many humans are poorly equipped to adequately protect against excess body weight and fat gain. Maintaining relatively high daily energy expenditure through ExEE and NEAT can help protect against unhealthy weight gain in the face of the current abundance of highly palatable food. Although body fat stores can be reduced by creating an energy deficit, severe energy restriction by dieting can result in metabolic adaptations that sabotage maintenance of lost weight and potentially may result in serious syndromes such as REDs. Increases in physical activity can contribute to increased energy expenditure, but the magnitude of this increase is often quite small for the beginning exerciser. Realistic expectations regarding energy intake and expenditure and their effects on body weight and composition must replace the often-mythical promises marketed to hopeful consumers by advertisements, gimmickry, and fad diets. Understanding the behavioral and metabolic features of the elite or recreational athlete is important in developing the most effective individualized approaches to facilitate their achievement of a healthy and competitive body weight and composition.

KEY TAKEAWAYS

Energy balance is, at its core, a simple concept: if energy availability from food and beverage intake exceeds expenditure, the excess energy will be stored in the body, primarily as fat, unless concomitant exercise or physical maturation favors greater storage as lean body mass; if energy expenditure exceeds intake, body energy stores will be lost.

Energy balance is best understood as a dynamic equation rather than a static one, wherein changes in energy expenditure often bring about compensatory voluntary or involuntary changes in energy intake. Conversely, changes in energy intake bring about compensatory changes in energy expenditure.

Total daily energy expenditure is the sum of the RMR, the TEF, and PAEE, including exercise and nonexercise activity thermogenesis.

Energy intake is influenced by neuroendocrine factors that regulate hunger and satiety. However, personal, social, and environmental factors, including the availability of high-energy-density foods and low levels of physical activity, can override the homeostatic regulation of body weight and contribute to increased body fat.

Weight loss is usually associated with an increase in hunger and a reduction in energy expenditure—called the energy gap—which is a major contributor to the common occurrence of weight regain. Regular exercise may help attenuate the energy gap by contributing to increased energy expenditure and enabling higher energy intake without accompanying weight gain.

Understanding the behavioral and metabolic features of the elite or recreational athlete is important in developing the most effective individualized approaches to facilitate their achievement of a healthy and competitive body weight and composition.

REFERENCES

1. Schutz Y. Dietary fat, lipogenesis and energy balance. *Physiol Behav.* 2004;83(4):557-564. doi:10.1016/j.physbeh.2004.09.015
2. Harper M-E, Green K, Brand MD. The efficiency of cellular energy transduction and its implications for obesity. *Annu Rev Nutr.* 2008;28:13-33. doi:10.1146/annurev.nutr.28.061807.155357
3. Chow CC, Hall KD. Short and long-term energy intake patterns and their implications for human body weight regulation. *Physiol Behav.* 2014;134:60-65. doi:10.1186/s40798-017-0076-1
4. Emanuela F, Grazia M, Marco de R, Maria Paola L, Giorgio F, Marco B. Inflammation as a link between obesity and metabolic syndrome. *J Nutr Metab.* 2012;2012:476380. doi:10.1155/2012/476380
5. Wells JCK. The evolution of human adiposity and obesity: where did it all go wrong? *Dis Model Mech.* 2012;5(5):595-607. doi:10.1242/dmm.009613
6. Leibel RL, Rosenbaum M, Hirsch J. Changes in energy expenditure resulting from altered body weight. *N Engl J Med.* 1995;332(10):621-628. doi:10.1056/NEJM199503093321001
7. Virtanen KA, Lidell ME, Orava J, et al. Functional brown adipose tissue in healthy adults. *N Engl J Med.* 2009;360(15):1518-1525. doi:10.1056/NEJMoa0808949
8. Cypess AM, Lehman S, Williams G, et al. Identification and importance of brown adipose tissue in adult humans. *N Engl J Med.* 2009;360(15):1509-1517. doi:10.1056/NEJMoa0810780
9. Petrovic N, Walden TB, Shabalina IG, Timmons JA, Cannon B, Nedergaard J. Chronic peroxisome proliferator-activated receptor γ (PPARγ) activation of epididymally derived white adipocyte cultures reveals a population of thermogenically competent, UCP1-containing adipocytes molecularly distinct from classic brown adipocytes. *J Biol Chem.* 2010;285(10):7153-7164. doi:10.1074/jbc.M109.053942
10. Mu W-J, Zhu J-Y, Chen M, Guo L. Exercise-mediated browning of white adipose tissue: its significance, mechanism and effectiveness. *Int J Mol Sci.* 2021;22(21):11512. doi:10.3390/ijms222111512
11. Bostrom P, Wu J, Jedrychowski MP, et al. A PGC1-α-dependent myokine that drives brown-fat-like development of white fat and thermogenesis. *Nature.* 2012;481(7382):463-468. doi:10.1038/nature10777
12. Norheim F, Langleite TM, Hjorth M, et al. The effects of acute and chronic exercise on PGC-1α, irisin and browning of subcutaneous adipose tissue in humans. *FEBS J.* 2014;28(3)1:739-749. doi:10.1111/febs.12619
13. Vosselman MJ, Hoeks J, Brans B, et al. Low brown adipose tissue activity in endurance-trained compared with lean sedentary men. *Int J Obes (Lond).* 2015;39(12):1696-1702. doi:10.1038/ijo.2015.130
14. Kerstholt N, Ewert R, Nauck M, et al. Association of circulating irisin and cardiopulmonary exercise capacity in healthy volunteers: results of the Study of Health in Pomerania. *BMC Pulm Med.* 2015;15:41. doi:10.1186/s12890-015-0035-x
15. Lagzdina R, Rumaka M, Gersone G, Tretjakovs P. Circulating irisin in healthy adults: changes after acute exercise, correlation with body composition, and energy expenditure parameters in cross-sectional study. *Medicina (Kaunas).* 2020;56(6):274. doi:10.3390/medicina56060274
16. Jedrychowski MP, Wrann CD, Paulo JA, et al. Detection and quantitation of circulating human irisin by tandem mass spectrometry. *Cell Metab.* 2015;22(4):734-740. doi:10.1016/j.cmet.2015.08.001
17. Albuquerque D, Stice E, Rodríguez-López R, Manco L, Nóbrega C. Current review of genetics of human obesity: from molecular mechanisms to an evolutionary perspective. *Mol Genet Genomics.* 2015;290(4):1191-1221. doi:10.1007/s00438-015-1015-9
18. Friedman JM. Modern science versus the stigma of obesity. *Nat Med.* 2004;10(6):563-569. doi:10.1038/nm0604-563
19. Morton GJ, Schwartz MW. The NPY/AgRP neuron and energy homeostasis. *Int J Obes Relat Metab Disord.* 2001;25(suppl 5):S56-S62. doi:10.1038/sj.ijo.0801915
20. Hagan MM, Rushing PA, Schwartz MW, et al. Role of the CNS melanocortin system in the response to overfeeding. *J Neurosci.* 1999;19(6):2362-2367. doi:10.1523/JNEUROSCI.19-06-02362.1999
21. Considine RV, Sinha MK, Heiman ML, et al. Serum immunoreactive-leptin concentrations in normal-weight and obese humans. *N Engl J Med.* 1996;334(5):292-295. doi:10.1056/NEJM199602013340503
22. Polonsky KS, Given BD, Van Cauter E. Twenty-four-hour profiles and pulsatile patterns of insulin secretion in normal and obese subjects. *J Clin Invest.* 1988;81(2):442-448. doi:10.1172/JCI113339
23. Friedman JM. A tale of two hormones. *Nat Med.* 2010;16(10):1100-1106. doi:10.1038/nm1010-1100
24. Funahashi H, Yada T, Suzuki R, Shioda S. Distribution, function, and properties of leptin receptors in the brain. *Int Rev Cytol.* 2003;224:1-27. doi:10.1016/s0074-7696(05)24001-9
25. Elias CF, Aschkenasi C, Lee C, et al. Leptin differentially regulates NPY and POMC neurons projecting to the lateral hypothalamic area. *Neuron.* 1999;23(4):775-786. doi:10.1016/s0896-6273(01)80035-0
26. Schwartz MW, Marks JL, Sipols AJ, et al. Central insulin administration reduces neuropeptide Y mRNA expression in the arcuate nucleus of food-deprived lean (Fa/Fa) but not obese (fa/fa) Zucker rats. *Endocrinology.* 1991;128(5):2645-2647. doi:10.1210/endo-128-5-2645
27. Keijer J, Hoevenaars FP, Nieuwenhuizen A, van Schothorst EM. Nutrigenomics of body weight regulation: a rationale for careful dissection of individual contributors. *Nutrients.* 2014;6(10):4531-4551. doi:10.3390/nu6104531

28. Keesey RE, Powley TL. Body energy homeostasis. *Appetite.* 2008;51(3):442-445. doi:10.1016/j.appet.2008.06.009
29. Schwartz MW, Baskin DG, Kaiyala KJ, Woods SC. Model for the regulation of energy balance and adiposity by the central nervous system. *Am J Clin Nutr.* 1999;69(4):584-596. doi:10.1093/ajcn/69.4.584
30. Schwartz MW, Niswender KD. Adiposity signaling and biological defense against weight gain: absence of protection or central hormone resistance? *J Clin Endocrinol Metab.* 2004;89(12):5889-5897. doi:10.1210/jc.2004-0906
31. Niswender KD, Baskin DG, Schwartz MW. Insulin and its evolving partnership with leptin in the hypothalamic control of energy homeostasis. *Trends Endocrinol Metab.* 2004;15(8):362-369. doi:10.1016/j.tem.2004.07.009
32. Schwartz MW, Woods SC, Seeley RJ, Barsh GS, Baskin DG, Leibel RL. Is the energy homeostasis system inherently biased toward weight gain? *Diabetes.* 2003;52(2):232-238. doi:10.2337/diabetes.52.2.232
33. Major GC, Doucet E, Trayhurn P, Astrup A, Tremblay A. Clinical significance of adaptive thermogenesis. *Int J Obes (Lond).* 2007;31(2):204-212. doi:10.1038/sj.ijo.0803523
34. Melby CL, Schmidt WD, Corrigan D. Resting metabolic rate in weight-cycling collegiate wrestlers compared with physically active, noncycling control subjects. *Am J Clin Nutr.* 1990;52(3):409-414. doi:10.1093/ajcn/52.3.409
35. Ravussin E, Bogardus C. Energy balance and weight regulation: genetics versus environment. *Br J Nutr.* 2000;83(suppl 1):S17-S20. doi:10.1017/s0007114500000908
36. Bullough RC, Melby CL. Effect of inpatient versus outpatient measurement protocol on resting metabolic rate and respiratory exchange ratio. *Ann Nutr Metab.* 1993;37(1):24-32. doi:10.1159/000177745
37. Levine JA. Measurement of energy expenditure. *Public Health Nutr.* 2005;8(7A):1123-1132. doi:10.1079/phn2005800
38. National Academies of Sciences, Engineering, and Medicine; Health and Medicine Division; Food and Nutrition Board; Committee on the Dietary Reference Intakes for Energy. *Dietary Reference Intakes for Energy*. National Academies Press; January 17, 2023.
39. Roberts SB, Dallal GE. Energy requirements and aging. *Public Health Nutr.* 2005;8(7A):1028-1036. doi:10.1079/phn2005794
40. Nieman DC, Trone GA, Austin MD. A new handheld device for measuring resting metabolic rate and oxygen consumption. *J Am Diet Assoc.* 2003;103(5):588-592. doi:10.1053/jada.2003.50116
41. Schoeller DA, van Santen E. Measurement of energy expenditure in humans by doubly labeled water method. *J Appl Physiol Respir Environ Exerc Physiol.* 1982;53(4):955-959. doi:10.1152/jappl.1982.53.4.955
42. Westerterp KR. Exercise, energy expenditure and energy balance, as measured with doubly labelled water. *Proc Nutr Soc.* 2018;77(1):4-10. doi:10.1017/S0029665117001148
43. Lifson N, Gordon GB, McClintock R. Measurement of total carbon dioxide production by means of D_2O^{18}. *J Appl Physiol.* 1955;7(6):704-710. doi:10.1152/jappl.1955.7.6.704
44. Harris JA, Benedict FG. A biometric study of human basal metabolism. *Proc Natl Acad Sci U S A.* 1918;4(12):370-373. doi:10.1073/pnas.4.12.370
45. Cunningham JJ. Body composition as a determinant of energy expenditure: a synthetic review and a proposed general prediction equation. *Am J Clin Nutr.* 1991;54(6):963-969. doi:10.1093/ajcn/54.6.963
46. Owen OE, Holup JL, D'Alessio DA, et al. A reappraisal of the caloric requirements of men. *Am J Clin Nutr.* 1987;46(6):875-885. doi:10.1093/ajcn/46.6.875
47. Owen OE, Kavle E, Owen RS, et al. A reappraisal of caloric requirements in healthy women. *Am J Clin Nutr.* 1986;44(1):1-19. doi:10.1093/ajcn/44.1.1
48. Liu HY, Lu YF, Chen WJ. Predictive equations for basal metabolic rate in Chinese adults: a cross-validation study. *J Am Diet Assoc.* 1995;95(12):1403-1408. doi:10.1016/S0002-8223(95)00369-X
49. Thompson J, Manore MM. Predicted and measured resting metabolic rate of male and female endurance athletes. *J Am Diet Assoc.* 1996;96(1):30-34. doi:10.1016/S0002-8223(96)00010-7
50. Mifflin MD, St Jeor ST, Hill LA, Scott BJ, Daugherty SA, Koh YO. A new predictive equation for resting energy expenditure in healthy individuals. *Am J Clin Nutr.* 1990;51(2):241-247. doi:10.1093/ajcn/51.2.241
51. Bullough RC, Gillette CA, Harris MA, Melby CL. Interaction of acute changes in exercise energy expenditure and energy intake on resting metabolic rate. *Am J Clin Nutr.* 1995;61(3):473-481. doi:10.1093/ajcn/61.3.473
52. Bell C, Day DS, Jones PP, et al. High energy flux mediates the tonically augmented beta-adrenergic support of resting metabolic rate in habitually exercising older adults. *J Clin Endocrinol Metab.* 2004;89(7):3573-3578. doi:10.1210/jc.2003-032146
53. Melby C, Scholl C, Edwards G, Bullough R. Effect of acute resistance exercise on postexercise energy expenditure and resting metabolic rate. *J Appl Physiol (1985).* 1993;75(4):1847-1853. doi:10.1152/jappl.1993.75.4.1847
54. van Baak MA. Meal-induced activation of the sympathetic nervous system and its cardiovascular and thermogenic effects in man. *Physiol Behav.* 2008;94(2):178-186. doi:10.1016/j.physbeh.2007.12.020
55. Caspersen CJ, Powell KE, Christenson GM. Physical activity, exercise, and physical fitness: definitions and distinctions for health-related research. *Public Health Rep.* 1985;100(2):126-131.
56. Ainsworth BE, Haskell WL, Whitt MC, et al. Compendium of physical activities: an update of activity codes and MET intensities. *Med Sci Sports Exerc.* 2000;32(suppl 9):S498-S504. doi:10.1097/00005768-200009001-00009
57. Levine JA, Vander Weg MW, Hill JO, Klesges RC. Non-exercise activity thermogenesis: the crouching tiger hidden dragon of societal weight gain. *Arterioscler Thromb Vasc Biol.* 2006;26(4):729-736. doi:10.1161/01.ATV.0000205848.83210.73
58. Levine JA. Nonexercise activity thermogenesis—liberating the life-force. *J Intern Med.* 2007;262(3):273-287. doi:10.1111/j.1365-2796.2007.01842.x

59. Levine JA, Lanningham-Foster LM, McCrady SK, et al. Interindividual variation in posture allocation: possible role in human obesity. *Science.* 2005;307(5709):584-586. doi:10.1126/science.1106561
60. Levine JA, Schleusner SJ, Jensen MD. Energy expenditure of nonexercise activity. *Am J Clin Nutr.* 2000;72(6):1451-1454. doi:10.1093/ajcn/72.6.1451
61. Lewis ZH, Lyons EJ, Jarvis JM, Baillargeon J. Using an electronic activity monitor system as an intervention modality: a systematic review. *BMC Public Health.* 2015;15:585. doi:10.1186/s12889-015-1947-3
62. Lee J-M, Kim Y, Welk GJ. Validity of consumer-based physical activity monitors. *Med Sci Sports Exerc.* 2014;46(9):1840-1848. doi:10.1249/MSS.0000000000000287
63. Ferguson T, Rowlands AV, Olds T, Maher C. The validity of consumer-level, activity monitors in healthy adults worn in free-living conditions: a cross-sectional study. *Int J Behav Nutr Phys Act.* 2015;12:42. doi:10.1186/s12966-015-0201-9
64. Hongu N, Orr BJ, Roe DJ, Reed RG, Going SB. Global positioning system watches for estimating energy expenditure. *J Strength Cond Res.* 2013;27(11):3216-3220. doi:10.1519/JSC.0b013e31828bae0f
65. Hall KD, Hammond RA, Rahmandad H. Dynamic interplay among homeostatic, hedonic, and cognitive feedback circuits regulating body weight. *Am J Public Health.* 2014;104(7):1169-1175. doi:10.2105/AJPH.2014.301931
66. Kojima M, Hosoda H, Date Y, Nakazato M, Matsuo H, Kangawa K. Ghrelin is a growth-hormone-releasing acylated peptide from stomach. *Nature.* 1999;402(6762):656-660. doi:10.1038/45230
67. le Roux CW, Neary NM, Halsey TJ, et al. Ghrelin does not stimulate food intake in patients with surgical procedures involving vagotomy. *J Clin Endocrinol Metab.* 2005;90(8):4521-4524. doi:10.1210/jc.2004-2537
68. le Roux CW, Patterson M, Vincent RP, Hunt C, Ghatei MA, Bloom SR. Postprandial plasma ghrelin is suppressed proportional to meal calorie content in normal-weight but not obese subjects. *J Clin Endocrinol Metab.* 2005;90(2):1068-1071. doi:10.1210/jc.2004-1216
69. Rogers RC, Hermann GE. Mechanisms of action of CCK to activate central vagal afferent terminals. *Peptides.* 2008;29(10):1716-1725. doi:10.1016/j.peptides.2008.06.023
70. Moran TH. Gut peptides in the control of food intake. *Int J Obes (Lond).* 2009;33(suppl 1):S7-S10. doi:10.1038/ijo.2009.9
71. King NA, Lluch A, Stubbs RJ, Blundell JE. High dose exercise does not increase hunger or energy intake in free living males. *Eur J Clin Nutr.* 1997;51(7):478-483. doi:10.1038/sj.ejcn.1600432
72. Thompson DA, Wolfe LA, Eikelboom R. Acute effects of exercise intensity on appetite in young men. *Med Sci Sports Exerc.* 1988;20(3):222-227. doi:10.1249/00005768-198806000-00002
73. Pomerleau M, Imbeault P, Parker T, Doucet E. Effects of exercise intensity on food intake and appetite in women. *Am J Clin Nutr.* 2004;80(5):1230-1236. doi:10.1093/ajcn/80.5.1230
74. King NA, Snell L, Smith RD, Blundell JE. Effects of short-term exercise on appetite responses in unrestrained females. *Eur J Clin Nutr.* 1996;50(10):663-667.
75. Imbeault P, Saint-Pierre S, Alméras N, Tremblay A. Acute effects of exercise on energy intake and feeding behaviour. *Br J Nutr.* 1997;77:511-521. doi:10.1079/bjn19970053
76. Bilski J, Manko G, Brzozowski T, et al. Effects of exercise of different intensity on gut peptides, energy intake and appetite in young males. *Ann Agric Environ Med.* 2013;20(4):787-793.
77. Stubbs RJ, Harbron CG, Murgatroyd PR, Prentice AM. Covert manipulation of dietary fat and energy density: effect on substrate flux and food intake in men eating ad libitum. *Am J Clin Nutr.* 1995;62(2):316-329. doi:10.1093/ajcn/62.2.316
78. Goldberg GR, Black AE, Jebb SA, et al. Critical evaluation of energy intake data using fundamental principles of energy physiology: 1. Derivation of cut-off limits to identify under-recording. *Eur J Clin Nutr.* 1991;45(12):569-581.
79. Melby CL, Ho RC, Jeckel K, Beal L, Goran M, Donahoo WT. Comparison of risk factors for obesity in young, nonobese African-American and Caucasian women. *Int J Obes Relat Metab Disord.* 2000;24(11):1514-1522. doi:10.1038/sj.ijo.0801413
80. Turnbaugh PJ, Ley RE, Mahowald MA, Magrini V, Mardis ER, Gordon JI. An obesity-associated gut microbiome with increased capacity for energy harvest. *Nature.* 2006;444(7122):1027-1031. doi:10.1038/nature05414
81. Lau E, Carvalho D, Pina-Vaz C, Barbosa JA, Freitas P. Beyond gut microbiota: understanding obesity and type 2 diabetes. *Hormones (Athens).* 2015;14(3):358-369. doi:10.14310/horm.2002.1571
82. Monteleone AM, Troisi J, Fasano A, et al. Multiomics data integration in anorexia nervosa patients before and after weight regain: a microbiome-metabolomics investigation. *Clin Nutr.* 2021;40(3):1137–1146. doi:10.1016/j.clnu.2020.07.021
83. Aurigemma NC, Koltun KJ, VanEvery H, Rogers CJ, De Souza MJ. Linking the gut microbiota to bone health in anorexia nervosa. *Curr Osteoporos Rep.* 2018;16(1):65–75. doi:10.1007/s11914-018-0420-5
84. Prince SA, Adamo KB, Hamel ME, Hardt J, Connor Gorber S, Tremblay M. A comparison of direct versus self-report measures for assessing physical activity in adults: a systematic review. *Int J Behav Nutr Phys Act.* 2008;5:56. doi:10.1186/1479-5868-5-56
85. Hall KD, Sacks G, Chandramohan D, et al. Quantification of the effect of energy imbalance on bodyweight. *Lancet.* 2011;378(9793):826-837. doi:10.1016/S0140-6736(11)60812-X
86. Wing RR, Hill JO. Successful weight loss maintenance. *Annu Rev Nutr.* 2001;21:323-341. doi:10.1146/annurev.nutr.21.1.323
87. Rosenbaum M, Hirsch J, Gallagher DA, Leibel RL. Long-term persistence of adaptive thermogenesis in subjects who have maintained a reduced body weight. *Am J Clin Nutr.* 2008;88(4):906-912. doi:10.1093/ajcn/88.4.906

88. Goldsmith R, Joanisse DR, Gallagher D, et al. Effects of experimental weight perturbation on skeletal muscle work efficiency, fuel utilization, and biochemistry in human subjects. *Am J Physiol Regul Integr Comp Physiol.* 2010;298(1):R79-R88. doi:10.1152/ajpregu.00053.2009
89. Jequier E. Energy metabolism in obese patients before and after weight loss, and in patients who have relapsed. *Int J Obes.* 1990;14(suppl 1):59-64; discussion 64-67.
90. Maclean PS, Bergouignan A, Cornier MA, Jackman MR. Biology's response to dieting: the impetus for weight regain. *Am J Physiol Regul Integr Comp Physiol.* 2011;301(3):R581-R600. doi:10.1152/ajpregu.00755.2010
91. Paris HL, Foright RM, Werth KA, et al. Increasing energy flux to decrease the biological drive toward weight regain after weight loss - A proof-of-concept pilot study. *Clinical Nutrition ESPEN.* 2016;11:e12-e120. doi:10.1016/j.clnesp.2015.11.005
92. Levine JA, Eberhardt NL, Jensen MD. Role of nonexercise activity thermogenesis in resistance to fat gain in humans. *Science.* 1999;283(5399):212-214. doi:10.1126/science.283.5399.212
93. Bouchard C, Tremblay A, Després JP, et al. The response to long-term overfeeding in identical twins. *N Engl J Med.* 1990;322(21):1477-1482. doi:10.1056/NEJM199005243222101
94. Christiansen T, Paulsen SK, Bruun JM, Ploug T, Pedersen SB, Richelsen B. Diet-induced weight loss and exercise alone and in combination enhance the expression of adiponectin receptors in adipose tissue and skeletal muscle, but only diet-induced weight loss enhanced circulating adiponectin. *J Clin Endocrinol Metab.* 2010;95(2):911-919. doi:10.1210/jc.2008-2505
95. Bouchard C, Tremblay A, Nadeau A, et al. Long-term exercise training with constant energy intake. 1: effect on body composition and selected metabolic variables. *Int J Obes.* 1990;14(1):57-73.
96. King NA, Hopkins M, Caudwell P, Stubbs RJ, Blundell JE. Individual variability following 12 weeks of supervised exercise: identification and characterization of compensation for exercise-induced weight loss. *Int J Obes (Lond).* 2008;32(1):177-184. doi:10.1038/sj.ijo.0803712
97. Donnelly JE, Hill JO, Jacobsen DJ, et al. Effects of a 16-month randomized controlled exercise trial on body weight and composition in young, overweight men and women: the Midwest Exercise Trial. *Arch Intern Med.* 2003;163(11):1343-1350. doi:10.1001/archinte.163.11.1343
98. Goran MI, Poehlman ET. Endurance training does not enhance total energy expenditure in healthy elderly persons. *Am J Physiol.* 1992;263(5 pt 1):E950-E957. doi:10.1152/ajpendo.1992.263.5.E950
99. Oshida Y, Yamanouchi K, Hayamizu S, Nagasawa J, Ohsawa I, Sato Y. Effects of training and training cessation on insulin action. *Int J Sports Med.* 1991;12(5):484-486. doi:10.1055/s-2007-1024718
100. Miller MA, Croft LB, Belanger AR, et al. Prevalence of metabolic syndrome in retired National Football League players. *Am J Cardiol.* 2008;101(9):1281-1284. doi:10.1055/s-2007-1024718
101. Booth FW, Roberts CK. Linking performance and chronic disease risk: indices of physical performance are surrogates for health. *Br J Sports Med.* 2008;42(12):950-952. doi:10.1136/bjsm.2008.052589
102. Phelain JF, Reinke E, Harris MA, Melby CL. Postexercise energy expenditure and substrate oxidation in young women resulting from exercise bouts of different intensity. *J Am Coll Nutr.* 1997;16(2):140-146. doi:10.1080/07315724.1997.10718664
103. Sedlock DA, Fissinger JA, Melby CL. Effect of exercise intensity and duration on postexercise energy expenditure. *Med Sci Sports Exerc.* 1989;21(6):662-666. doi:10.1249/00005768-198912000-00006
104. Osterberg KL, Melby CL. Effect of acute resistance exercise on postexercise oxygen consumption and resting metabolic rate in young women. *Int J Sport Nutr Exerc Metab.* 2000;10(1):71-81. doi:10.1123/ijsnem.10.1.71
105. Melby CL, Osterberg KL, Resch A, Davy B, Johnson S, Davy K. Effect of carbohydrate ingestion during exercise on post-exercise substrate oxidation and energy intake. *Int J Sport Nutr Exerc Metab.* 2002;12(3):294-309. doi:10.1123/ijsnem.12.3.294
106. Donnelly JE, Herrmann SD, Lambourne K, Szabo AN, Honas JJ, Washburn RA. Does increased exercise or physical activity alter ad-libitum daily energy intake or macronutrient composition in healthy adults? A systematic review. *PLoS One.* 2014;9(1):e83498. doi:10.1371/journal.pone.0083498
107. Mountjoy M, Sundgot-Borgen J, Burke L, et al. The IOC consensus statement: beyond the female athlete triad—relative energy deficiency in sport (RED-S). *Br J Sports Med.* 2014;48(7):491-497. doi:10.1136/bjsports-2014-093502
108. Mountjoy M, Sundgot-Borgen JK, Burke LM, et al. IOC consensus statement on relative energy deficiency in sport (RED-S): 2018 update. *Br J Sports Med.* 2018;52(11):687-697. doi:10.1136/bjsports-2018-099193
109. Cabre HE, Moore SR, Smith-Ryan AE, Hackney AC. Relative energy deficiency in sport (RED-S): scientific, clinical, and practical implications for the female athlete. *Dtsch Z Sportmed.* 2022;73(7):225-234. doi:10.5960/dzsm.2022.546
110. Nattiv A, De Souza MJ, Koltun KJ, et al. The male athlete triad—a consensus statement from the Female and Male Athlete Triad Coalition part 1: definition and scientific basis. *Clin J Sport Med.* 2021;31(4):345-353. doi:10.1097/JSM.0000000000000946
111. De Souza MJ, Nattiv A, Joy E, et al. 2014 Female Athlete Triad Coalition Consensus Statement on Treatment and Return to Play of the Female Athlete Triad: 1st International Conference held in San Francisco, California, May 2012 and 2nd International Conference held in Indianapolis, Indiana, May 2013. *Br J Sports Med.* 2014;48(4):289. doi:10.1136/bjsports-2013-093218

CHAPTER 11

Weight Management

Melissa L. Brown, PhD, RD, CSSD, LD

LEARNING OBJECTIVES

- Describe weight goals and expected performance outcomes for athletes.
- Differentiate optimal performance weight and body composition ranges for various types of athletes.
- Design an effective, comprehensive nutrition action plan for the weight management of athletes.
- Explain the purpose of evaluating athletes' goals and reassessing athletes' original assessment measures.

INTRODUCTION

Performance goals for athletes are often intertwined with weight goals and can be highly influenced by sport-specific expectations. Athletes are also not immune to societal expectations of body image considering that many people have their own ideas of what athletes should look like. Weight management can be a highly challenging and frustrating concept for athletes, and they often seek guidance from members of the sports medicine team, including the sports registered dietitian nutritionist (RDN). Collectively, body size and composition, as well as body shape, can be referred to as *physique*. Multiple factors impact an athlete's physique, only some of which are within the athlete's control. Sex, age, and genetics all contribute to physique and are not controllable factors. Physique can play a role in successful athletic performance, but it is critical for anyone working with athletes to understand that body weight and composition alone cannot accurately predict how an athlete will perform.[1,2]

Athletes seeking a performance edge should not be provided with an exact body composition to achieve. A sports RDN can implement an athlete-centered approach that can help assess weight and body composition and compare the measures to those of successful athletes in their sport who have similar, but not identical, physiques. Changing the amount of weight, skeletal muscle, or body fat of an athlete has potential performance advantages if goals are set appropriately. Unfortunately, athletes may set inappropriate weight and body composition goals or try to achieve their goals too quickly or during the wrong part of the training cycle. Significant changes to any part of an athlete's physique should ideally occur in the offseason to avoid detrimental effects to health and performance and to allow an appropriate time frame for changes to occur.[1,2] Sports RDNs can help athletes set weight ranges and body composition goals that support performance without negatively affecting training, recovery, and health. Once appropriate goals have been established, the sports RDN can also help the athlete develop an eating plan well matched to their sport, training schedule, and food preference. This chapter reviews the factors that should be considered when establishing weight and body composition goals and describes the evidence-based relationships that exist between physique and athletic performance. A case study illustrating how to practically apply this information concludes the chapter. For the purposes of this chapter, the standards discussed apply to sex assigned at birth. Research is emerging in some areas of practice regarding athletes who are transgender; however, the evidence available at this point is insufficient for general conclusions to be drawn. Future editions of this text will need to reevaluate and include the evidence as it emerges.

WEIGHT MANAGEMENT GOALS OF ATHLETES

Depending on their individual characteristics and the demands of their sport, an athlete may want to (1) increase skeletal muscle mass, (2) increase skeletal muscle mass and slightly increase body fat, (3) increase skeletal muscle mass while simultaneously decreasing body fat, (4) decrease body fat, or (5) increase body fat. As shown in Box 11.1, these changes can result in increased or decreased size and improved strength, power, speed, or cardiovascular endurance, which may enhance performance.[1,3-6]

BOX 11.1 Body Composition Goals and Expected Performance Outcomes[1,3-6]

Goal	Expected performance outcomes	Examples
Increase skeletal muscle mass	Increase strength and power	Sprinters, bodybuilders
Increase skeletal muscle mass and slightly increase body fat	Increase size and strength; provide a better physical match to opponents	Athletes in contact sports, especially as they progress to elite levels
Increase skeletal muscle mass and decrease body fat simultaneously	Increase strength and power; increase power-to-weight ratio	Athletes in "ball" sports (eg, basketball, baseball), cyclists, rowers, wrestlers
Decrease body fat	Increase speed; improve vertical or horizontal distance	Long-distance runners, gymnasts, figure skaters, high jumpers
Increase body fat	Increase size (mass)	Powerlifters, sumo wrestlers

Most athletes engage in some form of resistance training to maintain or increase muscular strength, power, and endurance. Novice athletes and those moving to more demanding levels of competition (eg, high school to college, college to professional) generally benefit from substantially increasing their skeletal muscle size, which often coincides with increased strength and muscle endurance. However, for many athletes, muscular strength and endurance are more important than increased size because too much muscle can result in decreased speed or perceived decreases in flexibility or agility. For example, a distance runner who gains too much skeletal muscle mass may find that speed is actually decreased because more effort must be made to transport the extra body weight associated with the extra muscle.

Changes in body fat can also substantially influence performance. Excess body fat is detrimental for many athletes because it reduces speed.[3] Excess body fat represents "dead weight" because the excess weight must be carried but does not contribute to muscle power. Decreasing excess body fat may have a positive effect on performance. However, trying to achieve an ever-lower percentage of body fat is a performance *disadvantage* because lean body mass (LBM) and strength may be lost and health problems can develop (eg, disrupted hormonal balance or disordered eating behaviors).[2] Although not mentioned as frequently as fat loss, some athletes may need to increase body mass by gaining body fat. Physical size alone can be a performance advantage, especially in contact sports. In these cases, additional body fat may aid the athlete's performance.

Regardless of the evidence supporting performance advantages at a certain body composition level, societal pressure also plays a role that cannot be ignored. Athletes often feel pressure to achieve a certain body weight or body fat percentage that is not only unrealistic but may be dangerous. Societal pressure results in some athletes being vulnerable and highly likely to participate in extreme weight loss measures or chronic dieting. Chronic dieting may result in long periods of low energy availability and nutrient deficiencies, and extreme weight loss measures can be detrimental to overall health.[1] Therefore, achievement of a particular weight or body composition is ideally done through a program promoting gradual changes without detrimental effects on health and performance.

DETERMINING OPTIMAL PERFORMANCE WEIGHT AND BODY COMPOSITION RANGES

Optimal performance weight and body composition are unique to each individual. Factors to consider when determining an optimal performance weight range are listed in Box 11.2 and discussed further in this section, but all may not apply to a particular athlete.[1-4]

Sport-Related Characteristics

Certain physical characteristics are associated with success in particular sports, including the following examples:

- All competitive bodybuilders have a high percentage of skeletal muscle mass and a low percentage of body fat.
- Conversely, sumo wrestlers are large-bodied, with a considerable amount of body fat.
- Strength and power sports emphasize lean muscle mass through periodized muscle hypertrophy cycles throughout the year. Goals for the gain in LBM vary. Some athletes attempt to optimize the power-to-weight ratio (discussed in a later section) because they must move their own body mass; others are more focused on gaining mass for absolute power.[7-9]
- Power athletes often prefer low body fat levels.
- Athletes participating in weight-class sports attempt to be as lean as possible while meeting the criteria for the lowest body weight category possible.[1,2,10]
- Athletes may also focus on an overall low body mass with low body weight and low body fat.[6] For example, elite distance runners tend to be lightweight and light-boned, and they have a relatively low percentage of body fat because these characteristics are associated with a low energy cost of movement with an optimal weight-to-surface area ratio for dissipation of heat.
- Athletes in sports such as gymnastics benefit from the mechanical advantages of a smaller, more compact body able to move in small spaces with ease.[1,2,7-9] In gymnastics, as well as figure skating and other similar aesthetic sports, appearance may be a factor in scoring.
- Athletes participating in light-contact team sports such as soccer tend to desire to be lean in order to increase agility and speed.[1,2]
- In contrast, in heavy-contact sports, such as football, rugby, and ice hockey, being physically well matched to one's opponents is often key to success, but physical size alone is not the determining factor in most sports.[1,2]

BOX 11.2 Factors to Consider in Setting Weight-Management Goals[1-4]

Sport-related characteristics

Sport
Position played
Relative need for power and endurance
Power-to-weight ratio
Relative need for speed, flexibility, agility, and mobility
Weight certification requirements

Physique-related characteristics

Body weight
Body composition
Body size
Body build
Metabolic syndrome phenotype
Body appearance

The relative need for power, speed, or endurance as well as the need to be agile, flexible, or mobile may be particularly important keys to an individual's success. The physical characteristics of the sport's successful athletes should be considered as a guideline, but in many sports, there is room for tremendous individual variability. Thus, some sports have greater physical uniformity among competitors, especially at the elite levels of competition, whereas other sports are more varied. For example, successful athletes in individual noncontact sports such as tennis and golf are of many body weights, sizes, and shapes.[2] Box 11.3 illustrates body weight and composition uniformity among athletes.

BOX 11.3 Weight and Body Composition Uniformity Among Athletes[2]

More body composition uniformity

Baseball catchers
Basketball centers, point guards
Bodybuilders
Figure skaters
Football linemen
Gymnasts
Long-distance cyclists
Long-distance runners
Powerlifters
Rhythmic gymnasts

Less body composition uniformity

Baseball pitchers
Divers
Golfers
Recreational triathletes
Tennis players

POSITION PLAYED

Table 11.1 provides information on sport-specific data (height, weight, age, BMI) for all-male rostered players for 6 professional sports leagues in the United States from 2022.[11-16] (Similar data for female professional athletes are not readily available, as body weight is not typically reported publicly.) The information in Table 11.1 demonstrates that physical uniformity may be associated with position played. For example, a football defensive end tends to be physically similar to other defensive ends but different in weight and body composition compared to running backs, defensive backs, and receivers. Defensive ends, tackles, linemen, centers, and guards tend to have a higher percentage of body fat than the other players on the team so that they are less easily pushed around by opposing players.[17-21] In contrast, wide receivers have less body fat than lineman because of their need for superior running speed.[21] Linebackers benefit from quick running speed and the agility to change direction quickly, but they also need enough mass to stop a run. Particularly in contact sports, position may dictate the need for an athlete to be of a particular size, weight, or body composition.[2]

In many team sports, a range of weights and body compositions can be suitable for a given position. For example, in soccer, some defenders are more muscular and weigh more than others who are lighter weight and have comparatively less muscle, yet each can succeed as a defender.[2] Weight and body composition vary in baseball outfielders in part because of their offensive skills[2]; some hit for power, whereas others hit to get on base, steal bases, and score on base hits. Power hitters benefit from greater body weight, whereas fast base runners are likely to have a body composition associated with speed (eg, relatively low percentage of body fat). Most of the professional sports listed in Table 11.1 exhibit some variation by position played. Interestingly, there is striking consistency among all players within the National Hockey League, suggesting that position played depends less on weight and body composition characteristics in this sport.

RELATIVE NEED FOR POWER AND ENDURANCE

Athletes are often characterized as strength and power or endurance athletes. Some sports depend predominantly on power, as shown on the left side of the continuum in Figure 11.1 on page 256, whereas others depend to a large degree on endurance capacity, as shown on the right in the same figure. Many sports require a blend of power and endurance. A sports RDN may find it helpful to determine the relative position of the athlete's sport on this continuum so that realistic weight and body composition goals can be established. For example, short-distance runners, such as 100-m and 200-m runners, depend primarily on explosive power. They have substantial upper- and lower-body skeletal muscle mass and a relatively heavy body weight. For middle-distance runners (eg,1,500 m), body composition begins to change as the race

TABLE 11.1 Sport-Specific Averages for All-Male Rostered Players for Six Professional Sports Leagues in 2022[11-16]

Professional league	Position	Height (in)	Weight (lb)	Age (y)	BMI
Major League Baseball (MLB)	Overall	73.7 ± 0.5	205.9 ± 3.8	27.0 ± 0.8	26.7 ± 0.5
	Pitchers	74.6 ± 0.6	209.5 ± 3.6	27.9 ± 0.7	26.5 ± 0.4
	Catchers	72.5 ± 0.9	207.8 ± 4.8	28.0 ± 1.8	27.6 ± 1.1
	Infielders	73.2 ± 0.7	205.6 ± 6.1	25.7 ± 0.8	26.6 ± 0.6
	Outfielders	72.7 ± 1.3	202.8 ± 10.9	25.8 ± 1.3	27.0 ± 0.6
	Designated hitter	74 ± 1.7	215.7 ± 13.7	28 ± 3.6	27.7 ± 1.7
Major League Lacrosse/ Premiere League Lacrosse	Overall	72.5 ± 0.4	195.3 ± 1.8	32.4 ± 4.9	26.1 ± 0.3
	Defensemen	72.3 ± 1.0	198.8 ± 4.4	34.9 ± 4.7	26.0 ± 0.6
	Midfielders	73.3 ± 0.7	200.9 ± 6.3	34.2 ± 6.0	26.4 ± 0.5
	Attackers	71.7 ± 0.4	191.7 ± 4.3	33.3 ± 4.8	26.3 ± 0.7
	Goalkeepers	72.7 ± 2.8	194.4 ± 14.5	36.7 ± 7.5	25.9 ± 0.3
Major League Soccer (MLS)	Overall	71.1 ± 2.9	164.9 ± 18.4	25.7 ± 4.8	22.9 ± 1.6
	Defenders	71.8 ± 2.6	167.9 ± 16.5	26.4 ± 4.9	22.9 ± 1.5
	Midfielders	69.7 ± 2.6	156.5 ± 15.4	25.0 ± 4.6	22.7 ± 1.5
	Forwards	70.8 ± 2.6	163.2 ± 16.1	25.3 ± 4.6	22.9 ± 1.5
	Goalkeepers	74.5 ± 1.7	186.7 ± 15.4	26.7 ± 5.2	23.9 ± 1.9
National Basketball Association (NBA)	Overall	78.6 ± 0.5	216.1 ± 4.4	25.7 ± 1.6	24.7 ± 0.7
	Guards	75.7 ± 0.3	194.5 ± 4.7	24.1 ± 1.3	23.9 ± 1.0
	Centers	82.9 ± 0.9	249.3 ± 10.7	25.4 ± 1.8	25.6 ± 0.6
	Forwards	80.2 ± 0.4	222.7 ± 4.9	25.5 ± 1.9	24.3 ± 0.9
National Football League (NFL)	Overall	74.1 ± 0.3	243.9 ± 3.1	26.2 ± 0.9	31.3 ± 0.3
	Quarterbacks	74.1 ± 0.9	215.4 ± 9.0	27.5 ± 2.6	27.7 ± 1.5
	Centers	76.1 ± 1.2	310.5 ± 8.6	26.7 ± 2.9	37.8 ± 1.6
	Offensive linemen	76.0 ± 1.1	309.3 ± 11.6	26.0 ± 1.8	37.7 ± 0.7
	Offensive guards	76.9 ± 0.9	318.1 ± 13.6	26.2 ± 2.9	37.8 ± 1.6
	Wide receivers	71.3 ± 0.3	193.9 ± 3.2	25.9 ± 3.2	26.8 ± 0.5
	Tight ends	76.1 ± 0.7	245.6 ± 10.6	26.5 ± 1.5	29.9 ± 1.1
	Running backs	70.8 ± 0.9	213.6 ± 11.7	26.4 ± 0.9	29.9 ± 0.9
	Fullbacks	73.8 ± 1.5	246.0 ± 11.9	25.5 ± 2.1	31.9 ± 2.2
	Safeties	71.8 ± 1.1	203.6 ± 10.0	26.4 ± 1.8	27.8 ± 1.6
	Cornerbacks	71.8 ± 0.6	192.1 ± 3.7	25.4 ± 0.5	26.3 ± 0.4
	Defensive ends	77.4 ± 1.8	286.3 ± 20.2	28.6 ± 4.6	33.6 ± 1.2
	Defensive tackles	76.1 ± 0.9	311.8 ± 4.7	26.2 ± 1.7	37.9 ± 1.1
	Defensive linebackers	74.7 ± 0.8	244.2 ± 9.2	25.9 ± 1.1	30.8 ± 1.1

Continued on next page

TABLE 11.1 Sport-Specific Averages for All-Male Rostered Players for Six Professional Sports Leagues in 2022[11-16] (CONTINUED)

Professional league	Position	Height (in)	Weight (lb)	Age (y)	BMI
National Football League (NFL) Continued	Long snappers	74.5 ± 1.7	231.3 ± 19.8	31.8 ± 3.1	29.4 ± 2.5
	Place kickers	72.5 ± 1.7	198 ± 18.4	30.5 ± 6.1	26.5 ± 2.1
	Punters	73.0 ± 2.1	201.3 ± 14.8	28.7 ± 4.2	26.6 ± 0.7
National Hockey League (NHL)	Overall	73.4 ± 0.5	199.0 ± 4.0	27.6 ± 1.1	25.9 ± 0.4
	Forwards	73.2 ± 0.3	195.6 ± 2.6	27.4 ± 3.3	25.9 ± 0.1
	Centers	73.0 ± 0.3	195.5 ± 1.3	27.4 ± 3.2	25.8 ± 0.1
	Defensemen	74.2 ± 0.6	201 ± 9.7	27.7 ± 3.4	25.9 ± 0.2
	Goalkeepers	74.0 ± 0.4	199.4 ± 5.7	27.9 ± 1.2	25.6 ± 0.6

The author acknowledges Hanna Pryhazhayeva, RD, CDN, and Morgan McDonald, RD, CDN, for their assistance in compiling the data for this table.

favors endurance rather than power. The 1,500-m runner is less muscular and lighter in weight than the 100-m runner. Long-distance runners, such as marathon runners, tend to be light in weight and to have a relatively low percentage of body fat because these characteristics are associated with efficiently moving the body quickly over a long distance. Cycling and swimming are other sports in which the distance covered influences the relative need for power and endurance and, therefore, weight and body composition.[1-3]

Athletes who rely only on strength or explosive power include bodybuilders, powerlifters, and certain field athletes, such as shot-putters and discus, hammer, and javelin throwers. Powerlifters and throwers benefit from being large-bodied and strong. Body fat adds to total body weight, which can be a performance advantage because it adds mass. However, too high a percentage of body fat can be a health disadvantage, particularly if the excess fat is abdominal fat.[18,20,22-28]

Most sports require a combination of power and endurance. For example, basketball and soccer require intermittent short bursts of power (eg, fast break, breakaway play) as well as cardiovascular endurance. Body weight and composition must be fine-tuned for the athlete to be able to do both well. Particularly challenging are those sports that require several power and endurance events, such as decathlon. Decathletes must have a body composition that is not too muscular (a disadvantage when running the 1,500-m race) or too low in weight (a disadvantage when shot-putting).[2]

Body composition is also a factor in cardiovascular conditioning. Reducing excess body fat may improve cardiovascular endurance and allow athletes to continue to perform well near the end of a game or event. This is especially important in sports with overtime periods, such as basketball, soccer, and lacrosse.[29] Although conditioning is important for all athletes, improved cardiovascular endurance may be the primary goal for performance-focused recreational athletes and older players who are competing for playing time with younger players. Such players often try to reduce excess body fat as a way to improve endurance and performance.[30]

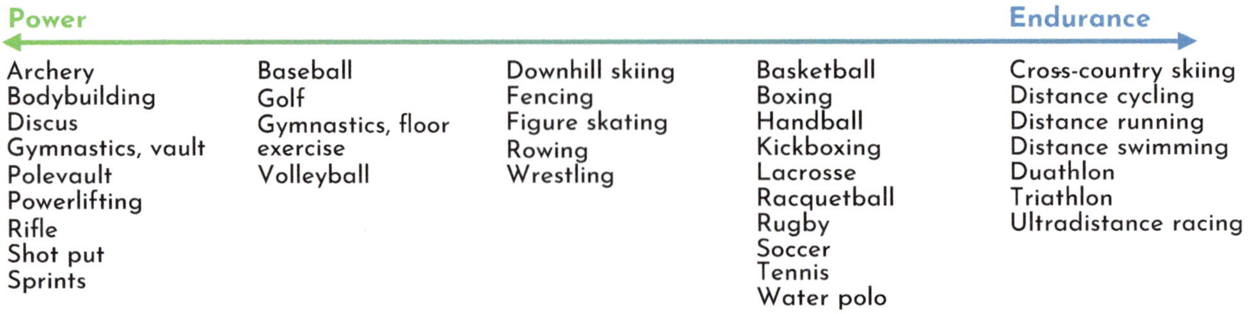

FIGURE 11.1 The power-endurance continuum

POWER-TO-WEIGHT RATIO

Power-to-weight ratio refers to the amount of power (eg, cycling power measured in watts or horsepower) that can be generated per pound or kilogram of body weight. A high power-to-weight ratio is a performance advantage in many sports, the result of a relatively low percentage of body fat and a relatively high percentage of skeletal muscle for the total amount of body weight. For example, male professional distance cyclists tend to have approximately 7% to 10% body fat. Excess body fat is dead weight because it must be moved but does not contribute to muscle power.[2,3]

Examples of sports that benefit from a high power-to-weight ratio include boxing, wrestling, martial arts, rowing (crew), high jumping, pole vaulting, distance running, gymnastics, swimming, diving, and cycling. A high power-to-weight ratio is also advantageous for athletes in positions that cover a large area of the field, rink, or court and depend on speed, such as some positions in basketball, ice hockey, lacrosse, rugby, figure skating, and soccer.[2,3]

Power-to-weight ratio can be changed by increasing skeletal muscle mass to increase power or decreasing body fat to decrease body weight. Unless an athlete has a large amount of excess body fat, maximizing power by increasing muscle mass is more likely to benefit performance than minimizing body fat. Athletes need to be aware that extreme changes in either direction can be detrimental to performance. For example, too great an increase in skeletal muscle mass can increase body weight too much, which can reduce speed. Conversely, decreasing body fat too much can hurt performance because there is not enough body fat to support rigorous training and competition. Health-related problems can also be brought on by these changes, such as joint problems or changes in hormone concentrations as a result of an eating disorder.[2]

RELATIVE NEED FOR SPEED, MOBILITY, FLEXIBILITY, AND AGILITY

An athlete's need for speed and mobility influences goals for body weight and composition. Some athletes may benefit from an increase in lower-body muscle mass and a decrease in body fat to increase sprint speed. Others may benefit from maintenance of muscle mass but a decrease in excess body fat. Because speed is easily measured, the impact of changes in weight and body composition on speed can be easily assessed. Some athletes feel that too much muscle reduces their flexibility and agility.[2]

WEIGHT CERTIFICATION REQUIREMENTS

Sporting events with weight divisions are divided as such to avoid possible injuries related to differences in strength and body mass. Athletes often attempt to manipulate the weight-class system by implementing rapid weight loss (RWL) strategies to compete at a lower weight class. Patterns of RWL followed by rapid weight gain are referred to as *weight cycles*. Boxing, wrestling, some martial arts, and lightweight crew (rowing) are examples of sports with weight categories. Weight-regulated sports put considerable emphasis on scale weight because the athlete cannot compete until body weight is certified. There is a theoretical performance advantage to being at the top rather than the bottom of the weight category, and this may influence an athlete to choose to compete in a weight category that is below a biologically comfortable weight.[2,8,10,27,31]

The need to have one's weight be certified cannot be overlooked as a significant factor in the athlete's preparation for competition. Unfortunately, the fastest way to manipulate scale weight is to reduce body water; therefore, RWL is a common practice that can be dangerous to an athlete's health. RWL practices include excessive exercise and severe dehydration through restrictions on fluid and food, as well as the use of laxatives, diuretics, or bowel preparation formulas and sauna suits to decrease body water.[32-37] Other practices may not be as extreme, such as temporarily attempting to decrease gut contents by consuming a low-sodium, low-fiber, and low-residue diet.[1,2,32-37]

Practicing RWL to meet certain weight criteria is often referred to as "making weight" or "cutting weight." Experts believe that up to 80% of athletes in combat sports practice some form of cutting weight, with a typical loss of 2% to 10% of body weight in the 2 to 3 days leading up to a competition.[35,36] The most common method of RWL in these athletes involves extreme dehydration, which can be dangerous and lead to acute kidney damage and even death.[38] The impact on health and performance is seen most frequently when the athlete is not allowed a refeed and/or rehydration period after weigh-in, which can vary from a few hours to 1 day.[39-41] In a 2022 meta-analysis, Mauricio et al[40] found that an RWL of up to

5% of body mass in less than 7 days does not adversely affect performance in adult male Olympic judo, tae kwon do, boxing, and wrestling athletes as long as a refeed period is allowed before competition. However, losing more than 5% of body mass raises the risk for serious adverse effects on health and performance. Given the current dearth of knowledge in this area, more research is needed, as very few studies are available and most do not include female subjects.[32,41,42]

Wrestling is a sport that has become synonymous with "making weight"; indeed, it came under increased scrutiny after multiple deaths occurred due to high-risk practices. To make weight, wrestlers were restricting water intake, losing excessive fluid and electrolytes through sweating, and taking diuretics. These practices are dangerous, especially when combined, as body temperature can be elevated to a medically unsafe and sometimes fatal level.[1,2,43,44] In response, the National Collegiate Athletic Association[45] put regulations into place to guide safe weight loss practices. The regulations set a minimum weight category for collegiate athletes before the beginning of the season based on body composition and proper hydration. However, not all weight-regulated sports have adopted such rule changes, and athletes in those sports remain at risk for potential medical problems and detrimental acute performance outcomes ranging from lack of concentration to more serious outcomes like fainting, kidney damage, and death.[1,2,43-45] For those athletes who use RWL practices, the sports RDN must provide accurate and evidence-based guidelines. For additional information on wrestling, see the Wrestling At A Glance section on page 752.

Physique-Related Characteristics

The challenge for both athletes and the professionals who work with them is to determine ranges for weight and body composition that are compatible with excellent performance, good health, *and* the individual's genetic potential and unique characteristics.

BODY WEIGHT

Weight is usually expressed as a single number, although it should be stated as a range. Use of a weight range helps to account for the error inherent in any form of measurement and also helps prevent misinterpretations due to natural day-to-day fluctuations in body weight, especially in water weight. A baseline weight is one of the first assessment measures taken, but an appropriate weight range cannot be established until information is known about the individual athlete's height, body build, and body composition, as well as the sport and position played.[1,2]

BODY COMPOSITION

A body composition assessment is necessary to set an appropriate weight range and to monitor changes in LBM and storage fat. An accurate assessment is critical, as explained in Chapter 9. However, the most accurate measures are not readily accessible or affordable to most athletes. Many have access to only 1 method, which will need to be repeated over time to track any changes. Body composition cannot predict success in any sport, but it can affect optimal performance.[1] Table 11.2 lists the estimated body compositions of competitive athletes in some sports as reported in the scientific literature.[2] These figures are only guidelines and should be used cautiously.

BODY BUILD

Body build, also referred to as somatotype, may be useful when discussing the influence of genetic predisposition on body composition. The classification of body builds is based on 3 categories: endomorphic, mesomorphic, and ectomorphic. Endomorphs tend to be stocky and have wide hips; they are at risk for easily gaining body fat, particularly in the abdominal area. Mesomorphs tend to gain skeletal muscle mass relatively easily and generally do not gain excessive amounts of body fat. Ectomorphs appear to be thin. Some individuals clearly fall into 1 of the 3 categories, but many reflect more than 1 somatotype.[2]

Body build is associated with certain sports. For example, shot-putters tend to be endomorphs, bodybuilders tend to be mesomorphs, and distance runners tend to be ectomorphs.[5] Visual appraisal does not quantify body dimensions, but it is one way to draw general observations about successful performance related to physique. Until an individual reaches full physical maturity, it may be difficult to accurately assess their physique.

TABLE 11.2 Estimated Body Composition of Selected Well-Trained Athletes[2]

Sport	Position or distance	Body fat (%)
Men		
Baseball, college	All positions	11.0-17.0
Baseball, professional	All positions	8.5-12.0
Basketball, professional	Centers	9.0-20.0
	Forwards	7.0-14.0
	Guards	7.0-13.0
Cycling, road, professional	Long distance	7.0-10.0
Football (American), college (NCAA Division I)	Defensive backs	7.0-14.5
	Receivers	9.0-16.5
	Quarterbacks	14.0-22.0
	Linebackers	12.5-23.5
	Defensive linemen	14.5-25.0
	Offensive linemen	18.5-28.5
Ice hockey, elite	Forwards and defensemen	10.0-11.5
Judo, national team	All weight classes	8.5-19.0
Rugby, professional	All positions	9.0-20.0
Running, elite	Middle distance	8.0-16.5
	Long distance	12.0-18.0
Soccer, college	All positions	13.0-19.0
Soccer, professional	All positions	7.5-18.0
Swimming or diving, college	Middle distance or diving	17.0-30.0
	Long distance	20.0-34.0
Tennis, elite		8.0-18.0
Water polo, national team		6.5-17.5
Wrestling, college		6.5-16.0
Women		
Ice hockey, elite	All positions	14.0-18.0
Running, elite	Middle distance	8.0-16.5
	Long distance	12.0-18.0
Soccer, college	All positions	13.0-19.0
Swimming or diving, college	Middle distance or diving	17.0-30.0
Swimming or diving, masters	Long distance	20.0-34.0
Tennis, elite		15.0-25.0

Abbreviation: NCAA, National Collegiate Athletic Association

BODY SIZE

Body size refers to height, weight, and body build. Although there are exceptions, many athletes need to increase body size as they move to the next level of competition (eg, from high school to collegiate sports and then from collegiate sports to professional sports). In many cases, this means an increase in skeletal muscle mass and body weight. It may also mean a small increase in body fat; in some positions, such as a defensive end in football, it can mean a substantial increase in fat. Although body size can be manipulated, it is ultimately determined by genetics. It is important to note that in the United States, puberty generally occurs between the ages of 11 and 19, so there is wide variety in when an athlete achieves full physical maturity. Body size has increased in many high school, collegiate, and professional athletes over the past 55 years, including in the sports of football, basketball, ice hockey, baseball, and tennis.[2,19,46-48] A dramatic increase has been seen in the weight of football players at every level from professional to youth.[19,20] Some of this change can be attributed to an increase in abdominal fat, a known health risk.

In sports in which a high body mass is coveted and categorized as optimal for performance, athletes should be counseled to avoid rapid and excessive gains in body fat. Excessive gains in body fat place athletes at risk for obesity and cardiometabolic disorders.[1,2,22-28,49] The use of BMI in athletes is widely acknowledged to be flawed because the presence of increased LBM among athletes tends to skew the results toward the overweight and obese categories, for the most part invalidating the utility of the BMI as a surrogate for body composition and as a predictor of health risks. However, in certain situations, BMI should not be ignored. As can be seen in Table 11.2, with the exception of athletes in Major League Soccer, the average BMI for all sports and positions meets the criteria for either overweight or obesity.[50]

In a 2018 publication, Churchill et al[27] described the weight gain and health affliction among former players from the National Football League (NFL). NFL players are among the largest athletes in modern-day sporting competitions, and in the NFL, the practice of gaining extreme amounts of body weight and body fat is common. The researchers described cardiovascular disease, cardiometabolic disease, neurocognitive impairment, sleep apnea, and chronic pain as the most common health afflictions of former NFL players (see Box 11.4). In addition, Owara et al[26] reported that all-cause and cause-specific mortality is higher in athletes with a BMI of 30 and greater. The data in Table 11.2 clearly indicate that players in the NFL are at risk, with an overall average BMI of 31.3 ± 0.3, and certain positions are associated with an even higher risk. Centers, offensive linemen, guards, and defensive tackles all have average BMIs of greater than 37. Of all of the professional sports leagues included in Table 11.2, only the NFL appears to fall at such high risk. Football-associated weight gain with BMI meeting the definition of obesity is a critical predictor of post-career health. Churchill et al[27] went on to describe the relationship between early-career weight gain and post-career health. The authors suggested that weight gained from the time the athlete was in high school until middle age (with the majority of the weight gained during the active years of football participation) is associated with a higher prevalence of the described health afflictions in middle age, including metabolic syndrome.

METABOLIC SYNDROME PHENOTYPE

Metabolic syndrome is characterized by a clustering of metabolic disorders and risk factors: abdominal obesity; hypertension; dyslipidemia, including elevated triglycerides and low high-density lipoprotein cholesterol; glucose intolerance; and insulin resistance (see Box 11.5 on page 262).[22] Sports RDNs should be aware of athletes who typically fall into the most extreme obesity categories and be aware of the sports that promote extremely large bodies, including excessive body fat, placing athletes at risk. Screening for metabolic disorders should be common practice for sports RDNs.

These features are associated with a higher risk for cardiovascular disease and type 2 diabetes. The prevalence of metabolic syndrome in the US adult population is approximately 25%, but the percentage increases with age.[22] Small studies of high school, collegiate, and professional football linemen have found a high incidence of metabolic syndrome, perhaps as high as 50% of linemen. Early screening is recommended, particularly for large-bodied, heavyweight athletes prone to increased abdominal fat.[23,24] In 1 study of collegiate football players, 62% had prehypertension and 20% were diagnosed with hypertension.[25]

BOX 11.4 Clinical Afflictions of Former National Football League Players

Cardiovascular disease

At least 1 of the following conditions:

- Prior myocardial infarction
- Prior stroke
- Prior coronary revascularization intervention (bypass surgery, angioplasty, or stent)

Cardiometabolic disease

Prior or current prescription of medication for 2 or more of the following conditions:

- Hypertension
- Hyperlipidemia
- Diabetes mellitus

Sleep apnea

Clinician-generated diagnosis of sleep apnea

Neurocognitive impairment

Clinician-generated diagnosis of dementia or chronic traumatic encephalopathy

OR

Prior or current prescription of medication to treat memory loss

Chronic pain

Prior or current prescription of medication for pain

AND

Ongoing daily use of pain medications

Reproduced with permission from reference 31: Churchill T, Krishnan S, Weisskopf M, et al. Weight gain and health affliction among former National Football League players. *Am J Med.* 2018;131(12):1491-1498. doi:10.1016/j.amjmed.2018.07.042

Evidence suggests that some female athletes in sports emphasizing strength may have hyperandrogenism, resulting in menstrual dysfunction, such as amenorrhea, and a tendency to abdominal obesity with accompanying insulin resistance and dyslipidemia. Some of these individuals meet the criteria for polycystic ovary syndrome. Menstrual dysfunction in female athletes as a result of a long-term energy deficit has been well studied as part of the female athlete triad. In contrast to those athletes, female athletes with hyperandrogenism typically do not suffer from an energy deficit or reduced bone mineral density and have a higher ratio of luteinizing hormone to follicle-stimulating hormone.[51]

BODY APPEARANCE

Body appearance cannot be overlooked when setting weight and body composition goals. An obvious example is the sport of bodybuilding, where competitors are scored based on body appearance. Weight and body composition are part of the subjective scoring of other aesthetic sports, such as gymnastics and figure skating. Dissatisfaction with weight, body shape, or body image can lead to disordered eating and eating disorders in both males and females.[52-54]

BOX 11.5 Diagnostic Criteria for Metabolic Syndrome[a,26]

Waist circumference	Greater than 102 cm (>40 in) in males Greater than 88 cm (>35 in) in females
Triglycerides	Greater than 150 mg/dL (1.7 mmol/L) Or drug treatment for elevated triglycerides
High-density lipoprotein cholesterol (HDL-C)	Less than 40 mg/dL (0.9 mmol/L) in males Less than 50 mg/dL (1.1 mmol/L) in females Or drug treatment for reduced HDL-C
Blood pressure	Greater than 130 mmHg systolic blood pressure Or greater than 85 mmHg diastolic blood pressure Or drug treatment for hypertension
Fasting blood glucose	Greater than 100 mg/dL (5.6 mmol/L) Or drug treatment for elevated glucose

[a] The combination of any 3 of the 5 criteria constitutes a diagnosis of metabolic syndrome.

For most athletes, body appearance is not part of the scoring. However, popular athletes featured in visual media may feel pressure to attain and maintain an athletic physique. Some sports, such as women's high jump, pole vaulting, and beach volleyball, feature tight-fitting clothing that reveals the body's contour. In general, female athletes are more concerned than male athletes with physical appearance, particularly perceived fatness, and are more likely to restrict energy intake and use weight-loss supplements.[55] Appearance is 1 reason that athletes of both sexes may use anabolic steroids. Interestingly, an athletic appearance is so socially powerful that some high school nonathletes use anabolic steroids to achieve a body composition associated with rigorous athletic training.[55]

FOUR-STEP PROCESS FOR ACHIEVING WEIGHT AND BODY COMPOSITION GOALS

The goal for an athlete is the appropriate weight range to support optimal performance and reflects a healthy body composition. Although the specific goals will depend on the individual, the process used to achieve the goals is universal. Four steps are critical:

1) Assessment
2) Goal setting
3) Action plan
4) Evaluation and reassessment

Step 1: Assessment

No two athletes are the same. Assessment is the starting point for any successful plan designed to achieve body weight and body composition goals. A proper assessment creates a picture of an individual athlete's current status, providing baseline information that is used for setting realistic and achievable goals. This information also becomes the basis for individual action plans designed to reach desired weight and body composition ranges and serves as a point of comparison. The more information an assessment provides, the better the sports RDN and the athlete are able to create a successful action plan and to gauge progress. Box 11.6 summarizes the assessment measurements used to create an individualized and targeted nutrition plan geared to help athletes set goals, design effective action plans, and evaluate and reassess progress.[1,2]

BOX 11.6 Assessment Measurements[1,2]

Physical assessment measures

Height

Weight

BMI, if appropriate

Girth measurements

Predominant somatotype (body build)

Waist circumference

Body composition (% lean mass, % body fat)

Physiological assessment measures

Medical physical examination (including laboratory tests)

Health history

Diet analysis (≥3 days)

Resting metabolic rate (measured or estimated)

Energy expenditure analysis (including intensity, frequency, and duration of exercise)

Performance measurements (eg, relative peak power, running speed)

PHYSICAL ASSESSMENT

Height and weight measurements are easy to take and necessary for determining optimal performance weight. Athletes in some sports and positions are similar in height and weight. Height measurements are necessary when assessing weight because many formulas for predicting body weight include height as a factor. Stadiometers provide the most accurate height measurement and make measuring quick and simple. However, in the absence of a stadiometer, height can be measured by having the athlete stand barefoot on a hard surface and against a wall, looking straight ahead with the head, shoulders, buttocks, and heels touching the wall. The athlete should stand as tall and straight as possible. With a ruler or other flat straightedge placed on the head of the athlete, the wall is marked at the underside of the 90° angle where the ruler meets the wall. Then, the distance from the ground to the marking on the wall is measured.[1,2]

Optimal weight is relative to height. Weight-class sports specify weight categories with specific weight ranges, so weight is a key issue for these athletes. To some degree, body weight is an important factor for all athletes. Weight measurements should be taken in the morning, using the same properly calibrated scale, after the athlete has urinated and before they have had anything to eat or drink and with the athlete wearing minimal clothing. Note that 1 weight measurement does not tell the whole story. To most accurately assess progress toward one's goal, serial weights should be taken regularly and uniformly. Regular weight checks also help an athlete keep tabs on hydration status and provide athletes with a basis for rehydration strategies.[1,2]

BMI is not typically used with athletes to determine overweight or obesity status. However, for those athletes who strive for a low body weight and low body fat or who appear to have excessive amounts of body fat, BMI may be a necessary assessment measure as an indicator of health status. The World Health Organization defines underweight in adults as a BMI of less than 18.5, which may indicate malnutrition, the presence of an eating disorder, or other health problems. In those younger than 20 years of age, underweight is defined as a BMI below the 5th percentile.[50]

Girth measurements provide a tool for measuring body size and proportion and for screening for excessive abdominal fat accumulation. Although not a direct measure of body composition, measuring the girth, or circumference, at 6 body sites is helpful in tracking change in body composition over time.[2] Girth measurements are inexpensive and easy to take. For the most accuracy, a flexible but inelastic tape measure is used to measure circumference, typically at the waist, hips, thighs, calves, arms, and chest. Changes in girth measurements can indicate whether the current plan is working. Waist circumference is 1 diagnostic criterion for metabolic syndrome (see Box 11.5).[22]

Body composition is an important factor in determining optimal performance weight. Accurate determination of an athlete's body composition is necessary for a comprehensive nutrition assessment because body weight is only 1 part of the picture. The composition of that weight is often the more important part. For practical purposes, the body is divided into 2 major compartments: fat and lean mass.

- Body fat is either essential fat or storage fat.
  - Essential fat, present in the heart, lungs, liver, spleen, and lipid-rich tissues of the central nervous system, is necessary for normal physiological functioning. In females, there is additional sex-specific essential fat that has reproductive and other hormonal functions. Essential fat in females is approximately 4 times that in males.
  - Storage fat is primarily in adipose tissue, including visceral fat that protects organs from trauma as well as fat beneath the skin. To maintain health and normal body function, lower limits for body fat percentage are set at 3% for males and 12% for females (or a body fat percentage that allows for the continuation of menstruation). These lower limits are for reference only, and even the leanest athletes typically exceed these percentages of body fat.[2]
- Fat-free mass (FFM) and LBM, although often used interchangeably, are not the same. Lean body mass contains a small percentage of non–sex-specific essential fat (approximately 3% of body mass), whereas FFM contains no fat (FFM = body mass – fat mass). In fully hydrated, healthy adults, the main difference between FFM and LBM is essential fat. LBM is generally the term used in body composition measurements. Lean body mass is often employed in the equations used to determine energy needs.[2]

Accurately determining an individual's body composition is not as easy as measuring body weight, height, and girth. For a detailed explanation of body composition methods and their strengths and weaknesses, refer to Chapter 9.

PHYSIOLOGICAL ASSESSMENT

Physiological measurements provide valuable baseline information about the athlete and include those obtained at a physical exam, such as biochemical assays and clinical assessments, as well as measurements of metabolic rate, nutrient intake, and exercise expenditure. For a detailed explanation of how to conduct a comprehensive sports nutrition assessment, refer to Chapter 8.

When available, laboratory tests allow the sports RDN to evaluate the nutritional status of the athlete by ascertaining whether biochemical parameters are within healthy ranges. Once collected, this information can be used as a target for dietary modifications and as a measure of progress. A clinical examination includes past and present medical history; family history; signs of disease or illness; and habits that may affect health, such as sleep patterns.[2]

An understanding of an athlete's usual dietary intake is an indispensable part of a comprehensive assessment. The more complete and accurate the diet record, the more likely that the prescribed meal plan will be precisely tailored to the athlete's energy and nutrient needs. A detailed 3- to 5-day diet record and nutrient analysis is the preferable method of collecting dietary information if time allows and the athlete is willing to record all foods and beverages consumed for this duration. This method of diet assessment not only provides a view of the athlete's usual eating patterns but also affords a measure of the quantity and quality of the food intake. This information provides the basis for a nutrition plan designed to help the athlete reach body weight and body composition goals. Dietary intake studies reveal that people routinely underestimate portions when recording food intake.[56] Therefore, it is crucial for the sports RDN to instruct athletes to eat as they usually do and to record portions as accurately and completely as possible so that the information reflects their typical food intake and meal patterns. Nutrient analysis software can be used to analyze the nutrient content of a food record, but the resulting analysis is only as good as the database on which the program is based. For the most complete information, the US Department of Agriculture National Nutrient Database for Standard Reference should form the foundation of the nutrient analysis program used.[57] When time or unwillingness prohibits the collection of a 3- to 5-day diet record, other methods of collecting dietary intake information can be employed, including a 24-hour recall, a food frequency questionnaire, or a usual diet intake pattern. In any case, sports RDN must explain how this information will be used in designing a personalized and precise meal plan.

Knowledge of metabolic rate provides an energy baseline that forms the foundation for a targeted, realistic, and effective weight-management plan. Resting metabolic rate (RMR) refers to the amount of energy needed for all metabolic processes of the active cell mass required to maintain normal regulatory balance and body functions at rest.[2] As explained in Chapter 10, RMR can be estimated by measuring oxygen consumption via indirect calorimetry or by using prediction equations (refer to Box 10.2 in Chapter 10).

Physical activity, also referred to as exercise energy expenditure, has a profound effect on total daily energy expenditure (TDEE). For athletes, the energy needed for training, conditioning, and performance represents a substantial proportion of total daily energy needs. World-class athletes, for instance, can almost double their TDEE with 3 to 4 hours of intense training.[2] Athletes should be educated on the importance of recording their daily exercise and noting both the intensity and duration of the exercise. An accurate determination of TDEE is difficult because of the variability of the contribution of physical exercise. Refer to Chapter 10 for information on how best to estimate TDEE.

Performance measurements, such as running speed and relative peak power, allow athletes to determine a baseline and track improvements in performance. Running speed is easy to measure. Relative peak power measures power-to-weight ratio. The 30-second Wingate test measures both average and peak power of the lower body. Upper-body power can be measured by using a modified Wingate test or an arm ergometer.[3]

Step 2: Goal Setting

Careful interpretation of the assessment measures will indicate whether the athlete's current weight and body composition are appropriate. The sports RDN should begin by determining whether the athlete's body composition is well matched to their sport (refer to Tables 11.1 and 11.2) and the athlete's genetic predisposition for leanness.

Although athletes may want to focus only on weight or body composition goals, it is important that they set multiple related goals. For example, an athlete could set a goal in each of these areas: performance, weight and body composition, and health.

- Performance-based goals may range from simply finishing an event (such as a marathon or triathlon) to very specific goals, such as improving performance time by 10 seconds.
- Weight range goals should be set to reflect an appropriate body composition range. As shown in Box 11.7, a formula can be used to help set the weight range.[58]

BOX 11.7 Calculating Target Weight[62]

The following formula, calculated using both lower and higher values for percentage body fat, is used to establish a weight range. To use this formula, an assessment of body composition must be performed because fat-free mass must be known. This formula assumes that the athlete is adequately hydrated.

Target body weight = current fat-free mass ÷ (1 - desired body fat percentage)

Example

A long-distance male cyclist currently weighs 187 lb. His body composition is 87% fat-free mass (163 lb) and 13% body fat. His goal is 8% to 10% body fat with no change in lean mass. An appropriate weight range to reflect this body composition goal is 177 to 181 lb (assuming that all weight is lost from adipose tissue).

Target body weight = 163 lb ÷ (1 - 0.08) = 163 lb ÷ 0.92 = 177 lb

Target body weight = 163 lb ÷ (1 - 0.1) = 163 lb ÷ 0.9 = 181 lb

This same formula can be used no matter how the athlete wants to change their body composition. For example, if this cyclist wanted to increase muscle mass by 5 lb to 168 lb and decrease body fat at the same time, his estimated weight range would be 183 to 187 lb (168 lb ÷ 0.92 and 168 lb ÷ 0.9).

» Health goals may include continued good health, but some athletes may need to set specific goals, such as continuing to menstruate, decreasing abdominal fat, or bringing a biochemical parameter into a healthy range.

In each case, goals need to be SMART. SMART, an acronym that athletes can easily remember, signifies the essential qualities of effective goals: **s**pecific, **m**easurable, **a**chievable, **r**ealistic, and **t**ime driven.

Step 3: Action Plan

The fundamental features of an effective action plan should place priority on the health and nutrition needs of the athlete first with athletic performance second and should include the following components:

» appropriate energy intake;
» adequate amounts of protein, carbohydrate, and fat;
» a variety of foods to ensure adequate amounts of vitamins, minerals, fiber, and water;
» proper timing of nutrient intake to aid in performance and recovery;
» appropriate training plan and daily physical activity;
» proper timing of weight changes (ideally not during a competition phase or season);
» consistent access to healthy foods; and
» personal food preferences, cost, and convenience.

ENERGY INTAKE

The number of calories needed daily cannot be predicted with precision, but an assessment of RMR and usual physical activity can help establish an estimate. For those who want to gain weight by increasing skeletal muscle mass, a general guideline for males is baseline calorie intake plus 400 to 500 kcal/d. For females, the recommendation is to add 300 to 400 kcal/d more than baseline. However, individuals vary to a great degree, and sports RDNs should individualize recommended daily energy intake.[1,2]

To reduce weight by reducing body fat, the guidelines are baseline intake minus 300 to 500 kcal/d for males and baseline intake minus 200 to 300 kcal/d for females. Greater reductions in daily energy intake may leave the athlete unable to maintain or increase energy output from physical activity and exercise. A reasonable weight-loss goal for athletes is to lose approximately 0.7% (0.5%–1.0%) of body weight per week, which helps to ensure the preservation of lean mass and performance.[1]

To gain skeletal muscle mass and lose body fat simultaneously, energy intake and nutrient timing must be as precise as possible. A starting point for daily intake is baseline requirements plus 300 kcal/d for males and baseline plus 200 kcal/d for females. However, close monitoring is needed, and total energy intake may need to be adjusted in 50- to 100-kcal increments daily until the desired outcome is reached. For those who wish to increase body fat, energy intake greater than baseline is necessary.[1]

PROTEIN INTAKE

In general, the amount of protein recommended for athletes daily is 1.4 to 2.0 g per kilogram of body weight.[1,2,59-64] The recommended protein intake to increase skeletal muscle mass in strength athletes is typically 1.7 to 2.0 g per kilogram of body weight per day, assuming that caloric intake is adequate. A common question asked by health professionals is whether athletes should use a high-protein diet when attempting weight loss. The literature has established that low-calorie diets in humans can lead to negative nitrogen balance and a significant loss of LBM.[1,2] Several studies in women who are overweight or obese have shown that the loss of LBM can be reduced (but not prevented entirely) with diets containing higher amounts of protein.[59]

Unfortunately, the amount of protein in a high-protein diet is often not clearly defined. A common recommendation for athletes consuming a moderately calorie-restricted diet (loss of ~0.7% of body weight per week with a range of 0.5%–1.0%) is a protein intake of approximately 1.5 g/kg/d, in an effort to protect against the loss of LBM. Maximizing the amount of body fat lost and protecting LBM is considered quality weight loss.[1,60-65] A study by Mettler and colleagues[60] found that a diet containing protein at a high level (~2.3 g/kg or ~35% of total caloric intake) helped to preserve LBM, but this diet was consumed for a very short time (2 weeks), and other levels of protein or other time frames were equally effective. A position paper on nutrition and athletic performance from the Academy of Nutrition and Dietetics, Dietitians of Canada, and the American College of Sports Medicine stated that during energy restriction, protein needs can be greater than 2.0 g/kg, but at this time, a definitive amount is not known.[1] It is prudent for athletes to work with a sports RDN when they are attempting to lose weight, protect against the loss of LBM, maintain their level of training, and/or maintain or improve their performance. Determining the amount of protein needed to achieve all of these goals is likely to require some trial and error. The other macronutrients—carbohydrate and fat—will also need to be fine-tuned.

The major concern with high-protein, calorie-reduced diets is carbohydrate content, which may not be sufficient to restore muscle glycogen and support training and performance over many weeks or months. Another issue is the amount of leucine consumed. Leucine is a branched-chain amino acid that activates a key signaling pathway needed to build and maintain skeletal muscle mass. Leucine, along with resistance exercise, is essential for optimal muscle protein synthesis. Both the amount and timing of leucine ingestion impact the maximal synthesis of skeletal muscle protein. Recommendations for adult athletes include 20 to 25 g (0.25 g per kilogram of body weight) of high-quality protein per meal with at least 2.2 g of leucine per meal (700–3,000 mg of leucine) distributed in doses every 3 to 4 hours. Whey protein and cow's milk are examples of excellent sources of protein and leucine. Older athletes may be anabolically resistant to optimal skeletal muscle protein synthesis and may benefit from 30 to 40 g (0.4 g per kilogram of body weight) of high-quality protein per meal, which should also provide sufficient leucine.[1,57] (For more information on older athletes, see Chapter 14.)

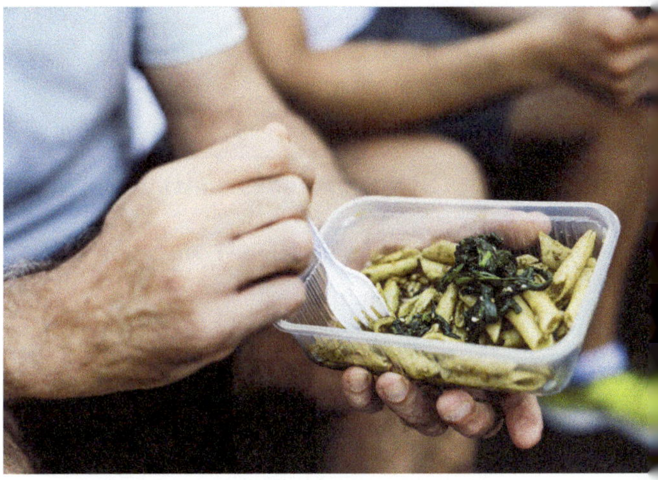

CARBOHYDRATE AND FAT INTAKE

Regardless of an athlete's weight management goals, their carbohydrate intake should be sufficient to resynthesize muscle glycogen stores daily (~3 to 12 g/kg). Fat restriction should be moderate. A general guideline for moderate fat intake is approximately 1 g per kilogram of body weight per day, or about 25% to 30% of total energy intake. Experts do not recommend restricting fat intake to less than 20% of total energy intake.[1] Current body weight is typically used to make calculations about the necessary intake in grams per kilogram per day. As body weight decreases, especially to a large degree, recalculations are needed to reflect the athlete's current (now lower) body weight.[2]

ACTION PLAN SUMMARY

Generally, athletes are encouraged to distribute food and beverage intake throughout the day by eating 3 meals and 2 or 3 snacks, ensuring energy and nutrient availability when most needed.[62] This distribution of calories and nutrients helps athletes begin exercise when adequately fueled and fully recover after exercise. Some postexercise carbohydrate and high-quality protein are necessary for the adequate resynthesis of muscle glycogen and the repair and synthesis of skeletal muscle, respectively. Consuming high-quality protein throughout the day may be beneficial for athletes restricting caloric intake because protein is associated with increased satiety as well as providing some protection against loss of skeletal muscle mass due to energy restriction.[1,2] Food intake and training must be coordinated. Each diet plan should be individualized, incorporating personal food preferences, religious beliefs, convenience, and cost.

Step 4: Evaluation and Reassessment

Even a plan that seems perfect on paper needs evaluation. Evaluation allows the athlete to determine if goals are being met. If progress is too slow or too fast, adjustments can be made before training, performance, or health is impacted. Reassessment of many of the original assessment measures is invaluable for tracking progress and, at times, adjusting the original goals. A case study illustrating a comprehensive plan for a linebacker in the National Football League appears in Box 11.8 on page 268.

BOX 11.8 Case Study of a National Football League Linebacker

An outside linebacker who is 6 ft 1 in (1.85 m) tall and weighs 226 lb (102.7 kg), with 19% body fat (43 lb [19.5 kg]) and 183 lb (83.2 kg) of lean mass, wants to be "ripped" by training camp. During his first 2 years in the National Football League (NFL), this athlete struggled to maintain his weight during the season. He lives alone and prepares his own meals. During the season, the team provides breakfast and lunch, but he often finds that he is too tired after a day of intense training to prepare a full dinner, and he is concerned that his nutrition may be lacking.

The athlete's goal is to earn a starting linebacker position in the upcoming season. To do this, he needs to gain strength and increase speed and agility. Wanting to be in peak condition when he reports to the team for conditioning, the athlete is engaged in an intense 6-hour workout 4 days per week at a high-level training facility during the break between the end of the season and offseason workouts.

Together, the athlete and the sports registered dietitian nutritionist (RDN) collected the necessary nutrition assessment data, set realistic achievable goals, planned an effective nutrition strategy to support his training regimen, and set benchmarks for evaluation and reassessment.

Step 1: Assessment

In the assessment, the sports RDN collected the following data:

- Height: 6 ft 1 in (1.85 m)
- Weight: 226 lb (102.7 kg)
- Somatotype: Mesomorph/ectomorph
- Body composition (BOD POD):
- ~19% body fat
  - ~43 lb (19.5 kg) of body fat
  - ~183 lb (83.2 kg) of lean mass
- Resting metabolic rate: 2,510 kcal
- Average daily energy intake: 2,805 kcal
- Average daily physical activity: 1,828 kcal

The assessment reveals that this athlete's weight and percentage of lean body mass are lower than those of many of his competitors. His mesomorphic/ectomorphic body build suggests that he can gain skeletal mass, but perhaps not as easily as a true mesomorph. A detailed 3-day record of dietary intake reveals that his average daily energy intake is 2,805 kcal.

Because of his large body size and large amount of skeletal muscle mass, the energy needed to support his resting metabolic rate is substantial, approximately 2,500 kcal/d. In addition, he expends more than 1,800 kcal/d, due in large part to his rigorous workouts. Total daily energy expenditure is therefore 4,338 kcal/d. The sports RDN quickly determines that the athlete's current intake does not meet the predicted amount of calories he needs daily to maintain his current weight and body composition. This is predominantly due to his fatigue after hours of working out and his lack of cooking skills. However, he likes to eat and enjoys a wide variety of foods. He will need to consume substantially more calories if he wishes to increase skeletal muscle mass.

Step 2: Goal setting

When asked, the athlete could quickly state his goal: to earn a starting position by being stronger and quicker than the other linebackers on the team. However, he was not able to translate this goal into measurable objectives. For example, when the sports RDN asked him how much he thought he should weigh or how quickly he expected to gain skeletal muscle mass, his answers suggested weight and body composition goals that were unrealistic. The sports RDN helped him establish some realistic goals and an appropriate time frame in which to meet them (see the accompanying chart). The athlete wanted to increase body mass as well as lean mass for greater bulk and strength. A goal weight of 230 to 233 lb was established by calculating a realistic gain of lean mass (0.5 to 0.75 lb/wk gain over 8 weeks) and adding it to his current weight. In working with the sports RDN, the athlete was able to establish goals that were SMART—specific, measurable, achievable, realistic, and time driven.

Goal	Objective
Earn a starting position.	Gain 0.75 lb/wk. After 8 weeks, reach goal weight range of 230 to 233 lb.
Gain strength to be able to compete with the other athletes in his position.	Gain 0.5 to 0.75 lb of lean mass per week. After 8 weeks, increase lean mass by 6 lb.
Gain speed and agility.	After 8 weeks, achieve a body fat percentage of 18% to 19%.

Step 3: Action plan

The athlete's action plan had 4 basic objectives:

- Increase calorie intake.
- Consume a high-carbohydrate, moderate-protein, moderate-fat diet.
- Distribute food intake over the course of the day to fuel activity and reduce fatigue.
- Consume a recovery snack immediately after exercise.

The athlete's initial meal plan of 4,800 kcal/d was based on his total energy expenditure of approximately 4,338 kcal plus an additional 500 kcal to cover the metabolic cost of building additional skeletal muscle tissue. Macronutrient distribution was based on 1.7 g of protein per kilogram of body weight and 8 g of carbohydrate per kilogram of body weight. The 4,800 kcal were distributed in a meal pattern of 3 meals plus 2 snacks per day. Preexercise meals and postexercise snacks were designed to ensure adequate fuel, sufficient high-quality protein, and proper rehydration and to support maximum muscle growth.

Using the 3-day food records, the sports RDN made suggestions for increasing the portion sizes of certain foods and incorporating ready-to-eat or easy-to-prepare foods into meals and snacks. A supermarket tour proved helpful, as did a few basic cooking classes, a list of suggested dinner meals, preworkout and postworkout snack options, and several easy recipes.

Continued on next page

BOX 11.8 Case Study of a National Football League Linebacker (CONTINUED)

Step 4: Evaluation and reassessment

The evaluation and reassessment step involved the following tasks:

- Keep a food intake record and evaluate for energy intake, macronutrient balance, and nutrient adequacy.
- Record weight weekly.
- Measure body composition after 4 and 8 weeks; compare strength, power, and performance before and after the 8-week program.

The effectiveness of the initial meal plan was determined by monitoring the athlete's weight. After 2 weeks, the athlete and sports RDN decided that an additional 200 kcal/d might be needed to achieve the target weekly weight gain. When the additional calories were added, weekly weight gain stayed on target. At the end of 8 weeks, this athlete had reached his body weight goal of 232 lb (105.5 kg). A reassessment of his body composition indicated 18% body fat and a gain of 6 lb (2.7 kg) of lean body mass. Having reached his preseason goals, this athlete followed a modified plan during the season, and for the first time in his NFL career, he was able to maintain his target weight throughout the season. In addition, the athlete experienced an injury-free season, started 16 games at weak-side linebacker, and was ranked first on the team with a career-high 143 tackles. He moved from weak-side to middle linebacker, where he started the final 8 games of the season.

Follow-up

Two years later, the linebacker suffered a severe knee sprain midway through the season and was placed on injured reserve. He was committed to arriving at offseason workouts in peak condition. At the end of the season, he once again engaged in a rigorous strength and conditioning program, 6 hours per day, 4 days per week, at the same training facility where he had trained 2 years prior. During the time he was on injured reserve, his weight dropped to 229 lb (104.1 kg). A body composition assessment determined that he had 19% body fat and 185.5 lb (84.3 kg) of lean body mass. During the 8-week conditioning program, his goal was to increase his total weight to 232 lb (105.5 kg) with 18% body fat. With his starting weight of 229 lb (104.1 kg), this meant a gain of 4.7 lb (2.1 kg) of lean mass and a loss of 1.7 lb (0.8 kg) of body fat. Because he needed to slightly trim body fat and slowly gain muscle, his meal plan was modified to a 4,800-kcal meal plan with 1.9 g of protein per kilogram of body weight and 8 g of carbohydrate per kilogram of body weight. Weekly monitoring of his weight indicated a gain of just less than 0.5 lb per week. By the end of the conditioning program, this athlete had reached his goals.

SUMMARY

Weight management goals and plans must be highly individualized. Factors that determine optimal weight and body composition ranges include sports-related characteristics, such as position played; relative need for power and endurance; and need for speed, mobility, flexibility, and agility. Physique-related characteristics, such as body size, build, weight, composition, and appearance, must also be considered. Achieving optimal weight and body composition goals requires an assessment, goal setting, an action plan, and evaluation and reassessment.

KEY TAKEAWAYS

When counseling an athlete, the sports RDN should make a checklist of sport- and physique-related factors to review and prioritize.

The checklist serves as a teaching tool to help athletes understand the many factors to be considered when setting weight and body composition goals.

Before such goals can be set, the sports RDN must conduct a comprehensive nutrition assessment.

Using the results of the assessment, the sports RDN can help the athlete set reasonable, realistic, and achievable weight and body composition goals periodized to the performance season and the physical demands on the athlete.

To support the athlete's progress toward these goals, the sports RDN creates a nutrition plan with the athlete that is tailored to the athlete's preferences and personal circumstances.

Routine monitoring and assessment of the athlete's progress are essential and reveal when the nutrition plan may need to be adjusted to help the athlete successfully reach their goals.

REFERENCES

1. Thomas DT, Erdman KA, Burke LM. Position of the Academy of Nutrition and Dietetics, Dietitians of Canada, and the American College of Sports Medicine: nutrition and athletic performance. *J Acad Nutr Diet.* 2016;116(3):501-528. doi:10.1016/j.jand.2015.12.006
2. Dunford M, Doyle JA. *Nutrition for Sport and Exercise.* 3rd ed. Cengage Learning; 2015.
3. Kinney WL, Wilmore JH, Costill DL. *Physiology of Sport and Exercise.* 6th ed. Human Kinetics; 2015.
4. Manore MM. Weight management for athletes and active individuals: a brief review. *Sports Med.* 2015;45(suppl 1):S83-S92. doi:10.1007/s40279-015-0401-0
5. Pasiakos SM, McLellan TM, Lieberman HR. The effects of protein supplements on muscle mass, strength, and aerobic and anaerobic power in healthy adults: a systematic review. *Sports Med.* 2015;45(1):111-131. doi:10.1007/s40279-014-0242-2
6. Zillmann T, Knechtle B, Rüst CA, Knechtle P, Rosemann T, Lepers R. Comparison of training and anthropometric characteristics between recreational male half-marathoners and marathoners. *Chin J Physiol.* 2013;56(3):138-146. doi:10.4077/CJP.2013.BAB105
7. Stellingwerff T, Maughan RJ, Burke LM. Nutrition for power sports: Middle distance running, track cycling, rowing, canoeing/kayaking, and swimming. *J Sport Sci.* 2011;29(suppl 1):S79-S89. doi:10.1080/02640414.2011.589469
8. Slater G, Rice A, Jenkins D, Hahn A. Body mass management of lightweight rowers: Nutritional strategies and performance implications. *Br J Sports Med.* 2014;48(21):1529-1533. doi:10.1136/bjsports-2014-093918
9. Garthe I, Raastad T, Refsnes PE, Koivisto A, Sundgot-Borgen J. Effect of two different weight-loss rates on body composition and strength and power-related performance in elite athletes. *Int J Sport Nutr Exerc Metab.* 2011;21(2):97-104. doi:10.1123/ijsnem.21.2.97
10. Sundgot-Borgen J, Meyer NL, Lohman TG, et al. How to minimise the health risks to athletes who compete in weight-sensitive sports review and position statement on behalf of the Ad Hoc Research Working Group on Body Composition, Health and Performance, under the auspices of the IOC Medical Commission. *Br J Sports Med.* 2013;47(16):1012-1022. doi:10.1136/bjsports-2013-092966
11. Major League Baseball Teams. Accessed December 4, 2022. www.mlb.com/team
12. Premier Lacross League Teams. Accessed December 4, 2022. https://premierlacrosseleague.com/teams
13. Major League Soccer Clubs. Accessed December 4, 2022. www.mlssoccer.com/clubs
14. National Basketball Association Teams and Rosters. Accessed December 4, 2022. www.nba.com/teams
15. National Football League Teams. Accessed December 4, 2022. www.nfl.com/teams
16. National Hockey League Teams. Accessed December 4, 2022. www.nhl.com/info/teams
17. Melvin MN, Smith-Ryan AE, Wingfield HL, Ryan ED, Trexler ET, Roelofs EJ. Muscle characteristics and body composition of NCAA Division I football players. *J Strength Cond Res.* 2014;28(12):3320-3329. doi:10.1519/JSC.0000000000000651
18. Bosch TA, Burruss TP, Weir NL, et al. Abdominal body composition differences in NFL football players. *J Strength Cond Res.* 2014;28(12):3313-3319. doi:10.1519/JSC.0000000000000650
19. Anzell AR, Potteiger JA, Kraemer WJ, Otieno S. Changes in height, body weight, and body composition in American football players from 1942 to 2011. *J Strength Cond Res.* 2013;27(2):277-284. doi:10.1519/JSC.0000000000000650
20. Skinner AC, Hasty SE, Turner RW II, Dreibelbis M, Lohr JA. Is bigger really better? Obesity among high school football players, player position, and team success. *Clin Pediatr (Phila).* 2013;52(10):922-928. doi:10.1177/0009922813492880
21. Santos DA, Dawson JA, Matias CN, et al. Reference values for body composition and anthropometric measurements in athletes. *PLoS ONE.* 2014;9(5):e97846. doi:10.1371/journal.pone.0097846
22. Steffes GD, Megura AE, Adams J, et al. Prevalence of metabolic syndrome risk factors in high school and NCAA division I football players. *J Strength Cond Res.* 2013;27(7):1749-1757. doi:10.1519/JSC.0b013e31827367cd
23. Helzberg JH, Camilo J, Waeckerle JF, O'Keefe JH. Review of cardiometabolic risk factors among current professional football and professional baseball players. *Phys Sportsmed.* 2010;38(3):77-83. doi:10.3810/psm.2010.10.1811
24. Buell JL, Calland D, Hanks F, et al. Presence of metabolic syndrome in football linemen. *J Athl Train.* 2008;43(6):608-616. doi:10.4085/1062-6050-43.6.608
25. Karpinos AR, Roumie CL, Nian H, Diamond AB, Rothman RL. High prevalence of hypertension among collegiate football athletes. *Circ Cardiovasc Qual Outcomes.* 2013;6(6):716-723. doi:10.1161/CIRCOUTCOMES.113.000463
26. Owora Ah, Kmush BL, Walia B, Sanders S. A systematic review of etiological risk factors associated with early mortality among National Football League players. *Orthop J Sports Med.* 2018;6(12):2325967118813312. doi:10.1177/2325967118813312
27. Churchill T, Krishnan S, Weisskopf M, et al. Weight gain and health affliction among former National Football League players. *Am J Med.* 2018;131(12):1491-1498. doi:10.1016/j.amjmed.2018.07.042
28. Ackland TR, Lohman TG, Sundgot-Borgen J, et al. Current status of body composition assessment in sport: Review and position statement on behalf of the ad hoc research working group on body composition health and performance, under the auspices of the I.O.C. Medical Commission. *Sports Med.* 2012;42(3):227-249. doi:10.2165/11597140-000000000-00000

29. Collins SM, Silberlicht M, Perzinski C, Smith SP, Davidson PW. The relationship between body composition and preseason performance tests of collegiate male lacrosse players. *J Strength Cond Res*. 2014;28(9):2673-2679. doi:10.1519/JSC.0000000000000454
30. Rüst CA, Knechtle B, Knechtle P, Rosemann T. Similarities and differences in anthropometry and training between recreational male 100-km ultra-marathoners and marathoners. *J Sports Sci.* 2012;30(12):1249-1257. doi:10.1080/02640414.2012.697182
31. Wilson G, Drust B, Morton JP, Close GL. Weight-making strategies in professional jockeys: Implications for physical and mental health and well-being. *Sports Med.* 2014;44(6):785-796. doi:10.1007/s40279-014-0169-7
32. Barley O, Chapman D, Abbiss C. Weight loss strategies in combat sports and concerning habits in mixed martial arts. *Int J Sports Physiol Perf.* 2018;13:933-939. doi:10.1123/ijspp.2017-0715
33. Reale R, Slater G, Burke LM. Acute-weight-loss strategies for combat sports and application to Olympic success. *Int J Sports Physiol Perf.* 2017;12:142-151. doi:10.1123/ijspp.2016-0211
34. Brechney G, Cannon J, Goodman S. Effects of weight cutting on exercise performance in combat athletes: a meta-analysis. *Int J Sport Nutr Exerc Metab.* 2022;17(7):995-1010. doi:10.1123/ijspp.2021-0104
35. Brito CJ, Roas AFCM, Brito ISS, et al. Methods of body mass reduction by combat sport athletes. *Int J Sport Nutr Exerc Metab.* 2012;22(2):89-97. doi:10.1123/ijsnem.22.2.89
36. Matthews JJ, Stanhope EN, Godwin MS, Holmes MEJ, Artioli GG. The magnitude of rapid weight loss and rapid weight gain in combat sport athletes preparing for competition: a systematic review. *Int J Sport Nutr Exerc Metabl.* 2019;29(4):441-452. doi:10.1123/ijsnem.2018-0165
37. Sundgot-Borgen J, Garthe I. Elite athletes in aesthetic and Olympic weight-class sports and the challenge of body weight and body compositions. *J Sport Sci.* 2011;29(suppl 1):S101-S114. doi:10.1080/02640414.2011.565783
38. Lakicevic N, Roklicer R, Bianco A, et al. Effects of rapid weight loss on judo athletes: a systematic review. *Nutrients.* 2020;12(5):1220. doi:10.3390/nu12051220
39. Artioli G, Iglesias R, Franchini E, et al. Rapid weight loss followed by recovery time does not affect judo-related performance. *J Sports Sci.* 2010;28(1):21-32. doi:10.1080/02640410903428574
40. Mauricio CDA, Merino P, Merlo R, et al. Rapid weight loss of up to five percent of the body mass in less than 7 days does not affect physical performance in official Olympic combat athletes with weight classes: A systematic review with meta-analysis. *Front Physiol.* 2022;13:830229. doi:10.3389/fphys.2022.830229
41. Coswig VS, Miarka B, Pires DA, et al. Weight regain, but not weight loss, is related to competitive success in real-life mixed martial arts competition. *Nutr Excer Metab.* 2019;29:1-8. doi:10.1123/ijsnem.2018-0034
42. Alwan N, Moss SL, Elliott-Sale KJ, Davies IG, Enright K. A narrative review on female physique athletes: the physiological and psychological implications of weight management practices. *Int J Sport Nutr Exerc Metab.* 2019;29:682-689. doi:10.1123/ijsnem.2019-0037
43. Davis S, Dwyer G, Reed K, et al. Preliminary investigation: the impact of the NCAA wrestling weight certification program on weight cutting. *J Strength Cond Res.* 2002;16(2):305-307. doi:10.1519/1533-4287(2002)016<0305:pitiot>2.0.co;2
44. Turocy PS, DePalma BF, Horswill CA, et al. National Athletic Trainers' Association position statement: safe weight loss and maintenance practices in sport and exercise. *J Athl Train.* 2011;46(3):322-336. doi:10.4085/1062-6050-46.3.322
45. Wrestling Rules Committee. NCAA Wrestling Rules. NCAA; 1999.
46. Yamamoto JB, Yamamoto BE, Yamamoto PP, Yamamoto LG. Epidemiology of college athlete sizes, 1950s to current. *Res Sports Med.* 2008;16(2):111-127. doi:10.1080/15438620802103320
47. Montgomery DL. Physiological profile of professional hockey players—a longitudinal comparison. *Appl Physiol Nutr Metab.* 2006;31(3):181-185. doi:10.1139/h06-012
48. Crotin RL, Forsythe CM, Bhan S, Karakolis T. Changes in physical size among major league baseball players and its attribution to elite offensive performance. *J Strength Cond Res.* 2014;28(10):2705-2708. doi:10.1519/JSC.0000000000000475
49. Grundy SM, Cleeman JI, Daniels SR, et al; American Heart Association; National Heart, Lung, and Blood Institute. Diagnosis and management of the metabolic syndrome: an American Heart Association/National Heart, Lung, and Blood Institute Scientific Statement. *Circulation.* 2005;112(17):2735-2752. doi:10.1161/CIRCULATIONAHA.105.169404
50. Graham R, Mancher M, Wolman DM, Greenfield S, Steinberg E, eds. *Clinical Practice Guidelines We Can Trust.* National Academies Press; 2011.
51. Javed A, Kashyap R, Lteif AN. Hyperandrogenism in female athletes with functional hypothalamic amenorrhea: a distinct phenotype. *Int J Womens Health.* 2015;7:103-111. doi:10.2147/IJWH.S73011
52. Goltz FR, Stenzel LM, Schneider CD. Disordered eating behaviors and body image in male athletes. *Braz J Psychiatry.* 2013;35(3):237-242. doi:10.1590/1516-4446-2012-0840
53. Kong P, Harris LM. The sporting body: body image and eating disorder symptomatology among female athletes from leanness focused and nonleanness focused sports. *J Psychol.* 2015;149(1-2):141-160. doi:10.1080/00223980.2013.846291
54. Muller SM, Gorrow TR, Schneider SR. Enhancing appearance and sports performance: are female collegiate athletes behaving more like males? *J Am Coll Health.* 2009;57(5):513-520. doi:10.3200/JACH.57.5.513-520
55. Calfee R, Fadale P. Popular ergogenic drugs and supplements in young athletes. *Pediatrics.* 2006;117(3):e577-e589. doi:10.1542/peds.2005-1429

56. Poslusna K, Ruprich J, de Vries JH, Jakubikova M, van't Veer P. Misreporting of energy and micronutrient intake estimated by food records and 24 hour recalls, control and adjustment methods in practice. *Br J Nutr.* 2009;101(suppl 2):S73-S85. doi:10.1017/S0007114509990602
57. Ahuja JK, Moshfegh AJ, Holden JM, Harris E. USDA food and nutrient databases provide the infrastructure for food and nutrition research, policy, and practice. *J Nutr.* 2013;143(2): 241S-249S. doi:10.3945/jn.112.170043
58. Rankin JW. Weight loss and gain in athletes. *Curr Sports Med Rep.* 2002;1(4):208-213. doi:10.1249/00149619-200208000-00004
59. Carbone JW, McClung JP, Pasiakos SM. Skeletal muscle responses to negative energy balance: effects of dietary protein. *Adv Nutr.* 2012;3(2):119-126. doi:10.3945/an.111.001792
60. Mettler S, Mitchell N, Tipton KD. Increased protein intake reduces lean body mass loss during weight loss in athletes. *Med Sci Sports Exerc.* 2010;42(2):326-337. doi:10.1249/MSS.0b013e3181b2ef8e
61. Doering TM, Reaburn PR, Phillips SM, Jenkins DG. Post-exercise dietary protein strategies to maximize skeletal muscle repair and remodeling in masters endurance athletes: a review. *Int J Sport Nutr Exerc Metab.* 2016;26(2):168-178. doi:10.1123/ijsnem.2015-0102
62. Ivy J, Ferguson-Stegall LM. Nutrient timing: the means to improving exercise performance, recovery, and training adaptation. *Am J Lifestyle Med.* 2014;8(4):246-259. doi:10.1177/1559827613502444
63. Jäger R, Kerksick CM, Campbell BI, et al. International Society of Sports Nutrition Position Stand: protein and exercise. *J Int Soc Sports Nutr.* 2017;14:20. doi:10.1186/s12970-017-0177-8
64. Hector AJ, Phillips SM. Protein recommendations for weight loss in elite athletes: a focus on body composition and performance. *Int J Sport Nutr Exerc Metab.* 2018;28(2):170-177. doi:10.1123/ijsnem.2017-0273
65. Ruiz-Castellano C, Espinar S, Contreras C, et al. Achieving optimal fat loss phase in resistance-trained athletes: a narrative review. *Nutrients.* 2021;13:3255. doi:10.3390/nu13093255

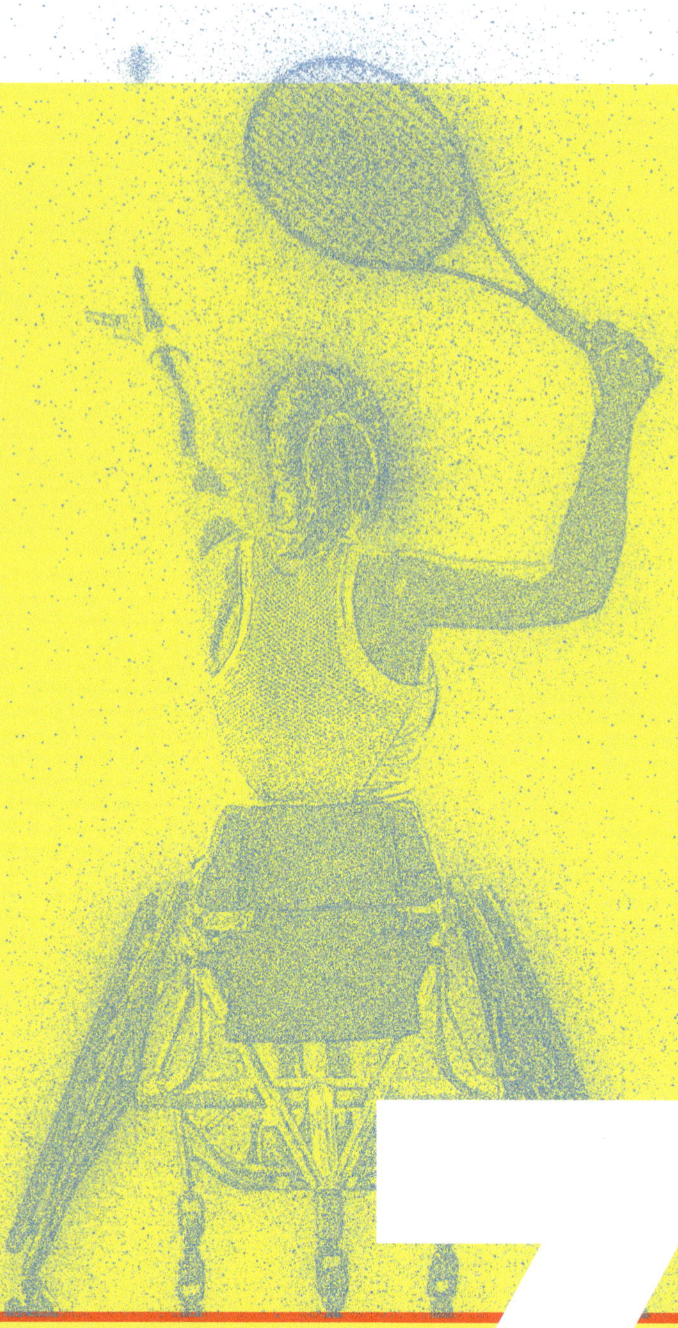

SECTION 3

PRINCIPLES IN PRACTICE

Athletics is not restricted to the young elite or the professional athlete. Today, children participate in competitive sports, as do older adults. This section provides the sports dietitian with insight into the physiological and health-related issues of diverse populations. Understanding the unique needs of these populations will help the sports dietitian develop plans to meet the needs of each athlete, whether it is a collegiate athlete who is challenged by a lack of cooking skills or an athlete with diabetes who needs medical nutrition therapy. In this section, lifecycle issues are discussed in chapters dealing with youth, college-aged, and older athletes (Chapters 12, 13, and 14, respectively). A chapter on elite athletes (Chapter 15) is included to highlight the opportunities and challenges faced by the sports dietitian when planning nutrition strategies for high-performing athletes. The unique nutritional needs of vegetarian athletes, pregnant athletes, athletes with disordered eating, and those with type 1 and type 2 diabetes are also included in this section (Chapters 16 through 19).

CHAPTER 12

Child and Adolescent Athletes

Roberta Anding, MS, RDN/LD, CSSD, CDCES, FAND

LEARNING OBJECTIVES

- Outline the unique physiological changes that occur during growth and development.
- Highlight the role of Tanner staging in determining energy and protein requirements during adolescence.
- Compare and contrast the thermoregulatory processes in children and adolescents vs adults.
- Identify nutrients of concern in childhood and adolescence.
- Discuss the strengths and limitations of dietary supplements for child and adolescent athletes.

INTRODUCTION

The popularity of youth sports is robust in the United States. Data from the 2020 Census estimates that more than 50 million children and adolescents participate in youth sports.[1] The knowledge regarding the impact of the COVID-19 pandemic on youth sports is evolving. According to the Aspen Institute's Project Play, participation in organized sports decreased during the pandemic in 2020, with a greater impact on families whose incomes were less than $25,000.[2] The National Federation of State High School Associations (NFHS) reported the following in their 2021–2022 participation survey[3]:

- Youth sports participation peaked during the 2017–2018 school year, with high school sports participation at approximately 7.9 million youth (58% male and 42% female).
- However, during the 2018–2019 school year, participation decreased by approximately 44,000. (These data do not reflect the impact of the pandemic on school sports.) The largest declines were in 2 historically popular sports: football and basketball.
- Throughout the United States, 11-player football has seen a decline of 30,829 participants, to the lowest participation rate since 1999 (1,006,013). Despite the decline in numbers, 11-player football remains the most popular sport for boys, and despite the decrease in absolute numbers, the number of schools offering football has increased. Publicity on the physical impact of football and the inherent danger of collision sports may be driving the decrease in participation.
- Outdoor track and field ranks second in participation (605,354 participants), followed by basketball (540,769 participants) and baseball (482,740 participants) for boys.
- Combined boys' and girls' basketball has also declined and is at its lowest participation rate since 1992.

- The most popular sports programs for girls include outdoor track and field (488,267 participants), volleyball (452,808 participants), basketball (399,067 participants), soccer (394,105 participants), and fast-pitch softball (362,038 participants).
- Absent from this data set are statistics regarding cheerleading, which has experienced a surge in popularity over the past decade.

The survey by NFHS estimated that more than 400,000 females were participating in cheerleading in the United States during the 2021–2022 school year, making it as popular as other traditional sports for girls. Of this cohort, 123,836 were involved in competitive spirit squads. In addition, although uniform data are lacking, many high school programs are also expanding into adaptive sports.[3]

Sports dietitians should stay abreast of current trends in sports participation for a variety of reasons. Nutritional guidance may vary based on the sport, the timing of the game, and the level of coaching available. Parents and volunteer coaches are often responsible for guidance on hydration, nutrition, and training in younger athletes. In high school, the coaches often assume more than 1 role, and their expertise in nutrition varies. Given the prevalence of youth sports and expanding sports options, the expertise of a sports dietitian is needed to promote evidence-based principles for performance and proper nutrition for growth and development.

BENEFITS OF YOUTH SPORTS

The plethora of benefits of youth sports are beyond the scope of this chapter but include both physical and psychosocial benefits. Physical activity should be considered an essential component of normal growth and development and be routinely assessed. Sports can provide an outlet for young people to begin and maintain physical activity. Regular physical activity in the formative years has been shown to be a predictor of a healthier body weight and regular exercise patterns in adulthood.[4,5] Not surprisingly, children who participate in sports have greater levels of cardiovascular fitness, lower levels of abdominal fat, and reduced arterial stiffness.[5,6] In addition to improving cardiorespiratory fitness, regular physical activity has been shown to improve lipid profiles in youth, most notably triglyceride and high-density lipoprotein cholesterol levels, although the improvement is often modest. The dose of exercise to improve lipids is a minimum of 40 minutes per day 5 days per week for a 4-month period.[7] This level of exercise is consistent with 1 sports season for children and teens.

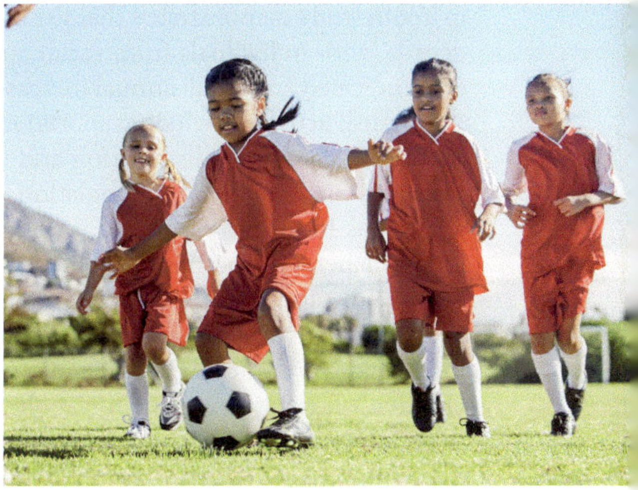

The psychological benefits of regular exercise for children and teens include improved self-esteem, increased social interaction, and a decrease in depressive symptoms.[8,9] Research from the Young-HUNT study suggests that physical activity improves indices of mental health and that participation in team sports also reduces psychological stress in senior high school girls.[9]

Improvements in Bone Density

Regular physical activity is also essential for the development and maintenance of bone mineral density. The osteogenic force of physical activity is related to the local and specific mechanical loading of the bone. The tensile and compressive forces of specific resistance or strength-producing programs can promote bone development. According to a National Strength and Conditioning Association position paper, when properly performed and supervised, a comprehensive strength and conditioning program is safe to initiate in children as young as 5 years old, although a strength program more typically begins at 12 years of age.[10] In addition, numerous sport-specific studies have demonstrated targeted areas of bone development based on the loading forces. Studies with gymnasts have shown improved bone density in wrists and the proximal portion of the femur given the nature of the sport.[11,12] Although research results vary, consistent load-bearing exercise in the prepubertal phase of adolescence can promote an increase in bone accrual of 0.6% to 1.7% per year.[13] In a review article by Hind and Burrows,[14] prepubertal children who exercised regularly experienced mean percent increases of 0.9% to 4.9% in bone parameters over 6 months in early pubertal development. Less bone accrual was realized in late adolescence or young adulthood, indicating the important role of exercise in bone accrual during childhood and early puberty.[8]

A longitudinal study of soccer players demonstrated that the osteogenic benefits of exercise in adolescents can have a positive impact on bone health after they complete their competitive years. Thirty years after they stopped playing, former soccer players were found to have a higher bone mineral density and greater bone mass compared with sedentary counterparts, indicating that playing sports during adolescence may have long-lasting health benefits.[15] In a review article, Tenforde and Fredericson[16] characterized the loading of bone in sports as high impact (gymnastics, hurdling), odd impact (soccer, basketball), and nonimpact (swimming, cycling). Sports with higher-impact loadings were found to result in favorable improvements in bone geometry, whereas nonimpact sports were found to be either neutral or detrimental to bone accrual. Optimal bone development during childhood and adolescence is predicated on energy availability and a normal hormonal milieu.

Impact on Obesity, Prediabetes, and Type 2 Diabetes

Multiple studies have highlighted the known benefits of physical fitness and nutrition on pediatric health, including lower body fat, improved lipid levels, lower blood pressure, and improved insulin sensitivity.[6,7] The prevalence of obesity in 6- to 11-year-olds increased from 16.4% in 2014 to 17.4% in 2016. During this same time frame, the prevalence of obesity in 12- to 19-year-olds remained consistent at 20.6%.[17] The relationship between obesity and diabetes is well known. The incidence of type 2 diabetes is steadily increasing in pediatrics. In a 2020 study, Andes et al[18] reported that the prevalence of prediabetes was 18%, that is, approximately 1 in 5 adolescents have a risk of type 2 diabetes. Data from the 2018 SEARCH for Diabetes in Youth study demonstrated that the incidence of type 2 diabetes had increased considerably over the past decade, with individuals from racial and ethnic minorities displaying the largest increase. The SEARCH data indicated an overall annual increase in pediatric type 2 diabetes of 4.8%.[19]

Physical activity (including sports) is an integral component of obesity and type 2 diabetes prevention. Increased visceral fat distribution and hepatic steatosis have been shown to be directly related to insulin resistance in the pediatric population.[20,21] The prevailing mechanism for the development of type 2 diabetes has historically centered on peripheral insulin resistance. Although the exact pathophysiology of type 2 diabetes in youth is yet to be completely elucidated, consistent, vigorous exercise (>80% of maximal heart rate) can improve the markers of insulin sensitivity, irrespective of changes in body composition.[22] In children, increased adiposity, including increased visceral fat, has been linked with the development of metabolic syndrome. A Finnish pediatric prospective study showed higher baseline fasting insulin levels in children who later developed metabolic syndrome.[23] The results of this study suggest that insulin resistance in children who are obese precedes metabolic and atherogenic complications.

Adolescents who were overweight and who participated in a structured exercise program for 3 to 5 days per week for 3 to 8 months experienced improved insulin sensitivity by up to 50%.[24] In this context, organized sport can be considered a public health strategy for preventing diabetes in youth. With increasing pressure to have larger linemen in football, prepubertal boys or boys in early puberty may seek to gain weight but may lack the androgen to add significant lean mass. Therefore, increasing body weight is likely to increase adipose tissue and not lean body mass, thus increasing the likelihood of insulin resistance. The progressive assessment of abdominal girth among adolescents and screening for acanthosis nigricans in athletes is critical for preventing type 2 diabetes in this vulnerable population. Waist circumference cutoffs for the diagnosis of metabolic syndrome have been established based on age, sex, and ethnicity; they can be useful for the practicing sports registered dietitian nutritionist (RDN) (refer to Table 12.1).[25] Given the magnitude of the pediatric obesity epidemic, sports RDNs will regularly encounter young athletes with metabolic syndrome.

Globally, pediatric obesity has profound individual, family, societal, and economic impacts. In 2009, the direct financial cost of pediatric obesity was estimated as $14.1 billion per year.[26] Data regarding the impact of the COVID-19 pandemic are emerging. A study of 432,032 children found that the rate of pediatric obesity doubled during the pandemic. The causes are multifactorial and include social isolation, stress, and decreased opportunities for activity.[27] In addition to the increased risk of type 2 diabetes, a teen who is obese is more likely to become an adult who is overweight or obese and has an increased risk of heart

TABLE 12.1 Optimal Waist Circumference Thresholds (cm) for Predicting Cardiovascular Risk Clustering in Adolescents Based on Ethnicity[25]

Age, y	Hispanic boys	Hispanic girls	Non-Hispanic White boys	Non-Hispanic White girls	Non-Hispanic Black boys	Non-hispanic Black girls
12	76.5	77.1	73.1	71.5	66.8	74.6
13	81.6	79.1	74.2	78.0	72.6	75.6
14	80.3	79.6	76.1	74.8	75.0	80.0
15	83.5	79.8	77.2	77.6	76.5	82.7
16	83.7	81.2	82.1	78.5	74.7	84.6
17	85.0	82.4	85.1	77.6	77.9	86.8
18	87.1	82.5	83.5	78.0	79.0	86.9
19	87.5	86.4	86.3	85.0	78.6	87.2

disease, hypertension, cancer, and osteoarthritis. Type 2 diabetes that develops among teens and young adults results in a much faster progression of the disease compared with type 2 diabetes with onset in middle age. Moreover, type 2 diabetes diagnosed in teens and young adults is a much more severe disease than type 1 diabetes diagnosed in the same age range. Diabetes complications such as nephropathy, retinopathy, and neuropathy come earlier and more frequently, and together, these factors result in a much higher mortality rate.[28]

It is incumbent on practicing sports RDNs to screen for prediabetes or type 2 diabetes risk factors. Health concerns include nonalcoholic fatty liver disease, sleep apnea, dyslipidemia, and asthma.[29] The complex physiological changes underlying pediatric obesity are underpinned by a low-grade inflammatory response. As the adipocytes increase in size, there is an increase in the secretion of proinflammatory cytokines including tumor necrosis factor α, resistin, and retinol-binding protein. The alteration in endocrine function can also increase the likelihood of other autoimmune diseases such as multiple sclerosis and type 1 diabetes.[30]

In obesity prevention and management, it is difficult to separate the distinct roles of exercise and diet. Although the causes of obesity are multifactorial, the factors driving the current epidemic include a steady increase in calories coupled with decreases in physical activity.[31]

Reduced intake of sugar-sweetened beverages has been highlighted as a specific dietary intervention to reduce pediatric obesity, and a 2015 study by Mesirow and Welsh[32] found that children and adolescents have reduced their intake of sugar-sweetened sodas and fruit drinks with added sugar. However, as the intake of these beverages has decreased, consumption of sweetened coffees, teas, energy drinks, and sports drinks has increased. Sports RDNs must keep abreast of the changing beverage consumption patterns of children and teens to provide guidance for athletes. Although genetics and inherited predispositions to body morphology ultimately influence body size, musculature, and body fatness, positive energy balance is the major contributor to excess body fatness.[33]

The sports RDN has a critical role to play in weight management in this vulnerable population. Considering the role of inflammation in excess body fatness, sports RDNs can provide an emphasis on nutritional principles to reduce inflammation, possibly by promoting a Mediterranean-style dietary approach. Nutrition recommendations should be designed to reduce body fat and maintain adequate energy for activity. Table 12.2 on page 282 provides guidance on the energy needs for children and adolescents.[34]

The Psychosocial Stigma of Obesity

The psychosocial stigma for children or adolescents who are overweight or obese can be substantial. Bullying and teasing regarding weight are pervasive in today's society. Neumark-Sztainer et al[35] measured the prevalence of reported weight teasing in a sample of more than 4,700 youths who were overweight or obese. Of the sample, 63% of the girls and 58% of the boys who were obese (BMI > 95th percentile) reported weight teasing.

TABLE 12.2 Summary of Estimated Energy Requirement Equations by Age, Sex, Physical Activity, and Energy Cost of Growth

Age group	Sex	Physical activity level category	EER equation (kcal/d)[a]
3 to 13.99 y	Male[b]	Inactive	EER = −447.51 + (3.68 × age) + (13.01 × height) + (13.15 × weight) + 20/15/25
		Low active	EER = 19.12 + (3.68 × age) + (8.62 × height) + (20.28 × weight) + 20/15/25
		Active	EER = −388.19 + (3.68 × age) + (12.66 × height) + (20.46 × weight) + 20/15/25
		Very active	EER = −671.75 + (3.68 × age) + (15.38 × height) + (23.25 × weight) + 20/15/25
	Female[c]	Inactive	EER = 55.59 − (22.25 × age) + (8.43 × height) + (17.07 × weight) + 15/30
		Low active	EER = −297.54 − (22.25 × age) + (12.77 × height) + (14.73 × weight) + 15/30
		Active	EER = −189.55 − (22.25 × age) + (11.74 × height) + (18.34 × weight) + 15/30
		Very active	EER = −709.59 − (22.25 × age) + (18.22 × height) + (14.25 × weight) + 15/30
14 to 18.99 y	Male	Inactive	EER = −447.51 + (3.68 × age) + (13.01 × height) + (13.15 × weight) + 20
		Low active	EER = 19.12 + (3.68 × age) + (8.62 × height) + (20.28 × weight) + 20
		Active	EER = −388.19 + (3.68 × age) + (12.66 × height) + (20.46 × weight) + 20
		Very active	EER = −671.75 + (3.68 × age) + (15.38 × height) + (23.25 × weight) + 20
	Female	Inactive	EER = 55.59 − (22.25 × age) + (8.43 × height) + (17.07 × weight) + 20
		Low active	EER = −297.54 − (22.25 × age) + (12.77 × height) + (14.73 × weight) + 20
		Active	EER = −189.55 − (22.25 × age) + (11.74 × height) + (18.34 × weight) + 20
		Very active	EER = −709.59 − (22.25 × age) + (18.22 × height) + (14.25 × weight) + 20

Abbreviation: EER = estimated energy requirement

[a] Age is in years, weight is in kilograms, and height is in centimeters.

[b] Energy cost of growth for boys: 3 y, 20 kcal/d; 4-8 y, 15 kcal/d; 9-13 y, 25 kcal/d.

[c] Energy cost of growth for girls: 3 y, 15 kcal/d; 4-8 y, 15 kcal/d; 9-13 y, 30 kcal/d.

Adapted with permission from reference 34: National Academies of Sciences, Engineering, and Medicine; Health and Medicine Division; Food and Nutrition Board; Committee on the Dietary Reference Intakes for Energy. Dietary *Reference Intakes for Energy*. National Academies Press; 2023. doi:10.17226/26818

In a 2022 meta-analysis, children and adolescents with obesity and overweight in schools were more likely to be the targets of bullying than their normal weight peers. In addition, being obese was significantly associated with different types of bullying, including physical, verbal, emotional, and cyberbullying. In contrast to the Neumark-Sztainer study, boys who were overweight or obese were more likely to have bullying experiences than girls. The study subjects also reported weight teasing within their families. Weight teasing was associated with an increase in binge eating and placed the youth at greater risk of further obesity.[36] In addition, research indicates that body dissatisfaction in youth who are overweight is an additional risk factor for eating disorders and disordered eating behaviors.[37]

Although the exact prevalence of weight-related teasing in youth sports is unknown, in a study of adolescents enrolled in weight loss camps, 42% reported being bullied by their physical education teachers and/or coaches.[38] The impact of weight-related teasing is also a predictor of adult increases in BMI. Data were collected from Project EAT-IV (Eating and Activity in Teens and Young Adults), a longitudinal cohort study conducted from 1999 through 2015. Weight-based teasing at baseline was examined as a predictor of weight, binge eating, dieting, eating as a coping strategy, unhealthy weight control, and body image at the 15-year follow-up, which was completed for 1,830 of the original study participants. The study revealed that weight-based teasing in adolescence predicted higher BMI and obesity 15 years later. For females, teasing from both family and peers had an impact on BMI, but for males, only peer-based teasing predicted higher BMI.[39]

The Psychological Impact of Sports

Youth sports can promote healthy psychosocial development and positive attributes in children. Physical activity in children and adolescents is thought to be a key determinant of cognitive development. *Cognitive development* is broadly defined as the ability to acquire knowledge through a variety of mechanisms, including experiences and sensory input. High cognitive function is an important determinant of health, and conversely, poor cognitive functioning is linked to increased morbidity and mortality.[40] Studies suggest that active children and teens have higher levels of cognitive function, reported as improved memory and concentration and better classroom behavior, leading to better academic performance.[41-43] Well-structured sports participation has been specifically linked to the learning of values, skills, self-control, persistence, and responsibility.[44] Sports can also promote resilience and the ability to rebound from disappointment.[45] Sports participation in high school has been associated with improved mental health and reduced depression. A 2022 meta-analysis showed significant mental health benefits associated with physical activity even when the dose of activity, in terms of time and intensity, was below public health recommendations.[46] Proposed mechanisms for this effect are complex but include neurobiological factors and improved social factors, such as a sense of connectedness and belonging.[47]

Despite the noted benefits, sports participation can also have negative consequences. Most children and teens report having fun as a primary reason for participation. Conversely, when a sport is no longer enjoyable, children and teens report becoming less active or finding something else that is more fun. A comprehensive review by the International Olympic Committee cautioned against early sports specialization, which is a contributor to increased injury rates and burnout.[48,49] Sports RDNs should be attuned to the signs and symptoms of depression and burnout as part of an initial assessment. Children and adolescents are especially vulnerable to inappropriate coaching and instructions. Of note, children and adolescents who live at the coaching facility, such as those in world class ballet, gymnastics, and figure skating, are at particular risk given their young age and potential social isolation from family and friends.

PHYSICAL GROWTH AND DEVELOPMENT

Prepubertal Stage

In the prepubertal phase or sexual maturity rating stage 1, boys and girls share many physical attributes. Body composition analyses are similar, with a body fat percentage of 16% to 17% and relatively similar amounts of lean weight.[50] Height, weight, injury risks, hemoglobin levels, and physical attributes of strength and endurance are also similar.[51,52] During the prepubertal phase, rate of growth is about 5 cm/y in both boys and girls. The activation of the pituitary-gonadal axis signals the onset of puberty, and the physiological changes become sex-specific. During early puberty, linear growth increases markedly in both sexes from approximately 5 cm/y in prepubertal boys and girls to 8.3 cm/y in pubertal girls and 9.5 cm/y in pubertal boys. Weight velocity increases from 3 kg/y in prepubertal boys to 9 kg/y during puberty; less is known about the weight velocity in pubertal girls. The changes in biological landmarks are sex specific.

Pubertal Development

Puberty is the process of physical and psychological maturation between childhood and adulthood. It is characterized by physical and psychological changes that influence nutritional needs and food choices. The biological changes include increases in height and weight, body composition changes, increases in energy and protein needs, sexual development, and increases in skeletal mass and density. Although the biological changes during puberty are consistent, the timing and tempo of these landmarks can vary and are influenced by genetics, sex, and nutritional status (eg, malnutrition and obesity). The impact of genetics in determining the cascade of pubertal events is estimated to be between 41% and 71%.[53] Therefore, pubertal development is the interaction of genetic traits with components of the environment.

The age of menarche has declined steadily in the United States over the past 50 years. Overweight and obesity are part of the etiology of this decline, but other variables are emerging as well.[54] Researchers have found that brominated flame retardants, phytoestrogens, phenols, and phthalates have the potential to affect the timing of puberty.[55] The alteration of normal pubertal development has the potential to impact body composition and nutritional needs. Girls who experience early menarche (age < 11 years) are more likely to become overweight and are less sensitive to insulin than girls who experience menarche later in adolescence (age > 14 years).[56,57]

Given the variability in timing and tempo of pubertal events, chronological age is not a reliable marker for predicting growth and nutritional requirements. Tanner stages (also known as sexual maturity ratings) are the best gauge of the current stage of growth and development. In females, the sexual maturity rating is based on appearance and development of breasts and pubic hair. In males, Tanner stages are characterized by testicular and penile development, along with the development and patterning of pubic hair. Although it is not within the scope of the sports RDN to conduct this level of physical examination, these biological landmarks can be identified as part of an adolescent self-assessment. The self-assessment of sexual maturity ratings does not replace a physical examination by a trained pediatrician, but it can be useful in distinguishing the prepubertal and pubertal phase.[58] Because energy and protein needs are determined by Tanner stages, this assessment can guide the RDN in the development of an appropriate nutrition plan. Box 12.1 presents the Tanner staging process and its nutritional implications, which are further expanded upon in the following sections.[59]

PUBERTAL DEVELOPMENT IN GIRLS

The first hallmark of puberty in girls is the development of breast buds at an average age of 10.6 years, signaling the onset of Tanner stage 2. Peak weight velocity occurs in girls before peak height velocity. In practical terms, girls "grow out and then grow up." Peak height velocity follows early in the pubertal process for girls during Tanner stage 2 and slows during Tanner stage 3. Menarche occurs during Tanner stage 4, which, on average, occurs at age 12.5 years in the United States. About 98% of adult height is achieved by Tanner stage 4. As part of a nutrition assessment, all sports RDNs should assess the individual's age of menarche to gauge the phase of growth and development, as this ultimately influences energy needs. However, ethnic and racial differences in pubertal timing exist. Research indicates that African American girls may enter puberty earlier than their White and Hispanic peers.[60] In a large practice-based study, 48% of African American girls had reached Tanner stage 2 by age 8 years, contrasting with the average age of onset of 10.6 years. In addition, obesity during the prepubescent phase can hasten the onset of puberty. In a study of Chinese girls, the girls who were obese entered Tanner stage 2 at 8.8 years of age, whereas the girls who were lean entered this phase of growth and development at 9.3 years of age.[61] Childhood obesity hastens the onset of puberty as a result of increased estradiol. Girls who experience early puberty will have a slightly extended period of growth compared with girls who experience a more typical pattern. Just as overnutrition can hasten the onset of puberty in girls, undernutrition may delay the onset and tempo of the pubertal cascade.

Evidence from developing countries shows that menarche occurs at an older age in malnourished teens, suggesting that food insecurity or energy restriction may delay menarche through nutritional

BOX 12.1 Sexual Maturity Ratings (Tanner Stages) and Nutritional Implications

Tanner stage	Development	Nutritional implications
Girls		
1	No pubic hair or maturation of genitalia	Calories based on Dietary Reference Intakes
2	Sparse pubic hair Small breast buds Increased sweat gland activity Initiation of peak height velocity (PHV); growth spurt of 3 to 5 in Average age: 10.6 years	Calories increase to their highest levels in adolescence Girls experience an increased peak in weight velocity around 6 to 9 months before PHV; they "grow out, then up"
3	Pubic hair increases, is darker and curly Breasts become larger Acne may occur End of PHV	Nutritional guidance needed to improve nutrient density
4	Menarche begins at an average age of 12.5 years 98% of adult height is achieved	May occur earlier in girls who are obese May be delayed with malnutrition or decreased energy availability
5	Adult breasts and pubic hair Increase in fat and muscle mass	Calorie and protein needs equal to those of an adult female
Boys		
1	No pubic hair or maturation of genitalia	Calories based on Dietary Reference Intakes
2	Penile enlargement Scrotum reddens and changes texture Increased activity of sweat glands	Lack of androgen limits lean mass accrual Strength training can improve neuromuscular control and strength without increase in mass
3	Faint noticeable mustache Voice begins to change Acne may occur Beginning of PHV; growth spurt of 6 to 8 in	Peak weight velocity and peak height velocity coincide Calories and protein increase to their highest levels
4	Voice deepens Acne may be severe	Muscle mass increases
5	Able to grow full beard Linear growth ceases between ages 18 and 21 years	Muscle mass increases Calorie and protein needs equal to those of an adult male

Adapted with permission from reference 59: Tanner JM. *Growth at Adolescence: With a General Consideration of the Effects of Hereditary and Environmenal Factors Upon Growth and Maturation from Birth to Maturity.* Blackwell Scientific Publications; 1962.

mechanisms.[62] Although there is controversy in the literature, data on underfueled young athletes indicate that intensive training may delay the onset of puberty, suggestive of low energy availability. In response to this growing concern in gymnasts, the Scientific Commission of the International Gymnastics Federation convened a committee to review the literature on the effects of intensive training on the growth and development of female gymnasts. The short stature and later maturation of female gymnasts have often been attributed to the demands of training and the emphasis on leanness; however, after extensive review, these characteristics were determined to be within the normal range of variability for the population.[63] Less information is available regarding other sports. Sports RDNs should take a detailed menstrual history to assess for the possibility of low energy availability.

After puberty, young females develop less strength than their male counterparts. Strength-trained female athletes can achieve approximately 70% of the total strength of their male counterparts and 30% to 50% of the upper body strength secondary to a relative decrease in lean mass compared with their male counterparts. Estrogen and progesterone promote the deposition of more body fat than muscle, possibly limiting strength gains. Females increase body fat levels from approximately 16% during the prepubertal phase to about 23% in adulthood. Muscle fiber types are not sex specific; however, females have an overall smaller muscle fiber size. Therefore, many of the physiological changes during puberty affecting sports performance can be attributed to hormonal and body composition changes.[50,51,55,63-66] Pubertal changes and performance changes in females are summarized in Box 12.2.[67]

BOX 12.2 Pubertal Changes Affecting Sports Performance in Females[67]

- Increase in percent body fat
- Reduced hemoglobin levels
- Reduced lung volume and aerobic capacity
- Increased levels of adiposity in those who mature early
- Improved balance and flexibility

PUBERTAL DEVELOPMENT IN BOYS

In boys, the first physical signs of maturation include testicular enlargement and a change in scrotal color. The average age of onset of Tanner stage 2 in boys is 11.6 years. Peak height velocity in boys occurs in Tanner stage 3, about the same time as peak weight velocity, with the coinciding increase in energy requirements. Height velocity increases from approximately 5 cm/y to 9.5 cm/y. Compared with girls, boys have a prolonged period of growth, resulting in a height about 13 cm greater than that of girls. As androgen levels increase, there is a considerable increase in lean body mass. Weight velocity increases from 3 kg/y in prepubertal boys to 9 kg/y during puberty. Lean mass doubles from about the age of 10 years through 17 years and is accompanied by the maturation of bone, further increasing energy requirements.[66] The increase in androgen not only increases lean weight but also allows for muscular hypertrophy with strength training. In the absence of adequate androgen, increasing energy and protein increases the likelihood of weight gain, which can lead to obesity. The sports RDN should assess the individual's stage of growth and development and provide education on typical growth and development. During adolescence, boys often struggle to gain weight secondary to the needs of growth and development and fueling their sport. As a result, a late-maturing boy is more likely to use or abuse performance-enhancing supplements to improve body composition.[68]

Obesity has an impact on growth parameters, although agreement on the effect is not universal. Pubertal boys who are obese have lower serum sex-hormone–binding globulin and, consequently, lower total testosterone levels compared with healthy-weight peers. In addition, obesity can cause an increase in the aromatization of testosterone to estradiol, which can increase the rate of skeletal maturation and increase the risk of gynecomastia.[69] Although the role of obesity and sexual maturation is established in girls, the role of obesity and sexual maturation in boys is less clear. Biro et al[54] found that, in a population-based cohort of 346 boys, the boys who had a greater fat mass as measured by the sum of skinfolds had less advanced sexual maturation by the age of 12 years, unlike what is seen in girls. Boys who had a higher BMI and greater adiposity reached a maturation stage at an older age. In a longitudinal, population-based study, Lee et al reported that a higher BMI *z*-score trajectory during early to middle childhood may be associated with later onset of puberty among boys.[70] These findings suggest that greater body fat mass is not linked to an earlier onset of puberty among boys. However, not all research supports this finding. De Leonibus et al[71] suggested that obesity in males may result in an earlier onset and completion of puberty in boys. More research is needed to determine the role of obesity and excess fatness on pubertal timing in males.

It is important to note that, in both girls and boys with obesity, the level of sex-hormone–binding globulin decreases, which is an independent risk factor for type 2 diabetes. Even in youth who are normal weight, a physiological insulin resistance appears at approximately Tanner stage 2. It is important for sports RDNs to assist with healthy eating patterns, encourage sustained physical activity, and focus on disease prevention for youth in sport.[72]

Normal Psychological Development

The transition from childhood to adolescence also marks a period of psychosocial development. This chapter does not examine this development in depth, but the sports RDN should recognize the hallmarks of this transition because they can impact the nutrition care process. The 3 major areas of psychological development for the adolescent include cognition, psychosocial relationships, and emotional development.[73]

The transition from concrete to abstract thinking is a normal developmental task of adolescence. Younger children often think in a concrete manner. Concrete thinkers rely on what they see or objects that are physically present and struggle with the extrapolation from a known item to an unknown. The world exists as good or bad and right or wrong; concrete thinkers struggle with shades of gray. As a simple example, consider a sports RDN counseling a young individual on reducing their intake of sugar-sweetened beverages to achieve an improved nutritional status. If the sports RDN counsels a concrete thinker on reducing lemonade consumption, they may see the concrete thinker reduce their intake of only this specific beverage. Reducing consumption of a single beverage is what was heard, and the inability to think abstractly may limit how the child comprehends the recommendation. Often, the perceived noncompliance is a failure of the provider to use developmentally appropriate language. Nutrition education for the concrete thinker needs to be precise and succinct, with clear instructions. Nutrition concepts should be prescriptive and have limited choices. Youths who remain concrete thinkers in high school may be frustrated with higher-functioning abstract concepts, such as advanced mathematics or too many choices in meal planning.[74]

Abstract thinking implies the ability to imagine things not yet experienced. Adolescents who can think abstractly can speculate about all possibilities, not just the known. Abstract thinkers may want to understand the "why" and may require more time and effort in a counseling session.[73] The emergence of abstract thinking allows the adolescent to develop more comprehensive thought, possibly through the development of the personal fable or the imaginary audience. This concept is based on the belief that an imaginary audience, often peers, is always watching or thinking about the individual. Also viewed as adolescent egocentrism, the concept of the personal fable may contribute to the belief that they are invincible. This belief can predispose the adolescent to increased risk-taking behavior because they believe that consequences only happen to others, not to them.[75] Among athletes, this can translate into use of anabolic steroids, abuse of diet pills for weight loss, and drinking and driving. In addition, the adolescent brain appears more sensitive to reward, including sweet substances, during early adolescence. This enhanced reward sensitivity in adolescence may increase the likelihood of succumbing to the rewarding properties of drugs and alcohol at this stage of life.[74,76]

The psychosocial development of normal adolescence includes identity formation and autonomy. Erickson postulated that identity formation is an essential developmental task of adolescence.[76] *Identity* is defined as who the adolescent is, separate and apart from the family of origin. Some risk-taking is central to the formation of an identity. During this critical stage of development, teens may experiment with dietary trends, lifestyles, and mannerisms. An identity related to sports is often formed during this phase. Jessor suggested that appropriate risk-taking can serve as a key social and personal determinant of self-confidence.[77] This developmental task progresses through adolescence, and in early adolescence (age 12–14 years) it is characterized by forming same-sex peer groups with less interest in family activities and parental guidance. During middle adolescence (age 15–17 years), the peer group becomes mixed and becomes the primary social group for the teen; family conflict can escalate. Sports RDNs may be valuable educators at this time, as the adolescent still seeks guidance from responsible adults other than their parents. In late adolescence (age 18–21 years), separation from the family of origin has developed. Conflict with family may decline. Additionally, during this phase, the sports RDN should consider interviewing older teens separate from their parents.

EXERCISE PHYSIOLOGY IN CHILDREN AND TEENS

Nutritional requirements for athletes are determined based on the type, intensity, and duration of the sport as well as the athlete's stage of physiological development. Most nutrition guidelines set for adults use well-established concepts of exercise physiology. However, growth, development, and pubertal status can influence muscular function and fuel utilization. The surge in the hormones associated with puberty (growth hormone, insulin-like growth factor, catecholamines, and sex steroid hormones) may indeed affect nutritional requirements. For ethical reasons, limited studies exist outlining the physiological differences among children, adolescents, and adults. Sports RDNs should use adult guidelines for calculating nutrient needs when the athlete reaches Tanner stage 5.

Children and young adolescents have limited endogenous carbohydrate stores. Glycogen storage capacity and the response to diets of different macronutrient distributions have not been studied extensively in children and adolescents because of the invasive nature of intervention studies. The regulation of glucose metabolism is mediated in part through insulin metabolism. Puberty is considered an insulin-resistant state secondary to a rise in growth hormone and sex steroid hormones.[78] Prepubertal children have insulin responses similar to those of adults. However, during Tanner stages 2 through 4, insulin sensitivity can be reduced by 30%. Metabolic flexibility, or the ability to efficiently adapt to substrate availability, is impaired during exercise in children who are obese. A 2021 study by Chu et al[79] found that the ability to oxidize oral carbohydrate was reduced by more than 23% in children who were obese compared to controls. More research is needed to assess the impact of a reduced ability to oxidize carbohydrate on body fat accumulation and exercise tolerance in children who are obese.

Although conflicting reports on substrate metabolism between children and adults exist, the majority of research studies indicate that children exhibit higher fat oxidation than adults.[80] Therefore, children are biologically equipped for sustained aerobic activity as opposed to anaerobic sports based on maturation landmarks. One study of five 11-year-old boys found that their phosphofructokinase (glycolytic) activity was approximately 40% of reported adult values.[81] In an additional study, Kaczor et al[82] reported that lactate dehydrogenase activity in skeletal muscle of 3- to 11-year-old children was only about 28% of the value determined for adults. Given the predominance of fat oxidation and the limited ability to store carbohydrate in childhood, as well as enzymatic immaturity, carbohydrate recommendations during exercise may be less than those for adults, although practical guidelines are lacking.[83]

It is unclear exactly when during adolescence the shift occurs favoring an adult metabolic pattern. This uncertainty may contribute to the conflicting study results in teens. In addition, less is known regarding the metabolic differences between girls and boys. Given the increase in lean mass, particularly in boys, it may be prudent to evaluate enzymatic activity based on fat-free mass (FFM).[84] A study by Stephens et al[85] suggested that the enhanced metabolism of fat appears to be dominant through midpuberty. In a conflicting study by Couto et al,[86] a higher-carbohydrate diet (70%) given to boys aged 13 through 18 years resulted in an improved overall performance compared to a low-carbohydrate diet (25%); the performance included a 400-m end-of-race sprint. This may be due to maturational changes or the impact of training on glucose disposal. There may also have been a difference in training as a result of the altered diets. Although there appears to be some difference between adolescents and adults, international experts have suggested that the carbohydrate needs of teens can be calculated using adult guidelines based on the intensity and duration of their sports.[87]

THERMOREGULATION AND FLUID REQUIREMENTS

The belief that children and adolescents are physiologically impaired in regulating temperature compared with adults has been challenged by more recent science. The capacity of young individuals to deal with thermal loads and exercise tolerance time in the heat appears to be similar to that of adults, although the physiological modes of action differ. Children have higher levels of relative evaporative cooling and sweating efficiency, thus yielding lower mass-dependent heat storage.[88] Therefore, the current perspective is that adequately hydrated youth athletes are not at a thermoregulatory disadvantage compared with similarly fit, hydrated, and acclimatized adults during exercise in the heat.[89]

Although children and teens can tolerate thermal loads in a similar fashion as adults, there are pubertal-related differences in the dissipation of heat loads. Children and teens rely less on sweating to promote thermal equilibrium and more on blood flow redistribution, with heat dissipation occurring through radiative and conductive cooling. Children rely more on dry heat dissipation by their larger relative skin surface areas than on evaporative heat loss, which controls thermoregulation in adults. With training, children and teens become more efficient at peripheral vasodilation as opposed to exhibiting alterations in sweat rate.[90] In essence, this means a lower sweat rate and accompanying lower sodium losses.

The link between dehydration and athletic performance in children is limited. In adults, dehydration levels of 2% to 7% can cause a decrement of performance in distance events lasting more than an hour. Wilk et al[91] found that dehydration levels of 1% negatively affected endurance performance in 10- to 12-year-old boys. As with other maturational landmarks, the transition from radiant cooling to evaporative cooling is driven by puberty, and this transition appears to be complete by the end of puberty, at about Tanner stage 5.[90]

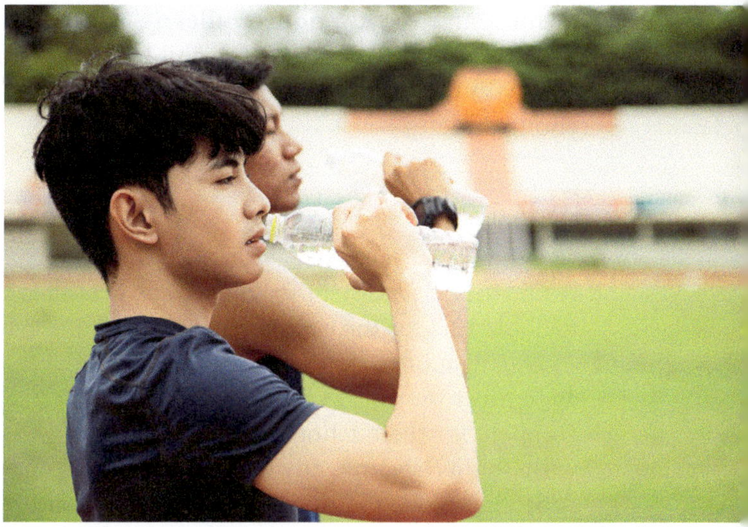

Fluid replacement guidelines for children can be calculated on the basis of body weight as an hourly fluid intake of 13 mL/kg (6 mL/lb). Postexercise rehydration requirements have been estimated at 4 mL per kilogram of body weight (2 mL per pound of body weight) for each hour of exercise to avoid initiating subsequent exercise in a dehydrated state.[92] Alternatively, the policy statement from the American Academy of Pediatrics (AAP) on climatic heat stress and the exercising child and adolescent suggests the intake of 100 to 250 mL every 20 minutes for 9- to 12-year-olds and 1 to 1.5 L/h for 13- to 18-year-olds, assuming adequate hydration status prior to activity.[93] The guidelines for preventing dehydration in children and adolescence are similar to those for adults. This includes beginning exercise well-hydrated, developing individualized drinking plans using pediatric sweat rate guidelines, limiting body mass losses during activity to 2% or less from preexercise values, and avoiding weight gain through overdrinking.

Preexisting illness, along with fitness level, may predispose children and adolescents to heat-related illnesses. Chronic illnesses such as diabetes insipidus, poorly controlled type 1 and type 2 diabetes, obesity, cystic fibrosis, febrile illnesses, and Graves disease are examples of illnesses that may alter fluid balance.[94-96] In addition, a recent bout of a gastrointestinal illness is a risk factor for dehydration if fluid balance is not corrected before initiation of activity.

The cause of heat-related illness in children and adolescents may be due not to impaired thermoregulatory response but rather to compromised preactivity hydration status.[97] Researchers have estimated that approximately 75% of children do not consume adequate amounts of water and more than 54% are dehydrated based on urine osmolality as a measure of hydration.[98] Young children may have less access to fluid during a school day than a teen who can drink during class changes. Other barriers to hydration can include clean and organized toilet facilities, lack of promotion of water intake in the classroom, and fear of bullying in the restroom.[99] Alcohol and some dietary supplements may also increase this risk and should be included in the assessment. The sports RDN should assess young athletes for preexisting chronic illness, school polices on drinking in class, and medication use as risk factors for dehydration. Education should focus on drinking hallmarks, such as consuming water when waking up and drinking water with meals and during class changes at school.

In practical terms, although children and teens are not at a unique metabolic disadvantage, the level of coaching and training in the pediatric population compared to older populations may increase the risk of a heat-related illness. In addition, many youth sports are supervised by parents, and a qualified professional may not be available to provide on-field guidance on fluid intake and supervision. Sports RDNs can educate teams, parent groups, booster clubs, and inexperienced coaches at the middle school and high school levels on evidence-based guidelines for proper hydration.[100] Assessment of hydration in children should focus on the use of urine color charts that have been validated in a pediatric population.[101]

As with adults, consideration of the type of beverage consumed is important. According to the American College of Sports Medicine (ACSM) guidelines, as well as the policy statement from the AAP, the use of a sports drink may be indicated for exercise longer than 1 hour to promote adequate fluid consumption and rehydration.[93,102] If exercise lasts longer than 1 hour in the heat, a sports drink provides the necessary electrolytes, carbohydrates, and fluid. Water is recommended for exercise lasting less than 1 hour. Children and teens should be educated on the proper use of sports drinks and avoid consumption during meals when either low-fat milk or water is the preferable option. A beverage hydration index has been developed to provide insight into the best beverages to promote rehydration.[103] Although not tested in a pediatric population, full-fat milk, skim milk, orange juice, and oral rehydration solutions were found to provide the best retention of fluid and rehydration profiles in an adult population. Milk and orange juice are valuable, cost-effective nutrition options for children and teens that also provide specific nutrients at risk for deficiency in this population (including calcium, vitamin D, and potassium) and promote rehydration for young athletes.

NUTRITION ASSESSMENT AND NUTRIENT NEEDS

A nutrition assessment for the pediatric athlete should be comprehensive and age and sex specific. Refer to Table 12.2 for the estimated energy requirement equations for children and adolescents.

During adolescence, energy needs are increased to promote normal growth and development, as well as to meet the energy demands of sports participation. In middle school and high school, athletes may compete for their school and participate in club sports outside of school. Given the inherent challenges with Tanner staging, any energy calculation for an adolescent athlete should be considered an estimate. Although group estimates of energy expenditure in adolescent athletes have been reported (ie, ~3,640 ± 830 kcal/d for males and ~3,100 ± 720 kcal/d for females), defining the individual energy requirements of an adolescent athlete with accuracy is difficult, given the individual variation in growth trajectories.[104]

During midpuberty, the increase in sex steroids enhances the ability to add lean mass. For young athletes, the accrual of lean mass through puberty and strength and conditioning increases overall energy needs. The ACSM and the Academy of Nutrition and Dietetics position paper recommend the prediction equations developed by Cunningham and by Harris and Benedict for estimating resting metabolic rate (RMR) in athletes.[105,106] The Cunningham prediction model incorporates FFM and differences in body composition between athletes and nonathletes. In contrast, the Harris-Benedict prediction equations do not include FFM but instead include total body weight and sex. Given the higher percentages of lean weight of most athletes, an equation that includes FFM may be advantageous, but FFM may not be readily available. Research by Thompson et al[107] suggested that the Cunningham equation is highly accurate for endurance athletes. The Cunningham equation has also been validated in recreational athletes.[108] However, in heavily muscled athletes, it may underestimate energy needs.[109] If FFM is available, the Cunningham equation for calculating RMR is:

$$\text{RMR} = 500 + [22 \times \text{FFM (kg)}]$$

Refer to Chapter 10 for sex-specific Cunningham equations.

Recent research suggests that adult prediction equations can underestimate energy expenditure in adolescent athletes by up to 300 kcal per day. A new prediction equation has been developed from a cohort (N = 126) of male and female adolescent athletes participating in a variety of sports. The mean age was 16.5 years, and the RMR was measured by indirect calorimetry. The predictive equation developed from indirect calorimetry assessment is[110]:

$$\text{RMR (kcal/d)} = 11.1 \times \text{body mass (kg)} + 8.4 \times \text{height (cm)} - [340\ \text{(male) or } 537\ \text{(female)}]$$

Researchers have also studied estimates for additional needs for growth and development. For example, Torun[111] estimated the caloric burden for synthesizing new tissue in well-nourished children and teens at 2 kcal/g of daily weight gain, although there is no practical way to assess this value. The calorie burden for growth and development is small but not irrelevant. However, the demands of training and competition have the greatest impact on overall energy needs beyond resting energy expenditure.

Low Energy Availability

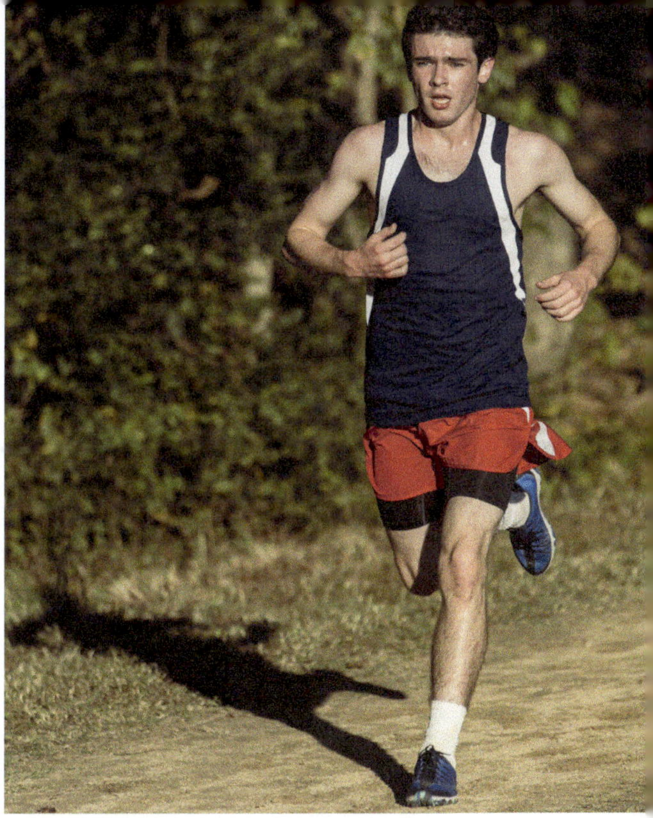

More recently, the concept of energy availability has emerged as a strategy for estimating energy needs and identifying energy deficits. Although any athlete can be at risk of low energy availability (LEA), athletes competing in high-training-volume sports; weight-class sports; or sports and activities that promote a low body weight such as ballet, dance, and figure skating are at particular risk.[112] A study of female athletes and performing artists indicated that approximately 75% of all female athletes exhibited LEA and were at increased risk of eating disorders.[113]

Energy availability is defined as dietary intake minus exercise energy expenditure using kilograms of FFM and is the amount of energy available to the body to perform all other functions after the cost of exercise is subtracted. The concept was first studied in females as part of the female athlete triad, where an energy availability of 45 kcal per kilogram of FFM per day was found to be associated with energy intake for optimal health and performance. Inadequate energy availability is considered to be a chronic reduction in energy availability below 30 kcal per kilogram of FFM per day and is associated with a loss or impairment of physiological function.[114] Chronic energy deficiency is often not reliably indicated by low body weight, and energy balance cannot be assumed by stable body weight.[115] Most of the research on LEA has focused on female athletes. A 2021 consensus paper highlighted the prevalence of and the differences in the female and male athlete triads. The definition of LEA in males is unclear but is often given as an intake of less than 15 kcal/kg of FFM. At this level of intake, there is a compensatory reduction of leptin and insulin. In addition, there appears to be a drive for muscularity and leanness in males, indicating that disordered eating patterns may manifest differently in females vs males.[116]

An additional factor to consider when using energy prediction equations is the role of growth and development. The Harris-Benedict equation has been used to predict resting energy expenditure (REE) in adult females who are underweight.[117-119] A reduced ratio of REE value measured to that predicted by the Harris-Benedict equation is often in the range of 60% to 80% in clinical models of starvation, such as anorexia nervosa. Less is known about the impact of the underfueled child athlete. The construct of energy availability has limited validity in childhood, and as such, clear guidelines on the use of this calculation in pediatric practice are lacking.

A 2019 study showed that decreased training and endurance response, decreased coordination, impaired judgment and concentration, irritability, and depression were demonstrated in adolescent and young adult female athletes (n = 1,000, mean age = 18.9 years), with self-reported LEA compared to those with adequate energy availability.[115] Emerging data suggest links between reduced performance and adaptation to training and the presence of menstrual irregularity and amenorrhea when compared to eumenorrheic peers. Lack of training adaptation may be an educational tool for the young athlete to understand the significance of amenorrhea.[119]

Physiological alterations at the metabolic level in underfueled athletes include decreased REE; suppressed triiodothyronine (T_3), insulin-like growth factor-1, and leptin concentrations; and elevated reverse T_3, ghrelin, peptide YY, and cortisol concentrations.[120-123] The underfueled athlete will often experience a downregulation of metabolic rate to compensate for chronic reduction in energy. In a clinical setting, the downregulation of metabolic rate can be manifested by bradycardia, hypothermia, and postural orthostatic tachycardia syndrome (POTS). Therefore, sports RDNs should regularly consider body temperature (<97°), heart rate (<50 bpm), and orthostatic dizziness as part of their assessment. Gastroparesis is also common and can alter normal hunger and satiety cues; the concept of intuitive eating may be flawed in athletes. Sports RDNs can use these surrogate measures of body temperature, heart rate, and POTS to objectively assess or augment the determination of energy availability when FFM data are not available. Box 12.3 on page 292 outlines considerations included in the assessment of an adolescent athlete.

BOX 12.3 Nutrition Assessment Checklist: Adolescent Athlete

Ask questions to determine if the athlete is a concrete or abstract thinker

- Dictates education style

Assess body composition

- Changes dependent on Tanner stage
- Percent body fat

Look for signs of acanthosis nigricans

- Indicative of insulin resistance
- Assess menstrual status, as amenorrhea may be present

Assess consumption of sugar-sweetened beverages (including sports drinks)

- Coffee drinks
- Energy drinks
- Inappropriate use of sports drinks

Assess daily eating pattern

- Is breakfast consumed daily?
- Snacks—frequency, what type of items?
- Fast-food consumption

Ask about enjoyment of sports

- Overtraining
- Monopolizes all free time

Ask about age of menarche

- Mother's age of menarche
- Inquire about alcohol use
- Consider interviewing adolescent alone

Inquire about supplement use

- Late-developing males at higher risk
- Team sports indicate higher risk

Dietary Assessment

The dietary assessment of an athlete's energy intake can be derived from weighed or measured food records (typically measuring intake for 3 to 7 days), 24-hour recalls, or food frequency questionnaires. An inherent challenge in the pediatric population is the poor historical recalls of children and adolescents. Parents should be part of the interview process with children. Children may need 6 to 9 24-hour recalls to establish recall reliability, and teens may require 3 to 6 recalls.[124] Given the limited amount of time in a clinical sports nutrition practice, dietary recalls may provide insight on food patterning but not necessarily energy intake. Athletes often consume sports nutrition foods, energy drinks, and sports drinks during practice, and the amount they consume is difficult to estimate. It is not surprising that adolescent athletes report intakes lower than those suggested by calculations.[125] Digital dietary histories may prove particularly useful in a younger athlete population.[126]

As with all populations, the pediatric population has unique vitamin and mineral needs. RDNs are well equipped to assess and screen for nutrient deficiencies. Nutrients of concern identified in the pediatric population include vitamin D, calcium, iron, potassium, and dietary fiber. Inadequate intakes of calcium, potassium, and dietary fiber can be alleviated by including dairy foods, vegetables, fruits, and whole grains.[127] However, given the limited food sources of vitamin D, this can be an especially vulnerable nutrient.

Alcohol may also be a source of calories for children and adolescents and is rarely assessed in an underage population. Not surprisingly, high school is a time when drinking rates increase sharply, given the propensity for risk-taking behaviors. In 2021, 23% of high school students reported current alcohol use, 47% reported use at some point in their lives, and 10.5% reported current episodes of binge drinking (drinking 5 or more drinks on 1 occasion for males or 4 or more drinks on 1 occasion for females). Females reported a higher prevalence of current and lifetime alcohol use than males. Current alcohol use was highest in students who identified as White (25.9%), followed by those identifying as Hispanic (22.9%) and Black (13.2%).[128] In studies of adolescent athletes, approximately 24% reported binge drinking.[129] Athletes involved in team sports are more likely to abuse alcohol than those in individual sports.[130]

Adolescents who use alcohol are also at risk for abusing anabolic steroids.[131,132] Teens who abuse anabolic steroids are more likely to experience polysubstance abuse.[133] Sports RDNs should routinely screen for alcohol use or abuse and consider it a risk factor for abuse of other illicit substances. Nutritional status, particularly related to B vitamins, magnesium, and other trace minerals, can be compromised by excessive alcohol intake.

PROTEIN NEEDS IN THE CHILD AND ADOLESCENT ATHLETE

A key component in the evaluation of protein needs in adolescents is the assumption of caloric adequacy. The consumption of inadequate calories allows for the production of energy from noncarbohydrate precursors, such as protein, via gluconeogenesis. All estimates of protein requirements are predicated on adequate energy balance. In addition to determining how to meet the demands of often-intensive training regimens, estimates of protein needs in the adolescent athletic population must account for increased needs for growth and development.[134] Nitrogen balance studies conducted in select adolescent athletes indicated that positive nitrogen balance is achieved with a protein intake ranging between 1.35 and 1.6 g of protein per kilogram per day.[135,136] Dietary intake patterns have shown that the protein intake of adolescent male athletes is about 1.5 g/kg/d. Among all adolescents, protein intake as a percentage of calories has increased in all ethnic groups with the exception of African American adolescents. From 1999 to 2000 and from 2009 to 2010, protein intake as a percentage of calories increased from 13.5% to 14.7% in boys and from 13.4% to 14.3% in girls.[137] Experts know little about the protein needs of female adolescent athletes. Given the research restrictions in the pediatric population, the physiology of protein metabolism and synthesis comes from data on the adult population.

Participation in sports, particularly team sports, may improve nutritional status, eating patterns, and nutrient intakes in teens, including overall protein intake.[138] Although overall protein intake is important, RDNs should also consider protein distribution patterns. Many high school athletes struggle with protein at breakfast, and the consumption of protein equally spaced throughout the day may be an additional predictor of adequate muscle protein synthesis.[139] This conclusion is further supported by RDN-observed fueling before, during, and after sports. Male dietary patterns often closely mimic the dietary recommendations, whereas females are less likely to meet the recommendations. Both boys and girls often fall short of carbohydrate needs.[140]

Protein status may be compromised in adolescents following restrictive diets, dietary fads, or inappropriately planned vegetarian diets. The EPIC-Oxford study highlighted the nutritional benefits and risks of a plant-based diet, identifying nutrients at risk of low intakes. Although parents may express concern regarding protein adequacy for the young athlete, the dietary components at risk include but are not limited to calcium, iron, iodine, long-chain omega-3 fatty acids, creatine, and vitamins D and B12.[141]

Sports RDNs are crucial in planning diets adequate in calories to ensure that protein is spared from being used as an energy source, protein consumption is spaced throughout the day, and fad diets are avoided by this vulnerable population. Lean sources of protein should be stressed to limit animal-based saturated fat.

DIETARY FAT IN THE CHILD AND ADOLESCENT ATHLETE

Quality sources of dietary fat can serve as valuable energy sources in children and adolescents struggling with energy adequacy. Often an athlete who is underweight is encouraged to consume high-fat fried foods or foods of poor nutrient density to gain weight. Dietary habits are formed and preferences are developed in childhood and adolescence; therefore, it is imperative to provide guidance on the appropriate food sources of dietary fat. High-fat diets, ketogenic diets, and low carbohydrate availability are concepts that have not been studied in the healthy pediatric population. Data from the HELENA study suggest that as dietary fat increases, there is an increase in truncal fat, regardless of the level of physical activity in adolescents.[142] The research on the role of dietary fat and adiposity in children is contradictory. Ambrosini et al[143] demonstrated a relationship between increasing dietary fat and total body fatness. However, a large study of Australian children suggested no relationship between macronutrient percentages and BMI.[144] The role of fat and adiposity in adolescent athletes is unclear, but RDNs should be careful not to promote high-fat diets, especially those that include food sources of *trans* and saturated fats. Researchers have also not yet determined whether all fatty acids stimulate the same physiological response.

Although fats can be a valuable source of energy, promoting the optimal type and amount of fat is important. In a study by Bachman et al,[145] major sources of dietary fats in the United States included oils from potato chips, salad dressing, and nuts and seeds. Major contributors of solid fats were grain-based desserts, cheeses, and sausages for all Americans. Among children and adolescents, major contributors of solid fats included pizza, grain-based desserts, and whole milk. In addition, these sources of solid fat also serve as sources of added sugars. Solid fats and added sugars comprise 30% of the added calories in the diets of children and adolescents[146]; the recommendation from the *Dietary Guidelines for Americans, 2020–2025*, is for less than 15% of total calories.[127] Sports RDNs should provide anticipatory guidance on reducing added solid fats and added sugars.

Dietary fat has a protein-sparing effect, provided that adequate energy is consumed. Additions of unsaturated oils in a variety of foods, such as nuts, nut butters, avocados, salad dressings, and mayonnaise can provide valuable calories. RDNs are in a position to provide helpful guidance on increasing dietary fats. Controlling the ratio of omega-6 to omega-3 fatty acids is also a central issue for optimal brain development. In an international review of fatty acid intake in children and adolescents, most children and teens worldwide exceeded the recommended limits for saturated fat and fell short of the recommended intake of polyunsaturated fatty acids (PUFAs).[147] The mean consumption of intakes of total eicosapentaenoic acid (EPA) and docosahexaenoic acid (DHA) varied between 45 and 150 mg in children and between 40 and 160 mg in adolescents. Given the suboptimal intake in children and adolescents, supplementation may be indicated.

The brain continues to grow postnatally, and myelinogenesis remains incomplete until early adulthood. The role of DHA in brain development and cognitive function is well established. The composition of the brain is about 60% fat, making it one of the highest-fat organs in the body. The majority of the fats are polyunsaturated: EPA, DHA, and arachidonic acid.[148] DHA is the dominant long-chain omega-3 PUFA in the brain and has been shown to accumulate in areas of the brain associated with learning and memory, such as the cerebral cortex and hippocampus.[149,150] The fatty acid content of the brain is dietary dependent; the phospholipids in the brain can be modified by diet.[151] Given the central role of long-chain fats, omega-3 fatty acids deserve special attention in pediatrics. Research has shown that DHA improves cognition, learning, memory, and school performance.[152] Given the limited food sources of DHA, children and teens who do not consume cold-water fish will most likely not meet target guidelines.[153] Research by Ritz et al[154] demonstrated that omega-3 intake by National Collegiate Athletic Association Division I athletes across 21 sports was low. The omega-3 status of these athletes was assessed by the objective measure, the omega-3 index (O3i). This index represents the sum of EPA + DHA as a percentage of the total fatty acid in erythrocyte cell membranes. In this cohort, the average O3i was 4.33%. Although an optimum percentage has not been defined, 8% is associated with the lowest risk of cardiovascular disease. The implications of this study are important for sports RDNs who design training tables. Planning more meals containing cold-water fish with a minimum of 2 per week may increase the omega-3 levels in the blood. The use of the O3i in adolescents also demonstrated that a higher O3i is predictive of a healthier eating pattern and reduced cardiovascular risk.[155]

A survey of adolescents' knowledge regarding omega-3 fatty acids demonstrated that teens could recognize the role of omega-3 fatty acids in heart health but lack knowledge on the roles of these long-chain PUFAs in brain, cognitive function, or athletic performance. Additionally, most teens (79%) were not educated by their health care providers on the roles of omega-3 fatty acids.[156] RDNs can provide valuable education on this important dietary fat and should plan diets with optimal health in mind. Supplementation with omega-3 fatty acids (EPA and DHA) should be considered to optimize their beneficial effects on health and athletic performance and recovery. Box 12.4 lists the age-specific recommended Adequate Intake of omega-3 fatty acids.[157]

VITAMIN D

Vitamin D deficiency continues to be a global nutritional issue. An analysis of data from the 2015–2016 National Health and Nutrition Examination Survey (NHANES) found that average daily vitamin D intakes from foods and beverages were 5.1 mcg (204 IU) in adult males, 4.2 mcg (168 IU) in adult females, and 4.9 mcg (196 IU) in children aged 2 to 19 years. In

BOX 12.4 Recommended Adequate Intake of Omega-3 Fatty Acids for Children and Adolescents[157]

4 to 8 years: 0.9 g/d

9 to 13 years (boys): 1.2 g/d

9 to 13 years (girls): 1.0 g/d

14 to 18 years (boys): 1.6 g/d

14 to 18 years (girls): 1.1 g/d

addition, NHANES data from 2013 through 2016 showed that 92% of adult males, more than 97% of adult females, and 94% of people aged 1 year and older ingested less than the estimated average requirement of 10 mcg (400 IU) of vitamin D from food and beverages.[158] Using the Institute of Medicine criteria with the end point of fracture, approximately 10.3% of US children aged 6 to 18 years (among an estimated population of 5.5 million) have 25-hydroxyvitamin D [25(OH)D] levels of less than 16 ng/mL, based on NHANES data.[159] Although there may be controversy in the literature on optimum levels, the Institute of Medicine, the AAP, and the Pediatric Endocrine Society define the parameters for 25-hydroxyvitamin D adequacy as follows[159,160]:

» Sufficient: more than 20 ng/mL
» Insufficient: 15 to 20 ng/mL
» Deficient: less than 15 ng/mL

However, other studies, most notably from the orthopedic literature on adults, suggest the following parameters for vitamin 25(OH)D[161,162]:

» Sufficient: 32 ng/mL or greater
» Insufficient: 20 to 32 ng/mL
» Deficient: less than 20 ng/mL

These values are based on cutoffs believed to optimize intestinal calcium absorption and prevent hyperparathyroidism. The role of vitamin D in bone mineral accrual is well established and beyond the scope of this chapter. Bone formation peaks during puberty, and the establishment of adequate bone density in childhood is critical for long-term bone health throughout adulthood. Pubertal girls with hypovitaminosis D seem to be at risk of not reaching maximum peak bone mass, particularly at the lumbar spine. Maintaining vitamin D blood levels at or above 20 ng/mL throughout the entire year may be needed to improve the bone markers in adolescents.[163,164]

Vitamin D is most closely aligned with bone health; however, the presence of vitamin D receptors throughout the body suggests an extraskeletal role for vitamin D. Research investigating the relationship between vitamin D deficiency and muscular status in the pediatric population is sparse. Ward et al assessed serum 25(OH)D levels in girls aged 12 to 14 years and measured muscle power. Vitamin D levels were significantly associated with muscle power and force in adolescent girls.[165] Inadequate vitamin D status may result in fatigue and diminished muscle oxygenation, consequently negatively affecting muscle strength and causing weakness.[166] Sport performance criteria, such as higher jump velocities and jump heights, are significantly improved with adequate levels of vitamin D.[167] Muscle biopsies from adult athletes with low vitamin D levels have demonstrated atrophic changes in fast-twitch type II muscle fibers, which are crucial to most athletes.[168] However, the supplementation of adolescents with vitamin D in a randomized controlled trial indicated that, despite improvements in 25-hydroxyvitamin D status, treatment with vitamin D was not shown to increase bone mineral accretion, bone geometry or strength, muscle force, or power. Improvements were found in jump velocity in girls with the lowest baseline 25-hydroxyvitamin D concentrations.[165]

Vitamin D deficiency may also increase the risk of injury and infection. Adolescent athletes with low vitamin D levels have been shown to have an increased risk of injury.[169] Heavy training can also increase the risk of upper respiratory infection. Research by He et al[170] on a study population of healthy male athletes demonstrated that supplementation with 5,000 IU of vitamin D per day increased the participants' saliva levels of antimicrobial peptides, which can reduce the risk of viral illnesses.

Accumulating data suggest that a deficiency of vitamin D may also contribute to iron deficiency anemia. One reason for this association is the pro-inflammatory effect of a vitamin D deficit, which eventually leads to an increase in hepcidin production via stimulation of pro-inflammatory cytokines. This anti-inflammatory effect of vitamin D has been confirmed by studies pointing to the reduction in hepcidin levels and increase in 25-hydroxyvitamin D concentration in vitamin D–deficient athletes when supplementation was provided.[171] Research by Sim et al[172] established the link between vitamin D deficiency and increased prevalence of anemia in adults, likely due to the role of vitamin D in erythropoiesis. Atkinson et al[173] demonstrated that, among White children, 25-hydroxyvitamin D levels in the upper quartiles (≥20 ng/mL) were associated with a nearly 0.2 g/dL higher hemoglobin concentration compared with those less than 20 ng/mL. In African American children, hemoglobin was higher among those with 25-hydroxyvitamin D levels greater than 11 ng/mL, highlighting ethnic differences.

CALCIUM

Calcium requirements are 1,000 mg/d for children (4–8 years) and 1,300 mg/d for preadolescents and adolescents (ages 9–13 and 14–18 years, respectively).[174] Although it is possible to meet these requirements through diet alone, the calcium intake of children and adults in the United States is generally lower than daily recommendations, especially for children aged 9 to 18 years and those who are Hispanic or African American.[175] The 2021 Youth Risk Behavior Surveillance System reported that 45.4% of high school girls and 26.4% of high school boys had not had milk in the past 7 days. Milk consumption decreased at the same time that soda intake increased. Over a period of 7 days, 64.9% of girls and 73% of boys had drunk regular soda.[176]

Adequate calcium is important for the development of peak bone mass in children and adolescents, especially during puberty. Inadequate calcium intake in adolescence may also increase the likelihood of bone disease in adults.[177] Approximately half of total body calcium is laid down during puberty in girls and up to two-thirds in boys by the end of puberty.[178,179] Although calcium-fortified foods are available, milk and milk products provide about 50% of total calcium intake within the United States and are the leading sources of dietary calcium for children aged 2 years and older. Plant-based milks have emerged on the market, and the majority, but not all, are calcium fortified. In contrast to the calcium naturally found in cow's milk, calcium must be added to plant-based milks and often precipitates out of solution. Smith et al[180] found that the shaking of plant-based milks improves the bioavailability of calcium. Specifically, unshaken almond and soy samples had 14% and 18% lower calcium contents than their well-mixed samples, whereas the unshaken rice and oat samples had 96% and 97% lower calcium contents than the well-mixed samples, respectively.

During pubertal growth, bone growth outpaces bone mineralization, which, in essence, decreases bone mineral deposition. A research study by Faulkner et al[181] demonstrated that the nadir of bone mineral density coincides with peak height velocity in both boys and girls. This also coincides with an increase in distal radius fractures during periods of rapid growth and development, suggesting that the relative lack of bone mineral density is clinically significant. In contrast to other biological processes where recovery is possible, the lack of calcium and poor bone mineralization during puberty may permanently impact bone development and increase the risk of osteoporosis in adulthood.[182] Recently, the role of the dietary fiber inulin has been shown to improve calcium absorption. Inulin has significant functions, such as improving calcium absorption through passive diffusion, expanding the absorption surface of the colon by stimulating cell growth, and promoting an increase in beneficial bacteria. The role of the gut microbiome in improving bone health is an area of expanding research.[183] RDNs should plan diets with a focus on adequate dietary sources of calcium, highlighting the importance of calcium bioavailability. Sources of dietary calcium are listed in Table 12.3.[184]

IRON

Iron needs during adolescence are increased primarily because of the rapid expansion of blood volume. Menarche also significantly impacts iron needs. Iron deficiency is the most prevalent mineral deficiency in the United States, affecting 9% to 16% of female adolescents.[185] In an athletic population, the documented prevalence is 15% to 35% of female athletes and 3% to 11% of male athletes.[186] In a study of German teens, the incidence of iron deficiency was found to be 10.9% in young male athletes and 35.9% in young female athletes.[187]

The causes of iron deficiency and subsequent anemia in young athletes are multifactorial and include increased needs, lack of dietary iron, coexistence of vitamin D deficiency, and such chronic illnesses as undiagnosed celiac disease or *Helicobacter pylori* infection. Among athletes, overuse of nonsteroidal anti-inflammatory drugs can also contribute to low iron status. Athletes participating in weight-class sports or sports emphasizing leanness are at increased risk as a result of low energy intake and, therefore, suboptimal iron intake. Athletes participating in endurance sports are presumed to have higher rates of iron turnover secondary to losses through sweat, gastrointestinal bleeding, hematuria, and hemolysis.[188,189]

In the American diet, the richest sources of heme iron (the most bioavailable form) include lean red meats and seafood. Dietary sources of nonheme iron include some vegetables, nuts, beans, and fortified grain products, including sports bars. The absorption of nonheme iron can be enhanced by the intake of vitamin C–rich foods and decreased with intake of tannins. Approximately half of dietary iron comes from fortified cereals, bread, and grain products. Poorly planned vegetarian or vegan diets can increase the risk of iron deficiency. Diets that eliminate breads, fortified grains, or cereals can also reduce the intake of nonheme iron.

TABLE 12.3 Calcium Content of Selected Foods[184]

Food	Serving size	Calcium content per serving (mg)
Almond milk, vanilla, sweetened	8 oz	451
Yogurt, plain, low fat	8 oz	415
Mozzarella, part skim	1.5 oz	333
Sardines, canned in oil, with bones	3 oz	325
Yogurt, fruit, low fat	8 oz	313-384
Cheddar cheese	1.5 oz	307
Milk, nonfat	8 oz	299
Soy milk, calcium fortified	8 oz	299
Milk, reduced fat (2% milk fat)	8 oz	293
Milk, buttermilk, low fat	8 oz	284
Milk, whole (3.25% milk fat)	8 oz	276
Orange juice, calcium fortified	6 oz	261
Tofu, firm, made with calcium sulfate	½ cup	253
Salmon, pink, canned, solids with bone	3 oz	181
Cottage cheese, 1% milk fat	1 cup	138
Tofu, soft, made with calcium sulfate	½ cup	138
Ready-to-eat cereal, calcium fortified	1 cup	100-1,000
Frozen yogurt, vanilla, soft serve	½ cup	103
Kale, raw, chopped	1 cup	100
Turnip greens, fresh, boiled	½ cup	99
Ice cream, vanilla	½ cup	84
Chinese cabbage, bok choy, raw, shredded	1 slice	74
Bread, white	1 slice	73
Pudding, chocolate, ready to eat, refrigerated	4 oz	55
Tortilla, corn, ready to bake/fry	1, 6-in diameter	46
Tortilla, flour, ready to bake/fry	1, 6-in diameter	32
Sour cream, reduced fat, cultured	2 Tbsp	31
Bread, whole wheat	1 slice	30
Broccoli, raw	½ cup	21
Cream cheese, regular	1 Tbsp	14

Undiagnosed chronic illnesses can contribute to iron deficiency. In cases of iron deficiency anemia that are refractory to treatment, celiac disease is diagnosed in 1.8% to 14.6% of patients.[188] *H pylori* is often an undiagnosed cause of iron deficiency. *H pylori* is more common in females. A study of female high school athletes found the prevalence of *H pylori* immunoglobulin G antibodies to be 14% and that of iron deficiency to be about 50%.[189]

The assessment of iron deficiency and iron deficiency anemia in pediatric practice are routinely done by measuring hemoglobin and hematocrit, and neither of these methods is sensitive or specific. The use of ferritin levels is not routine in general pediatrics. Female athletes may experience an elevated risk of iron deficiency and iron deficiency anemia and show declines in physical and cognitive performance.[190] In response to intense training, hepcidin, a peptide hormone that inhibits intestinal iron absorption and sequesters iron in macrophages, increases. The inflammatory response and the synthesis of proinflammatory cytokines, such as interleukin-6, act to stimulate hepcidin expression, in turn reducing iron absorption and sequestering iron in the macrophages. Ferritin levels may be reduced.[191] Hepcidin release may also be a marker of overreaching and overtraining.[192] Hepcidin is not routinely assessed in clinical practice. Sim et al[193] and others have developed a staged assessment of iron deficiency using commonly obtained serum measures as follows:

- Stage 1: Iron deficiency—iron stores in the bone marrow, liver, and spleen are depleted (ferritin < 35 mcg/L, hemoglobin > 115 g/L, transferrin saturation > 16%).
- Stage 2: Iron deficient nonanemia—erythropoiesis diminishes as the iron supply to the marrow is reduced (ferritin < 20 mcg/L, hemoglobin > 115 g/L, transferrin saturation < 16%).
- Stage 3: Iron deficiency anemia—hemoglobin levels decrease, resulting in frank anemia (ferritin < 12 mcg/L, hemoglobin < 115 g/L transferrin < 16%).

Athletes with iron deficiency can experience fatigue, decreased work capacity, immunosuppression, and depressed mood, as well as the inability to train appropriately and compete at a high level.[194] Table 12.4 lists dietary sources of iron.[184]

ERGOGENIC AIDS AND ADOLESCENT ATHLETES

Surveys indicate that dietary supplement use in 12- to 19-year-olds has increased in a linear fashion. In 2009–2010, NHANES data indicated that 22.1% of adolescents used a dietary supplement. This percentage increased to 29.7% by 2017–2018. The percentage of teens using 2 or more supplements also increased from 3.2% to 8.5%. The most common supplement was a multivitamin, followed by a single-vitamin preparation of vitamin D.[195]

Motivation for supplement use is dependent on age, sex, and sport. In a survey of preadolescent runners, researchers found that one-quarter of the athletes took dietary supplements. Females reporting a bone stress injury, following a vegetarian diet, or having a history of weight loss in the preceeding year were more likely to use supplements. Male runners were more likely to use creatine and sport foods, such as energy bars and sports drinks.[196] The nutritional supplementation practices of 32 national track and field athletes competing at the 2004 World Junior Championships were studied using an anonymous questionnaire. Approximately 62% of respondents reported using dietary supplements. Reasons for use included health, immune support, and improved performance. Although most athletes had access to a sports RDN, they reported that coaches (65%) were the most important source of supplementation education, followed by sports RDNs (30%) and doctors (25%) as other sources of information.[197]

The rates of use of ergogenic aid to enhance body composition have been reported to be as high as 58% among high school athletes.[198] A study by Dodge and Jaccard[199] found that, in the transition from adolescence to adulthood, young adult males who played a sport in high school were 15.6% more likely to use performance-enhancing supplements than their nonathletic peers. In addition, Eisenberg et al[200] reported that male high school athletes were more likely to try to increase muscle mass by changing their diets, increasing exercise, or using protein supplements than students who do not participate in sports. This time period thus provides an excellent opportunity for sports RDNs to educate clients on appropriate fueling strategies to achieve those goals within the limits of Tanner staging.

Research in the adult population has illustrated the effectiveness of dietary supplements to augment sports performance (for further discussion, refer to Chapter 7). Recently, the International Olympic

TABLE 12.4 Iron Content of Selected Foods[184]

Food	Serving size	Iron content per serving (mg)
Breakfast cereals, fortified with 100% of the daily value for iron	1 serving (size varies)	18
Oysters, eastern, cooked with moist heat	3 oz	8
White beans, canned	1 c	8
Chocolate, dark, 45%-69% cacao solids	3 oz	7
Beef liver, pan fried	3 oz	5
Lentils, boiled and drained	½ c	3
Spinach, boiled and drained	½ c	3
Tofu, firm	½ c	3
Kidney beans, canned	½ c	2
Sardines, Atlantic, canned in oil, drained solids with bones	3 oz	2
Chickpeas, boiled and drained	½ c	2
Tomatoes, canned, stewed	½ c	2
Beef, braised bottom round, trimmed to 1/8″ fat	3 oz	2
Potato, baked, flesh and skin	1 medium	2
Cashew nuts, oil roasted	1 oz (~18 nuts)	2
Green peas, boiled	½ c	1
Chicken, roasted, meat and skin	3 oz	1
Rice, white, long grain, enriched, parboiled, drained	½ c	1
Rice, brown, long, or medium grain, cooked	1 c	1
Bread, whole wheat	1 slice	1
Bread, white	1 slice	1
Raisins, seedless	¼ c	1
Spaghetti, whole wheat, cooked	1 c	1
Tuna, bluefin, fresh	3 oz	1
Turkey, roasted, breast meat and skin	3 oz	1
Nuts, pistachio, dry roasted	1 oz (~49 nuts)	1
Broccoli, boiled and drained	½ c	1
Egg, hard boiled	1 large	1

Committee outlined the evidence for dietary supplements for elite athletes. Although the focus was on adult athletes, this evidence on effectiveness can guide the sports RDN in working with children and adolescents.[201] Because of ethical constraints, less research is available in the pediatric population on the safety of these products.

Creatine is one of the most popular supplements used by teenagers. In 2019, Jovanov et al[202] surveyed 348 male and female adolescent athletes who were competing at an international level for their respective countries. The authors reported that 25.3% of these athletes indicated using creatine. In agreement with other studies, a significantly higher proportion of male athletes reported using creatine compared to female athletes. The ACSM and the AAP have stated that the evidence on potential side effects of creatine supplementation in people younger than 18 years is inadequate to formulate valid conclusions as to the risk-to-benefit ratio of creatine supplementation. Therefore, creatine supplementation is not advised for the pediatric population according to these organizations.[203,204] However, the safety and efficacy of creatine have been established in multiple studies. Creatine has been shown to improve exercise performance, enhance recovery, and improve the ability to tolerate heavy loads and training.[205] Nevertheless, sports RDNs, coaches, and athletes should note that professional organizations support establishing proper fueling strategies and physical activity before supplementation.

Evidence exists that the use of legal ergogenic aids may predict anabolic steroid use in young adults.[206] Sports RDNs should exercise caution in recommending sports-enhancing supplements in the pediatric population. Sports RDNs also play a critical role in educating student athletes, coaches, and parents on the potential for supplements to be contaminated with unknown and potentially banned substances.

SUMMARY

The popularity of youth sports is increasing, and sports RDNs should be well versed to provide culturally and developmentally appropriate nutritional care and education. The nutritional needs of the child and adolescent are based on sex, pubertal growth, and development. Tanner stages can guide the sports RDN in planning appropriate nutrition education based on the physiological and psychological needs of this population. A comprehensive nutrition assessment may reveal nutritional educational needs including about the roles of carbohydrate, protein, and fat in health and performance. Children and adolescents can be at risk for nutrient deficiencies in micronutrients that include calcium, iron, and vitamin D. Hydration strategies should also be addressed. Underfueling, or low energy availability, is a common concern and may be the result of food insecurity, a knowledge deficit, or the consequence of disordered eating or an eating disorder. Sports RDNs should exercise caution in recommending performance enhancing supplements and can play a key role in the education of athletes, parents, and coaches on the potential of adulterated and banned substances.

KEY TAKEAWAYS

The nutritional needs of the child and adolescent athlete are based on sex and stages of growth and development.

Tanner staging, or sexual maturity ratings, should guide the sports RDN in planning appropriate nutrition education.

Sports RDNs should assess developmental learning stages to determine the best education strategy.

When educating young athletes, sports RDNs should include key recommendations for carbohydrate, protein, fat, vitamin and mineral intake, and hydration goals.

Vitamin D, calcium, and iron are nutrients of concern in children and adolescents.

Sports RDNs should exercise caution in recommending performance-enhancing supplements to children and adolescent athletes.

REFERENCES

1. Mayol-Garcia Y. Girls take lessons, join clubs more often than boys but boys play more sports. United States Census Bureau. July 22, 2022. Accessed January 20, 2023. www.census.gov/library/stories/2022/07/children-continue-to-be-involved-in-extracurricular-activities.html
2. Project Play, Aspen Institute. Youth Sports Facts: Participation Rates. July 2023. Accessed January 15, 2024. https://projectplay.org/youth-sports/facts/participation-rates
3. National Federation of State High School Associations. 2021-2022 High School Athletics Participation Survey. 2022. Accessed January 15, 2024. www.nfhs.org/media/5989280/2021-22_participation_survey.pdf
4. Singh AS, Mulder C, Twisk JW, van Mechelen W, Chinapaw MJ. Tracking of childhood overweight into adulthood: a systematic review of the literature. *Obes Rev.* 2008;9(5):474-488. doi:10.1111/j.1467-789X.2008.00475.x
5. Mamun AA, Hayatbakhsh MR, O'Callaghan M, Williams G, Najman J. Early overweight and pubertal maturation—pathways of association with young adults' overweight: a longitudinal study. *Int Obes (Lond).* 2009;33(1):14-20. doi:10.1038/ijo.2008.220
6. Stigman S, Rintala P, Kukkonen-Harjula K, Kujala U, Rinne M, Fogelholm M. Eight-year-old children with high cardiorespiratory fitness have lower overall and abdominal fatness. *Int Pediatr Obes.* 2009;4(2):98-105. doi:10.1080/17477160802221101
7. Thackray AE, Barrett LA, Tolfrey K. Acute high-intensity interval running reduces postprandial lipemia in boys. *Med Sci Sports Exerc.* 2013;45(7):1277-1284. doi:10.1249/MSS.0b013e31828452c1
8. Eime RM, Young JA, Harvey JT, Charity MJ, Payne WR. A systematic review of the psychological and social benefits of participation in sport for adults: informing development of a conceptual model of health through sport. *Int Behav Nutr Phys Act.* 2013;10:135. doi:10.1186/1479-5868-10-135
9. Guddal MH, Stensland SØ, Småstuen MC, Johnsen MB, Zwart JA, Storheim K. Physical activity and sport participation among adolescents: associations with mental health in different age groups. Results from the Young-HUNT study: a cross-sectional survey. *BM Open.* 2019;9(9):e028555. doi:10.1136/bmjopen-2018-028555
10. Faigenbaum AD, Kraemer WJ, Blimkie CJ, et al. Youth resistance training: updated position statement paper from the National Strength and Conditioning Association. *Strength Cond Res.* 2009;23(5 suppl):S60-S79. doi:10.1519/JSC.0b013e31819df407
11. MacKelvie KJ, Petit MA, Khan KM, Beck TJ, McKay HA. Bone mass and structure are enhanced following a 2-year randomized controlled trial of exercise in prepubertal boys. *Bone.* 2004;34(4):755-764. doi:10.1016/j.bone.2003.12.017
12. Morris FL, Naughton GA, Gibbs JL, Carlson JS, Wark JD. Prospective ten-month exercise intervention in premenarcheal girls: positive effects on bone and lean mass. *Bone Miner Res.* 1997;12(9):1453-1462. doi:10.1359/jbmr.1997.12.9.1453
13. Specker B, Thiex NW, Sudhagoni RG. Does exercise influence pediatric bone? A systematic review. *Clin Orthop Relat Res.* 2015;473(11):3658-3672. doi:10.1007/s11999-015-4467-7
14. Hind K, Burrows M. Weight-bearing exercise and bone mineral accrual in children and adolescents: a review of controlled trials. *Bone.* 2007;40(1):14-27. doi:10.1016/j.bone.2006.07.006
15. Tveit M, Rosengren BE, Nilsson JÅ, Karlsson MK. Exercise in youth: high bone mass, large bone size, and low fracture risk in old age. *Scand Med Sci Sports.* 2015;25(4):453-461. doi:10.1111/sms.12305
16. Tenforde AS, Fredericson M. Influence of sports participation on bone health in the young athlete: a review of the literature. *PM R.* 2011;3(9):861-867. doi:10.1016/j.pmrj.2011.05.019
17. Hales CM, Fryar CD, Carroll MD, Freedman DS, Ogden CL. Trends in obesity and severe obesity prevalence in US youth and adults by sex and age, 2007-2008 to 2015-2016. *JAMA.* 2018;319(16):1723-1725. doi:10.1001/jama.2018.3060
18. Andes LJ, Cheng YJ, Rolka DB, Gregg EW, Imperatore G. Prevalence of prediabetes among adolescents and young adults in the United States, 2005-2016. *JAMA Pediatr.* 2020;174(2):e194498. doi:10.1001/jamapediatrics.2019.4498
19. Jensen ET, Dabelea D. Type 2 Diabetes in youth: new lessons from the SEARCH study. *Curr Diab Rep.* 2018;18(6):36. doi:10.1007/s11892-018-0997-1
20. Wittmeier KD, Wicklow BA, MacIntosh AC, et al. Hepatic steatosis and low cardiorespiratory fitness in youth with type 2 diabetes. *Obesity (Silver Spring).* 2012;20(5):1034-1040. doi:10.1038/oby.2011.379
21. Fabbrini E, Sullivan S, Klein S. Obesity and nonalcoholic fatty liver disease: biochemical, metabolic, and clinical implications. *Hepatology.* 2010;51(2):679-689. doi:10.1002/hep.23280
22. Garber CE, Blissmer B, Deschenes MR, et al; American College of Sports Medicine. American College of Sports Medicine position stand. Quantity and quality of exercise for developing and maintaining cardiorespiratory, musculoskeletal, and neuromotor fitness in apparently healthy adults: guidance for prescribing exercise. *Med Sci Sports Exerc.* 2011;43(7):1334-1359. doi:10.1249/MSS.0b013e318213fefb
23. Magnussen CG, Koskinen J, Chen W, et al. Pediatric metabolic syndrome predicts adulthood metabolic syndrome, subclinical atherosclerosis, and type 2 diabetes mellitus but is no better than body mass index alone: the Bogalusa Heart Study and the Cardiovascular Risk in Young Finns Study. *Circulation.* 2010;122(16):1604-1611. doi:10.1161/CIRCULATIONAHA.110.940809

24. Kang HS, Gutin B, Barbeau P, et al. Physical training improves insulin resistance syndrome markers in obese adolescents. *Med Sci Sports Exerc*. 2002;34(12):1920-1927. doi:10.1097/00005768-200212000-00010
25. Messiah SE, Arheart KL, Lipshultz SE, Miller TL. Body mass index, waist circumference, and cardiovascular risk factors in adolescents. *Pediatr.* 2008;153(6):845-850. doi:10.1016/j.jpeds.2008.06.013
26. Trasande L, Chatterjee S. The impact of obesity on health service utilization and costs in childhood. *Obesity (Silver Spring)*. 2009;17(9):1749-1754. doi:10.1038/oby.2009.67
27. Lange SJ, Kompaniyets L, Freedman DS, et al. Longitudinal trends in body mass index before and during the Covid-19 pandemic among persons aged 2-19 years — United States, 2018-2020. *MMWR Morb Mortal Wkly Rep*. 2021;70(37):1278-1283. doi:10.15585/mmwr.mm7037a3
28. Sattar N, Rawshani A, Franzén S, et al. Age at diagnosis of type 2 diabetes mellitus and associations with cardiovascular and mortality risks. *Circulation*. 2019;139(19):2228-2237. doi:10.1161/CIRCULATIONAHA.118.037885
29. Andersen LB, Sardinha LB, Froberg K, Riddoch CJ, Page AS, Anderssen SA. Fitness, fatness and clustering of cardiovascular risk factors in children from Denmark, Estonia and Portugal: the European Youth Heart Study. *Int Pediatr Obes*. 2008;3(suppl 1):58-66. doi:10.1080/17477160801896366
30. Marcus C, Danielsson P, Hagman E. Pediatric obesity—Long-term consequences and effect of weight loss. *Intern Med*. 2022;292(6):870-891. doi:10.1111/joim.13547
31. Abbott RA, Davies PS. Habitual physical activity and physical activity intensity: their relation to body composition in 5.0–10.5-y-old children. *Eur Clin Nutr.* 2004;58(2):285-291. doi:10.1038/sj.ejcn.1601780
32. Mesirow MS, Welsh JA. Changing beverage consumption patterns have resulted in fewer liquid calories in the diets of US children: National Health and Nutrition Examination Survey 2001-2010. *Acad Nutr Diet.* 2015;115(4):559-566.e4. doi:10.1016/j.jand.2014.09.004
33. Woodruff SJ, Hanning RM, Barr SI. Energy recommendations for normal weight, overweight and obese children and adolescents: are different equations necessary? *Obes Rev*. 2009;10(1):103-108. doi:10.1111/j.1467-789X.2008.00525.x
34. National Academies of Sciences, Engineering, and Medicine; Health and Medicine Division; Food and Nutrition Board; Committee on the Dietary Reference Intakes for Energy. *Dietary Reference Intakes for Energy*. National Academies Press; January 17, 2023. doi:10.17226/26818
35. Neumark-Sztainer D, Falkner N, Story M, Perry C, Hannan PJ, Mulert S. Weight-teasing among adolescents: correlations with weight status and disordered eating behaviors. *Int Obes Relat Metab Disord*. 2002;26(1):123-131. doi:10.1038/sj.ijo.0801853
36. Cheng S, Kaminga AC, Liu Q, et al. Association between weight status and bullying experiences among children and adolescents in schools: An updated meta-analysis. *Child Abuse Negl.* 2022;134:105833. doi:10.1016/j.chiabu.2022.105833
37. Goldschmidt AB, Wall MM, Loth KA, Neumark-Sztainer D. Risk factors for disordered eating in overweight adolescents and young adults. *Pediatr Psychol.* 2015;40(10):1048-1055. doi:10.1093/jpepsy/jsv053
38. Puhl RM, Peterson JL, Luedicke J. Weight-based victimization: bullying experiences of weight loss treatment-seeking youth. *Pediatrics*. 2013;131(1):e1-e9. doi:10.1542/peds.2012-1106
39. Puhl RM, Wall MM, Chen C, Bryn Austin S, Eisenberg ME, Neumark-Sztainer D. Experiences of weight teasing in adolescence and weight-related outcomes in adulthood: A 15-year longitudinal study. *Prev Med*. 2017;100:173-179. doi:10.1016/j.ypmed.2017.04.023doi:10.1542/peds.2012-1106
40. Gale CR, Cooper R, Craig L, et al. Cognitive function in childhood and lifetime cognitive change in relation to mental wellbeing in four cohorts of older people. *PLoS One*. 2012;7(9):e44860. doi:10.1371/journal.pone.0044860
41. Gottfredson LS, Deary IJ. Intelligence predicts health and longevity, but why? *Curr Dir Psychol Sci*. 2004;13(1):1-4. doi:10.1111/j.0963-7214.2004.01301001.x
42. Zarrett N, Fay K, Li Y, Carrano J, Phelps E, Lerner RM. More than child's play: variable- and pattern-centered approaches for examining effects of sports participation on youth development. *Dev Psychol.* 2009;45(2):368-382. doi:10.1037/a0014577
43. Oberle E, Ji XR, Kerai S, Guhn M, Schonert-Reichl KA, Gadermann AM. Screen time and extracurricular activities as risk and protective factors for mental health in adolescence: a population-level study. *Prev Med.* 2020;141:106291. doi:10.1016/j.ypmed.2020.106291
44. Jewett R, Sabiston CM, Brunet J, O'Loughlin EK, Scarapicchia T, O'Loughlin J. School sport participation during adolescence and mental health in early adulthood. *Adolesc Health*. 2014;55(5):640-644. doi:10.1016/j.jadohealth.2014.04.018
45. Dishman RK, Hales DP, Pfeiffer KA, et al. Physical self-concept and self-esteem mediate cross-sectional relations of physical activity and sport participation with depression symptoms among adolescent girls. *Health Psychol.* 2006;25(3):396-407. doi:10.1037/0278-6133.25.3.396
46. Pearce M, Garcia L, Abbas A, et al. Association between physical activity and risk of depression: a systematic review and meta-analysis. *JAMA Psychiatry.* 2022;79(6):550-559. doi:10.1001/jamapsychiatry.2022.0609
47. Pluhar E, McCracken C, Griffith KL, Christino MA, Sugimoto D, Meehan WP 3rd. Team sport athletes may be less likely to suffer anxiety or depression than individual sport athletes. *Sports Sci Med*. 2019;18(3):490-496. PMID: 31427871
48. Bergeron MF, Mountjoy M, Armstrong N, et al. International Olympic Committee consensus statement on youth athletic development. *Br Sports Med.* 2015;49(13):843-851. doi:10.1136/bjsports-2015-094962
49. DiFiori JP, Benjamin HJ, Brenner J, et al. Overuse injuries and burnout in youth sports: a position statement from the American Medical Society for Sports Medicine. *Clin Sport Med*. 2014;24(1):3-20. doi:10.1097/JSM.0000000000000060

50. Spear BA. Adolescent growth and development. *Am Diet Assoc.* 2002;102(3 suppl):S23-S29. doi:10.1016/s0002-8223(02)90418-9
51. Wilmore JH. The application of science to sport: physiological profiles of male and female athletes. *Can Appl Sport Sci.* 1979;4(2):103-115. PMID: 533623
52. Patel DR, Nelson TL. Sports injuries in adolescents. *Med Clin North Am.* 2000;84(4):983-1007, viii. doi:10.1016/s0025-7125(05)70270-4
53. Tanner JM. *Fetus Into Man: Physical Growth From Conception to Maturity.* Harvard University Press; 1989.
54. Biro FM, Khoury P, Morrison JA. Influence of obesity on timing of puberty. *Int Androl.* 2006;29(1):272-277; discussion 286-290. doi:10.1111/j.1365-2605.2005.00602.x
55. Wolff MS, Teitelbaum SL, Pinney SM, et al. Investigation of relationships between urinary biomarkers of phytoestrogens, phthalates, and phenols and pubertal stages in girls. *Environ Health Perspect.* 2010;118(7):1039-1046. doi:10.1289/ehp.0901690
56. Zhang Z, Hu X, Yang C, Chen X. Early age at menarche is associated with insulin resistance: a systemic review and meta-analysis. *Postgrad Med.* 2019;131(2):144-150. doi:10.1080/00325481.2019.1559429
57. Elks CE, Ong KK, Scott RA, et al; InterAct Consortium. Age at menarche and type 2 diabetes risk: the EPIC-InterAct study. *Diabetes Care.* 2013;36(11):3526-3534. doi:10.2337/dc13-0446
58. Rasmussen AR, Wohlfahrt-Veje C, Tefre de Renzy-Martin K, et al. Validity of self-assessment of pubertal maturation. *Pediatrics.* 2015;135(1):86-93. doi:10.1542/peds.2014-0793
59. Tanner JM. *Growth at Adolescence: With a General Consideration of the Effects of Hereditary and Environmenal Factors Upon Growth and Maturation from Birth to Maturity.* Blackwell Scientific Publications; 1962.
60. Ramnitz MS, Lodish MB. Racial disparities in pubertal development. *Semin Reprod Med.* 2013;31(5):333-339. doi:10.1055/s-0033-1348891
61. Zhai L, Liu J, Zhao J, et al. Association of obesity with onset of puberty and sex hormones in Chinese girls: a 4-year longitudinal study. *PLoS One.* 2015;10(8):e0134656. doi:10.1371/journal.pone.0134656
62. Belachew T, Hadley C, Lindstrom D, Getachew Y, Duchateau L, Kolsteren P. Food insecurity and age at menarche among adolescent girls in Jimma Zone Southwest Ethiopia: a longitudinal study. *Reprod Biol Endocrinol.* 2011;9:125. doi:10.1186/1477-7827-9-125
63. Malina RM, Baxter-Jones ADG, Armstrong N, et al. Role of intensive training in the growth and maturation of artistic gymnasts. *Sports Med.* 2013;43(9):783-802. doi:10.1007/s40279-013-0058-5
64. Malina RM. Physical activity and training: effects on stature and the adolescent growth spurt. *Med Sci Sports Exerc.* 1994;26(6):759-766. doi:10.1249/00005768-199406000-00016
65. Hermassi S, Hayes LD, Bartels T, Schwesig R. Differences in body composition, static balance, field test performance, and academic achievement in 10-12-year-old soccer players. *Front Physiol.* 2023;14:1150484. doi:10.3389/fphys.2023.1150484
66. Gong EJ, Spear BA. Adolescent growth and development: Implications for nutritional needs. *Nutr Educ.* 1988;20(6):273-279. doi:10.1016/S0022-3182(88)80003-7
67. Greydanus DE, Omar H, Pratt HD. The adolescent female athlete: current concepts and conundrums. *Pediatr Clin North Am.* 2010;57(3):697-718. doi:10.1016/j.pcl.2010.02.005
68. Yager Z, O'Dea JA. Relationships between body image, nutritional supplement use, and attitudes towards doping in sport among adolescent boys: implications for prevention programs. *Int Soc Sports Nutr.* 2014;11(1):13. doi:10.1186/1550-2783-11-13
69. Vandewalle S, De Schepper J, Kaufman JM. Androgens and obesity in male adolescents. *Curr Opin Endocrinol Diabetes Obes.* 2015;22(3):230-237. doi:10.1097/MED.0000000000000160
70. Lee JM, Kaciroti N, Appugliese D, Corwyn RF, Bradley RH, Lumeng JC. Body mass index and timing of pubertal initiation in boys. *Arch Pediatr Adolesc Med.* 2010;164(2):139-144. doi:10.1001/archpediatrics.2009.258
71. De Leonibus C, Marcovecchio ML, Chiavaroli V, de Giorgis T, Chiarelli F, Mohn A. Timing of puberty and physical growth in obese children: a longitudinal study in boys and girls. *Pediatr Obes.* 2014;9(4):292-299. doi:10.1111/j.2047-6310.2013.00176.x
72. Nokoff N, Thurston J, Hilkin A, et al. Sex differences in effects of obesity on reproductive hormones and glucose metabolism in early puberty. *Clin Endocrinol Metab.* 2019;104(10):4390-4397. doi:10.1210/jc.2018-02747
73. Sturdevant MS, Spear BA. Adolescent psychosocial development. *Am Diet Assoc.* 2002;102(3 suppl):S30-S31. doi:10.1016/s0002-8223(02)90419-0
74. Spear LP. Adolescent neurodevelopment. *Adolesc Health.* 2013;52(2 suppl 2):S7-S13. doi:10 .1016/j.jadohealth.2012.05.006
75. Vartanian LR. Revisiting the imaginary audience and personal fable constructs of adolescent egocentrism: a conceptual review. *Adolescence.* 2000;35(140):639-661. PMID: 11214204
76. Erikson EH. *Identity: Youth and Crisis.* WW Norton Company; 1968.
77. Jessor R. Successful adolescent development among youth in high-risk settings. *Am Psychol.* 1993;48(2):117-126. doi:10.1037//0003-066x.48.2.117
78. Bloch CA, Clemons P, Sperling MA. Puberty decreases insulin sensitivity. *Pediatr.* 1987;110(3):481-487. doi:10.1016/s0022-3476(87)80522-x
79. Chu L, Morrison KM, Riddell MC, Raha S, Timmons BW. Metabolic flexibility during exercise in children with obesity and matched controls. *Med Sci Sports Exerc.* 2021;53(1):159-164. doi:10.1249/MSS.0000000000002428
80. Riddell MC. The endocrine response and substrate utilization during exercise in children and adolescents. *Appl Physiol (1985).* 2008;105(2):725-733. doi:10.1152/japplphysiol.00031.2008
81. Eriksson O, Saltin B. Muscle metabolism during exercise in boys aged 11 to 16 years compared to adults. *Acta Paediatr Belg.* 1974;28(suppl):257-265. PMID: 4446986
82. Kaczor JJ, Ziolkowski W, Popinigis J, Tarnopolsky MA. Anaerobic and aerobic enzyme activities in human skeletal muscle from children and adults. *Pediatr Res.* 2005;57(3):331-335. doi:10 .1203/01.PDR.0000150799.77094.DE

83. Foricher JM, Ville N, Gratas-Delamarche A, Delamarche P. Effects of submaximal intensity cycle ergometry for one hour on substrate utilisation in trained prepubertal boys versus trained adults. *Sports Med Phys Fitness.* 2003;43(1):36-43. PMID: 12629460

84. Brandou F, Savy-Pacaux AM, Marie J, Brun JF, Mercier J. Comparison of the type of substrate oxidation during exercise between pre and post pubertal markedly obese boys. *Int Sports Med.* 2006;27(5):407-414. doi:10.1055/s-2005-865751

85. Stephens BR, Cole AS, Mahon AD. The influence of biological maturation on fat and carbohydrate metabolism during exercise in males. *Int Sport Nutr Exerc Metab.* 2006;16(2):166-179. doi:10.1123/ijsnem.16.2.166

86. Couto PG, Bertuzzi R, de Souza CC, et al. High carbohydrate diet induces faster final sprint and overall 10,000-m times of young runners. *Pediatr Exerc Sci.* 2015;27(3):355-363. doi:10.1123/pes.2014-0211

87. Desbrow B, McCormack J, Burke LM, et al. Sports Dietitians Australia position statement: sports nutrition for the adolescent athlete. *Int Sport Nutr Exerc Metab.* 2014;24(5):570-584. doi:10.1123/ijsnem.2014-0031

88. Inbar O, Morris N, Epstein Y, Gass G. Comparison of thermoregulatory responses to exercise in dry heat among prepubertal boys, young adults and older males. *Exp Physiol.* 2004;89(6):691-700. doi:10.1113/expphysiol.2004.027979

89. Bergeron MF. Youth sports in the heat: recovery and scheduling considerations for tournament play. *Sports Med.* 2009;39(7):513-522. doi:10 .2165/00007256-200939070-00001

90. Falk B, Dotan R. Children's thermoregulation during exercise in the heat: a revisit. *Appl Physiol Nutr Metab.* 2008;33(2):420-427. doi:10.1139/H07-185

91. Wilk B, Yuxiu H, Bar-Or O. Effect of hypohydration on aerobic performance of boys who exercise in the heat. *Med Sci Sports Exerc.* 2002;34(5):S48. doi:10.1097/00005768-200205001-00265

92. Rowland T. Fluid replacement requirements for child athletes. *Sports Med.* 2011;41(4):279-288. doi:10.2165/11584320-000000000-00000

93. Council on Sports Medicine and Fitness and Council on School Health; Bergeron MF, Devore C, Rice SG; American Academy of Pediatrics. Policy statement—Climatic heat stress and exercising children and adolescents. *Pediatrics.* 2011;128(3):e741-e747. doi:10.1542/peds.2011-1664

94. Karet FE. Disorders of water and acid-base homeostasis. *Nephron Physiol.* 2011;118(1):p28-p34. doi:10.1159/000320885

95. Bar-Or O, Blimkie CJ, Hay JA, MacDougall JD, Ward DS, Wilson WM. Voluntary dehydration and heat intolerance in cystic fibrosis. *Lancet.* 1992;339(8795):696-699. doi:10.1016/0140-6736(92)90597-v

96. Yardley JE, Stapleton JM, Carter MR, Sigal RJ, Kenny GP. Is whole-body thermoregulatory function impaired in type 1 diabetes mellitus? *Curr Diabetes Rev.* 2013;9(2):126-136. doi:10.2174/1573399811309020004

97. Suh H, Kavouras SA. Water intake and hydration state in children. *Eur Nutr.* 2019;58(2):475-496. doi:10.1007/s00394-018-1869-9

98. Drewnowski A, Rehm CD, Constant F. Water and beverage consumption among children age 4-13y in the United States: analyses of 2005-2010 NHANES data. *Nutr J.* 2013;12:85. doi:10.1186/1475-2891-12-85

99. Bottin JH, Morin C, Guelinckx I, Perrier ET. Hydration in children: what do we know and why does it matter? *Ann Nutr Metab.* 2019;74(suppl 3):11-18. doi:10.1159/000500340

100. Bass SL, Inge K. Thermoregulation in young athletes exercising in hot environments. *Int SportMed J.* 2001;2(5):1-6.

101. Kavouras SA, Johnson EC, Bougatsas D, et al. Validation of a urine color scale for assessment of urine osmolality in healthy children. *Eur Nutr.* 2016;55(3):907-915. doi:10.1007/s00394-015-0905-2

102. American College of Sports Medicine, Sawka MN, Burke LM, Eichner ER, Maughan RJ, Montain SJ, Stachenfeld NS. American College of Sports Medicine position stand. Exercise and fluid replacement. *Med Sci Sports Exerc.* 2007;39(2):377-390. doi:10.1249/mss.0b013e31802ca597

103. Maughan RJ, Watson P, Cordery PA, et al. A randomized trial to assess the potential of different beverages to affect hydration status: development of a beverage hydration index. *Am Clin Nutr.* 2016;103(3):717-723. doi:10.3945/ajcn.115.114769

104. Carlsohn A, Scharhag-Rosenberger F, Cassel M, Weber J, de Guzman A, Mayer F. Physical activity levels to estimate the energy requirement of adolescent athletes. *Pediatr Exerc Sci.* 2011;23(2):261-269. doi:10.1123/pes.23.2.261

105. Mifflin MD, St Jeor ST, Hill LA, Scott BJ, Daugherty SA, Koh YO. A new predictive equation for resting energy expenditure in healthy individuals. *Am Clin Nutr.* 1990;51(2):241-247. doi:10.1093/ajcn/51.2.241

106. Owen OE, Kavle E, Owen RS, et al. A reappraisal of caloric requirements in healthy women. *Am Clin Nutr.* 1986;44(1):1-19. doi:10.1093/ajcn/44.1.1

107. Thompson J, Manore MM. Predicted and measured resting metabolic rate of male and female endurance athletes. *Am Diet Assoc.* 1996;96(1):30-34. doi:10.1016/S0002-8223(96)00010-7

108. ten Haaf T, Weijs PJM. Resting energy expenditure prediction in recreational athletes of 18-35 years: confirmation of Cunningham equation and an improved weight-based alternative. *PLoS One.* 2014;9(9):e108460. doi:10.1371/journal.pone.0108460

109. Carlsohn A, Scharhag-Rosenberger F, Cassel M, Mayer F. Resting metabolic rate in elite rowers and canoeists: difference between indirect calorimetry and prediction. *Ann Nutr Metab.* 2011;58(3):239-244. doi:10.1159/000330119

110. Reale RJ, Roberts TJ, Lee KA, Bonsignore JL, Anderson ML. Metabolic rate in adolescent athletes: the development and validation of new equations, and comparison to previous models. *Int Sport Nutr Exerc Metab.* 2020;30(4):249-257. doi:10.1123/ijsnem.2019-0323

111. Torun B. Energy requirements of children and adolescents. *Public Health Nutr.* 2005;8(7A):968-993. doi:10.1079/phn2005791

112. Jagim AR, Fields J, Magee MK, Kerksick CM, Jones MT. Contributing factors to low energy availability in female athletes: a narrative review of energy availability, training demands, nutrition barriers, body image, and disordered eating. *Nutrients.* 2022;14(5):986. doi:10.3390/nu14050986

113. Torres-McGehee TM, Emerson DM, Pritchett K, Moore EM, Smith AB, Uriegas NA. Energy availability with or without eating disorder risk in collegiate female athletes and performing artists. *Athl Train.* 2021;56(9):993-1002. doi:10.4085/JAT0502-20

114. Heikura IA, Stellingwerff T, Areta JL. Low energy availability in female athletes: From the lab to the field. *Eur Sport Sci.* 2022;22(5):709-719. doi:10.1080/17461391.2021.1915391

115. Ackerman KE, Holtzman B, Cooper KM, et al. Low energy availability surrogates correlate with health and performance consequences of Relative Energy Deficiency in Sport. *Br Sports Med.* 2019;53(10):628-633. doi:10.1136/bjsports-2017-098958

116. Nattiv A, De Souza MJ, Koltun KJ, et al. The male athlete triad—a consensus statement from the female and male athlete triad coalition part 1: definition and scientific basis. *Clin Sport Med.* 2021;31(4):335-348. doi:10.1097/JSM.0000000000000946

117. Leibel RL, Rosenbaum M, Hirsch J. Changes in energy expenditure resulting from altered body weight. *N Engl Med.* 1995;332(10):621-628. doi:10.1056/NEJM199503093321001

118. Marra M, Polito A, De Filippo E, et al. Are the general equations to predict BMR applicable to patients with anorexia nervosa? *Eat Weight Disord.* 2002;7(1):53-59. doi:10.1007/BF03354430

119. Tornberg ÅB, Melin A, Koivula FM, et al. Reduced neuromuscular performance in amenorrheic elite endurance athletes. *Med Sci Sports Exerc.* 2017;49(12):2478-2485. doi:10.1249/MSS.0000000000001383

120. Polito A, Fabbri A, Ferro-Luzzi A, et al. Basal metabolic rate in anorexia nervosa: relation to body composition and leptin concentrations. *Am Clin Nutr.* 2000;71(6):1495-1502. doi:10.1093/ajcn/71.6.1495

121. Danforth E Jr, Burger AG. The impact of nutrition on thyroid hormone physiology and action. *Annu Rev Nutr.* 1989;9:201-227. doi:10.1146/annurev.nu.09.070189.001221

122. De Souza MJ, Lee DK, VanHeest JL, Scheid JL, West SL, Williams NI. Severity of energy-related menstrual disturbances increases in proportion to indices of energy conservation in exercising women. *Fertil Steril.* 2007;88(4):971-975. doi:10.1016/j.fertnstert.2006.11.171

123. Laughlin GA, Yen SS. Nutritional and endocrine-metabolic aberrations in amenorrheic athletes. *Clin Endocrinol Metab.* 1996;81(12):4301-4309. doi:10.1210/jcem.81.12.8954031

124. Ollberding NJ, Couch SC, Woo JG, Kalkwarf HJ. Within- and between-individual variation in nutrient intake in children and adolescents. *Acad Nutr Diet.* 2014;114(11):1749-58.e5. doi:10.1016/j.jand.2014.03.016

125. Aerenhouts D, Deriemaeker P, Hebbelinck M, Clarys P. Energy and macronutrient intake in adolescent sprint athletes: a follow-up study. *Sports Sci.* 2011;29(1):73-82. doi:10.1080/02640414.2010.521946

126. Baker LB, Heaton LE, Stein KW, Nuccio RP, Jeukendrup AE. Validity and relative validity of a novel digital approach for 24-h dietary recall in athletes. *Nutr J.* 2014;13:41. doi:10.1186/1475-2891-13-41

127. US Department of Agriculture and US Department of Health and Human Services. *Dietary Guidelines for Americans, 2020-2025.* 9th ed. December 2020. Accessed January 15, 2024. www.DietaryGuidelines.gov

128. Hoots BE, Li J, Hertz MF, et al. Alcohol and other substance use before and during the COVID-19 pandemic among high school students — youth risk behavior survey, United States, 2021. *MMWR Suppl.* 2023;72(1):84-92. doi:10.15585/mmwr.su7201a10

129. Chung T, Creswell KG, Bachrach R, Clark DB, Martin CS. Adolescent binge drinking. *Alcohol Res.* 2018;39(1):5-15. PMID: 30557142

130. Kulesza M, Grossbard JR, Kilmer J, Copeland AL, Larimer ME. Take one for the team? Influence of team and individual sport participation on high school athlete substance use patterns. *Child Adolesc Subst Abuse.* 2014;23(4):217-223. doi:10.1080/1067828X.2013.786928

131. Diehl K, Thiel A, Zipfel S, Mayer J, Schneider S. Substance use among elite adolescent athletes: findings from the GOAL Study. *Scand Med Sci Sports.* 2014;24(1):250-258. doi:10.1111/j.1600-0838.2012.01472.x

132. Bahrke MS, Yesalis CE, Kopstein AN, Stephens JA. Risk factors associated with anabolic-androgenic steroid use among adolescents. *Sports Med.* 2000;29(6):397-405. doi:10.2165/00007256-200029060-00003

133. Schneider KE, Webb L, Boon D, Johnson RM. Adolescent anabolic-androgenic steroid use in association with other drug use, injection drug use, and team sport participation. *Child Adolesc Subst Abuse.* 2020;29(4-6):246-251. doi:10.1080/1067828x.2022.2052219

134. Aerenhouts D, Zinzen E, Clarys P. Energy expenditure and habitual physical activities in adolescent sprint athletes. *Sports Sci Med.* 2011;10(2):362-368. PMID: 24149884

135. Aerenhouts D, Van Cauwenberg J, Poortmans JR, Hauspie R, Clarys P. Influence of growth rate on nitrogen balance in adolescent sprint athletes. *Int Sport Nutr Exerc Metab.* 2013;23(4):409-417. doi:10.1123/ijsnem.23.4.409

136. Mazzulla M, Volterman KA, Packer JE, et al. Whole-body net protein balance plateaus in response to increasing protein intakes during post-exercise recovery in adults and adolescents. *Nutr Metab (Lond).* 2018;15:62. doi:10.1186/s12986-018-0301-z

137. Kim OY, Kim EM, Chung S. Impacts of dietary macronutrient pattern on adolescent body composition and metabolic risk: current and future health status-a narrative review. *Nutrients.* 2020;12(12):3722. doi:10.3390/nu12123722

138. Croll JK, Neumark-Sztainer D, Story M, Wall M, Perry C, Harnack L. Adolescents involved in weight-related and power team sports have better eating patterns and nutrient intakes than non–sport-involved adolescents. *Am Diet Assoc.* 2006;106(5):709-717. doi:10.1016/j.jada.2006.02.010

139. Yasuda J, Tomita T, Arimitsu T, Fujita S. Evenly distributed protein intake over 3 meals augments resistance exercise–induced muscle hypertrophy in healthy young men. *Nutr.* 2020;150(7):1845-1851. doi:10.1093/jn/nxaa101

140. Baker LB, Heaton LE, Nuccio RP, Stein KW. Dietitian-observed macronutrient intakes of young skill and team-sport athletes: adequacy of pre, during, and postexercise nutrition. *Int Sport Nutr Exerc Metab.* 2014;24(2):166-176. doi:10.1123/ijsnem.2013-0132

141. Key TJ, Papier K, Tong TYN. Plant-based diets and long-term health: findings from the EPIC-Oxford study. *Proc Nutr Soc.* 2022;81(2):190-198. doi:10.1017/S0029665121003748

142. Labayen I, Ruiz JR, Ortega FB, et al. High fat diets are associated with higher abdominal adiposity regardless of physical activity in adolescents; the HELENA study. *Clin Nutr.* 2014;33(5):859-866. doi:10.1016/j.clnu.2013.10.008

143. Ambrosini GL, Emmett PM, Northstone K, Howe LD, Tilling K, Jebb SA. Identification of a dietary pattern prospectively associated with increased adiposity during childhood and adolescence. *Int Obes (Lond).* 2012;36(10):1299-1305. doi:10.1038/ijo.2012.127

144. Elliott SA, Truby H, Lee A, Harper C, Abbott RA, Davies PS. Associations of body mass index and waist circumference with: energy intake and percentage energy from macronutrients, in a cohort of Australian children. *Nutr J.* 2011;10:58. doi:10.1186/1475-2891-10-58

145. Bachman JL, Reedy J, Subar AF, Krebs-Smith SM. Sources of food group intakes among the US population, 2001-2002. *Am Diet Assoc.* 2008;108(5):804-814. doi:10.1016/j.jada.2008.02.026

146. Wambogo EA, O'Connor LE, Shams-White MM, Herrick KA, Reedy J. Top sources and trends in consumption of total energy and energy from solid fats and added sugars among youth aged 2-18 years: United States 2009-2018. *Am Clin Nutr.* 2022;116(6):1779-1789. doi:10.1093/ajcn/nqac238

147. Harika RK, Cosgrove MC, Osendarp SJ, Verhoef P, Zock PL. Fatty acid intakes of children and adolescents are not in line with the dietary intake recommendations for future cardiovascular health: a systematic review of dietary intake data from thirty countries. *Br Nutr.* 2011;106(3):307-316. doi:10.1017/S0007114511001528

148. Gharami K, Das M, Das S. Essential role of docosahexaenoic acid towards development of a smarter brain. *Neurochem Int.* 2015;89:51-62. doi:10.1016/j.neuint.2015.08.014

149. Bos DJ, van Montfort SJT, Oranje B, Durston S, Smeets PAM. Effects of omega-3 polyunsaturated fatty acids on human brain morphology and function: what is the evidence? *Eur Neuropsychopharmacol.* 2016;26(3):546-561. doi:10.1016/j.euroneuro.2015.12.031

150. Stonehouse W, Conlon CA, Podd J, et al. DHA supplementation improved both memory and reaction time in healthy young adults: a randomized controlled trial. *Am Clin Nutr.* 2013;97(5):1134-1143. doi:10.3945/ajcn.112.053371

151. Anding RH, Hwang DH. Effects of dietary linolenate on the fatty acid composition of brain lipids in rats. *Lipids.* 1986;21(11):697-701. doi:10.1007/BF02537243

152. Richardson AJ, Burton JR, Sewell RP, Spreckelsen TF, Montgomery P. Docosahexaenoic acid for reading, cognition and behavior in children aged 7-9 years: a randomized, controlled trial (the DOLAB Study). *PLoS One.* 2012;7(9):e43909. doi:10.1371/journal.pone.0043909

153. Rahmawaty S, Charlton K, Lyons-Wall P, Meyer BJ. Dietary intake and food sources of EPA, DPA and DHA in Australian children. *Lipids.* 2013;48(9):869-877. doi:10.1007/s11745-013-3812-4

154. Ritz PP, Rogers MB, Zabinsky JS, et al. Dietary and biological assessment of the omega-3 status of collegiate athletes: a cross-sectional analysis. *PLoS One.* 2020;15(4):e0228834. doi:10.1371/journal.pone.0228834

155. O'Sullivan TA, Ambrosini GL, Mori TA, Beilin LJ, Oddy WH. Omega-3 index correlates with healthier food consumption in adolescents and with reduced cardiovascular disease risk factors in adolescent boys. *Lipids.* 2011;46(1):59-67. doi:10.1007/s11745-010-3499-8

156. Roke K, Rattner J, Brauer P, Mutch DM. Awareness of omega-3 fatty acids and possible health effects among young adults. *Can Diet Pract Res.* 2018;79(3):106-112. doi:10.3148/cjdpr-2018-005

157. Panel on Macronutrients; Panel on the Definition of Dietary Fiber; Subcommittee on Upper Reference Levels of Nutrients; Subcommittee on Interpretation and Uses of Dietary Reference Intakes; Standing Committee on the Scientific Evaluation of Dietary Reference Intakes; Food and Nutrition Board, Institute of Medicine. *Dietary Reference Intakes for Energy, Carbohydrate, Fiber, Fat, Fatty Acids, Cholesterol, Protein, and Amino Acids.* National Academies Press; 2002. doi:10.17226/10490

158. Vitamin D Fact Sheet for Health Professionals. National Institutes of Health, Office of Dietary Supplements. September 18, 2023. Accessed January 16, 2024. https://ods.od.nih.gov/factsheets/VitaminD-HealthProfessional/#h8

159. Fischer PR, Johnson CR, Leopold KN, Thacher TD. Treatment of vitamin D deficiency in children. *Expert Rev Endocrinol Metab.* 2023;18(6):489-502. doi:10.1080/17446651.2023.2270053

160. Wagner CL, Greer FR; American Academy of Pediatrics Section on Breastfeeding; American Academy of Pediatrics Committee on Nutrition. Prevention of rickets and vitamin D deficiency in infants, children, and adolescents. *Pediatrics.* 2008;122(5):1142-1152. doi:10.1542/peds.2008-1862

161. Mitchell DM, Henao MP, Finkelstein JS, Burnett-Bowie SA. Prevalence and predictors of vitamin D deficiency in healthy adults. *Endocr Pract.* 2012;18(6):914-923. doi:10.4158/EP12072.OR

162. Bischoff-Ferrari HA, Giovannucci E, Willett WC, Dietrich T, Dawson-Hughes B. Estimation of optimal serum concentrations of 25-hydroxyvitamin D for multiple health outcomes. *Am Clin Nutr.* 2006;84(1):18-28. doi:10.1093/ajcn/84.1.18

163. Saggese G, Baroncelli GI, Bertelloni S. Puberty and bone development. *Best Pract Res Clin Endocrinol Metab.* 2002;16(1):53-64. doi:10.1053/beem.2001.0180

164. Smith TJ, Tripkovic L, Lanham-New SA, Hart KH. Vitamin D in adolescence: evidence-based dietary requirements and implications for public health policy. *Proc Nutr Soc.* 2018;77(3):292-301. doi:10.1017/S0029665117004104
165. Ward KA, Das G, Berry JL, et al. Vitamin D status and muscle function in post-menarchal adolescent girls. *Clin Endocrinol Metab.* 2009;94(2):559-563. doi:10.1210/jc.2008-1284
166. Wiciński M, Adamkiewicz D, Adamkiewicz M, et al. Impact of vitamin D on physical efficiency and exercise performance—a review. *Nutrients.* 2019;11(11):2826. doi:10.3390/nu11112826
167. Close GL, Russell J, Cobley JN, et al. Assessment of vitamin D concentration in non-supplemented professional athletes and healthy adults during the winter months in the UK: implications for skeletal muscle function. *Sports Sci.* 2013;31(4):344-353. doi:10.1080/02640414.2012.733822
168. Bartoszewska M, Kamboj M, Patel DR. Vitamin D, muscle function, and exercise performance. *Pediatr Clin North Am.* 2010;57(3):849-861. doi:10.1016/j.pcl.2010.03.008
169. Şenışık S, Köyağasıoğlu O, Denerel N. Vitamin D levels on sports injuries in outdoor and indoor athletes: a cross-sectional study. *Phys Sportsmed.* 2022;50(2):164-170. doi:10.1080/00913847.2021.1969217
170. He CS, Fraser WD, Tang J, et al. The effect of 14 weeks of vitamin D3 supplementation on antimicrobial peptides and proteins in athletes. *Sports Sci.* 2016;34(1):67-74. doi:10.1080/02640414.2015.1033642
171. Malczewska-Lenczowska J, Sitkowski D, Surała O, Orysiak J, Szczepańska B, Witek K. The association between iron and vitamin D status in female elite athletes. *Nutrients.* 2018;10(2):167. doi:10.3390/nu10020167
172. Sim JJ, Lac PT, Liu IL, et al. Vitamin D deficiency and anemia: a cross-sectional study. *Ann Hematol.* 2010;89(5):447-452. doi:10.1007/s00277-009-0850-3
173. Atkinson MA, Melamed ML, Kumar J, et al. Vitamin D, race, and risk for anemia in children. *Pediatr.* 2014;164(1):153-158.e1. doi:10.1016/j.jpeds.2013.08.060
174. Committee to Review Dietary Reference Intakes for Vitamin D and Calcium, Food and Nutrition Board, Institute of Medicine. Ross AC, Taylor CL, Yaktine AL, Del Valle *HB, eds. Dietary Reference Intakes for Calcium and Vitamin D.* National Academies Press; 2011. doi:10.17226/13050
175. Bailey RL, Dodd KW, Goldman JA, et al. Estimation of total usual calcium and vitamin D intakes in the United States. *Nutr.* 2010;140(4):817-822. doi:10.3945/jn.109.118539
176. Centers for Disease Control and Prevention. Youth Risk Behavior Survey Data. 2021. Accessed on May 8, 2023. www.cdc.gov/yrbs/dstr/index.html
177. Abrams SA. Calcium and vitamin D requirements for optimal bone mass during adolescence. *Curr Opin Clin Nutr Metab Care.* 2011;14(6):605-609. doi:10.1097/MCO.0b013e32834b2b01
178. Golden NH, Abrams SA; Committee on Nutrition. Optimizing bone health in children and adolescents. *Pediatrics.* 2014;134(4):e1229-e1243. doi:10.1542/peds.2014-2173
179. Bonjour JP, Chevalley T. Pubertal timing, bone acquisition, and risk of fracture throughout life. *Endocr Rev.* 2014;35(5):820-847. doi:10.1210/er.2014-1007
180. Smith NW, Dave AC, Hill JP, McNabb WC. Nutritional assessment of plant-based beverages in comparison to bovine milk. *Front Nutr.* 2022;9:957486. doi:10.3389/fnut.2022.957486
181. Faulkner RA, Davison KS, Bailey DA, Mirwald RL, Baxter-Jones AD. Size-corrected BMD decreases during peak linear growth: implications for fracture incidence during adolescence. *Bone Miner Res.* 2006;21(12):1864-1870. doi:10.1359/jbmr.060907
182. Kalkwarf HJ, Khoury JC, Lanphear BP. Milk intake during childhood and adolescence, adult bone density, and osteoporotic fractures in US women. *Am Clin Nutr.* 2003;77(1):257-265. doi:10.1093/ajcn/77.1.257
183. Bakirhan H, Karabudak E. Effects of inulin on calcium metabolism and bone health. *Int Vitam Nutr Res.* 2023;93(1):85-96. doi:10.1024/0300-9831/a000700
184. US Department of Agriculture, Agricultural Research Service, Nutrient Data Laboratory. USDA National Nutrient Database for Standard Reference, Release 28. September 2015. Accessed July 3, 2017. www.ars.usda.gov/northeast-area/beltsville-md/beltsville-human-nutrition-research-center/nutrient-data-laboratory/docs/usda-national-nutrient-database-for-standard-reference
185. Sekhar DL, Murray-Kolb LE, Kunselman AR, Paul IM. Identifying factors predicting iron deficiency in United States adolescent females using the ferritin and the body iron models. *Clin Nutr ESPEN.* 2015;10(3):e118-e123. doi:10.1016/j.clnesp.2015.03.001
186. Parks RB, Hetzel SJ, Brooks MA. Iron deficiency and anemia among collegiate athletes: a retrospective chart review. *Med Sci Sports Exerc.* 2017;49(8):1711-1715. doi:10.1249/MSS.0000000000001259
187. Roy R, Kück M, Radziwolek L, Kerling A. Iron deficiency in adolescent and young adult German athletes-a retrospective study. *Nutrients.* 2022;14(21):4511. doi:10.3390/nu14214511
188. Fernández-Bañares F, Monzón H, Forné M. A short review of malabsorption and anemia. *World Gastroenterol.* 2009;15(37):4644-4652. doi:10.3748/wjg.15.4644
189. Sandström G, Rödjer S, Kaijser B, Börjesson M. *Helicobacter pylori* antibodies and iron deficiency in female adolescents. *PLoS One.* 2014;9(11):e113059. doi:10.1371/journal.pone.0113059
190. Peeling P, Blee T, Goodman C, et al. Effect of iron injections on aerobic-exercise performance of iron-depleted female athletes. *Int Sport Nutr Exerc Metab.* 2007;17(3):221-231. doi:10.1123/ijsnem.17.3.221
191. McClung JP, Karl JP. Iron deficiency and obesity: the contribution of inflammation and diminished iron absorption. *Nutr Rev.* 2009;67(2):100-104. doi:10.1111/j.1753-4887.2008.00145.x
192. Ziemann E, Kasprowicz K, Kasperska A, Zembroń-Lacny A, Antosiewicz J, Laskowski R. Do high blood hepcidin concentrations contribute to low ferritin levels in young tennis players at the end of tournament season? *Sports Sci Med.* 2013;12(2):249-258. PMID: 24149803

193. Sim M, Garvican-Lewis LA, Cox GR, et al. Iron considerations for the athlete: a narrative review. *Eur Appl Physiol.* 2019;119(7):1463-1478. doi:10.1007/s00421-019-04157-y

194. Garvican LA, Lobigs L, Telford R, Fallon K, Gore CJ. Haemoglobin mass in an anaemic female endurance runner before and after iron supplementation. *Int Sports Physiol Perform.* 2011;6(1):137-140. doi:10.1123/ijspp.6.1.137

195. Stierman B, Mishra S, Gahche JJ, Potischman N, Hales CM. Dietary supplement use in children and adolescents aged ≤19 years — United States, 2017-2018. *MMWR Morb Mortal Wkly Rep.* 2020;69(43):1557-1562. doi:10.15585/mmwr.mm6943a1

196. Barrack MT, Sassone J, Dizon F, et al. Dietary supplement intake and factors associated with increased use in preadolescent endurance runners. *Acad Nutr Diet.* 2022;122(3):573-582. doi:10.1016/j.jand.2021.07.013

197. Nikolaidis PT, Son'kin VD. Sports physiology in adolescent track-and-field athletes: a narrative review. *Open Access Sports Med.* 2023;14:59-68. doi:10.2147/OAJSM.S417612

198. Chorley JN, Anding RH. Performance-enhancing substances. *Adolesc Med State Art Rev.* 2015;26(1):174-188. PMID: 26514038

199. Dodge TL, Jaccard JJ. The effect of high school sports participation on the use of performance-enhancing substances in young adulthood. *Adolesc Health.* 2006;39(3):367-373. doi:10.1016/j.jadohealth.2005.12.025

200. Eisenberg ME, Wall M, Neumark-Sztainer D. Muscle-enhancing behaviors among adolescent girls and boys. *Pediatrics.* 2012;130(6):1019-1026. doi:10.1542/peds.2012-0095

201. Maughan RJ, Burke LM, Dvorak J, et al. IOC consensus statement: dietary supplements and the high-performance athlete. *Br Sports Med.* 2018;52(7):439-455. doi:10.1136/bjsports-2018-099027

202. Jovanov P, Đorđić V, Obradović B, et al. Prevalence, knowledge and attitudes towards using sports supplements among young athletes. *Int Soc Sports Nutr.* 2019;16(1):27. doi:10.1186/s12970-019-0294-7

203. Gomez J; American Academy of Pediatrics Committee on Sports Medicine and Fitness. Use of performance-enhancing substances. *Pediatrics.* 2005;115(4):1103-1106. doi:10.1542/peds.2005-0085

204. Terjung RL, Clarkson P, Eichner ER, et al. American College of Sports Medicine roundtable. The physiological and health effects of oral creatine supplementation. *Med Sci Sports Exerc.* 2000;32(3):706-717. doi:10.1097/00005768-200003000-00024

205. Kreider RB, Kalman DS, Antonio J, et al. International Society of Sports Nutrition position stand: safety and efficacy of creatine supplementation in exercise, sport, and medicine. *Int Soc Sports Nutr.* 2017;14:18. doi:10.1186/s12970-017-0173-z

206. Nagata JM, Ganson KT, Gorrell S, Mitchison D, Murray SB. Association between legal performance-enhancing substances and use of anabolic-androgenic steroids in young adults. *JAMA Pediatr.* 2020;174(10):992-993. doi:10.1001/jamapediatrics.2020.0883

CHAPTER 13

College Athletes

Jennifer Ketterly, MS, RD, CSSD, LDN, and Caroline Mandel, MS, RD, CSSD

LEARNING OBJECTIVES

- Describe the unique personal, performance, and health concerns of college student-athletes.
- Recognize the role of athletic department stakeholders in successful implementation of nutrition services.
- Understand and interpret the importance of National Collegiate Athletic Association food- and nutrition-related legislation.
- Examine the various roles and responsibilities of a dietitian practicing in the college athletics environment.
- Develop appropriate nutrition education approaches for student-athletes.

INTRODUCTION

Over the past 30 years, interest and investment in sports dietetics services within athletic departments across National Collegiate Athletic Association (NCAA) member institutions has increased dramatically. The first collegiate sports dietitian in the United States, Kristine Clark, PhD, RD, FACSM, began serving Penn State student-athletes in 1991.[1] What has followed has been a growing respect for and recognition of the role that sports nutrition plays in the health and success of the student-athlete. As of this writing, there are more than 200 full-time registered dietitian nutritionists (RDNs) providing nutrition services to NCAA Division I athletic departments[2] and nearly 500,000 student-athletes participating in 43 sports at more than 1,100 NCAA member institutions (see Table 13.1).[3] Because of the rigorous demands of athletic participation, academic pressures, and the realities of college life, student-athletes can be at risk for complications heightened by poor nutrition. These may include inadequate recovery, fatigue, injury, and illness due to poor eating habits, lack of resources, or rigid training diets. Serving as a sports dietitian in the rapidly changing college environment requires a breadth and scope of practice unique in the field of nutrition.

THE STUDENT-ATHLETE

Collegiate athletes are a diverse group of students ranging in age from 17 to 24 years. They are considered postadolescent young adults or emerging adults.[4,5] Research suggests that this age group is still developing mentally and physically. They are known for taking more risks, being more self-centered, being vulnerable to addiction, and being less insightful or concerned about consequences than adults.[6] The student-athlete population at most NCAA institutions is typically diverse in terms of sex, race, culture, religion, nutrition knowledge, and socioeconomic status.[7] Student-athletes are required to be full-time students during their

TABLE 13.1 Division I, II, and III National Collegiate Athletic Associate Member Institutions (2020-2021)[a,3]								
	Division I		Division II		Division III		National Collegiate Athletic Association total	
Total members	350		309		443		1,102	
	Teams	Athletes	Teams	Athletes	Teams	Athletes	Teams	Athletes
Men	3,008	99,950	2,230	71,396	3,984	107,642	9,222	278,988
Women	3,700	87,425	2,697	52,979	4,336	78,773	10,733	219,177
Total	6,708	187,375	4,927	124,375	8,320	186,415	19,955	498,165

[a] Participation includes championship, nonchampionship, emerging, and other sports.

years of athletic eligibility, but not all are awarded a full athletic scholarship that includes money for food, and many do not have access to a sports dietitian.

Student-athletes nutritional needs evolve throughout their college careers based on living situation, athletic performance goals, health concerns, personal needs, and other factors. Box 13.1 lists examples of nutrition-related concerns by year of eligibility. In addition to learning about sports nutrition requirements to augment training and improve athletic performance, many student-athletes learn practical life skills regarding meal planning, grocery shopping, and proper food handling and safety, as well as nutrition guidelines for lifelong health and the prevention of chronic disease. Box 13.2 lists nutrition-related concerns of college student-athletes related to athletic performance, health, and personal needs.[8]

BOX 13.1 Nutrition-Related Concerns of College Student-Athletes by Year of Eligibility

Freshman

Transitioning to college life, including the dining hall meal plan, alcohol, stress, and time management

Adapting to a new team and training program

Facing the "freshman 15," along with issues of weight management, body composition, and body image

Finding one's social identity

Facing the increased competitiveness of collegiate sports

Experiencing continued physical growth and development

Moving toward emotional maturity and developing confidence

Sophomore

Transitioning to off-campus living, including menu planning, grocery shopping, and cooking skills

Preventing overtraining

Periodizing training and nutrition practices for year-round training and competition

Balancing sports with academics and social life

Perfecting the taper for endurance sports

Continued on next page

BOX 13.1 Nutrition-Related Concerns of College Student-Athletes by Year of Eligibility (CONTINUED)

Junior

Moving out of dormitory housing into a house or apartment

Finding easy meal preparation ideas and recipes

Preventing boredom or staleness with one's diet

Maintaining nutritional variety and interest for the long haul

Maintaining consistency with habits for continued success

Meeting the growing demands of the academic major

Senior or fifth year

Demonstrating leadership on and off the field of competition

Planning life after college athletics

Transitioning from collegiate athlete to professional athlete or recreational exerciser

Facing increased focus on healthful eating for a lifetime

Nutrition Knowledge and Sources of Information

College athletes are often misinformed about their fueling requirements and arrive on campus with nutrition information from multiple sources, including parents, friends, teammates, coaches, the internet, and social media. Although not all college student-athletes have access to a collegiate sports dietitian to provide guidance on their performance training diet and a healthy lifestyle, many student-athletes take advantage of the sports nutrition programs and services when available through the athletic department or campus health services. These services are often unlimited and available at no cost for the duration of an athlete's eligibility.

The following studies showcase the different levels of nutrition knowledge and sources of information among college athletes.

- Rosenbloom et al[9] assessed the nutrition knowledge of athletes at 1 NCAA Division I institution and found that many collegiate athletes have misconceptions about the roles of specific nutrients, such as carbohydrates, protein, vitamins, minerals, and supplements in sports performance. The students reported that their sources of sports nutrition information included coaches, athletic trainers, strength and conditioning staff, physicians, teammates, nutrition classes, sports dietitians, parents, and popular media. They concluded that athletes who make food choices based on inaccurate nutrition information could experience negative consequences in their performance.
- Pawlak et al[10] found that the factors with the greatest impact on collegiate baseball players' intention to eat healthy food included the athletes' daily schedules and their perception of a healthful diet's effects on their focus and concentration.
- Hornstrom et al[11] reported the nutrition knowledge scores, nutrition choice scores, and nutrition practice scores for 185 softball players from 11 Mid-American Conference teams. Two-thirds of the athletes had a failing knowledge score. Their choice score suggested that they made poor nutrition choices, with 17% reporting that they ate fast food every day or most days and more than half reporting that they occasionally, rarely, or never had a set meal schedule. Respondents who said they ate using the US Department of Agriculture's (USDA's) Food Guide Pyramid graphic for guidance had healthier diets; however, only 10% indicated that they used the Food Guide Pyramid to make food choices every day or most days.

BOX 13.2 General Nutrition-Related Concerns of College Student-Athletes[8]

Health

Nutrition support for medical diagnoses: food allergies and intolerances, gastrointestinal diseases, disordered eating or eating disorders, type 1 diabetes, metabolic disorders, chronic disease, and mental health diagnoses

Nutrition for injury prevention and rehabilitation

Nutrition habits to support immunity; what to eat when sick

Learning about the role of nutrition in lifelong health and wellness

Personal needs

Life transitions

- Transition to college life: new food resources (campus dining halls, fueling stations, training tables), dining out, frequent travel
- Transition to off-campus living: menu planning, grocery shopping, cooking, quick and easy meal preparation, food safety, food storage
- Transition to life after college athletics: life skills to support personal nutrition needs; nutrition-related health risks across the life cycle; and nutrition skills to plan, shop, cook, and fuel for lifelong wellness

Impact of academic and athletic time demands on food choices, timing, and frequency

Access to affordable, nutritious, and culturally appropriate foods

Weight management, body composition, and body image

Ability to find familiar foods or willingness to try new foods

Ability to match nutrition resources to personal concerns (eg, sustainability)

Continued physical, emotional, and cognitive growth and development

Ability to balance sports participation with academics and down time (eg, socializing, self-care, sleep)

- Valliant et al[12] found that, among 11 NCAA Division I volleyball players, nutrition knowledge scores ranged from 16 to 37 out of a possible 55 points prior to a nutrition intervention. At baseline, participants did not meet the sport-specific recommended requirements for energy (24.0 ± 8.6 kcal/kg/d vs the recommended 37–41 kcal/kg/d), carbohydrate (3.08 ± 1.1 g/kg/d vs the recommended 6-10 g/kg/d), protein (0.9 ± 0.3 g/kg/d vs the recommended 1.2–1.7 g/kg/d), or fat (77% of estimated needs). This was possibly due to meal skipping and the high number of study subjects (50%) trying to lose weight. The athletes improved in all areas of knowledge and intake after the intervention.
- Andrews et al[13] evaluated student-athletes' sports nutrition knowledge at a Division I mid-major program. The overall mean sports nutrition knowledge score for all student-athletes was 56.9%, with only 12 student-athletes having an adequate score of 75% or higher. No differences were seen by sex, class level, team, or completion of prior nutrition coursework. The authors concluded that inadequate sports nutrition knowledge increases the risk of inadequate nutrition and impaired performance.

» Riviere et al[14] conducted a narrative review of 14 studies that assessed current nutrition knowledge and practices and the impact of sports dietitians on nutrition outcomes and reported that sports nutrition knowledge among NCAA student-athletes was poor. The authors provided several examples of the positive correlation between athlete nutrition knowledge and eating behaviors, supporting nutrition education provided by the collegiate sports dietitian, instead of coaches and other staff, to help decrease the risk of low energy availability (LEA), micronutrient deficiencies, injury, disordered eating, and long-term risk of chronic disease.

Performance Concerns

College athletes are concerned about nutrition as it relates to the enhancement of performance, prevention of fatigue, recovery from training and competition, safe and legal use of dietary supplements, illness and injury, weight management, and altering or maintaining body composition.[15] Training and competing at the collegiate level may be vastly different for many athletes compared with high school, resulting in altered nutritional requirements. Wade et al[16] surveyed college strength and conditioning coaches and reported that, when freshman student-athletes arrive on campus, many have difficulty enduring collegiate sports training because they lack lower-extremity and core strength, flexibility, proper training technique, and mental toughness, coupled with a lack of performance nutrition knowledge. Educating student-athletes about the nutritional demands of sport at the collegiate level is paramount.

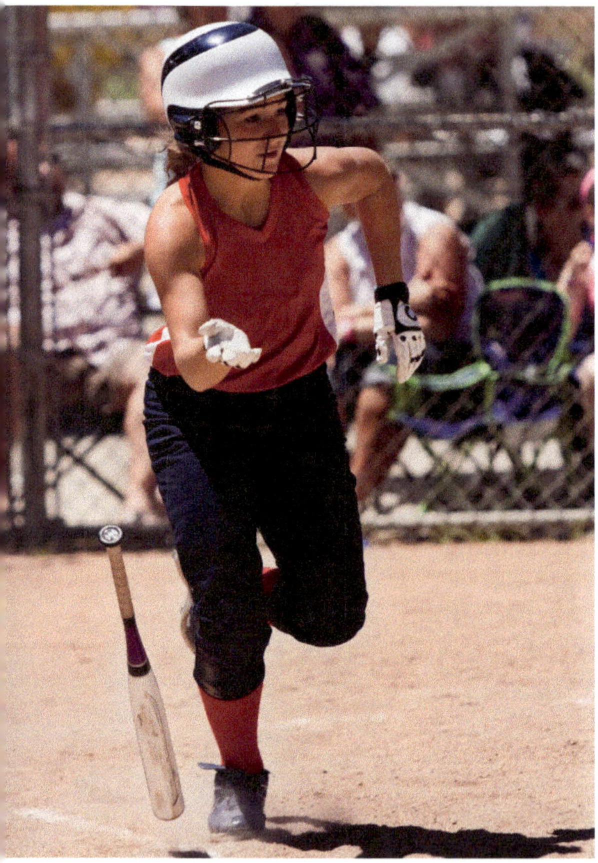

FUELING PERFORMANCE

Inadequate energy and carbohydrate intake, glycogen depletion, dehydration, and poor iron status are nutritional causes of fatigue, inadequate adaptation, and poor performance. Pairing nutrition education with fueling resources and identifying high-risk athletes for referral to the collegiate sports dietitian for individualized counseling and support can help athletes meet their fueling needs for training and competition.

Iron deficiency is most common in female athletes (15%–35% of female athletes), and approximately 5% to 11% of male athletes may also be at risk.[17] In 2003, Cowell et al[18] reported that only 24 of 55 NCAA Division I institutions (44%) screened their female athletes for iron deficiency. Twenty-two of the 24 institutions doing iron screening also provided nutrition advice to female student-athletes who were iron deficient. A great deal of variability existed among the institutions in terms of diagnostic criteria, treatment protocols, and follow-up procedures. The authors stated the need to develop standardized protocols for assessment and treatment of iron deficiency in female college athletes. In a retrospective chart review covering 5,674 blood draws for 2,749 student-athletes over a period of 12 years (2002–2014), Parks et al[18] reported the overall prevalence of iron deficiency anemia among incoming female student-athletes at preparticipation physical exams to be 5.7% (ranging from 1% –11%) with no team differences at the preparticipation physical exams as compared to the group mean. Iron deficiency anemia was defined as a hemoglobin (Hgb) level of less than 11.6 g/dL for females and less than 13.6 g/dL for males. Overall, 2.2% of female athletes indicated iron deficiency anemia, and 30.9% indicated iron deficiency without anemia. For male athletes, 1.2% indicated iron deficiency anemia, and 2.9% indicated iron deficiency without anemia. Factors that contribute to poor iron status in athletes include inadequate energy and dietary iron intakes, increased blood losses (eg, menstruation, gastrointestinal bleeding), foot-strike hemolysis, sweat loss, iron malabsorption, and possible impact of inflammation. The consequences of iron deficiency include impairments in athletic performance, immune function, and cognitive function.[18-20] Nutrition education by a collegiate sports dietitian can be used to prevent and treat iron deficiency.

The following are stages of iron deficiency for athletes based on laboratory results from Sim et al[17]:

- Stage 1 iron deficiency
  - serum ferritin less than 35 mcg/L
  - Hgb greater than 115 g/L
  - transferrin saturation greater than 16%
- Stage 2 iron deficiency (nonanemic)
  - serum ferritin less than 20 mcg/L
  - Hgb greater than 115 g/L
  - transferrin saturation less than 16%
- Stage 3 iron deficiency anemia
  - serum ferritin less than 12 mcg/L
  - Hgb less than 115 g/L
  - transferrin saturation less than 16%

RECOVERY

Strategies for recovery from training and competition include adequate nutrition, hydration, sleep, and stress management, as well as the use of training room modalities such as ice baths, contrast showers, massage, stretching, and foam roller exercises. Nutritional recovery includes the refueling and rehydration strategies used in the immediate postexercise period to gain training adaptations and prevent fatigue in subsequent exercise sessions.[15]

It can take anywhere from 24 to 72 hours for the body to recover from a bout of training depending on the volume and intensity of exercise performed. For athletes training at low intensity once a day, no special recovery recommendations are required. However, for athletes who need speedy refueling (less than 8 hours between 2 fuel-demanding sessions), consuming 1.0 to 1.2 g of carbohydrate per kilogram of body weight plus 0.25 to 0.3 g of protein per kilogram of body weight, along with adequate rehydration in the immediate postexercise period (within 60 minutes), improves glycogen resynthesis and muscle rebuilding and repair.[15] Emerging evidence suggests that nutrients such as vitamin D, omega-3 polyunsaturated fatty acids, creatine, and collagen with vitamin C may help support recovery.[21] For more information on postworkout carbohydrate and protein recommendations, refer to Chapters 2 and 3.

ERGOGENIC AIDS AND DIETARY SUPPLEMENTS

Although many athletes understand the relationship between optimal nutrition and athletic performance, the pressure to use ergogenic aids and dietary supplements may be overwhelming and can lead to athletes prioritizing these products over food and fluid intake. Ergogenic aids are defined as external influences that claim to enhance athletic performance and may include performance-enhancing drugs and dietary supplements.

Athletes are a major target of the multibillion-dollar supplement industry. The dietary supplement industry is underregulated by the US Food and Drug Administration, which has led to multiple reports of tainted supplements and athletes testing positive for banned substances. Many athletes use dietary supplements that claim to enhance athletic performance, increase muscle mass, decrease body fat, or improve health and immune function.[22] Even though dietary supplements may expose athletes to dangerous ingredients and banned substances that can put their health and eligibility at risk, 45.2% of 557 Division 1 student-athletes reported taking dietary supplements at least 2 days per week during the past year.[23] Froiland et al[24] reported on nutritional supplement use among 203 college athletes (115 male and 88 female) and their sources of information and found that 89% of the student-athletes had used or were currently using nutritional supplements. Females were more likely to take calcium and multivitamins, and males reported significant intakes of ginseng, β-hydroxy-β-methylbutyric acid (HMB), amino acids, glutamine, weight-gain products, and whey protein. Females were more likely to obtain information from family members, whereas males were more likely to obtain information from nutrition store staff, fellow athletes, friends, or coaches. Female athletes were more likely to take supplements for their health or to make up for an inadequate diet; males took supplements to improve speed and agility or strength and power or to gain weight or muscle. The 2017 NCAA National Study on Substance Use Habits of College Athletes reported that, whereas 89% of 23,028 student-athletes surveyed said that they had not taken any NCAA banned performance enhancers in the past year, a small percentage of student-athletes reported taking androstenedione or norandrostenedione (0.1%), HMB (0.1%), clenbuterol (0.1%), dehydroepiandrosterone (0.1%), erythropoietin (EPO) (0.1%), human growth hormone (0.1% injected, 0.2% oral), and testosterone boosters (0.7%). Seventy-five percent of student-athletes reported using dietary supplements. The most commonly used substances reported included protein products, multivitamins, energy drinks, and preworkout products, with growing interest in and use of fish oil, probiotics, and both prescription and nonprescription sleep aids.[22]

The NCAA recommends that athletes review dietary supplements and receive guidance with a qualified athletics department staff member before consuming any nutritional or dietary supplement product.[25] The Drug Free Sport AXIS (www.drugfreesport.com/education/axis) is a valuable resource for collegiate sports dietitians and athletes, where users can submit questions about banned substances in dietary supplements.[26] The United States Anti-Doping Agency (USADA) provides an online dietary supplement safety education and awareness resource called Supplement Connect (www.usada.org/athletes/substances/supplement-connect).[27] This tool can be adapted for use for NCAA student-athletes to help reduce their risk of taking dietary supplements contaminated with harmful or NCAA-banned substances. More information on dietary supplements and ergogenic aids can be found in Chapter 7.

ILLNESS, INJURY PREVENTION, AND REHABILITATION

In 1982, the National Athletic Trainers' Association and the NCAA created an ongoing collegiate sports injury database called the NCAA Injury Surveillance Program. Between 1988 and 2004, more than half of all athletic injuries to collegiate athletes were to the lower extremities. Preseason practice injury rates were 2 to 3 times higher than those recorded during the regular season. During the regular season, more injuries were reported during competition than during practice. Relatively few injuries occurred in weight rooms. Rates of concussion and injuries to anterior cruciate ligaments increased significantly between 1988 and 2004, likely because of improved reporting and identification. Several sports showed decreased competition injury rates, including women's gymnastics, basketball, and field hockey. Spring football and women's basketball exhibited decreased practice injury rates. Sports involving collision and contact (eg, football and wrestling) had the highest injury rates in both games and practice, whereas men's baseball had the lowest rate of injuries in practice, and women's softball had the lowest rate in games. Sports considered noncontact (eg, men's and women's soccer and basketball) have a substantial number of injuries caused by player contact.[28]

Coaches and RDNs must give special nutritional consideration to the injured athlete, including altered energy and protein needs, nutritional requirements presurgery and postsurgery, and discontinuation of select dietary supplements before surgery. In addition, the injured athlete may have increased concerns about weight and body composition during periods of inactivity and rehabilitation. Although exercise injuries vary, many athletes may experience a reduction or complete cessation in sports participation during the injury and rehabilitation phases. During this period of relative inactivity, the sports nutrition practitioner should screen athletes for malnutrition and make recommendations to avoid nutritional deficiencies, specifically in energy, carbohydrates, protein, fat, vitamins, and minerals. An athlete's nutrition requirements will change as the injury heals and rehabilitation exercises and sports participation progress toward a return to play. Wall et al[29] recommended dietary and rehabilitation goals that aim to limit the loss of muscle mass and strength following injury. Carbohydrate and fat requirements are determined on a case-by-case basis depending on each athlete's resting metabolic rate, daily activity level, and body composition goals. Recent evidence suggests that higher protein intakes of 2.0 to 2.5 g per kilogram of body weight per day postsurgery and during periods of immobilization may help mitigate the loss of muscle mass and muscular strength. In addition, growing evidence supports the use of omega-3 fatty acid and creatine supplements to help reduce inflammation, prevent muscle loss, and promote muscle protein synthesis during recovery from an exercise-induced injury.[30]

WEIGHT MANAGEMENT

Many student-athletes will consult with the sports dietitian about weight management, whether the goal is to gain or lose weight. This is an excellent opportunity to evaluate the student-athlete's nutritional status and identify areas of need for sports nutrition education while counseling the athlete on appropriate weight management strategies. The position of the Academy of Nutrition and Dietetics, Dietitians of Canada, and the American College of Sports Medicine is stated as follows[15]:

> *Body weight and composition should not be the sole criterion for participation in sports; daily weigh-ins are discouraged. Optimal body fat levels depend on the sex, age, and heredity of the athlete and may be sport-specific. Body fat assessment techniques have inherent variability and limitations. Preferably weight loss (fat loss) should take place in the off-season or begin before the competitive season and involve a qualified sports dietitian.*

The preferred time for periodizing weight change efforts is during the athlete's offseason. For weight loss, the sports dietitian must ensure adequate nutrient intake, provide a meal plan that minimizes loss of lean mass, and evaluate the student-athlete for risk of disordered eating. For weight gain, special care must be taken to help the athlete find ways to increase energy intake with energy-dense foods, ensure adequate nutrient intake, and avoid foods high in saturated fat and cholesterol that may increase risk of chronic disease. Athletes seeking to gain or lose weight are at risk of taking dietary supplements that may be tainted with harmful or banned substances. More information on weight management can be found in Chapter 11.

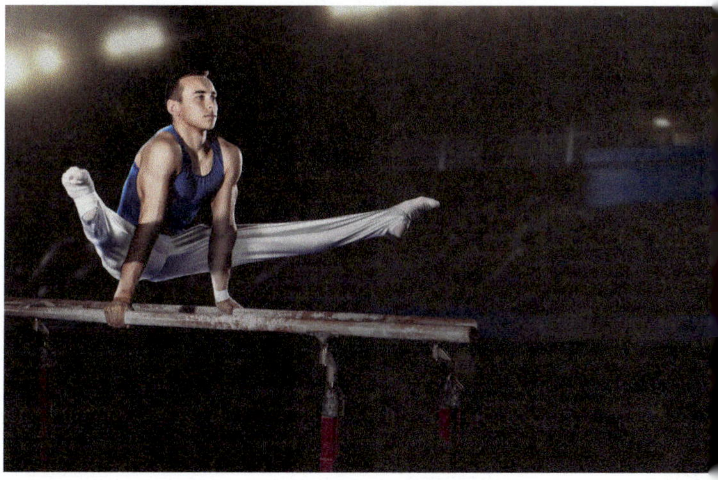

BODY COMPOSITION

Body composition is a measure of the ratio of lean mass to fat mass. For a review of techniques for measuring body composition, see Chapter 9. Methods that have been used in the collegiate setting include hydrostatic weighing, skinfold measurements, air displacement plethysmography, bioelectrical impedance analysis, and dual-energy x-ray absorptiometry (DXA). All methods have a degree of error associated with them that must be considered when interpreting results. Although the assessment of body composition can be a useful tool in helping the student-athlete track changes that may occur as a result of nutrition or training modifications, the *2014–15 NCAA Sports Medicine Handbook* points out the following factors to consider[31]:

- The weight on the scale does not tell an athlete what changes are occurring to their lean and fat mass.
- Comparing body composition with that of other athletes is not useful because of differences in age, weight, height, sex, and genetics, and may lead to unhealthy nutrition and exercise practices.
- A very low level of body fat has serious consequences on health and performance, including increased risk of injury and illness. Minimum body composition standards exist for both male and female athletes.
- Changes in body composition occur slowly over time, and reassessment twice per year is sufficient except in rare circumstances.

There is no ideal body composition for any one athlete or sport. Tracking changes in lean and fat mass over time can be useful. Education must be provided to student-athletes, coaches, and athletics staff, emphasizing that body composition is primarily a measure of nutrition status, not performance, and that many factors including genetics, training, coaching, preparation, nutrition, recovery, sleep, and mental health are determinants of performance. For example, lean body mass can be used to estimate an athlete's resting metabolic rate and daily energy expenditure that the collegiate sports dietitian can then use to evaluate an athlete's energy availability and nutrient needs for training and competition. Many collegiate athletics departments have developed weight and body composition policies outlining who will perform body composition assessments, when and how results will be presented to the athlete, who will have access to the data, how these data will be used, and how often measurements will be repeated. These policies help to ensure that athletes will be adequately educated about body composition assessment, that the data will not be abused or used punitively, and that the health and safety of the athlete will be prioritized. For information on weight management for athletes, refer to Chapter 11.

Health Concerns

Health concerns for the college student-athlete may include gastrointestinal disorders, risk of metabolic diseases, and risk of disordered eating or eating disorders. Although specific health assessment data on college athletes do not exist, health data reported in Box 13.3 from the 2022 American College Health Association-National College Health Assessment III (ACHA-NCHA III) can help the collegiate sports

BOX 13.3 Acute, Chronic, and Mental Health Concerns of College Students[32]

Acute health concerns

- Bronchitis
- Chicken pox
- Chlamydia
- Cold or virus (or other respiratory illness)
- Concussion
- Gonorrhea
- Influenza
- Mumps
- Mononucleosis
- Orthopedic injury
- Pelvic inflammatory disease
- Shingles
- Stomach or gastrointestinal virus, food poisoning, gastritis
- Urinary tract infection

Chronic health concerns

- Acne
- Allergies (food, animals/pets, environmental)
- Asthma
- Cancer
- Celiac disease
- Chronic pain
- Diabetes/insulin resistance
- Endometriosis
- Gastroesophageal reflux disease (GERD)
- Heart or vascular disorders
- Hypertension
- Hyperlipidemia
- Irritable bowel syndrome
- Migraine headache
- Polycystic ovary syndrome
- Sleep apnea
- Thyroid condition or disorder
- Urinary system disorder

Mental health concerns

- ADD/ADHD
- Alcohol- or drug-related abuse or addiction
- Anxiety
- Autism spectrum disorder
- Bipolar disorder and related conditions
- Depression
- Eating disorder
- Gambling disorder
- Insomnia
- OCD and related conditions
- Personality disorder
- PTSD
- Schizophrenia and other psychotic conditions
- Tourette syndrome
- Traumatic brain injury

dietitian understand the acute, chronic, and mental health concerns experienced by college students, many of which are tied to nutritional status or can be managed using medical nutrition therapy.[32]

GENERAL HEALTH AND WELLNESS

During the COVID-19 pandemic, collegiate sports dietitians played a major role in supporting the health and wellness of college student-athletes in the following ways:

- RDNs offered nutrition and hydration strategies to help athletes with the COVID-19 virus maintain adequate food and fluid intake despite symptoms such as fever, cough, and loss of taste and/or smell.
- RDNs modified fueling programs to protect the safety of student-athletes and staff.
- RDNs helped dispel nutrition and immunity myths and misinformation, calling on a wealth of evidence and experience to use sports nutrition to fuel athletes for health and wellness as they continued to train, compete, travel, and attend virtual classes.

Many college sports dietitians elevated their value to their departments and the sports medicine team by using nutrition strategies to promote health and support the nutrition needs of athletes when sick and during return-to-play protocols.

GASTROINTESTINAL DISORDERS

Student-athletes may present with gastrointestinal issues, including gastroesophageal reflux, gastritis, nausea, constipation, diarrhea, irritable bowel syndrome, food allergies and intolerances, celiac disease, and inflammatory bowel disease (ie, Crohn's disease and ulcerative colitis). The collegiate sports dietitian needs to be knowledgeable about medical nutrition therapy for these diagnoses and must also know how to balance an adequate training diet with the rigors of an academic and athletic training schedule.

RISK FOR CARDIOVASCULAR DISEASE

Although cardiovascular disease (CVD) risk factors, such as high cholesterol, high blood pressure, and diabetes, are not the first topic on the collegiate student-athlete's mind, it is well documented that heart disease is the number one cause of morbidity and mortality for all Americans.[33] Emerging science suggests that increased CVD risk is a reality for some collegiate student-athletes. The American Heart Association recommends screening college athletes for heart disease risk with the main goal of preventing sudden cardiac death and injury.[34] Muñoz et al[35] studied 135 NCAA Division II student-athletes from 11 sports and found that a significant number of college athletes had 1 or more risk factors for CVD, including increased waist circumference, elevated blood pressure, high total cholesterol, and low high-density lipoprotein cholesterol, despite participation in sports. These factors may predispose college athletes to cardiac risk later in life when exercise regimens are reduced. Borchers et al[36] reported that, of 104 NCAA Division I football players, 21% were obese (body fat > 25%), 21% had insulin resistance, and 9% had metabolic syndrome. All of the study participants who were obese were offensive and defensive linemen, and they were at a significantly increased risk of insulin resistance and metabolic syndrome compared with other position players. These data suggest that, although Division I collegiate football players participate in high-intensity training, they are at risk of developing metabolic syndrome. In the Trojan Lifetime Champions Health Study, Sorenson et al[37] reported that, among 496 former college athletes and nonathletes, the athletes had greater joint health concerns but comparable cardiopulmonary health compared with nonathletes. The authors concluded that being a college athlete as a young adult is not protective against heart disease. Counseling and education on lifestyle modification, exercise, and diet for reduced CVD risk are needed for all athletes, especially as they transition from NCAA sports participation to life after college athletics.

DIABETES

Athletes with diabetes compete at the highest level in every sport.[38] The collegiate sports dietitian should be part of the treatment team providing nutrition education and lifestyle strategies to optimize glycemic control.[39,40] The collegiate sports dietitian will more likely encounter athletes with type 1 diabetes because of the demographics of college students and should be prepared to address those cases. Refer to Chapter 19 for detailed information on diabetes management in athletes.

DISORDERED EATING, EATING DISORDERS, AND THE MALE AND FEMALE ATHLETE TRIADS

Disordered eating and eating disorders negatively impact health and performance. Athletes are at greater risk for developing eating disorders than nonathletes. Although experts do not know the exact prevalence of college athletes with eating disorders, studies on elite athletes show that approximately 18% to 25% of female athletes and 8% to 22% of male athletes met the criteria for eating disorders.[41] Reasons for this increased risk may include the stress of transitioning to college; critical comments from coaches, parents, judges, peers, or teammates; increased academic demands; the stress of losing scholarship or financial aid if they are injured or not able to participate in the sport; and pressures due to the technical, aesthetic, and other demands of sport.[42] Eating disorders and disordered eating are associated with serious health problems such as dehydration, electrolyte imbalance, depression, decreased bone density, cardiac arrhythmia, and death. Anorexia nervosa is a common eating disorder with the highest mortality rate of all psychiatric diseases. Greenleaf et al[43] studied 204 NCAA Division I female college athletes from 3 universities within the United States and found that 25.5% were symptomatic for eating disorders (some symptoms were reported but they were insufficient to warrant a clinical diagnosis) and 2% had eating disorders. These findings are consistent with other research on the prevalence of disordered eating and eating disorders in female college athletes. Reseachers observed no relationship between sport type and eating disorder classification, suggesting that eating disorders occur fairly consistently across different sports.

The NCAA collected information on 1,445 male and female student-athletes from 11 NCAA Division I schools and reported that, although the rates of clinical eating disorders based on *Diagnostic and Statistical Manual IV* criteria were low (0% for anorexia nervosa for both female and male athletes; 1.1% and 0% for bulimia for female and male athletes, respectively), the percentage of athletes at risk for disordered eating was significant (25% of female athletes and 9.5% of male athletes).[44] Eating disorders continue to be a problem that predominantly affects female athletes, but this study was unique in that it reported on the prevalence of eating disorders and the risk of disordered eating in male college student-athletes as well.

In 2014, DeSouza et al[45] published the 2014 Female Athlete Triad Coalition Consensus Statement defining the female athlete triad as a medical condition that involves 3 components: (1) LEA with or without disordered eating, (2) menstrual dysfunction, and (3) low bone mineral density. Although the prevalence of clinical eating disorders is low in female college athletes, many are at risk for disordered eating, which places them at increased risk for menstrual irregularity and bone injuries. Beals and Hill[46] examined the prevalence of the female athlete triad as characterized by disordered eating, menstrual dysfunction, and low bone mineral density among 112 female college athletes in 7 sports. They found that only 1 athlete met the criteria for all 3 disorders of the triad, but 28 athletes met the criteria for disordered eating, 29 athletes met the criteria for menstrual dysfunction, and 2 athletes had low bone mineral density.

Collegiate athletic departments know that disordered eating and the female athlete triad may have begun in athletes during the high school years and gone undiagnosed and untreated until the athlete reaches college. Kroshus et al[47] found that only 19% of high school nurses in the United States were able to identify the 3 components of the female athlete triad and only 25% said they work with coaches to help prevent health issues among female athletes. When determining awareness and knowledge of the triad and its health implications among female high school athletes and their coaches, Brown et al[48] found that triad risk factors were prevalent among athletes, but coach knowledge of the triad was limited.

The 2014 International Olympic Committee consensus statement: beyond the Female Athlete Triad—Relative Energy Deficiency in Sport (RED-S)[49] discussed the impact of inadequate energy intake on health and performance for female athletes and potentially for male athletes, including metabolic rate, menstrual function, bone health, immunity, protein synthesis, cardiovascular health, and psychological health caused by relative energy deficiency. The consensus statement reviews prevention, screening, diagnosis, treatment, and return-to-play recommendations and also includes information on male athletes.[49,50] In 2021, Nattiv et al[51] defined the male athlete triad as a medical condition that involves 3 components: (1) LEA with or without disordered eating, (2) functional hypothalamic hypogonadism, and (3) osteoporosis or low bone mineral density with or without bone stress injury. It is within the scope of care for collegiate sports dietitians to provide prevention, screening, and treatment for athletes with disordered eating and eating disorders.[52] *The NCAA Coaches Handbook: Managing the Female Athlete Triad* is a useful tool for educating athletic department coaches and staff about prevention, detection, and treatment of the female athlete triad.[53] Refer to Chapter 18 for more information on eating disorders in athletes.

Personal Concerns

The student-athlete may have a variety of personal, athletic, and health concerns that can affect nutritional status and, in turn, success as a college student. Personal concerns include transitioning to college life; struggling with the increased time demands of collegiate academics and athletics; navigating new food resources; managing budgets (depending on scholarship status and family resources); managing multiple relationships with coaches, teammates, teachers, family, and friends; and experiencing a lack of downtime for socializing and sleep. For many college athletes, this is the first time that they have lived without parents or guardians and have been solely responsible for their own food choices.

FOOD HABITS

College student-athletes bring with them 17 to 18 years of food and nutrition beliefs, preferences, and behaviors, some of which may help their health and athletic performance, and some of which may hinder them. Many individuals enter the adult life stage with an unhealthy dietary pattern already established from childhood and adolescence. *The Dietary Guidelines for Americans, 2020–2025 (DGA 2025),* describes the average fruit, vegetable, and dairy intakes for adolescent (14–18 years) and adult (19–30 years) individuals. Adolescents were shown to underconsume the recommended daily servings for fruits (1 serving per day; recommended 2–3 cups per day), vegetables (1 serving per day; recommended 3–4 cups per day), and dairy (1.5 servings for females and 2.5 servings for males per day; recommended 3 cups per day). Similar food-group consumption patterns were found for adults aged 19 through 59 years, with inadequate intake of fruit, vegetables, and dairy foods. Intakes of added sugars, sodium, and saturated fat exceeded the recommended guidelines for both age groups.[54]

The Healthy Eating Index (HEI) score is an overall measure of how well intakes align with *DGA 2025* as well as the components (food groups) of a healthy diet. The HEI score for adolescents and adults was found to be 51% and 56%, respectively. This low HEI score and underconsumption of fruits, vegetables, and dairy seen in adolescents increases the risk for nutrient deficiencies during a period of rapid growth and development. Balancing school and sport with other commitments, food cost, availability, and access are perceived barriers to healthy eating.[54]

FOOD AVAILABILITY AND INSECURITY

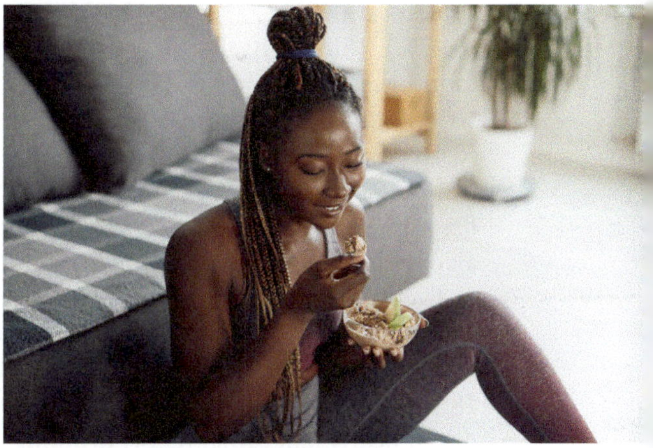

For students on campus for the first time, acclimating to dining hall food choices as a freshman may affect their nutritional status. Of note, international student-athletes may experience unique challenges in acclimating to the dining hall food choices. The sports dietitian may need to provide additional support in finding food choices with which the athlete is comfortable and that are part of their cultural food preferences. Students who move off-campus into a house or apartment in subsequent years and have to manage meal planning, grocery shopping, meal preparation, and food handling and storage for the first time may also face challenges. Athletes who live off-campus but do not have transportation may have decreased access to food, which can make it challenging for them to follow a sound training diet. In addition, an athlete on a limited budget may opt to use food money for other purposes, leaving little money for healthy meals. Because of a lack of published peer-reviewed studies and a wide variability in food resources available from school to school, limited data are available on food insecurity (FI) (defined as the lack of consistent access to safe and healthy food) in college student-athletes. Using the validated US Adult Food Security Survey Module, the USDA reported that 10.2% of US households in 2021 were food insecure.[55] Data on college students reported by Broton and Goldrick-Rab[56] suggested that more than half experienced some level of FI such as worry about not having enough to eat, not being able to afford balanced meals, and feeling hungry but not having enough to eat. In the ACHA-NCHA III survey, 10% of students surveyed responded that it was "often true" that "[i]n the last 30 days, the food I bought didn't last and I didn't have money to get more"; 13.1% said that it was "often true" that "[i]n the last 30 days, I couldn't afford to eat balanced meals"; and

4% answered affirmatively to the statement "[i]n the last 30 days, I cut the size of my meals or skipped meals because there wasn't enough money for food."[32]

One study found that the overall prevalence of FI in NCAA Division III student-athletes was 14.7%.[57] Poll et al[58] reported that, for male student-athletes at 1 Division I NCAA institution, FI during high school correlated with a preoccupation with food in college. Food insecurity during college was found to be significantly related to preoccupation with food and food hoarding in college, both risks for disordered eating. The authors concluded that FI among collegiate student-athletes exists and increases the risk for mental and physical health issues in addition to decreasing academic and athletic performance. More research using a validated tool to evaluate FI in collegiate student-athletes living outside of the traditional household referenced in the USDA survey model used in most studies is needed. Poll et al[58] recommended that student-athletes be evaluated for food security as part of annual screenings and that education and resources be provided for those at risk for or identified with FI.

NAME, IMAGE, AND LIKENESS (NIL)

New to the NCAA landscape is an interim policy, effective as of July 1, 2021, called Name, Image, and Likeness (NIL). This policy, which remains in effect until federal legislation is enacted, allows collegiate student-athletes to receive money for use of their name, image, and likeness when promoting a product or providing a service such as signing autographs or making a personal appearance.[59] This ability to make money needs to be balanced with the student-athlete's health and safety. For example, getting paid to promote a dietary supplement brand is now legal in the NCAA; however, student-athletes are still responsible for what they put in their bodies and are subject to testing for banned substances and drugs.

ALCOHOL AND DRUGS

Alcohol and drug use by college athletes is a major concern for athletic departments. Social pressures to use alcohol and drugs can jeopardize a student-athlete's athletic performance, health, and eligibility. Individuals involved in athletics are more likely to engage in a wide range of risky behaviors than are nonathletes.[60] According to the 2022 ACHA-NCHA III, alcohol use during the previous year by NCAA student-athletes (77%) was higher than alcohol use during the preceding 3 months by nonathletes (66.7%).[32] Similarly, the NCAA's 2018 National Study of Substance Use Habits of College Student-Athletes found that the overall use of alcohol during the preceding year by student-athletes decreased across all NCAA divisions from 83.1% in 2009 to 80.4% in 2013 and again to 77.1% in 2017.[22] Binge drinking (defined as 4 or more drinks for females or 5 or more drinks for males in 1 sitting) similarly decreased from 55% in 2009, to 51% in 2013, to 42% in 2017. More than half of NCAA student-athletes reported that first-time use of alcohol occurred in high school or earlier. Table 13.2 reports NCAA findings regarding alcohol use by NCAA Division I, II, and III student-athletes from 1993 to 2017.[22]

Even though some student-athletes continue to believe that their use of alcohol has no effect on athletic performance or general health and well-being, student-athletes are known to be at greater risk for abusing alcohol than their nonathlete peers, and they experience more frequent negative consequences. Interestingly, 18.1% of college student-athletes say they have never used alcohol, whereas for those student-athletes who drink, nearly half (46%) report drinking alcohol during both the offseason and the competitive season. Athletes who abstained from alcohol attributed their abstention mainly to concerns about health and athletic performance, to a desire to avoid alcohol's effects, or to their beliefs and values. The NCAA recommends prioritizing educational programming regarding the impact of alcohol use on athletic performance, academics, and health.[22,61] Box 13.4 describes the consequences of alcohol use on athletic performance.[62,63]

Excluding alcohol use, student-athletes are less likely to engage in social drug use than other college students. Self-reported drug use is highest among student-athletes who are male, play men's or women's lacrosse, or attend a Division III school.[22] Table 13.3 on page 324 reports the prevalence of substance use among student-athletes within the last year.

The hazards of tobacco use are well known. The NCAA bans the use of any tobacco product by all game personnel and all student-athletes during both practice and competitions. The 2022 ACHA-NCHA Undergraduate Student Reference Group Executive Summary reported that 21.2% of college students had used cigarettes in the preceding 3 months.[32] However, the NCAA's 2018 National Study of Substance Use Habits of College Student-Athletes reported that cigarette and marijuana use were lower in NCAA athletes compared to

TABLE 13.2 Alcohol Use (%) by National Collegiate Athletic Association Student-Athletes, 1993-2017[22]

Division	1993	1997	2001	2005	2009	2013	2017
Division I	86.3	79.2	80.5	74.3	81.7	78.4	74.5
Division II	89.1	79.7	78.8	74.9	81.5	79.3	74.5
Division III	93.2	82.6	83.3	81.6	85.3	83.3	81.1

BOX 13.4 Consequences of Alcohol Use on Athletic Performance[62,63]

Hydration	Alcohol is a powerful diuretic that increases urine output, leading to dehydration, and can delay rehydration. Dehydration weakens the pumping force of the heart, impairs temperature regulation, and accelerates fatigue, all of which contribute to decreased performance. Increased health risks of alcohol use during prolonged exercise in hot environments are also a concern.
Motor skills	Alcohol is a well-known depressant. It slows reaction time and impairs precision, equilibrium, hand-eye coordination, accuracy, balance, judgment, information processing, focus, stamina, strength, power, and speed; impairments can last up to 72 hours after alcohol intake.
Strength and power	Alcohol use can lead to decreased strength and power, decreased grip strength, decreased jump height, and faster time to fatigue during high-intensity exercise.
Recovery	Alcohol is a poor source of nutrients and may replace carbohydrates in the pre- and posttraining times, leading to impaired glycogen resynthesis, as well as decreased muscle protein synthesis and recovery. Alcohol disrupts sleep quality, further impairing recovery.
Risk of illness and injury	Athletes who drink alcohol have an elevated risk of injury. Regular alcohol consumption depresses immune function, increases swelling upon injury, and contributes to delayed healing.
Body composition and weight management	Body-fat accumulation due to the storage of ethanol as fat and the appetite stimulation effect of alcohol may lead to negative body composition changes and overall weight gain.
Effects of heavy, chronic alcohol consumption	Heavy alcohol consumption can cause nutritional deficiencies; altered digestion, absorption, and metabolism of nutrients; muscle damage, wasting, and weakness; and impaired ability to gain muscle mass and strength.
Long-term health	Long-term excessive alcohol consumption can cause pathological changes in the liver, heart, brain, and muscles that can lead to disability; nutritional deficiencies; altered digestion, absorption, and metabolism of nutrients; muscle damage, wasting, and weakness; and impaired ability to gain muscle mass and strength.

TABLE 13.3 Student-Athlete Substance Use Within the Last Year[22]

Substance	Rate of use
Marijuana	24.7%
Spit tobacco	13.4%
Cigarettes	10.5%
Cocaine	3.8%
Ecstasy	1.9%
LSD	1.7%
Amphetamines	1.5%
Heroin	0.2%

nonathletes. Moreover, cigarette use among Division I student-athletes decreased from 16% in 2009 to 10% in 2017. Marijuana use was higher among student-athletes who identified as living in a state in which it is legal for recreational or medical use. Self-reported reasons for marijuana use included social reasons, to aid sleep, anxiety or depression, and pain management. Spit tobacco use was also found to decrease slightly from 17% in 2009 to 13% in 2017 among all Division I college athletes. Spit tobacco use was greater in male than female athletes (22% and <1%, respectively) and highest in Division III athletes (14% in 2017). The most frequent spit tobacco users were found to be male athletes in ice hockey (46%), baseball (44%), lacrosse (35%), wrestling (33%), golf (23%), and football (22%).[22] Spit tobacco can lead to periodontal disease, loss of tooth structure, tooth staining, bad breath, and gum disease, as well an increased risk of oral cancer and leukoplakia.[64] Tobacco education and substance abuse prevention and intervention resources are available on the NCAA website (www.ncaa.org/health-and-safety/policy/drug-testing).[65]

THE ATHLETIC DEPARTMENT

Stakeholders

The NCAA sponsors 43 different sports that compete throughout the academic year in the fall, winter, and spring seasons. Sport profiles vary among Divisions I, II, and III as well as between conferences and individual campuses. Box 13.5 provides a list of men's and women's college sports.[66] On the campus level, a variety of services, operations, and personnel in and around the athletic department serve as strategic partners for the collegiate sports dietitian. Medical services personnel, coaching staff, athletic administrators, support service staff, and academic faculty can all be important sports nutrition stakeholders. Depending on the scope of service being provided, some or all of the department and campus stakeholders may be critical to the successful implementation of the nutrition mission or objectives. Key stakeholders are illustrated in Figure 13.1 on page 326.

MEDICAL SERVICES

Team physicians, orthopedic physicians, athletic trainers, and sport psychologists are important allies of the sports dietitian. Athletic trainers are an especially vital connection given their day-to-day involvement in student-athletes' medical care and overall team management. Establishing positive working relationships with these providers is crucial for the sports dietitian, as they can subsequently support and facilitate the collegiate sports dietitian's work with the individual athletes and teams. Similarly, campus health services often have clinical laboratories and onsite pharmacies with staff members who can become valuable colleagues for collaboration on nutrition-related biochemical screening protocols and over-the-counter dietary supplement or product purchasing. Some health centers may also have counseling and psychological services staff who can assist with the initial assessment and diagnosis of athletes with disordered eating. These providers can help identify proper referral outlets and bridge short-term and long-term care as needed.

COACHES

Coaching staffs, consisting of a head coach and assistant coaches, operations staff, and strength and conditioning coaches, are all obvious partners for the collegiate sports dietitian's work. Once these relationships

BOX 13.5 National Collegiate Athletic Association Championship and Nonchampionship Sponsored Sports

Men's championship sports

- Baseball
- Basketball
- Cross country
- Fencing (co-ed)
- Football
  - Football Bowl Subdivision (Division I only)
  - Football Championship Subdivision (Division I only)
- Golf
- Gymnastics (Division I and Division III only)
- Ice hockey
- Lacrosse
- Rifle (co-ed)
- Skiing (co-ed)
- Soccer
- Swimming/Diving
- Tennis
- Track, indoor
- Track, outdoor
- Volleyball
- Water polo
- Wrestling

Women's championship sports

- Basketball
- Beach volleyball
- Bowling
- Cross country
- Fencing (co-ed)
- Field hockey
- Golf
- Gymnastics
- Ice hockey
- Lacrosse
- Rifle (co-ed)
- Rowing
- Skiing (co-ed)
- Soccer
- Softball
- Swimming/diving
- Tennis
- Track, indoor
- Track, outdoor
- Volleyball
- Water polo

Men's nonchampionship sports

- Archery
- Badminton
- Bowling
- Equestrian
- Esports
- Rowing
- Rugby
- Sailing
- Squash

Women's emerging sports

- Acrobat and tumbling
- Equestrian
- Rugby
- Triathlon
- Wrestling

Other women's Sports

- Archery
- Badminton
- Esports
- Squash
- Synchronized swimming

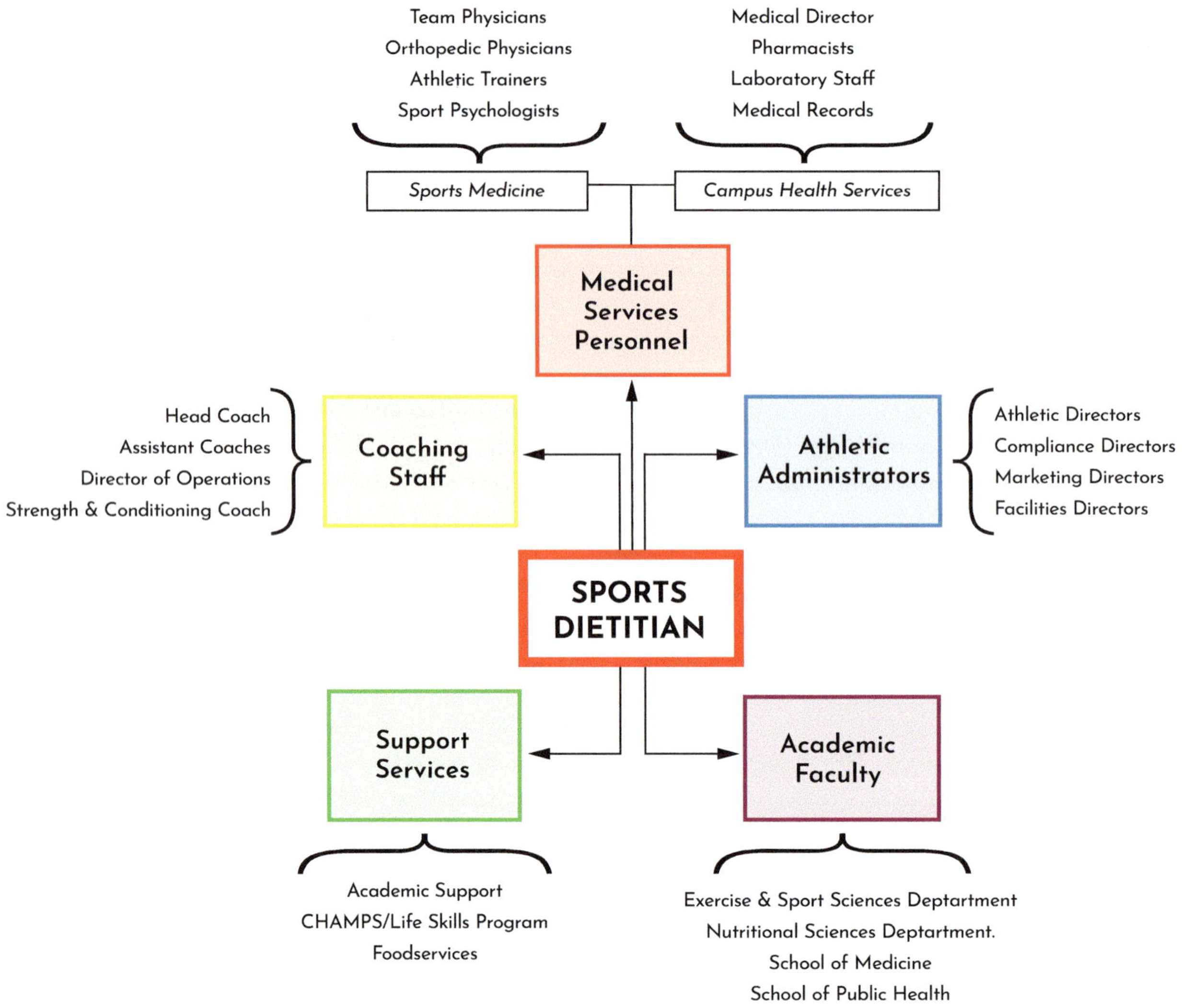

FIGURE 13.1 **Stakeholders in college athletics**

have been established, coaches will be more willing to allocate practice time to nutrition education, offer budgetary support toward nutrition priorities, and help facilitate a positive nutrition culture within the program. They can be vocal advocates of nutrition services and champion enhancement efforts to administration. In addition, coaches can promote sports nutrition in the recruiting process in an effort to set apart the comprehensive services offered by the college or university to help develop their student-athletes. Parents are often impressed when a nutrition program is part of the athletic environment and is available to support their young adults as they transition to campus life.

ADMINISTRATORS

Athletic administrators are key stakeholders in establishing and committing to nutrition services, as well as including food and nutrition practitioners in their department's philosophies. Athletic directors make the decision to invest in nutrition services and to offer them as part of the department's plan to carry out its mission. Compliance directors interpret and apply nutrition-related NCAA legislation at the campus level. They can also help identify available funding sources for special projects or needs (eg, student-athlete opportunity funds or NCAA grant monies). Marketing administrators can be especially valuable when considering contractual agreements with grocery, food retail, and supplement companies. Elements of these contracts can often be negotiated and structured to provide appropriate products or a level of support for nutrition services. These terms can potentially provide financial relief for team operating budgets, sports medicine supply lines, or nutrition department line items. Moreover, some administrators specifically oversee the construction or renovation of athletic facilities. The collegiate sports dietitian can suggest the inclusion of nutrition-related spaces, such as meal and training table spaces, easily accessible spaces for fueling stations, an area for cooking demonstrations, nutrition office and counseling space, and pre- and postworkout recovery spaces that include adequate food and product storage and food safety measures. Finally, most athletic departments work with a fundraising office and have a high-ranking administrator in the organizational structure who oversees the donor support relationships and funds. These administrators can identify potential program donors who may want to contribute to the development of nutrition-related projects or service growth.

UNIVERSITY SUPPORT SERVICES

Connecting with support services, such as academic support, the NCAA Life Skills program (www.ncaa.org/sports/2014/10/20/life-skills.aspx), and campus food services, can enhance and assist the collegiate sports dietitian in their goal of educating and feeding the student-athlete. In 2014, the NCAA reached out to its members to engage in collaborative efforts to renew the mission of the NCAA Life Skills program, namely, student-athlete wellness. Nutrition knowledge, skill, and education are priorities in the personal enhancement component of the program. Sports dietitians can support these institutional competencies by offering a variety of educational programming across classes and skill levels.

Because planning and coordinating meals is a major function of a collegiate sports dietitian, the campus foodservice vendor is a clear collaborator for the sports dietitian. The work of creating and implementing training tables and catered meals, as well as purchasing and distributing other food provisions, can be eased with strong relationships with foodservice personnel. The foodservice staff can also benefit from the RDN's involvement in providing expertise in recipe analysis and appropriate menu design.

ACADEMIC UNITS

Finally, interfacing with academic units on campus can provide cooperative associations with many benefits. For example, the RDN may be interested in and able to teach a class or lecture or to serve as a preceptor for nutrition students in return for the opportunity to create internships, independent studies, or experiential learning experiences. The intern and other students participating in these learning experiences can help the collegiate sports dietitian research special projects, create team education materials, manage fueling stations, and more. Moreover, the collegiate sports dietitian may be able to work collectively with the athletic and academic departments to create graduate assistant positions for students accepted into graduate programs and interested in gaining work experience as a sports dietitian. These positions can help train aspiring sports dietitians and provide additional staff support for service delivery. All of these undergraduate and graduate experiences supplement dietetics curricula and improve industry-specific readiness.

National Collegiate Athletic Association Compliance

To work in the field of sports nutrition at the collegiate level, sports dietitians need an understanding of NCAA rules and regulations. The NCAA, through various committee structures, incorporates legislative actions into adopted bylaws. These bylaws serve as the rules and regulations that govern the conduct of intercollegiate member institutions relating to athletic issues such as admissions, financial aid, eligibility, recruiting, and meals. Individual athletic departments are obligated to apply, adhere to, and enforce NCAA legislation. Each institution employs a compliance staff that oversees this function to ensure operational integrity. Most of the NCAA's nutrition-related legislation falls within the bylaws on financial aid, housing and meals, the banned drug list, and nutritional supplements. Box 13.6 on page 328 outlines the major nutrition-related bylaws.[67]

STUDENT-ATHLETE MEALS

Substantial changes in NCAA legislation surrounding athlete meals took place in 2014 and again in 2022. The NCAA removed restrictions on meals and snacks, effectively deregulating previous food limitations. Regulations governing meals and snacks provided by the athletic department were removed at the Division I level to offer more liberal use of whole foods to meet the unique nutritional needs of student-athletes. Meals were previously considered an extra benefit and limited to 1 meal per day per athlete, and snacks were limited to fruits, nuts, and bagels. Article 16 (Awards, Benefits, and Expense for Enrolled Student-Athletes, Bylaw 16.5 Housing and Meals) includes and defines applications related to allowable meals for student-athletes.

BOX 13.6 Division I Major Nutrition-Related Legislation of the National Collegiate Athletic Association[67]

Article 9.2.2 Division I Legislative Process

Bylaw 9.2.2.1.1 Authority to Adopt or Amend Legislation. The Atlantic Coast Conference, Big Ten Conference, Big 12 Conference, Pac-12 Conference, and Southeastern Conference and their member institutions shall have the authority to adopt or amend legislation that is identified as an area of autonomy.

Bylaw 9.2.2.1.2 Areas of Autonomy. The Atlantic Coast Conference, Big Ten Conference, Big 12 Conference, Pac-12 Conference, and Southeastern Conference and their member institutions are granted autonomy in the following areas to permit the use of resources to advance the legitimate educational or athletics-related needs of student-athletes and for legislative changes that will otherwise enhance student-athlete well-being:

(i) Health and Wellness. Legislation related to the health and wellness of student-athletes, including insurance and other items to permit appropriate and sufficient care.

(j) Meals and Nutrition. Legislation related to meals and nutritional demands for student-athletes.

Article 12 Amateurism and Athletics Eligibility

Bylaw 12.02.2 Actual and Necessary Expenses. Actual and necessary expenses are limited to:

(a) Meals;

(b) Lodging;

(c) Apparel, equipment, and supplies;

(d) Coaching and instruction;

(e) Health/medical insurance;

(f) Transportation (expenses to and from practice and competition, cost of transportation from home to training/practice site at the beginning of the season, preparation for an event and from training/practice/event site to home at the end of season/event);

(g) Medical treatment and physical therapy;

(h) Facility usage;

(i) Entry fees; and

(j) Other reasonable expenses.

Article 15.2 Elements of Financial Aid

Bylaw 15.2. Room and Board. An institution may provide a student-athlete financial aid that includes the cost of room and board, based on the official allowance for a room as listed in the institution's official publication (eg, catalog) and a board allowance that consists of 3 meals per day or the institution's maximum meal plan that is available to all students, whichever is greater.

Bylaw 15.2.2.1 Room and Board Stipend. An institution may provide the student-athlete an amount equal to the institution's official on-campus room allowance, the average of the room costs of all of its students living on campus or the cost of room as calculated based on its policies and procedures for calculating the cost of attendance for all students. The institution also may provide the student-athlete an amount that is equivalent to the value of the maximum meal plan that is available to all students or the cost of meals as calculated based on its policies and procedures for calculating the cost of attendance for all students.

Bylaw 15.2.2.3 Food Stamps. A grant-in-aid recipient who lives and eats off-campus may use the money provided for board to obtain governmental food stamps, provided the stamps are available to the student body in general. Additionally, the student-athlete must be eligible for such stamps without any special arrangements on the part of athletics department personnel or representatives of the institution's athletics interests.

Article 16 Awards, Benefits, and Expenses for Enrolled Student-Athletes

Bylaw 16.5.2 Permissible. [A] An institution may provide housing and meal benefits incidental to a student's participation in intercollegiate athletics as identified in this bylaw. [R]

Bylaw 16.5.2.3 [A] Meals and Snacks. An institution may provide meals and snacks to a student-athlete at any time. An institution shall not provide cash for a meal unless authorized by NCAA legislation. [R]

Bylaw 16.5.2.3.1 Meal Expenses in Conjunction with Competition and Practice Activities. [A] An institution may provide a student-athlete with cash for a meal in conjunction with competition or a meal missed due to practice activities in a manner consistent with cash provided by the institution to institutional staff members on away-from campus trips.

Bylaw 16.5.2.4 Meals Provided by a Representative of Athletics Interests. [A] A student-athlete or the entire team in a sport may receive an occasional meal from a representative of athletics interests on infrequent and special occasions.

Bylaw 16.5.2.5 Vacation-Period Expenses. [A] An institution may provide meals and lodging expenses to student-athletes (during official institutional vacation periods) for a reasonable period when student-athletes are required to remain in the locale of the institution for organized practice sessions or competition. If an institution does not provide a meal to its student-athletes under such circumstances, a cash allowance may be provided, not to exceed the amount provided by the institution to institutional staff members on away-from-campus trips. If a student-athlete lives at home during the vacation period, lodging expenses may not be provided by the institution. [R]

Bylaw 16.5.2.7 Nutritional Supplements. [A] An institution may provide permissible nutritional supplements to a student-athlete for the purpose of providing additional calories and electrolytes. Permissible nutritional supplements do not contain any NCAA banned substances and are identified according to the following classes: carbohydrate/electrolyte drinks, energy bars, carbohydrate boosters, protein supplements, omega-3 fatty acids, vitamins, and minerals. [R]

Article 16.8 Expenses Provided by the Institution for Practice and Competition [A]

Bylaw 16.8.1 Permissible. [A] An institution, conference or the NCAA may provide actual and necessary expenses to a student athlete to represent the institution in practice and competition (including expenses for activities/travel that are incidental to practice or competition). In order to receive competition-related expenses, the student-athlete must be eligible for practice. [D]

Article 16.10 Provision of Expenses by Individuals or Organizations Other Than the Institution [A]

Bylaw 16.10.3 Luncheon Meeting Expenses. [A] A student-athlete may accept transportation and meal expenses in conjunction with participation in a luncheon meeting of a booster club or civic organization, provided the meeting occurs within a 30-mile radius of the institution's main campus and no tangible award is provided to the student-athlete. [R]

Continued on next page

BOX 13.6 Division I Major Nutrition-Related Legislation of the National Collegiate Athletic Association[6] (CONTINUED)

Article 20.2 Active Membership

Bylaw 20.2.4.8 Drug-Testing Program and Consent Form. An active member institution shall administer annually, a drug testing consent form for each student-athlete (per Bylaw 12.02.14) pursuant to Bylaw 12.7.3 and shall ensure compliance with the following elements of the NCAA Drug-Testing Program: [D]

(f) Designate an individual (or individuals) as the athletics department resource for questions related to NCAA banned drugs and the use of nutritional supplements;

(g) Educate athletics department staff members who have regular interaction with student-athletes that:

(1) The NCAA maintains a list of banned drug classes and provides examples of banned substances in each drug class on the NCAA website; and

(2) Any nutritional supplement use may present risks to a student-athlete's health and eligibility; and

(3) Questions regarding NCAA banned drugs and the use of nutritional supplements should be referred to the institution's designated athletics department resource individual (or individuals).

Note that, in Box 13.6, "[A]" denotes a legislative provision that is an area of autonomy; "[D]" denotes an institutional violation for which the involved prospective or enrolled student-athlete's eligibility is not affected; and "[R]" denotes an institutional violation for which restitution is required from the prospective or enrolled student athlete.

The NCAA does not restrict the choice of meal, foods, or cost for the designated training table meals. (Training tables refer to meals served only to student-athletes in a closed setting. Refer to the Foodservice Management Responsibilities section later in this chapter for more information.) Division I institutions can provide meals and snacks at any time. These can be offered for breakfast, lunch, or dinner and can be specifically designed to meet the needs of the athletes. Each institution, team, or coach, in conjunction with the sports dietitian, should determine which meal(s) provide the most nutritional benefit to the athletes while also considering their academic, practice, and extracurricular schedules and meeting departmental budget parameters. Scholarship, recruited nonscholarship, and walk-on athletes who are members of the team are all eligible to participate in designated training table meals.

Additionally, if student-athletes miss a meal as a result of practice activities or an institutional committee meeting, they can still receive a training table meal. Athletes can be provided with meals associated with competition through the time at which they are released at the close of competition. The NCAA also deregulated when institutions can offer meals and snacks, stating that institutions can offer provisions during vacation periods and that athletes are eligible to receive meals or the cash value of the meals. Along with meals, fueling stations with whole foods, beverages, and grab-and-go–type foods are now available in many locker rooms and central athletic facilities. More information about fueling stations can be found in the Foodservice Management section.

As Division I removed meal and snack restrictions, Divisions II and III also revised regulations. In 2015, the NCAA lifted food restrictions for Division II schools as part of an evolving package of benefits for student-athletes. Across Division III, rather than providing food only on game days and road trips, schools are now able to supply athletes with permissible snacks following workouts and practices even in the offseason.

Subsidizing meal costs, training tables, meals incidental to participation, and unlimited snacks requires substantial investment from the athletic department, in terms of both finances and facilities. Ideally, training table meals should be served in an athletic facility convenient and accessible to athletes. However, if a specific athletic dining facility does not exist, training table or other meals can be catered and brought onsite or to any location. Often, teams will have meals delivered to their locker room or team room. Meals can be provided by campus foodservice providers or outside caterers, or local restaurants or athletic departments can opt to support a self-operation foodservice. The landscape has progressed since 1991, when the training table meal was limited to 1 per day, and from 2009, when the NCAA Housing and Meal Bylaw, Article 16.5, was amended to include provision of fruit, nuts, and bagels at any time.

This legislative progress offers great flexibility and opportunity for appropriate, high-quality food choices. However, the regulatory changes also bring potential operational and budgetary challenges to the athletic department and the collegiate sports dietitian. Armed with a sharp skill set and a full complement of knowledge, the collegiate sports dietitian is an excellent professional to assist in designing solutions to these food-related costs and operational challenges.

DIETARY SUPPLEMENTS

The use, purchase, and provision of dietary supplements by athletic departments is regulated by the NCAA. The relevant bylaw states that only permissible supplements can be provided for additional calories and electrolytes. Permissible supplements do not contain banned substances and are identified in 1 of 6 classes. The NCAA defines the 6 classes of permissible supplements an institution can purchase as follows:

- carbohydrate or electrolyte beverages
- energy bars
- carbohydrate boosters
- protein supplements
- omega-3 fatty acids
- vitamins and minerals

An updated banned substance list is released each year by the NCAA and can be accessed on the NCAA website in the drug testing information portion of the legislative and governance section. Stimulants, anabolic agents, and diuretics are examples of classes of banned substances.[68] The list also provides examples of banned substances in each class, but the list is not comprehensive. The NCAA maintains that student-athletes are responsible for anything they ingest. Therefore, each institution is required to identify a resource person working on campus to answer dietary supplement (and banned drug) questions from student-athletes and staff. The NCAA provides access to the Drug Free Sport AXIS (www.drugfreesport.com) for all member institutions. The collegiate sports dietitian can play a role in helping safeguard an individual's eligibility, as well as their health and safety, by establishing sound supplement product evaluation and review processes and helping student-athletes assess their risk of consuming a banned substance.

Impermissible supplements or ingredients are anything other than those listed in the 6 permissible classes and are not permitted for purchase by athletic departments. The following are examples of impermissible ingredients or supplements:

- amino acids
- conjugated linoleic acid
- creatine
- ginseng
- green tea

COLLEGIATE SPORTS DIETITIANS

Today's full-time collegiate sports dietitian typically wears many hats, including administrator, clinician, educator, foodservice coordinator, and academician (refer to Figure 13.2 on page 332). Because each athletic department and sports nutrition program or department is unique, the responsibilities of the collegiate sports dietitian can vary. As described in the *Standards of Practice (SOP) and Standards of Professional Performance (SOPP) for Registered Dietitian Nutritionists (RDNs) (Competent, Proficient, and Expert) in Sports and Human Performance*, there are 3 levels of practice in sports and human performance nutrition. Each is associated with specific knowledge, skills, and abilities, including for the *competent* practitioner who is just starting in the field, the *proficient* practitioner with 3 or more years of training and experience, and the *expert* practitioner who has built the highest level of skills, knowledge, and credentials.[69] Box 13.7 on page 332 defines the skills, responsibilities, and characteristics of competent-, proficient-, and expert-level sports nutrition practitioners.

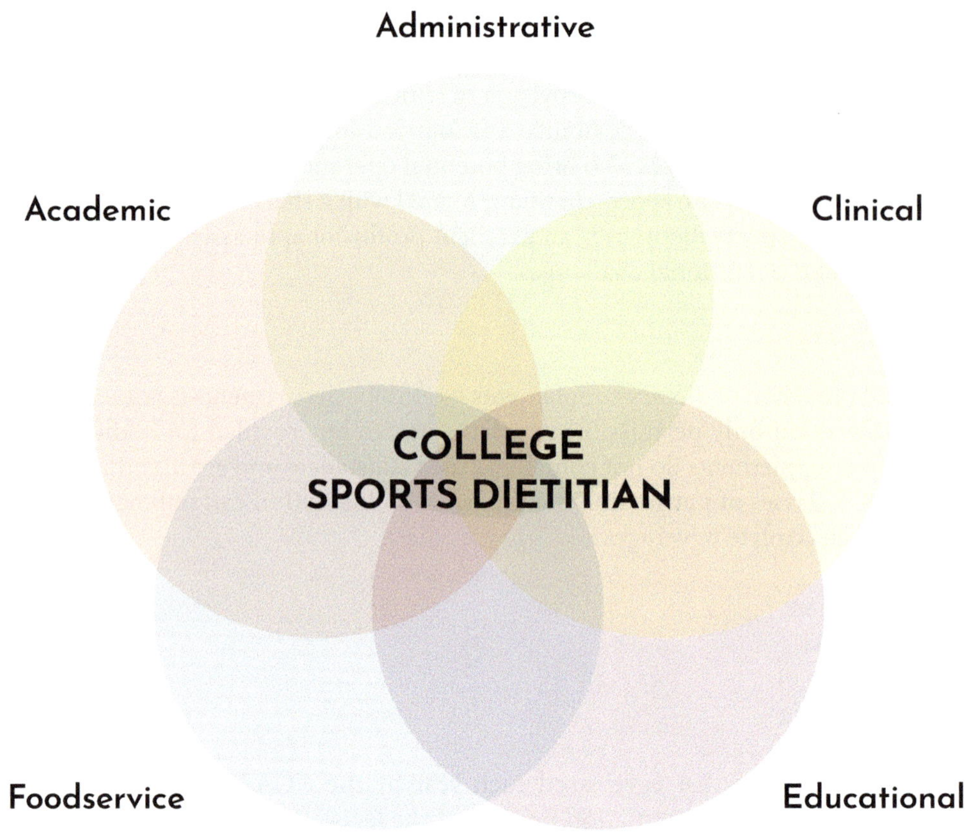

FIGURE 13.2 Roles and responsibilities of a full-time college sports dietitian

BOX 13.7 Definitions of Competent, Proficient, and Expert Sports Nutrition Practitioners[69]

Competent practitioner	A competent practitioner is a registered dietitian nutritionist (RDN) who is either just starting practice after having obtained RDN registration by the Commission on Dietetic Registration or an experienced RDN recently transitioning their practice to a new focus area of nutrition and dietetics.
Proficient practitioner	A proficient practitioner is an RDN who is generally 3 or more years beyond credentialing and consistently provides safe and reliable service, is successful in the RDN's chosen focus area of practice, and has obtained operational job performance skills. These RDNs demonstrate additional knowledge, skills, and experience. They may acquire specialist credentials to demonstrate proficiency in the focus area.
Expert practitioner	An expert practitioner is an RDN who is recognized within the profession and has mastered the highest degree of skill and knowledge in a focus area of nutrition and dietetics. The expert practitioner conducts and applies research to advance the body of knowledge and the development of best practices. As a recognized leader in the field, the expert RDN mentors students, other RDNs, and professionals and also advocates for the inclusion of nutrition concepts and professionals in sports and human performance. The expert-level practice is more complex, and the practitioner has a high degree of autonomy and responsibility.

As of 2024, a graduate degree (master's degree or doctorate) is required for all RDNs.[70] Additional coursework in exercise science, culinary nutrition, data science and research, and behavioral counseling can help the collegiate sports dietitian be successful. Many collegiate sports dietitians working with student-athletes have achieved the Board Certified Specialist in Sports Dietetics (CSSD) credential offered by the Commission on Dietetic Registration.

Competencies within the scope of practice of the collegiate sports dietitian that require lifelong learning and professional development include skill and experience in clinical nutrition, medical nutrition therapy, nutrition counseling, exercise physiology, foodservice management, and program administration. These competencies can help the sports dietitian successfully establish and manage the programming, operations, and management needs of collegiate sports nutrition programs and departments. The collegiate sports dietitian position is unique in that the role goes beyond clinical responsibilities and includes the administration and coordination of nutrition services compliant with NCAA guidelines and bylaws. These positions require a food and nutrition practitioner with experience working as part of a multidisciplinary team, counseling athletes on a variety of nutrition concerns ranging from medical diagnoses to everyday eating habits and performance fueling, and facilitating nutrition education seminars to diverse athletic groups. In addition, understanding sport-specific training schedules, the physiological demands of training and competing, common injuries, dietary supplement safety, body composition techniques, and team culture and beliefs of multiple sports teams is an important aspect of the collegiate sports dietitian position.

Collegiate sports dietitians provide nutrition programs and services for student-athletes competing in any of 43 different sports. Nutrition counseling, education, and fueling programs provided by collegiate sports dietitians to student-athletes can have the following benefits:

- enhanced adaptation to training
- prevention of fatigue
- optimized recovery from training and competition
- elevated exercise performance
- improved hydration status
- reduced risk of injury and illness
- achievement and maintenance of the desired body weight and body composition
- safe use of dietary supplements
- promotion of health and wellness

Although emphasizing sports nutrition strategies to enhance athletic performance, the collegiate sports dietitian is a jack-of-all-trades, both providing nutrition counseling and education for general health and providing nutrition intervention for medical diagnoses. The collegiate sports dietitian assists student-athletes in the following ways:

- advising food choices in the dining hall, at training table meals, before and after competition, and at the grocery store
- teaching menu planning, grocery shopping, and cooking skills for off-campus living
- providing medical nutrition therapy for individuals with diagnoses such as type 1 diabetes, celiac disease, gluten sensitivity, food allergies and intolerances, gastrointestinal disorders, and eating disorders

In addition to educating student-athletes, the collegiate sports dietitian educates coaches, athletic trainers, and other department personnel on the use of sports foods, drinks, and dietary supplements that are in compliance with the rules and bylaws of the NCAA.

The sports nutrition department model allows for the greatest impact and provision of a wider scope of services covering administrative, clinical, educational, foodservice management, and academic responsibilities.[52] The collegiate sports dietitian who works independently for a multisport athletic department (in either a full-time or part-time capacity) may narrow their focus to meeting the clinical and educational needs of the student-athlete population while serving only in a consultative manner on other administrative and foodservice projects. Some college and university athletic departments may choose, or may only be able to commit to, a consultant arrangement for collegiate sports dietitian services, in which case the collegiate sports dietitian most likely takes direction from the department's identified high-priority needs. The department's key stakeholders often help define these needs. In sum, collegiate sports dietitian services can be offered and delivered in a variety of arrangements based on the athletic department's resources and needs. The demand for high performers in these environments will likely continue to expand as student-athlete health and wellness are prioritized by the NCAA and athletic departments.

Administrative Responsibilities

Given the advancement of the collegiate athletics nutrition environment, full-time collegiate sports dietitians have assumed a great deal of administrative responsibilities in addition to carrying out the expected clinical and educational roles. Because collegiate sports nutrition programs frequently employ more than 1 sports dietitian, program- and people-management skills are critical to building an effective nutrition service model for the athletic department's multisport program. Leadership skills are needed to set mission, vision, values, and goals statements; participate in departmental strategic planning; and collaborate with campus programs (eg, campus dining, health services, academic departments). Some collegiate sports dietitians may hold the title of assistant or associate athletic director and serve on the athletic department leadership team. The nutrition program administrator manages personnel, including hiring and mentoring staff sports dietitians, delegating responsibilities to allow for staff autonomy, and serving as an expert in nutrition and dietetics.

Budget management responsibilities include developing an operating budget for the program, creating billing and invoice procedures, and monitoring department expenses. The collegiate sports dietitian negotiates and manages nutrition-related contracts with groups such as dietary supplement companies or local vendors to manage costs while ensuring optimal nutrition outcomes for the athletes. There may be potential for similar relationships and negotiations with laboratory services to test for iron deficiency, with grocery stores to become a primary vendor for preworkout and postworkout foods, and with distributors or nutritional supplement companies to provide practice and game-time hydration and recovery products. Being able to negotiate cost-effective purchases and contribute to sports marketing contract discussions allows the collegiate sports dietitian to offer added value to the athletic department and ultimately affect the delivery of high-quality, cost-effective nutrition to the student-athletes.

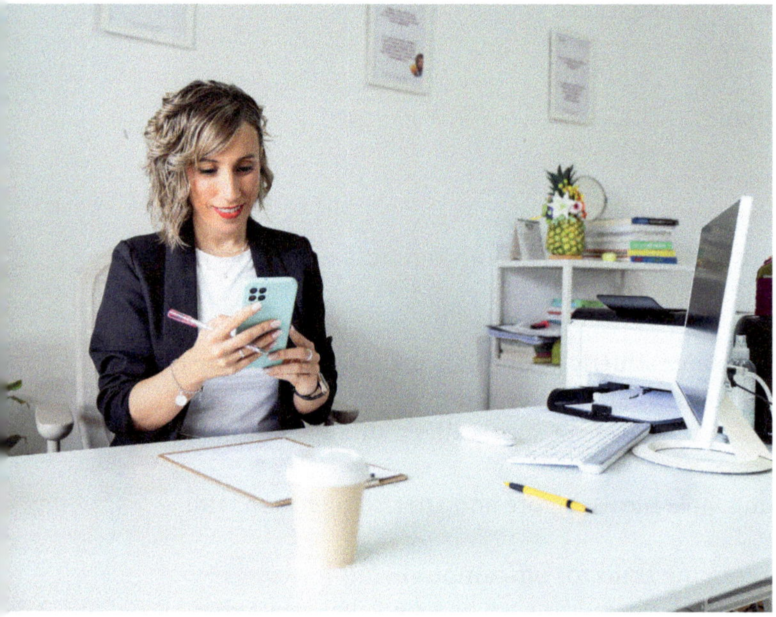

The management of clinical services includes supervising the provision of services and access to care, developing appropriate documentation processes, building secure and confidential services, and monitoring and implementing all federal and state regulatory requirements related to the practice of dietetics and foodservice. In addition, developing efficient appointment-scheduling procedures, identifying private nutrition counseling spaces, and determining consultation frequency and duration are part of managing clinical services. Services are used more often when athletes know where and how to find the collegiate sports dietitian and when services are offered. It is important to consider class schedules, treatment and practice times, and the athlete's path through campus when drafting an appointment schedule. For efficient scheduling, use an appointment service, online calendar and scheduling, and assistance from administrative support personnel and sports medicine clinics.

Collegiate sports dietitians develop policies and procedures that serve to standardize processes; educate coaches, student-athletes, and the performance team on evidence-based nutrition-related topics; and communicate programs and services to department staff. Relevant policies and procedures include:

- referrals to the collegiate sports dietitian;
- eating disorder prevention, detection, and treatment;
- dietary supplement review and education for NCAA compliance;

- weight and body composition assessment;
- iron deficiency prevention, screening, and treatment;
- relative energy deficiency in sport (REDs) screening, intervention, and monitoring;
- fueling station standard operating procedures;
- assessment of hydration status;
- nutrition intervention for bone health; and
- nutrition for injury rehabilitation and the return-to-play process.

The use of multidisciplinary treatment and performance teams can enhance communication and collaboration among providers and other support personnel to facilitate care for the student-athlete. Eating disorder treatment teams are crucial to managing the integrative nature of these diagnoses. Creating performance teams with coaches, athletic trainers, and strength and conditioning staff can be an effective way to communicate about an athlete's goals and progress while fostering respect for each discipline involved in the athlete's care. A body composition team may also be useful in some situations and with select teams.

The collegiate sports dietitian often functions as an athletic department representative. Recruiting events, campus committees, and community-sponsored functions are examples of situations in which the sports dietitian may be asked to participate and represent the athletic department. Serving as an ambassador for the department in a professional and collegial manner provides an opportunity to develop relationships inside and outside the department while building awareness of and furthering respect for the sports dietitian's expertise and services.

Clinical Responsibilities

In the clinical role, the sports dietitian provides medical nutrition therapy and individualized nutrition counseling to the student-athlete. Student-athletes self-refer for services or may be referred by another member of the athletic department. Reasons that a student-athlete may be referred to the sports dietitian include fatigue; poor eating habits; nutrient deficiencies (eg, iron, vitamin D); underhydration; weight management concerns; body composition assessment; iron deficiency; supplement questions; history of chronic dieting; food allergies and intolerances; vegan or vegetarian meal planning; gastrointestinal complaints; or medical diagnoses such as eating disorders, injury diabetes, high cholesterol, and hypertension. The collegiate sports dietitian can also refer student-athletes to the appropriate member of the athletic medicine team; campus resources; or off-campus resources, such as an eating disorder support group, as necessary. The collegiate sports dietitian assesses the student-athlete's dietary intake patterns and provides education and counseling to the student-athlete on appropriate nutrition strategies with the goals of managing medical diagnoses, optimizing performance, and promoting health. The dietitian works to develop rapport with the student-athlete and uses various counseling strategies, such as goal-setting, behavior modification, relapse prevention, cognitive behavioral therapy, and motivational interviewing. The sports dietitian has an arsenal of tools at their disposal, including evidence-based sports nutrition guidelines, medical nutrition therapy protocols for nutrition diagnoses, and best practices as determined by extensive practical experience in sports dietetics.

Collegiate sports dietitians participate in student-athlete preparticipation physicals by developing nutritional screening tools to identify athletes at risk for nutritional concerns. Screening questions can be used to identify weight and dieting history, meal and snack patterns, shopping habits and cooking skills, frequency of eating at restaurants, frequently consumed foods, and use of dietary supplements. The collegiate sports dietitian works closely with the athletic medicine staff to screen for nutrition-related issues such as iron deficiency anemia; weight management concerns; and risk for REDs, the female athlete triad, and eating disorders or disordered eating. Quatramoni[42] described collegiate athletes' vulnerability to nutritional risks due to the demands of sport and college life and recommended the Female Athlete Screening Tool to identify eating pathology for referral and intervention.[71]

Nutrition Education Responsibilities

As an educator, the collegiate sports dietitian develops and conducts nutrition education sessions encompassing nutrition for both general health and performance for sports teams, coaches, and athletic medicine staff, including athletic trainers, team physicians, physical therapists, and sports counselors. Providing nutrition education for coaches and athletic medicine staff helps to make sure everyone is on the same page and provides a consistent message to the student-athlete. Research has shown that nutrition knowledge plays an important role in adopting optimal nutrition practices, thus positively affecting athletic performance. Several studies have demonstrated that knowledge of correct performance nutrition and recovery principles among high school athletes, coaches, and incoming collegiate freshman student-athletes is limited or lacking.[72-75] Rockwell et al[76] assessed nutrition knowledge, opinions, and practices of coaches and athletic trainers from 21 sports at an NCAA Division I institution. Participants responded correctly to 67% of nutrition knowledge questions. Coaches and athletic trainers from women's sports gave more correct responses than those from men's sports. Coaches and athletic trainers who had 15 years or more of experience gave more correct responses than those with fewer years of experience. Torres-McGehee et al[77] reported that, of 579 Division I, II, and III participants surveyed, 77.8% of athletic trainers and 81.6% of strength and conditioning specialists had adequate sports nutrition knowledge, whereas 35.9% of coaches and 9% of student-athletes had adequate knowledge. Box 13.8 suggests topics for sports nutrition education relevant for student-athletes.[21,46,49,67,68,78-80]

Additional nutrition education approaches range from low to high tech and include the development of handouts and fact sheets, table tents, bulletin boards, newsletters, infographics, digital screens, websites, and blogs, as well as the use of social media platforms such as X (formerly Twitter), Instagram, Facebook, TikTok, Snapchat, and Pinterest. Handouts and fact sheets are great tools for team nutrition seminars, training tables, fueling stations, weight rooms, training rooms, and athletic medicine waiting rooms. Some collegiate sports dietitians develop their own handouts based on the needs of their student-athlete population, whereas others purchase or download resources from the internet. It is crucial for the collegiate sports dietitian to review all purchased or downloaded materials for credibility and appropriateness for the college student-athlete population. Fact sheets developed by RDNs through a collaboration between the NCAA, the Sports and Human Performance Nutrition (SHPN) dietetic practice group of the Academy of Nutrition and Dietetics, and the American Sports & Performance Dietitians Association (ASPDA) (formerly the Collegiate & Professional Sports Dietitians Association [CPSDA]) are available on the websites of the NCAA (www.ncaa.org), SHPN (www.shpndpg.org), and ASPDA/CPSDA (http://sportsrd.org). Additional sports nutrition-related websites can be found in Appendix B.

Collegiate sports dietitians can post high-visibility nutrition-themed articles or studies on a bulletin board in a training room, weight room, fueling station, training table, and/or medical clinic waiting area as another way to highlight relevant sports nutrition information. Actions such as posting recipes, resources, interactive quizzes, and contact information for the sports dietitian not only function to educate student-athletes and staff but also serve to market sports nutrition programs and services. Nutrition education topics to post in fueling stations are highlighted in Box 13.9 on page 338. Suggestions for point-of-service sports nutrition education topics for training tables are outlined in Box 13.10 on page 338.

Many collegiate sports dietitians have turned low-tech handouts and bulletin boards into electronic newsletters or blog topics. Some schools have their own nutrition channel through university television that can be posted at fueling stations, training tables, and other places around the athletic department such as the academic center or recruiting office. Posting information about sports nutrition services, hours, and contact information, as well as sports nutrition fact sheets on screens and departmental websites is a great way to leverage relevant technology. Videos of supermarket tours and cooking demos can also be included. Some schools have a password-protected website available for their student-athletes; for other schools, this information will be available to student-athletes and the general population who may be browsing the school's website. Allowing public access to these materials can be a useful recruiting tool. The combination of print and digital sports nutrition education and information adds to the athletic department's culture of performance improvement.

Foodservice Management Responsibilities

Foodservice management responsibilities for collegiate sports dietitians have increased dramatically because of changes in NCAA legislation (known commonly as "deregulation") on what types of foods and beverages athletic departments are permitted to provide to student-athletes and when they may provide them. The training table (meals served only to student-athletes in a closed setting) can be provided in an onsite athletic dining facility; in a residence dining hall; or catered to a locker room, team lounge, or other athletic space. In addition, athletic departments can now offer additional meals and unlimited snacks as part of athletic

BOX 13.8 Nutrition Education Topics for Student-Athletes[21,46,49,67,68,78-80]

Hydration	Provide education on hydration and performance as well as the signs and symptoms of dehydration. Weigh athletes privately before and after training. Inform athletes of their weight change and discuss sweating rate and daily fluid requirements. Reinforce ways to monitor hydration status, such as urine color and change in the weights measured before and after exercise.
Dining out	Collect menus for the team's favorite restaurants at home and on the road when traveling for competitions. Discuss how to make balanced meal choices, along with specific menu recommendations.
Dietary supplements	Review the National Collegiate Athletic Association (NCAA) banned drugs list and NCAA Bylaw 16.5.2 for lists of permissible supplement categories and impermissible ingredients.[67,68] Discuss the process used to evaluate dietary supplements for performance nutrition and NCAA compliance.[78,79] Bring products to evaluate, including examples that are banned, impermissible, and permissible. Encourage referrals to the team sports dietitian for dietary supplement evaluation to help the student-athlete make an informed choice about the safe and compliant use of dietary supplements.
Recovery nutrition	Present evidence on the role of nutrition in recovery. Show examples of foods, as well as permissible sports foods and supplements, that provide optimal carbohydrate, protein, micronutrients, and hydration for postexercise recovery.[21]
Eating disorders/ disordered eating	Provide annual education reviewing the prevention, detection, and management of eating disorders and disordered eating in athletes.[49,80] 1. Risk factors 2. Barriers to identifying disordered eating and eating disorders at an early stage 3. Signs and symptoms 4. Impact of disordered eating and eating disorders on health and performance 5. Resources available to help student-athletes 6. Ways to access treatment 7. What to say and what not to say 8. Best preemptive measures 9. Importance of optimal nutrition habits to reduce the risk of medical and performance consequences 10. Health and performance benefits of menstrual regularity for female athletes
Relative energy deficiency in sport (REDs)	Review the current literature on REDs and risk, including position statements from the Female Athlete Triad Coalition and the International Olympic Committee.[46,49] Discuss a multidisciplinary team approach to the prevention, screening, and treatment of REDs for athletes.
Iron screening protocol	Review why iron is important to health, cognition, and performance; symptoms of low iron; interpretation of iron laboratory results; iron-rich foods and foods that support or interfere with iron absorption; and iron supplement recommendations. Plan student-athlete education, follow-up, and documentation and reporting strategies.

BOX 13.9 Nutrition Education Topics for Fueling Stations

Fall

Navigating campus dining halls

The Freshman 15: is it real?

Meal planning for off-campus living

Grocery shopping 101

Fueling for preexercise

Are you hydrated?

Dining out

Winter

Vitamin D foods and supplements

What's new for the new year?

Eating disorders awareness week

March is National Nutrition Month

Quick and easy snack ideas

Nutrition for recovery

Spring/Summer

Sports foods and supplements

Breakfast is for champions

Frequently asked questions

Quick and easy meal solutions

Staying hydrated in the heat and humidity

BOX 13.10 Nutrition Education Topics for Training Tables

Weekly training table menus

Making the best choices at the training table

Are you hydrated?

The Athlete's Plate (from www.teamusa.org)

Hot topics in sports nutrition

Snack attack: how to fill nutrition gaps

Get the carbohydrate edge

Top 5 tips for fueling like a champion

Alcohol and performance do not mix

Fast food facts

Reading food labels: what athletes need to know

Dining out—world cuisine

Caffeine and athletic performance

Sports nutrition myths

participation. Many schools offer these additional foods and snacks at locations called fueling stations. Fueling stations can be set up as temporary or mobile food and supplement distribution points in locker rooms, weight rooms, concession stands, or other convenient locations, or they can be built into a fixed space to serve as a centralized location for multiple teams. Training tables and fueling stations are ideal locations for the collegiate sports dietitian to deliver nutrition education and help athletes select appropriate performance foods. Both are important examples of the planning, budgeting, and staffing responsibilities of the collegiate sports dietitian. Other examples of foodservice management responsibilities include:

- negotiating fair and appropriate meal costs for the training table;
- establishing food-quality and quantity standards;
- advocating for adequate staff and staffing patterns at the training table to provide optimal service;
- encouraging food-related data collection and forecasting models to achieve cost-effective operations;

- developing and reviewing cycle menus and suggesting alternative preparation methods or items to meet sports nutrition requirements and special dietary needs such as food allergies and intolerances, gastrointestinal diseases and other clinical diagnoses, and cultural and religious preferences;
- providing nutrition analysis of menu items and developing a format for posting nutrient and allergy information at point-of-sale;
- collaborating with training table staff to plan and deliver meals; and
- assisting operations staff in planning and coordinating foodservice needs for team travel and hotel stays, including menus, food quality, portion sizes, preparation methods, buffet arrangements, special dietary needs, and budget.

Academic Responsibilities

In addition to being an administrator, clinician, and educator, the proficient and expert dietitian working on a college campus has a unique opportunity to serve as a teacher and academician. The collegiate sports dietitian is often invited to provide guest lectures or teach a class for credit. Establishing working relationships with academic departments on campus can yield opportunities for sports nutrition research and publication, as well as collaborative equipment purchases, such as a BOD POD system for air displacement plethysmography or a DXA machine for body composition assessment. Additional academic opportunities include serving as a preceptor for students in dietetics or athletic training curricula, medical students in orthopedic rotations or sports medicine fellowships, and other sports medicine–related practicum experiences. As the demand for sports dietetics skills continues to increase, so does the need for additional training for this marketplace. Collegiate sports dietitians can establish and promote postgraduate fellowships, internships, and immersion experiences as important training grounds for the successful development of industry-specific skills.

SUMMARY

Student-athletes have unique personal, performance, and health-related concerns that can be challenging to balance. The collegiate sports dietitian can improve nutrition knowledge and help athletes eliminate nutrition-related barriers to optimal training, performance, and health. The role of the sports dietitian at the collegiate level has evolved into a recognized, accepted, and desired component of enhancing performance, assisting in health care needs, and safeguarding the student-athlete's eligibility. The sports dietitian has an opportunity to become highly involved throughout the athletic department and within the institution's academic environment. The athletic department houses many important stakeholders with whom collegiate sports dietitians need to collaborate to ensure success for nutrition services. College sports dietitians often do more than provide nutrition services to student-athletes; they also assume administrative, foodservice, and academic duties. The skills and experience needed to carry out full-time responsibilities and lead a department require an experienced RDN who is a proficient or expert practitioner. The opportunity to contribute to individual and team successes while becoming part of each sports team can be personally and professionally rewarding.

FUTURE DIRECTIONS

The demands and challenges for student-athletes and the scope of services for sports dietitians continue to evolve. The changing landscape of college athletics (eg, NIL, NCAA legislative and transfer changes, time demands) along with escalating mental health needs are present-day challenges that sports dietitians will need to find ways to incorporate and support. Additionally, much-needed attention on food insecurity concerns within this population should continue to be evaluated, promoted, and supported. An understanding of sports technology and of the interpretation of data from wearable devices will become critical for successful RDN integration into sport science and performance collaborations in the future. Behavior modification and communication skills will continue to be highly valuable in this sector. To help further develop future high-performing elite athletes, sports dietitians should aim for a well-prepared seat at the table.

Various nutrition service models ranging from full-time positions to consulting sports dietitians have emerged to meet the priority needs of departments across NCAA divisions and athletic departments. A variety of service models will be crucial to the continued growth and sustainability of the field. Differing models allow athletic administrators and departments to prioritize and scale their nutrition-related needs and budget allowances in today's economic climate. These same models will also allow pathways for development and opportunities for the evolution of practitioners across experience levels. The industry will strengthen its market by continuing to improve the depth and breadth of expertise and knowledge in all available opportunities. Postgraduate, expert-level training and experiences for RDNs will continue to be needed to keep pace with changing demands and to improve practitioner skill and readiness for the field.

As the market grows and the field is able to produce a steady flow of effective, well-rounded practitioners ready to continue accelerating the impacts of sports dietetics, industry standards need to be considered to reduce the variance in competency, skill, and RDN readiness for fully scoped roles. Additional advocacy efforts will continue to be needed to align sustainable staffing and scope-of-service models. Outcomes-based research and publication will greatly support field advancements and should be encouraged. Sports dietitians interested in working in the college athletics environment should focus on becoming experts in order to implement evidence-based recommendations for the health and human performance of groups and individuals.

KEY TAKEAWAYS

Student-athletes tackle the typical academic, social, health, and personal life stage concerns just like other college students, in addition to managing their training and competition schedules. Either of these domains can independently or collectively create a continuum of nutritional risk. RDNs can be an important resource while offering support and treatment for student-athletes.

Nutrition services can be more broadly implemented when the majority of athletic and campus stakeholder relationships are established and these individuals are engaged in the service's mission. Athletic trainers can be pivotal partners in the RDN's work.

Many NCAA meal and nutritional supplement bylaws govern the boundaries of these provisions. Collegiate sports dietitians should familiarize themselves with these regulations so they can recommend and implement appropriate services.

REFERENCES

1. Clark KL. Working with college athletes, coaches, and trainers at a major university. *Int Sport Nutr.* 1994;4(2):135-141. doi:10.1123/ijsn.4.2.135
2. American Sports and Performance Dietitians Association (ASPDA)/Collegiate & Professional Sports Dietitians Association (CPSDA). Full-Time Sports Dietitians list. Accessed November 6, 2022. https://sportsrd.org/career-development/full-time-sports-rds-working-with-usas-top-institutions
3. National Collegiate Athletic Association. NCAA Sports Sponsorship and Participation Rates Report (1956-57 through 2020-21). Posted December 1, 2021. Revised January 6, 2022. Accessed November 6, 2022. https://ncaaorg.s3.amazonaws.com/research/sportpart/2021RES_SportsSponsorshipParticipationRatesReport.pdf
4. Arnett JJ. Emerging adulthood: a theory of development from the late teens to the twenties. *Am Psychol.* 2000;55(5):469-480. doi:10.1037/0003-066X.55.5.469
5. Hochberg Z, Konner M. Emerging adulthood, a pre-adult life-history stage. *Front Endocrinol (Lausanne).* 2020;10:918. doi:10.3389/fendo.2019.00918
6. Knox R. The teen brain: it's just not grown up yet. Broadcast on Morning Edition, National Public Radio. Broadcast March 1, 2010. Accessed August 3, 2016. www.npr.org/templates/story/story.php?storyId=124119468
7. National Collegiate Athletic Association. NCAA Demographics Database 2011-12 through 2020-21. December 2021. Accessed November 20, 2022. www.ncaa.org/sports/2018/12/13/ncaa-demographics-database.aspx
8. Lee EC, Fragala M, Kavouras SA, Queen RM, Pryor JL, Casa DJ. Biomarkers in sports and exercise: tracking health, performance and recovery in athletes. *Strength Cond Res.* 2017;31(10):2920-2937. doi:10.1519/JSC.0000000000002122
9. Rosenbloom CA, Jonnalagadda SS, Skinner, R. Nutrition knowledge of collegiate athletes in a Division I National Collegiate Athletic Association institution. *Am Diet Assoc.* 2002;102(3):418-420. doi:10.1016/s0002-8223(02)90098-2
10. Pawlak R, Malinauskas B, Rivera D. Predicting intentions to eat a healthful diet by college baseball players: applying the theory of planned behavior. *Nutr Educ Behav.* 2009;41(5):334-349. doi:10.1016/j.jneb.2008.09.008
11. Hornstrom GR, Friesen CA, Ellery JE, Pike K. Nutrition knowledge, practices, attitudes and information sources of Mid-American Conference college softball players. *Food Nutr Sci.* 2011;2(2):109-117. doi:10.1016/s0002-8223(02)90098-2
12. Valliant MW, Emplaincourt HP, Wenzel RK, Garner BH. Nutrition education by a registered dietitian improves dietary intake and nutrition knowledge of a NCAA female volleyball team. *Nutrients.* 2012;4(6):505-516. doi:10.3390/nu4060506
13. Andrews A, Wojcik JR, Boyd JM, and Bowers CJ. Sports nutrition knowledge among mid-major Division I university student-athletes. *Nutr Metab.* 2016;2016:3172460. doi:10.1155/2016/3172460
14. Riviere AJ, Leach R, Mann H, et al. Nutrition knowledge of collegiate athletes in the United States and the impact of sports dietitians on related outcomes: a narrative review. *Nutrients.* 2021;13(6):1772. doi:10.3390/nu13061772
15. Thomas DT, Erdman KA, Burke LM. Position of the Academy of Nutrition and Dietetics, Dietitians of Canada, and the American College of Sports Medicine: nutrition and athletic performance. *Acad Nutr Diet.* 2016;116(3):501-528. doi:10.1016/j.jand.2015.12.006
16. Wade SM, Pope ZC, Simonson SR. How prepared are college freshman athletes for the rigors of strength and conditioning? A survey of college strength and conditioning coaches. *Strength Cond Res.* 2014;28(10):2746-2753. doi:10.1519/JSC.0000000000000473
17. Sim M, Garvican-Lewis LA, Cox GR, et al. Iron considerations for the athlete: a narrative review. *Eur Appl Physiol.* 2019;119:1463-1478. doi:10.1007/s00421-019-04157-y
18. Cowell BS, Rosenbloom CA, Skinner R, Summers SH. Policies on screening female athletes for iron deficiency in NCAA Division I-A institutions. *Int Sports Nutr Exerc Metab.* 2003;13(3):277-285. doi:10.1123/ijsnem.13.3.277
19. Rowland T. Iron deficiency in athletes: an update. *Am Lifestyle Med.* 2012;6(4):319-327. doi:10.1177/1559827611431541
20. Parks, RB, Hetzel SJ, Brooks MA. Iron deficiency and anemia among collegiate athletes: a retrospective chart review. *Med Sci Sports Exerc.* 2017;49(8):1711-1715. doi:10.1249/MSS.0000000000001259
21. Heaton LE, Davis JK, Rawson ES, et al. Selected in-season nutritional strategies to enhance recovery for team sport athletes: a practical overview. *Sports Med.* 2017;47:2201-2218. doi:10.1007/s40279-017-0759-2
22. National Collegiate Athletic Association. National Study on Substance Use Habits of College Student-Athletes. Executive Summary. June 2018. Accessed November 6, 2022. https://ncaaorg.s3.amazonaws.com/research/substance/2017RES_SubstanceUseExecutiveSummary.pdf
23. Barrack MT, Muster M, Nguyen J, Rafferty A, Lisagor T. An investigation of habitual dietary supplement use among 557 NCAA Division I athletes. *Am Coll Nutr.* 2020;39(7):619-627. doi:10.1080/07315724.2020.1713247
24. Froiland K, Koszewski W, Hingst J, Kopecky L. Nutritional supplement use among college athletes and their sources of information. *Int Sport Nutr Exerc Metab.* 2004;14(1):104-120. doi:10.1123/ijsnem.14.1.104
25. NCAA Sports Science Institute. NCAA Drug Testing Program 2022-23. National Collegiate Athletic Association. Summer 2022. Accessed November 24, 2022. https://ncaaorg.s3.amazonaws.com/ssi/substance/2022-23/2022-23SSI_DrugTestingProgram.pdf

26. Drug Free Sport International, The Drug Free Sport AXIS. Drug use prevention begins with expert education. Accessed October 20, 2023. www.drugfreesport.com/education/axis
27. United States Anti-Doping Agency (USADA). Supplement Connect. Accessed October 20, 2023. www.usada.org/athletes/substances/supplement-connect
28. Hootman JM, Dick R, Agel J. Epidemiology of collegiate injuries for 15 sports: summary and recommendations for injury prevention initiatives. *Athl Train.* 2007;42(2):311-319. PMID: 17710181
29. Wall BT, Morton JP, van Loon LJC. Strategies to maintain skeletal muscle mass in the injured athlete: nutritional considerations and exercise mimetics. *Eur Sport Sci.* 2015;15(1):53-62. doi:10.1080/17461391.2014.936326
30. Tipton K. Nutritional support for exercise-induced injuries. *Sports Med.* 2015;45(suppl 1):S93-S104. doi:10.1007/s40279-015-0398-4
31. Guideline 2e. Assessment of body composition. June 1991. Revised June 2002. In: *2014-15 NCAA Sports Medicine Handbook.* 25th ed. The National Collegiate Athletic Association; 2014:44-47. Accessed August 3, 2016. www.ncaapublications .com/productdownloads/MD15.pdf
32. American College Health Association. American College Health Association-National College Health Assessment III: Undergraduate Student Reference Group Executive Summary Spring 2022. American College Health Association; 2022. Accessed November 6, 2022. www.acha .org/NCHA/ACHA-NCHA_Data/Publications_and _Reports/NCHA/Data/Reports_ACHA-NCHAIII.aspx
33. Lloyd-Jones DM, Hong Y, Labarthe D, et al. Defining and setting national goals for cardiovascular health promotion and disease reduction: the American Heart Association's strategic Impact Goal through 2020 and beyond. *Circulation.* 2010;121(4):586-613. doi:10.1161/CIRCULATIONAHA.109.192703
34. Crawford M. Screening athletes for heart disease. *Heart.* 2007;93(7):875-879. doi:10.1136/hrt.2005.085365
35. Muñoz L, Norgan G, Rauschhuber M, et al. An exploratory study of cardiac health in college athletes. *Appl Nurs Res.* 2009;22(4):228-235. doi:10.1016/j.apnr.2008.02.008
36. Borchers JR, Clem KL, Habash DL, Nagaraja HN, Stokley LM, Best TM. Metabolic syndrome and insulin resistance in Division I collegiate football players. *Med Sci Sports Exerc.* 2009;41(12):2105-2110. doi:10.1249/MSS.0b013e3181abdfec
37. Sorenson SC, Romano R, Scholefield RM, et al. Holistic life span health outcomes among elite intercollegiate student athletes. *Athl Train.* 2014;49(5):684-695. doi:10.4085/1062-6050-49.3.18
38. Riddell MC, Scott SN, Fournier PA, et al. The competitive athlete with type 1 diabetes. *Diabetologia.* 2020;63(8):1475-1490. doi:10.1007/s00125-020-05183-8
39. American Diabetes Association position statement: standards of medical care in diabetes—2015. *Diabetes Care.* 2015;38(suppl 1):S1-S87. doi:10.2337/diaclin.33.2.97
40. Jimenez CC, Corcoran MH, Crawley JT, et al. National Athletic Trainers' Association position statement: management of the athlete with type 1 diabetes mellitus. *Athl Train.* 2007;42(4):536-545. PMID: 18176622
41. Joy E, Kussman A, Nattiv A. 2016 update on eating disorders in athletes: a comprehensive narrative review with a focus on clinical assessment and management. *Br Sports Med.* 2016;50(3):154-162. doi:10.1136/bjsports-2015-095735
42. Quatramoni PA. Clinical observations from nutrition services in college athletics. *Am Diet Assoc.* 2008;108(4):689-694. doi:10.1016/j.jada.2008.01.008
43. Greenleaf C, Petrie TA, Carter J, Reel JJ. Female collegiate athletes: prevalence of eating disorders and disordered eating behaviors. *Am Coll Health.* 2009;57(5):489-495. doi:10.3200/JACH.57.5.489-496
44. Johnson C, Powers PS, Dick R. Athletes and eating disorders: the National Collegiate Athletic Association study. *Int Eat Disord.* 1999;26(2):179-188. doi:10.1002 /(sici)1098-108x(199909)26:2<179::aid-eat7>3.0.co;2-z
45. DeSouza MJ, Nattiv A, Joy E, et al. 2014 Female Athlete Triad Coalition consensus statement on treatment and return to play of the female athlete triad: 1st international conference held in San Francisco, California, May 2012 and 2nd international conference held in Indianapolis, Indiana, May 2013. *Clin Sports Med.* 2014;48(4):289. doi:10.1136/bjsports-2013-093218
46. Beals KA, Hill AK. The prevalence of disordered eating, menstrual dysfunction and low bone mineral density among US collegiate athletes. *Int Sport Nutr Exerc Metab.* 2006;16(1):1-23. doi:10.1123/ijsnem.16.1.1
47. Kroshus E, Fischer AN, Nichols JF. Assessing the awareness and behaviors of U.S. high school nurses with respect to the female athlete triad. *Sch Nurs.* 2015;31(4):272-279. doi:10.1177/1059840514563760
48. Brown KN, Wengreen HJ, Beals KA. Knowledge of the female athlete triad and prevalence of triad risk factors among female high school athletes and their coaches. *Pediatr Adolesc Gynecol.* 2014;27(5):278-282. doi:10.1016/j.jpag.2013.11.014
49. Mountjoy M, Sundgot-Borgen J, Burke L, et al. The IOC consensus statement: beyond the Female Athlete Triad—Relative Energy Deficiency in Sport (RED-S). *Br Sports Med.* 2014;48(7):491-497. doi:10.1136/bjsports-2014-093502
50. Mountjoy, M, Sundgot-Borgen JK, Burke LM, et al. IOC consensus statement on relative energy deficiency in sport (RED-S): 2018 update. *Br Sports Med.* 2018;52:687-697. doi:10.1136/bjsports-2018-099193
51. Nattiv A, De Souza MJ, Koltun KJ, et al. The Male Athlete Triad-a consensus statement from the Female and Male Athlete Triad Coalition part 1: definition and scientific basis. *Clin Sport Med.* 2021;31(4):335-348. doi:10.1097/JSM.0000000000000946
52. Lambert V, Carbuhn A, Culp A, Ketterly J, Twombley B, White D. Interassociation consensus statement on sports nutrition models for the provision of nutrition services from registered dietitian nutritionists in collegiate athletics. *Athl Train.* 2022 Aug 1;57(8):717-732. doi:10.4085/1062-6050-0157.22
53. Sherman R, Thompson R; National Collegiate Athletic Association. NCAA Coaches Handbook: Managing the Female Athlete Triad. Accessed August 3, 2016. http://athletewellness.uncg.edu/wp-content /uploads/2014/05/Coaches-Handbook.pdf

54. US Department of Agriculture and US Department of Health and Human Services. *Dietary Guidelines for Americans, 2020-2025*. 9th ed. December 2020. Accessed November 6, 2022. www.dietaryguidelines.gov/sites/default/files/2021-03/Dietary_Guidelines_for_Americans_2020-2025.pdf
55. Coleman-Jensen A, Rabbitt MP, Gregory CA, Singh A. Household Food Security in the United States in 2021. US Department of Agriculture Economic Research Service. September 2022. Accessed November 30, 2022. www.ers.usda.gov/webdocs/publications/104656/err-309_summary.pdf?v=1688.4
56. Broton KM, Goldrick-Rab S. Going without: an exploration of food and housing insecurity among undergraduates. *Educ Res.* 2018;47(2):121-133. doi:10.3102/0013189x17741303
57. Brown ML, Karpinski C, Bragdon M, Mackenzie M, Abbey E. Prevalence of food insecurity in NCAA Division III collegiate athletes. *Am Coll Health.* 2023;71(5):1374-1380. doi:10.1080/07448481.2021.1942886
58. Poll KL, Holben DH, Valliant M, Joung HD. Food insecurity is associated with disordered eating behaviors in NCAA division 1 male collegiate athletes. *Am Coll Health.* 2020;68(2):105-109. doi:10.1080/07448481.2018.1529035
59. National Collegiate Athletic Association. NCAA adopts interim name, image and likeness policy. June 30, 2021. Accessed November 20, 2022. www.ncaa.org/news/2021/6/30/ncaa-adopts-interim-name-image-and-likeness-policy.aspx
60. Ford JA. Substance use among college athletes: a comparison based on sport/team affiliation. *Am Coll Health.* 2007;55(6):367-373. doi:10.3200/JACH.55.6.367-373
61. Bruce S, Wyrick DL. Best practices to address student-athlete alcohol abuse. Division III. National Collegiate Athletic Association Sport Science Institute. Accessed October 20, 2023. www.ncaa.org/sports/2014/10/10/best-practices-to-address-student-athlete-alcohol-abuse.aspx
62. American College of Sports position statement on the use of alcohol in sports. *Med Sci Sports Exerc.* 1982;14:ix-xi.
63. Vella LD, Cameron-Smith D. Alcohol, athletic performance and recovery. *Nutrients.* 2010;2(8):781-789. doi:10.3390/nu2080781
64. Burak LJ. Smokeless tobacco education for college athletes. *Phys Educ Recreat Dance.* 2001;72(1):37-45.
65. National Collegiate Athletic Association Sport Science Institute. Drug testing. Accessed October 20, 2023. www.ncaa.org/sports/2013/11/22/drug-testing.aspx
66. National Collegiate Athletic Association. NCAA Sports Sponsorship and Participation Rates Report. December 1, 2021. Revised Jan 6, 2022. Accessed November 6, 2022. https://ncaaorg.s3.amazonaws.com/research/sportpart/2021RES_SportsSponsorshipParticipationRatesReport.pdf
67. National Collegiate Athletic Association. 2022-2023 NCAA Division 1 Manual. NCAA. August 2022. Accessed November 14, 2022. www.ncaapublications.com/p-4657-2022-2023-ncaa-division-i-manual.aspx
68. National Collegiate Athletic Association. 2023-2024 NCAA Banned Substances. Accessed July 6, 2024. https://ncaaorg.s3.amazonaws.com/ssi/substance/2023-24/2023-24NCAA_BannedSubstances.pdf
69. Daigle K, Subach R, Valliant M. Academy of Nutrition and Dietetics: Revised 2021 Standards of Practice and Standards of Professional Performance for Registered Dietitian Nutritionists (Competent, Proficient, and Expert) in Sports and Human Performance Nutrition. *Acad Nutr Diet.* 2021;121(9):1813-1830.e55. doi:10.1016/j.jand.2021.04.018
70. Commission in Dietetic Registration (CDR). Accessed October 20, 2023. www.cdrnet.org
71. McNulty KY, Adams CH, Anderson JM, Affenito SG. Development and validation of a screening tool to identify eating disorders in female athletes. *Am Diet Assoc.* 2001;101(8):886-892. doi:10.1016/S0002-8223(01)00218-8
72. Alaunyte I, Perry JL, Aubrey T. Nutritional knowledge and eating habits of professional rugby league players: does knowledge translate into practice? *Int Soc Sports Nutr.* 2015;12:18. doi:10.1186/s12970-015-0082-y
73. Folasire OF, Akomolafe AA, Sanusi RA. Does nutrition knowledge and practice of athletes translate to enhanced athletic performance? Cross-sectional study amongst Nigerian undergraduate athletes. *Glob Health Sci.* 2015;7(5):215-225. doi:10.5539/gjhs.v7n5p215
74. Devlin BL, Belski R. Exploring general and sports nutrition and food knowledge in elite male Australian athletes. *Int Sport Nutr Exerc Metab.* 2015;25(3):225-232. doi:10.1123/ijsnem.2013-0259
75. Wade SM, Pope ZC, Simonson SR. How prepared are college freshman athletes for the rigors of college strength and conditioning? A survey of college strength and conditioning coaches. *Strength Cond Res.* 2014;28(10):2746-2753. doi:10.1519/JSC.0000000000000473
76. Rockwell SM, Nickols-Richardson SM, Thye F. Nutrition knowledge, opinions, and practices of coaches and athletic trainers at a Division I university. *Int Sports Nutr Exerc Metab.* 2001;11(2):174-185. doi:10.1123/ijsnem.11.2.174
77. Torres-McGehee TM, Pritchett KL, Zippel D, Minton DM, Cellamare A, Sibilia M. Sports nutrition knowledge among collegiate athletes, coaches, athletic trainers, and strength and conditioning specialists. *Athl Train.* 2012;47(2):205-211. doi:10.4085/1062-6050-47.2.205
78. Buell JL, Franks R, Ransone J, Powers ME, Laquale KM, Carlson-Phillips A. National Athletic Trainers' Association position statement: evaluation of dietary supplements for performance nutrition. *Athl Train.* 2013;48(1):124-136. doi:10.4085/1062-6050-48.1.16
79. Kersey RD, Elliot DL, Goldberg L, et al. National Athletic Trainers' Association position statement: anabolic-androgenic steroids. *Athl Train.* 2012;47(5):567-588. doi:10.4085/1062-6050-47.5.08
80. Bonci CM, Bonci LJ, Granger LR, et al. National Athletic Trainers' Association position statement: preventing, detecting, and managing disordered eating in athletes. *J Athl Train.* 2008;43(1):80–108. doi:10.4085/1062-6050-43.1.80

CHAPTER 14

Masters Athletes

Christine A. Rosenbloom, PhD, RDN, FAND

LEARNING OBJECTIVES

- Identify physiological changes associated with aging and describe why masters athletes are considered exemplars of optimal aging.
- Discuss considerations for determining energy requirements and macronutrient needs for masters athletes.
- Describe optimal protein intake for the masters athlete, including quantity, quality, and timing.
- Explain why water might be the most important nutrient for masters athletes and discuss challenges associated with euhydration.
- Review dietary supplements that may provide benefit to some masters athletes.

INTRODUCTION

What do athletes do when they get older and are no longer competitive in the sport they love? Many of them are taking on a new title: *masters athlete*. Events for masters athletes can range from sanctioned events provided through formal governing bodies, such as USA Track & Field, to the Huntsman World Senior Games held annually in Utah. In 2019, the World Senior Games hosted a record 11,119 athletes aged 50 years and older competing in 32 sports representing 32 countries, a substantial increase from the 500 athletes who competed in the inaugural senior games held in 1987. Almost every city and country in the world has an association devoted to masters athlete competitions. Box 14.1 provides an overview of some of the major organizations devoted to masters athletics.

WHO ARE MASTERS ATHLETES?

Many sports have masters divisions defined by the rules of the governing body (eg, USA Track & Field, World Masters Athletics, and the National Senior Games Association) or a separate organization designed to meet the needs of retired professional athletes (eg, the Professional Golfers' Association Tour Champions and the Association of Tennis Professionals Champions Tour). The age at which one becomes a "master" ranges from sport to sport and can be as young as 18 years (swimming) or as old as 50 years (golf). The World Masters Athletics organization defines the age for masters athletes as 35 years or older. Competition is also age-graded, usually in 5-year intervals. World Athletics (https://worldathletics.org) displays records for masters events in age-graded categories up to the 95- to 99-year-old group. The focus of this chapter is on masters athletes who are aged 50 years or older.

BOX 14.1 Examples of Masters Athlete Organizations

National Senior Games

www.nsga.com

History	Originated as the National Senior Olympics in 1985. First National Senior Olympics held in 1987 with 2,500 competitors. Name changed to the US National Senior Organization in 1990. Known today as the National Senior Games Association. Athletes must be aged 50 years or older and must qualify through National Senior Games Association State Games.
Sponsored activities	The National Games is a 20-sport biennial competition for men and women and is the largest multisport event in the world for seniors.

International Masters Games Association (IMGA)

www.imga.ch

History	The first World Masters Games was held in 1985. The governing body was reorganized in 1995 as the IMGA from member international federations to represent masters sports worldwide.
Sponsored activities	The World Masters Games, Winter World Masters Games, European Masters Games, Pan-American Masters Games, and Asia-Pacific Masters Games are held every 4 years. The inaugural Pan-American Masters Games, also called the Americas Masters Games, were held in 2016.

Huntsman World Senior Games

www.seniorgames.net

History	Began as the World Senior Games in 1987. Known today as the Huntsman World Senior Games. Open to any athletes aged 50 years or older.
Sponsored activities	Yearly competitions in St George, UT.

World Masters Athletics

https://world-masters-athletics.com

History	Started by middle-aged road runners; the first organized event was held in 1975. It has evolved into an international masters organization for track and field for those aged 35 years or older.
Sponsored activities	Area and world championships held in both stadia (within a stadium, such as track and field and track running events) and nonstadia (on the road, such as cross-country and longer-distance events).

AGING IN THE UNITED STATES

The US population is aging. In 2019, the number of people aged 65 years and older numbered 54.1 million, an increase of 14.4 million, or 36%, since 2009. In the US government–issued report *Profile of Older Americans 2020* the following statistics are presented[1]:

- In 2019, 3.8 million people celebrated their 65th birthdays, with population estimates of an annual net increase between 2018 and 2019 of 1.7 million people aged 65 years and older.
- People aged 65 years and older represented 16% of the population in 2019. This proportion is expected to increase to 21.6% by 2040.
- As of 2019, individuals reaching the age of 65 years had an average life expectancy of an additional 19.6 years (20.8 years for females and 18.2 years for males).
- There were more than 100,000 centenarians in 2019, more than triple the 1980 figure.

In 1900, there were 4.9 million people aged 60 years and older in the United States. That number had jumped to 45.8 million by 2000. Projections by the US Census Bureau estimate that there will be 94.7 million older adults in 2060.[1]

Aging is a global topic. Populations around the world are aging at a faster pace than in the past and this demographic transition will have an impact on almost all aspects of society. Already, more than 1 billion people are aged 60 years or older worldwide, leading the United Nations to declare 2021–2030 as the Decade of Healthy Ageing.[2]

The fitness industry is taking notice of the aging population. Gym and fitness memberships were previously concentrated in the 18- to 34-year-old range, but membership among those older than 50 years of age have increased. Gym franchises are finding it essential to appeal to older adults, and they have added amenities such as health maintenance services that include measuring and monitoring blood sugar, blood pressure, and bone density. The International Council on Active Aging challenges the fitness industry to see older adults not just as new customers but also as an abundant pool of talented people who are receptive to transitioning into a new career. Older adults can serve as personal trainers and provide a new wave of fitness entrepreneurs.[3]

Recent growth in masters competitions suggests increasing numbers of athletes in the future. In reviewing data for the New York City Marathon from 1983 through 1999, Jokl et al[4] showed that older age groups had the largest relative increase in participation and, as a group, masters athletes improved their performance times at a higher rate than younger athletes over the past 17 years. Older female athletes outpaced older male athletes in both participation and performance.

EXERCISE RECOMMENDATIONS AND BENEFIT OF EXERCISE IN ADULTS

In 1996, the US Surgeon General issued *Physical Activity and Health: A Report of the Surgeon General*,[5] the first report of its kind. In the same year, the World Health Organization issued *The Heidelberg Guidelines for Promoting Physical Activity Among Older Persons*,[6] stressing both the individual and the societal benefits of physical activity. The physical, mental, and societal benefits of a physically active lifestyle are summarized in Box 14.2.[5-8] These seminal reports concluded that regular physical activity induces higher cardiopulmonary fitness, which decreases overall mortality, reduces the risk of coronary heart disease and high blood pressure, reduces the risk of colon cancer, protects against the development of type 2 diabetes, builds bone mass, increases muscle strength and balance, helps control body weight, relieves the symptoms of depression and anxiety, and improves mood.[5,6]

Thirteen years after the initial government reports were released, the American College of Sports Medicine issued a position stand on exercise for older adults. The position stand concluded that older adults benefit from 4 types of physical activity: aerobic exercise training, resistance exercise, flexibility exercise to extend the range of motion in their joints, and balance training to strengthen the lower body to reduce the risk of falls. (Most of the evidence for this position stand was based on individuals aged 65 years and older, but younger adults were also included when relevant.)[7] The US Department of Health and Human Services has expanded the recommendations for physical activity to quantify that all adult Americans

BOX 14.2 Benefits of a Physically Active Lifestyle[5-8]

Physiological benefits

- Decreased resting blood pressure
- Increased cardiac output
- Increased blood flow to skeletal muscles and skin
- Increased maximal oxygen uptake (VO_2 max)
- Increased high-density lipoprotein cholesterol
- Increased components of the immune system, such as natural killer cells and circulating T lymphocytes and B lymphocytes
- Increased bone mass
- Increased strength and balance
- Normalized blood glucose levels

Health benefits

- Decreased overall mortality
- Decreased risk of cardiovascular disease
- Decreased risk of hypertension
- Decreased risk of thrombosis
- Decreased risk of colon cancer
- Decreased risk of type 2 diabetes
- Decreased risk of obesity
- Decreased risk of falls and fractures in older adults
- Decreased symptoms of depression and anxiety
- Improved sleep
- Enhanced relaxation
- Enhanced mood state
- Increased psychological well-being
- Enhanced social and cultural integration

Societal benefits

- Reduced health and social care costs
- Enhanced productivity of older adults
- A positive and active image of older adults

older than 65 years of age should get at least 150 minutes of moderate-intensity aerobic activity every week and perform muscle-strengthening activities that work the major muscles 2 or more times per week. Added health benefits are gained when older adults engage in physical activity beyond the equivalent of 300 minutes (5 hours) of moderate-intensity physical activity per week.[8] At every age, exercise induces beneficial physiological adaptations that improve functional abilities.

WHAT DO WE KNOW ABOUT AGING AND SPORT?

It is common to classify aging based on chronological age, but chronological age is a poor predictor of functional age. Someone may be 50 years old (chronological age), but because of a sedentary lifestyle, they may have difficulty performing activities of daily living (functional age). Maximal oxygen uptake (VO_2 max) is known to decrease with age and to decline further with advanced age. In addition to being a limiting factor of aerobic exercise performance, VO_2 max is a good predictor of cardiovascular and all-cause mortality. Declines in VO_2 max also contribute to frailty and functional decline.[9]

Peak performance in a sport depends on the key functional element required for success. For example, in sports such as gymnastics, for which flexibility is crucial, top athletes are usually in their teens. In aerobic sports, competitors usually peak in their mid-20s, when training improvements and competition experience help athletes; but, in general, most champions are not older than their middle to late 30s. In sports such as golf, the most successful athletes are generally in their 30s or 40s.

For some activities, aging may mean improved performance. For example, marathon times in older athletes have improved dramatically. Irishman Tommy Hughes set the over-60 marathon world record with a time of 2:30:02 in October 2020—a remarkable feat for the 60-year-old man, who averaged 5.75 minutes per mile over the 26.2-mile course.[10] Lepers and Cattagni[11] analyzed running times in the New York City Marathon from 1980 through 2009 and found that during that time period, not only did the participation of masters runners increase but the times of older runners also improved significantly (for men older than 64 years and women older than 44 years).The authors concluded that masters runners had "probably not yet reached their limits in marathon performance." In another example, Akkari et al[12] studied running and swimming times of masters athletes using data from masters organizations databases from 1975 through 2013. Age groups were separated into eight 5-year segments, spanning ages 40 to 79 years. They observed a progressive improvement in athletic event time that was significantly greater as age increased, leading them to conclude that not only was participation in masters competitions increasing but the performance of the athletes was also continuing to improve.

AGE-RELATED PHYSIOLOGICAL CHANGES

This section will review several age-related physiological changes and how these changes are attenuated in masters athletes. Research on masters athletes is frequently conducted on endurance athletes, and the physiological benefits of aerobic exercise are found in almost every body system. In general, the research on masters athletes shows that participation in competition at the masters level confers physical and psychological benefits.[12-19] Data are limited on many aspects of age changes in older athletes, but examples from the literature are cited when available.

Oxygen Uptake and Aerobic Capacity

VO_2 max decreases by about 10% per decade in healthy adults beginning at about the age of 30 years. In older endurance athletes, the decline is still evident, but it occurs at a lower rate of about 5% per decade.[13] Researchers note that it is hard to determine how much of this loss is due to the normal aging process or to the adoption of a more sedentary lifestyle. In addition, the rate of decline is not linear, with a 3% to 6% decline in early adulthood and a more rapid decline of more than 20% in those 70 years and older. In a longitudinal study of 42 athletes, Katzel et al[14] found a 22% decrease in VO_2 max in older endurance athletes during an 8-year follow-up period. The greatest decrease in VO_2 max occurred in athletes who could not maintain a high volume of training, suggesting that the decrease in VO_2 max is related less to aging and more to an inactive lifestyle. In this study, only 7 athletes (17% of study participants) were still training at high volume at the end of the study. The authors concluded that maintaining a high level of aerobic fitness, even for a highly motivated athlete, becomes more difficult with advancing age. Exercise can improve oxygen uptake, but even the most fit masters athlete will see some decline in oxygen uptake as they age.

Muscle Quantity and Quality

Muscle strength and function decline with age, termed *dynapenia* and *sarcopenia*, respectively. Although it is difficult to say exactly when these changes begin (as they depend on many factors, most importantly physical activity and general health), they are likely to begin in the fifth decade. Muscle loss proceeds at a rate of about 0.8% per year, and strength is lost at a rate of about 1% to 3% per year.[16] The average strength of individuals in their 80s is about 40% less than that of individuals in their 20s.[17] This difference is important because muscle strength is a strong predictor of several detrimental outcomes: slower gait speed, increased risk of falls, and increased risk of hospitalization and mortality. Compared to older adults with high muscle strength, older adults with low muscle strength have a 4.3-fold greater risk for slow gait speed and a 2.6-fold greater risk for severe mobility problems. Many changes at both the cellular and molecular levels appear to contribute to changes in aging muscle. These include a decrease in size and number of type II muscle fibers, a shift from fast to slow fiber type, reduced number of mitochondria, reduced number of satellite cells, infiltration of fat into muscle, reduction in myosin and protein content and function, and reduced elasticity of muscle.[18] Melov et al[19] reported that a 6-month resistance training program can reverse muscle weakness and improve muscle strength in healthy older adults. A Cochrane review of 121 randomized control trials including 6,700 participants showed that progressive resistance strength training is an effective intervention for improving physical functioning in older adults.[17] The relationship of these data to nutritional interventions is discussed later in this chapter.

Body Composition

As stated by Kuk et al[20] in their 2009 review, "[a]ging is a process that has deleterious effects in nearly every facet of human body composition." In general, aging results in:

- increases in belly (abdominal) fat;
- increases in fat deposits in skeletal and heart muscle, the liver, and bone marrow;
- increases in body weight until about the age of 70 years in both males and females; and
- the redistribution of body fat, with an increase in visceral fat and decreases in peripheral fat stores.

Many of these changes can be assessed with the typical anthropometric measures commonly available in outpatient settings (ie, body weight, waist circumference, skinfold measurements). What is unclear is if these changes are primarily due to lifestyle or mainly due to a combination of age-related physiological metabolic processes.

Researchers have not yet clearly demonstrated whether exercise negates all of these body composition changes because such an effect is not directly reported in the masters athlete literature. However, many studies on masters athletes designed to assess other physiological changes frequently report participants' weight, and percentages of body fat and lean mass as demographic information. A number of studies have shown that the body composition of masters athletes is more likely to have a higher percentage of lean body mass and less fat mass than that of their sedentary peers.[14,20-23]

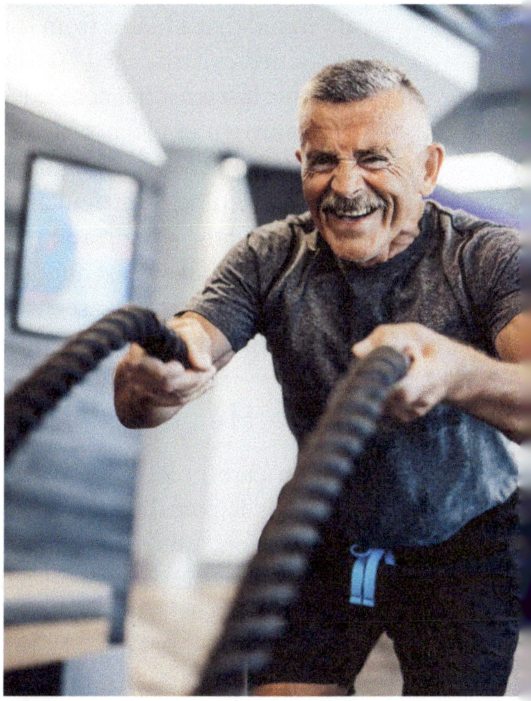

In addition to increases in adiposity that occur with aging, decreases in muscle mass are also observed. Wroblewski et al[21] were interested in determining whether chronic exercise practiced by masters athletes could attenuate changes in body composition. The researchers recruited 20 men and 20 women who trained for masters competitions at least 4 or 5 times per week. The athletes ranged in age from 40 years to older than 70 years (5 men and 5 women in each 10-year age group of 40–49 years, 50–59 years, 60–69 years, and 70 years and older). In this population, chronic exercise training preserved lean muscle mass while preventing fat infiltration into other tissues. Not all body composition changes were attenuated, as a slight increase in total body fat was observed. However, the study suggested that exercise training can help prevent some of the deleterious changes in body composition associated with aging. In a cross-sectional, observational study of 156 masters athletes (78 men aged 40–86 years and 78 women aged 40–77 years) participating in the Pan Pacific Masters Games, athletes volunteered to be evaluated for grip strength, gait speed, and anthropometrics, as well completing a general health questionnaire.[23] The primary results showed that both the male and female masters athletes had significantly better anthropometric, functional, and health characteristics than their age-matched peers in the general public.

Pratley et al[24] further elucidated changes in body composition, specifically waist-to-hip ratio, in masters athletes. Eleven aerobically trained men (aged 50–70 years) with average training (runners and triathletes) of 17 years were compared with 10 active but not regular exercisers. They showed that those who had participated in long-term aerobic exercise training were more insulin sensitive than sedentary individuals of similar age and body composition and that insulin sensitivity was independently related to a lower waist-to-hip ratio in the athletes. The researchers concluded that the higher insulin sensitivity related to

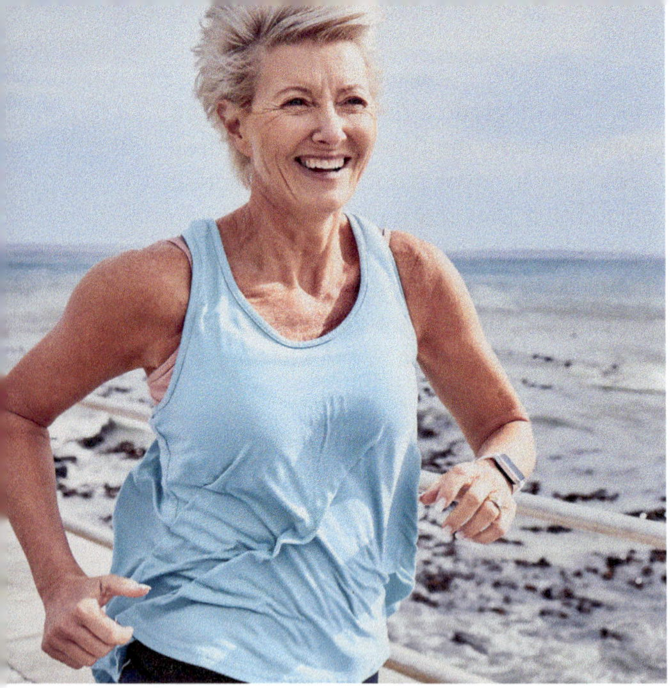

long-term exercise training prevents the accumulation of fat in abdominal sites.

Cardiovascular Health and Disease Risk

For years, aerobic exercise has been recommended to lower the risk of cardiovascular disease. Strong evidence shows that physical activity delays death from all causes. This includes the leading causes of death, such as heart disease and some cancers. Indeed, only a few lifestyle choices have as large an effect on mortality as physical activity. The most recent physical activity guidelines estimate that people who are physically active for approximately 150 minutes per week have a 33% lower risk of all-cause mortality than those who are not physically active.[8]

A longitudinal study on coronary heart disease (CHD) risk factors in older track athletes was reported by Mengelkoch et al.[15] Twenty-one participants aged 60 to 92 years were assessed at 3 evaluation points (initial, 10 years, and 20 years). Measurements included smoking history, blood pressure, resting electrocardiogram, total cholesterol, plasma glucose, body weight, percentage body fat, BMI, waist-to-hip ratio, and VO_2 max. All CHD risk factors remained low, and even after 20 years, all values for the variables measured were within normal limits. In this study, the prevalence of CHD risk factors remained low into old age in masters athletes, indicating that regular activity has a favorable effect on physical measurements that impact chronic disease risk.

Whereas exercise appears to offer benefits on lipid levels into old age in masters athletes, a study by Giada et al[25] found that a hiatus from training of just 2 months resulted in a reversal of the favorable lipid profile found in trained cyclists, aged 50 to 65 years. Similar to the decreases in VO_2 max found with decreased training volume, it seems that continued exercise is necessary to maintain a favorable lipid profile in older athletes.

Moorman et al[26] noted the potential double-edged sword for masters athletes related to heart health. The health benefits of regular physical activity are well documented; however, intense exercise can trigger life-threatening ventricular arrhythmias in the presence of underlying cardiovascular disease. Sudden cardiac death is the leading cause of sport- and exercise-related mortality in athletes, and about half of people who have heart attacks have no prior symptoms of heart disease. With newer technologies to detect underlying heart disease, Moorman et al[26] proposed a comprehensive risk assessment for older athletes, including tests such as coronary artery calcium scoring.

Bone Health

Health care practitioners are increasingly interested in bone health in the older population, and osteoporosis is considered a major public health concern. According to the Bone Health and Osteoporosis Foundation, approximately 54 million Americans 50 years of age and older are affected by low bone mass or osteoporosis. Half of all females and up to 1 in 4 males aged 50 years and older will break a bone due to osteoporosis.[27]

Exercise, especially weight-bearing exercise, confers benefits to bone mineral density (BMD). Loading the skeleton with weight improves the strength and density of bones.[7] Research with masters athletes has found that habitual physical exercise throughout life can help preserve bone health. Florindo et al[28] measured BMD in more than 300 Brazilian athletes 50 years of age and older and found significant positive associations between physical activity and bone mass density in older men.

Non–weight-bearing exercise, such as swimming, is thought to be less effective in protecting bone, but female runners and swimmers recruited from the 2005 National Senior Olympics were found to have *z* scores (which measure the difference between an individual's BMD and the average BMD for healthy people of the same age, ethnicity, and sex) that were much greater than the national average, suggesting that exercise has a positive effect on mediating bone loss in older women.[29]

To study bone health, 244 athletes (107 women and 137 men) were recruited at the World Masters Athletics Championship held in March 2019. The athletes were divided into 3 categories based on their events: endurance athletes, speed-power athletes, and throwing athletes. All athletes were regular participants in international athletic championships, had trained since their youth, and reported a current training frequency of at least 4 times per week. Dual-energy x-ray absorptiometry (DXA) was used to assess bone mass and BMD of the participants at 2 sites in the forearm. The results suggested that BMD and bone mass were strongly determined by the levels of lean body mass, intracellular water, and extracellular water and the type of training associated with the event. Regardless of sex, athletes from throwing sports had the highest body mass and BMD of the forearm bones. However, the prevalence of low DXA T-scores, representing greater decreases from the average peak BMD, especially among women, indicated a risk of fracture development in about half of this sample of masters athletes. The athletes involved in the strength-based sports had healthier BMDs, suggesting that participating in strength events slows the progress of bone loss and osteoporosis.[22]

Summary of Physiological Changes Associated With Aging

Currently, available research on all body systems and the benefits of physical activity in masters athletes is not abundant. Most of the studies involve athletes competing in endurance events (predominantly running and cycling), but research clearly shows that people who maintain an active lifestyle reap many physical health benefits. Chronic diseases such as cardiovascular disease, hypertension, and diabetes are less prevalent in masters athletes compared with age-matched sedentary persons. Changes considered typical consequences of aging, such as reduced muscle mass and strength, reduced aerobic capacity, bone loss, and deterioration of the insulin response to a glucose challenge, seem to be minimized in masters athletes because of their lifelong habit of physical activity.

In addition to physiological changes, cognitive function has become a topic of interest in masters athletes. Although studies have been limited to a small group of endurance masters athletes, those in middle and older age groups have been found to exhibit less cognitive decline and brain structural and functional deteriorations compared with age-matched sedentary adults.[30]

Masters athletes are seen as "exemplars" of successful aging and have much to teach about how to avoid the physical and mental deterioration that is often associated with typical aging.[30,31] As stated by Tanaka,[32] masters athletes "are the symbol of human strength, functional capacity, and resilience and might be the closest you can get to the fountain of youth!"

NUTRITIONAL CONSIDERATIONS IN MASTERS ATHLETES

Few studies exist that focus on nutrition in masters athletes. Sports dietitians and researchers in the field of sports medicine will find this area ripe for study to add to the scant body of literature. To support the contention for additional research, in 2019, Ratajczak et al[33] conducted a cross-sectional study during the 8th World Masters Indoor Athletics Championships held in Poland. They studied 86 male masters athletes (mean age of 50 years) from several European countries. Because masters athletes are thought to be exemplars of optimal aging, the authors expected the athletes' nutritional habits to align with their goals for peak performance. Diet quality was evaluated using food groups described as "healthy" and were representative of foods eaten in the athlete's country. Whereas 98% of the athletes described their diets as "good" or "very good," the results showed otherwise. Diet quality was based on the frequency of consuming 10 food groups noted in various guidelines for healthy dietary patterns. The results showed many "nutritional mistakes," which culminated in diets that did not support athletic performance. The authors noted that theirs was the first study to show that inappropriate food choices are also a common problem for masters athletes.

Energy Intake, Energy Expenditure, and Exercise

Evidence suggests that energy needs decrease with age. Approximately one-third of the decrease in energy needs is related to a decrease in basal metabolic rate (BMR) and the remainder is related to decreases in physical activity. However, most research on BMR in older adults does not include individuals who vigorously exercise. Even so, van Pelt et al[34] concluded that resting metabolic rate (RMR) decreases with age, even in highly active older men, but the decrease is related to age-associated decreases in exercise training volume and intensity.

The Dietary Reference Intakes (DRIs) for energy and macronutrient intakes established estimated energy requirements (EERs) at 4 levels of energy expenditure. However, even the category of "active" physical activity level, as described by the report *Dietary Reference Intakes for Energy*, may be too low for a masters athlete. Table 14.1 lists EERs for active older adults, which may be used to determine individualized energy needs.[35]

TABLE 14.1 Estimated Energy Requirements for Active Older Adults[35]

Age group, y	Males, kcal/d	Females, kcal/d
50-59	2,757	2,186
60-69	2,657	2,116
70-79	2,557	2,046
80-89	2,457	1,976

Few studies have assessed the energy needs of older athletes. In the studies that have tried to quantify energy needs, results have shown that energy needs do not differ for masters athletes compared with younger athletes.[36,37] The main factor predicting energy needs is the volume of exercise, not aging per se. Practitioners can use the same energy equations they use for younger athletes in assessing energy needs for older adults. However, practitioners must also accurately quantify activity when working with masters athletes because training tends to decrease in older athletes, and therefore, based on training volume, energy expenditure might not be as high. One review of energy expenditure and aging concluded that regular participation in physical activity (aerobic activities, primarily running) may attenuate the age-related decrease in RMR.[38] For a more detailed discussion on energy balance in athletes, refer to Chapter 10.

Studies have reported that exercise training increases the thermic effect of food (TEF) in older adults. Lundholm et al[39] studied active, well-conditioned men (mean age of 70 years) participating in aerobic exercise 3 to 5 times per week for at least 1 hour. Sedentary age- and weight-matched case controls were used for comparison. Participants were fed a liquid formula containing 500 kcal (56% carbohydrate, 24% protein, 20% fat), and BMR was measured. Higher oxygen uptake was found in the well-trained men compared with the sedentary control group, and the TEF of the former group was also significantly increased (by approximately 56%). The authors concluded that, in this study, physical activity seemed to have a potentiating effect on TEF in older people.

Although only a handful of studies on low energy intake in masters athletes have been published, the literature shows that many athletes underconsume energy for a variety of reasons. In older athletes, these reasons could include body composition concerns, not consuming enough calories for their specific sports energy requirements, or disordered eating behaviors. Low energy intake affects both male and female athletes. Low energy availability can lead to adverse physiological and psychological outcomes, potentially impairing an athlete's health and sports performance.[40] Masters athletes may be challenged to maintain sufficient energy intake to support training, competition, and recovery, leading to an energy deficit and low intakes of macronutrients and micronutrients.[41] Refer to Chapter 18, Eating Disorders in Athletes, for additional information.

Carbohydrate

Carbohydrate should provide the major source of energy in any athlete's diet (see Chapter 2). The DRIs suggest an intake of 45% to 65% of total energy from carbohydrate.[35] Although no ideal level of carbohydrate consumption has been defined for masters athletes, the guidelines used for younger athletes should be recommended: 3 to 5 g per kilogram of body weight per day for very light, low-intensity skill exercise; 5 to 7 g per kilogram of body weight per day for moderate-intensity exercise and for those training for about 1 hour per day; and 6 to 10 g per kilogram of body weight per day for endurance athletes who train at moderate intensity for 1 to 3 h/d. Flexibility is important in establishing carbohydrate goals, recognizing that individual preferences, as well as training and competition schedules, may necessitate adjustment of the carbohydrate intake. To meet fuel needs and general nutrition goals, athletes who exercise for less than 1 h/d with moderate-intensity activity or for several hours per day with low-intensity exercise should aim for 3 to 5 g per kilogram of body weight per day.[42] Currently, there is no reason to believe that masters athletes would not benefit from the same carbohydrate recommendations based on studies of younger adult athletes.[43] As discussed in Chapter 2, these recommendations should be adjusted for each athlete based on their energy needs, their specific training needs, and feedback from their training performance.

Many masters athletes may be confused about the role of carbohydrate in sport because they have been exposed to media messages that promote low-carbohydrate diets while extolling the virtues of protein. Drastically cutting carbohydrate intake may diminish an athlete's performance. Aiming for quality carbohydrates at every meal (whole grains, fruits, vegetables, and dairy) is one strategy to help athletes consume adequate carbohydrate to meet the demands of training and competition, maintain energy balance, and reduce risk for some chronic diseases.

Protein

The debate surrounding the protein needs of exercising individuals is not new, but the context of aging poses the question: What are the dietary protein requirements of masters athletes? Although research on protein metabolism has progressed over the past decade, there is still controversy on the exact amount of dietary protein needed to support optimal aging and the demands of masters athletics. Nutrition and resistance exercise are both needed to stimulate muscle protein synthesis (MPS); however, older adults may need higher intakes of protein than younger adults to stimulate MPS.[16,44,45] Aging is associated with dual issues of impairment in the muscle protein anabolic response to feeding and the synthesis of muscle protein in response to all types of exercise.[45]

The term *anabolic resistance* is used to describe the decreased sensitivity of muscle to small amounts of dietary protein in aging individuals.[44] Doering et al[46] have shown that masters athletes have lower integrated rates of MPS compared to younger athletes during intense endurance training when paired with high protein intake. Mounting evidence, supported by several consensus statements, suggests that the Recommended Dietary Allowance (RDA) for protein (0.8 g per kilogram of body weight) is inadequate to promote optimal health in older adults.[47] In addition, research indicates that the timing and distribution of protein throughout the day is important for stimulating MPS and maintaining muscle mass and function in older adults.[45,46]

In young men, 20 g of protein is the suggested amount per meal to stimulate MPS, but in older adults, the necessary amount appears to be greater, at about 35 to 40 g of protein per meal.[47] Moore et al[44] suggest 0.4 g of protein per kilogram if body weight per meal or 1.2 g of protein per kilogram of body weight per day, along with resistance exercise, to overcome anabolic resistance. In contrast, most adults consume less than 15 g of protein at breakfast, whereas the evening meal typically contains more than 60% of daily protein.[48] Ingesting specific quantities of protein at each meal, equally spaced throughout the day, appears to confer the greatest advantage for MPS for older adults.

The European Geriatric Medicine Society appointed an international study group to review dietary protein needs and aging. The PROT-AGE Study Group made the following recommendations[49]:

- To maintain and regain muscle, older adults (>65 years) should consume 1.0 to 1.2 g of protein per kilogram of body weight per day.
- The premeal anabolic threshold of dietary protein and amino acid intake is higher in older adults compared with younger adults, and recommended intake for healthy older adults is 25 to 30 g of protein per meal, including 2.5 to 2.8 g of leucine.

In addition, Doering et al[46] suggested that masters endurance athletes consume leucine-rich protein sources in the range of 35 to 40 g, or approximately 0.40 g per kilogram of body mass, after hard exercise to support muscle repair and remodeling. They suggested that it may be beneficial for masters athletes to spread protein evenly throughout the day in 4 meals. For more information on protein and the amino acid leucine as they relate to athletes, refer to Chapter 3.

Fat

The recommended daily intake of fat for athletes is approximately 1 g per kilogram of body weight. The recommended fat intake for active older adults does not differ from that for younger adults. An intake of 20% of energy from fat ensures adequate intake of essential fatty acids, with 30% to 35% of energy from fat as the upper limit recommended by most professional health organizations. The DRIs suggest fat ranges from 20% to 35% of total energy.[35] The *Dietary Guidelines for Americans, 2020–2025* recommends limiting saturated fats to 10% of calories and replacing saturated fats with unsaturated fats. The limits on dietary cholesterol are not emphasized; however, dietary cholesterol should be considered within the context of a healthy eating plan. Many foods that are high in cholesterol are also high in saturated fats. Two exceptions are eggs and shellfish, which, although high in cholesterol, are low in saturated fats and provide good sources of high-quality protein for aging athletes.[50]

Overview of Micronutrients

The DRIs recognize the need for differing amounts of some micronutrients in people older than 50 years of age. The DRIs for vitamins B6, B12, and D and the mineral calcium are higher for older adults, and the DRI for iron is decreased for older females.[51] Deficiencies in micronutrients can impair exercise tolerance, but little is known about the dietary intakes or requirements for masters athletes.

Few studies have assessed nutrient intakes in masters athletes. Nieman et al[52] studied completed 3-day food records from 291 masters men and 56 masters women who participated in the 1987 Los Angeles Marathon. Nieman et al found that the female runners had low intakes of vitamin D and zinc compared with the RDA.

A handful of other studies have found that even though masters athletes consume more calories than sedentary age-matched individuals and more than predicted energy intakes based on the national dietary guidelines, masters athletes are not meeting all of the nutrient intake targets. Specifically, they generally have low intakes of vitamins D and E, folic acid, calcium, zinc, and magnesium.[53,54] Additional studies to assess micronutrient intakes in masters athletes are needed.

Hydration

Masters athletes should pay particular attention to hydration status for the following reasons:

- Older adults have less body water than younger adults. Body water decreases to about 60% to 70% of total body mass in older adults, from a high of 80% in infancy.[55]
- Thirst sensation decreases with age with a blunting of thirst in response to dehydration. Body water regulation relies on thirst to control water intake.[56]
- After the age of 40 years, renal mass declines with a subsequent decrease in renal blood flow. The ability of an older person's kidneys to concentrate urine decreases, meaning that more water is needed to remove waste products.[56]
- Sweat glands change as the skin ages, with less sweat being produced per gland with aging.[57]
- An increase in plasma osmolality at rest occurs with aging, so that more time is required to restore body fluids in the face of dehydration.[56,57]

Normal age-related changes in thirst and fluid regulation, coupled with the increased need for fluids in the exercising individual, make this a focal topic for masters athletes. Box 14.3 provides hydration tips for older adults exercising in hot or humid conditions.[56-59]

In addition to normal age-related changes in hydration status, common medications used by older adults may affect total body water. Nonsteroidal anti-inflammatory drugs, commonly used for mild to moderate pain, inhibit not only the prostaglandins involved in pain and inflammation but also those involved in normal renal function. Some medications may blunt the thirst effect (such as selective serotonin reuptake inhibitors), and some drugs and herbal supplements increase urinary output (eg, thiazide diuretics, ginseng, saw palmetto, St John's wort, and wheatgrass).[60] Masters athletes should be aware of the effects of medications on hydration.

DIETARY SUPPLEMENTS

Dietary supplements are marketed to older adults for a variety of reasons, often as "antiaging" treatments. Although no dietary supplement is truly antiaging, a few supplements may be helpful to some masters athletes.

BOX 14.3 Fluid Tips for Older Athletes in Hot or Humid Conditions[56-59]

Acclimate	Perform about half of your usual exercise on the first few days of hot weather. Decrease the duration or slow the pace, and then gradually build back up.
Hydrate	Drink approximately 16 oz of fluid 30 to 40 minutes before exercise and at least 8 oz every 15 minutes during exercise. Weigh yourself before and after exercise. After exercise, drink enough fluid to get back to, or near, the preexercise weight over a 2-hour period. Eat foods with high water content. Use a sports drink to restore lost electrolytes and keep the "drive to drink" alive.
Use common sense	If you are concerned that it is too hot to exercise, consider foregoing the outdoor activity.
Learn about exercise in the heat	Pay attention to warning signs and symptoms of dehydration, heat exhaustion, and heat stroke.

Antioxidants

Antioxidant supplements are frequently touted to improve performance and help reduce oxidative damage resulting from exercise. If exercise *does* have a downside, it is the production of free radicals during strenuous activity. Although the body increases its natural antioxidant defense systems in the face of activity, it is unclear whether the body's natural defenses are sufficient to fight free-radical production without additional antioxidants obtained from supplements.[61] Increasing antioxidant-rich foods in the diet is one way to increase these nutrients. However, it is often difficult to get the DRI for vitamin E of 15 mg without including plant oils, seeds, and nuts. Although the evidence for using antioxidant supplements to combat free-radical production is equivocal, using the Tolerable Upper Intake Level (UL) established in the DRIs (2,000 mg of vitamin C and 1,000 mg of vitamin E) can provide guidance for a sports dietitian working with masters athletes.[51] This is not to suggest that the UL is the recommended intake, but if athletes supplement with these vitamins, the UL can be a guide to help the dietitian recognize if the level of supplementation is excessive. For more information on antioxidants, see Chapter 5 on vitamins, minerals, and exercise.

Creatine

Creatine is a dietary supplement popular with athletes (see Chapter 7). Some evidence supports adding creatine during strength training to augment physiological adaptations to exercise in older adults.[62,63] Levels of creatine and phosphocreatine in skeletal muscle decrease with aging, and phosphocreatine regeneration following exercise falls by about 8% per decade after the age of 30 years.[64] Candow et al[63] conducted a meta-analysis on creatine supplementation during resistance training in individuals 50 years of age and older. They concluded that creatine supplementation resulted in greater training capacity, leading to muscle accretion and strength gains in older adults who were strength training. Combining creatine with resistance training could be an effective lifestyle intervention to combat the sarcopenia of aging. Even though the literature on creatine supplementation for muscle function in older adults shows favorable effects, the effect is minimal without resistance training. There is research to suggest that creatine could be a therapeutic tool in combating age-related sarcopenia, but this does not apply to masters athletes, as exercise is the preferred way to avoid sarcopenia.[62-64]

Omega-3 Fatty Acids

An area of emerging research regarding older athletes is supplementation with omega-3 fatty acids. Sarcopenia is thought to be associated with chronic low-level inflammation, and omega-3 fatty acid supplementation can help reduce inflammation.[47] Whether supplementation will help older athletes maintain or build muscle has yet to be established, and supplementation with omega-3 fats in the prevention of inflammatory disorders has shown disappointing results. However, there is a theoretical basis for such supplementation.

In a study with a small sample size (N = 16), healthy older adults (>65 years) were randomized to receive 4 g of Lovaza (containing 1.86 g of eicosapentaenoic acid and 1.5 g of docosahexaenoic acid) or corn oil. The rate of muscle protein synthesis and anabolic signaling pathways were evaluated before and after the 8-week study. The group receiving the omega-3 fatty acids exhibited hyperaminoacidemia (high levels of amino acid in the blood) and an increase in the activation of muscle signaling pathways.[65]

Research on the role of omega-3 fatty acids and anabolic resistance and recovery from hard training in older athletes is also an area of interest. Even though the theoretical reasoning for supplementation is sound, there is little evidence to suggest that high doses of omega-3 fatty acids exceeding the current recommendations for the general population (250 to 500 mg of EPA + DHA per day) enhance exercise performance in older persons.[66] More research needs to be conducted before supplementation is recommended, but such supplementation could provide a relatively inexpensive way to support muscle mass with aging.

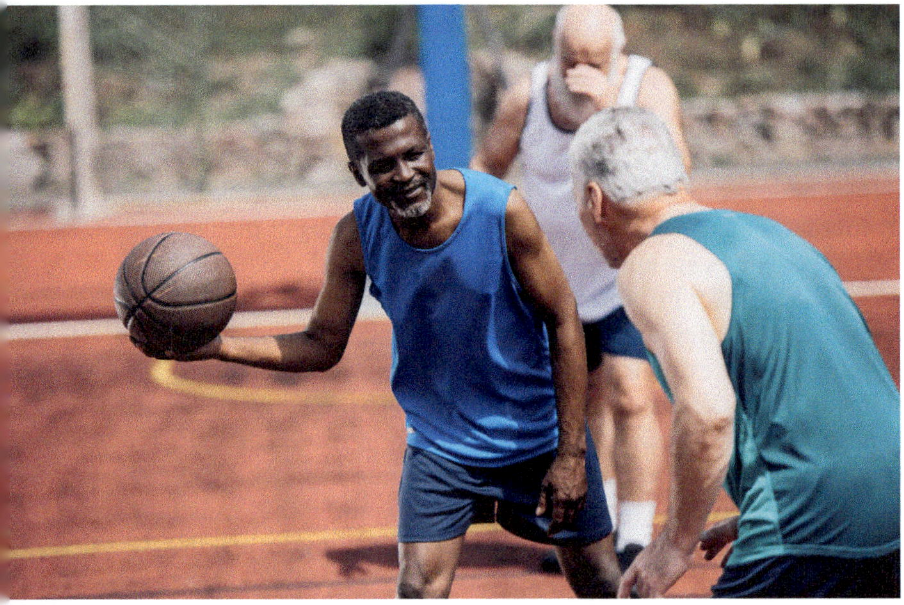

Nicotinamide ribose (NR) is an additional supplement of interest that can increase levels of the coenzyme nicotinamide adenine dinucleotide (NAD).[67,68] NAD is found in every cell of the body, and its levels decline with age. Exercise demands higher energy expenditure and, therefore, a higher turnover of adenosine triphosphate (ATP) and a higher demand for NAD to regenerate ATP. NR has gained attention because of its role as a direct precursor for NAD^+ synthesis in skeletal muscle and because it is thought to impact skeletal muscle mitochondrial function. To date, most research with NR has been performed in animal models and preclinical trials with small numbers of test subjects. However, a recent small randomized controlled trial using 500 mg of NR twice a day in healthy middle-aged and older adults found it to be well tolerated and effective in raising NAD levels (vs placebo). It is too early to say that NR supplementation will improve exercise tolerance in masters athletes, but preliminary research shows a benefit for reducing blood pressure and arterial stiffness, which could indirectly benefit exercise performance.[69] NR is generally recognized as safe by the US Food & Drug Administration.[68]

Banned Substances

As is the case for younger athletes, some governing bodies test masters athletes for banned substances. This practice is not without controversy because many of the drugs on banned substances lists are medications commonly used by older adults to treat disease. For example, aromatase inhibitors, including letrozole (Femara) and anastrozole (Arimidex), and selective estrogen receptor modulators, including tamoxifen, are on the banned substances list. These drugs are used by breast cancer survivors, and although athletes can apply for a therapeutic use exemption, many may not realize that a drug prescribed by a physician could be considered doping to gain an advantage in sport.

Dietary supplements claiming to boost testosterone can fall into the banned substances category, and some masters athletes may not realize that supplements can contain banned substances. Moreover, more than 30 US states have legalized cannabis for medical and/or recreational use, so masters athletes should know that it is considered a banned substance by the World Anti-Doping Agency.

For a complete list of banned substances, see the World Anti-Doping Agency website (www.wada-ama.org/en). In addition, Chapter 7 provides more information on supplements and sports foods.

ACCOMPLISHMENTS OF AGING ATHLETES

The aging of the population brings challenges and opportunities for athletes. Today, older people run marathons, climb mountains, sky dive, swim competitively, and hike the 2,160-mile Appalachian Trail. Consider these accomplishments by masters athletes:

- Diana Nyad, at the age of 64 years, swam 110 miles from Cuba to Florida, completing 53 hours of nonstop swimming after 4 previous failed attempts.
- Dara Torres is the first-ever US swimmer to compete in 5 Olympic Games, and she medaled 3 times in the 2008 Beijing Olympics at 41 years of age.
- Eamonn Coghlan, a dominating indoor runner in the mid-1970s and 1980s, was the first man older than 40 years to break the 4-minute mile.
- Randy Johnson, a pitcher for the Arizona Diamondbacks, threw a perfect game at 40 years of age—the oldest player to do so. His last pitch was clocked at 98 miles per hour.
- Priscilla Welch, a 58-year-old lifelong marathoner, was named the best female masters marathoner in history by *Runner's World*. At 42 years of age, she won the overall women's title at the New York City Marathon, the oldest woman to claim that honor.
- Gina Little, 77 years of age, of London, completed 602 marathons to become the oldest person to finish all 6 Abbott World Marathon Majors.
- Haile Sataylin of Israel made history when he competed in the 2008 Olympic Games in the men's marathon at 53 years of age.
- Phil Shipp of Arizona won the gold medal in the decathlon at the USA Track & Field Masters meet at 86 years of age.
- Sister Madonna Buder, known as the "Iron Nun," is the oldest person to finish an Ironman Triathlon within the 17-hour time limit, which she did in 2008 at 77 years of age. She is still active at the age of 91 years.
- Yuichiro Miura of Japan became the oldest person to summit Mount Everest at 80 years of age in 2013. He first set the record in 2003 at 70 years of age and reclaimed the record when he was 80 years old. In 2023, he successfully reached the summit of Mt Fuji when he was 90 years old, completing the 3-day trek in a specially-designed mountaineering wheelchair.

SUMMARY

Masters athletes may well be models of optimal aging. Engaging in physical activities into old age has protective effects on the body and erases what is often called usual aging. If a pill existed to preserve physical and mental function with aging, exercise might be it. To date, much of the research on masters athletes has been conducted with male athletes engaging in aerobic activities associated with track and field events. Diversity in studying masters athletes would be welcomed to help practitioners understand how to transfer knowledge on the benefits of exercise to a broader population.

Even though there is research on the physiological benefits of participating in masters athletics, very little is known on dietary intakes and recommendations for appropriate dietary patterns in a diverse population of older athletes. Sports dietitians are encouraged to seek out masters athletes groups to conduct research on dietary intakes to help inform recommendations for optimal macronutrient and micronutrient intakes.

KEY TAKEAWAYS

The evidence is clear that many older people can maintain a vigorous active lifestyle. Although research on the nutritional needs of masters athletes has been minimal, several conclusions can be drawn.

Aging has deleterious effects on almost all body systems, but regular physical activity appears to lessen most of these age-related changes.

Metabolic rate is driven by lean tissue and physical activity.

Older adults who remain physically active have the same needs for energy as active younger athletes. Energy intake should be adjusted when training volume decreases.

Fluid may be the most important nutrient for masters athletes. A programmed schedule of drinking can reduce the risk for dehydration without overconsumption of fluids.

Carbohydrate and fat recommendations are the same for older athletes as for younger athletes, and adjustments should be made based on duration and intensity of exercise.

Protein needs appear to be higher in older adults. Distributing protein intake throughout the day with approximately equal intakes at each meal may help to overcome the anabolic resistance of aging muscle.

Older adults should pay special attention to vitamin and mineral intakes. A multivitamin and mineral supplement formulated for seniors may be a good addition to supplement dietary intake. Senior-formulated vitamin and mineral supplements contain less iron and more vitamins B12, B6, and D compared with those targeted for younger adults.

Masters athletes in competition may be drug tested for banned substances. Several drugs commonly used to treat chronic diseases are on the banned substance list; therefore, masters athletes may need a therapeutic use exemption if they take certain prescription medications.

REFERENCES

1. Administration for Community Living, US Department of Health and Human Services. *2020 Profile of Older Americans.* May 2021. Accessed August 30, 2022. https://acl.gov/sites/default/files/Profile%20of%20OA/2020ProfileOlderAmericans_RevisedFinal.pdf
2. World Health Organization. WHO's Work on the UN Decade of Healthy Ageing (2021-2030). Accessed August 30, 2022. www.who.int/initiatives/decade-of-healthy-ageing
3. International Council on Active Aging. The older population is set to transform the fitness industry. ICAA blog. Posted July 2018. Accessed August 30, 2022. www.icaa.cc/blog/2018-07/The-older-population-is-set-to-transform-the-fitness-industry.htm
4. Jokl P, Sethi PM, Cooper AJ. Master's performance in the New York City Marathon 1983-1999. *Br Sports Med.* 2004;38(4):408-412. doi:10.1136/bjsm.2002.003566
5. Office of the Surgeon General. *Physical Activity and Health: A Report of the Surgeon General.* US Department of Health and Human Services, Centers for Disease Control and Prevention, National Center for Chronic Disease Prevention and Health Promotion; 1996.
6. Ageing and Health Programme, Division of Health Promotion, Education and Communication. *The Heidelberg Guidelines for Promoting Physical Activity Among Older Persons.* World Health Organization; 1996.
7. American College of Sports Medicine; Chodzko-Zajko WJ, Proctor DN, Fiatarone Singh MA, et al. American College of Sports Medicine position stand. Exercise and physical activity for older adults. *Med Sci Sports Exerc.* 2009;41(7):1510-1530. doi:10.1249/MSS.0b013e3181a0c95c
8. US Department of Health and Human Services. *Physical Activity Guidelines for Americans*, 2nd ed. US Department of Health and Human Services; 2018.
9. Valenzuela PL, Maffiuletti NA, Joyner MJ, Lucia A, Lepers R. Lifelong endurance exercise as a countermeasure against age-related decline: physiological overview and insights from masters athletes. *Sports Med.* 2020;50(4):703-716. doi:10.1007/s40279-019-01252-0
10. Dennehy C. Alcohol nearly killed Tommy Hughes. Now He Holds the Over-60 Half Marathon Record. *Runner's World.* September 22, 2020. Accessed August 31, 2022. www.runnersworld.com/runners-stories/a34062899/tommy-hughes-overcame-alcoholism-over-60-half-marathon-world-record
11. Lepers R, Cattagni T. Do older athletes reach limits in their performance during marathon running? *Age (Dordr).* 2012;34(3):773-781. doi:10.1007/s11357-011-9271-z
12. Akkari A, Machin D, Tanaka H. Greater progression of athletic performance in older Masters athletes. *Age Ageing.* 2015;44(4):683-686. doi:10.1093/ageing/afv023
13. Betik AC, Hepple RT. Determinants of VO2 max decline with aging: an integrated perspective. *Appl Physiol Nutr Metab.* 2008;33(1):130-140. doi:10.1139/H07-174
14. Katzel LI, Sorkin JD, Fleg JL. A comparison of longitudinal changes in aerobic fitness in older endurance athletes and sedentary men. *Am Geriatr Soc.* 2001;49(12):1657-1664. doi:10.1046/j.1532-5415.2001.t01-1-49276.x
15. Mengelkoch LJ, Pollock ML, Limacher MC, et al. Effects of age, physical training, and physical fitness on coronary heart disease risk factors in older track athletes at twenty-year follow-up. *Am Geriatr Soc.* 1997;45(12):1446-1453. doi:10.1111/j.1532-5415.1997.tb03194.x
16. Phillips SM. Current concepts and unresolved questions in dietary protein requirements and supplements in adults. *Front Nutr.* 2017;4:13. doi:10.3389/fnut.2017.00013
17. Liu CJ, Latham NK. Progressive resistance strength training for improving physical function in older adults. *Cochrane Database Syst Rev.* 2009;2009(3):CD002759. doi:10.1002/14651858.CD002759.pub2
18. Miljkovic N, Lim JY, Miljkovic I, Frontera WR. Aging of skeletal muscle fibers. *Ann Rehabil Med.* 2015;39(2):155-162. doi:10.5535/arm.2015.39.2.155
19. Melov S, Tarnopolsky MA, Beckman K, Felkey K, Hubbard A. Resistance exercise reverses aging in human skeletal muscle. *PLoS One.* 2007;2(5):e465. doi:10.1371/journal.pone.0000465
20. Kuk JL, Saunders TJ, Davidson LE, Ross R. Age-related changes in total and regional fat distribution. *Ageing Res Rev.* 2009;8(4):339-348. doi:10.1016/j.arr.2009.06.001
21. Wroblewski AP, Amati F, Smiley MA, Goodpaster B, Wright V. Chronic exercise preserves lean muscle mass in masters athletes. *Phys Sportsmed.* 2011;39(3):172-178. doi:10.3810/psm.2011.09.1933
22. Kopiczko A, Adamczyk JG, Gryko K, Popowczak M. Bone mineral density in elite masters athletes: the effect of body composition and long-term exercise. *Eur Rev Aging Phys Act.* 2021;18(1):7. doi:10.1186/s11556-021-00262-0
23. Fien S, Climstein M, Quilter C, et al. Anthropometric, physical function and general health markers of Masters athletes: a cross-sectional study. *PeerJ.* 2017; 5:e3768. doi:10.7717/peerj.3768
24. Pratley RE, Hagberg JM, Rogus EM, Goldberg AP. Enhanced insulin sensitivity and lower waist-to-hip ratio in master athletes. *Am Physiol.* 1995;268(3 Pt 1):E484-E490. doi:10.1152/ajpendo.1995.268.3.E484
25. Giada F, Vigna GB, Vitale E, et al. Effect of age on the response of blood lipids, body composition, and aerobic power to physical conditioning and deconditioning. *Metabolism.* 1995;44(2):161-165. doi:10.1016/0026-0495(95)90259-7
26. Moorman AJ, Dean LS, Yang E, Drezner JA. Cardiovascular risk assessment in the older athlete. *Sports Health.* 2021;13(6):622-629. doi:10.1177/19417381211004877
27. Bone Health and Osteoporosis Foundation Home page. Accessed November 11, 2022. www.bonehealthandosteoporosis.org

28. Florindo AA, Latorre Mdo R, Jaime PC, Tanaka T, Pippa MG, Zerbini CA. Past and present habitual physical activity and its relationship with bone mineral density in men aged 50 years and older in Brazil. *Gerontol A Biol Sci Med Sci.* 2002;57(10):M654-M657. doi:10.1093/gerona/57.10.m654
29. Velez NF, Zhang A, Stone B, Perera S, Miller M, Greenspan SL. The effect of moderate impact exercise on skeletal integrity in master athletes. *Osteoporos Int.* 2008;19(10):1457-1464. doi:10.1007/s00198-008-0590-6
30. Tanaka H, Tarumi T, Rittweger J. Aging and physiological lessons from master athletes. *Compr Physiol.* 2019;10(1):261-296. doi:10.1002/cphy.c180041
31. Geard D, Reaburn PRJ, Rebar AL, Dionigi RA. Masters athletes: exemplars of successful aging? *Aging Phys Act.* 2017;25(3):490-500. doi:10.1123/japa.2016-0050
32. Tanaka H. Aging of competitive athletes. *Gerontology.* 2017;63(5):488-494. doi:10.1159/000477722
33. Ratajczak J, Czerniak U, Wieliński D, et al. Pro-healthy diet properties and its determinants among aging masters athletes. *Int Environ Res Public Health.* 2021 17;18(14):7614. doi:10.3390/ijerph18147614
34. van Pelt RE, Dinneno FA, Seals DR, Jones PP. Age-related decline in RMR in physically active men: relation to exercise volume and energy intake. *Am Physiol Endocrinol Metab.* 2001;281(3):E633-E639. doi:10.1152/ajpendo.2001.281.3.E633
35. National Academies of Sciences, Engineering, and Medicine; Health and Medicine Division; Food and Nutrition Board; Committee on the Dietary Reference Intakes for Energy. *Dietary Reference Intakes for Energy.* The National Academies Press; January 17, 2023. doi:10.17226/26818
36. Bunyard LB, Katzel LI, Busby-Whitehead MJ, Wu Z, Goldberg AP. Energy requirements of middle-aged men are modifiable by physical activity. *Am Clin Nutr.* 1998;68(5):1136-1142. doi:10.1093/ajcn/68.5.1136
37. Wilmore JH, Stanforth PR, Hudspeth LA, et al. Alterations in resting metabolic rate as a consequence of 20 wk of endurance training: the HERITAGE Family Study. *Am Clin Nutr.* 1998;68(1):66-71. doi:10.1093/ajcn/68.1.66
38. Starling RD. Energy expenditure and aging: effects of physical activity. *Int Sport Nutr Exerc Metab.* 2001;11(suppl):S208-S217. doi:10.1123/ijsnem.11.s1.s208
39. Lundholm K, Holm G, Lindmark L, Larsson B, Sjöström L, Björntorp P. Thermogenic effect of food in physically well-trained elderly men. *Eur Appl Physiol Occup Physiol.* 1986;55(5):486-492. doi:10.1007/BF00421642
40. Logue D, Madigan SM, Delahunt E, Heinen M, Mc Donnell S-J, Corish CA. Low energy availability in athletes: a review of prevalence, dietary patterns, physiological health, and sports performance. *Sports Med.* 2018;48(1):73-96. doi:10.1007/s40279-017-0790-3
41. Louis J, Vercruyssen F, Dupuy O, Bernard T. Nutrition for master athletes: is there a need for specific recommendations? *Aging Phys Act.* 2019;28(3):489-498. doi:10.1123/japa.2019-0190
42. Burke LM, Hawley JA, Wong SHS, Jeukendrup AE. Carbohydrates for training and competition. *Sports Sci.* 2011;29(suppl 1):S17-S27. doi:10.1080/02640414.2011.585473
43. Tarnopolsky MA. Nutritional consideration in the aging athlete. *Clin Sport Med.* 2008;18(6):531-538. doi:10.1097/JSM.0b013e318187ac44
44. Moore DR, Churchward-Venne TA, Witard O, et al. Protein ingestion to stimulate myofibrillar protein synthesis requires greater relative protein intakes in healthy older versus younger men. *Gerontol A Biol Sci Med Sci.* 2015;70(1):57-62. doi:10.1093/gerona/glu103
45. Churchward-Venne TA, Breen L, Phillips SM. Alterations in human muscle protein metabolism with aging: protein and exercise as countermeasures to offset sarcopenia. *Biofactors.* 2014;40(2):199-205. doi:10.1002/biof.1138
46. Doering TM, Jenkins DG, Reaburn PR, Borges NR, Hohmann E, Phillips SM. Lower integrated muscle protein synthesis in masters compared with younger athletes. *Med Sci Sports Exerc.* 2016;48(8):1613-1618. doi:10.1249/MSS.0000000000000935
47. McKendry J, Currier BS, Lim C, Mcleod JC, Thomas ACQ, Phillips SM. Nutritional supplements to support resistance exercise in countering the sarcopenia of aging. *Nutrients.* 2020;12(7):2057. doi:10.3390/nu12072057
48. Layman DK, Anthony TG, Rasmussen BB, et al. Defining meal requirements for protein to optimize metabolic roles of amino acids. *Am Clin Nutr.* 2015;101(6):1330S-1338S. doi:10.3945/ajcn.114.084053
49. Bauer J, Biolo G, Cederholm T, et al. Evidence-based recommendations for optimal dietary protein intake in older people: a position paper from the PROT-AGE Study Group. *Am Med Dir Assoc.* 2013;14(8):542-559. doi:10.1016/j.jamda.2013.05.021
50. US Department of Agriculture and US Department of Health and Human Services. *Dietary Guidelines for Americans, 2020-2025.* 9th ed. December 2020. Accessed July 23, 2023. www.DietaryGuidelines.gov
51. Panel on Dietary Antioxidants and Related Compounds; Subcommittee on Upper Reference Levels of Nutrients; Subcommittee on Interpretation and Uses of Dietary Reference Intakes; Standing Committee on the Scientific Evaluation of Dietary Reference Intakes; Food and Nutrition Board, Institute of Medicine. *Dietary Reference Intakes: Recommended Intakes for Individuals.* National Academies Press; 1998.
52. Nieman DC, Butler JV, Pollett LM, Dietrich SJ, Lutz RD. Nutrient intake of marathon runners. *Am Diet Assoc.* 1989;89(9):1273-1278. PMID: 2549112
53. Chatard JC, Boutet C, Tourny C, Garcia S, Berthouze S, Guézennec CY. Nutritional status and physical fitness of elderly sportsmen. *Eur Appl Physiol Occup Physiol.* 1998;77(1-2):157-163. doi:10.1007/s004210050314
54. Beshgetoor D, Nichols JF. Dietary intake and supplement use in female master cyclists and runners. *Int Sport Nutr Exerc Metab.* 2003;13(2):166-172. doi:10.1123/ijsnem.13.2.166
55. Panel on Dietary Reference Intakes for Electrolytes and Water; Standing Committee on the Scientific Evaluation of Dietary Reference Intakes; Food and Nutrition Board, Institute of Medicine. *Dietary Reference Intakes for Water, Potassium, Sodium, Chloride, and Sulfate.* National Academies Press; 2004.

56. American College of Sports Medicine; Sawka MN, Burke LM, Eichner ER, Maughan RJ, Montain SJ, Stachenfeld NS. American College of Sports Medicine position stand. Exercise and fluid replacement. *Med Sci Sports Exerc.* 2007;39(2):377-390. doi:10.1249/mss.0b013e31802ca597
57. Kenney WL, Fowler SR. Methylcholine-activated eccrine sweat gland density and output as a function of age. *Appl Physiol (1985).* 1988;65(3):1082-1086. doi:10.1152/jappl.1988.65.3.1082
58. Notley SR, Meade RD, D'Souza AW, Friesen BJ, Kenny GP. Heat loss is impaired in older men on the day after prolonged work in the heat. *Med Sci Sports Exerc.* 2018;50(9):1859-1867. doi:10.1249/MSS.0000000000001643
59. Kenney WL, Anderson RK. Responses of older and younger women to exercise in dry and humid heat without fluid replacement. *Med Sci Sports Exerc.* 1988;20(2):155-160. doi:10.1249/00005768-198820020-00009
60. Walter AN, Lenz TL. Hydration and medication use. *Am Lifestyle Med.* 2011;5(4):332-335. doi:10.1177/1559827611401203
61. Powers SK, Criswell D, Lawler J, et al. Rigorous exercise training increases superoxide dismutase activity in ventricular myocardium. *Am Physiol.* 1993;265(6 Pt 2):H2094-H2098. doi:10.1152/ajpheart.1993.265.6.H2094
62. Candow DG, Chilibeck PD, Forbes SC. Creatine supplementation and aging musculoskeletal health. *Endocrine.* 2014;45(3):354-361. doi:10.1007/s12020-013-0070-4
63. Candow DG, Forbes SC, Kirk B, Duque G. Current evidence and possible future applications of creatine supplementation for older adults. *Nutrients.* 2021;13(3):745. doi:10.3390/nu13030745
64. Fleischman A, Makimura H, Stanley TL, et al. Skeletal muscle phosphocreatine recovery after submaximal exercise in children and young and middle-aged adults. *Clin Endocrinol Metab.* 2010;95(9):E69-E74. doi:10.1210/jc.2010-0527
65. Smith GI, Atherton P, Reeds DN, et al. Dietary omega-3 fatty acid supplementation increases the rate of muscle protein synthesis in older adults: a randomized controlled trial. *Am Clin Nutr.* 2011;93(2):402-412. doi:10.3945/ajcn.110.005611
66. Murphy CH, McGlory C. Fish oil for healthy aging: potential application to master athletes. *Sports Med.* 2021;51(suppl 1):31-41. doi:10.1007/s40279-021-01509-7
67. Close GL, Hamilton DL, Philp A, Burke LM, Morton JP. New strategies in sport nutrition to increase exercise performance. *Free Radic Biol Med.* 2016;98:144-158. doi:10.1016/j.freeradbiomed.2016.01.016
68. Custodero C, Saini SK, Shin MJ, et al. Nicotinamide riboside-A missing piece in the puzzle of exercise therapy for older adults? *Exp Gerontol.* 2020;137:110972. doi:10.1016/j.exger.2020.110972
69. Martens CR, Denman BA, Mazzo MR, et al. Chronic nicotinamide riboside supplementation is well-tolerated and elevates NAD^+ in healthy middle-aged and older adults. *Nat Commun.* 2018;9(1):1286. doi:10.1038/s41467-018-03421-7

CHAPTER 15

Elite Athletes

Louise Burke, OAM, PhD, APD, FACSM

LEARNING OBJECTIVES

- Discuss the role of a sports dietitian working with elite athletes.
- Identify the nutritional needs of elite athletes that are unique because of their schedules, lifestyle factors, and physiological demands.
- Appropriately apply the results of sports nutrition research to elite athletes.
- Develop key strategies for successfully working with elite athletes.

INTRODUCTION

The usual working definition of *elite* is "the best" or "the chosen few." This chapter addresses the nutritional needs of athletes who have reached the professional, world-class, or Olympic rank in their respective sports. These athletes have special nutritional requirements or challenges as a result of their extreme levels of training and competition, as well as the lifestyle that underpins their sporting involvement.

Sports dietitians are drawn to work with top athletes for many reasons, including the following:

- Elite athletes are often operating at the extremes of human nutrition and physiological capacity. It is fascinating to see what the human body can achieve and how it must be fueled to reach this level of operation.
- Elite athletes represent a motivated group of clients who seek and appreciate the nutrition advice that they are offered and usually adhere to recommendations.
- Sports dietitians have the opportunity to work with famous people and in high-profile situations, which can seem glamorous and can publicize a private practice.
- Sports dietitians are surrounded by inspired and inspiring people. They become participants in the excitement and emotion of high-level sports competitions.
- Funding and the culture of high-level sports can provide the sports dietitian with a well-resourced environment in which to work, with access to such advantages as advanced body composition and dietary assessment tools, chefs and high-quality meal support, and other high-level professionals. This may enhance practice and job satisfaction.
- The work can provide opportunities to travel.
- Sports nutrition is a precise discipline with tangible benefits. The athlete and the sports dietitian receive short-term rewards and rapid feedback about the success of their nutrition strategies.
- The work draws on the sports dietitian's creativity and ingenuity to find practical strategies to address the athlete's unique nutritional challenges. Finding individualized solutions to these problems is interesting and demanding.
- The work is fast-paced and high-stakes, which can attract people who work well in such conditions.

Of course, these and other ideas about working with elite athletes are usually just perceptions, and some ideas are ill founded. For example, many dietetics students are interested in sports nutrition as an alternative to a career in weight-loss counseling. Yet, a common reason for athletes to seek the help of a sports dietitian is to reduce weight or body fat.

This chapter provides an overview of some of the nutritional issues that are important to top-level athletes, as well as strategies for the sports dietitian to work successfully with such clients.

THE STRUCTURE OF HIGH-LEVEL SPORT: IMPLICATIONS FOR NUTRITIONAL NEEDS AND PRACTICE

Several characteristics of high-level sports create special nutritional needs or challenges for the athletes involved. These include:

- heavy training loads,
- demanding competition schedules,
- frequent travel,
- unusual environments for training adaptations or competition preparation (heat, altitude),
- the culture of sport (the price and rewards of fame and publicity), and
- the influence and power of coaches and other personnel involved with the athlete.

Although there are clear differences among sports, the training program of an elite or professional athlete typically involves 15 to 30 hours of highly periodized and specialized exercise sessions each week. Other activities related to recovery, injury treatment and prevention, media and sponsor commitments, and team tactical preparation may also be scheduled into the weekly timetable. The training program is likely to change but often calls for high energy requirements and targeted needs for carbohydrate and protein around key sessions to support high-quality training as well as recovery and adaptation, respectively. The sports care provider is likely to encounter increased requirements for some nutrients and the need to address substantial losses of fluids and electrolytes through sweating.[1] At this level of sport, athletes would be expected to have the support and incentive to implement cutting-edge sports nutrition practices, including many of the evolving themes in sports nutrition such as awareness of the benefits of periodizing nutrition strategies and nutrient intake as well as the strategic timing of nutrient intake in relation to exercise or postexercise recovery and adaptation.[2-4] Indeed, many professional sporting teams offer catering and specialized nutrition stations within the club environment to address the challenges of amplified nutrition needs and busy timetables. Highly paid athletes may also employ their own chefs to organize their nutritional needs at home. High-performance athletes may be more proactive with the use of sports supplements and other special strategies,[5] reflecting an amplified pressure and reward for opportunities with any potential to enhance performance as well as their status as targets for sponsorship by product manufacturers and salespeople. However, they also face greater penalties associated with the poor use of supplements, especially if this leads to an Anti-Doping Rule Violation resulting from the presence of banned substances (for more information, refer to Chapter 7, Supplements and Sports Foods).

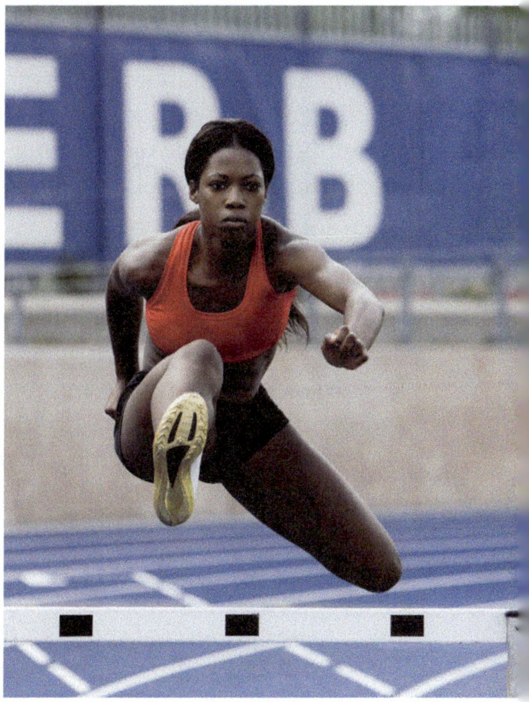

Elite Athlete Competition Schedules

The competition schedule of the elite athlete usually presents a set of nutritional and lifestyle challenges that differ from those of the training schedule. In general, athletes organize their training to peak at 1 to 3 major competitions yearly; however, most will compete in many other events each year. Athletes use these lesser competitions to practice and fine-tune their strategies for key events or to provide high-quality training sessions for more important competitions. In addition, each competition may involve more than 1 round of events (ie, heats, semifinals, and finals) that ultimately decide the outcome. Some sports, particularly team sports, can be played in a tournament format with a series of games every 24 to 72 hours. Team sports played seasonally, traditionally with a weekly game, have evolved to have even more demanding competitive schedules at the elite level. It is not unusual for professional soccer, baseball, and basketball players to play a match every 2 or 3 days, especially when the player or the team is entered into more than 1 association or league.[6,7]

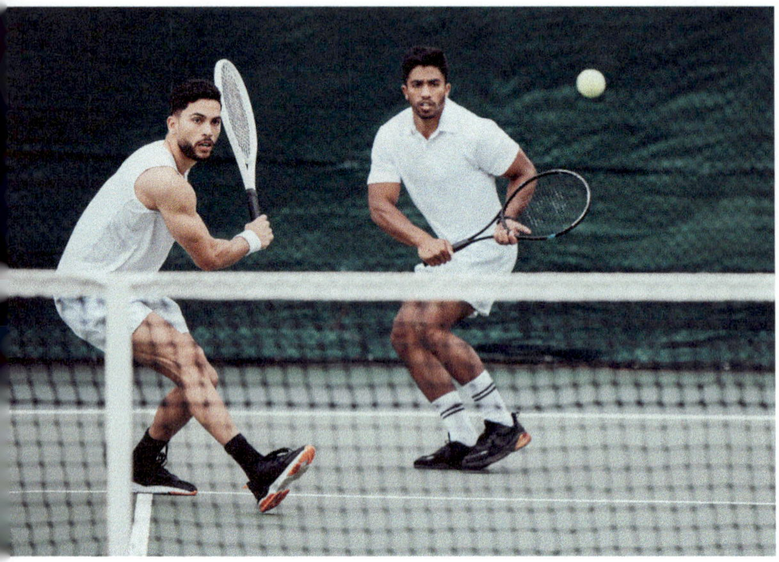

During each competition phase, athletes typically focus on acute eating strategies before, during, and between races, games, or events to meet the specialized requirements for optimal performance and recovery.[4,8,9] Travel and other factors that limit food availability can often challenge the athlete to meet immediate nutritional goals, not to mention big-picture issues of energy balance and overall macronutrient and micronutrient needs.[10] The sports dietitian needs to be creative in helping the athlete achieve strategies such as carbohydrate loading, an optimal preevent meal, adequate food and fluid intake during an event, and proactive recovery eating. In some sports, the switch between training and competition phases is ever changing. For example, professional football (soccer) players in Europe may play 1 to 3 matches per week depending on the number of leagues in which they are entered. Meanwhile, the schedule of each tennis tournament and the demands of each match are variable, and a loss can suddenly shift the player from competition mode into training mode until the next competition. The sports dietitian must be able to help an athlete pivot between the goals and mindset of each phase, particularly as they change rapidly and unpredictably. Furthermore, when competition makes up a substantial proportion of the elite athlete's life and total eating patterns—for example, professional cyclists who compete for 80 to 100 days each year and ride in stage races lasting up to 3 weeks[11]—there is a need for competition nutrition strategies that can include a wider set of dietary goals.

Elite Athlete Lifestyles

The lifestyles of most top-level athletes are busy and irregular. At the entry point into an elite sport, many younger athletes juggle training and events around the commitments of high school and college. Because many sports are not wholly professional or financially rewarding, some top-class athletes must continue to work part-time or full-time in addition to keeping their sporting commitments. Meals and snacks eaten during the day must fit into their lifestyles (eg, work, school, and family commitments). A chaotic or displaced eating pattern may challenge some athletes to meet the high energy and nutrient requirements associated with maturational and muscular growth, training, and recovery—in particular, prolonged sessions of high-intensity work or resistance-training programs designed to increase muscle size and strength.

The elite level of sport is a specialized environment, which includes not only the physical aspects of club rooms and training or competition venues but also the culture of each sport. The pressure to win often means that the athlete is desperate to find dietary shortcuts or "magic bullets," becoming an easy target for the unsupported claims made about fad diets, dietary supplements, and other unusual eating strategies. The athlete is often susceptible to and specifically targeted by companies and individuals who recognize the benefits of being associated with a high-profile individual or team. Many sports provide an insular world where high-level athletes swap ideas and theories with their peers, trainers, and coaches or are influenced by material on the internet and in sports magazines, without necessarily checking the credibility of their information sources. Sports dietitians need to break into these circles to be aware of the latest trends and ideas. They must also contend with a wide array of other, often influential sources of nutrition advice directed at the athlete. They may have to fight for the athlete's time, concentration, or resources, which are often limited and must be shared with other sports science and medical professionals, managers, coaching and training staff, and the media. On the positive side, most top-level athletes take a professional approach to preparing for their sport and will make effective use of information and practical advice. The structure of many high-level teams and sporting organizations is to surround their athletes with a group of professionals specializing in sports science and medicine as well as training and conditioning. It is both efficient and rewarding to be part of such a support network, and the sports dietitian should find ways to optimize their interaction in the multidisciplinary team.[12]

NUTRITIONAL ISSUES FOR ELITE ATHLETES

In an ideal world, elite athletes would meet their increased energy needs and nutrient requirements with well-chosen and varied diets. However, this may not always be the case. Very few studies have been conducted on the dietary practices of the world's top athletes, and much of the available literature fails to address the potential for biased data because of the limitations of dietary survey methodology. Even fewer studies have measured indexes of nutritional status among top athletes. Nevertheless, it seems most elite male athletes have the potential to consume diets that meet the guidelines for sports nutrition, although individuals (especially in "leanness" sports [eg, road cycling, distance running]) may restrict energy intake (and by association, other nutrients) to meet goals around body mass and composition. Elite female athletes are at greater general risk of such concerns.[13] Other athletes at risk are those involved in weight-controlled or weight-division sports, such as boxing, wrestling, weightlifting, and lightweight rowing, for which preparation for competition often involves severe energy restriction.[14]

Meeting Energy and Fuel Needs Across a Range of Extremes

An athlete's energy intake is of interest for several reasons:

- It sets the potential for achieving the athlete's requirements for energy-containing macronutrients (especially protein and carbohydrate) and the food needed to provide vitamins, minerals, and other non–energy-containing dietary compounds required for optimal function and health.
- It helps the athlete manipulate muscle mass and body-fat levels to achieve the specific body composition ideal for athletic performance.
- It affects the function of many body systems related to health and performance.
- It challenges the practical limits to food intake set by such issues as food availability and gastrointestinal comfort.

The total energy expenditure of each athlete is unique, arising from the contribution of their basal metabolic rate; the thermic effects of food and exercise; and in some cases, growth. Energy expenditure is increased by high levels of lean body mass, growth (including the desired adaptations to a resistance-training program), and a high-volume training program. (For more information on energy balance, refer to Chapter 10.) For some elite athletes, these 3 factors coexist to create very large energy demands—for example, the male swimmer or rower who faces an increase in training commitment during periods of adolescent growth spurts. Other elite athletes have very large energy requirements because of the extraordinary fuel demands of their competition programs. The energy and fuel costs of very strenuous exercise programs are impressively high. For example, professional cyclists in the Grand Tours have reported consuming mean daily intakes exceeding 5,500 kcal and 12 g of carbohydrate per kilogram of body weight for periods of 3 weeks during competition, with some exceptional fuel-demanding stages involving a carbohydrate intake of 18 g/kg for the day.[15-17] During the 2008 Beijing Olympic Games, media sources reported that 8-time gold-medal winning swimmer Michael Phelps consumed approximately 12,000 kcal/d. This news created considerable awe among the public but caused skepticism among sports nutrition experts. Phelps denied this information in his subsequent autobiography, claiming his true intake may be up to 8,000 to 10,000 kcal/d.[18] These figures may be estimates of his heaviest days of intake rather than a true average, but nevertheless, they illustrate the potential for high energy needs among athletes with heavy training loads.

At such extreme levels of energy demand, lack of nutrition knowledge, limited access to suitable foods, gastrointestinal discomfort, or inadequate time for preparing or eating food can prevent the athlete from consuming sufficient food or fluid over the day to meet their energy needs. Indeed, this scenario is now recognized as a cause of low energy availability (LEA), which, when it reaches problematic levels of exposure, can lead to the relative energy deficiency in sport (REDs) syndrome.[19] Even when overall energy needs can be met, the athlete may experience difficulty in achieving intake goals of specific nutrients (eg, carbohydrate and protein) around exercise sessions. In this case, the athlete may need to consume food and drink in greater quantities than would be provided in an everyday diet or dictated by appetite and thirst. Again, the availability of foods and fluids, or opportunities to consume them, may be limited, and the athlete may be distracted by other activities (eg, media commitments, drug testing, performance debriefs). To meet these challenges, the athlete will need to plan ahead to meet nutrient goals from foods convenient to store, prepare, and eat. Specialized advice from a sports dietitian is therefore useful to help address energy intake challenges faced by athletes, particularly to find actionable strategies for various practical challenges. (Refer to Chapter 11 for information on weight management.)

Body Composition for Optimal Performance

Physical characteristics, including height, limb lengths, total body mass (weight), muscle mass, and body fat can all play roles in sports performance. Many elite athletes are subjected to rigid criteria for an ideal physique based on the characteristics of other successful competitors. The pressure to conform to such an ideal comes from the athlete's own perfectionism and drive to succeed, as well as the influence of coaches, trainers, other athletes, and the media. Although athletes at all levels may battle to achieve their desired weight and body-fat level, a disadvantage of being an elite athlete is that this battle may be played out in the public arena; through commentary on websites, newspapers, and magazines; and in the discussions of sports reporters. Wearing tight-fitting clothing (such as those required as part of a team uniform) in public has been identified as a risk factor for the development of disordered eating among athletes.[20] One can imagine how this stress is amplified when the (largely sedentary) audience (measured in the millions) feels justified in criticizing an athlete for perceived pockets of fat made apparent by tight-fitting spandex. Case studies of such humiliation involving high-performance female swimmers,[21,22] tennis players,[23] distance runners,[24,25] and gymnasts[26] are well-known.

Although information about the physique of elite athletes is a source of fascination for the community as well as for other athletes, one should be cautious about making rigid prescriptions about the ideal physique based on the anthropometrics of successful competitors. The concept of a single ideal fails to take into account the considerable variability in the physical characteristics of people, even among individuals in the same sport. Furthermore, athletes periodize their body composition over the course of the training and competition year and take many years of training and maturation to finally achieve their optimal shape and body composition.[27] Finally, because a wide variety of techniques are used to assess characteristics such as body fat or lean mass, it is impractical to generalize an ideal body type from available data about specific athletes. Clinical experience shows a range of values for body fat and body weight consistent with long-term good performance and health within each sport. Sequential profiling of an athlete can monitor the development of physical characteristics associated with good performance for that individual and also identify the changes in physique expected over a season or period of specialized training. For additional information on nutrition assessment and body composition, see Chapters 8 and 9.

Nevertheless, in many sports in which a low body-mass or body-fat level offers distinct advantages to performance, fat loss has become a focus or even an obsession. The benefits of leanness can be seen in terms of the energy cost of movement (eg, distance running, cycling), the physics of movement in a tight space or against gravity (eg, gymnastics, diving, cycling uphill), or aesthetics (eg, gymnastics, bodybuilding). In many such weight-conscious (or body fat–conscious) sports, elite athletes strive to achieve minimum body-fat levels; some athletes try to reduce their body fat to levels less than what is considered natural or healthy. In the short term, this may improve performance. However, unsound weight loss methods, including disordered eating or eating disorders, are a principal cause of problematic LEA, leading to the REDs syndrome and its sequalae of health and performance impairments.[19] These can be career-ending for some athletes. Reproductive disorders and poor bone health were the first recognized outcomes of excessive training and/or restricted energy intake in female athletes within the female athlete triad.[20] However, experts now recognize that energy mismatches occur as a result of a number of scenarios in both males and females, with potential for disruption to an expanded number of body systems.[19,28]

Practitioners should put into place techniques for the early recognition and treatment of REDs in the elite athlete environment. Surprisingly, this can sometimes be challenging to implement in high-performance sports, despite the growing evidence that LEA impairs performance as well as health.[19] The perceived or real benefits of achieving very low levels of body fat and body mass have become so ingrained in some elite sports that unhealthy patterns of restrained eating are normalized or even regarded as heroic. Many biographies of the careers of elite athletes reveal stories of extreme eating behaviors that were considered simply part of their sport. For example, former professional road bicycle racer Tyler Hamilton noted a range of weight-loss techniques that he used in his constant battle to be as lean as possible, including a strategy shared by other riders: "[C]ome home from a training ride, chug a big bottle of fizzy water and take 2 or 3 sleeping pills. By the time you woke up, it would be dinner, or if you were lucky, breakfast."[29] Retired Danish professional cyclist Michael Rasmussen became obsessed with removing any excess weight (down to the milligram), such as peeling off unnecessary stickers from his bike; this carried over to his training diet. He was "famous for counting each grain of rice before eating and taking water—not milk—with his breakfast cereal."[30] These examples illustrate the clear need for a change in the culture around weight and body fat within many elite sports. A more sensible approach to weight management is covered elsewhere,[31] including in Chapter 11. It is noted here, however, that the sports dietitian must play a role in changing the culture of organizations to improve their consideration and management of physique, such as the work conducted by the Australian Institute of Sport in partnership with Australia's National Eating Disorders Collaboration.[32]

The Special Challenges of Travel

Travel plays a major role in the lifestyle of the elite athlete, and most world-class athletes often travel within their own state or country and sometimes internationally for competition or specialized training opportunities. The various challenges imposed by travel, whether domestic or international, are summarized in Box 15.1.[33] These include disruption to the athlete's normal eating routine and access to their preferred foods, as well as exposure to a different standard of food and water hygiene. The process of travel itself is also problematic, exposing the athlete to jet lag, interruption of the normal training program, and boredom eating when confined during travel.

Elite athletes need to become organized travelers, identifying the challenges of their intended locations before the trip and planning to circumvent potential problems. During travel, athletes should adjust their eating to suit a period of inactivity as well as any increases in fluid losses due to a dry atmosphere, such as on an airplane. As soon as the trip begins, they should also switch to a meal routine based on the time zone of their country of destination to assist with the change in body clock.[10] The travel plan may include organizing catering needs and menus before the trip. In addition, supplies of special foods and drinks may be taken on the trip to complement these catering plans or to make up for the absence of key nutrients or favorite foods.

Of course, these plans must be implemented with an understanding of some of the practical constraints

BOX 15.1 Challenges and Solutions for the Traveling Athlete[33]

Challenges of traveling

Disrupted training and lifestyle during transit to a new location

Jet lag and changes in time zones that require a new schedule

Changes in climate and altitude at a new location, creating different nutritional needs

Changes to food availability, including reliance on hotels, restaurants, and takeout rather than home cooking and 24/7 access to a kitchen

Excitement and distraction of a new location

Changes in training load and timetable requiring a new daily schedule

Continued on next page

BOX 15.1 Challenges and Solutions for the Traveling Athlete[33] (CONTINUED)

Change in food culture, including absence of important and familiar foods, and inability to understand menus and food labels

Temptations of all-you-can-eat meal options in some athletic settings or the desire to try a new food culture and new foods

Risk of gastrointestinal illnesses due to exposure to food and water that may have poor hygiene standards

---

Strategies to cope with the challenges of traveling

Plan ahead

Investigate food issues on travel routes (eg, airlines) and at the destination. Contact caterers and food organizers well ahead of the trip to let them know meal timing and menu needs.

Eat and drink well en route

Avoid boredom eating on planes, buses, trains. Eat according to real needs, taking into account the forced rest during travel.

Adopt eating patterns that suit the destination time zone as soon as the trip starts. This will help the body clock to adapt.

Be aware of unseen fluid losses in air-conditioned vehicles and pressurized airplanes.

Supplement the local fare with one's own supplies

Take (or send) a supply of portable, nonperishable foods to replace important items that may be missing. Useful items include breakfast cereals; cereal bars and crackers; dried fruit; and specialized sports products, such as powdered liquid meals and sports drinks.

Extend meal-only catering plans with locally purchased or one's own supplies of well-chosen snacks

Take care with food and water hygiene

Find out whether the local water supply is safe to drink. If not, stick to drinks from sealed bottles or hot drinks made from well-boiled water. Avoid ice added to drinks.

In high-risk environments, eat only at reputable hotels or restaurants. Avoid food from local stalls and markets, despite the temptation to enjoy an authentic cultural experience.

Stick to well-cooked foods. Avoid salads or unpeeled fruits that have been in contact with local water or soil.

Adhere to the food plan

Choose the best of the local cuisine to meet nutritional needs, supplementing with one's own supplies where needed.

Be assertive in asking for needed foods at catering outlets, for example, low-fat cooking styles or an extra carbohydrate choice.

Recognize the challenges of all-you-can-eat dining. Stick to the set meal plan and resist the temptation to eat what is there or what everyone else is eating.

involved. For example, quarantine laws in some countries or states may prevent the importation of some food products. In addition, the athlete should be aware that heightened security regulations and tighter weight restrictions on luggage have made it more difficult to travel with food supplies. Strategies to address these challenges include removing foodstuffs from packaging, taking powdered versions of sports foods to lighten luggage, and organizing supplies to be freighted over or delivered directly to travel destinations rather than transported with the athlete. Elite athletes can sometimes be fortunate enough to have personal or team-based sponsorships with airlines or other travel agencies that can facilitate the transport of their luggage. Being famous can be beneficial when presenting at check-in with special needs, but a good travel plan should not rely on special last-minute help. If sports foods or supplements are sourced from a local supplier, the athlete should take special caution regarding the potential for contamination with banned substances and seek batch-tested products.

Often, competitions or specialized training protocols occur in physiologically challenging environments. For example, recent hot-weather competitions have included the 2019 World Athletic Championships and the 2022 World Cup football tournament in Qatar, as well as the 2016 Rio de Janeiro and 2020 Tokyo Olympic Games. Football matches during the 2010 World Cup in Johannesburg, South Africa, were played at an altitude of approximately 1,700 m (5,600 feet). In such cases, the athlete usually undertakes acclimatization in a similar environment or in a chamber that can simulate the characteristics of the competition site. This is done as final preparation for the competition. However, on other occasions, the athlete may choose to train in hot conditions or at a high altitude (or simulated altitude) to gain physiological adaptations that can be applied to moderate weather or a sea-level environment. Nutritional requirements during these specialized periods will reflect both the type of training, ranging from a precompetition taper to a period of intensified training, and the additional needs posed by heat or altitude. In both hot and moderate- to high-altitude environments, the athlete can expect to incur an increase in needs for nutrients, including iron, energy, fluid, carbohydrate, and protein.[33,34]

Finally, some sporting competitions or environments involve cultural, religious, or practical limitations on the food supply that athletes must take into consideration. Athletes traveling to Muslim-based countries may find that they are unable to access pork products on menus, whereas beef may not be served in Hindu cultures, as was the case in the athletes' dining hall at the 2010 Commonwealth Games in New Delhi, India. Many institutions and catering services have enacted bans on nuts or other high-risk food allergens. When these foods play a large role in the athlete's diet, it can be difficult to find a sufficient range of alternative choices. The 2012 London Olympic Games overlapped with the month of Ramadan, bringing the practice of Ramadan fasting to the attention of many athletic and spectating communities for the first time. Such fasting, 1 of the 5 pillars of the Islamic faith, involves abstention from all fluid and food intake from first light to sunset, as well as prayer and food rituals involved with the breaking of the fast at sunset and throughout the night. This required a range of special catering activities and education strategies for the Olympic Games, which are practiced in different formats and scenarios on an annual basis in many major competitions[35]

Studies on Recreational Athletes vs Elite Athletes

Many people believe that sports nutrition strategies are targeted to the elite athlete. It is true that the pressures and rewards for optimal performance are greater at this level and may justify the expense or effort involved in addressing special nutritional needs. However, the majority of studies on sports nutrition strategies involve participants throughout the spectrum, from recreationally active individuals to well-trained athletes. In fact, few intervention studies have involved world-class or elite athletes. This is understandable, because, by definition, elite athletes are a rare population, and it is difficult to conduct a study that does not conflict with their commitments to training and competition. Furthermore, many studies have been conducted on populations that are described incorrectly or by nonstandardized nomenclature. For example, some scientists might be sufficiently impressed by the novelty of carrying out a study on a group of people who are dedicated to completing large volumes of running or cycling to consider them "elite" or "highly trained," whereas others involved in high-performance sport might assess the physiological and performance characteristics of the study participants and reach a more conservative description of their caliber and training status. To better assist in understanding the available and future sports science literature, a group of health care, fitness, and nutrition researchers recently developed a standardized system to describe performance levels of all athletes, which is summarized in Box 15.2.[36] This model can be applied retrospectively as well as prospectively to ensure that the attributes of elite athletes and their practices or their response to various sports nutrition strategies are appropriately appreciated. A group of researchers recently undertook several audits[37-40] of the sports nutrition literature that has contributed to many of the current guidelines according to a standardized format that used this tiering system as a reference point.[41] These surveys (discussed in more detail in the next section) found that, within the literature across a range of sports nutrition strategies, the proportion of study participants that could be classified within this framework as Tier 3 and higher (considered to be at least highly trained) ranged from 4% to 15% of the total pool.[37-40]

Given that most research is undertaken on subelite athletes, there is some interest in whether these results apply to elite and world-class performers. In fact, experts have suggested that some sports nutrition strategies that have been tested in cohorts from a variety of events and training/caliber tiers do not offer the same benefits to highly trained and elite athletes as they do to lesser-trained groups. These strategies include supplementation with beetroot juice (nitrate) and periodizing sessions with low carbohydrate availability within a training program. Box 15.3 on page 372 summarizes the findings of the current scientific literature on these themes, as examples of (1) proposed explanations for apparent differences in the true response of elite and lesser-trained cohorts, (2) the limitations of the current research in adequately testing this hypothesis, and (3) strategies to assist high-performance athletes in deciding whether to implement a strategy that may not have strict evidence of efficacy for their specific use.[42-57]

BOX 15.2 Athlete Classification Framework[36]

Tier	Criteria for classification
Tier 5: World class *Less than 0.00006% of the global population*	Olympic and/or world medalists World record holders and athletes achieving within 2% of world-record performance and/or world leading performance Top 3 to top 20 in world rankings and/or top 3 to top 10 at an Olympics or World Championships (ie, finalists in their event), with this number determined based on the size and depth of competition in the event Top players within top teams (teams that medal or are in the most competitive leagues) or athletes achieving individual accolades (ie, most valuable player, player of the year) Maximal, or nearly maximal, training within the given sports norms Exceptional skill level achieved (ie, running biomechanics, ball skills, acquired decision-making components)
Tier 4: Elite or international level *About 0.0025% of the global population*	Competing at the international level (individuals or team-sport athletes on a national team) Team-sport athletes competing in international leagues or tournaments Top 4 to top 300 in world rankings, with this number determined based on the size and depth of competition in the event Achievement of close to top 7% of world-record performance and/or world leading performance National Collegiate Athletic Association (NCAA) Division I athletes Maximal, or nearly maximal, training within the given sports norms, with the intention to participate in top-level competition Highly proficient in skills required to perform a sport (ie, biomechanics, ball skills, acquired decision-making components)

Tier 3: Highly trained or national level *(Provincial/State or Academy Programs)* *About 0.014% of the global population*	Competing at the national level Team-sport athletes competing in national and/or state leagues or tournaments Achievement of close to top 20% of world-record performance and/or world leading performance NCAA Division II and III athletes Completing structured and periodized training and developing toward (within 20%) maximal or nearly maximal norms within the given sport Developing proficiency in skills required to perform a sport (ie, biomechanics, ball skills, acquired decision-making components)
Tier 2: Trained or developmental *Around 12% to 19% of the global population*	Local level representation Regularly training around 3 times per week Identify with a specific sport Training with a purpose to compete Limited skill development
Tier 1: Recreationally Active *About 35% to 42% of the global population*	Meet World Health Organization minimum activity guidelines: adults aged 18 through 64 years completing at least 150 to 300 minutes of moderate-intensity activity or 75 to 150 minutes of vigorous intensity activity per week, plus muscle strengthening activities 2 or more days per week May participate in multiple sports or forms of activity

Adapted with permission from McKay AKA, Stellingwerff T, Smith ES, et al. Defining training and performance caliber: a participant classification framework. *Int J Sports Physiol Perform.* 2022;17(2):317-331. doi:10.1123/ijspp.2021-0451

Studies on Male vs Female Athletes

Despite growing interest in female sports and the corresponding improvements in media coverage, athletic salaries and prize money, and available events on the world stage (eg, Olympic program), surveys of the sports science literature across many themes show that females are vastly underrepresented as participants. Specific audits of the literature from which sports nutrition guidelines have been derived show that studies on all-male study participants outnumber those on females by at least 10 to 1.[37-40] This varies across topics, however, with a standardized audit protocol[37] finding that females make up 23% of the participants in research on evidence-based performance supplements (eg, caffeine, creatine),[37] 71% of participants in medical supplement studies (eg, iron, vitamin D),[38] 11% of participants in studies of acute strategies for carbohydrate intake around exercise (eg, carbohydrate loading, preexercise meals, in-event fueling),[39] and 16% of those in studies of chronic approaches to carbohydrate intake in the training diet.[40]

Very few studies have been set up to appropriately compare responses between males and females to see if outcomes derived from studies of male athletes can be applied equally to their female counterparts.[37-40] There are many potential explanations for this observation;[41] for example, high-performance female athletes may be less available to participate in studies if their lower levels of financial support mean that they are juggling study or work with their sporting commitments. Females in general may be less interested in participating in studies with certain protocols (eg, intervening to change their eating practices or requiring the collection of blood or muscle samples). Researchers may be more reluctant to undertake studies on females or include females in their study cohorts because of the additional expense and logistics needed to control or standardize

BOX 15.3 Principles of Comparing Research Between Elite and Lesser-Trained Competitors[42-57]

Background to the hypothesized benefit

The practitioner must understand the physiological and mechanistic basis of the nutrition strategy so that special features that may occur in the scenario of the elite athlete can be isolated. The applicability of the strategy may be due to features of the athlete or features of their specialized execution of training or competition.

Example from literature on nitrate supplementation

Acute intake of supplemental nitrate may increase the formation of nitric oxide (NO) via the nitrate-nitrite-NO pathway that begins with the reduction of nitrate in the mouth by commensal bacteria in the oral microbiome.[42] NO may enhance sports performance through direct effects on muscle contractility or by reducing the oxygen cost of exercise.[42]

Example from literature on periodized carbohydrate availability for training

Undertaking exercise with low glycogen stores (and, to a lesser extent, low exogenous carbohydrate [CHO] availability) may upregulate signaling cascades that underpin mitochondrial biogenesis and increased capacity for fuel oxidation that occurs with endurance training.[43] Prolonging the postexercise period before restoring muscle glycogen may extend the period during which such adaptations occur, enhancing the outcomes. A clever combination of training and dietary sequences that integrates some high-quality sessions with high CHO availability, delayed refueling ("sleep low"), and some low- to moderate-intensity sessions undertaken with low CHO availability may enhance the overall training outcomes, leading to enhanced performance.[43]

Evidence that elite and highly trained athletes might have different responses

Studies that directly compare the responses of elite vs recreational athletes or meta-analyses that can identify factors that contribute to performance benefits are of interest. Ideally, some of these studies will measure characteristics that provide a mechanism to explain different outcomes.

Example from literature on nitrate supplementation

A study of nitrate supplementation in athletes of different calibers reported that "individual aerobic fitness level affects the ergogenic benefits induced by dietary nitrate supplementation. The optimal nitrate loading regimen required elevates plasma nitrate and to enhance performance in elite athletes is different from that of low-fit subjects and requires further studies."[44] Furthermore, a meta-analysis of nitrate supplementation studies found that the benefits were only significantly observed in active individuals and recreational athletes.[45]

Example from literature on periodized carbohydrate availability for training

Studies of trained but sub-elite athletes have shown that strategic periodization of CHO availability over 1 or 3 weeks of training leads to a superior performance outcome,[46,47] in comparison to training undertaken with sustained high CHO availability. However, studies in highly trained and elite athletes have failed to show a superior performance outcome with periodized vs sustained high CHO availability.[48-50]

Explanation for apparent differences between lesser-trained or lower-caliber athletes and high-performance athletes

Aspects of the literature should be examined to identify whether studies were undertaken with a methodology that was likely to allow any real benefits to be detected. Type 2 errors (also called false negatives) are common in studies with small sample sizes, which are typical of sports nutrition interventions. Once this issue has been examined, specific characteristics of elite and highly trained athletes and their performance should be considered to explain any apparent differences from lower-level athletes in their response to the sports nutrition strategy.

Example from literature on nitrate supplementation

Many studies within the nitrate supplementation literature have failed to use adequate or optimal dosing protocols or have focused on a performance protocol that was highly variable or unlikely to be affected by NO availability.[51] Therefore, some studies involving high-performance athletes may not have been able to adequately test the efficacy of nitrate supplementation. However, elite athletes may also have characteristics that make them less likely to benefit from nitrate supplementation: a greater percentage of type II muscle fibers, greater muscle capillarization and adaptation (which reduces the development of hypoxia and metabolic acidosis), and a more developed pathway to produce NO from arginine. These conditions may reduce the benefit of enhancing the activity of the nitrate-nitrite-NO pathway.[42]

Example from literature on periodized carbohydrate availability for training

Very few published studies have focused on the effects of periodized vs sustained high CHO availability on training adaptation and performance outcomes, because of the difficulty of undertaking chronic training-nutrition studies. Nevertheless, elite competitors may exhibit a different response than lower-level athletes because they are already close to their training/performance ceiling so any changes will necessarily be small and small changes are hard to detect. Furthermore, the high volume and intensity of training sessions and the "tried-and-true" sequencing of sessions in the programs of elite competitors may already create fluctuations in muscle glycogen. Therefore, elite athletes may already achieve periodized CHO availability without special dietary strategies. Finally, the superimposition of these dietary strategies may cause additional fatigue that requires a specific taper before performance outcomes are evident.

Making a pragmatic decision: should the high-performance athlete use this strategy?

Pros and cons of using the strategy should be examined. Studies within the general literature that are more suited to the elite athlete, with optimal protocols, may be given more prominence. An approach focusing on an individual case study (involving the specific athlete and controlled observation of special training sessions or lower-level competition) could be implemented to confirm the benefit of the strategy and any fine-tuning that may promote benefits.

Example from literature on nitrate supplementation

Few side effects arise from nitrate supplementation other than pink stools or urine following the intake of beetroot juice. Some studies, and individuals within investigations involving high-performance athletes, show benefits of nitrate supplementation for specific events and dosing protocols.[52,53] This approach might be targeted toward high-performance athletes in events in which a higher-dose or preloading protocol is used and performance involves shorter, higher-intensity exercise that creates greater hypoxic and acidic stress, along with a relatively greater involvement of type II muscle fibers or small muscle groups.[42] The high-performance athlete could experiment with their use of nitrate supplementation in scenarios that have a plausible chance of benefiting and make an individualized decision.[54,55]

Example from literature on periodized carbohydrate availability for training

The high-performance endurance athlete should assess their current training and nutrition strategies to identify how well these appear to match fueling practices to the goals of each session. In some cases, they will find that "trial and error" or logistics/cultural practices have led them to sequences that already achieve periodization goals. There may be downsides to overemphasis on low CHO availability strategies, including fatigue and an increased risk of illness and injury.[43] Athletes typically change the emphasis of different training-nutrition strategies across the course of the season, with deliberate integration of some low CHO availability strategies in the base phase, and greater emphasis on fueling support for high-quality sessions, particularly during immediate preparation for competition.[56,57]

menstrual status (use of hormonal contraceptives, eumenorrheic, amenorrheic) or menstrual phase (in the case of naturally menstruating females). Indeed, very few studies on female athletes have adequate assessed or standardized menstrual characteristics, potentially reducing the validity of the results.[37-40] Clearly, more work needs to be done to improve the quantity and quality of research that can address whether special considerations apply to female athletes in regard to sports nutrition guidelines.

What Magnitude of Performance Change Is Important to an Elite Athlete?

In many sports, the outcomes are decided by milliseconds, millimeters, a single fumble, or an expert action; the difference between winning and losing is measured in millions of dollars and everlasting fame. Hallmarks of traditional intervention studies in sports nutrition—small sample sizes, performance protocols of modest reliability, and traditional probability statistics—make such studies unlikely to detect differences or changes in performance that could be worthwhile to the athlete.[58,59] Indeed, most scientific investigations of nutrition strategies, particularly supplement use, are biased toward rejecting the hypothesis that the product or tactic enhances performance.

Many elite athletes take a favorable attitude toward unproven supplements or other nutrition strategies on the basis that even a minuscule effect is worth the investment. This concept is often confirmed by the discussion in newer research papers in which the performance difference due to an intervention is directly compared with the outcome of a sporting event. For example, the researchers may note that the mean improvement in performance with supplement X was 2.3%, which would span the difference between the first-place winner and the eighth finisher in a particular race. Such results often give rise to the inference or misunderstanding that if the eighth athlete in this race had used supplement X, their performance would have been elevated to winning status. However, this simplistic approach misrepresents the real nature of sports performance because it focuses only on interindividual differences rather than the equally important issue of intraathlete variability or reliability. More specifically, it neglects the reality that the day-to-day performance of athletes varies across a range that overlaps with that of their fellow competitors, such that the rerunning of an event would likely lead to a different outcome without any intervention being applied.

Hopkins et al[58] have discussed alternative ways to detect worthwhile performance enhancements in elite sports, taking into account the margins in performance between and within highly competitive athletes. After modeling the results of various sporting events, they suggested that worthwhile changes to the outcome of most events require a performance difference equal to approximately 0.3 to 0.5 times the variability (coefficient of variation [CV]) of performance for that event. Furthermore, across a range of events, the CV of performance of top athletes is usually within the range of 0.5% to 3%, with differences according to the type of effect and the caliber of the performer.[60] Although an improvement of approximately 0.5% of the event CV does not guarantee clear movement of the athlete from finalist to winner, it may increase their likelihood of winning by about 10%.[60] Such a difference is still outside the realm of detection for many of the studies commonly published in scientific journals.

Individual Differences in Response to Nutrition Interventions

Many investigations of sports nutrition interventions now also report the results of individual participants as well as the mean group outcome and show that even when the mean response suggests a worthwhile improvement in performance, the experiences of individual participants can range from a negative effect to a very large performance gain. The occurrence of side effects can also be an individual experience. Such differences in response to the same intervention are often interpreted as evidence of a responder vs nonresponder phenomenon. Although this outcome undoubtedly occurs in the case of some products and individuals, care should be taken in distinguishing it from the previously discussed day-to-day variability in individual performance.

Part of the modern landscape of health and medicine includes the gathering appreciation that genetic differences may also account for a large fraction of the variability in health responsiveness. For example, researchers are interested in whether single nucleotide polymorphisms (SNPs) of genes involved in caffeine metabolism or its interaction with adenosine receptors might account for individual differences in the response to caffeine supplementation. Although various hypotheses have been raised and tested and some studies have apparently shown differences in performance outcomes following caffeine use that appear to favor a certain SNP, the findings from the overall literature are mixed and confusing.[61] Additional work is needed to identify whether the current interest in personalized medicine can be applied to sports nutrition with confidence.

Various sources of information should be used to explore or confirm the concept of individual responsiveness to a sports nutrition intervention.[58] Within research scenarios, the starting point is to control the situation so that the intervention is the only variable changing. Additional techniques include looking for a correlation between markers of altered biochemistry or physiology associated with an intervention and change in performance. Strategies such as enrolling large numbers of study participants and undertaking covariate analysis of various characteristics—including genetic profiling—provide a sophisticated, albeit resource-intensive, tactic. A simpler strategy is to undertake repeated interventions of the strategy within the trial to look for a consistent response.

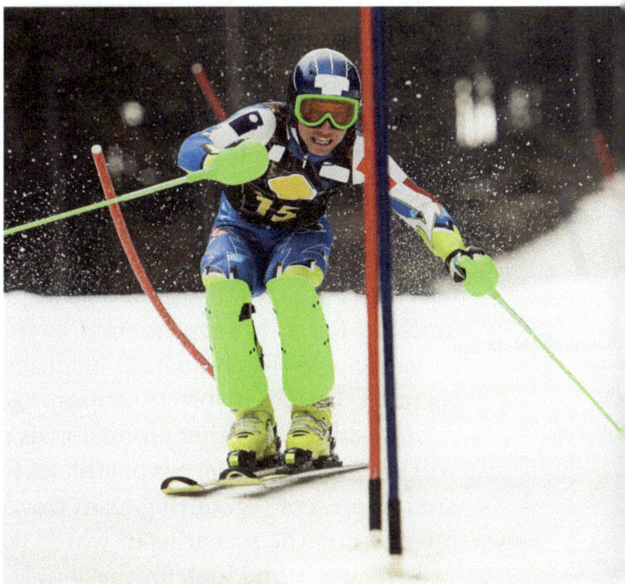

Within real-life practice, elite athletes who receive sports science support may have access to information about their specific physiological or biochemical responses to certain nutrition interventions that enable them to identify successful strategies or tweak characteristics. In the future, it may become possible to receive a genetic profiling report that could identify potential responsiveness to different kinds of strategies. For the moment, the most pragmatic way for an athlete to investigate a sports nutrition intervention is to consider best-practice guidelines as a starting point that will cover most individuals. They can also identify whether they are a nonresponder or responder to the intervention through trial and error, aided by standardized application and systematic reporting of the outcomes of their activities.

STRATEGIES FOR WORKING WITH ELITE ATHLETES

A successful practice working with elite athletes requires the sports dietitian to use certain strategies and to display a set of key personal characteristics. The following ideas can help the sports dietitian develop a rewarding career working with this select athlete population.

Getting Started

Be prepared to start at the bottom to gain experience. Look for opportunities to start with local teams and athletes rather than expecting to start with a job with a national sporting organization or major professional team.

Focus on the task at hand. Do well with your current project rather than seeking ways to reach the next level—if you do well where you are, the opportunities will take care of themselves.

Use your contacts and involvement in sports to develop a knowledge base and experience. Your own sporting experiences can earn credibility with athletes and coaches and provide an intimate understanding of what it is like to be an athlete.

Find a mentor. Set a professional development program for yourself that includes regular journal reading and conference attendance. Stay up to date with both the science and practice of sports nutrition.

Learn About a Sport and Its Special Features

Learn all you can about how a sport influences the nutritional needs of competitors, as well as current nutrition practices and beliefs. Get specific information about training practices, competition programs, and lifestyle patterns, including individual differences among players on a team and among different sports.

Attend training sessions and events to better understand the culture and experiences of athletes, coaches, and other team members. Let the athletes know that you are interested in their activities.

Stay in frequent communication with the athletes you work with. For example, if the team won a recent game, be sure to congratulate them to show that you care about their success.

Stay informed about supplements used or promoted within a sport. To stay abreast of current ideas and practices, monitor information from social media, the internet, sports magazines, health-food shops, and supplement stores, as well as the general talk among players.

Be a Team Player

Identify all the people who work with an individual athlete or team and already provide their nutrition ideas or implement their nutrition practice. This will include people in the organized support structure and in the personal network that each athlete may develop. Be prepared to listen to the approaches and input of these people and find a niche in which your services and ideas will be appreciated.

Know when to stand your ground (you are the nutrition expert) and when to be flexible (a compromise of your ideas may be necessary for athletes to accept). Look for middle ground. For example, a coach or trainer may insist that the athlete consume branched-chain amino acids after a training session to promote recovery. Rather than debating whether the present literature provides support for benefits of postexercise supplementation with amino acid supplements, consider setting up recovery snacks for the team, including fruit smoothies, flavored yogurt, and cereal with milk. Provide educational material showing the coach and athletes that these snacks provide a good source of branched-chain amino acids (similar to the amounts found in supplements), as well as carbohydrate and fluid for refueling and rehydration.

Participate (when invited) in all activities of the athlete or team support network, even if these do not seem to directly involve nutrition. Note that you may not be involved in all team activities. Cultivate relationships with other professionals or team support personnel so they are aware of what you can do and will provide early referrals of athletes for your specialty services and support your nutrition plan when you are not present (eg, during team travel). Note, of course, that other team support people may already be busy during the scenarios in which you are hoping to delegate some nutrition tasks. Be reasonable with your requests, and look for the simplest but most impactful way to be represented.

Be Creative With Nutrition Activities

Create educational resources that target the needs and interests of your individual athletes and teams. Use innovative ways to provide information rather than relying on standard lectures or interview and consultation formats. Be prepared to organize information or activities in bite-size chunks or address the issues that are of immediate interest to your athletes rather than following a standard script. Create individual messages or timelines if needed for each athlete.

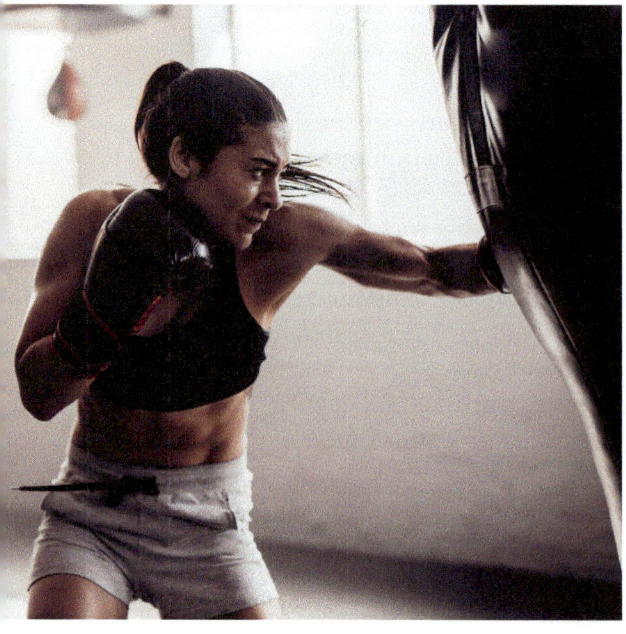

Make use of social media and the learning opportunities that appeal most to athletes. TikTok videos or Instagram posts may be the language spoken by younger people; old-school handouts are likely to be relegated to the floors of the training facilities. Short videos and changing displays in an environment in which the athletes are a captive audience—for example, around a coffee machine in the team kitchen or in the locker room—may mean they are consumed by osmosis to reinforce key nutrition messages and strategies.

Monitor behaviors and outcomes. If you are frequently delivering a message and behaviors are not changing in response, you may need to restructure how that message is being delivered.

Plan interactive activities, such as cooking classes or supermarket tours, or install recovery stations with suitable drinks and snacks at training or competition venues. These activities provide visibility and tangible outcomes. Many people learn better through practical activities.

It is possible that you will work with elite athletes from foreign countries, which may cause you to run into a language barrier. In this case, be prepared to find creative and interesting nutrition resources that are in the appropriate language, if possible, to ensure that all athletes have access to the valuable information you provide.

Remember, It Is Not All About You

Many people who become involved in the preparation of elite athletes start to identify closely with the success of these athletes. Although it is rewarding to feel that you contributed to a successful outcome or were part of a valued support team, it is important to maintain perspective about your role. High-level sports and high-profile athletes attract an entourage of people, many of whom use a cult of personality to make themselves seem indispensable. In some cases, members of this entourage can become as famous (or infamous) as the athlete. Although it is often important to be able to sell your message in a memorable way, it is more important to maintain an appropriate and ethical profile.

Stay Ethical

Sports are all about rules and regulations. There is a professional code of conduct that covers your role as a nutrition advisor or therapist. Sometimes, you may feel pressured to assist an athlete in a dangerous or unethical practice, such as excessive loss of body fat or weight or use of a supplement containing prohibited substances (see Chapter 7). Stay true to professional standards, even when the athlete threatens to undertake the practice without your assistance.

In addition, maintain confidentiality in your work with high-profile athletes. Even when opinions or information seem to be discussed as public conversation, guard your knowledge about the athletes with whom you work. This includes the nature of your nutrition work as well as other information, such as inside knowledge of injuries or other problems. At best, breaches of this information are an invasion of the athlete's privacy. At worst, they may be considered insider trading in a world where betting on sports is a highly lucrative industry.

Tips for Survival in a High-Pressure Environment

Be organized and have definite goals for your activities. Set up a contract with the appropriate person (medical director, head coach, athlete) in which the range of services you can provide is discussed and agreed upon. Provide feedback or summary information on completed services so that your input is documented and appreciated.

Set expectations with management and know what their priorities are. Ask how they measure success. Monitor and track actions and outcomes each year. Be prepared to provide supporting information to management at the end of the year to show the impact you are making.

Do not forget to build in ways of assessing and rewarding your own progress and achievement of goals. It is easy to overlook your own performance when the focus is on the athlete(s).

Finally, make sure to look after your own health and well-being. Sometimes, the service of athletes requires long hours and the elevation of their needs above your own. Be prepared for the politics of high-level sport. Coaches and medical staff are frequently abandoned by their athletes or suddenly dismissed from a team, often through no fault of their own. Expect that this will happen to you. Be prepared to pick yourself up and develop a new plan.

SUMMARY

Working with elite athletes provides an opportunity for the sports dietitian to test their sports science knowledge and creativity in solving practical challenges faced by athletes pushing to their extreme limits. The elite environment can be both high pressure and high return. The sports dietitian will need to remain up to date with the latest scientific information and adhere to a code of conduct that includes an understanding of the ethics of sport, a respect for confidentiality, and care for their own well-being. It can be rewarding to see that nutrition plays a role in the achievement of the highest levels of success in sport. However, the role is often specific to the needs of a gifted individual and a unique situation.

KEY TAKEAWAYS

Elite athletes train and compete at high intensity and undertake multiple training sessions; for most elite athletes, this is their job.

Elite athletes are highly motivated; they seek and appreciate the nutrition advice that they are offered and usually adhere to recommendations.

The increase in requirements for energy, carbohydrate, and other nutrients associated with high-performance sport is often supported by special catering opportunities that are provided in the athlete's environment. However, some athletes may need assistance in achieving their special nutrition needs.

Travel plays a major role for the elite athlete; domestic and international competitions disrupt the athlete's usual eating routine and access to their preferred foods and can expose them to different standards of food and water hygiene.

The margins of winning and losing in sport are small, which often motivates the athlete (and their entourage) to be aggressive with new strategies and ideas in sports nutrition. Unfortunately, few of the studies undertaken on most sports nutrition topics are carried out with populations of elite performers. Better research techniques and better ways to perform case studies on individual athletes may assist the athlete in making an informed decision about whether a strategy "works."

Sports dietitians who work with elite athletes should practice ethical behaviors in all dealings with the athletes.

REFERENCES

1. Garth AK, Burke LM. What do athletes drink during competitive sporting activities? *Sports Med.* 2013;43(7):539-564. doi:10.1007/s40279-013-0028-y
2. Thomas DT, Erdman KA, Burke LM. American College of Sports Medicine joint position statement. Nutrition and athletic performance. *Med Sci Sports Exerc.* 2016;48(3):543-568. doi:10.1249/MSS.0000000000000852
3. Mujika I, Halson S, Burke LM, et al. An integrated, multifactorial approach to periodization for optimal performance in individual and team sports. *Int Sports Physiol Perform.* 2018;13(5):538-561. doi:10.1123/ijspp.2018-0093
4. Burke LM. Nutrition for recovery after competition and training. In: Burke LM, Deakin V, Minehan M, eds. *Clinical Sports Nutrition.* 6th ed. McGraw-Hill 2021:375-416.
5. Garthe I, Maughan RJ. Athletes and supplements: prevalence and perspectives. *Int Sport Nutr Exerc Metab.* 2018;28(2):126-138. doi:10.1123/ijsnem.2017-0429
6. Davis JK, Oikawa SY, Halson S, et al. In-season nutrition strategies and recovery modalities to enhance recovery for basketball players: a narrative review. *Sports Med.* 2022;52(5):971-993. doi:10.1007/s40279-021-01606-7
7. Collins J, Maughan RJ, Gleeson M, et al. UEFA expert group statement on nutrition in elite football. Current evidence to inform practical recommendations and guide future research. *Br Sports Med.* 2021;55(8):416. doi:10.1136/bjsports-2019-101961
8. Burke LM, Hawley JA, Wong SHS, Jeukendrup AE. Carbohydrates for training and competition. *Sports Sci.* 2011;29(suppl 1):S17-S27. doi:10.1080/02640414.2011.585473
9. Burke LM. Nutritional approaches to counter performance constraints in high-level sports competition. *Exp Physiol.* 2021;106(12):2304-2323. doi:10.1113/EP088188
10. Halson SL, Burke LM, Pearce J. Nutrition for travel: from jet lag to catering. *Int Sport Nutr Exerc Metab.* 2019;29(2):228-235. doi:10.1123/ijsnem.2018-0278
11. Burke L. Road cycling and triathlon. In: Burke L, ed. *Practical Sports Nutrition.* Human Kinetics; 2007:71-107.
12. Burke L. Practical and cultural factors. In: Burke L, ed. *Practical Sports Nutrition.* Human Kinetics; 2007:27-39.
13. Burke LM, Cox GR, Culmmings NK, Desbrow B. Guidelines for daily carbohydrate intake: do athletes achieve them? *Sports Med.* 2001;31(4):267-299. doi:10.2165/00007256-200131040-00003
14. Burke LM, Slater GJ, Matthews JJ, Langan-Evans C, Horswil CA. ACSM Expert Consensus Statement on weight loss in weight-category sports. *Curr Sports Med Rep.* 2021;20(4):199-217. doi:10.1249/JSR.0000000000000831
15. Garcia-Roves PM, Terrados N, Fernandez SF, et al. Macronutrients intake of top level cyclists during continuous competition – change in the feeding pattern. *Int Sports Med.* 1998;19(1):61-67. doi:10.1055/s-2007-971882
16. Fordyce T. Chris Froome: Team Sky's unprecedented release of data reveals how British rider won Giro d'Italia. *BBC Sport.* July 4, 2018. Accessed July 22, 2023. www.bbc.com/sport/cycling/44694122
17. Plasqui G, Rietjens G, Lambriks L, et al. Energy expenditure during extreme endurance exercise: the Giro d'Italia. *Med Sci Sports Exerc.* 2019;51(3):568-574. doi:10.1249/MSS.0000000000001814
18. Phelps M, Abrahamson A. *No Limits: The Will to Succeed.* Simon and Schuster; 2008.
19. Mountjoy M, Ackerman KE, Bailey DM, et al. 2023 International Olympic Committee's (IOC) consensus statement on Relative Energy Deficiency in Sport (REDs). *Br Sports Med.* 2023;57(17):1073-1097. doi:10.1136/bjsports-2023-106994
20. Nattiv A, Loucks AB, Manore MM, et al. American College of Sports Medicine position stand. The female athlete triad. *Med Sci Sports Exerc.* 2007;39(10):1867-1882. doi:10.1249/mss.0b013e318149f111
21. Woods RM. Swimmers 'ruined' by culture of fat-shaming and bullying. BBC News. February 24, 2023. Accessed April 10, 2023. www.bbc.com/news/uk-england-64256659
22. Swimming Australia's ethics committee meets to discuss fresh reports of fat-shaming and abusive culture. SBS News. June 14, 2021. Accessed April 10, 2023. www.sbs.com.au/news/article/swimming-australias-ethics-committee-meets-to-discuss-fresh-reports-of-fat-shaming-and-abusive-culture/l4spe9da8
23. Ingles S. Why are we fat-shaming tennis players? *The Guardian.* May 31, 2014. Accessed April 10, 2023. www.theguardian.com/sport/shortcuts/2014/may/31/fat-shaming-tennis-players-taylor-townsend?CMP=share_btn_tw
24. Smothers H. The world's fastest women are still being body-shamed. *Vice.* November 15, 2019. Accessed July 22, 2023. www.vice.com/en/article/vb5abx/the-worlds-fastest-women-are-still-being-body-shamed
25. Cain M. I was the fastest girl in the world until I joined Nike. *New York Times.* November 7, 2019. Accessed July 22, 2023. www.nytimes.com/2019/11/07/opinion/nike-running-mary-cain.html
26. Whitehead J. Gymnast Katelyn Ohashi speaks out about body shaming. *The Independent.* August 13, 2019. Accessed April 10, 2023. www.independent.co.uk/life-style/health-and-families/katelyn-ohashi-viral-gymnast-body-shaming-weight-gain-a8927351.html
27. Stellingwerff T. Case study: body composition periodization in an Olympic-level female middle-distance runner over a 9-year career. *Int Sport Nutr Exerc Metab.* 2018;28(4):428-433. doi:10.1123/ijsnem.2017-0312
28. Nattiv A, De Souza MJ, Koltun KJ, et al. The male athlete triad—a consensus statement from the female and male athlete triad coalition part 1: definition and scientific basis. *Clin Sport Med.* 2021;31(4):345-353. doi:10.1097/JSM.0000000000000946

29. Coyle D, Hamilton T. *The Secret Race: Inside the Hidden World of the Tour de France: Doping, Cover-ups, and Winning at All Costs.* Random House, 2013.

30. Saddles B. Rasmussen blows whistle on a decade of dope. *Eurosport.* January 2, 2013. Accessed April 10, 2023. www.eurosport.com/cycling/rasmussen-blows-whistle-on-a-decade-of-dope_sto4706268/story.shtml

31. Sundgot-Borgen J, Meyer NL, Lohman TG, et al. How to minimise the health risks to athletes who compete in weight-sensitive sports review and position statement on behalf of the Ad Hoc Research Working Group on Body Composition, Health and Performance, under the auspices of the IOC Medical Commission. *Br Sports Med.* 2013;47(16):1012-1022. doi:10.1136/bjsports-2013-092966

32. Wells KR, Jeacocke NA, Appaneal R, et al. The Australian Institute of Sport (AIS) and National Eating Disorders Collaboration (NEDC) position statement on disordered eating in high performance sport. *Br Sports Med.* 2020;54(21):1247-1258. doi:10.1136/bjsports-2019-101813

33. Stellingwerff T, Peeling P, Garvican-Lewis LA, et al. Nutrition and altitude: strategies to enhance adaptation, improve performance and maintain health: a narrative review. *Sports Med.* 2019;49(suppl 2):169-184. doi:10.1007/s40279-019-01159-w

34. McCubbin AJ, Allanson BA, Caldwell Odgers JN, et al. Sports Dietitians Australia position statement: nutrition for exercise in hot environments. *Int Sport Nutr Exerc Metab.* 2020;30(1):83-98. doi:10.1123/ijsnem.2019-0300

35. Burke LM, King C. Ramadan fasting and the goals of sports nutrition around exercise. *Sports Sci.* 2012;30(suppl 1):S21-S31. doi:10.1080/02640414.2012.680484

36. McKay AKA, Stellingwerff T, Smith ES, et al. Defining training and performance caliber: a participant classification framework. *Int Sports Physiol Perform.* 2022;17(2):317-331. doi:10.1123/ijspp.2021-0451

37. Smith ES, McKay AKA, Kuikman M, et al. Auditing the representation of female versus male athletes in sports science and sports medicine research: evidence-based performance supplements. *Nutrients* 2022;14(5):953. doi:10.3390/nu14050953

38. Smith ES, McKay AKA, Kuikman M, et al. Managing female athlete health: auditing the representation of female versus male participants among research in supplements to manage diagnosed micronutrient issues. *Nutrients* 2022;14(16):3372. doi:10.3390/nu14163372

39. Kuikman MA, McKay AKA, Smith ES, et al. Female athlete representation and dietary control methods among studies assessing chronic carbohydrate approaches to support training. *Int Sports Nutr Exerc Metab.* 2023;33(4):198-208. doi:10.1123/ijsnem.2022-0214

40. Kuikman MA, Smith ES, McKay AKA, et al. Fueling the female athlete: auditing her representation in studies of acute carbohydrate intake for exercise. *Med Sci Sports Exerc.* 2023;55(3):569-580. doi:10.1249/MSS.0000000000003056

41. Smith ES, McKay AKA, Ackerman KE, et al. Methodology review: a protocol to audit the representation of female athletes in sports science and sports medicine research. *Int Sport Nutr Exerc Metab.* 2022;32(2):114-127. doi:10.1123/ijsnem.2021-0257

42. Jones AM. Dietary nitrate supplementation and exercise performance. *Sports Med.* 2014;44(suppl 1):35-45. doi:10.1007/s40279-014-0149-y

43. Burke LM, Hawley JA, Jeukendrup A, et al. Toward a common understanding of diet-exercise strategies to manipulate fuel availability for training and competition preparation in endurance sport. *Int Sport Nutr Exerc Metab.* 2018;28(5):451-463. doi:10.1123/ijsnem.2018-0289

44. Porcelli S, Ramaglia M, Bellistri G, et al. Aerobic fitness affects the exercise performance responses to nitrate supplementation. *Med Sci Sport Exerc.* 2015;47(8):1643-1651. doi:10.1249/MSS.0000000000000577

45. Hoon MW, Johnson NA, Chapman PG, Burke LM. The effect of nitrate supplementation on exercise performance in healthy individuals: a systematic review and meta-analysis. *Int Sport Nutr Exerc Metab.* 2013;23(5):522-532. doi:10.1123/ijsnem.23.5.522

46. Marquet LA, Brisswalter J, Louis J, et al. Enhanced endurance performance by periodization of carbohydrate intake: "sleep low" strategy. *Med Sci Sport Exerc.* 2016;48(4):663-672. doi:10.1249/MSS.0000000000000823

47. Marquet LA, Hausswirth C, Molle O, et al. Periodization of carbohydrate intake: short-term effect on performance. *Nutrients* 2016;8(12):755. doi:10.3390/nu8120755

48. Burke LM, Ross ML, Garvican-Lewis LA, et al. Low carbohydrate, high fat diet impairs exercise economy and negates the performance benefit from intensified training in elite race walkers. *Physiol.* 2017;595(9):2785-2807. doi:10.1113/JP273230

49. Burke LM, Sharma AP, Heikura IA, et al. Crisis of confidence averted: Impairment of exercise economy and performance in elite race walkers by ketogenic low carbohydrate, high fat (LCHF) diet is reproducible. *PLoS One.* 2020;15(6):e0234027. doi:10.1371/journal.pone.0234027

50. Gejl KD, Thams LB, Hansen M, et al. No superior adaptations to carbohydrate periodization in elite endurance athletes. *Med Sci Sport Exerc.* 2017;49(12):2486-2497. doi:10.1249/MSS.0000000000001377

51. Shannon OM, Allen JD, Bescos R, et al. Dietary inorganic nitrate as an ergogenic aid: an expert consensus derived via the modified Delphi technique. *Sports Med.* 2022;52(10):2537-2558. doi:10.1007/s40279-022-01701-3

52. Hoon MW, Jones AM, Johnson NA, et al. The effect of variable doses of inorganic nitrate-rich beetroot juice on simulated 2,000-m rowing performance in trained athletes. *Int Sport Physiol Perform.* 2014;9(4):615-620. doi:10.1123/ijspp.2013-0207

53. Peeling P, Cox GR, Bullock N, Burke LM. Beetroot juice improves on-water 500 m time-trial performance, and laboratory-based paddling economy in national and international-level kayak athletes. *Int Sport Nutr Exerc Metab.* 2015;25(3):278-2884. doi:10.1123/ijsnem.2014-0110

54. Jonvik KL, Nyakayiru J, van Loon LJC, Verdijk LB. Last Word on Viewpoint: Can elite athletes benefit from dietary nitrate supplementation? *Appl Physiol (1985).* 2015;119(6):770. doi:10.1152/japplphysiol.00622.2015

55. Jonvik KL, Nyakayiru J, van Loon LJC, Verdijk LB. Can elite athletes benefit from dietary nitrate supplementation? *Appl Physiol (1985).* 2015;119(6):759-761. doi:10.1152/japplphysiol.00232.2015

56. Stellingwerff T. Contemporary nutrition approaches to optimize elite marathon performance. *Int Sport Physiol Perform.* 2013;8(5):573-578. doi:10.1123/ijspp.8.5.573

57. Shaw G, Boyd KT, Burke LM, Koivisto A. Nutrition for swimming. *Int Sport Nutr Exerc Metab.* 2014;24(4):360-372. doi:10.1123/ijsnem.2014-0015

58. Hopkins WG, Hawley JA, Burke LM. Design and analysis of research on sport performance enhancement. *Med Sci Sport Exerc.* 1999;31(3):472-485. doi:10.1097/00005768-199903000-00018

59. Burke LM, Peeling P. Methodologies for investigating performance changes with supplement use. *Int Sport Nutr Exerc Metab.* 2018;28(2):159-169. doi:10.1123/ijsnem.2017-0325

60. Malcata RM, Hopkins WG. Variability of competitive performance of elite athletes: a systematic review. *Sports Med.* 2014;44(12):1763-1774. doi:10.1007/s40279-014-0239-x

61. Grgic J, Pickering C, Del Coso J, Schoenfeld BJ, Mikulic P. CYP1A2 genotype and acute ergogenic effects of caffeine intake on exercise performance: a systematic review. *Eur Nutr* 2021;60(3):1181-1195. doi:10.1007/s00394-020-02427-6

CHAPTER 16

Vegetarian Athletes

D. Enette Larson-Meyer, PhD, RD, CSSD, FACSM

LEARNING OBJECTIVES

- Define key terms related to plant-based eating patterns including vegan, lactovegetarian, lacto-ovo vegetarian, and plant-based.
- Identify the various reasons athletes elect to follow vegetarian, vegan, or plant-based diets and the possible reasons that interest in plant-based diets as a whole may be increasing.
- Describe the strategies that may help individual athletes meet their energy needs through consumption of a variety of foods, including whole grains, fruits, vegetables, legumes, nuts, seeds, and (if desired) dairy products and eggs.
- Identify the nutrients that tend to be found less abundantly in plant-based foods compared to animal-based foods and/or that are less well absorbed and describe the strategies for increasing intake and status of these nutrients.
- Explain the reasons that relative energy deficiency in sport (REDs) is often identified with higher prevalence in vegetarian athletes.

INTRODUCTION

Athletes may elect to follow vegetarian diets for health, environmental, ecological, religious, or spiritual reasons.[1,2] In addition, a dietary shift toward the adoption of plant-based diets is one of key strategies considered necessary to achieve the United Nations Sustainable Development Goals and the Paris Agreement[3] and to promote increased health for both planet and people, including athletes.[4] Currently, the number of athletes who follow vegetarian eating patterns is unknown, but such eating patterns are thought to be gaining popularity among athletes. A survey of 351 athletes participating in the 2010 Commonwealth Games suggested that as many as 8% followed vegetarian diets; 1% of those reported being vegan.[5] Similarly, a 2015 survey of 422 marathon finishers found that 9% reported following vegan, vegetarian, or pescatarian diets.[6] Among athletes, however, a 2018 survey suggested that principal motives for following vegetarian-based dietary patterns included animal rights, environmental concerns, health, and improved physical performance.[7] Box 16.1 explores the common terms used to classify vegetarian diets.[8]

Well-planned vegetarian diets are nutritionally adequate, appropriate for athletes at all ages and levels from recreational to elite, and provide health benefits in the prevention and treatment of chronic diseases.[9-14] Like most athletes, vegetarian athletes may benefit from education about food choices to optimize their health and peak performance. This chapter reviews the energy, macronutrient, vitamin, and mineral requirements of the plant-based athlete and provides tips for meeting nutritional needs with an exclusive (or near-exclusive) vegetarian diet. This chapter also includes tips for the sports dietitian working with plant-based athletes.

BOX 16.1 Definitions of Vegetarian and Plant-Based Diets[8]

Lacto-ovo vegetarian	Does not eat meat, fish, or fowl; eats dairy and egg products
Ovovegetarian	Does not eat meat, fish, fowl, or dairy; eats eggs
Lactovegetarian	Does not eat meat, fish, fowl, or eggs; eats dairy products
Vegan	Does not eat any animal products, including meat, fish, fowl, eggs, dairy, and honey; most vegans also do not use animal products such as silk, leather, and wool
Plant-based	A more recent term that may be used to define diets ranging from vegan to semivegetarian

SPORTS NUTRITION CONSIDERATIONS: ENERGY AND MACRONUTRIENTS

Energy

The energy needs of athletes and active individuals, whether consuming a plant-based diet or not, vary considerably and are dependent on body size, body composition, sex, training regimen, and nontraining physical activity patterns. Experts estimate that energy expenditure ranges from 2,600 kcal/d in female swimmers to 8,500 kcal/d in male cyclists participating in the Tour de France bicycle race.[15] In practice, the total daily energy expenditure of individual athletes can be estimated using a variety of methods, as discussed in detail in Chapter 10.

Meeting energy needs is a priority for all athletes. Inadequate energy intake relative to energy expenditure negates the benefits of training and compromises performance. Although some athletes who follow vegetarian and vegan diets may have difficulty meeting energy requirements because of the high fiber content or low energy density of plant-based diets, sports dietitians are likely to encounter vegetarian athletes with a variety of energy needs.[16] To meet their energy requirements and maintain body weight, some athletes may need to consume 6 to 8 meals and snacks per day while managing their dietary fiber intake.[17] High-fiber diets, given their bulky nature, often reduce overall energy consumption. Others may require lower energy intakes to promote weight reduction for health or performance. Sports dietitians should work with individual athletes to help meet their energy needs through the consumption of a variety of foods, including whole grains, fruits, vegetables, legumes, nuts, seeds, and (if desired) dairy products and eggs.[11] Both the US Department of Agriculture's MyPlate, which has adjustments for different energy requirements and tips for vegetarians,[18] and the guidelines developed by Larson-Meyer and Ruscigno[11] specifically for vegetarian athletes may be useful when educating athletes about healthy eating patterns. Furthermore, the same group that developed and validated the Athlete's Plate Nutrition Education Tool has recently created a vegetarian version that models easy, moderate, and hard training days (http://swell.uccs.edu/vegetarianvegan-athletes-plate).[19] Eating plans developed for individuals who consume vegetarian or vegan diets may also provide a useful framework if the number of servings is increased appropriately for athletes.[20,21] Another recent resource is that of Guest and Lynch.[22]

Box 16.2 on page 384 contains sample menus for a 3,000-kcal/d vegetarian diet and a 4,600-kcal/d vegan diet. These energy levels may be required to meet the needs of individuals who train or exercise regularly. Vegetarian athletes who struggle to consume adequate energy may benefit from consuming only one-third to one-half of their grains and fruit in the whole, unprocessed form.[11] This will reduce excessive fiber intake and lessen early onset of satiety. Additionally, vegetarian athletes struggling to meet energy demands may benefit from selecting more energy-dense foods, such as nuts, seeds, and avocados, and decreasing the amount of fiber in the diet.

BOX 16.2 Sample 3,000 kcal Vegetarian Menu and 4,600 kcal Vegan Menu[a]

3,000 KCAL VEGETARIAN MENU[b]	4,600 KCAL VEGAN MENU[c]
Breakfast	
1 cup raisin bran cereal	1½ cups raisin bran cereal
1 cup fat-free milk	1 cup fortified soy milk
2 slices mixed-grain toast	3 slices mixed-grain toast
2 tsp margarine	3 tsp vegan butter
1 medium banana	1 medium banana
8 oz fruit juice	8 oz fruit juice
Lunch	
Whole-wheat pita stuffed with shredded spinach, sliced tomato, 2 oz feta cheese, 2 Tbsp olive oil	Tofu salad on a 4-oz hoagie roll (1 cup firm tofu, 2 tsp mustard, 2 tsp soy mayonnaise, lettuce, tomato)
1 large apple	1 large apple
2 small oatmeal cookies	3 small oatmeal cookies
	8 oz carrot juice
Snack	
Sesame seed bagel	Sesame seed bagel
1 Tbsp peanut butter	1 Tbsp peanut butter
1 Tbsp jam	1 Tbsp jam
	1 cup fortified soy milk
Dinner	
Lentil spaghetti sauce	Lentil spaghetti sauce (1½ cup cooked lentils, ½ onion, 1½ cups canned tomatoes, 1 Tbsp olive oil)
(1 cup cooked lentils, ½ onion, 1½ cups canned tomatoes, 1 Tbsp olive oil)	
3 oz dry pasta, cooked	4 oz dry pasta, cooked
1 Tbsp parmesan cheese	3 (1-oz) slices French bread dipped in 2 Tbsp olive oil
2 (1-oz) slices French bread dipped in 1 Tbsp olive oil	1½ cups steamed collards
1 cup steamed broccoli	
Snack	
1 cup fruit yogurt	1 cup fruit sorbet
	1 oz toasted almonds

[a] Both menus assume that grain products are made from enriched flour.
[b] Vegetarian menu: 3,066 kcal, 106 g of protein, 469 g of carbohydrate, 85 g of fat (14% protein, 25% fat, 61% carbohydrate), 1,600 mg of calcium, 29 mg of iron, 14 mg of zinc.
[c] Vegan menu: 4,626 kcal, 146 g of protein, 704 g of carbohydrate, 136 g of fat (13% protein, 26% fat, 61% carbohydrate), 1,133 mg of calcium, 60 mg of iron, 15 mg of zinc.

Carbohydrate

Carbohydrates should make up the bulk of the athlete's diet. Adequate carbohydrate intake maintains muscle and liver glycogen stores.[16,23-25] Further, it optimizes mood and performance during prolonged, moderate-intensity exercise and intermittent, short-duration, high-intensity exercise,[26-33] which includes team sports.[34] Thus, for many athletes, maintaining sufficient carbohydrate intake will result in a delayed time to fatigue during training or competition or better sprinting potential at the end of a race or sporting event. The benefit of carbohydrate consumption, however, is not limited to the maintenance of muscle and liver glycogen stores and the preservation of blood glucose. Dietary carbohydrate is important for maintaining intermediates of the tricarboxylic acid cycle (Krebs cycle),[35] preserving the bioenergetic state of skeletal muscle,[30] and preventing a decline in exercise economy (oxygen cost at a given pace or speed).[36,37] Oral exposure to carbohydrates through consumption or mouth rinsing may enhance performance through stimulation of the central nervous system.[33,38] (For more information on carbohydrate, refer to Chapter 2.)

Active individuals should be able to meet their carbohydrate needs easily on a vegetarian diet by consuming a variety of sources such as cereals, grains, legumes, starchy vegetables, fruits, and some meat analogues such as tempeh (made from fermented soybeans). The carbohydrate recommendations for athletes range from as low as 3 to 5 g per kilogram of body weight per day to as high as 12 g per kilogram of body weight per day.[16,39] The amount recommended within this range depends on the athlete's total daily energy expenditure, training intensity and training periodization, and training goals. For example, elite, college, or other competitive athletes undergoing extreme training (>4 h/d) may benefit from a higher carbohydrate intake and should strive for the higher recommended range of 8 to 12 g per kilogram of body weight per day. Conversely, athletes participating at a level that demands less training (eg, skill-based activity or recreational exercisers) or those attempting to reduce body weight or fat stores may require only 3 to 5 g per kilogram of body weight per day.[39] Sports dietitians may find that the concept of carbohydrate exchanges and label-reading exercises are useful for educating athletes about meeting their carbohydrate needs.[11] Knowledge of carbohydrate sources is also useful in planning carbohydrate intake before, during, and after exercise.

Protein

The protein needs of athletes vary according to the sport or activity, intensity of training, and level of experience.[40] The protein needs of active vegetarians who engage in light to moderate activity several times per week are likely to be met by the Recommended Dietary Allowance (RDA) of 0.8 g per kilogram of body weight per day.[17,41] The protein requirements of those who train more intensely may be higher than the RDA to support a positive nitrogen balance and promote postexercise muscle protein synthesis. Whereas the most current guidelines recommend protein intake in the range 1.2 to 2.0 g per kilogram of body weight per day for athletes regardless of dietary pattern,[16] a recent meta-analysis found that protein intakes of greater than approximately 1.6 g per kilogram of body weight per day did not promote further training-induced gains in either strength or fat-free mass.[42] In a 2021 study, researchers provided 1.6 g of protein per kilogram of body weight to young men undergoing a 12-week supervised resistance training regimen. They found no differences in the gains in strength or lean mass between those following an exclusively plant-based diet consisting of plant-based whole foods supplemented with soy protein isolate compared to their athletic counterparts following a mixed whole foods diet supplemented with whey protein isolate.[43] Higher protein (and essential amino acids) needs for athletes during routine endurance and resistance training are needed to cover enhanced protein deposition during muscle development and increased protein utilization as an auxiliary fuel during exercise.[44] Moreover, inadequate intake of total energy or carbohydrate increases protein needs. During prolonged endurance activity, for example, athletes with low glycogen stores metabolize twice as much protein as those with adequate stores, primarily as a result of increased gluconeogenesis.[45]

Dietary protein—particularly the amino acid leucine—may play a role beyond the supply of building blocks and energy and serve as an important trigger for muscle protein synthesis induced by training.[40] More specifically, increases in the plasma leucine concentration to a critical threshold after a meal (through the consumption of protein containing about 2–3 g of leucine) are thought to "turn on" muscle protein synthesis (see Chapter 3 for additional details on the leucine trigger hypothesis). Research further suggests that the peak in leucine concentration varies by the content and absorbability of leucine in individual proteins. For example, researchers have shown that whey induces a much greater spike in plasma leucine than soy or casein proteins. Soy, particularly fiber-free isolated protein, is a rich source of leucine, as are pea (and other legumes), brown rice, corn, and potato proteins.[46] The leucine in some of these products, however, may not be as rapidly absorbable as the leucine in whey.

There is currently no research to suggest that protein recommendations are different for athletes following a vegetarian diet than for those consuming an omnivorous diet. Although some experts have suggested (and periodically misstated) that vegetarians may need approximately 10% more protein than omnivores to account for the lower digestibility of plant proteins compared with animal proteins, available evidence does not support a separate requirement for vegetarians consuming complementary plant proteins.[17,41] In addition, a meta-analysis of nitrogen balance studies found that the source of dietary protein did not significantly affect the protein needs of healthy individuals.[47] However, sports dietitians should be aware that protein needs might be slightly higher in athletes whose dietary protein sources come mainly from whole plant food sources that are harder to digest, such as legumes and whole grains, rather than plant sources that are easier to digest, such as soy protein.[48] Protein needs may also be higher in athletes with low energy intakes.[46]

Vegetarian athletes can easily meet their protein needs if their diets are adequate in energy and contain a variety of plant-based protein foods, such as legumes (including soy foods), nuts, seeds, and grains. Based on extensive research, Young and Pellett[49] have emphasized that vegetarians do not need to be overly concerned with protein complementing—that is, eating specific combinations of plant-based proteins in the same meal—but they should strive to consume a variety of plant foods during the course of a day. This pattern should provide all essential amino acids and ensure adequate nitrogen retention and utilization in healthy adults.[10,13,49] Emphasizing amino acid balance at individual meals is not necessary because amino acids that are modest in 1 meal are buffered by amino acid pools found primarily in skeletal muscle and supported by the turnover of endogenous gut proteins.[49,50] Some plant foods do tend to be low in certain amino acids, including methionine and lysine. However, typical combinations of protein foods[49] or what are now commonly termed "protein blends,"[46,51,52] such as beans and rice or peas and barley, create more balanced amino acid profiles. Milk, cheese, and eggs can also supplement plant protein sources for athletes following vegetarian diets.[53-55] Note, however, that cereal grains tend to be low in lysine, so athletes who do not consume dairy or eggs should incorporate beans and soy products into their diets to ensure adequate lysine intake.[49] The protein content of selected vegetarian foods are presented in Table 16.1.[56]

Data from 2013 suggest that plant-based diets, including both vegetarian and vegan diets, contain an average of about 14% of energy as protein.[57] Thus, an 80-kg male athlete consuming 3,600 kcal would receive 1.58 g of protein per kilogram of body weight from the average vegetarian diet. Similarly, a 50-kg female gymnast consuming 2,200 kcal would receive 1.54 g of protein per kilogram of body weight. Although these data suggest that plant-based athletes should, in theory, consume protein within the suggested range without special meal planning, a 2019 study in a small group of endurance athletes using actual intake data and digestible indispensable amino acid scores (DIAAS) suggested that an additional 10 to 20 g of protein may be needed to meet intake in the range of 1.2 to 1.4 g of protein per kilogram of body weight.[58] Thus, some athletes, including those actively restricting energy intake and those desiring intake in the upper range of the recommendation (ie, 1.7–2.0 g per kilogram of body weight), may need to focus on increasing protein intake according to training needs.[16,40] This is easily accomplished by encouraging the athlete to incorporate protein-rich vegetarian foods into their regular meals or snacks. Specific examples include adding soy milk, cottage cheese, or yogurt to fruit; lentils to spaghetti sauce; tofu to stir-fry; and garbanzo beans or a hard- or soft-cooked egg to a salad or grain dish. Athletes should also be educated that not all milk alternatives (ie, almond and rice milks) are rich sources of proteins and that it is therefore important to read nutrition labels on such beverages to make optimal choices. Furthermore, research has suggested that there may be additional benefit to protein consumption in proximity to strength or endurance exercise and to spreading protein throughout the course of the day (ie, consuming 20–25 g at regular meals and snacks vs consuming all protein in an evening meal).[59,60] Both strategies may enhance maintenance of and net gains in skeletal muscle.[60,61] Overall, ample data demonstrate that protein supplementation with plant-derived proteins can support gains in muscle mass and strength when combined with habitual resistance-type training.[43,46,62-64]

TABLE 16.1 Approximate Protein Content of Selected Vegetarian Food Sources[56]

Food	Portion	Protein, g/portion
Bread, most types	1 oz (1 slice)	2-3
Rice, pasta, other grains, cooked	~½ cup	2-3
Pasta (lentil-based), cooked	~½ cup	4-6
Cheese, medium to hard	1 oz	7
Cheese, cottage	½ cup	16
Egg, whole	1 large	7
Legumes (most beans, peas, and lentils)	½ cup	7
Milk, all types	1 cup	8
Nuts, most types	2 Tbsp	7
Peanut butter	2 Tbsp	7
Tempeh	½ cup	15
Tofu, firm	1 cup	20
Tofu, soft	1 cup	10
Vegetables, most	½ cup	2-3
Vegetarian "burgers"	1 patty	6-20
Vegetarian "chicken"	1 patty	9-12
Vegetarian "dogs"	1 dog	9-12
Yogurt, Greek/Greek-style	1 cup	~10-16
Yogurt, most types	1 cup	8-10

Adapted from selected food labels and reference 56: US Department of Agriculture. FoodData Central. Accessed September 30, 2024. https://fdc.nal.usda.gov

Fat

Dietary fat should make up the remainder of energy needs after carbohydrate and protein requirements are met. In a joint statement, the Academy of Nutrition and Dietetics, the American College of Sports Medicine, and Dietitians of Canada recommended that fat intake guidelines align with the *Dietary Guidelines for Americans, 2020–2025*.[16] Consumption of less than 20% of energy from fat, however, is not recommended and has the potential to impair endurance performance, unfavorably alter one's lipid profile, and interfere with normal menstrual function in female athletes.[16,65-72] Fat is particularly important in an athlete's diet because it provides energy, essential fatty acids, and other essential elements of cell membranes and is needed for absorption of fat-soluble vitamins. Dietary fat may be necessary for maintaining intramyocellular triglyceride stores, which serve as an important fuel source during prolonged, moderate-intensity exercise.[69,73-75] Studies to date, however, have not demonstrated that low intramyocellular triglyceride stores are responsible for the reduced performance associated with very low-fat diets.

Careful assessment of the amount and type of fat consumed may be useful. Some vegetarian athletes, particularly endurance-trained athletes (runners and triathletes), may consume excessive carbohydrate and inadequate fat, possibly with the misconception that dietary fat increases body fat and impairs performance. Similarly, recreational athletes with cardiovascular disease or type 2 diabetes (eg, an active vegetarian following a heart attack) may be following extremely low-fat vegetarian diet plans (<10% of energy from fat), as recommended by Ornish and Barnard and their respective colleagues,[76-80] which have been shown to promote the regression of coronary atherosclerosis and improve glycemic control. Such low-fat diets, however, may be too restrictive for athletes during heavy training. On the other hand, other vegetarian athletes may consume diets that are too rich in saturated fat (from excessive intakes of full-fat dairy, coconut oil, and/or bakery products) or choose to follow low-carbohydrate, high-fat (LCHF) diets. A 2019 case report of a world-class long-distance triathlete who followed a LCHF diet for 32 weeks (instead of his typical lacto-ovo vegetarian diet) highlights the potential detriments of such diets on performance and psychological outcomes.[81] Additional information on LCHF diets can be found in Chapter 4. The reader is also referred to key research by Hawley and Leckey[82] and Burke and colleagues[36,37] on this topic.

The type of fat included in the diet of vegetarian athletes is important.[83] The proportion of energy from the various fatty acids should be in accord with national guidelines, contain less than 10% of energy from saturated fat, and also meet the Dietary Reference Intakes (DRIs) of 1.6 and 1.1 g/d of α-linolenic acid (ALA) for males and females, respectively.[84] Vegetarian diets are generally rich in sources of omega-6 polyunsaturated fatty acids but may be low in omega-3 fatty acids.[57,85] Omega-3 fatty acids may be important for inflammation modulation[86,87] and dampening exercise-induced muscle damage.[88] Vegetarian athletes may therefore benefit from incorporating more foods that are rich in omega-3 fatty acids (walnuts; flaxseed; and canola, flax, hemp, and walnut oils) into the diet in place of some oils rich in omega-6 fatty acids (corn, cottonseed, sunflower, and safflower).[11] Although studies have suggested that less than 10% of ALA is elongated to eicosapentaenoic acid (EPA) in humans, this conversion may be improved when the omega-6 concentrations in the diet or blood are not high or excessive.[89] Athletes who may benefit from increased omega-3 consumption, including athletes who are pregnant and those with chronic inflammatory injuries or cardiovascular disease, can consider microalgae supplements rich in docosahexaenoic acid (DHA).[90] These supplements are vegan and well absorbed, and they positively influence blood concentrations of both DHA and EPA.[91]

SPORTS NUTRITION CONSIDERATIONS: VITAMINS AND MINERALS

Calcium and Vitamin D

CALCIUM

Regular exercise has not been shown to increase calcium requirements. Thus, athletes and active individuals should strive to meet the DRI of 1,000 mg for those between ages 19 and 50 years, 1,200 mg for those older than 50 years, and 1,300 mg for those younger than 18 years.[17] Limited evidence also suggests that athletes with amenorrhea may benefit from an additional 500 mg of calcium per day to retain calcium balance.[92] Low dietary calcium intake, along with reduced vitamin D status, is associated with decreased bone density and increased risk for stress fractures, particularly in athletes who are amenorrheic.[93,94] One study found that 8 weeks of supplementation with 800 IU of vitamin D plus 2,000 mg of calcium reduced the incidence of stress fracture in female naval recruits by 20%.[95] In addition, emerging evidence suggests a benefit to incorporating calcium-rich foods into the pretraining meal because intake at this time may be advantageous in dampening the fall of serum ionized calcium and markers of bone resorption (breakdown) observed during training.[96,97] More information on calcium, vitamin D, and bone health can be found in Chapter 5.

In general, vegetarian athletes who are eumenorrheic can meet daily calcium recommendations by including several servings of dairy products or about 5 to 8 servings of calcium-containing plant foods daily (see Box 16.3). Those following vegetarian (but not vegan diets), however, may consume more calcium than omnivores.[98] Nondairy foods rich in well-absorbed calcium include low-oxalate green leafy vegetables (kale; broccoli; Chinese cabbage; and collard, mustard, and turnip greens), calcium-set tofu, textured vegetable protein, fortified plant-based milks, tahini, fortified orange juice, blackstrap molasses, and some calcium-fortified cereals.[13,21] Laboratory studies have determined that the calcium bioavailability of most of these plant foods is as good as or better than that of cow's milk, which has a fractional absorption of close to 32%.[99-102] The exceptions include soy milk fortified with tricalcium phosphate, most legumes, nuts, and seeds, which have fractional absorptions of 17% to 24%.[102] Other plant foods, including spinach, beet greens, rhubarb, and Swiss chard, are not well-absorbed sources of calcium because of their high oxalate or phytate contents.

Interestingly, a clinical study found that young sedentary adult vegetarians maintained a positive calcium balance and appropriate bone resorption (measured by urinary deoxypyridinoline) when calcium was provided from dairy products or plant foods, despite a lower calcium intake on the plant-based diet

BOX 16.3 Vegetarian Sources of Select Vitamins and Minerals[56]

Calcium	Calcium-set tofu, calcium-fortified beverages (orange juice and other fruit juices, soy and other nondairy or plant-based milks), broccoli, Chinese cabbage, kale, collard greens, mustard greens, turnip greens, almonds, tahini, texturized vegetable protein, blackstrap molasses, cow's milk, certain cheeses, legumes
Iron	Legumes, nuts and seeds, whole and enriched grains, enriched and fortified cereals and pasta, leafy green and root vegetables, dried fruits
Iodine	Iodized salt and sea vegetables (kombu, arame, dulse, and other types of seaweed), dairy products and eggs (because of agriculture feed and industrial processes)
Magnesium	Legumes, nuts and seeds, whole grains, green leafy vegetables, blackstrap molasses
Riboflavin (Vitamin B2)	Whole-grain and fortified breads and cereals, legumes, tofu, nuts and seeds, tahini, bananas, asparagus, figs, dark green leafy vegetables, avocado, most sea vegetables (kombu, arame, dulse, and other types of seaweed), dairy products
Vitamin B12	Yeast flakes (eg, Redstar T6635); fortified foods such as ready-to-eat cereals, meat analogues, and some types/brands of soy and rice milks; dairy products; eggs
Vitamin D[a]	Fatty fish (salmon, sardines, mackerel); fortified foods such as cow's milk, plant-based milks, orange juice, ready-to-eat breakfast cereals, margarines, and yogurt; egg yolks; sun-dried mushrooms
Zinc	Legumes, nuts and seeds, whole-grain products, fortified ready-to-eat cereals, soy products, commercial meat analogues, hard cheeses

[a] Sun exposure (~5–30 min on the arms and legs between 10 AM and 2 PM according to non-daylight savings time, several times per week) is another source of vitamin D.

(843 ± 140 mg) compared with the dairy-containing diet (1,322 ± 03 mg).[103] However, a 2019 systematic review and meta-analysis of more than 37,000 men and women in the general population found evidence of lower bone mineral density in the lumbar spine and hip (femoral neck) among vegetarians and vegans compared to omnivores.[104] In contrast, a 2020 review by Hsu[105] found no evidence that carefully chosen plant-based diets that provide adequate calcium along with sufficient vitamin D have detrimental effects on bone health. As the impact of diet on bone is complex and influenced additionally by the intake of many nutrients including protein, magnesium, vitamin K, zinc, and bioactive components found in plant foods,[10] athletes following vegetarian diets should ensure that they reach adequate intakes of bone-specific nutrients to avoid negative consequences on bone health.[104]

Although it is possible to maintain one's calcium balance on a Western plant-based diet, some athletes may find it convenient to use fortified foods or calcium supplements to achieve calcium balance, particularly when their requirements are elevated because of growth, amenorrhea, or menopause.[13,21,101] Because vitamin D is also required for adequate calcium absorption and the promotion of bone health, a calcium supplement containing vitamin D may be advised depending on the vitamin D status of the individual athlete. Research has shown that only 10% to 15% of dietary calcium is absorbed in the vitamin D–deficient state, whereas 30% to 35% is absorbed when the vitamin D status is sufficient.[106,107] Higher vitamin D status promotes higher bioavailability of calcium through the vitamin D–induced expression of calbindin (an intestinal calcium-binding protein) and an epithelial calcium channel protein that increases the efficiency of calcium and phosphorus absorption by active transport across the intestinal mucosa.[108]

VITAMIN D

Beyond bone health, vitamin D is involved in many physiological functions important to an athlete's health and performance, including immune function, inflammatory modulation, and skeletal muscle function.[109-113] Athletes at risk for poor vitamin D status include those living at northern or southern latitudes (>32°) with dark pigmented skin or excess body fat and those who train primarily indoors or in the early morning or late afternoon throughout the year.[110,111,114,115] These athletes would benefit from supplementation with enough vitamin D to maintain serum 25-hydroxyvitamin D (25[OH]D) concentration within the normal range (>30 ng/mL) or the optimal range (40–70 ng/mL).[116] Both vitamins D3 (cholecalciferol) and D2 (ergocalciferol) are used in supplements and to fortify foods, including cow's milk and some brands and types of plant-based milks, orange juice, breakfast cereals, margarines, and yogurt. Individuals who follow a vegan diet should note that vitamin D3 that is obtained through the ultraviolet radiation of 7-dehydrocholesterol from lanolin (a waxy substance made by the sebaceous glands of animals with wool) is not vegan. However, vitamin D3 derived from lichen and vitamin D2 produced through the irradiation of ergosterol from yeast should be acceptable to vegans.[107] Research has suggested that, at lower doses (ie, 1,000 IU), vitamin D2 is as effective as vitamin D3, but when taken in higher doses (>4,000 IU), vitamin D2 is less effective at increasing and maintaining endogenous 25(OH)D concentrations.[117-120] Vitamin D2 supplementation has been associated with some side effects including amplified eccentric exercise-induced muscle damage.[121] Natural and fortified sources of vitamin D are listed in Box 16.3.

Iron

Iron depletion is one of the most prevalent nutrient deficiencies in athletes, especially in female athletes[122,123] and those with low energy availability.[124] Iron depletion both with anemia (stage 3) and without anemia (stage 2) can impair muscle function and maximal oxygen uptake and can also decrease endurance performance.[123,125] Whereas iron depletion among athletes is most commonly attributed to insufficient energy or low intakes of absorbable iron, other factors can affect iron status including acute inflammation; periods of rapid growth; high-altitude training; and increased iron losses through gastrointestinal bleeding, heavy sweating, foot strike, intravascular hemolysis, hematuria, or heavy menstrual blood losses.[16,123,125-128] Following a vegetarian diet may be a risk factor for some athletes based on dietary intake patterns and iron losses.

Most of the iron in a vegetarian diet is nonheme iron, which has a lower absorption rate (5%–10%) than heme iron (15%–30%) and is sensitive to inhibitors and enhancers of iron absorption.[10,13,17] Inhibitors of iron absorption include phytates; dietary or supplemental calcium; and the polyphenolic compounds (including tannins) in tea, coffee, herbal teas, and cocoa. Fiber has only a slight impact on impairing iron absorption.[129] Enhancers of iron absorption include vitamin C and other organic acids such as citric, malic, lactic, tartaric, and erythorbic (used in food processing) acids, which can significantly enhance iron absorption and reduce the inhibitory effects of tannins and phytates.[17,130,131] Vitamin C is by far the most potent plant-based factor for iron absorption; research has shown that ingesting 25 mg of vitamin C increases the absorption of iron from foods consumed at the same meal by threefold to fourfold.[132] Furthermore, individuals with low iron stores or a higher physiological need for iron will tend to absorb more iron and excrete less.[17] Recent research has highlighted that enhanced iron absorption associated with low iron stores is driven by the peptide hormone hepcidin.[125,133] Because of increased iron losses and the lower bioavailability of iron from a vegetarian diet, there is some indication that vegetarian athletes may have higher iron needs. In fact, the recommended iron intake for such athletes may be 1.3 to 1.8 times higher than the RDA.[10,17] Therefore, it may be prudent for vegetarian athletes to aim for iron intakes that are slightly higher than the RDA.

In most cases, vegetarians who eat a varied and well-balanced diet that is rich in whole grains, legumes, nuts, seeds, dried fruits, iron-fortified cereals, and green leafy vegetables can achieve adequate iron status without iron supplementation.[134] Studies of vegetarian athletes and nonathletes have found that vegetarians commonly have average iron intakes similar to or higher than those of nonvegetarians, yet they often have a lower iron status.[57,134,135] However, evidence in nonathletes suggests that, although vegetarians tend to have lower serum ferritin than nonvegetarians, they are at no greater risk for iron deficiency anemia.[136] Vegetarian athletes should, therefore, be educated about plant sources of iron (see Box 16.3), along with factors that

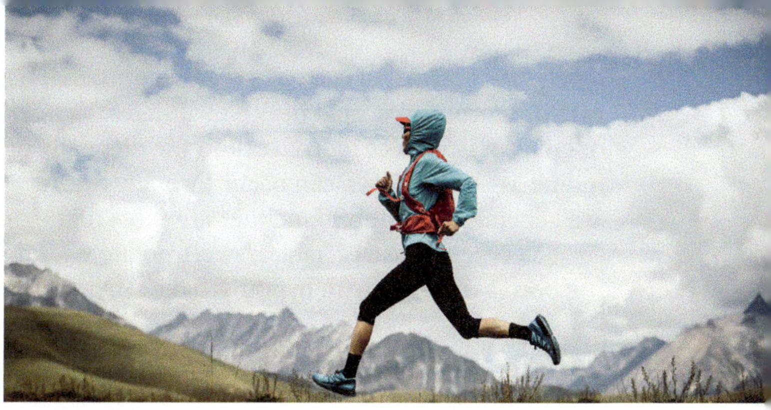

enhance and interfere with its absorption.[11] For example, an athlete who drinks coffee, tea, or milk with legume-containing meals could be advised to drink citrus fruit juice or water instead and ensure that the meal is served with a plethora of vitamin C–rich fruits and vegetables to enhance the iron absorbed from that meal. Even though iron supplementation has been shown to improve energy efficiency (energy expended relative to external work performed) and endurance performance in iron-depleted athletes who are not anemic, supplements should be recommended only for those with compromised stores, as indicated by a low serum ferritin concentration, elevated total iron-binding capacity, or elevated serum transferrin receptor.[137-139] Athletes taking iron supplements should have their iron status monitored because of the prevalence of hereditary hemochromatosis and other iron-overload abnormalities in the United States, as well as the potential association between excess iron and chronic disease.[17,140] Information on iron supplementation protocols is reviewed in Chapter 5.

Zinc

Vegetarian athletes, female athletes, and athletes in heavy training often have serum zinc concentrations on the lower end of the normal range or below the recommended level.[141,142] In vegetarians, a lower zinc status is most likely due to the reduced bioavailability of zinc from plant foods compared with animal foods, but it may also be related to the selection of zinc-poor foods.[17,131] The lower bioavailability of zinc in vegetarian diets is due mainly to the higher phytic acid content of many plant foods, including phytate-rich unrefined grains and legumes.[143] Lower bioavailability in foods may increase the dietary zinc requirement by 50%.

Although overt zinc deficiencies are typically not present in Western vegetarians, experts do not know the significance of marginal deficiencies because of the difficulty of evaluating zinc status.[13] Serum zinc concentrations are often altered by increases in training intensity and may not reflect tissue zinc stores or zinc status.[142,144,145] Although additional research is needed, zinc supplementation has not been shown to influence serum zinc concentrations during training or to offer performance benefits.[144,145]

Because of the potential negative effects of zinc deficiency on health and performance, sports dietitians should work with vegetarian athletes to ensure that the RDA for zinc is met or exceeded through consumption of zinc-containing plant foods. Consumption of zinc-containing foods with organic acids, including citric acid (found in many fruits and vegetables), may enhance zinc absorption.[131,146] In support of this recommendation, a study from the US Department of Agriculture found that nonathletic women consuming a diet that regularly contained legumes and whole grains for 8 weeks maintained their zinc status within normal limits even though the diet was lower in total zinc and higher in both phytate and fiber than a control omnivorous diet.[147] Another study of women who habitually followed a plant-based diet found that adding milk and yogurt to a plant-based diet high in phytate increased zinc bioavailability by more than 70% without altering iron bioavailability.[148] Soaking and sprouting beans, grains, nuts, and seeds are other methods that can improve zinc bioavailability by reducing binding to phytic acid.[13,131] The zinc contents of selected protein-containing plant foods are included in Box 16.3.

Iodine

Iodine status has not generally been a concern for athletes living in industrialized countries. Evidence is mounting, however, that individuals following vegan or vegetarian diets may be at increased risk for iodine deficiency.[149-154] One study that assessed the iodine status of 81 nonathletic adults found that 25% of the vegetarians and 80% of the vegans had iodine deficiency (as indicated by a urinary iodine excretion value of less than 100 mcg/L) compared with 9% of the nonvegetarians.[149] Major dietary sources of iodine include cow's milk and other dairy products, eggs, and iodized salt.[10] Small amounts of iodine (ie, several micrograms) are also found in plant foods, but the amount depends on the soil iodine content, as well as irrigation and fertilizer use.[17] Seaweed provides variable amounts of iodine.[10] In 2020, Larson-Meyer and Gostas[155] exposed a need for more research addressing the possible effects of iodine deficiency on thyroid function, performance, and overall health in athletes. Vegetarian athletes can meet the RDA for iodine by consuming one-half teaspoon of iodized salt in the diet daily or by taking a multivitamin containing iodine. Significant iodine losses, however, can occur through sweat.[156] Sea salt, kosher salt, and salty seasonings such as tamari are generally not iodized; neither are most high-sodium processed foods. In addition, whereas plant foods such as cruciferous vegetables, sweet potatoes, and soybeans naturally contain goitrogens, these foods have not been associated with hypothyroid or thyroid insufficiency if iodine status is adequate.[157]

Magnesium

Experts widely believe most people in the United States have suboptimal magnesium status, mainly because of the limited intake of magnesium-rich foods including whole grains, legumes, nuts, seeds, and leafy vegetables and excess intake of processed foods.[158] Consuming less than the recommended amount of magnesium may also be common in athletes,[159] with those participating in sports that require weight control (eg, wrestling, ballet, and gymnastics) being especially vulnerable.[16,159] Athletes participating in strenuous exercise may also be at risk because of increased magnesium losses in urine and sweat that may increase magnesium requirements by 10% to 20%.[160] As a whole, however, plant-based diets may offer an advantage[57] because seeds, nuts, legumes, unmilled cereal grains, dark green vegetables, and dark chocolate are high in magnesium. Marginal magnesium deficiency impairs exercise performance and amplifies the negative consequences of strenuous exercise including oxidative stress. In athletes with a suboptimal magnesium status, increased dietary intake of magnesium or magnesium supplementation may have beneficial effects on blood pressure and exercise performance.[160] Foods rich in magnesium, which come mostly from unprocessed plant-based sources, are listed in Box 16.3.

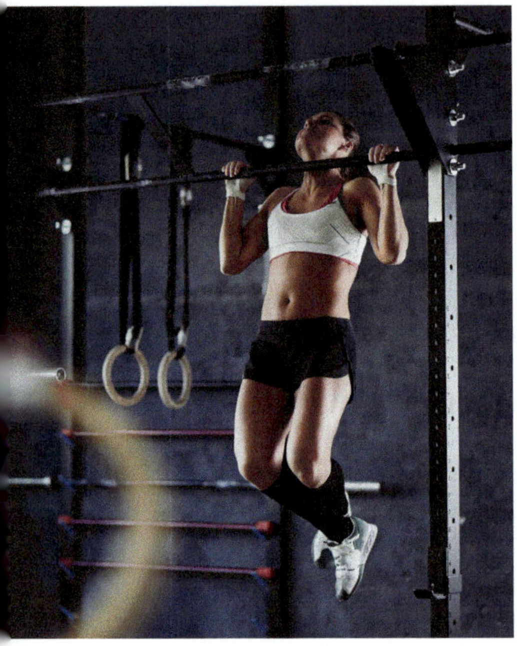

B Vitamins

Vegetarian diets can easily satisfy the requirements for most B vitamins.[13,161] However, diets containing little to no eggs or dairy and those low in energy may not supply adequate vitamin B12 and riboflavin.[133] Similarly, ketogenic plant-based diets that are devoid of grain products may also be low in thiamin, niacin, and riboflavin.

VITAMIN B12

Cobalamin, the active form of vitamin B12, is found almost exclusively in animal products.[17,162] Therefore, vegan athletes should make an effort to consume vitamin B12–fortified foods daily or take a multivitamin containing vitamin B12. Vegetarian food sources of vitamin B12 include yeast flakes, soy milk and other fortified plant-based milks, breakfast cereals, and meat analogues that are vitamin B12–fortified.[13,163] Although some discussion in the lay literature suggests that fermented soy products, seaweeds, and spirulina (and other algae) can supply bioavailable vitamin B12, research does not consistently support this concept. This is due to the fact that the standard assay for determining vitamin B12 content does not distinguish between biologically active forms and analogues.[164-166]

Vegetarians who consume dairy products or eggs are likely to have adequate intakes of vitamin B12; however, both vegans and vegetarians may be at risk for low B12 status.[13,162,164] Because of the irreversible neurologic damage that can occur with vitamin B12 deficiency, markers of vitamin B12 status (homocysteine, methylmalonic acid, and holotranscobalamin II) should be measured if there is concern that an individual's diet may be lacking in reliable sources of vitamin B12.[162,167] The typical manifestation of vitamin B12 deficiency as macrocytic anemia can be masked by high folate intake, a probable finding in vegan or vegetarian athletes who consume ample legumes and dark green leafy and other vegetables.

RIBOFLAVIN

Riboflavin intake may be low in athletes who avoid dairy products, particularly when energy intake is restricted to promote weight loss.[16,161] There is some evidence that riboflavin needs may be increased in individuals who are habitually physically active and in those who begin an exercise program, particularly if riboflavin status was marginal prior to exercise initiation.[18,168,169] Because dairy products are rich sources of riboflavin, education on the plant sources of riboflavin may help ensure adequate intake. This may be particularly true for plant-based athletes who also avoid grain products, which are natural or enriched sources of riboflavin as well as thiamin and niacin. Good plant sources of riboflavin are listed in Box 16.3.[56]

SPORTS NUTRITION CONSIDERATIONS: SUPPLEMENTS

Vegetarian athletes, similarly to other athletes, may inquire about nutritional supplements or ergogenic aids to assist their athletic training and performance. As with all athletes, vegetarian athletes should first be encouraged to follow a balanced diet before considering supplements.[139] Vegetarian and vegan athletes might be concerned about whether the ingredients are animal or plant derived, which may vary by manufacturer (see *Vegan Journal's Guide to Food Ingredients* in the Vegetarian Resources section at the end of this chapter). A discussion on supplements can be found in Chapter 7, but the supplements of particular interest to vegetarian athletes—protein, creatine, carnitine, and carnosine—are briefly discussed here.

Protein Supplements

Protein from supplements is not needed if the athlete is consuming adequate energy and making proper food choices.[40] For convenience, protein-containing sports beverages and bars can be used occasionally to supplement the diet and may be particularly useful in the postexercise period. Such products are typically formulated with protein isolates or concentrates containing whey, casein, soy, or pea proteins. Blends of other plant proteins are presently in development and will continue to appear on the sports supplement market.[52] Although research has suggested that supplemental beverages that contain only soy protein are not as effective as cow's milk at promoting postexercise muscle protein synthesis over the short term, not all studies are in agreement,[170] and longer-term studies (of at least 6 weeks in duration) indicate that soy protein is as effective as whey protein.[63]

Creatine, Carnitine, and Carnosine

Creatine, carnitine, and carnosine are supplied mostly by meat and other animal products in the diet. Even though these molecules can be synthesized endogenously from amino acid precursors, serum concentrations of creatine and carnitine and skeletal muscle concentrations of creatine and carnosine are generally lower in those following vegetarian diets.[171-178] Substantial evidence suggests that supplementation with creatine monohydrate can increase the creatine content of skeletal muscle and improve performance in repeated bouts of maximal and endurance sprinting; supplementation can also provide potential gains in fat-free mass, muscle force, and power output with resistance training.[179] Several, but not all, studies have noted that vegetarians who take creatine supplements experience greater increases in skeletal muscle total creatine, phosphocreatine, lean tissue mass, and work performance during weight-training and anaerobic bicycle performance than their nonvegetarian teammates.[172,176,180,181] A 2020 systematic review supports the greater benefit of creatine supplementation in vegetarians compared to omnivorous athletes at enhancing creatine phosphate stores in muscle but not in the brain. Overall, creatine supplementation was found to have a beneficial effect at increasing lean mass, type II fiber area, insulin-like growth factor 1, muscular strength, muscular endurance, Wingate mean power output, and memory.[182]

In contrast to the case of creatine, little evidence suggests that vegetarian athletes should take supplements of carnitine, carnosine, or β-alanine (the rate-limiting precursor of carnosine synthesis) because of their plant-based diet alone. Carnitine is an essential cofactor that aids the transport of long-chain fatty acids into the mitochondria; however, its ergogenic potential has not proven effective, likely because of its low bioavailability and the high doses required to produce only minimal changes in the carnitine levels in skeletal muscle.[183] A study in male vegetarians and omnivores found that 12 weeks of carnitine supplementation had no influence on energy metabolism or exercise performance despite increases in the carnitine levels in both plasma and skeletal muscle.[184]

Carnosine is an important intracellular buffer in skeletal muscle and one of the immediate defenses against accumulation of proteins during exercise.[183] Although vegetarians have been found to have lower carnosine levels, this does not seem to negatively affect muscle buffering capacity.[185] Additionally, switching to a vegetarian diet for as long as 3 months was found not to alter carnitine homeostasis or result in lower muscle carnosine content.[177,185] whereas sprint-interval training increased the muscle carnosine content in vegetarian men.[186] Taking β-alanine supplementation, however, is known to increase muscle carnosine in both vegetarians and omnivores and to effectively buffer muscle pH in some athletes.[177,179,187] Refer to Chapter 7 for further information.

NUTRITION BEFORE, DURING, AND AFTER EXERCISE

Athletes following vegetarian diets should follow the same guidelines as athletes eating mixed diets for food and fluid consumption before, during, and after exercise.[16] These guidelines are reviewed in detail in Chapters 2 (carbohydrates), 3 (protein), and 6 (fluids and electrolytes). Information specific to vegetarian athletes is presented here.

Preexercise Nutrition

The meal or snack eaten before a competition or exercise session should be high in carbohydrate (to maintain blood glucose and top off glycogen stores), provide fluids, and prevent hunger and gastrointestinal distress. Athletes should be encouraged to consume familiar, well-tolerated, high-carbohydrate meals that are low in fiber, simple sugars, and sodium.[16] Vegetarian athletes accustomed to eating gas-producing foods such as legumes, which are not typically recommended in the preevent meal, may tolerate these foods without complications. Some studies,[20] although not all, suggest that low–glycemic-index (low-GI) foods compared with high-GI foods (eg, lentils vs mashed potatoes) may offer a performance advantage, particularly during prolonged submaximal exercise.[188-190] Nonetheless, plant-based athletes may desire preworkout products that are void of processed ingredients.[191]

Nutrition During Exercise

Adequate carbohydrate and fluid intakes are also essential during certain types of exercise. Intake of carbohydrate and fluid should be initiated shortly after the start of exercise to maximize time for sugar and nutrients to reach the bloodstream. Although commercial sports drinks and gels consumed with water work well for delivering easily absorbed carbohydrate, some vegetarian athletes may prefer natural, less processed, or noncommercial sources of carbohydrate. In this case, fruit juices diluted with water (4 oz of juice in 4 oz of water makes a 6% solution); low-sodium vegetable juices, such as carrot juice (7% solution); and honey or solid foods ingested with water (8 oz of water for every 15 g of carbohydrate corresponds to 6.3% intake) may be appropriate. Research has shown that solid food and honey are as effective as liquids for increasing blood glucose and enhancing performance and are easily digested.[192-194] A pinch (or two) of table salt can also be added to juices or low-sodium solids as necessary for longer events (ie, lasting more than about 3–4 hours).[195] Honey may be of particular interest to some plant-based athletes because it is perceived as a natural sugar and is a mixture of glucose and fructose; however, honey is considered an animal product and is not consumed by most vegans.

Postexercise Nutrition

All athletes—including vegetarian athletes—should consume a mixed meal or snack providing carbohydrates, protein, fat, and fluid soon after a strenuous competition or training session. This may be particularly beneficial following prolonged or strenuous exercise, when athletes should consume carbohydrate and protein immediately after exercise to promote recovery, particularly when engaging in multiple daily practices or if exercise training is to be resumed the following day.[39,40] Including sources of sodium and potassium in the recovery meal is also important for replacing sweat losses of these electrolytes,[196] whereas dietary fat may be needed for the replacement of intramyocellular lipid stores following high-volume endurance training.[68,69] Multi-ingredient sports foods and admixtures containing vegan protein sources are becoming increasingly available for use in the postworkout period. A recent study in 10 trained men found that such admixtures were more effective than maltodextrose in promoting the recovery of muscle function.[197] Sports dietitians can expect to educate vegetarian athletes on the selection and use of such sports nutrition products in comparison with whole foods during the recovery period, as well as the selection of fluids for efficient rehydration.[198]

SPECIAL CONCERN: RELATIVE ENERGY DEFICIENCY IN SPORT

Low energy availability—with or without eating disorders—reduces bone density, alters menstrual function, and provides a significant health risk for female and male athletes.[200,201] Some studies have indicated that this condition, more recently termed relative energy deficiency in sport (REDs) and formerly identified as the female athlete triad, may be higher in vegetarian athletes, but the findings are not consistent.[200,202-204] In some cases, the apparent increased prevalence of REDs or its components among vegetarians can be explained by study design or recruitment bias.[201] For example, some studies have defined "vegetarians" as those having a low-meat diet and not necessarily a vegetarian diet and have not differentiated between the 2 distinct types of eating patterns.[135] Studies may also recruit a biased sample of vegetarians (eg, those with menstrual cycle disturbances may be more likely to volunteer for a study on menstrual cycle disturbances).[201] Furthermore, as reviewed in the next section, proclaiming to be vegetarian may be perceived as a socially acceptable way to mask an eating disorder.[204-207] Professionals should be cautioned to assess each athlete, including those following plant-based diets, and not to make generalizations based on dietary preferences.[16] Overall, the selected energy and nutrient composition of some vegetarian diets can predispose vegetarian athletes to amenorrhea and reduced bone density rather than the vegetarian diet itself.

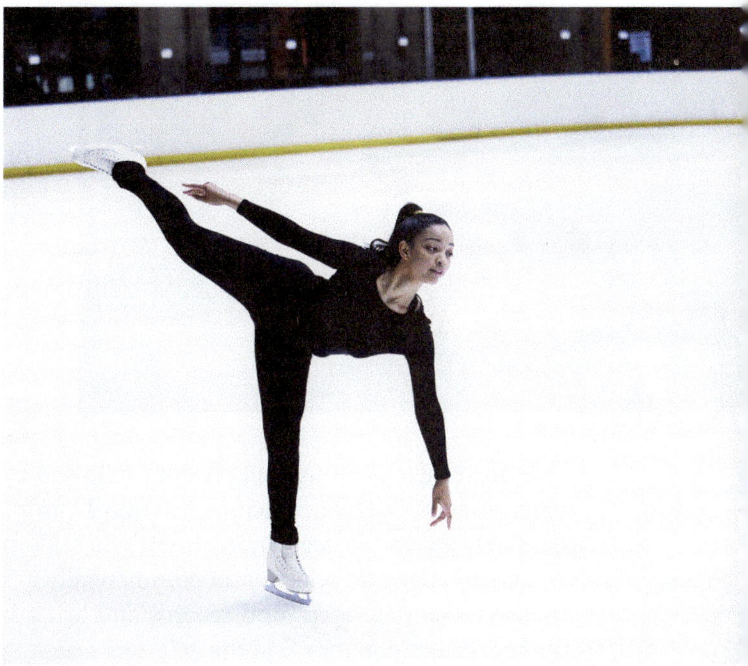

Because available research suggests that reproductive disruption typically occurs when energy availability (dietary energy intake minus exercise energy expenditure) is less than a threshold of 30 kcal per kilogram of lean body mass, vegetarian athletes who are amenorrheic should be counseled on how to meet energy needs on a vegetarian diet, which may include reducing fiber intake, increasing the frequency of meals and snacks,[200,203,208] and/or learning to select and prepare vegetarian-based meals. For athletes in heavy training, a diet with excessive fiber may lead to lower energy intake and potentially reduce the enterohepatic circulation of sex steroid hormones.[209,210] Refer to Chapter 18 for more information on REDs.

ASSESSING, COUNSELING, AND WORKING WITH VEGETARIAN ATHLETES

Assessment

The body size and composition of vegetarian athletes varies, as do their dietary practices, food choices, and reasons for being vegetarian. The sports dietitian should first obtain and evaluate anthropometric measures, biochemical (laboratory) values, pertinent clinical information, and dietary and environmental factors, as outlined by Larson-Meyer, Woolf, and Burke.[139] Although the laboratory and clinical data collected will vary, evaluation of the mean corpuscular volume, hemoglobin, hematocrit, ferritin, and 25(OH)D concentrations (including total and unbound)[211] may be helpful. For female athletes, it is important to assess energy intake, menstrual function, training load, fatigue, history of injuries, and exercise performance to look for signs of the female athlete triad or REDs.[200] Unintended weight or muscle loss, tiredness, fatigue, reduced strength gains, reduced performance, and loss of menstrual cycle function are signs that the diet may be lacking in total energy and possibly in certain macronutrients or micronutrients.[139] Assessment of vitamin B12 intake and status is also advised in athletes adhering to vegan diets; this is particularly important because symptoms of vitamin B12 deficiency can occur even when serum concentrations are not below the "cut-off" for deficiency.[163]

The dietary assessment should begin by determining which foods the athlete eliminates from their diet and which foods they consider acceptable. This will help assess nutrient adequacy and ensure that the nutrients in omitted foods (such as dairy products) can be met with acceptable plant-based foods. Although a variety of terms, including plant-based, lacto-ovo vegetarian, lactovegetarian, vegan, and strict vegetarian, are commonly used to describe vegetarians[212] (see Box 16.1 on page 383), recent evidence-based analysis suggests that these very broad categories mask important variations within vegetarian diets and dietary practices.[13] For example, 2 lacto-ovo vegetarian athletes may have different philosophies about dairy products that would require different treatment plans. One may consume several servings of dairy products per day, whereas the other may eat only cheese and small amounts of dairy found in processed foods. Similarly, some vegans may be extremely strict, eliminating all commercially available foods that contain any ingredient that is derived from an animal or processed with an animal derivative (eg, commercial bread), whereas others will avoid only foods of obvious animal origin. Furthermore, some individuals claim to follow vegetarian diets when they mean that they avoid red meat but occasionally eat fish or poultry.

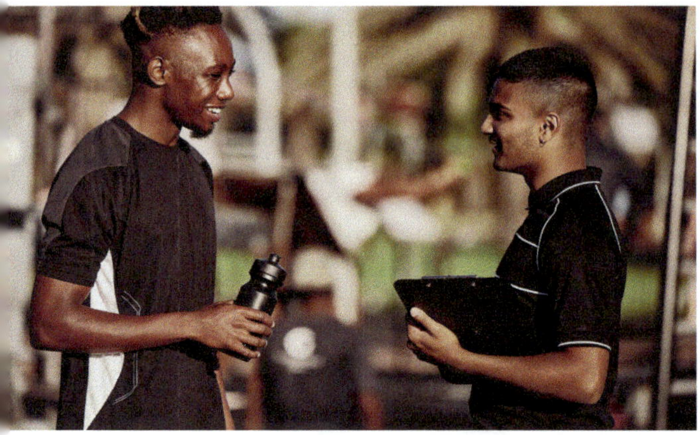

Performing a thorough diet history followed by an analysis of energy and key nutrients, such as carbohydrate, protein, fat, fiber, calcium, vitamin D, iron, zinc, iodine, riboflavin, and vitamin B12, is the best way to reliably assess the vegetarian athlete's diet. Computer nutrient databases may be helpful, but many do not contain an adequate selection of commercially available vegetarian food products. In many cases, it is useful to have the athlete keep food records and bring in food labels from the vegetarian products they consume. The sports dietitian may find the 369-item vegan-specific questionnaire developed by Sabate's group useful for some athletic populations and situations.[213]

Information collected about the environment should include a discussion of the athlete's belief system[139] (ie, why they have chosen to follow a vegetarian diet) and barriers to healthy eating. Although health, planetary sustainability, ecology, animal and human welfare, and religion are admirable reasons for following a vegetarian diet, desire to lose weight or to create a certain social image may raise a red flag. Individuals who lack a solid philosophy, which is what typically drives many vegetarians in their desire to eat well, may be at higher nutritional risk. A final concern is that vegetarianism may be used as a convenient and socially acceptable way for individuals with disordered eating tendencies to reduce energy intake and thus mask their disordered eating behaviors.[204-207] Some evidence suggests that individuals who report weight control as a reason for following a vegetarian diet may be at particular risk compared to those who report other motives.[205] Occasionally, vegetarianism may therefore be a red flag for disordered eating and increased risk for the female athlete triad and REDs.[16,200] Refer to Chapter 8 for more information on nutrition assessment.

Counseling and Nutrition Treatment

The role of the nutrition professional during counseling, nutrition education, and treatment is to work with the athlete to ensure adequate nutritional status given their lifestyle, income, and vegetarian belief system. Guidelines initially developed for counseling vegetarians who are pregnant are useful when working with the vegetarian population in general and include establishing rapport, reinforcing positive nutrition practices, prioritizing nutrition concerns, and providing individualized dietary recommendations.[214,215] Work by Iwasa-Madge and Sesbreno[216] further suggests that messaging to encourage a flexible rather than a strict view of plant-based diets may be a more feasible and acceptable approach when educating athletes on plant-based diets. It is also important to remember that nutritional requirements are for essential nutrients (eg, protein, calcium, and iron) rather than for specific foods (eg, meat or milk) or food groups (eg, meat group or dairy group). Given the position of the Academy of Nutrition and Dietetics on vegetarian diets, a vegetarian athlete should never be advised to consume meat or dairy to be healthy.[13] Box 16.4 contains tips for helping vegetarian athletes select a well-balanced vegetarian diet.

BOX 16.4 Tips for Vegetarian Athletes

Choose a variety of foods, including those that are whole and minimally processed, enriched grains, fruits, vegetables, legumes, nuts, seeds, and if desired, dairy products and eggs.

Consume adequate energy to optimize performance and help meet other nutrient needs, including needs for protein, iron, zinc, magnesium, and riboflavin. Decrease fiber and increase energy intake by consuming one-third to one-half of cereal or grain servings from refined rather than whole-grain sources and replace some high-fiber fruit or vegetable servings with juice servings on high training days.

To help meet energy needs, consume small, frequent meals and snacks, and strive to obtain one-third to one-half of grains, fruits, and vegetables from more refined sources such as enriched pasta, white rice, and fruit juice, rather than whole-food sources on high training days.

Strive to consume a variety of protein-rich foods during the course of the day. Consumption of protein-rich foods along with carbohydrate foods in the 30 minutes after strenuous exercise may enhance recovery.

Incorporate healthful fats in cooking and seasoning foods, and limit foods that are high in saturated and *trans* fats.

Include foods that are rich in omega-3 fatty acids, such as flax, hemp, and chia seeds; walnuts; and canola, flax, hemp, and walnut oils.

If dairy products are not consumed, choose 8 or more servings per day of calcium-rich foods. Refer to to Box 16.3.

Obtain adequate vitamin D through regular sun exposure or from fortified foods or supplements. In the absence of adequate sun exposure, intake of vitamin D between 1,000 and 1,500 IU is needed daily to maintain optimal vitamin D status. Larger athletes may require higher daily intakes.

To meet iron and zinc needs, consume a variety of iron-rich grains and legumes daily. Aim to consume a fruit or vegetable that contains vitamin C and/or other organic acids along with most meals to boost absorption. Allium spices, including onions and garlic, may also enhance iron absorption.

Incorporate legumes and 1 to 2 servings of nuts into the diet almost daily. These foods provide protein and an abundance of other nutrients, including iron, zinc, magnesium, and some calcium. Nuts also provide additional energy and healthful fats.

Use iodized salt when cooking and in salting foods. Remember that the sodium needs of athletes are often increased as a result of sodium losses in sweat.

Incorporate sources of vitamin B12 in the diet each day. Vegan sources include 1 Tbsp of nutritional yeast, 1 cup (8 oz) of fortified soy milk, 1 oz (28 g) of fortified cereal, and 1.5 oz (42 g) of fortified meat analogue. Servings for vegetarians include ½ cup (4 oz) of cow's milk, 6 oz (172 g) of yogurt, and 1 egg.

Limit consumption of overly processed (ultraprocessed) foods, which typically contain added sugars and unhealthful fats.

ENCOURAGING AN OPTIMAL VEGETARIAN DIET

Some athletes or active individuals—vegetarian or omnivore—may find it difficult to select a healthy well-balanced diet with adequate variety.[214] Factors such as a lack of knowledge about food preparation, lack of time, and economic constraints may lead to a monotonous diet. Vegetarian cookbooks (particularly with pictures), videos, and credible websites can be used to provide ideas for increasing dietary variety and preparing simple meals. A tour of a supermarket or natural foods store may help identify products that are suitable for vegetarians. Vegetarian cooking classes for teams or individual athletes are also a great way to provide hands-on education and introduce new vegetarian foods and recipes.

SUMMARY

Athletes at all levels of performance can meet their energy and nutrient needs on a vegetarian diet that contains a variety of plant foods.[11,16] Depending on their food patterns, however, some athletes may have trouble meeting their dietary needs for certain key nutrients, including total energy, carbohydrate, protein, fat, calcium, vitamin D, iron, zinc, iodine, riboflavin, and vitamin B12. Therefore, vegetarian athletes, like most athletes, may benefit from education on food choices that provide adequate energy and nutrients, thereby promoting optimal training, optimal performance, and good health.

Sports dietitians who work with vegetarian and vegan athletes and their trainers and coaches need to be sensitive to and knowledgeable about vegetarianism and exercise training. Athletes should be encouraged to eat a wide variety of plant foods; they should not be told that they need poultry, fish, or dairy products to obtain adequate nutrition. It is the position of the Academy of Nutrition and Dietetics,[13] as well as the nutrition and dietetics societies of most other European countries,[163] that appropriately planned vegetarian (and vegan) diets "are healthful, nutritionally adequate, and may provide health benefits in the prevention and treatment of certain diseases" and can "meet the needs of competitive athletes."[13]

VEGETARIAN RESOURCES

Consumer Publications

» Davis B, Melina V. *Becoming Vegan, Express Edition: The Everyday Guide to Plant-Based Nutrition.* 2nd ed. Book Publishing Co; 2013.

» Larson-Meyer DE, Ruscigno M. *Plant-Based Sports Nutrition: Expert Fueling Strategies for Training, Recovery, and Performance.* Human Kinetics; 2006.

» USDA MyPlate. Enjoy Vegetarian Meals. www.myplate.gov/tip-sheet/enjoy-vegetarian-meals

» *Vegan Journal (previously Vegetarian Journal).* Bimonthly publication by the Vegetarian Resource Group. www.vrg.org/journal

» *Vegan Journal's Guide to Vegetarian and Vegan Restaurants in the US and Canada* (online version). Vegetarian Resource Group. www.vrg.org/restaurant/index.php

» Yacoubou J. *Vegetarian Journal's Guide to Food Ingredients* (online version). Vegetarian Resource Group. www.vrg.org/ingredients/index.php

» Wasserman D, Stahler C. *Meatless Meals for Working People: Quick and Easy Vegetarian Recipes.* 5th ed. Vegetarian Resource Group; 2009.

» Wasserman D, Mangels R. *Simply Vegan: Quick Vegetarian Meals.* 5th ed. Vegetarian Resource Group; 2013.

Professional Publications

» Mangels R, Messina V, Messina M. *The Dietitian's Guide to Vegetarian Diets: Issues and Applications.* 4th ed. Jones & Bartlett Learning; 2023.
» Raj S, Guest NS, Landry MJ, Mangels AR, Pawlak R, Rozga M. Vegetarian Dietary Patterns for Adults: A Position Paper of the Academy of Nutrition and Dietetics. *J Acad Nutr Diet.* 2025;125(6):831-846.e2. doi:10.1016/j.jand.2025.02.002
» Carlson P, ed. *The Complete Vegetarian: The Essential Guide to Good Health.* University of Illinois Press; 2009.
» Sabaté J. *Vegetarian Nutrition.* CRC Press; 2001.

Quantity Recipes for Feeding Groups of Vegetarian Athletes

» Berkoff N. *Vegan in Volume: Vegan Quantity Recipes for Every Occasion.* Rev ed. Vegetarian Resource Group; 2007.
» *Vegetarian Journal's FoodService Update and Quantity Cooking Information.* Vegetarian Resource Group. www.vrg.org//fsupdate/index.htm

Resource Groups

» Vegetarian Nutrition Dietetic Practice Group of the Academy of Nutrition and Dietetics. www.vndpg.org/home
» The Vegetarian Resource Group. www.vrg.org

KEY TAKEAWAYS

A well-balanced vegetarian or vegan diet can support athletes at all levels of training and performance.

Meeting energy needs is a nutrition priority for all athletes, including vegetarian athletes.

A varied and well-balanced diet rich in whole grains, legumes, nuts, seeds, dried fruits, iron-fortified cereals, and green leafy vegetables can help ensure that vegetarian athletes meet their needs for most nutrients.

Educating vegetarian athletes on food sources of carbohydrate, protein, fat, calcium, vitamin D, iron, zinc, iodine, riboflavin, and vitamin B12 will help ensure adequate health and performance.

REFERENCES

1. Loker A, Francis C. Urban food sovereignty: urgent need for agroecology and systems thinking in a post-COVID-19 future. *Agroecol Sust Food.* 2020;44(9):1118-1123. doi:10.1080/21683565.2020.1775752
2. Kaminski DM, Caputo V, McKendree MGS. The US public's attitudes on animal and worker welfare in the dairy and poultry industries. *Agric Resour Econ.* 2024;49(1):23-38. doi:10.22004/ag.econ.330845
3. Willett W, Rockström J, Loken B, et al. Food in the Anthropocene: the EAT-Lancet Commission on healthy diets from sustainable food systems. *Lancet.* 2019;393(10170):447-492. doi:10.1016/S0140-6736(18)31788-4
4. Meyer N, Reguant-Closa A. "Eat as if you could save the planet and win!" Sustainability integration into nutrition for exercise and sport. *Nutrients.* 2017;9(4):412. doi:10.3390/nu9040412
5. Pelly FE, Burkhart SJ. Dietary regimens of athletes competing at the Delhi 2010 Commonwealth Games. *Int Sport Nutr Exerc Metab.* 2014;24(1):28-36. doi:10.1123/ijsnem.2013-0023
6. Wilson PB. Nutrition behaviors, perceptions, and beliefs of recent marathon finishers. *Phys Sportsmed.* 2016;44(3):242-251. doi:10.1080/00913847.2016.1177477
7. Craddock JC, Neale EP, Peoples GE, Probst YC. Examining dietary behaviours, diet quality, motives and supplementation use in physically active individuals following vegetarian-based eating patterns. *Nutr Bull.* 2022;47(4):473-487. doi:10.1111/nbu.12592
8. Most Frequently Asked Questions. The Vegetarian Resource Group. Accessed October 24, 2023. www.vrg.org/nutshell/faq.htm#types
9. Burke LM, Castell LM, Casa DJ, et al. International Association of Athletics Federations consensus statement 2019: nutrition for athletics. *Int Sport Nutr Exerc Metab.* 2019;29(2):73-84. doi:10.1123/ijsnem.2019-0065
10. Craig WJ, Mangels AR, Fresán U, et al. The safe and effective use of plant-based diets with guidelines for health professionals. *Nutrients.* 2021;13(11):4144. doi:10.3390/nu13114144
11. Larson-Meyer DE, Ruscigno M. *Plant-Based Sports Nutrition: Expert Fueling Strategies for Training, Recovery, and Performance.* Human Kinetics; 2020
12. Lynch H, Johnston C, Wharton C. Plant-based diets: considerations for environmental impact, protein quality, and exercise performance. *Nutrients.* 2018;10(12):1841. doi:10.3390/nu10121841
13. Melina V, Craig W, Levin S. Position of the Academy of Nutrition and Dietetics: vegetarian diets. *Acad Nutr Diet.* 2016;116(12):1970-1980. doi:10.1016/j.jand.2016.09.025
14. Rudloff S, Bührer C, Jochum F, et al. Vegetarian diets in childhood and adolescence: Position paper of the nutrition committee, German Society for Paediatric and Adolescent Medicine (DGKJ). *Mol Cell Pediatr.* 2019;6(1):4. doi:10.1186/s40348-019-0091-z
15. Goran MI, Poehlman ET, Johnson RK. Energy requirements across the life span: new findings based on measurement of total, energy-expenditure with doubly labeled water. *Nutr Res.* 1995;15(1):115-150. doi:10.1016/0271-5317(95)91657-X
16. Thomas DT, Erdman KA, Burke LM. Position of the Academy of Nutrition and Dietetics, Dietitians of Canada, and the American College of Sports Medicine: Nutrition and Athletic Performance. *Acad Nutr Diet.* 2016;116(3):501-528. doi:10.1016/j.jand.2015.12.006
17. Otten JJ, Hellwig JP, Meyers LD, eds. *Dietary Reference Intakes: The Essential Guide to Nutrient Requirements.* National Academies Press; 2006.
18. US Department of Agriculture. USDA MyPlate: Enjoy Vegetarian Meals. March 2022. Accessed January 17, 2023. www.myplate.gov/tip-sheet/enjoy-vegetarian-meals
19. Reguant-Closa A, Harris MM, Lohman TG, Meyer NL. Validation of the athlete's plate nutrition educational tool: phase I. *Int Sport Nutr Exerc Metab.* 2019;29(6):628-635. doi:10.1123/ijsnem.2018-0346
20. Mangels R, Messina V, Messina M. *The Dietitian's Guide to Vegetarian Diets: Issues and Applications.* 4th ed. Jones & Bartlett; 2023
21. Messina V, Melina V, Mangels AR. A new food guide for North American vegetarians. *Am Diet Assoc.* 2003;103(6):771-775. doi:10.1053/jada.2003.50141
22. Guest NS, Lynch H. Plant-based diets and athletic performance. *Aspetar Sports Med J.* 2021;10:12-16. https://journal.aspetar.com/en/archive/volume-10-targeted-topic-sports-nutrition/plant-based-diets-and-athletic-performance
23. Casey A, Mann R, Banister K, et al. Effect of carbohydrate ingestion on glycogen resynthesis in human liver and skeletal muscle, measured by ^{13}C MRS. *Am Physiol Endocrinol Metab.* 2000;278(1):E65-E75. doi:10.1152/ajpendo.2000.278.1.E65
24. Nilsson LH, Hultman E. Liver glycogen in man—the effect of total starvation or a carbohydrate-poor diet followed by carbohydrate refeeding. *Scand Clin Lab Invest.* 1973;32(4):325-330. doi:10.3109/00365517309084355
25. Bergström J, Hermansen L, Hultman E, Saltin B. Diet, muscle glycogen and physical performance. *Acta Physiol Scand.* 1967;71(2):140-150. doi:10.1111/j.1748-1716.1967.tb03720.x
26. Achten J, Halson SL, Moseley L, Rayson MP, Casey A, Jeukendrup AE. Higher dietary carbohydrate content during intensified running training results in better maintenance of performance and mood state. *Appl Physiol (1985).* 2004;96(4):1331-1340. doi:10.1152/japplphysiol.00973.2003
27. Brewer J, Williams C, Patton A. The influence of high carbohydrate diets on endurance running performance. *Eur Appl Physiol Occup Physiol.* 1988;57(6):698-706. doi:10.1007/BF01075991

28. Coggan AR, Swanson SC. Nutritional manipulations before and during endurance exercise: effects on performance. *Med Sci Sports Exerc.* 1992;24(9 suppl):S331-S335.

29. Hargreaves M, Costill DL, Coggan A, Fink WJ, Nishibata I. Effect of carbohydrate feedings on muscle glycogen utilization and exercise performance. *Med Sci Sports Exerc.* 1984;16(3):219-222.

30. Larson DE, Hesslink RL, Hrovat MI, Fishman RS, Systrom DM. Dietary effects on exercising muscle metabolism and performance by 31P-MRS. *Appl Physiol (1985).* 1994;77(3):1108-1115. doi:10.1152/jappl.1994.77.3.1108

31. Pizza FX, Flynn MG, Duscha BD, Holden J, Kubitz ER. A carbohydrate loading regimen improves high intensity, short duration exercise performance. *Int Sport Nutr.* 1995;5(2):110-116. doi:10.1123/ijsn.5.2.110

32. Sugiura K, Kobayashi K. Effect of carbohydrate ingestion on sprint performance following continuous and intermittent exercise. *Med Sci Sports Exerc.* 1998;30(11):1624-1630. doi:10.1097/00005768-199811000-00011

33. Stellingwerff T, Cox GR. Systematic review: carbohydrate supplementation on exercise performance or capacity of varying durations. *Appl Physiol Nutr Metab.* 2014;39(9):998-1011. doi:10.1139/apnm-2014-0027

34. Williams C, Rollo I. Carbohydrate nutrition and team sport performance. *Sports Med.* 2015;45(suppl 1):S13-S22. doi:10.1007/s40279-015-0399-3

35. Spencer MK, Yan Z, Katz A. Carbohydrate supplementation attenuates IMP accumulation in human muscle during prolonged exercise. *Am Physiol.* 1991;261(1 pt 1):C71-C76. doi:10.1152/ajpcell.1991.261.1.C71

36. Burke LM, Ross ML, Garvican-Lewis LA, et al. Low carbohydrate, high fat diet impairs exercise economy and negates the performance benefit from intensified training in elite race walkers. *Physiol.* 2017;595(9):2785-2807. doi:10.1113/JP273230

37. Burke LM, Sharma AP, Heikura IA, et al. Crisis of confidence averted: impairment of exercise economy and performance in elite race walkers by ketogenic low carbohydrate, high fat (LCHF) diet is reproducible. *PLoS One.* 2020;15(6):e0234027. doi:10.1371/journal.pone.0234027

38. Jeukendrup AE. Oral carbohydrate rinse: placebo or beneficial? *Curr Sports Med Rep.* 2013;12(4):222-227. doi:10.1249/JSR.0b013e31829a6caa

39. Burke LM, Hawley JA, Wong SHS, Jeukendrup AE. Carbohydrates for training and competition. *Sports Sci.* 2011;29(suppl 1):S17-S27. doi:10.1080/02640414.2011.585473

40. Phillips SM, Van Loon LJ. Dietary protein for athletes: from requirements to optimum adaptation. *Sports Sci.* 2011;29(suppl 1):S29-S38. doi:10.1080/02640414.2011.619204

41. Panel on Macronutrients; Panel on the Definition of Dietary Fiber; Subcommittee on Upper Reference Levels of Nutrients; Subcommittee on Interpretation and Uses of Dietary Reference Intakes; Standing Committee on the Scientific Evaluation of Dietary Reference Intakes; Food and Nutrition Board, Institute of Medicine. *Dietary Reference Intakes for Energy, Carbohydrate, Fiber, Fat, Fatty Acids, Cholesterol, Protein, and Amino Acids.* National Academies Press; 2005. doi:10.17226/10490

42. Morton RW, Murphy KT, McKellar SR, et al. A systematic review, meta-analysis and meta-regression of the effect of protein supplementation on resistance training-induced gains in muscle mass and strength in healthy adults. *Br Sports Med.* 2018;52(6):376-384. doi:10.1136/bjsports-2017-097608

43. Hevia-Larraín V, Gualano B, Longobardi I, et al. High-protein plant-based diet versus a protein-matched omnivorous diet to support resistance training adaptations: a comparison between habitual vegans and omnivores. *Sports Med.* 2021;51(6):1317-1330. doi:10.1007/s40279-021-01434-9

44. Tipton KD, Witard OC. Protein requirements and recommendations for athletes: relevance of ivory tower arguments for practical recommendations. *Clin Sports Med.* 2007;26(1):17-36. doi:10.1016/j.csm.2006.11.003

45. Lemon PW, Mullin JP. Effect of initial muscle glycogen levels on protein catabolism during exercise. *Appl Physiol Respir Environ Exerc Physiol.* 1980;48(4):624-629. doi:10.1152/jappl.1980.48.4.624

46. Pinckaers PJM, Trommelen J, Snijders T, van Loon LJC. The anabolic response to plant-based protein ingestion. *Sports Med.* 2021;51(suppl 1):59-74. doi:10.1007/s40279-021-01540-8

47. Rand WM, Pellett PL, Young VR. Meta-analysis of nitrogen balance studies for estimating protein requirements in healthy adults. *Am Clin Nutr.* 2003;77:109-127. doi:10.1093/ajcn/77.1.109

48. Joint FAO/WHO/UNU Expert Consultation on Protein and Amino Acid Requirements in Human Nutrition. *Protein and Amino Acid Requirements in Human Nutrition: Report of a Joint FAO/WHO/UNU Expert Consultation.* Food and Agriculture Organization of the United Nations, World Health Organization, and United Nations University; 2002. WHO Technical Report Series No. 935.

49. Young VR, Pellett PL. Plant proteins in relation to human protein and amino acid nutrition. *Am Clin Nutr.* 1994;59(5 suppl):1203S-1212S. doi:10.1093/ajcn/59.5.1203S

50. Bergström J, Fürst P, Vinnars E. Effect of a test meal, without and with protein, on muscle and plasma free amino acids. *Clin Sci (Lond).* 1990;79(4):331-337. doi:10.1042/cs0790331

51. Gorissen SHM, Crombag JJR, Senden JMG, et al. Protein content and amino acid composition of commercially available plant-based protein isolates. *Amino Acids.* 2018;50(12):1685-1695. doi:10.1007/s00726-018-2640-5

52. van Loon L. Plant versus animal-based proteins to support muscle conditioning. *Sports Sci Exch.* 2021;34(220):1-7.

53. Abou Sawan S, van Vliet S, West DWD, et al. Whole egg, but not egg white, ingestion induces mTOR colocalization with the lysosome after resistance exercise. *Am Physiol Cell Physiol.* 2018;315(4):C537-C543. doi:10.1152/ajpcell.00225.2018
54. Pinckaers PJM, Kouw IWK, Hendriks FK, et al. No differences in muscle protein synthesis rates following ingestion of wheat protein, milk protein, and their protein blend in healthy, young males. *Br Nutr.* 2021;126(12):1832-1842. doi:10.1017/S0007114521000635
55. Wilkinson SB, Tarnopolsky MA, Macdonald MJ, Macdonald JR, Armstrong D, Phillips SM. Consumption of fluid skim milk promotes greater muscle protein accretion after resistance exercise than does consumption of an isonitrogenous and isoenergetic soy-protein beverage. *Am Clin Nutr.* 2007;85(4):1031-1040. doi:10.1093/ajcn/85.4.1031 [Erratum: *Am Clin Nutr.* 2013;98(2):512. doi:10.3945/ajcn.113.067389]
56. US Department of Agriculture. FoodData Central. Accessed September 30, 2024. https://fdc.nal.usda.gov
57. Rizzo NS, Jaceldo-Siegl K, Sabate J, Fraser GE. Nutrient profiles of vegetarian and nonvegetarian dietary patterns. *Acad Nutr Diet.* 2013;113(12):1610-1619. doi:10.1016/j.jand.2013.06.349
58. Ciuris C, Lynch HM, Wharton C, Johnston CS. A comparison of dietary protein digestibility, based on DIAAS scoring, in vegetarian and non-vegetarian athletes. *Nutrients.* 2019;11(12):3016. doi:10.3390/nu11123016
59. Mamerow MM, Mettler JA, English KL, et al. Dietary protein distribution positively influences 24-h muscle protein synthesis in healthy adults. *Nutr.* 2014;144(6):876-880. doi:10.3945/jn.113.185280
60. Tipton KD, Rasmussen BB, Miller SL, et al. Timing of amino acid-carbohydrate ingestion alters anabolic response of muscle to resistance exercise. *Am Physiol Endocrinol Metab.* 2001;281(2):E197-E206. doi:10.1152/ajpendo.2001.281.2.E197
61. Tipton KD, Elliott TA, Cree MG, Aarsland AA, Sanford AP, Wolfe RR. Stimulation of net muscle protein synthesis by whey protein ingestion before and after exercise. *Am Physiol Endocrinol Metab.* 2007;292(1):E71-E76. doi:10.1152/ajpendo.00166.2006
62. Babault N, Païzis C, Deley G, et al. Pea proteins oral supplementation promotes muscle thickness gains during resistance training: a double-blind, randomized, placebo-controlled clinical trial vs. whey protein. *Int Soc Sports Nutr.* 2015;12(1):3. doi:10.1186/s12970-014-0064-5
63. Messina M, Lynch H, Dickinson JM, Reed KE. No difference between the effects of supplementing with soy protein versus animal protein on gains in muscle mass and strength in response to resistance exercise. *Int Sport Nutr Exerc Metab.* 2018;28(6):674-685. doi:10.1123/ijsnem.2018-0071
64. Lim MT, Pan BJ, Toh DWK, Sutanto CN, Kim JE. Animal protein versus plant protein in supporting lean mass and muscle strength: a systematic review and meta-analysis of randomized controlled trials. *Nutrients.* 2021;13(2):661. doi:10.3390/nu13020661
65. Brown RC, Cox CM. Effects of high fat versus high carbohydrate diets on plasma lipids and lipoproteins in endurance athletes. *Med Sci Sports Exerc.* 1998;30(12):1677-1683. doi:10.1097/00005768-199812000-00004
66. Hoppeler H, Billeter R, Horvath PJ, Leddy JJ, Pendergast DR. Muscle structure with low- and high-fat diets in well-trained male runners. *Int Sports Med.* 1999;20(8):522-526. doi:10.1055/s-1999-8838
67. Horvath PJ, Eagen CK, Ryer-Calvin SD, Pendergast DR. The effects of varying dietary fat on the nutrient intake in male and female runners. *Am Coll Nutr.* 2000;19(1):42-51. doi:10.1080/07315724.2000.10718913
68. Larson-Meyer DE, Borkhsenious ON, Gullett JC, et al. Effect of dietary fat on serum and intramyocellular lipids and running performance. *Med Sci Sports Exerc.* 2008;40(5):892-902. doi:10.1249/MSS.0b013e318164cb33
69. Larson-Meyer DE, Newcomer BR, Hunter GR. Influence of endurance running and recovery diet on intramyocellular lipid content in women: a 1H NMR study. *Am Physiol Endocrinol Metab.* 2002;282(1):E95-E106. doi:10.1152/ajpendo.2002.282.1.E95
70. Muoio DM, Leddy JJ, Horvath PJ, Awad AB, Pendergast DR. Effect of dietary fat on metabolic adjustments to maximal VO_2 and endurance in runners. *Med Sci Sports Exerc.* 1994;26(1):81-88.
71. Thompson PD, Cullinane EM, Eshleman R, Kantor MA, Herbert PN. The effects of high-carbohydrate and high-fat diets on the serum lipid and lipoprotein concentrations of endurance athletes. *Metabolism.* 1984;33(11):1003-1010. doi:10.1016/0026-0495(84)90228-2
72. Laughlin GA, Yen SS. Nutritional and endocrine-metabolic aberrations in amenorrheic athletes. *Clin Endocrinol Metab.* 1996;81(12):4301-4309. doi:10.1210/jcem.81.12.8954031
73. Décombaz J, Schmitt B, Ith M, et al. Postexercise fat intake repletes intramyocellular lipids but no faster in trained than in sedentary subjects. *Am Physiol Regul Integr Comp Physiol.* 2001;281(3):R760-R769. doi:10.1152/ajpregu.2001.281.3.R760
74. Romijn JA, Coyle EF, Sidossis LS, et al. Regulation of endogenous fat and carbohydrate metabolism in relation to exercise intensity and duration. *Am Physiol.* 1993;265(3 pt 1):E380-E391. doi:10.1152/ajpendo.1993.265.3.E380
75. Romijn JA, Coyle EF, Sidossis LS, Rosenblatt J, Wolfe RR. Substrate metabolism during different exercise intensities in endurance-trained women. *Appl Physiol (1985).* 2000;88(5):1707-1714. doi:10.1152/jappl.2000.88.5.1707
76. Gould KL, Ornish D, Kirkeeide R, et al. Improved stenosis geometry by quantitative coronary arteriography after vigorous risk factor modification. *Am Cardiol.* 1992;69(9):845-853. doi:10.1016/0002-9149(92)90781-s
77. Gould KL, Ornish D, Scherwitz L, et al. Changes in myocardial perfusion abnormalities by positron emission tomography after long-term, intense risk factor modification. *JAMA.* 1995;274(11):894-901. doi:10.1001/jama.1995.03530110056036

78. Ornish D, Brown SE, Scherwitz LW, et al. Can lifestyle changes reverse coronary heart disease? The Lifestyle Heart Trial. *Lancet*. 1990;336(8708):129-133. doi:10.1016/0140-6736(90)91656-u

79. Barnard ND, Cohen J, Jenkins DJ, et al. A low-fat vegan diet and a conventional diabetes diet in the treatment of type 2 diabetes: a randomized, controlled, 74-wk clinical trial. *Am Clin Nutr*. 2009;89(5):1588S-1596S. doi:10.3945/ajcn.2009.26736H

80. Barnard ND, Katcher HI, Jenkins DJA, Cohen J, Turner-McGrievy G. Vegetarian and vegan diets in type 2 diabetes management. *Nutr Rev*. 2009;67(5):255-263. doi:10.1111/j.1753-4887.2009.00198.x

81. Mujika I. Case study: Long-term low-carbohydrate, high-fat diet impairs performance and subjective well-being in a world-class vegetarian long-distance triathlete. *Int Sport Nutr Exerc Metab*. 2019;29(3):339-344. doi:10.1123/ijsnem.2018-0124

82. Hawley JA, Leckey JJ. Carbohydrate dependence during prolonged, intense endurance exercise. *Sports Med*. 2015;45(suppl 1):S5-S12. doi:10.1007/s40279-015-0400-1

83. Elliott PS, Kharaty SS, Phillips CM. Plant-based diets and lipid, lipoprotein, and inflammatory biomarkers of cardiovascular disease: a review of observational and interventional studies. *Nutrients*. 2022;14(24):5371. doi:10.3390/nu14245371

84. US Department of Agriculture and US Department of Health and Human Services. *Dietary Guidelines for Americans, 2020-2025*. 9th ed. December 2020. Accessed January 17, 2023. www.dietaryguidelines.gov/sites/default/files/2021-03/Dietary_Guidelines_for_Americans_2020-2025.pdf

85. Reid MA, Marsh KA, Zeuschner CL, Saunders AV, Baines SK. Meeting the nutrient reference values on a vegetarian diet. *Med Aust*. 2013;199(S4):S33-S40. doi:10.5694/mja11.11510

86. Jeromson S, Gallagher IJ, Galloway SD, Hamilton DL. Omega-3 fatty acids and skeletal muscle health. *Mar Drugs*. 2015;13(11):6977-7004. doi:10.3390/md13116977

87. Da Boit M, Hunter AM, Gray SR. Fit with good fat? The role of n-3 polyunsaturated fatty acids on exercise performance. *Metabolism*. 2017;66:45-54. doi:10.1016/j.metabol.2016.10.007

88. Jakeman JR, Lambrick DM, Wooley B, Babraj JA, Faulkner JA. Effect of an acute dose of omega-3 fish oil following exercise-induced muscle damage. *Eur Appl Physiol*. 2017;117(3):575-582. doi:10.1007/s00421-017-3543-y

89. Williams CM, Burdge G. Long-chain n-3 PUFA: plant v. marine sources. *Proc Nutr Soc*. 2006;65(1):42-50. doi:10.1079/pns2005473

90. Geppert J, Kraft V, Demmelmair H, Koletzko B. Docosahexaenoic acid supplementation in vegetarians effectively increases omega-3 index: a randomized trial. *Lipids*. 2005;40(8):807-814. doi:10.1007/s11745-005-1442-9

91. Conquer JA, Holub BJ. Supplementation with an algae source of docosahexaenoic acid increases (n-3) fatty acid status and alters selected risk factors for heart disease in vegetarian subjects. *Nutr*. 1996;126(12):3032-3039. doi:10.1093/jn/126.12.3032

92. Heaney RP, Recker RR, Saville PD. Menopausal changes in calcium balance performance. *Lab Clin Med*. 1978;92(6):953-963.

93. Myburgh KH, Hutchins J, Fataar AB, Hough SF, Noakes TD. Low bone density is an etiologic factor for stress fractures in athletes. *Ann Intern Med*. 1990;113(10):754-759. doi:10.7326/0003-4819-113-10-754

94. Wolman RL, Clark P, McNally E, Harries MG, Reeve J. Dietary calcium as a statistical determinant of spinal trabecular bone density in amenorrhoeic and oestrogen-replete athletes. *Bone Miner*. 1992;17(3):415-423. doi:10.1016/0169-6009(92)90790-k

95. Lappe J, Cullen D, Haynatzki G, Recker R, Ahlf R, Thompson K. Calcium and vitamin D supplementation decreases incidence of stress fractures in female navy recruits. *Bone Miner Res*. 2008;23(5):741-749. doi:10.1359/jbmr.080102

96. Lundy B, McKay AKA, Fensham NC, et al. The impact of acute calcium intake on bone turnover markers during a training day in elite male rowers. *Med Sci Sports Exerc*. 2023;55(1):55-65. doi:10.1249/MSS.0000000000003022

97. Barry DW, Hansen KC, van Pelt RE, Witten M, Wolfe P, Kohrt WM. Acute calcium ingestion attenuates exercise-induced disruption of calcium homeostasis. *Med Sci Sports Exerc*. 2011;43(4):617-623. doi:10.1249/MSS.0b013e3181f79fa8

98. Clarys P, Deliens T, Huybrechts I, et al. Comparison of nutritional quality of the vegan, vegetarian, semi-vegetarian, pesco-vegetarian and omnivorous diet. *Nutrients*. 2014;6(3):1318-1332. doi:10.3390/nu6031318

99. Heaney RP, Dowell MS, Rafferty K, Bierman J. Bioavailability of the calcium in fortified soy imitation milk, with some observations on method. *Am Clin Nutr*. 2000;71(5):1166-1169. doi:10.1093/ajcn/71.5.1166

100. Weaver CM, Plawecki KL. Dietary calcium: adequacy of a vegetarian diet. *Am Clin Nutr*. 1994;59(5 suppl):1238S-1241S. doi:10.1093/ajcn/59.5.1238S

101. Weaver CM, Proulx WR, Heaney R. Choices for achieving adequate dietary calcium with a vegetarian diet. *Am Clin Nutr*. 1999;70(3 suppl):543S-548S. doi:10.1093/ajcn/70.3.543s

102. Zhao Y, Martin BR, Weaver CM. Calcium bioavailability of calcium carbonate fortified soymilk is equivalent to cow's milk in young women. *Nutr*. 2005;135(10):2379-2382. doi:10.1093/jn/135.10.2379

103. Kohlenberg-Mueller K, Raschka L. Calcium balance in young adults on a vegan and lactovegetarian diet. *Bone Miner Metab*. 2003;21(1):28-33. doi:10.1007/s007740300005

104. Iguacel I, Miguel-Berges ML, Gómez-Bruton A, Moreno LA, Julián C. Veganism, vegetarianism, bone mineral density, and fracture risk: a systematic review and meta-analysis. *Nutr Rev*. 2019;77(1):1-18. doi:10.1093/nutrit/nuy045

105. Hsu E. Plant-based diets and bone health: sorting through the evidence. *Curr Opin Endocrinol Diabetes Obes*. 2020;27(4):248-252. doi:10.1097/MED.0000000000000552

106. Heaney RP, Dowell MS, Hale CA, Bendich A. Calcium absorption varies within the reference range for serum 25-hydroxyvitamin D. *Am Coll Nutr*. 2003;22(2):142-146. doi:10.1080/07315724.2003.10719287

107. Holick MF. Sunlight and vitamin D for bone health and prevention of autoimmune diseases, cancers, and cardiovascular disease. *Am Clin Nutr.* 2004;80(6 suppl):1678S-1688S. doi:10.1093/ajcn/80.6.1678S
108. Holick MF. The vitamin D epidemic and its health consequences. *Nutr.* 2005;135(11):2739S-2748S. doi:10.1093/jn/135.11.2739S
109. Cannell J. Peak athletic performance and vitamin D. *The Vitamin D Newsletter.* March 11, 2007. The Vitamin D Council; 2007. Accessed April 18, 2017. www.vitamindcouncil.org
110. Larson-Meyer DE. The importance of vitamin D for athletes. *Sports Sci Exch.* 2015;28(148):1-8.
111. Larson-Meyer DE, Willis KS. Vitamin D and athletes. *Curr Sports Med Rep.* 2010;9(4):220-226. doi:10.1249/JSR.0b013e3181e7dd45
112. Yoon S, Kwon O, Kim J. Vitamin D in athletes: focus on physical performance and musculoskeletal injuries. *Phys Act Nutr.* 2021;25(2):20-25. doi:10.20463/pan.2021.0011
113. Owens DJ, Allison R, Close GL. Vitamin D and the athlete: current perspectives and new challenges. *Sports Med.* 2018;48(suppl 1):3-16. doi:10.1007/s40279-017-0841-9
114. Zürcher SJ, Quadri A, Huber A, et al. Predictive factors for vitamin d concentrations in Swiss athletes: a cross-sectional study. *Sports Med Int Open.* 2018;2(5):E148-E156. doi:10.1055/a-0669-0791
115. Heller JE, Thomas JJ, Hollis BW, Larson-Meyer DE. Relation between vitamin D status and body composition in collegiate athletes. *Int Sport Nutr Exerc Metab.* 2015;25(2):128-135. doi:10.1123/ijsnem.2013-0250
116. Cannell JJ, Hollis BW. Use of vitamin D in clinical practice. *Altern Med Rev.* 2008;13(1):6-20.
117. Armas LA, Hollis BW, Heaney RP. Vitamin D2 is much less effective than vitamin D3 in humans. *Clin Endocrinol Metab.* 2004;89(11):5387-5391. doi:10.1210/jc.2004-0360
118. Trang HM, Cole DE, Rubin LA, Pierratos A, Siu S, Vieth R. Evidence that vitamin D3 increases serum 25-hydroxyvitamin D more efficiently than does vitamin D2. *Am Clin Nutr.* 1998;68(4):854-858. doi:10.1093/ajcn/68.4.854
119. Holick MF, Biancuzzo RM, Chen TC, et al. Vitamin D2 is as effective as vitamin D3 in maintaining circulating concentrations of 25-hydroxyvitamin D. *Clin Endocrinol Metab.* 2008;93(3):677-681. doi:10.1210/jc.2007-2308
120. Logan VF, Gray AR, Peddie MC, Harper MJ, Houghton LA. Long-term vitamin D3 supplementation is more effective than vitamin D2 in maintaining serum 25-hydroxyvitamin D status over the winter months. *Br Nutr.* 2013;109(6):1082-1088. doi:10.1017/S0007114512002851
121. Nieman DC, Gillitt ND, Shanely RA, Dew D, Meaney MP, Luo B. Vitamin D2 supplementation amplifies eccentric exercise-induced muscle damage in NASCAR pit crew athletes. *Nutrients.* 2013;6(1):63-75. doi:10.3390/nu6010063
122. Malczewska J, Raczynski G, Stupnicki R. Iron status in female endurance athletes and in non-athletes. *Int Sport Nutr Exerc Metab.* 2000;10(3):260-276. doi:10.1123/ijsnem.10.3.260
123. Sim M, Garvican-Lewis LA, Cox GR, et al. Iron considerations for the athlete: a narrative review. *Eur Appl Physiol.* 2019;119(7):1463-1478. doi:10.1007/s00421-019-04157-y
124. Finn EE, Tenforde AS, Fredericson M, et al. Markers of low-iron status are associated with female athlete triad risk factors. *Med Sci Sports Exerc.* 2021;53(9):1969-1974. doi:10.1249/MSS.0000000000002660
125. Peeling P, Dawson B, Goodman C, Landers G, Trinder D. Athletic induced iron deficiency: new insights into the role of inflammation, cytokines and hormones. *Eur Appl Physiol.* 2008;103(4):381-391. doi:10.1007/s00421-008-0726-6
126. Eichner ER. Runner's macrocytosis: a clue to footstrike hemolysis. Runner's anemia as a benefit versus runner's hemolysis as a detriment. *Am Med.* 1985;78(2):321-325. doi:10.1016/0002-9343(85)90443-7
127. Barney DE, Ippolito JR, Berryman CE, Hennigar SR. A prolonged bout of running increases hepcidin and decreases dietary iron absorption in trained female and male runners. *Nutr.* 2022;152(9):2039-2047. doi:10.1093/jn/nxac129
128. Pedlar CR, Brugnara C, Bruinvels G, Burden R. Iron balance and iron supplementation for the female athlete: A practical approach. *Eur Sport Sci.* 2018;18(2):295-305. doi:10.1080/17461391.2017.1416178
129. Coudray C, Bellanger J, Castiglia-Delavaud C, Rémésy C, Vermorel M, Rayssignuier Y. Effect of soluble or partly soluble dietary fibres supplementation on absorption and balance of calcium, magnesium, iron and zinc in healthy young men. *Eur Clin Nutr.* 1997;51(6):375-380. doi:10.1038/sj.ejcn.1600417
130. Hallberg L, Hulthén L. Prediction of dietary iron absorption: an algorithm for calculating absorption and bioavailability of dietary iron. *Am Clin Nutr.* 2000;71(5):1147-1160. doi:10.1093/ajcn/71.5.1147
131. Platel K, Srinivasan K. Bioavailability of micronutrients from plant foods: an update. *Crit Rev Food Sci Nutr.* 2016;56(10):1608-1619. doi:10.1080/10408398.2013.781011
132. Monsen ER, Balintfy JL. Calculating dietary iron bioavailability: refinement and computerization. *Am Diet Assoc.* 1982;80(4):307-311.
133. Badenhorst CE, Black KE, O'Brien WJ. Hepcidin as a prospective individualized biomarker for individuals at risk of low energy availability. *Int Sport Nutr Exerc Metab.* 2019;29(6):671-681. doi:10.1123/ijsnem.2019-0006
134. Saunders AV, Craig WJ, Baines SK, Posen JS. Iron and vegetarian diets. *Med Aust.* 2013;199(S4):S11-S16. doi:10.5694/mja11.11494
135. Snyder AC, Dvorak LL, Roepke JB. Influence of dietary iron source on measures of iron status among female runners. *Med Sci Sports Exerc.* 1989;21(1):7-10. doi:10.1249/00005768-198902000-00002
136. Haider LM, Schwingshackl L, Hoffmann G, Ekmekcioglu C. The effect of vegetarian diets on iron status in adults: A systematic review and meta-analysis. *Crit Rev Food Sci Nutr.* 2018;58(8):1359-1374. doi:10.1080/10408398.2016.1259210

137. Woolf K, St Thomas MM, Hahn N, Vaughan LA, Carlson AG, Hinton P. Iron status in highly active and sedentary young women. *Int Sport Nutr Exerc Metab.* 2009;19(5):519-535. doi:10.1123/ijsnem.19.5.519

138. Hinton PS, Sinclair LM. Iron supplementation maintains ventilatory threshold and improves energetic efficiency in iron-deficient nonanemic athletes. *Eur Clin Nutr.* 2007;61(1):30-39. doi:10.1038/sj.ejcn.1602479

139. Larson-Meyer DE, Woolf K, Burke L. Assessment of nutrient status in athletes and the need for supplementation. *Int Sport Nutr Exerc Metab.* 2018;28(2):139-158. doi:10.1123/ijsnem.2017-0338

140. Herbert V. Everyone should be tested for iron disorders. *Am Diet Assoc.* 1992;92(12):1502-1509.

141. Lukaski HC. Micronutrients (magnesium, zinc, and copper): are mineral supplements needed for athletes? *Int Sport Nutr.* 1995;5(suppl):S74-S83.

142. Micheletti A, Rossi R, Rufini S. Zinc status in athletes: relation to diet and exercise. *Sports Med.* 2001;31(8):577-582. doi:10.2165/00007256-200131080-00002

143. Hunt JR. Bioavailability of iron, zinc, and other trace minerals from vegetarian diets. *Am Clin Nutr.* 2003;78(3 suppl):633S-639S. doi:10.1093/ajcn/78.3.633S

144. Lukaski HC. Vitamin and mineral status: effects on physical performance. *Nutrition.* 2004;20(7-8):632-644. doi:10.1016/j.nut.2004.04.001

145. Manore MM, Helleksen JM, Merkel J, Skinner JS. Longitudinal changes in zinc status in untrained men: effects of two different 12-week exercise training programs and zinc supplementation. *Am Diet Assoc.* 1993;93(10):1165-1168. doi:10.1016/0002-8223(93)91653-8

146. Lönnerdal B. Dietary factors influencing zinc absorption. *Nutr.* 2000;130(5S suppl):1378S-1383S. doi:10.1093/jn/130.5.1378S

147. Hunt JR, Matthys LA, Johnson LK. Zinc absorption, mineral balance, and blood lipids in women consuming controlled lactoovovegetarian and omnivorous diets for 8 wk. *Am Clin Nutr.* 1998;67(3):421-430. doi:10.1093/ajcn/67.3.421

148. Rosado JL, Díaz M, González K, Griffin I, Abrams SA, Preciado R. The addition of milk or yogurt to a plant-based diet increases zinc bioavailability but does not affect iron bioavailability in women. *Nutr.* 2005;135(3):465-468. doi:10.1093/jn/135.3.465

149. Krajcovicová-Kudlácková M, Bucková K, Klimes I, Seboková E. Iodine deficiency in vegetarians and vegans. *Ann Nutr Metab.* 2003;47(5):183-185. doi:10.1159/000070483

150. Remer T, Neubert A, Manz F. Increased risk of iodine deficiency with vegetarian nutrition. *Br Nutr.* 1999;81(1):45-49. doi:10.1017/s0007114599000136

151. Groufh-Jacobsen S, Hess SY, Aakre I, Folven Gjengedal EL, Blandhoel Pettersen K, Henjum S. Vegans, vegetarians and pescatarians are at risk of iodine deficiency in Norway. *Nutrients.* 2020;12(11):3555. doi:10.3390/nu12113555

152. Leung AM, Lamar A, He X, Braverman LE, Pearce EN. Iodine status and thyroid function of Boston-area vegetarians and vegans. *Clin Endocrinol Metab.* 2011;96(8):E1303-E1307. doi:10.1210/jc.2011-0256

153. Lightowler HJ, Davies GJ. Iodine intake and iodine deficiency in vegans as assessed by the duplicate-portion technique and urinary iodine excretion. *Br Nutr.* 1998;80(6):529-535. doi:10.1017/s0007114598001627

154. Waldmann A, Koschizke JW, Leitzmann C, Hahn A. Dietary intakes and lifestyle factors of a vegan population in Germany: results from the German Vegan Study. *Eur Clin Nutr.* 2003;57(8):947-955. doi:10.1038/sj.ejcn.1601629

155. Larson-Meyer DE, Gostas DE. Thyroid function and nutrient status in the athlete. *Curr Sports Med Rep.* 2020;19(2):84-94. doi:10.1249/JSR.0000000000000689

156. Smyth PP, Duntas LH. Iodine uptake and loss-can frequent strenuous exercise induce iodine deficiency? *Horm Metab Res.* 2005;37(9):555-558. doi:10.1055/s-2005-870423

157. Messina M, Redmond G. Effects of soy protein and soybean isoflavones on thyroid function in healthy adults and hypothyroid patients: a review of the relevant literature. *Thyroid.* 2006;16(3):249-258. doi:10.1089/thy.2006.16.249

158. US Department of Agriculture, Agricultural Research Service. What we eat in America, NHANES 2017-March 2020 prepandamic. Accessed Sept 4, 2023. www.ars.usda.gov/northeast-area/beltsville-md-bhnrc/beltsville-human-nutrition-research-center/food-surveys-research-group/docs/wweia-data-tables

159. Volpe SL. Magnesium and the athlete. *Curr Sports Med Rep.* 2015;14(4):279-283. doi:10.1249/JSR.0000000000000178

160. Nielsen FH, Lukaski HC. Update on the relationship between magnesium and exercise. *Magnes Res.* 2006;19(3):180-189.

161. Woolf K, Manore MM. B-vitamins and exercise: does exercise alter requirements? *Int Sport Nutr Exerc Metab.* 2006;16(5):453-484. doi:10.1123/ijsnem.16.5.453

162. Herrmann W, Geisel J. Vegetarian lifestyle and monitoring of vitamin B-12 status. *Clin Chim Acta.* 2002;326(1-2):47-59. doi:10.1016/s0009-8981(02)00307-8

163. Niklewicz A, Smith AD, Smith A, et al. The importance of vitamin B_{12} for individuals choosing plant-based diets. *Eur Nutr.* 2023;62(3):1551-1559. doi:10.1007/s00394-022-03025-4

164. Pawlak R, Parrott SJ, Raj S, Cullum-Dugan D, Lucus D. How prevalent is vitamin B_{12} deficiency among vegetarians? *Nutr Rev.* 2013;71(2):110-117. doi:10.1111/nure.12001

165. Rauma AL, Törrönen R, Hänninen O, Mykkänen H. Vitamin B-12 status of long-term adherents of a strict uncooked vegan diet ("living food diet") is compromised. *Nutr.* 1995;125(10):2511-2515. doi:10.1093/jn/125.10.2511

166. Watanabe F, Yabuta Y, Bito T, Teng F. Vitamin B_{12}-containing plant food sources for vegetarians. *Nutrients.* 2014;6(5):1861-1873. doi:10.3390/nu6051861

167. Herrmann W, Schorr H, Obeid R, Geisel J. Vitamin B-12 status, particularly holotranscobalamin II and methylmalonic acid concentrations, and hyperhomocysteinemia in vegetarians. *Am Clin Nutr.* 2003;78(1):131-136. doi:10.1093/ajcn/78.1.131

168. Belko AZ, Obarzanek E, Kalkwarf HJ, et al. Effects of exercise on riboflavin requirements of young women. *Am Clin Nutr.* 1983;37(4):509-517. doi:10.1093/ajcn/37.4.509
169. Soares MJ, Satyanarayana K, Bamji MS, Jacob CM, Ramana YV, Rao SS. The effect of exercise on the riboflavin status of adult men. *Br Nutr.* 1993;69(2):541-551. doi:10.1079/bjn19930054
170. Churchward-Venne TA, Pinckaers PJM, Smeets JSJ, et al. Myofibrillar and mitochondrial protein synthesis rates do not differ in young men following the ingestion of carbohydrate with whey, soy, or leucine-enriched soy protein after concurrent resistance- and endurance-type exercise. *Nutr.* 2019;149(2):210-220. doi:10.1093/jn/nxy251
171. Balsom P, Ekblom B, Söderlund E, Sjödin D, Hultman E. Creatine supplementation and dynamic high-intensity intermittent exercise. *Scand Med Sci Sports.* 1993;3:143-149. doi:10.1111/j.1600-0838.1993.tb00378.x
172. Burke DG, Chilibeck PD, Parise G, Candow DG, Mahoney D, Tarnopolsky M. Effect of creatine and weight training on muscle creatine and performance in vegetarians. *Med Sci Sports Exerc.* 2003;35(11):1946-1955. doi:10.1249/01.MSS.0000093614.17517.79
173. Delanghe J, De Slypere JP, De Buyzere M, Robbrecht J, Wieme R, Vermeulen A. Normal reference values for creatine, creatinine, and carnitine are lower in vegetarians. *Clin Chem.* 1989;35(8):1802-1803.
174. Harris RC, Söderlund K, Hultman E. Elevation of creatine in resting and exercised muscle of normal subjects by creatine supplementation. *Clin Sci (Lond).* 1992;83(3):367-374. doi:10.1042/cs0830367
175. Lukaszuk JM, Robertson RJ, Arch JE, et al. Effect of creatine supplementation and a lacto-ovo-vegetarian diet on muscle creatine concentration. *Int Sport Nutr Exerc Metab.* 2002;12(3):336-348. doi:10.1123/ijsnem.12.3.336
176. Shomrat A, Weinstein Y, Katz A. Effect of creatine feeding on maximal exercise performance in vegetarians. *Eur Appl Physiol.* 2000;82(4):321-325. doi:10.1007/s004210000222
177. Blancquaert L, Baguet A, Bex T, et al. Changing to a vegetarian diet reduces the body creatine pool in omnivorous women, but appears not to affect carnitine and carnosine homeostasis: a randomised trial. *Br Nutr.* 2018;119(7):759-770. doi:10.1017/S000711451800017X
178. Everaert I, Mooyaart A, Baguet A, et al. Vegetarianism, female gender and increasing age, but not CNDP1 genotype, are associated with reduced muscle carnosine levels in humans. *Amino Acids.* 2011;40(4):1221-1229. doi:10.1007/s00726-010-0749-2
179. Maughan RJ, Burke LM, Dvorak J, et al. IOC consensus statement: dietary supplements and the high-performance athlete. *Int Sport Nutr Exerc Metab.* 2018;28(2):104-125. doi:10.1123/ijsnem.2018-0020
180. Clarys PM, Zinzen EM, Hebbelinck M. The effect of oral creatine supplementation on torque production in a vegetarian and non-vegetarian population: a double blind study. *Veg Nutr Int J.* 1997;1:100-105.
181. Maughan RJ, Greenhaff PL, Hespel P. Dietary supplements for athletes: emerging trends and recurring themes. *Sports Sci.* 2011;29(suppl 1):S57-S66. doi:10.1080/02640414.2011.587446
182. Kaviani M, Shaw K, Chilibeck PD. Benefits of creatine supplementation for vegetarians compared to omnivorous athletes: a systematic review. *Int Environ Res Public Health.* 2020;17(9):3041. doi:10.3390/ijerph17093041
183. Peeling P, Binnie MJ, Goods PSR, Sim M, Burke LM. Evidence-based supplements for the enhancement of athletic performance. *Int Sport Nutr Exerc Metab.* 2018;28(2):178-187. doi:10.1123/ijsnem.2017-0343
184. Novakova K, Kummer O, Bouitbir J, et al. Effect of l-carnitine supplementation on the body carnitine pool, skeletal muscle energy metabolism and physical performance in male vegetarians. *Eur Nutr.* 2016;55(1):207-217. doi:10.1007/s00394-015-0838-9
185. Baguet A, Everaert I, De Naeyer H, et al. Effects of sprint training combined with vegetarian or mixed diet on muscle carnosine content and buffering capacity. *Eur Appl Physiol.* 2011;111(10):2571-2580. doi:10.1007/s00421-011-1877-4
186. de Salles Painelli V, Nemezio KM, Pinto AJ, et al. High-intensity interval training augments muscle carnosine in the absence of dietary beta-alanine intake. *Med Sci Sports Exerc.* 2018;50(11):2242-2252. doi:10.1249/MSS.0000000000001697
187. Hobson RM, Saunders B, Ball G, Harris RC, Sale C. Effects of β-alanine supplementation on exercise performance: a meta-analysis. *Amino Acids.* 2012;43(1):25-37. doi:10.1007/s00726-011-1200-z
188. Karamanolis IA, Laparidis KS, Volaklis KA, Douda HT, Tokmakidis SP. The effects of pre-exercise glycemic index food on running capacity. *Int Sports Med.* 2011;32(9):666-671. doi:10.1055/s-0031-1277180
189. Thomas DE, Brotherhood JR, Brand JC. Carbohydrate feeding before exercise: effect of glycemic index. *Int Sports Med.* 1991;12(2):180-186. doi:10.1055/s-2007-1024664
190. Wu CL, Williams C. A low glycemic index meal before exercise improves endurance running capacity in men. *Int Sport Nutr Exerc Metab.* 2006;16(5):510-527. doi:10.1123/ijsnem.16.5.510
191. Gallien G, Bellar D, Davis GR. The efficacy of a pre-workout vegan supplement on high-intensity cycling performance in healthy college-aged males. *Diet Suppl.* 2017;14(6):697-705. doi:10.1080/19390211.2017.1310780
192. Lancaster S, Kreider RB, Rasmussen C, et al. Effects of honey supplementation on glucose, insulin, and endurance cycling performance. *FASEB J.* 2001;15:LB315.
193. Lugo M, Sherman WM, Wimer GS, Garleb K. Metabolic responses when different forms of carbohydrate energy are consumed during cycling. *Int Sport Nutr.* 1993;3(4):398-407. doi:10.1123/ijsn.3.4.398
194. Neufer PD, Costill DL, Flynn MG, Kirwan JP, Mitchell JB, Houmard J. Improvements in exercise performance: effects of carbohydrate feedings and diet. *Appl Physiol (1985).* 1987;62(3):983-988. doi:10.1152/jappl.1987.62.3.983
195. Gisolfi CV, Duchman SM. Guidelines for optimal replacement beverages for different athletic events. *Med Sci Sports Exerc.* 1992;24(6):679-687.
196. Maughan RJ, Leiper JB, Shirreffs SM. Restoration of fluid balance after exercise-induced dehydration: effects of food and fluid intake. *Eur Appl Physiol Occup Physiol.* 1996;73(3-4):317-325. doi:10.1007/BF02425493

197. Naclerio F, Seijo M, Earnest CP, Puente-Fernández J, Larumbe-Zabala E. Ingesting a post-workout vegan-protein multi-ingredient expedites recovery after resistance training in trained young males. *Diet Suppl.* 2021;18(6):698-713. doi:10.1080/19390211.2020.1832640

198. Maughan RJ, Watson P, Cordery PA, et al. A randomized trial to assess the potential of different beverages to affect hydration status: development of a beverage hydration index. *Am Clin Nutr.* 2016;103(3):717-723. doi:10.3945/ajcn.115.114769

199. Mountjoy M, Sundgot-Borgen J, Burke L, et al. The IOC consensus statement: beyond the Female Athlete Triad—Relative Energy Deficiency in Sport (RED-S). *Br Sports Med.* 2014;48(7):491-497. doi:10.1136/bjsports-2014-093502

200. Nattiv A, Loucks AB, Manore MM, et al. American College of Sports Medicine position stand. The female athlete triad. *Med Sci Sports Exerc.* 2007;39(10):1867-1882. doi:10.1249/mss.0b013e318149f111

201. Barr SI. Vegetarianism and menstrual cycle disturbances: is there an association? *Am Clin Nutr.* 1999;70(3 suppl):549S-554S. doi:10.1093/ajcn/70.3.549S

202. Slavin J, Lutter J, Cushman S. Amenorrhea in vegetarian athletes [letter]. *The Lancet.* 1984;1(8392):1474-1475. doi:10.1016/s0140-6736(84)91973-1

203. Cialdella-Kam L, Kulpins D, Manore MM. Vegetarian, gluten-free, and energy restricted diets in female athletes. *Sports (Basel).* 2016;4(4):50. doi:10.3390/sports4040050

204. Timko CA, Hormes JM, Chubski J. Will the real vegetarian please stand up? An investigation of dietary restraint and eating disorder symptoms in vegetarians versus non-vegetarians. *Appetite.* 2012;58(3):982-990. doi:10.1016/j.appet.2012.02.005

205. Zickgraf HF, Hazzard VM, O'Connor SM, et al. Examining vegetarianism, weight motivations, and eating disorder psychopathology among college students. *Int Eat Disord.* 2020;53(9):1506-1514. doi:10.1002/eat.23335

206. Martins Y, Pliner P, O'Connor R. Restrained eating among vegetarians: does a vegetarian eating style mask concerns about weight? *Appetite.* 1999;32(1):145-154. doi:10.1006/appe.1998.0185

207. Heiss S, Walker DC, Anderson DA, Morison JN, Hormes JM. Vegetarians and omnivores with diagnosed eating disorders exhibit no difference in symptomology: a retrospective clinical chart review. *Eat Weight Disord.* 2021;26(3):1007-1012. doi:10.1007/s40519-020-00903-w

208. Cialdella-Kam L, Guebels CP, Maddalozzo GF, Manore MM. Dietary intervention restored menses in female athletes with exercise-associated menstrual dysfunction with limited impact on bone and muscle health. *Nutrients.* 2014;6(8):3018-3039. doi:10.3390/nu6083018

209. Goldin BR, Adlercreutz H, Gorbach SL, et al. Estrogen excretion patterns and plasma levels in vegetarian and omnivorous women. *N Engl Med.* 1982;307(25):1542-1547. doi:10.1056/NEJM198212163072502

210. Raben A, Kiens B, Richter EA, et al. Serum sex hormones and endurance performance after a lacto-ovo vegetarian and a mixed diet. *Med Sci Sports Exerc.* 1992;24(11):1290-1297.

211. Rockwell MS, Kostelnik SB, McMillan RP, Lancaster M, Larson-Meyer DE, Hulver MW. An association between bioavailable 25-hydroxyvitamin D and bone mineral density in a diverse cohort of collegiate athletes. *Med Sci Sports Exerc.* 2022;54(3):371-376. doi:10.1249/MSS.0000000000002807

212. Shaw KA, Zello GA, Rodgers CD, Warkentin TD, Baerwald AR, Chilibeck PD. Benefits of a plant-based diet and considerations for the athlete. *Eur Appl Physiol.* 2022;122(5):1163-1178. doi:10.1007/s00421-022-04902-w

213. Dyett P, Rajaram S, Haddad EH, Sabate J. Evaluation of a validated food frequency questionnaire for self-defined vegans in the United States. *Nutrients.* 2014;6(7):2523-2539. doi:10.3390/nu6072523

214. Mangels A. Working with vegetarian clients. *Issues in Vegetarian Dietetics.* 1995;5:1-4.

215. Johnston PK. Counseling the pregnant vegetarian. *Am Clin Nutr.* 1988;48(3 suppl):901-905. doi:10.1093/ajcn/48.3.901

216. Iwasa-Madge K, Sesbreno E. A proposed conceptual sport nutrition approach for athlete development and assessment: the athlete nutrition development approach. *Sports Med Open.* 2022;8(1):142. doi:10.1186/s40798-022-00532-w

CHAPTER 17

Pregnant Athletes

Kaneen Gomez-Hixson, MS, RDN, CSSD, CD-N

LEARNING OBJECTIVES

- Understand the roles that exercise and nutrition play in the fertility of female athletes.
- Review the key physiological challenges for athletes during pregnancy.
- Explain the primary aspects of fueling during pregnancy, including energy requirements, macronutrients, key micronutrients, and hydration.
- Identify contraindicated foods, products, substances, and supplements in pregnancy.
- Summarize the weight gain recommendations for pregnant athletes based on prepregnancy BMI.
- Recognize the recommendations for exercise during pregnancy with regard to safety, environment, growth and development, mode, and intensity.
- Describe postpartum recommendations for athletes regarding nutrition and lactation, healthy weight-loss strategies, and safe return to sport.

INTRODUCTION

With the growing number of females participating in sports, many face the challenges of navigating pregnancy, caring for a child, and being an athlete, feeling as though they need to choose between parenting and being an athlete. Common concerns include how to properly fuel fetal development while maintaining a healthy weight gain, what volume and intensity of exercise are appropriate and safe during each stage of pregnancy, and how intensive training will impact fertility. Although many remarkable female athletes have demonstrated that these roles do not need to conflict and that fertility, pregnancy, motherhood, and sport can coexist, some sports organizations and sports sponsors still do not create an environment or network that values or supports pregnancy and motherhood in sport. Consider the remarkable stories of elite athletes such as Serena Williams, Allyson Felix, Alysia Montaño, Alex Morgan, Sydney Leroux, and Paula Radcliffe, who have all been outspoken regarding their abilities to perform at the highest levels of sport during and after pregnancy. Whereas female athletes were previously advised to "take it easy" during pregnancy, that is neither a necessary nor an evidence-based approach. During the past few years, more female athletes have been vocal regarding the feats and challenges involved in balancing pregnancy and motherhood in athletics. Moreover, meaningful organizations such as For All Mothers (www.forallmothers.org) have been established with the intention of supporting and celebrating females and mothers in sports. Despite this progress, much more research involving females from all levels of athletics during and after pregnancy is needed to fully understand the unique needs of this population during this incredible life stage. Overall, registered dietitian nutritionists (RDNs), alongside a team of health professionals, play an integral role in helping female athletes by providing menu-planning and nutrition guidance that works with their fitness and training routines in the prepregnancy period, through each stage of pregnancy, and during the postpartum period.

FERTILITY IN FEMALE ATHLETES

According to the US Centers for Disease Control and Prevention, for the years 2015 through 2019, nearly 16.3% of females aged 15 to 49 years were unable to become pregnant or to carry a child to term, a condition known as impaired fecundity. Another 8.5% experienced infertility, defined as the inability to become pregnant after 12 months of trying.[1] However, most females who present with fertility problems do not face *absolute* impaired fecundity and infertility—in which case there would be *no* chance of conception. Rather, they are living with *subfecundity* or *subfertility*, where the likelihood of conception is good, especially when issues contributing to reproductive complications are remedied.

Experts report that subfertility and subfecundity are higher among athletic females than among their nonathletic counterparts. The combination of intense training routines and insufficient energy intake trigger unhealthy aberrations in the athlete's weight and body fat or imbalances in hormones essential to the regulation of the menstrual cycle that may negatively influence fertility.[2-10] Even subtle menstrual disturbances such as luteal phase defects, characterized by poor endometrial maturation secondary to inadequate progesterone production and short luteal phases, have been linked to infertility and spontaneous abortions and are estimated to affect nearly half of all athletic females.[11] Although other factors such as age also affect infecundity and infertility, this chapter focuses on modifiable changes, including exercise routine, energy intake, weight status, and overall nutrition. Reducing infertility is a top priority of many health organizations, including Healthy People 2030.[12] RDNs and other health professionals have a unique opportunity to provide the guidance needed to help make significant headway in attaining this goal and to make a positive difference in the life of an athlete who aspires to have a baby.

Exercise and Reproductive Health

Exercise can reduce the risk of many adverse health outcomes, including infertility. Females who exercise regularly benefit from improvements in overall hormonal and metabolic profiles; increased blood flow to the uterus and ovaries; enhanced insulin sensitivity and glucose homeostasis; reduced blood pressure; and decreased body fat or weight, especially in the abdominal region.[6,13,14,15] In addition, gestational weight gain and odds of cesarean delivery are lower in individuals engaged in a prenatal exercise program, thereby helping to speed postpartum recovery. Prenatal exercise can also reduce the odds of having a newborn who is large for gestational age (defined as having a birth weight greater than the 90th percentile for gestational age and sex) by 31% without altering the risk of having a newborn who is small for gestational age (defined as having a birth weight less than the 10th percentile for gestational age and sex). Both high and low birth weights are typically associated with health risks for the newborn.[16] Despite these benefits, conflicting views remain regarding the optimal frequency, duration, and intensity of exercise during the prenatal period.[17]

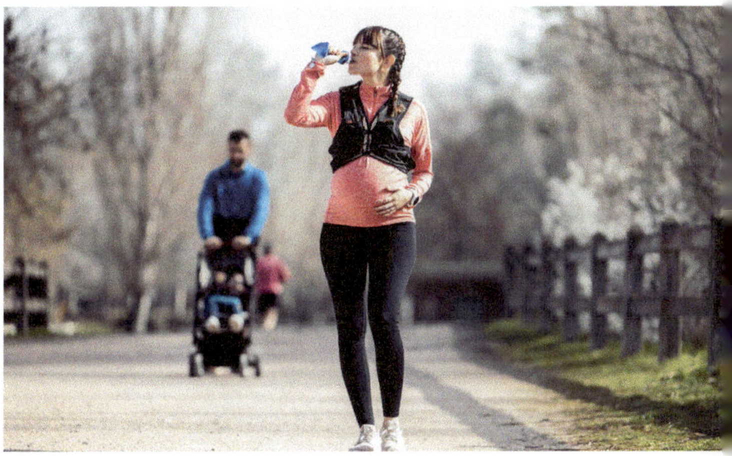

Current evidence-based physical activity guidelines for adults established by the US Department of Health and Human Services, called *Physical Activity Guidelines for Americans,* recommend a minimum of 150 minutes per week of moderate-intensity activity, 75 minutes per week of vigorous-intensity activity, or an equivalent combination of moderate- and vigorous-intensity aerobic activity in conjunction with moderate- to high-intensity muscle-strengthening exercises on 2 or more days per week. Additional amounts are encouraged to extend health benefits. Vigorous intensity is defined in absolute terms as 6.0 metabolic equivalents (METs) or in relative terms as 60% to 84% of one's aerobic capacity reserve (or heart rate reserve). The second edition of the *Physical Activity Guidelines for Americans,* published in 2018, also specifically states that pregnant females should complete at least 150 minutes of moderate-intensity aerobic activity per week and may continue vigorous-intensity aerobic activity if having done so habitually.[18] However, many reproductive specialists believe that competitive sporting activity and exercise at an extreme (vigorous) level facilitates reproductive complications and elevates the risk for infecundity and infertility, and therefore, they often recommend reductions in training volume and intensity to support conception.[17]

Research specific to the competitive athlete is generally lacking, and early data evaluating exercise patterns and fertility have been equivocal; some studies show a lower risk of infecundity and infertility among vigorous exercisers,[19,20] whereas others show increased risk at the highest levels of exercise frequency or intensity.[21,22] Evidence indicates that the stress of exercise coupled with insufficient nutrition to meet the metabolic demands of exercise may result in conditions under which conception is not possible (see Box 17.1).[23-27]

Exercise, especially energy-exhaustive endurance exercise such as long-distance running, cycling, and triathlon, can impose significant stress on a female's homeostasis, lead to the release of excess cortisol into the bloodstream, and disturb reproductive function. Additionally, there has been long-standing concern among experts that the redistribution of blood flow to the muscles of pregnant athletes during exercise may result in inadequate oxygen to the fetus, which could lead to miscarriage. However, currently, only low to moderate levels of evidence suggest a negative effect of strenuous exercise on risk of miscarriage. For example, limited evidence suggests that the risk of miscarriage is increased in situations when intense exercise occurs at the time of implantation. Some experts have also expressed concern that changes to the pelvic floor muscles during strenuous exercise may increase the need for cesarean section, yet conflicting evidence shows that individuals who exercise actually have a lower risk of cesarean delivery.[28] The focus of nutrition professionals caring for this population should be to ensure adequate energy intake to support baseline metabolic demands as well as the metabolic demands of exercise to maintain menstrual and reproductive integrity. Nutrition guidance from an RDN is important for the female athlete transitioning into pregnancy, in addition to support from other medical professionals.

BOX 17.1 Signs That Exercise Stress May Be Too High[23-27]

Low energy availability	BMI less than 18.5
Menstrual dysfunction	Body fat lower than 12%
Low bone mineral density	Elevated blood pressure
Substantial loss of weight	

Nutrition and Reproductive Health

Appropriate preconception nutrition and weight status help set the stage for a healthy pregnancy. Poor nutritional habits, especially when combined with aberrant weight status, are associated with compromised reproductive health and poor pregnancy outcomes for both the birth parent and the child.[29,30] The focus of care during the preconception period should be to modify biomedical, behavioral, and social risks to support a healthy pregnancy.[15]

Preconception Weight Status

The World Health Organization has defined what constitutes a "healthy" BMI (refer to Table 17.1).[31] According to the American Society for Reproductive Medicine, 12% of primary infertility results from deviations from a healthy weight status.[32]

OVERWEIGHT STATUS

Overweight and obesity are conditions exhibited by females aged 18 years and older at rates of 44% and 16%, respectively.[33] Evidence demonstrates that these conditions favor the development of ovulatory dysfunction and infertility, likely as a result of elevated insulin levels and insulin resistance.[34,35] One study reported a decrease in the probability of natural conception of 4% per unit of BMI greater than 29.[36] Prepartum obesity is associated with several adverse reproductive outcomes, including gestational diabetes, hypertension, preeclampsia, miscarriage, cesarean delivery, preterm delivery, postpartum weight retention, and fetal growth disorders.[23,34,36]

TABLE 17.1 Weight Status According to BMI[31]	
Classification	**BMI**
Severe thinness	<16.00
Moderate thinness	16.00-16.99
Mild thinness	17.00-18.49
Underweight	<18.5
Healthy	18.50-24.99
Overweight	25.00-29.99
Obese	≥30.00
Moderate obesity	30.00-34.99
Severe obesity	35.00-39.99
Morbid obesity	≥40.00

Fortunately, ovulatory function and pregnancy rates, as well as pregnancy outcomes, show significant improvement after weight loss in females who are obese.[37] For example, a randomized controlled study of 49 women who were obese and undergoing fertility treatment demonstrated that, among the 27 participants in the intervention group who completed a 12-week intervention consisting of a very low-energy diet for the initial 6 weeks followed by a hypocaloric diet combined with weekly group coaching sessions incorporating dietary, exercise, and behavioral guidance yielded greater anthropometric changes and significant improvements in pregnancy rate compared to the 22 participants in the control group (48% vs 14%), as well as a marked increase in the number of live births (44% vs 14%). The number of fertility treatment cycles to achieve pregnancy also decreased by 50%. In this study, the only intervention that the participants in the control group received was receiving a recommendation to lose weight and printed material for weight loss.[38] Similarly, meaningful weight loss (≥10% of body weight) was shown to significantly improve the rates of conception (88% vs 54%) and live birth (71% vs 37%) in women who were overweight and struggling with infertility compared to those with minimal or no weight loss.[39] Thus, weight-loss counseling should be encouraged for females who are overweight and planning to conceive, with a focus on replacing nutrient-poor and calorie-dense foods such as soda and refined grains with lower-calorie, nutrient-rich alternatives such as fruits, vegetables, whole grains, and legumes.

UNDERWEIGHT STATUS

Underweight status (BMI < 18.5) contributes to an estimated 6% of infertility cases.[30] For the female athlete, a low body weight is often the result of chronic low energy availability (when energy expenditure exceeds dietary energy intake) driven by strenuous exercise and conscious or subconscious restrictive eating patterns. This, in turn, can trigger hypothalamic dysfunction and suppress hormones (particularly gonadotropin-releasing factor) necessary for normal menstruation, ovulation, and conception.[40] Deficiencies in leptin, a hormone produced by fat cells in the body, may be a compounding factor in the development of reproductive dysfunction among female athletes. During periods of reduced or low energy availability, an individual's leptin concentration decreases independent of adiposity.[41]

Research has shown that negative effects on reproductive health occur when one's energy availability falls below a threshold of 30 kcal per kilogram of fat-free mass daily.[42] Even a reduced energy availability of less than 45 kcal per kilogram of fat-free mass daily can lead to menstrual irregularities and negatively impact bone mass, and it can also slow metabolic rate, trigger hypoglycemia, and elevate blood cholesterol.[28,43] The combination of low energy availability (with or without an eating disorder), menstrual dysfunction, and diminished bone health is a condition known as the female athlete triad. This triad is estimated to affect up to 15% of female athletes, with a greater number experiencing at least one of the conditions involved.[44] In 2014, the International Olympic Committee coined a new term, relative energy deficiency in sport (REDs), to describe a syndrome of impaired physiological functioning caused by low energy availability. Similarly to the female athlete triad, REDs encompasses impairments in menstrual function and bone health and also includes detriments in metabolic rate, immunity, protein synthesis, and cardiovascular health.[45,46] Females who compete in sports in which thinness is perceived to enhance performance such as gymnastics, figure skating, ballet, and long-distance running seem to be at greater risk for exhibiting symptoms of the female athlete triad and REDs.[3,4,43,47-50] However, it is important to note that any athlete can be impacted by REDs. (Refer to Chapter 10, Energy Balance, and Chapter 18, Eating Disorders in Athletes, for more information on these topics.)

ENERGY BALANCE AND REPRODUCTIVE HEALTH

Fortunately, more than 70% of females whose infertility stems from body weight disorders are likely to conceive spontaneously by restoring body weight to a healthy status.[32] RDNs, in conjunction with behavior therapists or other mental health professionals, can play a key role in helping athletes establish and maintain a healthy relationship with food. When necessary, this includes making corrections to energy balance for weight loss or gain as a means to facilitate a hormonal environment favorable for reproduction. For females who are overweight, especially those whose weight is greater than 120% of their predicted ideal body weight, increased energy output through increases in physical activity or decreases in energy intake is warranted. For athletes who are underweight, especially those with a body weight less than 95% of their predicted ideal body weight, experts advise an increase in energy intake or a reduction in energy expenditure through training.

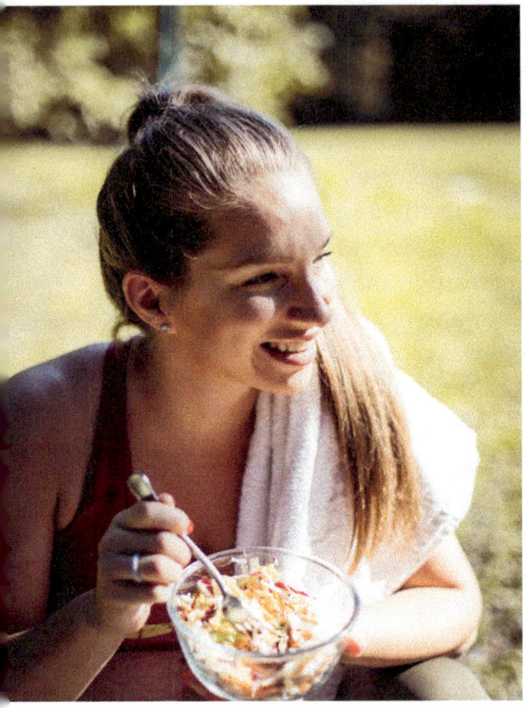

Optimizing energy availability (>45 kcal per kilogram of fat-free mass per day) through reductions in training or in energy intake is also crucial for female athletes of healthy weight who exhibit the symptoms of chronic anovulation, menstrual disorders, and secondary amenorrhea resulting from hypothalamic disorder. Screening tools such as the LEAF (Low Energy Availability in Females) questionnaire[51] and the RED-S CAT (Relative Energy Deficiency in Sport Clinical Assessment Tool)[46] can be helpful, especially when eating disorders are suspected. When menses fails to return after 5 months, practitioners may need to incorporate hormonal preparations as a therapeutic protocol to protect against further reproductive complications and bone loss. Restoration of reproductive function may take as long as 6 months.

Considering the impact of the female athlete triad and REDs on reproductive function, some female athletes may be concerned about their fertility and childbearing capabilities in the long term, even after menstrual dysfunction is resolved. Although many female athletes have chosen to bear children and return to their sports career, not all choose to do so. Therefore, both athletes and sports health care practitioners must understand the long-term impact of the consequences of REDs and the female athlete triad on fertility and pregnancy. Evidence in this area remains in its infancy, but 2 studies from 2023 attempted to examine the association between menstrual dysfunction during sports careers and the impact of such dysfunction on reproductive function, or fertility, after sports retirement. The first study aimed to estimate the relative amount of menstrual abnormalities, infertility, and other pregnancy- and childbirth-related problems in a group of 137 former elite long-distance runners in Japan. Among the group of female athletes surveyed, being amenorrheic or underweight during their athletic career was not associated with problems related to pregnancy or childbirth. Instead, older age at the time of pregnancy appeared to be the main factor that influenced fertility.[52] Of the 137 participants, 11 had previously required infertility treatment. The second study aimed to investigate the association between menstrual dysfunction during one's active sports career and postretirement infertility among a group of 613 female former athletes in Japan. The infertility rate among the sample of female athletes was 11.9%, and researchers found that menstrual dysfunction that continued from active sports participation to postretirement may impact fertility for retired female athletes.[53] Although both studies were limited in their cross-sectional study designs, the findings are promising. They also illustrate the need for female athletes to address their menstrual dysfunction in order to improve fertility and pregnancy outcomes even if they plan to become pregnant after their sports career ends. Moreover, these studies highlight how important it is for female athletes who experience REDs or the female athlete triad during their sports careers to receive support from RDNs and other health professionals even after their sports careers end to best support health and well-being. Future studies should continue to investigate the long-term reproductive repercussions of the female athlete triad and REDs on female athletes.

Eating Disorders and Pregnancy

The athletic population has a higher risk of eating disorders than nonathletes (refer to Chapter 18, Eating Disorders in Athletes). Pregnant athletes with eating disorders are at a very high nutritional risk because of the competition for nutritional resources between the birth parent and the fetus.[15] There is currently no evidence regarding the prevalence of eating disorders in pregnant individuals. In pregnant females with anorexia nervosa and bulimia nervosa, complications such as hyperemesis gravidarum, anemia, spontaneous abortion, preterm birth, cesarean section, low fetal birth weight, and postpartum depression have been found. Additional complications related to bulimia nervosa include vaginal bleeding, hypertension, fetal abnormalities, breech delivery, and stillbirth.[15,54] Moreover, developmental disturbances, anxiety, depression, and substance abuse have been found in children born to individuals with anorexia nervosa during pregnancy.[15,55,56] Given the potentially life-threatening complications related to pregnancy and eating disorders, if there is any concern that a pregnant athlete is exhibiting signs of an eating disorder, they should be referred to the appropriate interdisciplinary team of professionals, including an RDN, for appropriate treatment. Any female athlete exhibiting signs of a clinical eating disorder or disordered eating behaviors should be considered at a higher risk of pregnancy complications if pregnancy occurs before effective eating disorder treatment is implemented. Even if a pregnant athlete has a history of an eating disorder that was previously treated, they should still be closely monitored in case such abnormal eating behaviors return during pregnancy.

NUTRITION QUALITY

RDNs can assess and help implement positive diet and lifestyle changes to improve reproductive function and fertility results in female athletes.[57,58] Beyond sufficient energy consumption to support the metabolic demands of daily living and exercise and the establishment of a healthy preconception weight status, evidence suggests that the quality of nutrition during the preconception period has implications for fertility and pregnancy outcomes. For example, a diet focused on plant-based rather than animal-based protein and fat has been shown to dramatically reduce the risk of impaired ovulation.[59,60] Impaired ovulation is estimated to contribute to 25% to 50% of infertility cases.[61] Furthermore, avoidance of *trans* fats is likely effective in protecting against infertility.[62] *Trans* fats can be found in some commercially produced cakes and other sweets; potato chips, corn chips, and other snack foods; fast foods; powdered soups; and hard margarines containing hydrogenated vegetable oil. Beginning in 2018, the US Food and Drug Administration issued a requirement that manufacturers no longer add partially hydrogenated oils—the primary source of *trans* fats in processed foods—to foods because of the strong evidence of their negative health effects.[63]

For the female athlete undergoing in vitro fertilization and intracytoplasmic sperm injection, research has shown that consumption of a Mediterranean-style diet rich in vegetables, fruits, fish, whole grains, and vegetable-based oils increases blood folate and vitamin B6 levels, which correlates with successful fertility.[64] For all athletes, the benefits of healthy eating during the preconception period carry through pregnancy as well. Adherence to the alternate Mediterranean diet or the Alternative Healthy Eating Index, both of which exclude wine, as well as the Dietary Approaches to Stop Hypertension (DASH) diet, has been shown to reduce the risk for developing gestational diabetes by 24%, 34%, and 46%, respectively. Following such dietary patterns may thus help protect against obstetrical complications and birth defects associated with gestational diabetes.[65]

The use of a prenatal vitamin has been associated with a 73% lower incidence of infertility in women, likely as a result of improved ovarian function.[66-68] Inadequate folate intake can reduce the ovarian response to internal gonadotropin, resulting in impaired ovulation and infertility. In addition, a higher intake of folate prepregnancy is also associated with a reduced risk of miscarriage.[69] Research has shown that supplements containing B vitamins, especially folic acid, reduce the risk of fetal neural defects such as spina bifida and anencephaly, congenital heart disease, and cleft lip and palate by 70%.[70-72] Beyond eating foods rich in folic acid, all females of childbearing age should consume 400 mcg of folic acid daily from fortified foods or dietary supplements. For planned pregnancies, experts recommend daily supplementation with prenatal vitamins for several months in advance of conception to help achieve these goals.[66]

Frequent and excessive use of caffeine and alcohol are potentially detrimental to fertility. Intake of 300 mg or less of caffeine per day does not seem to affect the risk of infertility or the risk of adverse pregnancy outcomes, including miscarriage.[73] Research has shown that a daily intake of more than 500 mg of caffeine, however, plays a significant role in the development of subfecundity in a first pregnancy.[74] Yet a slightly lower dose of 455 mg/d (range: 3.71–3,561 mg/d) did not significantly impact the success rate of pregnancy (positive pregnancy test and blood ß-human chorionic gonadotropin levels 14 days after embryo transfer and ultrasound confirmation 5 weeks after embryo transfer) after in vitro fertilization. Even so, the authors of this study did note that an increase in caffeine consumption was positively associated with the number of miscarriages.[75] Consequently, the current American College of Obstetricians and Gynecologists recommendation (first released in 2010 and reaffirmed in 2015 and 2023) is that all females attempting conception avoid exceeding 200 mg of caffeine per day.[76]

Consumption of alcohol can trigger hypogonadism. More frequent drinking will worsen this condition and interfere with hormonal homeostasis and fertility. Research demonstrates that consumption of more than 2 alcoholic beverages per day increases the relative risk of infertility by 60% in females.[77] For females undergoing in vitro fertilization, consumption of more than 25 g of ethyl alcohol (equivalent to approximately 18 oz of beer, 7.5 oz of wine, or 2.2 oz 80-proof vodka) daily has been strongly associated with poorer-quality embryos.[78] As a result, abstinence from alcohol is recommended when one is attempting to conceive.[79]

A FEMALE ATHLETE'S PREGNANCY JOURNEY

Pregnancy triggers a cascade of hormonal aberrations that elicits physical and biomechanical changes in metabolic, cardiovascular, and musculoskeletal makeup. These changes, which are essential for the optimal growth and development of the fetus, affect the nutritional demands and exercise capacity of the female athlete. As was true before pregnancy, maintaining fitness with an exercise program and making wise food choices during pregnancy are proven to provide a wealth of benefits. Maternal benefits include enhanced cardiovascular fitness, prevention of urinary incontinence, healthy gestational weight gain, decreased musculoskeletal discomfort, reduced incidence of muscle cramps and edema, mood stability, and better management of blood sugars and blood pressure.[80-82] Fetal benefits include improved stress tolerance and advanced neurobehavioral maturation.[80,83,84] However, failure to take certain precautions when exercising and being negligent of nutritional needs can be devastating to fetal growth and development and potentially dangerous to the athlete as well. This section breaks down the key physiological challenges associated with each trimester of pregnancy and explores the recommended nutrient and exercise modifications that support a healthy pregnancy.

Key Physiological Challenges for Female Athletes

During the first trimester of pregnancy, athletes may experience fatigue, abnormal eating habits, dyspnea, nausea, bouts of dizziness, heartburn, and constipation. As fetal growth accelerates in the second and third trimesters, increasing pressure on the bladder from the expanding uterus can lead to a frustrating and uncomfortable need to urinate multiple times during a workout as well as at rest. Furthermore, heartburn and reflux can escalate. Toward the end of pregnancy, fatigue returns, and musculoskeletal dysfunctions, such as lower back pain, pelvic pain, and leg cramps, can arise, making weight-bearing movement increasingly uncomfortable. Education on the causes of these common physiological challenges and guidance on remedies can help improve overall maternal well-being throughout the pregnancy and can also improve pregnancy outcomes.[85]

FATIGUE

Although fatigue can be caused by many things, including lack of sleep and poor nutrition, the unusual fatigue experienced by individuals early in pregnancy is generally the result of surging progesterone levels acting in concert with other hormonally driven changes within the cardiovascular system.[85] In the first few weeks of gestation, a notable rise in the pregnant woman's resting heart rate occurs.[86] From around week 6 to the end of the first trimester, blood volume expands approximately 10% to 15%, causing a 30% to 40% increase in cardiac output, as well as increases in pulse rate and stroke volume.[86,87] These cardiovascular changes can make a routine workout feel more difficult. Dyspnea driven by a 30% to 35% rise in tidal volume may also hinder workouts. Additionally, some athletes experience reductions in blood pressure and consequent bouts of dizziness when standing up during the early weeks of pregnancy. These episodes result from increased blood flow to the uterus and a substantial decrease in systemic vascular resistance.[88,89] Fortunately, as the body adapts to the hormonal and cardiovascular changes occurring during early pregnancy, fatigue tapers. In fact, many individuals report surging energy levels and consequent increases in exercise patterns during the second trimester. Accelerating fetal growth patterns late in the second trimester and well into the third trimester place a greater energy demand on the body, and as a result, fatigue often returns. Proper nutrition and hydration, continued exercise, and additional rest can be helpful in offsetting some of the fatigue experienced in late-stage pregnancy.[85,90]

MORNING SICKNESS

An estimated 70% of pregnant individuals worldwide are affected by nausea or vomiting, a condition known as morning sickness.[91,92] This can hamper a female athlete's ability to train, as well as their overall well-being during the first trimester and, in rare cases, throughout the pregnancy. Morning sickness and fatigue are common reasons for a pregnant athlete to consult a health professional. Severe nausea and vomiting, termed *hyperemesis gravidarum* (HG), is the number one cause of hospitalization in the first trimester, impacting 1.1% to 1.2% of pregnancies in the United States and worldwide.[91-93] Although the exact cause of morning sickness is unknown, changes in ovarian and placental hormones, including a surge in postconception estrogen levels, are likely responsible.[94]

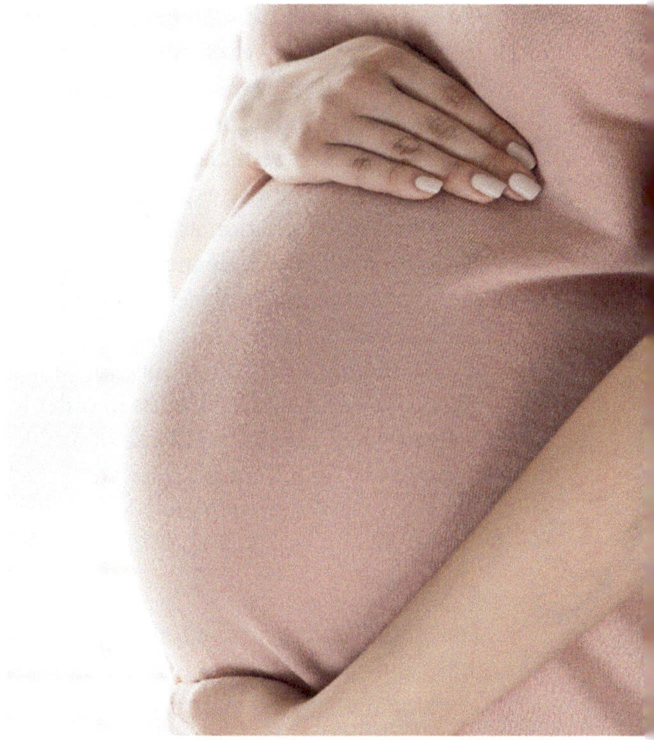

The first 10 weeks of pregnancy are a delicate time for the developing embryo. Essential growth patterns occur that facilitate the development of every essential organ, including the brain, spinal cord, heart, lungs, and gastrointestinal tract. Failure to treat HG during the first trimester can have negative fetal consequences. For example, there is evidence that HG increases the risk for low birth weight (<2.5 kg) and restricts fetal growth throughout pregnancy, a condition called intrauterine growth restriction.[95-97] Preliminary evidence also suggests that HG may have health ramifications for children long after birth, including childhood insulin resistance and psychological disorders in adulthood.[98]

In cases of HG, hospitalization should be considered. Intravenous intervention is often required to address fluid and nutrition concerns, including dehydration, electrolyte imbalances, blood volume depletion, and nutrient deficiencies, and to ensure overall positive outcomes.[99,100] Nutrition treatment via nasogastric tube feedings is also an effective means of promoting optimal maternal weight gain and favorable pregnancy outcomes.[101]

Some female athletes experiencing morning sickness, especially those with severe cases, may experience unnecessary or dramatic weight loss (>5% of body weight), nutrient deficiency driven by an aversion to nutrient-dense foods, undernutrition, dehydration, electrolyte imbalances, and blood volume depletion.[93] In addition, a rare, dangerous complication of prolonged vomiting in pregnancy is Wernicke encephalopathy. This condition is initiated by an acute deficiency of thiamin resulting from body stores and intake being unable to meet increased metabolic demands and is marked by confusion, ocular abnormalities, and ataxia. Thiamin replacement is indicated for those with Wernicke's encephalopathy.[102]

Treatment protocols for morning sickness should be tailored to the individual. Mild to moderate cases of morning sickness are most commonly addressed with diet and lifestyle changes, as well as nonpharmacologic supplements, such as vitamin B6 and ginger.[99] Although science-based evidence to support these practices is lacking, common dietary recommendations based on anecdotal reports of relief include the following[99,100]:

- Eat small, frequent meals to avoid an empty stomach or feelings of hunger.
- Eat dry, salty, and bland foods, such as crackers.
- Incorporate protein-rich foods, such as eggs, yogurt, nuts, and cheese, at each feeding.

To aid rehydration in cases of vomiting, the pregnant athlete can use an electrolyte-enhanced effervescent in water (eg, Nuun), a homemade oral rehydration solution (6 tsp sugar, ½ tsp salt, 1 L water), or a sports drink (eg, Gatorade). Vitamin B6 has more than 50 years of evidence-based support from randomized controlled studies and placebo-controlled clinical trials and can be safely taken during pregnancy at doses up to 200 mg/d.[103] The use of ginger products, which carry antiemetic qualities, has been supported in several studies at doses of up to 1,000 mg/d,[104,105] and some data suggest that it is more effective than vitamin B6 in relieving the severity of nausea and decreasing the frequency of vomiting.[106]

CONSTIPATION

Constipation includes infrequent or painful bowel movements, at times leading to anorectal hemorrhoids. Approximately 13% of individuals experience these symptoms during pregnancy. Surging levels of progesterone, which relax the smooth muscles of the digestive tract, and lower levels of the hormone motilin in early pregnancy cause food to travel much more slowly through the intestines, thus predisposing pregnant females to increased risk of constipation. In addition, increased water absorption from the intestines can make evacuation difficult because of dried-out stools. A prepregnancy BMI greater than 24 and advanced maternal age (>35 years) seem to increase this risk. Diet can also play a large role. Dietary supplementation with prenatal vitamins (which contain iron, a mineral that negatively impacts gut flora when consumed in excess) and calcium (a mineral that has a mild binding effect) can contribute to constipation. It is also common to see reduced fiber intake and decreased physical activity (both factors that can exacerbate constipation) in those experiencing pronounced cases of fatigue and morning sickness.[107]

A simple explanation as to why constipation may be occurring can provide comfort to the affected athlete. Easy resolutions include increasing fluid and dietary fiber intake; staying as active as possible throughout the day; and practicing postmeal defecation, when colonic activity is greatest.[107] Individuals who struggle with diet and exercise modifications may find it necessary to supplement their meals with fiber, such as by adding 4 to 6 Tbsp of bran, or to ingest bulk-forming agents such as psyllium, methylcellulose, or polycarbophil with 1 or 2 glasses of water on a daily basis in order to help increase fecal water content, decrease colonic transit time, and increase stool weight.[108] The use of probiotic supplements, especially *Bifidobacterium lactis*, has been found to improve whole gut transit time, stool frequency, and stool consistency.[109] Athletes may need a combination of interventions to have regular bowel movements and prevent constipation and discomfort.

GASTROESOPHAGEAL REFLUX DISEASE

Heartburn and regurgitation are symptoms of gastroesophageal reflux disease (GERD) and are estimated to affect upward of 80% of pregnant individuals. In early pregnancy, GERD symptoms are often associated with hormonal changes that initiate alterations in gastrointestinal transit time and reductions in lower esophageal sphincter pressure. Nausea and vomiting caused by GERD can occur later in pregnancy. Intragastric and intra-abdominal pressure increasing secondary to the enlarged (gravid) uterus may exacerbate GERD symptoms.[110,111] The first line of defense should be implementing appropriate lifestyle and dietary adjustments. Using a food log to identify dietary triggers is helpful. The most common avoidable dietary triggers include acidic foods such as citrus and tomatoes, spicy foods, caffeine, carbonated beverages, peppermint, and chocolate. A high intake of animal fats has also been correlated with increased incidence of GERD symptoms; therefore, plant-based diets are often encouraged as a dietary remedy. In addition, eating smaller meals, not eating too close to bedtime, and wearing loose-fitting clothes have been explored as natural remedies.[112] When symptoms do not resolve with implementation of dietary and lifestyle changes, antacids, histamine-2 receptor antagonists, and proton pump inhibitors can be used safely under the guidance of a physician.[110]

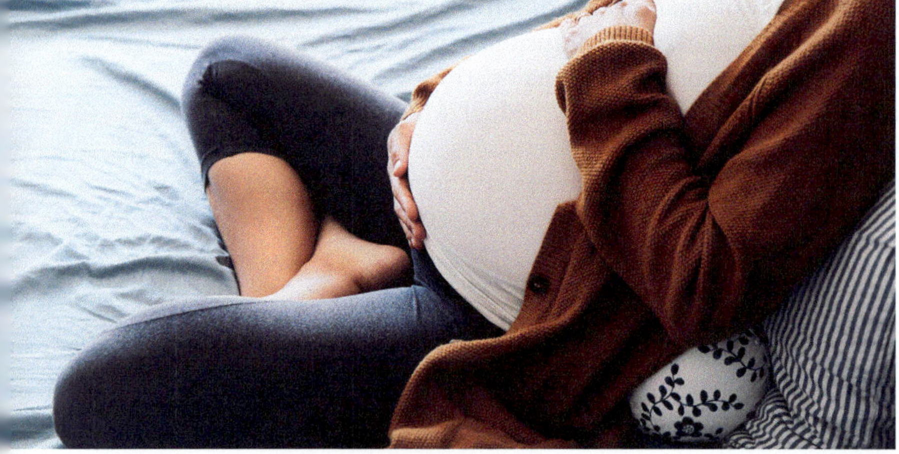

FREQUENT URINATION

Early in pregnancy, human chorionic gonadotropin increases the rate of blood flow through the kidneys, filling the bladder more rapidly and increasing urination frequency. Throughout the entirety of pregnancy, and especially late in the second trimester and through the third trimester, the expanding uterus increases pressure on the bladder, thus enhancing the urge to urinate. Symptoms tend to crest when the baby drops to the pelvic area in preparation for delivery in the third trimester.[113] To alleviate some of the discomfort associated with frequent urination in pregnancy, the following strategies can be offered[114]:

- Reduce fluid intake before bedtime.
- Do not resist the need to urinate.
- Wear a sanitary pad to absorb leaks caused by coughing, sneezing, or physical activity.

MUSCULOSKELETAL DYSFUNCTION

Musculoskeletal dysfunction is a common problem in pregnancy, especially during the second and third trimesters when the body's center of mass shifts anteriorly, causing an increase in lumbar lordosis and consequent pain in the lower back and pelvic girdle. Studies have estimated that 33% to 85% of pregnant females experience lower back pain[115,116] and 20% to 37% experience pelvic girdle pain.[116,117] Other common musculoskeletal issues include calf muscle cramping, foot pain, and restless leg syndrome, impacting an estimated 47% to 64%, 37%, and 26% of pregnant females, respectively.[116,118] The exact mechanism for muscle cramping and pain is unknown, but it is thought to be triggered by muscle fatigue and nerve dysfunction rather than electrolyte deficiency or other abnormalities.[119] Fortunately, there does not seem to be a relationship between musculoskeletal dysfunction and complications during pregnancy or unfavorable fetal outcome. Musculoskeletal dysfunction can, however, make a pregnant athlete's comfort level decline, especially during the final few weeks of pregnancy.

When the athlete's body is experiencing pain, muscles tighten and compensate, which can cause asymmetry and misalignment of joints.[120,121] Continuing to train while exhibiting these misalignments can exacerbate them, prolong an athlete's postpartum recovery, and negatively influence their ability to safely return to competition.[121] Thus, education on proper body mechanics and safe, effective treatment options for pain management are important. Physical therapy is a proven effective and safe treatment option for musculoskeletal dysfunction in pregnancy and may include soft-tissue mobilization or massage, postural exercises, and strengthening and stabilization exercises to improve support of the pelvic girdle and pelvic floor.[122] Bracing or external supports can provide additional aid and help manage pain during exercise and daily activities.[123,124] Although a wide range of oral interventions are marketed for leg cramps, including magnesium, calcium, vitamin B, and vitamin C, the evidence to support their use is inconclusive.[125] The support for passive stretching and deep tissue massage is equivocal, but both are harmless strategies that can be recommended to temporarily relieve cramps during pregnancy.[119]

Fueling During Pregnancy

Maintaining a good nutritional status throughout pregnancy is important for optimal fetal development and pregnancy outcome, as well as the long-term health of the child. Evidence suggests that maternal dietary inadequacies early in pregnancy can impair placental development and function, which consequently can affect the maternal-fetal transfer of nutrients and contribute to intrauterine growth restriction. Maternal dietary inadequacies that continue throughout pregnancy can also impact fetal growth and organ development through effects on the endocrine system or imprinted gene expression.[126] These developmental inadequacies increase risk for stillbirth; premature birth; low birth weight; perinatal mortality; infant neurologic, intestinal, respiratory, and circulatory disorders; birth defects; underdevelopment of some organs; cretinism; and brain damage.[127] Therefore, providing optimal nutrition and fueling guidance to pregnant athletes is important. Nutritional components leading to a healthy pregnancy include the consumption of a wide variety of foods, prenatal vitamin and mineral supplementation, appropriate pregnancy weight gain, consistent moderate exercise unless contraindicated, adequate hydration, the avoidance of alcohol and other harmful substances, and safe food handling.[128]

ENERGY REQUIREMENTS

Adequate calorie intake is required during pregnancy to accommodate energy deposition in maternal and fetal tissues, increases in the maternal basal metabolic rate (BMR), and changes in the energy cost of physical activity.[128-131] As previously discussed, for athletes with a recent history of eating disorders, close monitoring by a team of health professionals including an RDN, a physician, and a mental health specialist may be warranted throughout pregnancy to protect against relapse and the development of pregorexia, a term coined by the media to describe women who have an intense fear of gaining weight during pregnancy. Customized dietary guidance, including the possibility of reducing energy intake from targeted guidelines, and close physician monitoring are likely to be necessary for someone who is overweight or obese and who is gaining (or wishes to gain) less weight than recommended but has an appropriately growing fetus.[132-135]

First Trimester During early gestation, the energy demands of pregnancy are minimal, with BMR increasing by only about 5% compared with the prepregnancy state in individuals with a healthy BMI. The increase in energy demands is slightly higher, 7%, in females with high BMIs.[129] As a result, significant adjustments to calorie intake are not required to accommodate the energy demands of pregnancy during the first trimester.[130] In fact, for many athletes, especially those engaged in energy-exhaustive endurance exercise, overall daily calorie needs may actually decrease in pregnancy as a result of dramatic reductions in their overall training load, the presence of nausea, and intense fatigue brought on by hormonal changes. A target energy intake of 45 kcal per kilogram of prepregnancy fat-free mass per day plus the amount of energy exhausted during exercise should be encouraged during the first trimester of pregnancy.[128,136]

Second Trimester In the second trimester, most of the energy costs of pregnancy are attributed to maternal factors such as expansion of the blood volume, growth of the uterus and breasts, and fat storage. BMR gradually increases to a value that is approximately 11% greater than the prepregnancy value in those with healthy BMIs. For females who are overweight or obese, BMR rises by approximately 16% from the prepregnancy value.[129] Female athletes often report better energy levels and less nausea during the second trimester, and thus, they often increase exercise patterns, further driving up daily calorie needs. To support the energy demands of pregnancy in the second trimester, a target energy intake of 45 kcal per kilogram of prepregnancy fat-free mass per day, plus an additional 340 kcal to accommodate increased pregnancy BMR, plus the amount of energy exhausted during exercise should be encouraged.[128,136]

Third Trimester Fetal growth patterns peak during the third trimester, driving up BMR substantially from prepregnancy values. For individuals with BMI values in the healthy and overweight category, BMR increases by approximately 24% from prepregnancy values. For those with BMI values in the obese category, BMR increases by approximately 38% from prepregnancy values.[129] Pregnancy weight hits a peak in the third trimester, making some physical activities awkward. Additionally, fatigue returns for many athletes late in their pregnancy, and energy output from physical activity often decreases from second-trimester norms. Thus, total daily energy demands, for some, may not change much from second to third trimester. To support the energy demands of pregnancy in the third trimester, a target energy intake of 45 kcal per kilogram of prepregnancy fat-free mass per day, plus an additional 452 kcal to accommodate increased pregnancy BMR, plus the amount of energy exhausted during exercise should be encouraged.[128,136]

Labor and Delivery The overall energy cost of reproduction, from conception through delivery, has been estimated at 75,000 to 85,000 kcal.[131] The actual energy cost of labor and delivery is dependent on its duration, which can range between 13 and 17 hours for first-time pregnancies and is typically substantially less for each subsequent pregnancy. A 2015 meta-analysis of 385 studies focused on individuals giving birth in hospitals that had been published in 1990 and subsequent years examined the caloric needs of hospital births and revealed that the energy demands for giving birth are similar to those of marathon runners.[137] The greatest rate of energy expenditure occurs during the final transitional phase of labor in the course of active pushing. This phase typically lasts between 30 minutes and 2 hours.

Although there are currently no formal prelabor nutrition recommendations, health care practitioners would be prudent to consider that a carbohydrate-loading protocol in healthy individuals with noncomplicated pregnancies may be of possible benefit to performance, given that labor and delivery have been shown to be as metabolically demanding as continuous moderate exercise. Carbohydrate loading entails meeting a high carbohydrate intake (9 to 12 g per kilogram of body weight per day) for 24 to 48 hours while simultaneously reducing exercise to an easy taper as a means of enhancing muscle glycogen stores and protecting against premature muscle fatigue during exercise.[136,138] A more modest carbohydrate intake of 8 g per kilogram of body weight per day is likely to provide a similar loading benefit provided that the overall energy intake is sufficient.[139] An individual's prepregnancy weight should be used in the calculation of prelabor carbohydrate targets. Because it is hard to pinpoint the date of labor (unless an induction or cesarean section is scheduled), practitioners may simply encourage their patients to favor carbohydrate-rich foods as they near their due dates. Low-residue carbohydrate choices are preferable once labor begins to help minimize fecal matter and secretions in the intestines that may otherwise contribute to unpleasant gastrointestinal issues and other complications.[140]

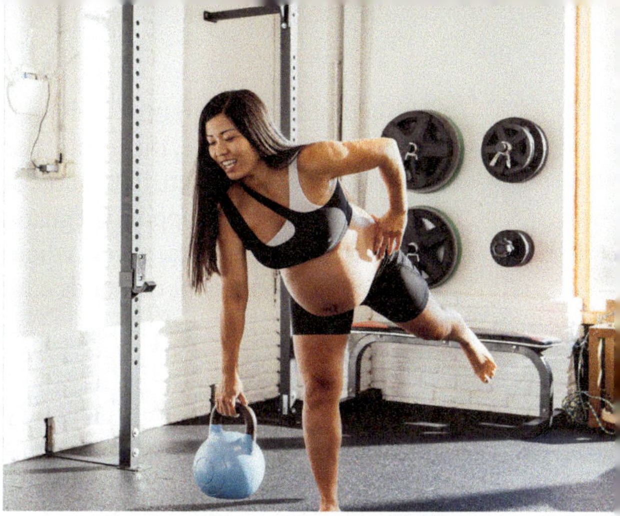

As is the case with prolonged exercise, a body in labor begins to use fat as an energy source when deprived of energy. This may cause an accumulation of fatty acids and ketones in both the birth parent and the fetus. Although this situation is well tolerated in the short term, left unmanaged during prolonged labor, ketosis can lead to ketoacidosis, which may reduce uterine contractions and lead to a longer than typical labor, an increased need for induction, an increased need for forceps delivery, increased peripartum blood loss, and lower Apgar scores in newborns.[137,141] Furthermore, energy deprivation is a form of maternal stress that may shunt blood away from the uterus and placenta and contribute to fetal distress.[137] Thus, traditional guidelines that advised against eating or drinking during labor because of concerns regarding aspiration (which can lead to pneumonia) have since been modified by the American College of Obstetricians and Gynecologists to allow low-risk individuals in the active phase of labor to ingest small quantities of clear fluids and foods, such as water, fruit juice without pulp, broth, gelatin products, carbonated beverages, tea, black coffee, sports drinks, and ice pops.[142] For example, an isotonic sports drink has been shown to lead to a statistically significant reduction in maternal ketone production compared with water and is thus a viable option for protecting against ketoacidosis and improving pregnancy outcomes during prolonged labor.[143] Clear liquids also facilitate optimal hydration, which can be of concern in those who are not given intravenous fluids during labor.

The practice of restricting intake during labor to a clear liquid diet was initiated in the 1940s as a safeguard against aspiration by a pregnant person under general anesthesia. As improvements in anesthesia care make the use of general anesthesia during labor much less common and pain control during labor safer, the risks related to aspiration indicate that fasting for healthy individuals is unnecessary. As a result, some practitioners believe that the extra energy associated with eating a light meal, including some solids, early in labor should be allowed because of the extra energy provided.[137] Studies defining the adequate nutritional diet and quantity to be ingested during labor as a means to optimize energy, comfort levels, and recovery are currently lacking. However, in accordance with individual tolerance and obstetrician and anesthesiologist approval, easy-to-digest foods such as bananas, applesauce, broth-based soups, toast, crackers, light sandwiches, yogurt, rice, quinoa, and cereal may be offered as fueling options. Contraindications for food intake during labor include eclampsia, preeclampsia, obesity, and the use of opioids to manage labor pain.[142]

Macronutrient Requirements

A balanced diet providing adequate carbohydrate, protein, fat, and essential fatty acids is important for both healthy fetal development and protection against the development of conditions that compromise maternal health, such as gestational diabetes and preeclampsia.

CARBOHYDRATE

Because the fetus uses glucose almost exclusively as its metabolic fuel, ensuring adequate maternal dietary intake of carbohydrate is a key factor in facilitating optimal fetal growth patterns throughout pregnancy. The current Recommended Dietary Allowance (RDA) for carbohydrate intake during pregnancy is 175 g/d, a slight increase from 130 g/d for nonpregnant females.[130] However, female athletes require 5 to 7 g of carbohydrate per kilogram of body weight to sustain muscle energy reserves and meet the metabolic demands of exercise.[136] Therefore, those maintaining a moderate exercise program in pregnancy should be instructed to consume carbohydrate in the amount of 5 to 7 g per kilogram of prepregnancy body weight per day plus an additional 45 g to support pregnancy.[130,136] Choosing nutrient-dense and fiber-rich carbohydrate sources, such as fruits, vegetables, beans, whole grains, seeds, and nuts, should be encouraged to help accommodate increased micronutrient demands and to reduce constipation, a common side effect early in pregnancy.

PROTEIN

The availability of adequate protein during pregnancy is essential to support fetal growth and development (eg, through tissues such as the placenta and the extraembryonic membranes), as well as the accretion of maternal tissues such as the heart, blood, and breasts. Even though the majority of protein weight gain in the fetus occurs during the second and third trimesters of pregnancy, additional protein above the prepregnancy recommendations of 0.8 g per kilogram of body weight per day is warranted during the first trimester to accommodate maternal adaptations involving protein and nitrogen metabolism that occur before there is a significant increase in fetal demand.[144] However, current recommendations do not support increasing intake until the second trimester, when intake is advised at 1.1 g per kilogram of prepregnancy weight per day or an additional 25 g of protein for singleton pregnancies and 1.4 g per kilogram of prepregnancy weight per day or 50 g of protein for twin pregnancies.[130] Protein intake recommendations for strength- and endurance-trained athletes are already 1.2 to 2.0 g per kilogram of body weight per day; therefore, the health care practitioner would be prudent to advise pregnant athletes who will continue training routines during pregnancy to consume an additional 25 g daily (50 g for twin pregnancies) during the second and third trimesters to accommodate increased protein turnover during exercise as well as pregnancy demands.[136,138] Encourage high-quality sources of protein that include all essential amino acids, such as meat, eggs, poultry, dairy, and fish with a low mercury content (refer to the section Contraindicated Food Products, Substances, and Supplements in Pregnancy). Careful monitoring, including screening for protein deficiency, may be needed for female athletes who follow vegan or vegetarian dietary patterns to ensure that all essential amino acids are available for optimal fetal development and growth (see Chapter 16 for more about vegetarian diets).

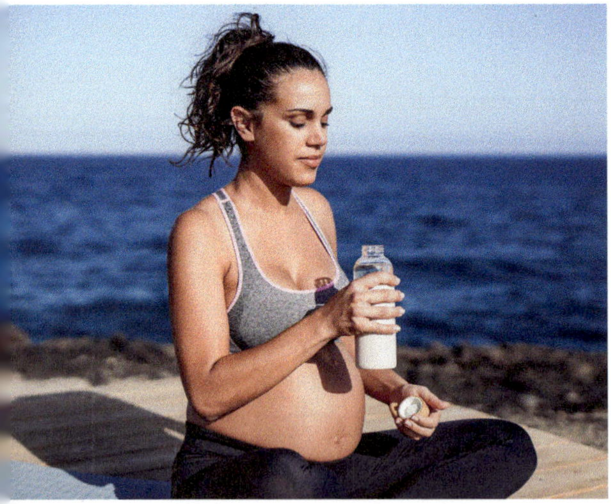

FAT

Although the recommendations for fat intake during pregnancy remain the same as those for the general population (20% to 35% of total daily energy intake), choosing healthy sources that are rich in essential fatty acids, such as omega-3 and omega-6 polyunsaturated fatty acids (PUFAs), is particularly important because it can help support the rapid cellular growth and activity of the developing fetus early in pregnancy. The omega-3 and omega-6 PUFAs carry particular biological importance, with docosahexaenoic acid (DHA), eicosapentaenoic acid (EPA), dihomo-γ-linolenic acid, and arachidonic acid playing metabolic, structural, and signaling roles.[145] Data have demonstrated that maternal dietary supplementation with DHA and EPA increases gestation length, enhances fetal growth, and reduces the risk of pregnancy complications.[146] Furthermore, enhanced maternal consumption of dietary omega-3 long-chain PUFAs seems to exert long-term favorable effects on fetal immune function, especially in relation to allergic and respiratory diseases.[147,148] Current intake recommendations for omega-3 and omega-6 fatty acids during pregnancy are 1.4 and 13 g/d, respectively, representing 27% and 8% increases from the corresponding prepregnancy values.[130] According to the *Dietary Guidelines for Americans, 2020–2025*, during pregnancy, females should eat 8 to 12 oz of seafood that is low in methyl mercury per week.[79] To accommodate these recommendations, pregnant individuals and those attempting to conceive should aim to consume 1 or 2 portions of fish per week, including oily fish.[149] The health care practitioner should also encourage additional healthy sources of fat, such as avocados, nuts, seeds, and olives, whereas intake of *trans* fatty acids and animal-based saturated fats should be discouraged. The latter 2 types of fats appear to promote deleterious metabolic effects during early-stage fetal development that increase the long-term risk of developing metabolic disorders later in life.[150]

Micronutrient Requirements

Although deficiencies of any required nutrients during fetal development can result in health problems for the child, several nutrients are of particular importance because maternal inadequacies during pregnancy may contribute to devastating birth defects. Therefore, in addition to helping pregnant athletes achieve a balanced dietary intake, encouraging the use of multivitamins or prenatal vitamins is key to ensuring a healthy first trimester.

IRON

Although a pregnant person's hemoglobin mass does not significantly expand until the second and third trimesters of pregnancy, increased dietary intake of iron is recommended from the time of conception to accommodate normal iron losses, support fetal and placental growth, and build iron stores before demands become more pronounced.[151] The current RDA for iron during pregnancy is 27 mg/d, representing a 50% increase from the prepregnancy value.[152] Female athletes may be at elevated risk for iron deficiency and iron deficiency anemia because of heightened levels of hepcidin, a peptide hormone that inhibits iron absorption and sequesters iron in macrophages. Research indicates that hepcidin concentrations increase in response to exercise, which makes early screening of added importance for this population.[153] Iron deficiency and iron deficiency anemia exacerbate feelings of fatigue and compromise overall maternal health in the first trimester; they can also contribute to poor pregnancy outcomes, including preterm delivery, prematurity, and a small-for-gestational-age birth weight.[151,154] In some cases, iron deficiency may escalate the risk for pica, the act of craving substances (often nonfood substances, such as ice, dirt, and clay) that contain little to no nutritional value. Pica can be harmful for both the birth parent and the child, especially when the cravings include nonfood substances that increase the risk of exposure to toxic and parasitic ingredients. Iron deficiency is also correlated with restless leg syndrome, making inclusion of questions regarding history of restless leg syndrome and pica of possible benefit when screening for iron deficiency.[155] In addition to incorporating iron-rich foods such as lean meat, seafood, edamame, white beans, nuts, fortified grain products, and spinach, supplemental iron is recommended if an individual's ferritin levels drop below 70 mcg/L. Suggested supplement guidelines are as follows[154]:

- For ferritin greater than 70 mcg/L, no iron supplementation is needed.
- For ferritin between 31 and 70 mcg/L, supplement with 30 to 40 mg of ferrous iron per day.
- For ferritin between 30 and 15 mcg/L, supplement with 60 to 80 mg of ferrous iron per day.
- For ferritin less than 15 mcg/L and/or iron deficiency anemia, supplement with therapeutic doses of 100 mg of ferrous iron per day.

FOLATE

Folate plays an integral role in the transformation of the neural tube into the brain and spinal cord during the first 28 days of pregnancy and consequently provides protection against neural tube defects such as spina bifida and anencephaly. Folate requirements increase from preconception values of 200 to 600 mcg/d during the first trimester.[156,157] Continued supplementation with 400 mcg/d in the second and third trimesters has been shown to increase maternal and cord-blood folate status and prevent the increase in homocysteine concentration that otherwise occurs in late pregnancy; thus, supplementation may be of added benefit to pregnancy outcomes and health in early childhood.[158] Ensuring adequate dietary consumption from natural food sources such as avocados, oranges, asparagus, green leafy vegetables, dried beans, and peas, as well as fortified grain products, should serve as the first line of defense. However, over-the-counter supplemental folate is often needed to achieve red blood cell folate levels associated with maximal protection against neural defects, especially when maternal nutrition is compromised secondary to morning sickness, a common first-trimester symptom.[157] Multivitamin tablets with folate are generally found in 3 formulations:

- regular over-the-counter multivitamins with 400 to 600 mcg of folate
- prenatal over-the-counter multivitamins with 1,000 mcg of folate
- prescription multivitamins with 5,000 mcg of folate

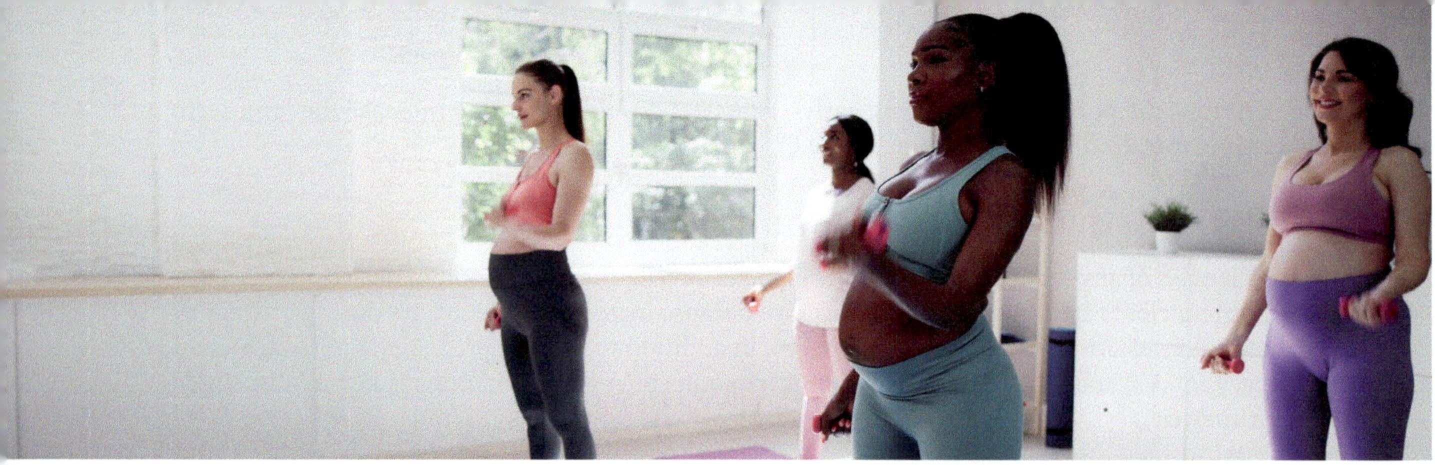

The higher doses of folate found in prenatal over-the-counter supplements are designed to protect against maternal folate deficiency as a result of fetal demand for the nutrient being satisfied at the expense of maternal demand. Prescription doses of folate are primarily reserved for females with a high risk for primary or recurrent neural tube or other folic acid–sensitive congenital anomalies. To help mitigate possible concerns that high supplemental intakes of folate may mask pernicious anemia, prescription doses of folate should be consumed in conjunction with 2.6 mcg of vitamin B12 per day.[157]

VITAMIN B12

Adequate intake of vitamin B12 is critical during pregnancy, as this vitamin plays a fundamental role in neural myelination, brain development, and growth of the fetus. A dietary deficiency early in pregnancy is considered a risk factor for neural tube closure defects. Furthermore, maternal vitamin B12 insufficiency (<200 pmol/L) can lead to adverse pregnancy outcomes including preeclampsia, intrauterine growth restriction, impaired fetal brain function, preterm delivery, and low birth weight (<2,500 g).[159] The RDA for vitamin B12 increases by 8% from the nonpregnancy value to 2.6 mcg/d to accommodate an increase in the production of red blood cells, the manufacturing of genetic material, and healthy functioning of the nervous system. Some data suggest that doses as high as 3 times the RDA are of benefit to maternal and fetal health during pregnancy.[156,160] Health care practitioners should encourage daily intake of good dietary sources of vitamin B12, such as eggs, cheese, milk products, meat, fish, shellfish, and poultry, as well as fortified grains and soy foods. To ensure optimal intake, supplemental vitamin B12 may be warranted for vegans as well as individuals experiencing food insecurity.[161,162]

ZINC

Zinc is a key micronutrient during pregnancy, particularly in the first trimester when organs begin to form and the immune system develops. To help accommodate fetal growth and development, the RDA for zinc increases from 8 to 11 mg/d during pregnancy.[152] Because a suboptimal zinc status in pregnancy may elevate the risk for numerous adverse outcomes including preeclampsia, gestational hypertension, low birth weight (<2,500 g), premature delivery, labor and delivery complications, and congenital anomalies, supplemental zinc at doses up to 30 mg/d may be warranted for individuals who fail to fulfill the increased RDA for zinc through food intake.[163-165] Those who follow plant-based diets often have difficulty acquiring sufficient zinc both because the most abundant sources of zinc are animal based and because the dietary phytates found in plant foods can interfere with zinc absorption.[166] In addition, females in low-income settings seem to be at greater risk for zinc deficiency and are thus likely to benefit from supplementation.[167]

CHOLINE

Choline helps support the structure and function of the brain and spinal cord during fetal development. It is also necessary for the synthesis of both lecithin, an essential constituent of the human brain and nervous system, and acetylcholine, an important neurotransmitter. Results from both animal- and human-based studies suggest that maternal choline supplementation during pregnancy may help improve cognitive function, stress response, and cerebral inhibition in children.[168-170] The current Adequate Intake recommendation for choline during all 3 trimesters of pregnancy is 450 mg/d, a 25 mg/d increase from prepregnancy values.[156] Good dietary sources of choline include cow's milk, egg yolk, liver, and peanuts.

VITAMIN D

Vitamin D is a key nutrient for establishing and maintaining optimal fetal and maternal bone health. It also aids in the uptake and metabolism of calcium and phosphorus and is consequently a critical component of bone mineralization and growth.[171-175] Poor maternal vitamin D status during pregnancy has been associated with fetal health complications, such as disordered skeletal homeostasis, congenital rickets, and fractures in newborns, with much of this damage being irreversible.[175-177] In addition, evidence is mounting that low maternal serum vitamin D levels may predispose the child to lifelong chronic disease, including certain types of cancers, autoimmune disease, neurologic disease, insulin resistance, and cardiovascular disease.[178,179]

Some studies have suggested a tenuous link between suboptimal maternal vitamin D status and undesirable pregnancy outcomes, including infection, preeclampsia, gestational diabetes, preterm birth, and small-for-gestational-age status.[179-184] In addition, researchers have estimated that anywhere from 5% to 84% of pregnant females across the globe either fail to consume the current RDA for vitamin D, 15 mcg/d (600 IU/d), or have inadequate serum vitamin D levels (<20 ng/mL).[183,185] Experts estimate that 33% of the population in the United States has a vitamin D deficiency.[186] Research among athletic populations suggests that maintaining a concentration of serum 25-hydroxyvitamin D greater than or equal to 30 ng/mL (preferably ≥40 ng/mL) protects against common infectious illness, impaired muscle function, and stress fractures, all of which are important to the well-being of the female athlete during pregnancy, as well as to the return to sport after pregnancy.[187] Because vitamin D is found in very few foods and the contribution of sun exposure to vitamin D status depends on many factors, including latitude, skin color, amount of skin exposed, duration of exposure, and use of sunscreens, vitamin D supplementation throughout pregnancy may be needed to achieve concentrations that are supportive of fetal and maternal health. Most prenatal vitamins contribute 10 mcg (400 IU) of vitamin D.

Some data suggest that supplementation with 25 to 50 mcg/d (1,000 to 2,000 IU of vitamin D) throughout gestation may be warranted as a means to offer the infant substantial protection against vitamin D deficiency during the first 2 months of life.[188,189] However, the health care practitioner should note that an excessive serum 25-hydroxyvitamin D concentration (>50 ng/mL) can be equally dangerous because it can breach the placental barrier and adversely affect the total amount of calcium stored in fetal bones, which may ultimately lead to neonatal death. Thus, supplementation with vitamin D is unnecessary in females with healthy serum 25-hydroxyvitamin D concentrations of 20 to 50 ng/mL, and supplementation at levels greater than 2,000 IU/d should be approached with caution.[190]

IODINE

Adequate intake of iodine throughout pregnancy is essential for fetal brain development and growth. It is also essential for maternal thyroid function. Maternal dietary inadequacies have been shown to put a child at elevated risk for intellectual disabilities, as well as growth, hearing, and speech problems, and to also put the birth parent at elevated risk for hypothyroidism. Pregnancy hypothyroidism has been linked to several adverse pregnancy outcomes, including prematurity, low birth weight, miscarriage, preeclampsia, fetal death, and impaired fetal neurocognitive development.[191] Therefore, pregnant individuals should be advised to meet the current iodine RDA of 220 mcg daily through dietary intake and supplementation.[192]

Hydration Needs

To accommodate substantial gestational blood water expansion, the adequate intake of fluid suggested to achieve a euhydrated state increases from 2.7 to 3 L/d during pregnancy.[193] However, because the amount of fluid needed to reach a euhydrated state can be highly variable, especially in athletes, urine color may be a valid alternative for assessing urine concentration and overall hydration status in pregnant athletes. Current data suggest that pregnant individuals who present with a urine color of 4 or greater are likely to have a urine osmolality of less than or equal to 500 mOsm/kg; thus, increased fluid intake is warranted to improve hydration status.[194] Female athletes should be advised to always carry fluids with them during workouts as well as during the day to avoid dehydration, which has been demonstrated to negatively affect amniotic fluid levels and initiate premature labor. In addition, pregnant athletes exercising in what would generally be considered extreme environments need to be even more cognizant of their fluid intake. For example, environments with excess heat and humidity and high-altitude environments both increase fluid requirements. Box 17.2 provides further recommendations for pregnant individuals exercising at altitude.[15,195-197]

BOX 17.2 Exercising at Altitude During Pregnancy[15,195-197]

Whereas not all athletes will need to consider the safety of exercising at altitude when pregnant, many elite endurance athletes regularly train in these environments. Inevitably, it is important to determine whether pregnant athletes exercising at altitude need to take certain precautions. The greatest concern for pregnant athletes training at altitude is that hypoxia and exercise can reduce blood flow to the uterus, resulting in reduced oxygen availability to the fetus. Because of safety and ethical concerns, research studies investigating this topic are rare. Indeed, no study has investigated the upper limits when maximal exercise and altitude exposure are combined during pregnancy.[195] Moreover, no studies have involved elite athletes. One study examined fetal tolerance to an oxygen-reduced environment among 7 healthy pregnant females between 33- and 34-weeks' gestation at sea level and at an altitude of 6,000 feet, using symptom-limited maximal oxygen uptake (VO_2 max) exercise tests. Cardiopulmonary and metabolic variables from the 2 environments were compared, and no threatening fetal responses to the oxygen-reduced environment were found.[196] Despite these initial findings, given the significant lack of data, it is recommended that pregnant athletes avoid high-intensity training at altitudes greater than 5,000 to 6,500 ft to prevent adverse pregnancy outcomes.[197]

CONTRAINDICATED FOOD PRODUCTS, SUBSTANCES, AND SUPPLEMENTS IN PREGNANCY

Hormonal changes during pregnancy compromise the cell-mediated immune function of both pregnant females and their fetuses, making exposure to foodborne pathogens that can be passed to the fetus, such as *Salmonella enterica* and *Listeria monocytogenes,* of particular concern during pregnancy. Whereas maternal infection may be asymptomatic or present with mild flulike symptoms, including fever, muscle aches, and gastrointestinal symptoms, fetal or neonatal infection is often severe and potentially fatal.[198,199] In addition, substances such as alcohol and caffeine and certain dietary supplements can penetrate the placenta and reach the fetus, where they are only partially metabolized by the child's immature digestive system and may thus increase the risk for adverse pregnancy outcomes, such as fetal alcohol spectrum disorder.[200-202] Therefore, pregnant individuals should be advised to take special precaution with the intake of certain food and drink products, substances, and ingredients during pregnancy, including the following:

- raw fish and shellfish
- undercooked meat and poultry
- raw or soft-cooked eggs
- raw sprouts
- seafood with a high mercury content
- unpasteurized foods
- unwashed fruits and vegetables
- caffeine
- alcohol
- dietary supplements

Raw Fish and Shellfish

Raw fish, including oysters, clams, mussels, and scallops, and refrigerated, uncooked seafood, such as lox and Nova-style salmon, as well as any kippered or smoked seafood, pose a greater threat of parasitic and bacterial infection than cooked fish and should be avoided during pregnancy. During preparation, fish should be cooked to an internal temperature of 145°F (63°C), at which point it will separate into flakes and appears opaque throughout. Shrimp, lobster, and scallops should be cooked until they are milky white. Clams, mussels, and oysters should be cooked until their shells open.[198,199]

Undercooked Meat and Poultry

Like raw seafood, undercooked meat and poultry are at greater risk of being contaminated with foodborne pathogens than their cooked counterparts. A meat thermometer can be a helpful at-home tool to ensure that meat and poultry are cooked thoroughly. When dining out, meats should be requested well-done. Because hot dogs and lunch meat are carriers of the foodborne pathogen *L monocytogenes,* they should be cooked until steaming hot before consumption.[198,199]

Raw or Soft-Cooked Eggs

A carrier of *S enterica,* eggs are among the most common causes of *Salmonella* infection. Therefore, consumption of raw or undercooked eggs is discouraged during pregnancy. Food products containing raw or partially cooked eggs, such as eggnog; custard; cookie dough; cake batter; and any hollandaise, mayonnaise, or Caesar salad dressing made with raw eggs, should also be avoided during pregnancy.[198,199] Eggs that have been pasteurized to reduce the risk of foodborne illness in dishes that are not cooked or are only lightly cooked, such as liquid egg products or eggs pasteurized in the shell, are safe for consumption.

Raw Sprouts

Raw sprouts, such as alfalfa, clover, radish, and mung bean, are vulnerable to bacteria entering through cracks in their seeds before sprouting. Thus, consumption is risky and discouraged during pregnancy.[198,199]

Seafood High in Mercury

Because high levels of the organometallic compound methyl mercury can be toxic to the nervous system of a fetus, certain fish, such as tilefish from the Gulf of Mexico, king mackerel, shark, and swordfish, should be avoided during pregnancy. As a safe alternative, consuming up to 12 oz of fish and shellfish with lower counts of methyl mercury such as shrimp, canned light tuna, salmon, catfish, pollock, anchovies, and trout is recommended.[198,199] However, as previously mentioned, omega-3 fatty acids are incredibly important during pregnancy to support fetal health and development. Thus, RDNs should be sure that their clients do not avoid seafood completely (unless this is not part of their food preferences or eating patterns) because of concerns over mercury content.

Unpasteurized Foods

Whereas many grocery store chains do not carry unpasteurized foods such as milk, soft cheeses (eg, queso blanco, queso fresco, queso panela, Camembert, Brie, feta, and blue), and juices because of heightened risk that they carry foodborne pathogens, some stores do sell them. Pregnant individuals should read labels when food shopping, especially when at a nonchain or farmers market, and they should buy and consume only pasteurized products. When dining out, pregnant individuals are advised to check with the kitchen before ordering certain types of cheeses and juices.[198,199]

Caffeine

Caffeine crosses the placenta, and the developing fetus is ill-equipped to fully metabolize the stimulant, which creates the potential adverse pregnancy outcomes of miscarriage, preterm labor, and low-birth-weight babies. Therefore, individuals are advised to limit their caffeine intake to less than 200 mg/d during pregnancy, with abstinence indicated for those with known caffeine sensitivities before pregnancy.[201] Education on common caffeine-containing products, including coffee, tea, energy drinks, and some soft drinks, along with their caffeine doses should be provided early in pregnancy. Health care practitioners should also be sure to educate clients on the lesser-known contributors to dietary caffeine intake including dietary supplement ingredients such as guarana, yerba mate, kola and kola nut, cocoa, and citrus aurantium (bitter orange), as well as various sports foods that contain caffeinated gels and blocks.

Alcohol

Because alcohol passes freely through the placenta to the fetus, no level of consumption is verified safe during pregnancy. Abuse of alcohol during pregnancy is linked to fetal alcohol syndrome, characterized by malformations of the skeletal system, heart, and brain; growth deficiencies; problems with the central nervous system; poor motor skills; increased mortality; and problems with learning, memory, social interaction, attention span, problem solving, speech, and hearing. Even moderate intake (eg, a 5-oz glass of wine or a 12-oz beer for females) can elicit fetal alcohol effects marked by mental and behavioral impairments.[200] Thus, all health care practitioners should advise pregnant individuals to avoid alcohol throughout pregnancy.

Dietary Supplements

Dietary ingredients found in dietary supplements, including vitamins, minerals, herbs or other botanicals, and amino acids, are not subject to the premarket safety evaluations required of food ingredients and medications. As a result, the general efficacy and safety of these products is questionable at all times and is especially not to be trusted during pregnancy. Thus, their use is discouraged unless specifically recommended by a health care practitioner for pregnancy health. Ingredients found in dietary supplements reach the fetus primarily by crossing the placenta. Exposure during pregnancy to some ingredients and substances in dietary supplements can indirectly impact the fetus by initiating uterine contractions and premature labor or by lowering maternal blood pressure, which, in turn, may reduce blood flow to the placenta and the consequent supply of oxygen and nutrients to the fetus, increasing the risk of the child being born at a low birth weight.[201,202] Exposure during pregnancy to some ingredients found in dietary supplements may also directly cause damage, abnormal development, and death of the fetus.[202]

WEIGHT GAIN RECOMMENDATIONS

The optimal quantity of weight gain in pregnancy for both maternal and fetal health is the subject of some debate. The current guidelines of the Institute of Medicine (IOM) and the American College of Obstetricians and Gynecologists (reaffirmed in 2023) recommend a total weight gain of 25 to 35 lb for singleton pregnancies in individuals with a healthy BMI (18.5 through 24.9).[132,133] A slightly greater weight gain of 28 to 40 lb for singleton pregnancies is recommended for female athletes who enter pregnancy underweight (BMI < 18.5).[130,131] Those who are overweight (BMI = 25 through 29.9) are encouraged to minimize pregnancy weight gain to 15 to 25 lb for singleton pregnancies.[132,133] Individuals who are obese (BMI > 30) should minimize pregnancy weight gain to 11 to 20 lb for singleton pregnancies.[131,132] For twin pregnancies, the IOM recommends a total gestational weight gain of 37 to 54 lb for individuals of normal weight, 31 to 50 lb for those who are overweight, and 25 to 42 lb for those who are obese.[132]

Singleton pregnancy–associated weight gain during the first trimester of 1.1 to 4.4 lb can be attributed to the expanding uterus, growing breasts, and increased blood volume. This amount makes up only a small percentage of the total recommended pregnancy weight gain. Slightly more weight gain is attributed to the same causes for twin pregnancies. During the second and third trimesters, when fetal growth increases dramatically, a weekly weight gain of approximately 1 lb for singleton pregnancies and 1.5 lb for twin pregnancies is recommended for individuals with underweight and healthy prepregnancy BMIs. The recommended weekly weight gains during the second and third trimesters for those who are overweight and obese are 0.6 and 0.5 lb, respectively, for singleton pregnancies and slightly higher for twin pregnancies.[132] Some experts speculate that, if adequate fetal growth is occurring, even lower rates of pregnancy weight gain in those who are overweight and obese may be warranted to help optimize the long-term health of the child.[134,135] Maintaining a healthy rate of weight gain in pregnancy has been shown to decrease the risk for several adverse maternal and neonatal outcomes, including gestational diabetes, hypertension, cesarean birth, fetal macrosomia, preterm birth, stillbirth, small- or large-for-gestational-age status, and low birth weight.[132-135,203-205]

Especially relevant for female athletes interested in making a postpartum comeback is the finding that staying within the IOM weight-gain guidelines during pregnancy helps reduce the risk of retaining more than 2 kg of pregnancy weight at 18 months postpartum and beyond, regardless of prepregnancy weight status.[206] Therefore, it is important for RDNs and other health professionals working with pregnant athletes to discuss the IOM pregnancy weight-gain guidelines and to provide appropriate diet and exercise guidance to help achieve these goals.

EXERCISE DURING PREGNANCY

Some female athletes fear that their training may trigger miscarriage or cause harm to their child, so they stop exercise completely upon discovery of their pregnancy. Current evidence does not substantiate these concerns. In fact, the evidence demonstrates that moderate resistance and cardiovascular exercise during pregnancy is not a direct cause of miscarriage and instead may help support a healthy pregnancy and offset some of the discomforts associated with nurturing fetal growth.[4,206-208]

For a competitive athlete, the excitement of pregnancy may be overshadowed by concern about how pregnancy weight gain will affect their body, sport performance, and ability to return to competition. Helping the athlete transition from a "train to win" or "train to perform" attitude to a "train for health" mindset is not always easy. Education on exercise tolerance and contraindications and benefits can go a long way in providing comfort to the athlete and establishing the framework for a healthy pregnancy (see Box 17.3).[208]

BOX 17.3 Exercise During Pregnancy[208]

For pregnant individuals who want to exercise throughout pregnancy, the American College of Sports Medicine provides the following recommendations.

Safety

As changes in weight distribution occur, balance and coordination may be affected. Avoid activities with increased fall risk, contact sports, and activities with increased risk of abdominal trauma.

Environment

Temperature regulation is highly dependent on hydration and environmental conditions. Ensure adequate fluid intake before, during, and after exercise. Avoid physical activity in the heat, especially with high humidity.

Growth and development

Monitor the level of exercise and adjust dietary intake to ensure proper weight gain. Stop exercising if the following occurs: persistent shortness of breath, severe chest pain, regular and painful contractions, vaginal bleeding, persistent dizziness or faintness.

Mode and intensity

Weight-bearing and nonweight-bearing exercise are thought to be safe during pregnancy. Improved maternal fitness is a well-known benefit of nonweight-bearing exercise, such as swimming and cycling. Weight-bearing exercises are similarly beneficial as long as they are comfortable. Aim to accumulate 150 minutes of moderate physical activity per week.

Consult with a health care provider if considering competitive athletics or volume significantly above recommended levels, or when exercising at altitude.

Exercise

A healthy individual with a normal pregnancy may either continue a regular exercise regimen or begin a new exercise program during pregnancy.

POSTPARTUM RECOMMENDATIONS

After welcoming a new baby, many athletes are eager to resume exercise activities and are motivated to eat healthfully as a means to help shed their pregnancy weight and facilitate a strong return to competition. There is some anecdotal evidence to suggest that athletic performance may improve postpartum. Comparatively, a recent study among 150 female marathon runners found that, when age is considered, maternity does not have an impact on postpartum athletic performance development.[209] A complete disregard for the physiological changes that occur in the body after childbirth, however, is unwise. The transition after having a baby presents unique challenges that an athlete must consider, such as the high energy cost of lactation or the repercussions of pelvic floor injury. Disregarding these new obstacles can place an athlete at heightened risk for injury, compromise their overall health, and hinder their ability to successfully return to sport. Health practitioners working with athletes after childbirth can play an integral role in facilitating a successful return to sport by providing education and guidance on proper nutrition during lactation, nutrition and fitness strategies to promote healthful weight loss, and appropriate precautions to take when returning to sport activity.

Nutrition and Lactation

It is the position of the Academy of Nutrition and Dietetics that exclusive breastfeeding provides optimal nutrition and health protection for the first 6 months of life and that breastfeeding with complementary foods from 6 months until at least 12 months of age is the ideal feeding pattern for infants.[210]

Many female athletes express concern about their milk production and composition being negatively affected by exercise training and consequently choose to supplement with formula or delay their return to fitness activity until after weaning. However, there is currently no evidence to support the notion that exercise training, even at moderate to high intensity, hurts the production or composition of breast milk, including important immune factors (eg, secretory immunoglobulin A, lactoferrin, and lysozyme).[211,212]

Ensuring adequate nutrition to support the metabolic demands of lactation is critical. For an athlete, the combined energetic costs of lactation and physical training can be extremely demanding. Failure to consume adequate calories can exacerbate postpartum fatigue and interfere with both nursing and fitness performance. Mean milk production of 749 g/d (~26 oz/d) requires an additional 453 kcal/d or approximately 17 kcal per ounce of milk produced to support the metabolic demands of lactation.[213] Given the variability of daily milk production, additional caloric intake in the range of 300 to 500 kcal is often recommended to support lactation. Thus, the health care practitioner should encourage a target energy intake of 45 kcal per kilogram of fat-free mass per day, plus an additional 300 to 500 kcal to accommodate lactation, plus the amount of energy needed for physical activity.[136,213]

Because lactation may reduce bone density by as much as 5% as a result of osteoclastic activity, it is prudent to encourage lactating athletes to regularly consume foods that are rich in calcium to ensure that they acquire the RDA of 1,000 mg of calcium.[214] Although bone mass is generally recovered once the child is weaned, the rate and extent of recovery can be influenced by the duration of lactation and postpartum amenorrhea and may differ by skeletal site.[215]

Healthy Weight-Loss Strategies

Body composition and body weight are 2 of many factors that contribute to optimal exercise performance and overall health. Returning to prepregnancy form is a goal that most athletes strive to achieve postpartum. However, it is important to mention that every individual's pregnancy and postpartum experience is different. Weight-loss interventions may not produce immediate results, but positive lifestyle changes can support long-term health and may eventually lead to weight loss. Practitioners can play a key role in providing the tools needed to promote healthy fat loss, optimized health, and enhanced performance in a time frame that is realistic and appropriate for the individual athlete. Research has shown that the average weight retention at 1 year postpartum falls to around 2.0 kg, with the greatest rate of weight loss occurring in the first 3 months postpartum and then continuing at a slow and steady rate until about 6 months postpartum.[216] Females who exclusively breastfeed for at least 3 months have been shown to exhibit significantly less weight retention than those who supplement or discontinue breastfeeding before 3 months.[217] Recent studies demonstrated that exercise programs with objectively defined goals, such as heart rate or total steps, and those with intensive dietary intervention, including self-monitoring through the use of food journals, are highly effective in aiding sustained postpartum weight loss.[218,219] For individuals who began their pregnancy at a healthy weight and gained the recommended amount of weight during pregnancy, a gradual weight loss not to exceed 4.5 lb/mo should be encouraged after the first month postpartum and until prepregnancy weight is achieved.[220]

Return to Sport

Obstetricians often recommend waiting to exercise until after the first postpartum checkup, generally scheduled 4 to 6 weeks after delivery. However, according to the American College of Obstetricians and Gynecologists, an earlier return to physical training is usually safe, provided that no medical or surgical complications occurred during labor and delivery.[221] Athletes should note that hormonal and physiological changes occur in the body postpartum that can increase the risk for injury when too much activity is taken on too soon. One of the greatest challenges results from a hormone called relaxin. For up to 6 months after childbirth, and even longer for individuals who are nursing, the body produces relaxin, which, as the name suggests, relaxes the muscles, joints, and ligaments, contributing to instability. These changes can make high-impact exercise, such as running, lifting heavy weights, and performing rapid changes of direction, potentially dangerous to an athlete postpartum. This is especially true for females with pelvic floor weakness, because constant and excessive downward pressure on the pelvic floor can increase the postpartum risk for hemorrhage, prolapse, and urine leakage.[222,223] Because of these concerns, lower-impact activities, such as swimming, elliptical, and bodyweight exercises, should be the focal point of any conditioning program during the early postpartum stages or until pelvic floor stability is established. Refer to Box 17.4 for information on postpartum recovery.[221,224-226]

BOX 17.4 The Pregnancy-Performance Connection[221,224-226]

Overcoming performance roadblocks is not an easy feat, but with perseverance, an athlete can experience key physiological benefits that can facilitate a successful return to sporting competition.

According to James Clapp III, MD,[224-226] a renowned researcher in the area of exercise and pregnancy, athletes who regularly train at a moderately hard level of perceived effort for about an hour a day throughout pregnancy and are able to resume a similar pattern soon after delivery will experience significant improvements in exercise economy, meaning that the cost of oxygen to perform a specific workload is lower, and an increase of about 10% in their maximum aerobic capacity, even if their overall training load is lighter than it was prepregnancy.

These benefits are thought to last for about a year postpartum, possibly longer. Although scientific evidence supporting the translation of these benefits to athletic performance in high-performing endurance athletes is lacking, it is thought to be one reason why so many female athletes come back stronger after giving birth.

In 2021, a group of researchers developed a framework, coined the *6 Rs Framework*,[227] to help multidisciplinary teams support athletes in their return to their sport (refer to Figure 17.1 on page 430).

EXPERIENCES OF ELITE ATHLETES DURING PREGNANCY

This chapter has been made clear throughout that research on elite athletes during pregnancy and postpartum is scarce. Despite the increased number of elite athletes publicly sharing their feats and challenges of pregnancy and postpartum, more research still needs to be conducted to better understand the unique needs of elite pregnant and postpartum athletes. Although this chapter covers nutrition and exercise

Reframing Return-to-Sport Postpartum: the 6 Rs Framework

Donnelly GM, Moore IS, Brockwell E, Rankin A, Cooke R. British Journal of Sports Medicine 2021

This framework is underpinned by a whole-systems, biopsychosocial approach that requires the safety of the mother and baby to be the overarching consideration.

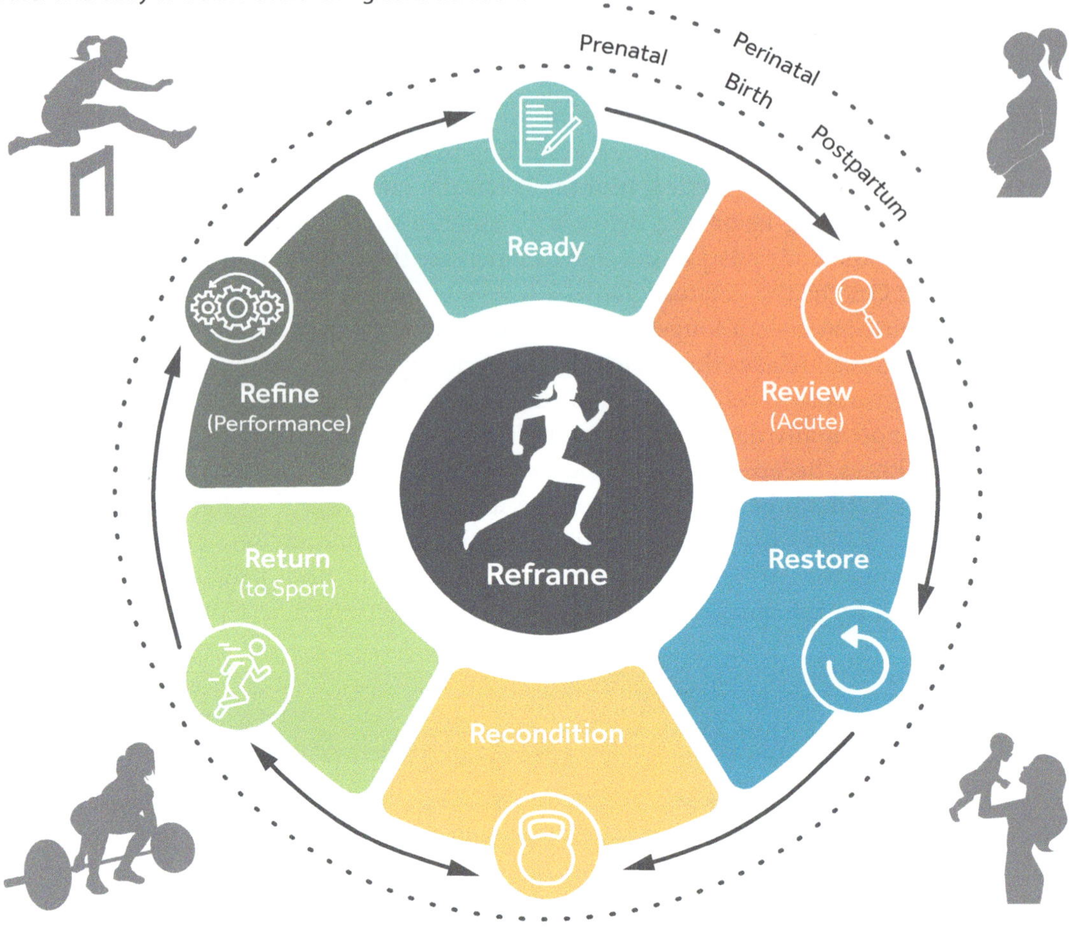

Ready

Ready the athlete for anticipated whole-systems, biopsychosocial changes by proactively educating them about perinatal health considerations during the transition into pregnancy and motherhood (e.g., weight-gain, pelvic floor function, perinatal mental health). Aim to maintain exercise throughout pregnancy (where it is safe to do so for the mother and baby), limit deconditioning and optimise postpartum recovery with forward planning.

Review

Review and evaluate the postpartum athlete and address acute musculoskeletal and pelvic health rehabilitation needs. Screen for whole-systems, biopsychosocial considerations.*

Restore

Restore physical and psychological wellbeing depending on individual needs and prepare the perinatal athlete for returning to structured training environments. Include pelvic floor rehabilitation and other relevant whole-systems considerations.

Recondition

Recondition the perinatal athlete for their required physical and psychological sporting demands. Commence graded exposure towards individual-specific training load requirements. Revisit whole-systems, biopsychosocial considerations and monitor symptoms as training increases.

Return

Return-to-sport through an individualised, evidence-informed and guided exposure to the competitive environment and re-evaluate regularly.

Refine

Refine whole-systems, biopsychosocial strategies (e.g., optimise sleep quality, monitor for signs of relative energy deficiency syndrome) to enhance athlete training and competition availability, retaining the athlete in their sport and optimising performance.

*Whole-systems, biopsychosocial considerations - childbirth related trauma (e.g., abdominal wall dysfunction, pelvic floor dysfunction or post-traumatic stress); menstrual health; breast health (e.g., review breast support particularly in the breastfeeding athlete); energy balance (e.g., relative energy deficiency in sport); psychological wellbeing (e.g., perinatal mental health); fear of movement; and sleep (e.g., sleep routine and quality).

FIGURE 17.1 The 6 Rs Framework: a phased whole-systems, biopsychosocial approach[227] This framework is intended to help multidisciplinary teams effectively support female athletes in their return to their sport during the postpartum period. The focus is placed on the importance of viewing postpartum return-to-sport as part of a gradual progression that should not be rushed. Thus, athletes may move backward and forward among the 6 phases depending on their individual needs.
Reproduced with permission from reference 225: Donnelly GM, Moore IS, Brockwell E, Rankin A, Cooke R. Reframing return-to-sport postpartum: the 6 Rs framework. *Br J Sports Med.* 2022;56(5):244-245. doi:10.1136/bjsports-2021-104877

guidance for all levels of pregnant athletes, it is important to explore the limited data that do exist specifically for elite pregnant athletes and their experiences at the highest level of sport.

In 2022, 1 qualitative study explored the experiences of elite athletes during pregnancy.[228] Although this study included only 20 athletes, it provides a valuable glimpse into the lived experiences of elite athletes juggling the challenges of pregnancy and parenthood. Moreover, the insights offered by this report can help RDNs working with this population better understand some of the barriers these athletes may face during pregnancy and postpartum. All of the participants in this study trained and/or competed in elite athletics immediately before and during pregnancy within the preceding 5 years of when the study was conducted. The athletes went through a screening process that included completing a questionnaire describing their sporting background and an overview of their pregnancy experiences, followed by a 1-hour semistructured interview with each participant. The participants represented 11 Olympic sports (team and individual) and were generally from North America and Europe. "Mother vs athlete" was the overarching message found, with 5 main themes as described in Box 17.5. Many participants felt that they had to choose between motherhood and their sport. Importantly, several participants described their skepticism regarding the programs and guidelines put together by trainers, coaches, and health care practitioners because of the lack of evidence-based guidelines specific to pregnant athletes at their level. Although RDNs were not specifically included in these statements, RDNs working with this population should be aware of this potential skepticism, as it can serve as a barrier to building rapport with the athlete during nutrition counseling and motivational interviewing. The participants also shared concerns about the safety of training during pregnancy, as well as the need to have a supportive network to maintain a career as an elite athlete during pregnancy. Several of the athletes described some health care staff as part of their network, illustrating the importance of RDNs being part of the supportive network that guides athletes through their pregnancy and postpartum journeys. The most apparent reason that most participants experienced conflict between their identities as mothers and as athletes was financial concern. The participants reported that funding for pregnant athletes was inconsistent across various sporting organization, resulting in a lack of security.[228]

Although the data discussed in this section are anecdotal, the lived experiences presented here are incredibly important for health care practitioners to understand, as they reveal many of the challenges faced by this population. RDNs, other members of the interdisciplinary team, and sporting organizations and sponsors as a whole need to be better equipped to provide high-quality care and support through all stages of life for elite athletes, including during pregnancy and postpartum. Future research including elite female athletes must be conducted to support evidence-based guidelines for this population.

BOX 17.5 Actionable Steps to Support Elite Female Athletes

Pregnancy planning and fertility

Example supporting quotes	"We had tried to get pregnant but we weren't successful. We had a very specific timeline." "I wasn't having a regular menstrual cycle because of heavy training volumes, I have a leaner build. So it was a lot harder for me to get pregnant the first time around."
Policy recommendations and actionable steps to support pregnant athletes	Educate coaches, medical professionals, and athletes of reproductive age about the impact of training on the menstrual cycle and fertility. Develop clear maternity leave policies and support to allow athletes to plan for pregnancy.

Continued on next page

BOX 17.5 Actionable Steps to Support Elite Female Athletes (CONTINUED)

Pregnancy disclosure and discrimination	
Example supporting quotes	"I wouldn't discuss it with them [coaches] at all until I knew I had to . . . I was worried that they would question my commitment." "I think that more than anything, it was my own insecurities of thinking that as a female, if I get pregnant, they're not going to accept me anymore."
Policy recommendations and actionable steps to support pregnant athletes	Provide training sessions to athletes, coaches, medical professionals, and sporting organizations on promoting a supportive environment for pregnant athletes. Increase the visibility of athletes who have successfully navigated pregnancy and elite sport. Develop antidiscrimination laws to support athletes who become pregnant.
Training pregnant athletic bodies	
Example supporting quotes	"It was difficult to accept early on . . . I sort of saw my [training] plummet . . . I did have quite a hard time with reconciling in my own head that I was in a different place and that I was going to have to back off." "There may be guidelines that exist, but I'm not convinced that they apply to athletes."
Policy recommendations and actionable steps to support pregnant athletes	Increase high-quality research into the impact of elite-level training during pregnancy (eg, fertility, safety, limits, and health outcomes). Improve knowledge translation of evidence-based recommendations to athletes, coaches, and health care practitioners.
Safety concerns	
Example supporting quotes	"I got pregnant while I was competing and pulled out of a race because I thought I was pregnant. And just thought, 'Oh my gosh, I don't want to be like damaging the fetus.'" "I want there to be more concrete answers about what I can and can't do . . . can I actually harm the fetus . . . if it's going to harm the baby I'm not going to do it?"
Policy recommendations and actionable steps to support pregnant athletes	Increase high-quality research into the impact of elite-level training during pregnancy. Provide training and education to health care practitioners on evidence-based recommendations for training and competing during pregnancy.

Supportive network and equitable funding	
Example supporting quotes	"A supportive partner has been huge for me, a supportive coach, someone who can understand the woman's body and what it goes through [during pregnancy]." "I don't think it's very convenient for anybody when an elite woman becomes pregnant. But what is a support right now is more social media attention for pregnant athletes and more shaming of sponsors that don't treat their pregnant athletes or postpartum athletes properly, and the rewriting of a lot of sponsorship agreements."
Policy recommendations and actionable steps to support pregnant athletes	Normalize and value pregnancy and elite sport by developing best-practice policies and funding to support pregnancy. Promote and provide greater visibility of athletes who have successfully navigated pregnancy and elite sport. Develop networks for athletes considering pregnancy to speak with others about shared experiences.

Adapted with permission from reference 226: Davenport MH, Nesdoly A, Ray L, Thornton JS, Khurana R, McHugh TF. Pushing for change: a qualitative study of the experiences of elite athletes during pregnancy. *Br J Sports Med.* 2022;56(8):452-457. doi:10.1136/bjsports-2021-104755

SUMMARY

The transitions from preconception to pregnancy to lactation and the postpartum stage can be life-changing for athletes. Practitioners need to be equipped to support athletes throughout all of these transitions and to be aware of the unique nutrition considerations that come with them. Although an athlete may feel pressure to return to their prepregnancy body composition and exercise levels after pregnancy, it is important that an interdisciplinary team, including an RDN, help the athlete return to their sport safely. Understanding the individual nutrition-related barriers that an athlete may face before, during, and after pregnancy is key for providing person-centered care to athletes hoping to balance their sport with pregnancy and caring for a child.

KEY TAKEAWAYS

BEFORE PREGNANCY:

Female athletes who have struggled to maintain a normal menstrual cycle (defined as experiencing menstruation every 28 to 30 days) at any point during training or competition may need to reduce their overall training load or increase their energy intake.

Gains in both body weight and fat may be necessary for female athletes carrying very low body weights, defined as having a BMI of less than 18.5.

Developing healthy weight-loss strategies, including exercise, for athletes with BMIs greater than 25 will help boost fertility by enhancing insulin function and improving the body's overall hormone profile.

Consuming a balanced diet and supplementing with prenatal vitamins, which provide key fertility nutrients such as folate and iron, are nutrition strategies shown to boost fertility.

Limit caffeine intake to no more than 200 mg/d and abstain from alcohol preconception to support fertility.

DURING PREGNANCY:

Advising the pregnant athlete on how to achieve a balanced dietary intake, adhere to food safety recommendations, and take multivitamins or prenatal vitamins is key to ensuring a healthy pregnancy.

A target energy intake of 45 kcal per kilogram of prepregnancy fat-free mass per day plus the amount of energy burned during exercise should be encouraged during the first trimester of pregnancy, with an additional 340 and 452 kcal in the form of carbohydrate and protein being warranted during the second and third trimesters, respectively, to support increased fetal growth patterns.

Adequate intake of fluid suggested for maintaining a euhydrated state increases from 2.7 to 3 L/d during pregnancy to accommodate substantial gestational expansion of the pregnant person's blood volume.

For healthy individuals with a normal pregnancy, a regular exercise regimen should be encouraged under the supervision of their physician.

AFTER PREGNANCY:

It is the position of the Academy of Nutrition and Dietetics that exclusive breastfeeding provides optimal nutrition and health protection for the first 6 months of life and that breastfeeding with complementary foods from 6 months until at least 12 months of age is the ideal feeding pattern for infants.

A target energy intake of 45 kcal per kilogram of fat-free mass per day plus an additional 300 to 500 kcal to accommodate lactation plus the amount of energy needed for physical activity should be encouraged.

For athletes who began their pregnancy at a healthy weight and gained the recommended amount of weight during pregnancy, a gradual weight loss not to exceed 4.5 lb/mo should be encouraged after the first month postpartum and until the desired weight is achieved.

REFERENCES

1. Key statistics from the National Survey of Family Growth – I Listing: Infertility. Centers for Disease Control and Prevention. Last reviewed December 16, 2022. Accessed June 1, 2023. www.cdc.gov/nchs/nsfg/key_statistics/i-keystat.htm#infertility
2. Marquez S, Molinero O. Energy availability, menstrual dysfunction, and bone health in sports; an overview of the female athlete triad. *Nutr Hosp.* 2013;28(4):1010-1017. doi:10.3305/nh.2013.28.4.6542
3. De Souza MJ, Toombs RJ, Scheid JL, O'Donnell E, West SL, Williams NI. High prevalence of subtle and severe menstrual disturbances in exercising women: confirmation using daily hormone measures. *Hum Reprod.* 2010;25(2):491-503. doi:10.1093/humrep/dep411
4. Weinstein Y, Weinstein A. Energy balance, body composition and the female athlete triad syndrome. Article in Hebrew. *Harefuah.* 2012;151(2):97-126. PMID: 22741211
5. Ahrens KA, Vladutiu CJ, Mumford SL, etal. The effect of physical activity across the menstrual cycle on reproductive function. *Ann Epidemiol.* 2014;24(2):127-134. doi:10.1016/j.annepidem.2013.11.002
6. Orio F, Muscogiuri G, Ascione A, et al. Effects of physical exercise on the female reproductive system. *Minerva Endocrinol.* 2013;38(3):305-319. PMID: 24126551
7. Gibbs JC, Williams NI, Mallinson RJ, Reed JL, Rickard AD, De Souza MJ. Effect of high dietary restraint on energy availability and menstrual status. *Med Sci Sports Exerc.* 2013;45(9):1790-1797. doi:10.1249/MSS.0b013e3182910e11
8. Statuta SM, Asif IM, Drezner JA. Relative energy deficiency in sport (RED-S). *Br Sports Med.* 2017;51(21):1570-1571. doi:10.1136/bjsports-2017-097700
9. Cabre HE, Moore SR, Smith-Ryan AE, Hackney AC. Relative energy deficiency in sport (RED-S): scientific, clinical, and practical implications for the female athlete. *Dtsch Z Sportmed.* 2022;73(7):225-234. doi:10.5960/dzsm.2022.546
10. Mountjoy M, Sundgot-Borgen JK, Burke LM, et al. IOC consensus statement on relative energy deficiency in sport (RED-S): 2018 update. *Br Sports Med.* 2018;52(11):687-697. doi:10.1136/bjsports-2018-099193
11. De Souza MJ. Menstrual disturbances in athletes: a focus on luteal phase defects. *Med Sci Sports Exerc.* 2003;35(9):1553-1563. doi:10.1249/01.MSS.0000084530.31478.DF
12. Healthy People 2030. Office of Disease Prevention and Health Promotion, US Department of Health and Human Services. Accessed June 1, 2023. https://health.gov/healthypeople
13. Physical activity and exercise during pregnancy and the postpartum period: ACOG committee opinion, number 804. *Obstet Gynecol.* 2020;135(4):e178-e188. doi:10.1097/AOG.0000000000003772
14. Surehka T, Himabindu Y, Sriharibabu M, Pandey AK. Impact of physical activity on ovarian reserve markers in normal, overweight, and obese reproductive age women. *Indian Physiol Pharmacol.* 2014:58(2):162-165. PMID: 25509968
15. Bø K, Artal R, Barakat R, *et al.* Exercise and pregnancy in recreational and elite athletes: 2016 evidence summary from the IOC expert group meeting, Lausanne. Part 1—exercise in women planning pregnancy and those who are pregnant. *Br Sports Med.* 2016;50:571-589. doi:10.1136/bjsports-2016-096218
16. Wiebe HW, Boulé NG, Chari R, Davenport MH. The effect of supervised prenatal exercise on fetal growth: a meta-analysis. *Obstet Gynecol.* 2015;125(5):1185-1194. doi:10.1097/AOG.0000000000000801
17. Kehler AK, Heinrich KM. A selective review of prenatal exercise guidelines since the 1950s until present: written for women, health care professionals, and female athletes. *Women Birth.* 2015;28(4):e93-e98. doi:10.1016/j.wombi.2015.07.004
18. US Department of Health and Human Services. *Physical Activity Guidelines for Americans*, 2nd ed. Published November 2018. Accessed June 1, 2023. https://health.gov/sites/default/files/2019-09/Physical_Activity_Guidelines_2nd_edition.pdf
19. Chavarro JE, Rich-Edwards JW, Rosner BA, Willett WC. Diet and lifestyle in the prevention of ovulatory disorder infertility. *Obstet Gynecol.* 2007;110(5):1050-1058. doi:10.1097/01.AOG.0000287293.25465.e1
20. Rich-Edwards JW, Spiegelman D, Garland M, et al. Physical activity, body mass index, and ovulatory disorder infertility. *Epidemiology.* 2002;13(2):184-190. doi:10.1097/00001648-200203000-00013
21. Gudmundsdottir SL, Flanders WD, Augestad LB. Physical activity and fertility in women: the North-Trøndelag Health Study. *Hum Reprod.* 2009;24(12):3196-3204. doi:10.1093/humrep/dep337
22. Wise LA, Rothman KJ, Mikkelsen EM, Sorensen HT, Riis AH, Hatch EE. A prospective cohort study of physical activity and time to pregnancy. *Fertil Steril.* 2012;97(5):1136-1142.e4. doi:10.1016/j.fertnstert.2012.02.025
23. Maïmoun L, Georgopoulos NA, Sultan C. Endocrine disorders in adolescent and young female athletes: impact on growth, menstrual cycles, and bone mass acquisition. *Clin Endocrin Metab.* 2014;99(11):4037-4050. doi:10.1210/jc.2013-3030
24. Brooks KA, Carter JG. Overtraining, exercise, and adrenal insufficiency. *Nov Physiother.* 2013;3(125):11717. doi:10.4172/2165-7025.1000125
25. Kreher JB, Scwartz JB. Overtraining syndrome: a practical guide. *Sports Health.* 2012;4(2):128-138. doi:10.1177/1941738111434406

26. Meczekalski B, Katulski K, Czyzyk A, Podfigurna-Stopa A, Maciejewska-Jeske M. Functional hypothalamic amenorrhea and its influence on women's health. *Endocrinol Invest.* 2014;37(11):1049-1056. doi:10.1007/s40618-014-0169-3

27. Melin A, Tornberg ÅB, Skouby S, et al. Energy availability and the female athlete triad in elite endurance athletes. *Scand Med Sci Sports.* 2015;25(5):610-622. doi:10.1111/sms.12261

28. Bø K, Artal R, Barakat R, *et al.* Exercise and pregnancy in recreational and elite athletes: 2016 evidence summary from the IOC expert group meeting, Lausanne. Part 2—the effect of exercise on the fetus, labour and birth. *Br Sports Med.* 2016;50:1297-1305. doi:10.1136/bjsports-2016-096810

29. Sharma R, Biedenharn KR, Fedor JM, Agarwal A. Lifestyle factors and reproductive health: taking control of your fertility. *Reprod Biol Endocrinol.* 2013;11:66. doi:10.1186/1477-7827-11-66

30. Provost MP, Acharya KS, Acharya CR, et al. Pregnancy outcomes decline with increasing recipient body mass index: an analysis of 22,317 fresh donor/recipient cycles from the 2008-2010 Society for Assisted Reproductive Technology Clinic Outcome Reporting System registry. *Fertil Steril.* 2015;105(2):364-368. doi:10.1016/j.fertnstert.2015.10.015

31. World Health Organization. *Obesity: Preventing and Managing the Global Epidemic. Report of a WHO Consultation.* WHO Technical Report Series 894. World Health Organization; 2000.

32. American Society for Reproductive Medicine. Weight and Infertility. Revised 2023. Accessed October 3, 2024. www.reproductivefacts.org/globalassets/_rf/news-and-publications/bookletsfact-sheets/english-pdf/weight_and_fertility-factsheet.pdf

33. Obesity and overweight. World Health Organization website. Updated March 1, 2024. Accessed August 27, 2024. www.who.int/en/news-room/fact-sheets/detail/obesity-and-overweight

34. Marsh CA, Hecker E. Maternal obesity and adverse reproductive outcomes: reducing the risk. *Obestet Gynecol Surv.* 2014;69(10):622-628. doi:10.1097/OGX.0000000000000115

35. Jungheim ES, Travieso JL, Carson KR, Moley KH. Obesity and reproductive function. *Obstet Gynecol Clin North Am.* 2012;39(4):479-493. doi:10.1016/j.ogc.2012.09.002

36. van der Steeg JW, Steures P, Eijkemans MJ, et al. Obesity affects spontaneous pregnancy chances in subfertile, ovulatory women. *Hum Reprod.* 2008;23(2):324-328. doi:10.1093/humrep/dem371

37. Sim KA, Partridge SR, Sainsbury A. Does weight loss in overweight or obese women improve fertility treatment outcomes? A systematic review. *Obes Rev.* 2014;15(1):839-850. doi:10.1111/obr.12217

38. Sim KA, Dezarnaulds GM, Denyer GS, Skilton MR, Caterson ID. Weight loss improves reproductive outcomes in obese women undergoing fertility treatment: a randomized controlled trial. *Clin Obes.* 2014;4(2):61-68. doi:10.1111/obr.12217

39. Kort JD, Winget C, Kim SH, Lathi RB. A retrospective cohort study to evaluate the impact of meaningful weight loss on fertility outcomes in an overweight population with infertility. *Fertil Steril.* 2014;101(5):1400-1403. doi:10.1016/j.fertnstert.2014.01.036

40. Sowińska-Przepiera E, Andrysiak-Mamos E, Jarząbek-Bielecka G, et al. Functional hypothalamic amenorrhoea—diagnostic challenges, monitoring, and treatment. *Endokrynol Pol.* 2015;66(3):252-260. doi:10.5603/EP.2015.0033

41. Niedźwiedzka B1, Jagielska G, Bartoszewicz Z, Kondracka A, Brzozowska A, Karowicz-Bilińska A. Assessment of neuropeptide Y, leptin and leptin-receptor concentrations in teenagers suffering from anorexia nervosa. Article in Polish. *Ginekol Pol.* 2013;84(4):268-276. doi:10.17772/gp/1575

42. Loucks AB. Energy availability, not body fatness, regulates reproductive function in women. *Exerc Sport Sci Rev.* 2003;31(3):144-148. doi:10.1097/00003677-200307000-00008

43. Melin A, Tornberg AB, Skouby S, et al. Low-energy density and high fiber intake are dietary concerns in female endurance athletes. *Scand Med Sci Sports.* 2016;26(9):1060-1071. doi:10.1111/sms.12516

44. Gibbs JC, Williams NI, De Souza MJ. Prevalence of individual and combined components of the female athlete triad. *Med Sci Sports Exerc.* 2013;45(5):985-996. doi:10.1249/MSS.0b013e31827e1bdc

45. Mountjoy M, Sundgot-Borgen J, Burke L, et al. The IOC consensus statement: beyond the female athlete triad—relative energy deficiency in sport (RED-S). *Br Sport Med.* 2014;48(7):491-497. doi:10.1136/bjsports-2014-093502

46. Mountjoy M, Sundgot-Borgen J, Burke L, et al. RED-S CAT. Relative Energy Deficiency in Sport (RED-S) Clinical Assessment Tool (CAT). *Br Sport Med.* 2015;49(7):421-423. doi:10.1136/bjsports-2015-094873

47. Folscher L-L, Grant CC, Fletcher L, Janse van Rensberg DC. Ultra-marathon athletes at risk for the female athlete triad. *Sports Med Open.* 2015;1(1):29. doi:10.1186/s40798-015-0027-7

48. Bacchi E, Spiazzi G, Zendrini G, Bonin C, Moghetti P. Low body weight and menstrual dysfunction are common findings in both elite and amateur ballet dancers. *Endocrinol Invest.* 2013;36(5):343-346. doi:10.3275/8645

49. Gibbs JC, Williams NI, Scheid JL, Toombs RJ, De Souza MJ. The association of a high drive for thinness with energy deficiency and severe menstrual disturbances: confirmation in a large population of exercising women. *Int Sport Nutr Exerc Metab.* 2011;21(4):280-290. doi:10.1123/ijsnem.21.4.280

50. Doyle-Lucas AF, Akers JD, Davy BM. Energetic efficiency, menstrual irregularity, and bone mineral density in elite professional female ballet dancers. *Dance Med Sci.* 2010;14(4):146-154. doi:10.1177/1089313X1001400403

51. Melin A, Tornberg AB, Skouby S, et al. The LEAF questionnaire: a screening tool for the identification of female athletes at risk for the female athlete triad. *Br Sports Med.* 2014;48(7):540-545. doi:10.1136/bjsports-2013-093240

52. Fujita Y, Sasaki E, Yoneda K, et al. Menstrual status and pregnancy in former elite long-distance runners with menstrual disorders. *Clin Sport Med.* 2023;33(2):172-178. doi:10.1097/JSM.0000000000001083
53. Nose-Ogura S, Yoshino O, Kamoto-Nakamura H, et al. Age and menstrual cycle may be important in establishing pregnancy in female athletes after retirement from competition. *Phys Sportsmed.* 2024;52(2):175-180. doi:10.1080/00913847.2023.2199687
54. Cardwell MS. Eating disorders during pregnancy. *Obstet Gynecol Surv.* 2013;68:312-323. doi:10.1097/OGX.0b013e31828736b9
55. Park RJ, Senior R, Stein A. The offspring of mothers with eating disorders. *Eur Child Adolesc Psychiatry.* 2003;12(suppl 1):i110-i119. doi:10.1007/s00787-003-1114-8
56. Patel P, Wheatcroft R, Park RJ, et al. The children of mothers with eating disorders. *Clin Child Fam Psychol Rev.* 2002;5(1):1-19. doi:10.1023/a:1014524207660
57. Hammiche F, Laven JS, van Mil N, et al. Tailored preconceptional dietary and lifestyle counseling in a tertiary outpatient clinic in The Netherlands. *Hum Reprod.* 2011;26(9):2432-2441. doi:10.1093/humrep/der225
58. Walfisch A, Koren G. Preconception counseling: rational, practice and challenges. *Minerva Ginecol.* 2011;63(5):411-419.
59. Sińska B, Kucharska A, Dmoch-Gajzlerska E. The diet in improving fertility in women. Article in Polish. *Pol Merkur Lekarski.* 2014;36(216):400-402.
60. Chavarro JE, Rich-Edwards JW, Rosner BA, Willet WC. Protein intake and ovulatory infertility. *Am Obstet Gynecol.* 2008;198(2):210.e1-e7. doi:10.1016/j.ajog.2007.06.057
61. Weiss RV, Clapauch R. Female infertility of endocrine origin. *Arq Bras Endocrinol Metabol.* 2014;58(2):144-152. doi:10.1590/0004-2730000003021
62. Szostak-Węgierek D. Nutrition and fertility. Article in Polish. *Med Wieku Rozwoj.* 2011;15(4):431-436.
63. Center for Food Safety and Applied Nutrition. Final Determination Regarding Partially Hydrogenated Oils (Removing Trans Fat). US Food and Drug Administration. Published May 18, 2018. Accessed October 26, 2023. www.fda.gov/food/food-additives-petitions/final-determination-regarding-partially-hydrogenated-oils-removing-trans-fat
64. Vujkovic M, de Vries JH, Lindemans J, et al. The preconception Mediterranean dietary pattern in couples undergoing in vitro fertilization/intracytoplasmic sperm injection treatment increases the chance of pregnancy. *Fertil Steril.* 2010;94(6):2096-2101. doi:10.1016/j.fertnstert.2009.12.079
65. Tobias DK, Zhang C, Chavarro J, et al. Adherence to dietary patterns and lower risk of gestational diabetes mellitus. *Am Clin Nutr.* 2012;96(2):289-295. doi:10.3945/ajcn.111.028266
66. Wilson RD, Audibert F, Brock J-A, et al; Genetics Committee. Pre-conception folic acid and multivitamin supplementation for the primary and secondary prevention of neural tube defects and other folic acid-sensitive congenital anomalies. *Obstet Gynaecol Can.* 2015;37(6):534-552. doi:10.1016/s1701-2163(15)30230-9
67. Chavarro JE, Rich-Edwards JW, Rosner BA, Willett WC. Use of multivitamins, intake of B vitamins, and risk of ovulatory infertility. *Fertil Steril.* 2008;89(3):668-676. doi:10.1016/j.fertnstert.2007.03.089
68. Chavarro JE, Rich-Edwards JW, Rosner BA, Willett WC. Iron intake and risk of ovulatory infertility. *Obstet Gynecol.* 2006;108(5):1145-1152. doi:10.1097/01.AOG.0000238333.37423.ab
69. Gaskins AJ, Rich-Edwards JW, Hauser R, et al. Maternal prepregnancy folate intake and risk of spontaneous abortion and stillbirth. *Obstet Gynecol.* 2014;124(1):23-31. doi:10.1097/AOG.0000000000000343
70. Gardiner PM, Nelson L, Shellhaas CS, et al. The clinical content of preconception care: nutrition and dietary supplements. *Am Obstet Gynecol.* 2008;199(6 suppl 2):S345-S356. doi:10.1016/j.ajog.2008.10.049
71. De-Regil LM, Fernández-Gaxiola AC, Dowswell T, Peña-Rosas JP. Effects and safety of periconceptional folate supplementation for preventing birth defects. *Cochrane Database Syst Rev.* 2010;(10):CD007950. doi:10.1002/14651858.CD007950.pub2
72. Buhling KJ, Grajecki D. The effect of micronutrient supplements on female fertility. *Curr Opin Obstet Gynecol.* 2013;25(3):173-180. doi:10.1097/GCO.0b013e3283609138
73. Morgan S, Koren G, Bozzo P. Is caffeine consumption safe during pregnancy? *Can Fam Physician.* 2013;59(4):361-362.
74. Bolúmar F, Olsen J, Rebagliato M, Bisanti L; European Study Group on Infertility Subfecundity. Caffeine and delayed conception: a European multicenter study on infertility and subfecundity. *Am Epidemiol.* 1997;145(4):324-334. doi:10.1093/oxfordjournals.aje.a009109
75. Al-Saleh I, El-Doush I, Grisellhi B, Coskun S. The effect of caffeine consumption on the success rate of pregnancy as well as various performance parameters of in-vitro fertilization treatment. *Med Sci Monit.* 2010;16(12):CR598-CR605.
76. American College of Obstetrics and Gynecology, Committee on Obstetric Practice. ACOG committee opinion no. 462: Moderate caffeine consumption during pregnancy. *Obstet Gynecol.* 2010;116(2 pt 1):467-468. doi:10.1097/AOG.0b013e3181eeb2a1
77. Eggert J, Theobald H, Engfeldt P. Effects of alcohol consumption on female fertility during an 18-year period. *Fertil Steril.* 2004;81(2):379-383. doi:10.1016/j.fertnstert.2003.06.018
78. Wdowiak A, Sulima M, Sadowska M, Grzegorz B, Bojar I. Alcohol consumption and quality of embryos obtained in programmes of in vitro fertilization. *Ann Agric Environ Med.* 2014;21(2):450-453. doi:10.5604/1232-1966.1108623
79. US Department of Agriculture and US Department of Health and Human Services. *Dietary Guidelines for Americans, 2020-2025.* 9th ed. December 2020. Accessed August 8, 2025. www.dietaryguidelines.gov/sites/default/files/2021-03/Dietary_Guidelines_for_Americans-2020-2025.pdf
80. Symons Downs D, Chasan-Taber L, Evenson KR, Leiferman J, Yeo S. Physical activity and pregnancy: past and present evidence and future recommendations. *Res Q Exerc Sport.* 2012;83(4):485-502. doi:10.1080/02701367.2012.10599138

81. Sanabria-Martínez G, García-Hermosa A, Poyatos-León R, Álvarez-Bueno C, Sánchez-López M, Martínez-Vizcaíno V. Effectiveness of physical activity interventions on preventing gestational diabetes mellitus and excessive maternal weight gain: a meta-analysis. *BJOG.* 2015;122(9):1167-1174. doi:10.1111/1471-0528.13429
82. Hinman SK, Smith KB, Quillen DM, Smith MS. Exercise in pregnancy: a clinical review. *Sports Health.* 2015;7(6):527-531. doi:10.1177/1941738115599358
83. Sanabria-Martínez G, García-Hermoso A, Poyatos-León R, González-García A, Sánchez-López M, Martínez-Vizcaíno V. Effects of exercise-based interventions on neonatal outcomes: a meta-analysis of randomized controlled trials. *Am Health Promot.* 2016;30(4):214-223. doi:10.1177/0890117116639569
84. Szymanski LM, Satin AJ. Exercise during pregnancy: fetal responses to current public health guidelines. *Obstet Gynecol.* 2012;119(3):603-610. doi:10.1097/AOG.0b013e31824760b5
85. Nasik E, Eryilmaz G. Incidence of pregnancy-related discomforts and management approaches to relieve them among pregnant women. *Clin Nurs.* 2014;23(11-12):1736-1750. doi:10.1111/jocn.12323
86. Tan EK, Tan EL. Alterations in physiology and anatomy during pregnancy. *Best Pract Res Clin Obstet Gyenacol.* 2013;27(6):791-802. doi:10.1016/j.bpobgyn.2013.08.001
87. Bernstein IM, Ziegler W, Badger GJ. Plasma volume expansion in early pregnancy. *Obstet Gynecol.* 2001;97(5 pt 1):669-672. doi:10.1016/s0029-7844(00)01222-9
88. Hegewald MJ, Crapo RO. Respiratory physiology in pregnancy. *Clin Chest Med.* 2011;32(1):1-13. doi:10.1016/j.ccm.2010.11.001
89. Berry MJ, McMurray RG, Katz VL. Pulmonary and ventilator responses to pregnancy, immersion, and exercise. *Appl Physiol (1985).* 1989;66(2):857-862. doi:10.1152/jappl.1989.66.2.857
90. Gaston A1, Prapavessis H. Tired, moody, and pregnant? Exercise may be the answer. *Psychol Health.* 2013;28(12):1353-1369. doi:10.1080/08870446.2013.809084
91. Einarson TR, Piwko C, Koren G. Prevalence of nausea and vomiting of pregnancy in the USA: a meta analysis. *Popul Ther Clin Pharmacol.* 2013;20(2):e163-e170. Accessed May 11, 2023. Retrieved from www.jptcp.com/index.php/jptcp/article/view/386
92. Einarson TR, Piwko C, Koren G. Quantifying the global rates of nausea and vomiting of pregnancy: a meta analysis. *Popul Ther Clin Pharmacol.* 2013;20(2):e171-e183.
93. Ducarme G, Dochez V. *Hyperemesis gravidarum:* A review. Article in French. *Presse Med.* 2015;44(12 pt 1):1226-1234. doi:10.1016/j.lpm.2015.06.008
94. Sanu O, Lamont RF. *Hyperemesis gravidarum:* pathogenesis and the use of antiemetic agents. *Expert Opin Pharmacother.* 2011;12(5):737-748. doi:10.1517/14656566.2010.537655
95. Veenendaal MVE, van Abeelen AFM, Painter RC, van der Post JAM, Rosebloom TJ. Consequences of *hyperemesis gravidarum* for offspring: a systematic review and meta-analysis. *BJOG.* 2011;118(11):1302-1313. doi:10.1111/j.1471-0528.2011.03023.x
96. Fejzo MS, Poursharif B, Korst LM, et al. Symptoms and pregnancy outcomes associated with extreme weight loss among women with *hyperemesis gravidarum. Womens Health (Larchmt).* 2009;18(12):1981-1987. doi:10.1089/jwh.2009.1431
97. Hastoy A, Lien Tran P, Lakestani O, Barau G, Gérardin P, Boukerrou M. L'hyperémèse gravidique: quelles conséquences sur la grossesse? [*Hyperemesis gravidarum* and pregnancy outcomes]. Article in French. *Gynecol Obstet Biol Reprod (Paris).* 2015;44(2):154-163. doi:10.1016/j.jgyn.2013.12.003
98. Ayyavoo A, Derraik JGB, Hofman PL, Cutfield WS. *Hyperemesis gravidarum* and long-term health of the offspring. *Am Obstet Gynecol.* 2014;210(6):521-525. doi:10.1016/j.ajog.2013.11.035
99. Maltepe C, Koren G. The management of nausea and vomiting of pregnancy and hyperemesis gravidarum—a 2013 update. *Popul Ther Clin Pharmacol.* 2013;20(2):e184-e192. Retrieved from https://jptcp.com/index.php/jptcp/article/view/388
100. Herrell HE. Nausea and vomiting of pregnancy. *Am Fam Physician.* 2014;89(12):965-970.
101. Stokke G, Gjelsvik BL, Flaatten KT, Birkeland E, Flaatten H, Trovik J. *Hyperemesis gravidarum*, nutritional treatment by nasogastric tube feeding: a 10-year retrospective cohort study. *Acta Obstet Gynecol Scand.* 2015;94(4):359-367. doi:10.1111/aogs.12578
102. Kotha VK, De Souza A. Wernicke's encephalopathy following *hyperemesis gravidarum.* A report of three cases. *Neuroradiol J.* 2013;26(1):35-40. doi:10.1177/197140091302600106
103. Committee on Practice Bulletins-Obstetrics. ACOG Practice Bulletin No. 189: Nausea and vomiting of pregnancy. *Obstet Gynecol.* 2018;131(1):e15-e30. doi:10.1097/AOG.0000000000002456
104. Viljoen E, Visser J, Koen N, Musekiwa A. A systematic review and meta-analysis of the effect and safety of ginger in the treatment of pregnancy-associated nausea and vomiting. *Nutr J.* 2014;13:20. doi:10.1186/1475-2891-13-20
105. Saberi F, Sadat Z, Abedzadeh-Kalahroudi M, Taebi M. Effect of ginger on relieving nausea and vomiting in pregnancy: a randomized, placebo-controlled trial. *Nurs Midwifery Stud.* 2014;3(1):e11841. doi:10.17795/nmsjournal11841
106. Ensiyeh J, Sakineh M-AC. Comparing ginger and vitamin B-6 for the treatment of nausea and vomiting: a randomized controlled trial. *Midwifery.* 2009;25(6):649-653. doi:10.1016/j.midw.2007.10.013
107. Shi W, Xu X, Zhang Y, Guo S, Wang J, Wang J. Epidemiology and risk factors of functional constipation in pregnant women. *PLoS One.* 2015;10(7):e0133521. doi:10.1371/journal.pone.0133521
108. Longo SA, Moore RC, Canzoneri BJ, Robichaux A. Gastrointestinal conditions during pregnancy. *Clin Colon Rectal Surg.* 2010;23(2):80-89. doi:10.1055/s-0030-1254294
109. Dimidi E, Christodoulides S, Fragkos KC, Scott SM, Whelan K. The effect of probiotics on functional constipation in adults: a systematic review and meta-analysis of randomized controlled trials. *Am Clin Nutr.* 2014;100(4):1075-1084. doi:10.3945/ajcn.114.089151

110. Law R, Maltepe C, Bozzo P, Einarson A. Treatment of heartburn and acid reflux associated with nausea and vomiting of pregnancy. *Can Fam Physician.* 2010;56(2):143-144. doi:10.1016/j.jogc.2016.08.009
111. Ramu B, Mohan P, Rajasekaran MS, Jayanthi V. Prevalence and risk factors for gastroesophageal reflux in pregnancy. *Trop Gastroenterol.* 2011;30(3):144-147. doi:10.1007/s12664-010-0067-3
112. Vazquez JC. Heartburn in pregnancy. *BM Clin Evid.* 2015;2015:1411.
113. Liang C-C, Chang S-D, Lin S-J, Lin Y-J. Lower urinary tract symptoms in primiparous women before and during pregnancy. *Arch Gynecol Obstet.* 2012;285(5):1205-1210. doi:10.1007/s00404-011-2124-2
114. Boyle R, Hay-Smith EJ, Cody JD, Mørkved S. Pelvic floor muscle training for prevention and treatment of urinary and fecal incontinence in antenatal and postnatal women: a short version Cochrane review. *Neurourol Urodyn.* 2014;33(3):269-276. doi:10.1002/nau.22402
115. Stuber KJ, Wynd S, Weiss CA. Adverse events from spinal manipulation in the pregnant and postpartum periods: a critical review of the literature. *Chiropr Man Therap.* 2012;20:8. doi:10.1186/2045-709X-20-8
116. Ramachandra P, Maiya AG, Kumar P, Kamath A. Prevalence of musculoskeletal dysfunctions among Indian pregnant women. *Pregnancy.* 2015;2015:437105. doi:10.1155/2015/437105
117. Aldabe D, Ribeiro DC, Milosavljevic S, Dawn Bussey M. Pregnancy-related pelvic girdle pain and its relationship with relaxin levels during pregnancy: a systematic review. *Eur Spine J.* 2012;21(9):1769-1776. doi:10.1007/s00586-012-2162-x
118. Hensley JG. Leg cramps and restless legs syndrome during pregnancy. *Midwifery Womens Health.* 2009;54(3):211-218. doi:10.1016/j.jmwh.2009.01.003
119. Allen RE, Kirby KA. Nocturnal leg cramps. *Am Fam Physician.* 2012;86(4):350-355.
120. Bhardwaj A, Nagandla K. Musculoskeletal symptoms and orthopaedic complications in pregnancy: pathophysiology, diagnostic approaches and modern management. *Postgrad Med J.* 2014;90(1066):450-460. doi:10.1136/postgradmedj-2013-132377
121. Noon ML, Hoch AZ. Challenges of the pregnant athlete and low back pain. *Curr Sports Med Rep.* 2012;11(1):43-48. doi:10.1249/JSR.0b013e31824330b6
122. Tseng P-C, Puthussery S, Pappas Y, Gau M-L. A systematic review of randomised controlled trials on the effectiveness of exercise programs on lumbo pelvic pain among postnatal women. *BMC Pregnancy Childbirth.* 2015;15:316. doi:10.1186/s12884-015-0736-4
123. Flack NA, Hay-Smith EJ, Stringer MD, Gray AR, Woodley SJ. Adherence, tolerance and effectiveness of two different pelvic support belts as a treatment for pregnancy-related symphyseal pain – a pilot randomized trial. *BMC Pregnancy Childbirth.* 2015;15:36. doi:10.1186/s12884-015-0468-5
124. Cakmak B, Inanir A, Nacar MC, Filiz B. The effect of maternity support belts on postural balance in pregnancy. *PM R.* 2014;6(7):624-628. doi:10.1016/j.pmrj.2013.12.012
125. Zhou K, West HM, Zhang J, Xu L, Li W. Interventions for leg cramps in pregnancy. *Cochrane Database Syst Rev.* 2015;8:CD010655. doi:10.1002/14651858.CD010655.pub3
126. Belkacemi L, Nelson DM, Desai M, Ross MG. Maternal undernutrition influences placental-fetal development. *Biol Reprod.* 2010;83(3):325-331. doi:10.1095/biolreprod.110.084517
127. Ramakrishnan U, Grant F, Goldenberg T, Zongrone A, Martorell R. Effect of women's nutrition before and during early pregnancy on maternal and infant outcomes: a systematic review. *Paediatr Perinat Epidemiol.* 2012;26(suppl 1):285-301. doi:10.1111/j.1365-3016.2012.01281.x
128. Kaiser LL, Campbell CG; Academy Positions Committee Workgroup. Practice paper of the Academy of Nutrition and Dietetics abstract: nutrition and lifestyle for a healthy pregnancy outcome. *Acad Nutr Diet.* 2014;114(9):1447. doi:10.1016/j.jand.2014.07.001
129. Butte NF, Wong WW, Treuth MS, Elis KJ, O'Brian Smith E. Energy requirements during pregnancy based on total energy expenditure and energy deposition. *Am Clin Nutr.* 2004;79(6):1078-1087. doi:10.1093/ajcn/79.6.1078
130. Panel on Macronutrients; Panel on the Definition of Dietary Fiber; Subcommittee on Upper Reference Levels of Nutrients; Subcommittee on Interpretation and Uses of Dietary Reference Intakes; Standing Committee on the Scientific Evaluation of Dietary Reference Intakes; Food and Nutrition Board, Institute of Medicine. *Dietary Reference Intakes for Energy, Carbohydrate, Fiber, Fat, Fatty Acids, Cholesterol, Protein, and Amino Acids.* National Academies Press; 2002.
131. Butte NF, King JC. Energy requirements during pregnancy and lactation. *Public Health Nutr.* 2005;8(7A):1010-1027. doi:10.1079/phn2005793
132. Committee to Reexamine IOM Pregnancy Weight Guidelines; Food and Nutrition Board; Board on Children, Youth, and Families; Institute of Medicine; National Research Council. *Weight Gain During Pregnancy: Reexamining the Guidelines.* Rasmussen KM, Yaktine AL, eds. National Academies Press; 2009.
133. American College of Obstetrics and Gynecology, Committee on Obstetric Practice. ACOG committee opinion no. 548. Weight gain during pregnancy. *Obstet Gynecol.* 2013;121:210-212. doi:10.1097/01.aog.0000425668.87506.4c
134. Mehta SH, Kruger M, Sokol RJ. Institute of Medicine guidelines for appropriate pregnancy weight gain for obese women may be too high. *Reprod Med.* 2015;60(7-8):324-328.
135. Truong YN, Yee LM, Caughey AB, Cheng YW. Weight gain in pregnancy: does the Institute of Medicine have it right? *Am Obstet Gynecol.* 2015;212(3):362.e1-e8. doi:10.1016/j.ajog.2015.01.027
136. Maughan R, Burke L. *Nutrition for Athletes. A practical guide to eating for health and performance. Prepared by the Nutrition Working Group of the International Olympic Committee Based on an International Consensus Conference held at the IOC in Lausanne in October 2010.* International Olympic Committee; April 2012. Accessed December 1, 2015. https://library.olympics.com/Default/doc/SYRACUSE/74010

137. Most healthy women would benefit from light meal during labor. American Society of Anesthesiologists. Published November 6, 2015. Accessed December 1, 2015. www.asahq.org/about-asa/newsroom/news-releases/2015/11/eating-a-light-meal-during-labor
138. Thomas DT, Erdman KA, Burke LM. Position of the Academy of Nutrition and Dietetics, Dietitians of Canada, and the American College of Sports Medicine: nutrition and athletic performance. *Acad Nutr Diet.* 2016;116(3):501-528. doi:10.1016/j.jand.2015.12.006
139. Delidicque L, Francaux M. Recommendations for healthy nutrition in female endurance runners: an update. *Front Nutr.* 2015;2:17. doi:10.3389/fnut.2015.00017
140. Vanhauwaert E, Matthys C, Verdonck L, De Preter V. Low-residue and low-fiber diets in gastrointestinal disease management. *Adv Nutr.* 2015;6(6):820-827. doi:10.3945/an.115.009688
141. Maharaj D. Eating and drinking in labor: should it be allowed? *Eur Obstet Gynecol Reprod Biol.* 2009;146(1):3-7. doi:10.1016/j.ejogrb.2009.04.019
142. American College of Obstetricians and Gynecologists, Committee on Obstetric Practice. ACOG committee opinion no. 441. Oral intake during labor. *Obstet Gynecol.* 2009;114(3):714. doi:10.1097/AOG.0b013e3181ba0649
143. Kubli M, Scrutton MJ, Seed PT, O'Sullivan G. An evaluation of isotonic "sport drinks" during labor. *Anesth Analg.* 2002;94:404-408. doi:10.1097/00000539-200202000-00033
144. Kalhan SC. Protein metabolism in pregnancy. *Am Clin Nutr.* 2000;71(5 suppl):1249S-1255S. doi:10.1093/ajcn/71.5.1249 s
145. Haggarty P. Fatty acid supply to the human fetus. *Annu Rev Nutr.* 2010;30:237-255. doi:10.1146/annurev.nutr.012809.104742
146. Jones ML, Mark PJ, Waddell BJ. Maternal dietary omega-3 fatty acids and placental function. *Reproduction.* 2014;147(5):R143-R152. doi:10.1530/REP-13-0376
147. Rogers LK, Valentine CJ, Keim SA. DHA supplementation: current implications in pregnancy and childhood. *Pharmacol Res.* 2013;70(1):13-19. doi:10.1016/j.phrs.2012.12.003
148. Shek LP, Foong-Fong Chong M, Yi Lim J, Soh S-E, Chong Y-S. Role of dietary long-chain polyunsaturated fatty acids in infant allergic and respiratory diseases. *Clin Dev Immunol.* 2012; 2012:730568. doi:10.1155/2012/730568
149. Koletzko B, Boey CC, Campoy C, et al. Current information and Asian perspectives on long-chain polyunsaturated fatty acids in pregnancy, lactation, and infancy: systematic review and practice recommendations from an early nutrition academy workshop. *Ann Nutr Metab.* 2014;65(1):49-80. doi:10.1159/000365767
150. Mennitti LV, Oliveira JL, Morais CA, et al. Type of fatty acids in maternal diets during pregnancy and/or lactation and metabolic consequences of the offspring. *Nutr Biochem.* 2015;26(2):99-111. doi:10.1016/j.jnutbio.2014.10.001
151. Milman N. Iron in pregnancy. How do we secure an appropriate iron status in the mother and child? *Ann Nutr Metab.* 2011;59(1):50-54. doi:10.1159/000332129
152. Panel on Micronutrients, Subcommittee on Upper Reference Levels of Nutrients; Subcommittee of Interpretation and Use of Dietary Reference Intakes; Standing Committee on the Scientific Evaluation of Dietary Reference Intakes; Food and Nutrition Board, Institute of Medicine. *Dietary Reference Intakes for Vitamin A, Vitamin K, Arsenic, Boron, Chromium, Copper, Iodine, Iron, Manganese, Molybdenum, Nickel, Silicon, Vanadium, and Zinc.* National Academies Press; 2001. doi:10.17226/10026
153. McClung JP. Iron status and the female athlete. *Trace Elem Med Biol.* 2012;26(2-3):124-126. doi:10.1016/j.jtemb.2012.03.006
154. Alwan NA, Cade JE, McArdle HJ, Greenwood DC, Hayes HE, Simpson NA. Maternal iron status in early pregnancy and birth outcomes: insights from the baby's vascular health and iron in pregnancy study. *Br Nutr.* 2015;113(12):1985-1992. doi:10.1017/S0007114515001166
155. Singh A, Chaudhary R, Sonker A, Pandey HC. Importance of donor history of restless leg syndrome and pica to assess iron deficiency. *Transfus Apher Sci.* 2016;54(2):259-261. doi:10.1016/j.transci.2015.09.002
156. Standing Committee on the Scientific Evaluation of Dietary Reference Intakes and its Panel on Folate, Other B Vitamins, and Choline; Subcommittee on Upper Reference Levels of Nutrients; Food and Nutrition Board, Institute of Medicine. *Dietary Reference Intakes for Thiamin, Riboflavin, Niacin, Vitamin B_6, Folate, Vitamin B_{12}, Pantothenic Acid, Biotin, and Choline.* National Academies Press; 1998. doi:10.17226/6015
157. Genetics Committee; Wilson RD, Audibert F, Brock J-A, et al. Pre-conception folic acid and multivitamin supplementation for the primary and secondary prevention of neural tube defects and other folic acid sensitive congenital anomalies. *Obstet Gynaecol Can.* 2015;37(6):534-552. doi:10.1016/s1701-2163(15)30230-9
158. McNulty B, McNulty H, Marshall B, et al. Impact of continuing folic acid after the first trimester of pregnancy: findings of a randomized trial of folic acid supplementation in the second and third trimesters. *Am Clin Nutr.* 2013;98:92-98. doi:10.3945/ajcn.112.057489
159. Finkelstein JL, Layden AL, Stover PJ. Vitamin B-12 and perinatal health. *Adv Nutr.* 2015;6(5):552-563. doi:10.3945/an.115.008201
160. Bae S, West AA, Yan J, et al. Vitamin B-12 status differs among pregnant, lactating and control women with equivalent nutrient intakes. *Nutr.* 2015;145(7):1507-1514. doi:10.3945/jn.115.210757
161. Duggan C, Srinivasan K, Thomas T, et al. Vitamin B-12 supplementation during pregnancy and early lactation increases maternal, breast milk, and infant measures of vitamin B-12 status. *Nutr.* 2014;144(5):758-764. doi:10.3945/jn.113.187278
162. Kaiser L, Allen LH. Position of the American Dietetic Association: nutrition and lifestyle for a healthy pregnancy outcome. *Am Diet Assoc.* 2008;108(3):553-561. doi:10.1016/j.jada.2008.01.030
163. Ma Y, Shen X, Zhang D. The relationship between serum zinc level and preeclampsia: a meta-analysis. *Nutrients.* 2015;7(9):7806-7820. doi:10.3390/nu7095366

164. Tande DL, Ralph JL, Johnson LK, Scheett AJ, Hoverson BS, Anderson CM. First trimester dietary intake, biochemical measures, and subsequent gestational hypertension among nulliparous women. *Midwifery Womens Health.* 2013;58(4):423-430. doi:10.1111/jmwh.12007

165. Nossier SA, Naeim NE, El-Sayed NA, Abu Zeid AA. The effect of zinc supplementation on pregnancy outcomes: a double blind, randomized controlled trial, Egypt. *Br Nutr.* 2015;114(2):274-285. doi:10.1017/S000711451500166X

166. Foster M, Herulah UN, Prasad A, Petocz P, Samman S. Zinc status of vegetarians during pregnancy: a systematic review of observational studies and meta-analysis of zinc intake. *Nutrients.* 2015;7(6):4512-4525. doi:10.3390/nu7064512

167. Ota E, Mori R, Middleton P, et al. Zinc supplementation for improving pregnancy and infant outcomes. *Cochrane Database Syst Rev.* 2015;2015(2):CD000230. doi:10.1002/14651858.CD000230.pub5

168. Jiang X, West AA, Caudill MA. Maternal choline supplementation: a nutritional approach for improving offspring health. *Trends Endocrinol Metab.* 2014;25(5):263-273. doi:10.1016/j.tem.2014.02.001

169. Blustztajn JK, Mellott TJ. Neuroprotective actions of perinatal choline nutrition. *Clin Chem Lab Med.* 2013;51(3):591-599. doi:10.1515/cclm-2012-0635

170. Blusztajn JK, Mellott TJ. Choline nutrition programs brain development via DNA and histone methylation. *Cent Nerv Syst Agents Med Chem.* 2012;12(2):82-94. doi:10.2174/187152412800792706

171. Shin JS, Choi MY, Longtine MS, Nelson DM. Vitamin D effects on pregnancy and the placenta. *Placenta.* 2010;31(12):1027-1034. doi:10.1016/j.placenta.2010.08.015

172. Shaw NJ, Mughai MZ. Vitamin D and child health part 1 (skeletal aspects). *Arch Dis Child.* 2013;98(5):363-367. doi:10.1136/archdischild-2011-301264

173. Pettifor JM, Prentice A. The role of vitamin D in paediatric bone health. *Best Pract Res Clin Endocrinol Metab.* 2011;25(4):573-584. doi:10.1016/j.beem.2011.06.010

174. Marshall I, Mehta R, Petrova A. Vitamin D in the maternal-fetal-neonatal interface: clinical implications and requirements for supplementation. *Matern Fetal Neonatal Med.* 2013;26(7):633-638. doi:10.3109/14767058.2012.746306

175. Moon RJ, Harvey NC, Cooper C. Endocrinology in pregnancy: influence of maternal vitamin D status on obstetric outcomes and the fetal skeleton. *Eur Endocrinol.* 2015;173(2):R69-R83. doi:10.1530/EJE-14-0826

176. Zhu K, Whitehouse AJO, Hart PH, et al. Maternal vitamin D status during pregnancy and bone mass in offspring at 20 years of age: a prospective cohort study. *Bone Miner Res.* 2104;29(5):1088-1095. doi:10.1002/jbmr.2138

177. Specker BL. Does vitamin D during pregnancy impact offspring growth and bone? *Proc Nutr Soc.* 2012;71(1):38-45. doi:10.1017/S0029665111003053

178. Shaw NJ, Mughai MZ. Vitamin and child health: part 2 (extraskeletal and other aspects). *Arch Dis Child.* 2013;98(5):368-372. doi:10 .1136/archdischild-2012-302585

179. Olmos-Ortiz A, Avila E, Durand-Carbajal M, Diaz L. Regulation of calcitriol biosynthesis and activity: focus on gestational vitamin D deficiency and adverse pregnancy outcomes. *Nutrients.* 2015;7(1):443-480. doi:10.3390/nu7010443

180. Wagner CL, Baggerly C, McDonnell S, et al. Post-hoc analysis of vitamin D status and reduced risk of preterm birth in two vitamin D pregnancy cohorts compared with South Carolina March of Dimes 2009-2011 rates. *Steroid Biochem Mol Biol.* 2016;155(pt B):245-251. doi:10.1016/j.jsbmb.2015.10.022

181. Wei SQ. Vitamin D and pregnancy outcomes. *Curr Opin Obstet Gynecol.* 2014;26(6):438-447. doi:10.1097/GCO.0000000000000117

182. Schneuer FJ, Roberts CL, Guilbert C, et al. Effects of maternal serum 25-hydroxyvitamin D concentrations in the first trimester on subsequent pregnancy outcomes in an Australian population. *Am Clin Nutr.* 2014;99(2):287-295. doi:10.3945/ajcn.113.065672

183. Brannon PM. Vitamin D and adverse pregnancy outcomes: beyond bone health and growth. *Proc Nutr Soc.* 2012;71(2):205-212. doi:10.1017/S0029665111003399

184. Achkar M, Dodds L, Giguere Y, et al. Vitamin D status in early pregnancy and risk of preeclampsia. *Am Obstet Gynecol.* 2015;212(4):511.e1-e7. doi:10.1016/j.ajog.2014.11.009

185. Committee to Review Dietary Reference Intakes for Vitamin D and Calcium, Institute of Medicine. Ross AC, Taylor CL, Yaktine AL, Del Valle HB, eds. *Dietary Reference Intakes for Calcium and Vitamin D.* National Academies Press, 2011.

186. Ginde AA, Sullivan AF, Mansbach JM, Camargo CA Jr. Vitamin D insufficiency in pregnant and nonpregnant women of childbearing age in the United States. *Am Obstet Gynecol.* 2010;202(5):436.e1-e8. doi:10.1016/j.ajog.2009.11.036

187. Larson-Meyer E. Vitamin D supplementation in athletes. *Nestle Nutr Inst Workshop Ser.* 2013;75:109-121. doi:10.1159/000345827

188. March KM, Chen NN, Karakochuk CD, et al. Maternal vitamin D3 supplementation at 50 ug/d protects against low serum 25-hydroxyvitamin D in infants at 8-wk of age: a randomized controlled trial of 3 doses of vitamin D beginning in gestation and continued in lactation. *Am Clin Nutr.* 2015;102(2):402-410. doi:10.3945/ajcn.114.106385

189. Grant CC, Stewart AW, Scragg R, et al. Vitamin D during pregnancy and infancy and infant serum 25-hydroxyvitamin D concentration. *Pediatrics.* 2014;133(1):e143-e153. doi:10.1542/peds.2013-2602

190. Lieben L, Stockmans I, Moermans K, Carmeliet G. Maternal hypervitaminosis D reduces fetal bone mass and mineral acquisition and leads to neonatal lethality. *Bone.* 2013;57(1):123-131. doi:10.1016/j.bone.2013.07.029

191. Obican SG, Jahnke GD, Soldin OP, Scialli AR. Teratology public affairs committee position paper: Iodine deficiency in pregnancy. *Birth Defects Res A Clin Mol Teratol.* 2012;94(9):677-682. doi:10.1002/bdra.23051

192. Swanson C, Zimmerman M, Seaff S, et al. Summary of an NIH workshop to identify research needs to improve the monitoring of iodine status in the United States and to inform the DRI. *Nutr.* 2012;142(6):1175S-1185S. doi:10.3945/jn.111.156448
193. Panel on Dietary Reference Intakes for Electrolytes and Water; Standing Committee on the Scientific Evaluation of Dietary Reference Intakes; Food and Nutrition Board, Institute of Medicine of the National Academies. *Dietary Reference Intakes for Water, Potassium, Sodium, Chloride, and Sulfate.* National Academies Press; 2005.
194. McKenzie AL, Muñoz CX, Ellis LA, et al. Urine color as an indicator of urine concentration in pregnant and lactating women. *Eur Nutr.* 2017;56(1):355-362. doi:10.1007/s00394-015-1085-9
195. Huch R. Physical activity at altitude in pregnancy. *Semin Perinatol.* 1996;20:303-314. doi:10.1016/s0146-0005(96)80023-1
196. Artal R, Fortunato V, Welton A, et al. A comparison of cardiopulmonary adaptations to exercise in pregnancy at sea level and altitude. *Am J Obstet Gynecol.* 1995;172(4 pt 1):1170-1178; discussion 1178-1180. doi:10.1016/0002-9378(95)91475-7
197. Entin PL, Coffin L. Physiological basis for recommendations regarding exercise during pregnancy at high altitude. *High Alt Med Biol.* 2004;5:321-334. doi:10.1089/ham.2004.5.321
198. Tam C, Erebara A, Einarson A. Food-borne illness during pregnancy: prevention and treatment. *Can Fam Physician. 2010:*56(4):341-343.
199. *Food Safety for Pregnant Women, Their Unborn Babies, and Children Under Five.* US Food and Drug Administration; January 2022. Accessed July 25, 2024. www.fda.gov/media/83740/download
200. Williams JF, Smith VC; Committee on Substance Abuse. Fetal alcohol spectrum disorders. *Pediatrics.* 2015;136(5):e20153113. doi:10.1542/peds.2015-3113
201. American College of Obstetricians and Gynecologists, Committee on Obstetric Practice. ACOG committee opinion no. 462. Moderate caffeine consumption during pregnancy. *Obstet Gynecol.* 2010;116(2 part 1): 467-468. doi:10.1097/AOG.0b013e3181eeb2a1
202. Schweitzer AS. Dietary supplements during pregnancy. *Perinat Educ.* 2006;15(4):44-45. doi:10.1624/105812406X107834
203. Hung T-H, Chen S-F, Hsu J-J, Hsieh T-T. Gestational weight gain and risks for adverse perinatal outcomes: a retrospective cohort study based on the 2009 Institute of Medicine guidelines. *Taiwan Obstet Gynecol.* 2015;54(4):421-425. doi:10.1016/j.tjog.2015.06.010
204. Asvanarunat E. Outcomes of gestational weight gain outside the Institute of Medicine guidelines. *Med Assoc Thai.* 2014;97(11):1119-1125.
205. Haugen M, Brantsaeter AL, Winkvist A, et al. Associations of pre-pregnancy body mass index and gestational weight gain with pregnancy outcome and postpartum weight retention: a prospective observational cohort study. *BMC Pregnancy Childbirth.* 2014;14:201. doi:10.1186/1471-2393-14-201
206. Thorell E, Goldsmith L, Weiss G, Kristiansson P. Physical fitness, serum relaxin and duration of gestation. *BMC Pregnancy Childbirth.* 2015;15:168. doi:10.1186/s12884-015-0607-z
207. Petrov Fieril K, Glantz A, Fagevik Olsen M. The efficacy of moderate-to-vigorous resistance exercise during pregnancy: a randomized controlled trial. *Acta Obstet Gynecol Scand.* 2015;94(1):35-42. doi:10.1111/aogs.12525
208. American College of Sports Medicine. ACSM Information on Pregnancy Physical Activity. 2020. Accessed October 3, 2024. www.acsm.org/docs/default-source/files-for-resource-library/pregnancy-physical-activity.pdf?sfvrsn=12a73853_4
209. Forstmann N, Meignié A, De Larochelambert Q, et al. Does maternity during sports career jeopardize future athletic success in elite marathon runners? *Eur Sport Sci.* 2023;23(6):896-903. doi:10.1080/17461391.2022.2089054
210. Lessen R, Kavanaugh K. Position of the Academy of Nutrition and Dietetics: promoting and supporting breastfeeding. *Acad Nutr Diet.* 2015;115(3):444-449. doi:10.1016/j.jand.2014.12.014
211. Dewey KG, Lovelady CA, Nommsen-Rivers LA, McCrory MA, Lonnerdal B. A randomized study of the effects of aerobic exercise by lactating women on breast-milk volume and composition. *N Engl Med.* 1994;330(7):449-453. doi:10.1056/NEJM199402173300701
212. Lovelady CA, Hunter CP, Geigerman C. Effect of exercise on immunologic factors in breast milk. *Pediatrics.* 2003;111(2):E148-E152. doi:10.1542/peds.111.2.e148
213. Butte NF, King JC. Energy requirements during pregnancy and lactation. *Public Health Nutr.* 2005;8(7A):1010-1027. doi:10.1079/phn2005793
214. Oliveri B, Parisi MS, Zeni S, Maultalen C. Mineral and bone mass changes during pregnancy and lactation. *Nutrition.* 2004;20(2):235-240. doi:10.1016/j.nut.2003.10.011
215. Kim HJ, Kwon H, Oh SW, et al. Breast feeding is associated with postmenopausal bone loss: findings from the Korea National Health and Nutrition Examination Survey. *Korean Fam Med.* 2015;36(5):216-220. doi:10.4082/kjfm.2015.36.5.216
216. Ferrari RM, Siega-Riz AM, Evernson KR, Moos MK, Melvin CL, Herring AH. Provider advice about weight loss and physical activity in the postpartum period. *Womens Health.* 2010;19(3):397-406. doi:10.1089/jwh.2008.1332
217. López-Olmedo N, Hernández-Cordero S, Neufeld LM, Garcia-Guerra A, Mejia-Rodriguez F, Gómez-Humaran M. The associations of maternal weight change with breastfeeding, diet and physical activity during the postpartum period. *Matern Child Health J.* 2016;20(2):270-280. doi:10.1007/s10995-015-1826-7
218. Nascimento SL, Pudwell J, Surita FG, Adamo KB, Smith GN. The effect of physical exercise strategies on weight loss in postpartum women: a systematic review and meta-analysis. *Int Obes (Lond).* 2014;38(5):626-635. doi:10.1038/ijo.2013.183
219. Lim S, O'Reilly S, Behrens H, Skinner T, Ellis I, Dunbar JA. Effective strategies for weight loss in post-partum women: a systematic review and meta-analysis. *Obes Rev.* 2015;16(11):972-987. doi:10.1111/obr.12312

220. Subcommittee for a Clinical Application Guide, Committee on Nutritional Status During Pregnancy and Lactation, Food and Nutrition Board, Institute of Medicine. *Nutrition During Pregnancy and Lactation: An Implementation Guide.* National Academies Press; 1992.

221. American College of Obstetricians and Gynecologists, Committee on Obstetric Practice. ACOG committee opinion no. 650. Physical activity and exercise during pregnancy and the postpartum period. *Obstet Gynecol.* 2015;126:e135-e142. doi:10.1097/AOG.0000000000001214

222. Kahyoglu Sut H, Balkanli Kaplan P. Effect of pelvic floor muscle exercise on pelvic floor muscle activity and voiding functions during pregnancy and the postpartum period. *Neurourol Urodyn.* 2016;35(3):417-422. doi:10.1002/nau.22728

223. Zhou Y-n, Wu Q-k, Cheng H, Teng Y-c. Relationship between serum relaxin levels and female pelvic floor prolapse. *Shanghai Jiaotong Univ (Med Sci Ed) [Shanghai Jiaotong Daxue Xuebao, Yixueban].* 2012;32(4):393-395. doi:10.3969/j.issn.1674-8115.2012.04.004

224. Clapp JF 3rd. Long-term outcome after exercising throughout pregnancy: fitness and cardiovascular risk. *Am Obstet Gynecol.* 2008;199(5):489.e1-489.e4896. doi:10.1016/j.ajog.2008.05.006

225. Clapp JF 3rd, Capeless E. The VO2max of recreational athletes before and after pregnancy. *Med Sci Sports Exerc.* 1991;23(10):1128-1133.

226. Clapp JF 3rd, Capeless E. Cardiovascular function before, during, and after the first and subsequent pregnancies. *Am Cardiol.* 1997;80(11):1469-1473. doi:10.1016/s0002-9149(97)00738-8

227. Donnelly GM, Moore IS, Brockwell E, Rankin A, Cooke R. Reframing return-to-sport postpartum: the 6 Rs framework. *Br Sports Med.* 2022;56(5):244-245. doi:10.1136/bjsports-2021-104877

228. Davenport MH, Nesdoly A, Ray L, Thornton JS, Khurana R, McHugh T-LF. Pushing for change: a qualitative study of the experiences of elite athletes during pregnancy. *Br Sports Med.* 2022;56(8):452-457. doi:10.1136/bjsports-2021-104755

CHAPTER 18

Eating Disorders in Athletes

Christina Scribner, MS, RDN, CSSD, CEDS, and Katherine Beals, PhD, RD, FACSM, CSSD

LEARNING OBJECTIVES

- Describe the spectrum of disordered eating and eating disorders.
- Describe the prevalence of eating disorders among athletes.
- Recognize risk factors, signs, and symptoms of disordered eating and eating disorders.
- Identify therapeutic approaches to reestablish healthy eating patterns.
- Explain strategies to optimize nutrition therapy and engage in self-care.

INTRODUCTION

Participation in athletics confers a multitude of physical, physiological, and psychological benefits. Nonetheless, for some athletes, pressures within the sports environment (along with other predisposing factors) can increase the risk of developing disordered eating (DE). Whereas the prevalence of clinical eating disorders (EDs) in athletes is similar to that in nonathletes, DE behaviors appear to plague athletes at a greater rate, particularly in sports that emphasize leanness. The health consequences of DE and EDs are significant and can be severe. Thus, prompt identification, intervention, and treatment are critical. Registered dietitian nutritionists (RDNs) serve a critical role for athletes, blending their knowledge of medical nutrition with an understanding of behavior change and collaboration.

The purpose of this chapter is to provide an overview of theoretical and applied science related to the risk, identification, and care of athletes living with EDs and DE. This chapter provides background to aid in the development of a greater understanding of affected individuals, as well as an overall view of the spectrum of DE and EDs within the athletic population.

A variety of potential strategies can be considered based on the specific needs of the individual and the resources available to the practitioner for achieving nutritional rehabilitation as identified through the maintenance of weight within a healthy range. This is determined by a combination of BMI or growth trajectory, reproductive health, and predominantly healthful thoughts and behaviors related to food and body that result in an overall improved state of health. The RDN is an integral member of an interdisciplinary treatment team that, at its core, includes a physician, RDN, and licensed mental health therapist,[1] and potentially also a psychiatrist, physical therapist, athletic trainer, coach, and others in the athlete's entourage.[2]

An overview of therapeutic modalities and treatment models, the qualifications and therapeutic qualities of effective RDNs, and best-practice strategies in the provision of medical nutrition therapy as part of an interdisciplinary approach is provided. The knowledge and experience of veteran sports RDNs in treating athletes with EDs is offered as practical clinical suggestions. Skills and support for the RDN serving people who are living with DE and EDs is suggested. Finally, suggestions for preventing EDs and DE among athletes are shared.

With the increasing visibility of EDs and its preceeding DE in athletes has come the need to recruit personnel for programs that can identify, treat, manage, and help prevent EDs. Sports RDNs are often among the first to come into contact with an athlete with DE or an ED. It is essential that the sports RDN has a firm understanding of DE and EDs and is prepared to provide appropriate nutrition-based care.

EATING DISORDER CLASSIFICATIONS

Eating disorders are diagnosed and classified according to criteria published by the American Psychiatric Association (APA). The APA has published the *Diagnostic and Statistical Manual of Mental Disorders* (*DSM*) as a guide to the diagnosis of mental disorders affecting mood, personality, identity, and cognition for health care professionals around the world since 1952. The 5th edition, known as *DSM-5*, was published in 2013. Nine years later, new scientific advances warranted a revision (March 2022) rather than a new edition. *DSM-5-TR* (Text Revision) provides increased clarity to avoid misclassification of mental disorders.[3] Many of the changes in the current version reflect the issues that became more apparent during the COVID-19 pandemic and traumas around the world. These changes include the language used in relation to ethnoracial differences, racism, and discrimination that affect psychiatric diagnoses. Terms such as *Caucasian*, *race*, *racial*, and *minority* were dropped. *Ethnoracial* is used in alignment with US Census categories, such as Hispanic, White, and African American, that combine ethnic and racialized identifiers.[4]

The *International Classification of Disease (ICD)*, maintained by the World Health Organization (WHO), is an alphanumeric system used to code diseases and medical conditions. *DSM-5-TR* uses a modification of the 10th *ICD* revision (effective since 2015), known as *ICD-10-CM*, which is the clinical modification version of the WHO's *ICD-10*.[5] The clinical modification of the *ICD* by the Centers for Disease Control and Prevention's (CDC's) National Center for Health Statistics (NCHS) is used to code and classify morbidity data from inpatient and outpatient records, physician offices, and most NCHS surveys. Using the *DSM-5-TR* along with *ICD* codes and coding nutrition counseling and therapy using the current procedural terminology (CPT) coding system is fundamental to recordkeeping and insurance reimbursement. Furthermore, it allows practitioners to contribute to the collection of data and statistical information toward health-related statistics. Whereas *ICD-10* is still in use at the time of this writing, *ICD-11* was approved in 2019 and released by the WHO for global use on January 1, 2022. Nevertheless, it will likely take an additional 4 to 5 years for *ICD-11* to be fully implemented in the United States.[6] *ICD-11* is described as a more flexible system requiring less training to implement.[7]

Eating disorders are covered in *DSM-5* Chapter 10, titled Feeding and Eating Disorders. The chapter describes the variety of "persistent disturbance of eating or eating-related behavior that results in the altered consumption or absorption of food and that significantly impairs physical health or psychosocial functioning." Detailed and updated descriptions for each of the EDs are available online from the APA.[8] Box 18.1 summarizes the *DSM-5* criteria for EDs.[3,8-11]

Although coding according to the *DSM* is important, the regimented training diet, extreme levels of physical activity, attention to body weight and shape, and particulars of body composition relative to competitive sports complicates use of the *DSM-5* criteria among athletes,[2] leaving more to clinical interpretation.

The Spectrum of Disordered Eating and Eating Disorders

Although often used interchangeably, the terms *disordered eating* and *eating disorder* are not interchangeable. In fact, the term *disordered eating* is currently not specifically defined by authoritative organizations (eg, the Academy for Eating Disorders, the National Eating Disorders Association, or the International Association of Eating Disorders Professionals) but is generally used as an umbrella term to encompass a range of dysfunctional and disordered thoughts and behaviors surrounding food and eating, including (but not limited to) a clinical ED. On the other hand, the term *eating disorder* refers to one of the clinical conditions delineated by the *DSM-5-TR* (refer to Box 18.1).

BOX 18.1 Summary of Criteria for Identifying Feeding and Eating Disorders from the Diagnostic and Statistical Manual of Mental Disorders, 5th ed[3,8-11]

Anorexia nervosa (AN)

Dietary restriction of energy intake relative to requirements, leading to significantly low (less than minimally normal or, for youth, less than minimally expected) body weight in the context of age, sex, developmental trajectory, and physical health

Intense fear of gaining weight or of becoming fat, or persistent behavior that interferes with weight gain, even though at a significantly low weight

Disturbance in the way one's body weight or shape is experienced, undue influence of body weight or shape on self-evaluation, or persistent lack of recognition of the seriousness of low body weight

Subtype unspecified (*International Classification of Disease*, 10th ed [*ICD-10*], F50.0; *International Classification of Disease*, 11th ed [*ICD-11*], 6B80)

Subtypes include

- Restricting type (*ICD-10*, F50.01): During the past 3 months, the individual has not engaged in recurrent episodes of binge eating or purging behavior (ie, self-induced vomiting or the misuse of laxatives, diuretics, or enemas); this subtype describes individuals who engage in dieting or fasting and/or excessive exercise
- Anorexia nervosa with significantly low body weight, unspecified (*ICD-11*, 6B80.0Z)
- Anorexia nervosa with dangerously low body weight, unspecified (*ICD-11*, 6B80.1Z)
- Anorexia nervosa with significantly low body weight, restricting pattern (*ICD-11*, 6B80.00)
- Anorexia nervosa with dangerously low body weight, restricting pattern (*ICD-11*, 6B80.10)
- Anorexia nervosa in recovery with normal body weight (*ICD-11*, 6B80.2)
- Binge-eating/purging type (*ICD-10*, F50.02; *ICD-11*, 6B81): During the past 3 months, the individual has engaged in recurrent episodes of binge-eating or purging behavior (eg, self-induced vomiting or the misuse of laxatives, diuretics, or enemas)
- Anorexia nervosa with significantly low body weight, binge-purge pattern (*ICD-11*, 6B80.01)
- Anorexia nervosa with dangerously low body weight, binge-purge pattern (*ICD-11*, 6B80.11)

Current severity

Mild: BMI of 17 or greater

Moderate: BMI of 16 to 16.99

Severe: BMI of 15 to 15.99

Extreme: BMI less than 15

Remission types

Partial: After full criteria for AN were met, the individual no longer meets low body weight but continues to experience intense fear of gaining weight or becoming fat, exhibits behaviors that interfere with weight gain, or exhibits a disturbance in self-perception of weight and shape

Full: After full criteria for AN were met, none of the criteria have been met for a sustained period

Continued on next page

BOX 18.1 *Summary of Criteria for Identifying Feeding and Eating Disorders from the Diagnostic and Statistical Manual of Mental Disorders, 5th ed*[3,8-11] **(CONTINUED)**

Bulimia nervosa (BN)

Recurrent episodes of binge eating (eating in a discrete period [eg, 2 h] an amount of food that is definitely larger than what most people would eat in a similar time period and under similar circumstances with a feeling that one cannot stop or control what or how much is eaten)

Recurrent inappropriate compensatory behaviors or purging intended to prevent weight gain (eg, self-induced vomiting; misuse of laxatives, diuretics, or other medications; fasting; excessive exercise)

Self-evaluation is unduly influenced by body shape and weight

Behaviors occur on average once per week for 3 months

Disturbance does not occur exclusively during episodes of AN

(*ICD-10*, F50.2; *ICD-11*, 6B81)

Current severity

Mild: Average of 1 to 3 episodes of inappropriate compensatory behaviors per week

Moderate: Average of 4 to 7 episodes of inappropriate compensatory behaviors per week

Severe: Average of 8 to 13 episodes of inappropriate compensatory behaviors per week

Extreme: Average of 14 or more episodes of inappropriate compensatory behaviors per week

Remission types

Partial: After full criteria for BN were met, the individual no longer meets all of the criteria for a sustained period

Full: After full criteria for BN were met, none of the criteria have been met for a sustained period

Binge-eating disorder (BED)

Presence of recurrent binge-eating episodes (as described for BN)

Binge-eating episodes are associated with 3 or more of the following symptoms:

- eating much more rapidly than normal
- eating until uncomfortably full
- eating large amounts of food in the absence of physical hunger
- eating alone and feeling embarrassed by how much one is eating
- feeling disgusted with oneself, depressed, or very guilty afterward

Marked distress regarding binge eating

Binge eating occurs, on average, at least once per week for 3 months

Binge eating is not associated with recurrent use of inappropriate compensatory behavior and does not occur exclusively during AN or BN

(*ICD-10*, F50.8; *ICD-11*, 6B82)

Current severity

Mild: 1 to 3 binge-eating episodes per week

Moderate: 4 to 7 binge-eating episodes per week

Severe: 8 to 13 binge-eating episodes per week

Extreme: 14 or more binge-eating episodes per week

Remission types

Partial: After full criteria for BED were met, the individual engages in binge eating at an average frequency of less than once per week

Full: After full criteria for BED were met, none of the criteria have been met for a sustained period

Avoidant/restrictive food intake disorder (ARFID)

An eating or feeding disturbance that results in at least 1 of the following:

- significant weight loss or failure to achieve expected weight gain or faltering growth in children
- significant nutritional deficiency
- dependence on enteral feeding or oral nutritional supplements
- marked interference with psychosocial functioning

Disturbance is not better explained by a lack of available food or by a cultural practice

ARFID does not entail disturbance in body weight or shape, nor is it attributable to another eating disorder or mental disorder

The eating disturbance is not attributable to a concurrent medical condition and is not better explained by another mental disorder

When it co-occurs with another condition or disorder, the severity of the eating disturbance exceeds that routinely associated with the condition or disorder and warrants additional clinical attention

(*ICD-10*, F50.82; *ICD-11*, 6B83)

Full remission

After criteria for ARFID have been met, the criteria have not been met for a sustained period

Pica

Persistent eating of nonnutritive, nonfood substances that are not part of a culturally supported or socially normative practice over a period of at least 1 month

Inappropriate eating behavior for the developmental level of the individual that is typically not diagnosed prior to the age of 2 years; may occur among children who are otherwise developing normally

Pica in adults is frequently related to intellectual disability or other mental disorders

When pica occurs in the context of another mental disorder (eg, intellectual disability, autism, schizophrenia) or medical condition (eg, pregnancy), it is sufficiently severe to warrant additional clinical attention

Continued on next page

BOX 18.1 Summary of Criteria for Identifying Feeding and Eating Disorders from the Diagnostic and Statistical Manual of Mental Disorders, 5th ed[3,8-11] (CONTINUED)

(*ICD-10*, F98.3 [in children]; (*ICD-10*, F50.8 [in adults])

(*ICD-11*, 6B84)

Full remission

After criteria for pica have been met, the criteria have not been met for a sustained period

Rumination disorder

Repeated regurgitation of food (rechewed, reswallowed, or spit out) that is not related to another gastrointestinal or medical condition (eg, nausea or reflux), nor does it occur exclusively during AN, BN, BED, or ARFID, for at least 1 month

If the symptoms occur in the context of another mental disorder (eg, intellectual disability or another neurological disorder), they are sufficiently severe to warrant additional clinical attention

(*ICD-10*, F98.21; *ICD-11*, 6B85)

Full remission

After criteria for rumination disorder have been met, the criteria have not been met for a sustained period

Other specified feeding or eating disorder[a] (OSFED)

Applies to symptoms characteristic of a feeding and eating disorder that cause clinically significant distress or impairment in social, occupational, or other important areas of functioning but do not meet the full criteria for any of the other diagnostic classes

Clinicians identify the reason the disorder does not meet criteria for another feeding or eating disorder (eg, atypical anorexia nervosa: all criteria for AN met except abnormally low body weight)

(*ICD-10*, F 50.89, 6B8Y)

(Other specified anorexia nervosa *ICD-11*, 6B80.Y)

Atypical AN (eg, lacks the significant weight criteria for AN, yet may experience many of the physiological complications associated with AN)

BN (of low frequency and/or limited duration)

BED (of low frequency and/or limited duration)

Purging disorder: Recurrent purging behavior to influence weight or shape in the absence of binge eating

Night eating syndrome: Recurrent episodes of night eating manifested by awakening from sleep or by excessive food consumption after the evening meal that causes significant distress and/or impairment of functioning; disorder is not explained by other mental disorder or BED, including substance use or effect of medication

Unspecified feeding or eating disorder (UFED)

Applies to the presentation of symptoms characteristic of a feeding and eating disorder that cause clinically significant distress or impairment in social, occupational, or other important areas of functioning but do not meet the full diagnostic criteria for any of the other disorders in feeding and eating disorders

This category may also apply in situations when the practitioner does not specify why criteria do not meet a more specific diagnosis or has insufficient information to make a diagnosis of another specific feeding and eating disorder (eg, urgent care settings)

(*ICD-10*, F50.9; *ICD-11*, 6B8Y)

[a] Note that OSFED was previously known as "*eating disorder not otherwise specified (EDNOS)*." The name of this disorder was updated with the release of *DSM-5*.

When one is living with DE, changes in thoughts and behaviors occur that may be transient. For example, someone may engage in DE to lose weight, in response to grief over the loss of a loved one or relationship, in answer to the stress related to athletic events, or in reaction to an injury or illness. The food-related behaviors that result reflect a *temporary* change in eating patterns and critical self-evaluation. DE may also reflect long-term attitudes and behaviors and are sometimes described simply as "an unhealthy relationship with food" or subclinical ED. When DE occurs for prolonged periods, it may result in significant physical, psychological, and social damage or dysfunction and may progress into a clinical ED. Whereas less extreme forms of DE are much more prevalent than clinical EDs, both DE and EDs are worthy of serious attention and have the potential for medical instability or even death.

To be diagnosed with a clinical ED, an individual must meet a standard set of criteria as outlined in the *DSM-5-TR*.[9] An ED refers to a potentially life-threatening mental illness that can have long-standing adverse consequences on the individual's psychosocial and physical health and reduces their quality of life.[12,13] When someone has an ED, thoughts and behaviors related to food and body consume much of their life. An ED involves complex thought processes and typically affects numerous body systems, leading to multiple serious physical and psychosocial problems.

The *DSM* identifies clinical mental disorders based on criteria that define problematic behavioral disorders across the lifespan. The updated diagnostic criteria of *DSM-5* for *anorexia nervosa (AN)* and *bulimia nervosa (BN)* differ from diagnostic criteria in the previous edition by not requiring the overvaluation of weight, shape, or other body-image disturbance.[9,14] *Binge-eating disorder (BED)* was first included as its own category of ED in *DSM-5*[9] and is considered the most common ED in the United States.[15]

Avoidant/restrictive food intake disorder (ARFID) was also introduced in *DSM-5* and describes individuals who experience clinically significant struggles with food and eating.[9] Those with ARFID are diverse in terms of age, medical and psychiatric comorbidities, severity, nutritional status, motor skills, and psychosocial function. Neither BED nor ARFID require weight outside the "normal weight" range for diagnosis. It is not always immediately clear when an individual's decision to limit or avoid food is "disordered" because many public health problems of our time are related to food. Disordered eating can appear in many forms, including under the guise of following a healthy lifestyle. Von Essen and Mårtensson[16] reported on young adults in Sweden who attempted to use food choice as a means toward a healthy lifestyle. Their findings revealed that the preferred diet was typically organic and that their food practices included both "looking inward" for direction on food choice and using food as an "outward-bound" strategy toward making the world more understandable and friendly. It is common to see food choice reflecting an individual's knowledge or belief about how food affects physical, mental, or social health, as well as the health of the planet. However, there is a point at which trends in eating do not support optimal health, as with EDs.

Steven Bratman, MD, author of *Health Food Junkies: Orthorexia Nervosa: Overcoming the Obsession With Healthful Eating*,[17] coined the term *orthorexia* in a 1977 issue of *Yoga Journal*. Experts have proposed diagnostic criteria for orthorexia nervosa (ON) to identify the pathological eating pattern characterized by an extreme and unhealthy obsession to "eat right." The criteria included consumption of a nutritionally unbalanced diet related to preoccupation with food purity or the effect of food on physical or emotional health, rigid avoidance of foods deemed unhealthy, a sense of worry and guilt related to transgressions, intolerance of others' food beliefs, and spending excessive amounts on food relative to one's income. Additional criteria identify impaired physical health (eg, malnutrition) resulting from nutritional imbalance and severe distress. Finally, the obsessive preoccupation with food in ON is not an exacerbation of another disorder. People with ON avoid foods that they perceive as being unhealthy, that contain ingredients that they feel are undesirable, or that were prepared in a manner that violates their value system. Case reports among individuals with such preoccupations reveal severe medical findings similar to those found with malnutrition secondary to AN.[18]

It is important for health care practitioners to recognize that ED symptoms rarely exist in isolation and that individuals living with EDs often cross over between and among various specific disorders, presenting with changing symptoms over the course of the illness. Crossover is more common in the initial years of illness. For example, individuals with AN-restrictive subtype may develop symptoms of binge eating or purging AN and then cross over to BN. Transition between specific ED categories and unspecified EDs is common, with the movement to an unspecified ED often representing movement toward recovery.[19] Box 18.2 provides a case example of a teenager with ARFID.

BOX 18.2 Avoidant/Restrictive Food Intake Disorder Case Example

Anna is a 17-year-old girl with a history of picky eating since early childhood. She generally eats foods that are not mixed with others and fears that she will choke on foods that seem unfamiliar. In third grade, her best friend moved, and shortly thereafter, her grandmother died suddenly and unexpectedly. Her mother described these losses as a "turning point" when Anna was no longer responding to eating through bribery as she did when she was younger. Anna experiences anxiety, restless sleep, and facial tics. She has recently gotten her driver's license but is fearful of driving. Anna wants to graduate high school with straight A's. She procrastinates on homework and fears authority figures. She is using psychotherapy and psychiatry. She is motivated to make progress in nutrition therapy by her desire to be able to eat socially with friends.

Growth chart percentiles: Weight for age, 67th percentile; stature for age, 77th percentile; BMI for age, 54th percentile.

In this example, Anna created a hierarchy of foods that described her food preferences and comfort levels. Nutrition therapy focused on gradual food exposure and increasing combinations of new foods with various textures and sizes along with foods that are liked and accepted to successfully improve Anna's sense of safety and confidence in eating a wide variety of foods.

Excessive Exercise in Disordered Eating and Eating Disorders

Issues with physical activity often coexist with eating problems; some people avoid activity, and others depend on it. Whereas only about a quarter of American adults and youth met the recommendations outlined in the *Physical Activity Guidelines for Americans* for both aerobic and muscle-strengthening activities,[20] a subset of people engage in an unhealthy obsession with exercise, which can lead to a host of negative physical and mental effects including musculoskeletal injuries, metabolic derangements, cardiovascular stress, nutrient deficiencies, anxiety, and depression.[21,22] The term *exercise* falls under the umbrella of physical activity. *Physical activity* refers to a variety of types of bodily movement, whereas *exercise* is undertaken with a purpose and a structure that includes repetition.[23] Avoidance of exercise or excessive exercise alone do not qualify as an ED. (Exercise avoidance may be related to weight stigma, trauma, or bullying.) Excessive exercise may be a dysfunctional strategy toward feeling better or a means of purging unwanted energy intake, or it may present as a behavior related to another disorder that includes compulsive or obsessive behavior and coexists with the diagnosis of an ED. Excessive exercise is commonly explained by those who overexercise as their means of managing uncomfortable thoughts or emotions.

Obsession with exercise is important for health care practitioners to assess as it may be part of the pathology of an ED, where exercise is a secondary means of controlling body weight or shape.[22] Excessive exercise is often referred to in the literature as "exercise addiction." Landolfi[24] distinguished between healthy (committed) levels of exercise and exercise addiction. Criteria for exercise addiction included continued exercise regardless of physical injury or psychological or social consequences (eg, personal inconvenience or disruption to other areas of life, including marriage, employment, and lack of time for other activities that interfere with exercise). Exercise addiction is related to intrinsic rewards such as feeling greater self-esteem and confidence, as well as the experience of disturbing sensations of deprivation when unable to exercise. Committed exercisers are motivated by extrinsic rewards such as achieving an award or beating a time, distance, or competitor and do not experience severe withdrawal symptoms (as identified by Cook and Hausenblas[25] in their characterization of exercise dependence) when they cannot exercise. Excessive exercisers lack life balance characterized by rest and recovery and engage in a level of exercise that is not sustainable in terms of long-term physical, psychological, and social health outcomes.[24]

Identification of "excessive" exercise can be challenging in the athlete population. The training programs undertaken by many athletes (particularly elite and/or ultraendurance athletes) could be considered excessive but are necessary to achieve training and performance goals. This level of exercise could be considered excessive by the general population but may be necessary for training; the amount of exercise is not the issue. Exercise addiction is not included in *DSM-5* as there are no clinical criteria to make the diagnosis.[22] Thus, motivation for the exercise needs to be considered. Screening for risk of addiction to exercise in the Exercise Addiction Inventory-Revised (EAI-R) is based on symptoms of substance abuse and behavior-based addiction. The EAI-R is a 6-item questionnaire that rates constructs of addiction to exercise on a 5-point agree-disagree scale to assess risk. A total score of 24 to 30 suggests high risk of addiction.[22,26] See Box 18.3.[22]

BOX 18.3 Exercise Addiction Inventory-Revised (EAI-R) Core Symptoms of Exercise Addiction[22]

1. Exercise is the most important thing in my life.
2. I have conflicts with family or friends because I exercise so much.
3. I use exercise to change my mood (eg, to feel happier or forget about problems).
4. Over the last year, I have increased the amount of daily exercise that I do.
5. If I don't exercise every day, I get restless, upset, or sad.
6. I have tried to reduce the amount of exercise I do but end up exercising as much as I did before.

The EAI-R has been applied to a variety of active populations, from leisure exercisers to elite athletes. About 3% of leisure exercisers are thought to be at risk for exercise addiction, with the risk increasing for athletes in a variety of disciplines, reaching 17% to 34% among elite athletes. Lichtenstein et al[22] found no difference between the genders in terms of risk among elite athletes. However, younger age and acute or overuse injury were associated with higher risk. Increased risk of exercise addiction was also associated with an increased risk of EDs.

PREVALENCE OF DISORDERED EATING AND EATING DISORDERS IN ATHLETES

At the time of this publication, no large-scale, international epidemiological studies of DE and/or EDs among athletes have been published. Thus, the "true" prevalence of DE and EDs among athletes is currently unknown. Published data examining DE in elite Norwegian athletes, US collegiate athletes, and larger samples of single-sport athletes (most often endurance athletes) indicate prevalence ranges from 6% to 45% in female athletes and from 0% to 19% in male athletes. Prevalence estimates for the clinically recognized EDs among competitive athletes tend to be somewhat lower. Estimates for female athletes are as follows: AN, 0% to 6.7%; BN, 0% to 12.1%; and eating disorder not otherwise specified (EDNOS; now termed OSFED), 2% to 13.4%. For male athletes, the estimates are as follows: AN, 0%; BN, 0% to 7.5%; and EDNOS, 0% to 9.7%.[27] The ranges in the prevalence estimates are likely explained by discrepancies in 1 or more of the following: the screening instruments/assessment tools used, the definitions of DE and EDs employed, and the accuracy of self-reporting among the athlete populations studied.

Most studies examining the prevalence of EDs among athletes used 1 or more of the following self-report instruments: the Eating Attitudes Test (EAT), the Eating Disorder Inventory (EDI), the 3-Factor Eating Questionnaire, and/or the Bulimia Test Revised (BULIT-R). These questionnaires, although validated in the general population, have not been sufficiently validated in an athletic population; thus, any data on athletes derived from studies using them could be subject to error.[28,29] Screening tools specific to female athletes that have been validated and used to estimate the prevalence of DE/EDs among this population include the Female Athlete Screening Tool (FAST), the Athletic Milieu Direct Questionnaire (AMDQ), the Physiologic Screening Test, and the Survey of Eating Disorders among Athletes (SEDA). Because they were developed to screen for DE/EDs in female athletes, these instruments may or may not be valid and reliable tools to assess DE/EDs in male athletes. More recently, the Eating Disorders Screen for Athletes (EDSA) and the Disordered Eating Screen for Athletes (DESA-6) were created to assess eating pathology among both male and female athletes. Schaefer, Crosby, and Machado[30] summarized self-report and interview instruments for assessing DE and EDs among adults. Keep in mind that self-report questionnaires, regardless of their specificity to a given population, are subject to inaccuracies and reporting bias (which is especially true for those living with DE/EDs).[27,29] Finally, the variety of measures used in different prevalence studies makes inconsistencies in prevalence estimates more likely and comparisons between and among studies extremely difficult.

Studies have also varied widely in how they have defined EDs. Whereas some studies adhered to the strict *DSM* criteria and required rigorous interviews to diagnose EDs, others used only self-report questionnaires, symptom checklists, and/or risk factor identifiers that are more likely indicative of DE. The use of stricter criteria will result in lower prevalence estimates, whereas the use of more liberal criteria will result in higher prevalence estimates. Finally, studies have varied greatly in the sample populations studied, including the ages and sexes of athletes, the types of athletes (eg, recreational, high school, collegiate, and elite athletes, as well as physically active individuals), and the types of sports (endurance, strength, aesthetic, lean-build, non-lean-build, etc). The population studied can have a significant impact on the prevalence estimates generated.

Table 18.1 presents some of the more recent (post-2000) prevalence studies (along with 2 large-scale prevalence studies that have been widely cited).[31-57] From the data contained within the table, it is possible to make general conclusions regarding the prevalence of DE/EDs among athletes.

- Research consistently shows that the prevalence of DE is greater than the prevalence of clinical EDs among athletes. Whereas earlier studies seemed to suggest that athletes were at greater risk of DE/EDs than nonathletic controls, more recent studies do not always concur. The discrepancies again seem to be due to differences in the athletic population studied (eg, elite vs more recreational athletes, high school vs collegiate vs Olympic/professional athletes).[27]
- Although all athletes in any sport may be at risk for developing DE/EDs, the prevalence of DE has consistently been shown to be higher in those that participate in thin-build or weight-dependent sports.[27] These sports can be categorized into 3 groups: (1) aesthetic sports, such as diving, figure skating, gymnastics, and synchronized swimming; (2) sports in which low body mass and body-fat levels are considered a physical or biomechanical advantage, such as distance running, road cycling, and triathlon; and (3) sports that require weight categories for competition, such as lightweight rowing, weightlifting, and wrestling.[28]
- The prevalence of EDs and DE is higher among female athletes than among male athletes.[27] Interestingly, research suggests that there is an interaction between sex and sport in terms of DE prevalence. For example, Schaal and colleagues[31] reported that the prevalence of DE was highest in endurance sports among female athletes, whereas in males, it was most prevalent in the weight-dependent sports.

TABLE 18.1 Summary of Recent (Post-2000) Studies Examining the Prevalence of Disordered Eating in Athletes[31-57]

Study, country	Sample	Instrument	Prevalence
Berg et al (2022), United States[32]	146 female distance runners (participants in Olympic Marathon trials)	Questionnaire developed by the authors that included self-reported diagnosis of an ED and weight-control behaviors	32% of participants reported previous EDs, whereas 6% reported a current ED
Smith et al (2022), United States[33]	268 competitive female cheerleaders	EAT-26	34% scored above the cutoff for ED risk
Borgelt and Burmeister (2022), United States[34]	330 collegiate English equestrian athletes	EAT-26	35% of the athletes exceeded the cutoff for DE
Martínez-Rodríguez et al (2021), Spain[35]	69 elite male and female handball players from the Spanish national beach handball team	EAT-26	11% of females and 3% of males were classified as "at risk" for an ED
Joubert et al (2020), United States[36]	604 elite international male and female rock climbers	EAT-26	16.5% of female climbers and 6.3% of male climbers were scored above the cutoff for DE
Prather et al (2016), United States[37]	220 female soccer players (grade/middle school, high school, collegiate, and professional)	EAT-26	8.1% were considered "at risk" for an ED
Thiemann et al (2015), Germany[38]	108 German professional athletes (46 in aesthetic sports and 62 in ball-game sports) and 108 nonathletic control subjects	Self-report questionnaire and clinical interview	17% of athletes from aesthetic sports, 3% of athletes from ball-game sports, and 2% of nonathletes were classified as having an ED
Fortes et al (2014), Portugal[39]	580 male and female high school athletes and 362 age-matched nonathletes	EAT-26	18% of female athletes and 14% of male athletes showed ED symptoms based on EAT-26 scores compared with 26% and 15% of female and male nonathletes, respectively
Chatterton and Petrie (2013), United States[40]	732 male collegiate athletes	Q-EDD; 7 items from the BULIT-R	16% reported DE symptoms; 1% were classified as having an ED (EDNOS)

Continued on next page

TABLE 18.1 Summary of Recent (Post-2000) Studies Examining the Prevalence of Disordered Eating in Athletes[31-57] (CONTINUED)

Study, country	Sample	Instrument	Prevalence
Goltz et al (2013), Brazil[41]	150 male athletes in aesthetic and weight-dependent sports	EAT-26, BITE, BSQ	DE behaviors and body-image dissatisfaction were found in 43 athletes (28%) in aesthetic sports and 23 athletes (15%) in weight-dependent sports
Martinsen and Sundgot-Borgen (2013), Norway[42]	611 elite adolescent male and female athletes and 355 adolescent male and female control subjects	Two-stage screening process consisting of a questionnaire developed by the authors, including subscales of the EDI-2, weight history, and self-reported history of EDs (stage 1), followed by a clinical interview using the EDE and EDE-Q (stage 2)	After the initial screening, 51% of the control subjects and 25% of the athletes were classified as "at risk" for an ED. In stage 2, the prevalence of EDs among the total population of athletes was estimated to be 7% compared to an estimate of 2% among the total population of control subjects, with the ED prevalence higher for female athletes than male athletes (14% vs 3%, $P < .001$) and for female than male control subjects (5% vs 0%, $P < .001$)
Schaal et al (2011), France[31]	2,067 male and female elite athletes	Psychological evaluation using *DSM-IV* criteria for clinical EDs	6% of female athletes and 4% of male athletes indicated a current or ongoing ED; 11% of female athletes and 5.5% of male athletes reported a history of EDs
Thein-Nissenbaum et al (2011), United States[43]	311 female high school athletes	EDE-Q	35% of female athletes presented with symptoms of DE
Martinsen et al (2010), Norway[44]	606 elite male and female high school athletes and 355 male and female control subjects	Questionnaire developed by the authors, including dieting, use of pathogenic weight-control methods, and the drive for thinness and body dissatisfaction subscales from the EDI	45% of female athletes and 13% of male athletes reported symptoms of DE compared with 71% and 30% of female and male control subjects, respectively

Study, country	Sample	Instrument	Prevalence
Greenleaf et al (2009), United States[45]	204 female collegiate athletes	Q-EDD and BULIT-R	2% of athletes were classified as having an ED; 26% had symptoms consistent with DE
Rosendahl et al (2009), Germany[46]	576 male and female high school athletes and 291 adolescent male and female control subjects	EAT-26	27% of female athletes and 10% of male athletes met the criteria for DE based on EAT-26 scores compared with 36% of female and 12% of male controls
Petrie et al (2008), United States[47]	203 collegiate male athletes	Q-EDD and BULIT-R	None of the athletes presented with a clinical ED; 19% showed symptoms of EDs based on the 2 self-report instruments
Torstveit et al (2008), Norway[48]	186 adolescent and adult female elite athletes and 145 nonathletic female control subjects	EDE-Q and clinical interview	33% of athletes and 21% of nonathletic control subjects were classified as having an ED based on the clinical interview
Nichols et al (2007), United States[49]	423 female high school athletes	EDE-Q	20% of athletes met the EDE-Q criteria for DE
Nichols et al (2006), United States[50]	170 female high school athletes	In-depth interview developed by the authors using the EDE	18% met the criteria for DE
Beals and Hill (2006), United States[51]	112 female collegiate athletes	Questionnaire developed by the authors, including the EDE-Q and Eating Disorder Inventory Symptom Checklist	3% of athletes self-reported a clinical ED; 23% of athletes met the criteria for DE
Toro et al (2005), United Kingdom[52]	283 elite female athletes competing in 20 sports	EAT and CETCA (based on *DSM-III-R* criteria)	11% of the athletes exceeded the EAT cutoff score; 2.5% and 20% of the athletes met the CETCA criteria for AN and BN, respectively
Sundgot-Borgen and Torstveit (2004), Norway[53]	660 Norwegian elite female athletes	Two-stage screening process consisting of a questionnaire developed by the authors, including subscales of the EDI, weight history, and self-reported history of EDs (stage 1), followed by a clinical interview using the EDI (stage 2)	21% (*n* = 121) of the female athletes were classified as "at risk" after the initial screening; results of the clinical interview indicated that 2% met the criteria for AN, 6% for BN, 8% for EDNOS, and 4% for anorexia athletica

Continued on next page

TABLE 18.1 Summary of Recent (Post-2000) Studies Examining the Prevalence of Disordered Eating in Athletes[31-57] (CONTINUED)

Study, country	Sample	Instrument	Prevalence
Byrne and McClean (2002), Australia[54]	263 elite male and female athletes and 263 nonathletic male and female control subjects	CIDI and number of self-report questionnaires	22% of female athletes and 4% of male athletes were classified with an ED compared with 5.5% of female control subjects and no male control subjects
Beals and Manore (2002), United States[55]	425 female collegiate athletes	EAT-26 and EDI-BD	3% and 2% of the athletes self-reported a diagnosis of clinical AN and BN, respectively; 15% and 32% of the athletes scored above the designated cutoff scores on the EAT-26 and EDI-BD, respectively
Johnson et al (1999), United States[56]	562 female collegiate athletes	EDI-2 and questionnaire developed by the authors using *DSM-IV* criteria	None of the athletes met the *DSM-IV* criteria for AN, whereas 1% met the criteria for BN; 2% and 6% of the athletes believed they might have AN and BN, respectively Subclinical AN and BN were identified in 3% and 9% of the women, respectively; 35% to 38% demonstrated DE behaviors (eg, binge eating, vomiting, laxatives, diuretics, diet pills, elevated drive for thinness subscale score, elevated body dissatisfaction score)
Sundgot-Borgen (1993), Norway[57]	522 Norwegian elite female athletes	EDI and an in-depth interview developed by the author based on *DSM-III* criteria	1%, 8%, and 8% were diagnosed with AN, BN, and anorexia athletica, respectively

Abbreviations: AN, anorexia nervosa; BITE, Bulimic Investigatory Test, Edinburgh; BN, bulimia nervosa; BSQ, Body Shape Questionnaire; BULIT-R, Bulimia Test Revised; CETCA, Eating Disorders Assessment Questionnaire; CIDI, Composite International Diagnostic Interview; DE, disordered eating; *DSM-III*, *Diagnostic and Statistical Manual of Psychiatric Disorders*, 3rd ed; *DSM-IV*, *Diagnostic and Statistical Manual of Psychiatric Disorders*, 4th ed; EAT, Eating Attitudes Test; EAT-26, Eating Attitudes Test 26; ED, eating disorder; EDE, Eating Disorder Examination; EDE-Q, Eating Disorder Examination Questionnaire; EDI, Eating Disorder Inventory; EDI-2, Eating Disorder Inventory-2; EDI-BD, Eating Disorder Inventory, Body Dissatisfaction subscale; EDNOS, eating disorder not otherwise specified; Q-EDD, Questionnaire for Eating Disorder Diagnosis

HEALTH RISKS ACROSS THE SPECTRUM OF DISORDERED EATING AND EATING DISORDERS

All individuals suspected of having an ED or DE need to have a thorough medical assessment. Not only can an ED be misdiagnosed, but EDs also affect multiple organ systems and may lead to acute and potentially chronic complications throughout the body. The two extremes of disordered energy balance are represented by undernutrition on one end of the spectrum, characterized as semistarvation or starvation, and overnutrition on the other end. Significant and lasting health issues with or without weight loss or gain occur when energy intake is consistently mismatched with energy needs; individual responses to undernutrition and overnutrition vary, and some individuals lose weight or gain weight more or less than others. Individuals may be malnourished and dealing with an ED at any weight: low, average, or high. Although the energy-related responses to severe dietary restriction are not well understood, the body seems to strive to maintain consistency in terms of body composition as evidenced by the maintenance of the body fat percentage during weight cycling and after weight regain following semistarvation. Dual-energy x-ray absorptiometry (DXA) and magnetic resonance imaging (MRI) are tools currently used to determine changes in body composition.[58]

Undernutrition

Undernutrition indicates a deficit of 1 or more essential nutrients and threatens physical, cognitive, and social qualities of life.[59] Inadequate nutrition impairs growth; basic physiological functions such as thermogenesis, reproduction, and cellular maintenance; movement[60,61]; and mental function, as determined by poor cognitive flexibility/rigid thinking, irritability/moodiness, diminished memory, poor recall, and general problems with decision making.[59] Inadequate energy intake relative to energy needs may be acute or chronic, resulting from physical or psychological constraints. For example, athletes may experience a reduction in appetite with heavy training rather than the expected drive for more food to meet elevated energy needs. In addition, environmental factors may reduce the availability of food, such as travel, scheduling, or time.

In sports nutrition, *energy availability* (EA) is defined as the amount of dietary energy (kilocalories) available to support good health and normal physiological body functions after the energy cost of exercise is subtracted from energy intake and normalized to fat-free mass (or lean body mass). Inadequate energy intake to meet the needs of exercise and physical activity—otherwise known as low energy availability (LEA)—may result from a lack of understanding regarding nutritional needs, poor time management, poor food preparation or shopping skills, or intentional limits set on the type of food eaten or restrictions set on caloric intake under the pressure of achieving a body ideal associated with a sport.[13] LEA is typically defined as less than 30 kcal per kilogram of fat-free mass per day.[60,61] Determining and documenting LEA is often challenging for the RDN outside of research settings because the calculation is typically based on a self-report of dietary intake, physical activity, and body composition. Furthermore, the concept of LEA is fraught with a lack of clear guidelines for assessing each of the components of EA, energy intake, and body composition.[61] LEA resulting from a dietary restraint or exercise without sufficient food intake appears to be the start of the DE continuum, so it may be the common mechanistic factor underlying the onset of an ED.

Experts do not fully understand the reason that some athletes cross the line from dieting and use of extreme weight-loss methods to clinical EDs, but it seems that a genetic predisposition combined with vulnerability in terms of the athlete's age, the type of sport practiced, and the individual's mental health status and history are all involved. Researchers hypothesized that thoughts and emotions originating from fear of fatness or intense drive for thinness may lead to goal-oriented behaviors that then lead to changes in brain signaling that are similar to those seen with drug addiction and result in automatic, habitual disordered behaviors.[62] The difficulty in effectively treating EDs may be related to these neural changes that result in people engaging in behaviors unconsciously, commonly referred to as being "on autopilot."

Although adipose tissue appears to constitute most of the body mass lost under severe and prolonged dietary restriction, carbohydrate reserves are depleted after just 24 hours of starvation. Amino acids are mobilized from organs and skeletal muscle for gluconeogenesis to provide glucose for the brain. In extended periods of severe restriction, tissues will use fatty acids and ketones to spare glucose for the brain. In addition, prolonged starvation results in increased use of ketones by the brain.[63]

Assessments using the DXA and MRI methodologies in the population with EDs would provide greater insight regarding the effects of dietary restriction on energy expenditure and protein mobilization from low metabolic rate tissue (fat mass and skeletal muscle) vs high metabolic rate organs, such as the heart, liver, and kidneys.[58] The proportions of weight lost from adipose tissue and lean tissue depend in large part on the amount of stored adipose tissue available, such that a leaner person will lose a greater proportion from lean tissue during dietary restriction. Degenerative changes in lean tissue include compromise of the heart, reduced erythropoiesis, depression of the immune system, and impaired capacity of the liver to metabolize drugs or toxic substances in the diet.[64]

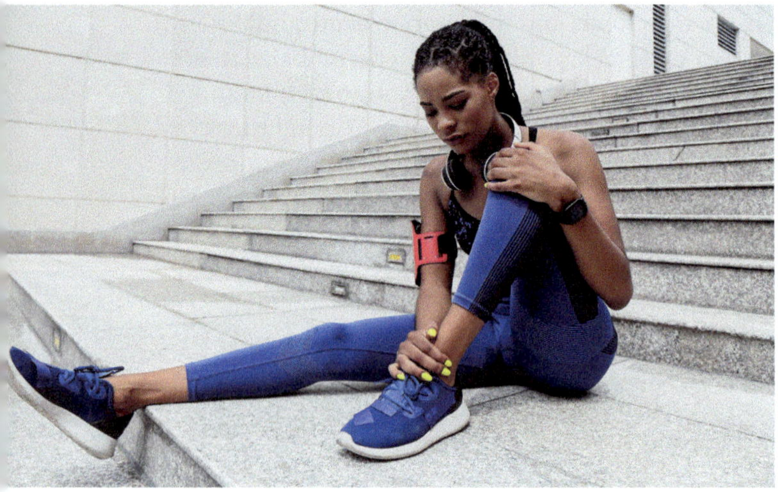

The depletion of fatty tissues and liver glycogen stores results in liver transaminase abnormalities (elevated aspartate transaminase [AST] and alanine transaminase [ALT]). Severe caloric restriction may result in fatal hypoglycemia as a result of the depletion of liver glycogen stores that could be used for gluconeogenesis to maintain safe blood glucose levels. Hypoglycemic risk seems to be higher among older individuals.[65] The depletion of substrates needed for hormone production—estrogen deficiency in females and testosterone deficiency in males—also occurs as a result of an energy-deficient diet.[66] Substrate depletion due to inadequate energy availability affects nerve conduction and results in muscle fiber atrophy and weakness. Thus, the neuromuscular system, which includes the brain, spinal cord, nerves, and all muscles in the body (including organ tissue), is often regarded as the most significantly affected system in severe AN.[67]

The vulnerable years of adolescence pose a special concern for those with DE and EDs, from the standpoints of both acute and chronic effects and the challenge of recognition. Young athletes may not present with the typical signs and symptoms and may be overlooked. The health care practitioner should be on the alert for growth stunting, failure to maintain growth trajectory, or pubertal delay.[68] Inadequate energy intake negatively affects growth and development, interfering with the accrual of bone density and the formation of organ systems. When LEA leads to the underdevelopment or wasting of skeletal, smooth, and/or cardiac muscle, numerous acute and chronic complications, including sudden death in severe cases, may result.[69]

Overnutrition

Overeating that leads to excessive food intake or being overweight may also affect health and performance. Some people restrict their intake early in the day and then find themselves overeating later. This behavior is commonly referred to as *back-loading* and may involve binge eating (as described in Box 18.1). The physical health risks of EDs that include binge eating include digestive and menstrual problems, joint and muscle pains, and headache. In addition, excessive eating, as in BED, may result in health risks that can include type 2 diabetes, heart disease, certain types of cancer, sleep disorders, digestive problems, and muscle and joint pain. Mental health risks include missing social activities, anxiety, depression, and suicidal thoughts.[70]

Although the health risks of overweight and obesity are important in nutrition assessment at the pediatric, adolescent, and adult levels, it is important to remember that a person's weight is an anthropometric measure that is just one part of the risk assessment. Unfortunately, individuals with DE/EDs often equate their weight with self-worth, ability, and overall health. Weight loss may be a desired consequence of health behavior change, but in and of itself, it is not necessarily a healthy behavior change. The practitioner should keep the following points in mind:

- Focus on behaviors rather than outcomes.[71]
- Place the person being served at the center of care, actively listening to their concerns, and refrain from judgmental language that perpetuates weight bias that stigmatizes the individual or family members.[71]

- Although commercially available apps are aimed at weight loss, they may not be valid or use evidence-based or expert recommendations, particularly for children and adolescents.[72]
- A significant increase in restrained eating after weight-focused treatment is an early indicator of ED pathology.[72]
- ED symptoms among children and adolescents often do not show up until more than 27 months after the onset of dieting.[72]
- Recognize the limits of your skills and knowledge. Seek assistance and expertise from others when necessary. Pediatric individuals with overweight or obesity should be referred to RDNs working in multicomponent programs and trained or specialized to treat EDs.[72]
- Mental health concerns (anxiety, depression, body shape concerns, low self-esteem, and EDs) underscore the need to screen and address psychological comorbidities when providing treatment for overweight or obesity.[71,72]
- Approach people, children, and their parents without judgment or blame.[71,72]
- Collaborate with families and use an interdisciplinary team to address the complex and multilevel factors that contribute to overweight and obesity at any age.[71,72]

Cardiovascular Abnormalities

Cardiovascular concerns include chest pain, abnormal heart rhythms (arrhythmia), an abnormally rapid heart rate (tachycardia), an abnormally slow resting heart rate (bradycardia), hypotension, and mitral valve prolapse, among others. Cardiovascular abnormalities warrant referral to a specialist for evaluation with an electrocardiogram.

Generally accepted norms for resting pulse are in the range from 60 to 100 beats per minute (bpm). However, a review of the literature did not reveal an authoritative source for defining heart rate limits for the application of these clinical terms. Spodick[73] suggests a lower threshold of 50 bpm and an upper threshold of 90 bpm as a red flag, alerting practitioners to potential cardiac abnormalities. Similarly, an adolescent with a heart rate of less than 50 bpm will be identified as being bradycardic.[74] Monitoring of an individual's heart rate does not require specialized instrumentation. RDNs may routinely monitor heart rate as an indicator of changes in health and dietary adequacy. Bradycardia is the most common cardiovascular complication of AN and should not be confused with the long-term sinus-node sickness that athletes often consider a confirmation of their cardiovascular fitness, the bradycardia commonly known as "athlete's pulse."[66] Even though neither type of bradycardia is well understood, the mechanism of bradycardia in a person with AN may be different from that in a well-nourished endurance athlete. Among those who are calorically restricted and underweight, bradycardia is thought to be a physiological downregulation of metabolism to conserve energy, seen in up to 95% of individuals with AN.[75] Research has indicated that increased vagal tone, decreased glycogen content of myocardial cells, and atrophy result from inadequate caloric intake.[76] The difference can be explained to the individual by checking their pulse at rest and then upon minimal exertion (walking down the hall or going from sitting or lying to standing). An abnormally rapid heart rate (tachycardia, >100 bpm) upon even minor exertion may be present among individuals who are exercising excessively, reflecting a malnourished heart that is not in good condition because of cardiac deconditioning and the weakness of malnutrition. The heart of a well-nourished athlete would have little response (increase of less than 20 bpm) to the energy demands of standing and walking a short distance.[77] The nutrition assessment helps determine whether bradycardia or tachycardia are due to malnutrition. Arrythmias, either tachycardia or bradycardia, should be viewed as a sign warranting physician evaluation.[78] Noncardiac causes of chest pain in an individual with an ED could be due to a gastrointestinal disorder, anxiety, or a host of other medical issues.[79]

Hypoglycemia and concomitant depletion of liver glycogen necessary to maintain blood glucose have been associated with sudden death in persons with severe AN.[75] Congestive heart failure and mitral valve prolapse may also result from malnutrition.[80] Even though the cardiac complications of AN may result in death, overall, they are largely considered (at least in the early stages) reversible and likely to result in full recovery with treatment.[81]

Changes in cardiovascular function among those living with EDs, as well as seemingly well-nourished, endurance-trained athletes, are not well understood. Whereas a reduction of the resting heart rate among athletes engaged in long-term training for ultraendurance events is typically considered a benign adaptation to maintain normal cardiac output and blood pressure concomitant with conditioning that increases stroke volume and vagal tone, some evidence suggests that it too may be pathological and indicative of remodeling of the heart, rather than being due to changes in resting autonomic tone.[82]

Gastrointestinal Issues

Individuals with EDs frequently complain of gastrointestinal (GI) distress. Common gut complaints include bloating, food intolerance, reflux, and constipation. These complaints may precede or accompany the diagnosis of an ED. GI issues are common among all medical disciplines, and this is perhaps why they are generally not specifically addressed in many ED treatment programs. The pathophysiology behind gut complaints is complicated and it is incompletely understood, and so may warrant a differential diagnosis.

Gastroparesis is diagnosed by documented delayed gastric emptying time, nausea, vomiting, early satiation, postprandial fullness, bloating, and upper abdominal pain.[83] Although gastrointestinal endoscopy and imaging are not generally performed to diagnose gastroparesis, individuals are often identified as "symptomatic for gastroparesis" based on GI complaints. Health care practitioners often explain to the individual that gastroparesis means "gastric paralysis" and results from ED behaviors, especially dietary restriction, that impair or slow the actions of the muscles of the stomach and intestines to conserve energy and that it will improve with recovery.

The gut microbiome has become a recent area of interest. The gut microbiome (also called microflora) is influenced by food choice, including the method of feeding as an infant and habitual diet.[84] Changes in microflora can result in changes in intestinal function, such as producing excess gas. These changes may be due to a host of factors, including immune function, alterations in the mucosal barrier, and the production of short-chain fatty acids and vitamins. GI distress has also been related to psychosocial distress, with perceived severity of bloating related to anxiety and depression. Thus, it comes as no surprise that the approximately 500 species of gut microbiota have gained recognition as a potential factor in ED development, maintenance, and recovery because of their impact on energy metabolism and body weight, as well as anxiety and depression.[84,85] This area is still largely unexplored, but preliminary evidence suggests that the intestinal microbiota may have biological and psychological effects.

Superior mesenteric artery (SMA) syndrome is a serious, although rare, complication of malnutrition. Symptoms include early satiety, nausea, and vomiting. SMA syndrome is characterized by partial blockage of the upper bowel caused by loss of the fatty tissue that normally serves as a pad between the gut and the superior mesenteric artery and aorta. Loss of this fat pad results in compression of the upper bowel. Individuals with SMA syndrome need medical supervision until the condition corrects with renourishment.[75,78]

Bone Issues

Athletes who participate in weight-bearing sports are expected to have higher bone mineral density (BMD) than nonathletes. Athletes who participate in high-impact sports, such as gymnastics and volleyball, and in odd-impact training, as in soccer and racquet sports, appear to have higher BMDs than as many as 41% to 45% of elite endurance athletes who experience low BMDs. The maximal rate of bone formation typically occurs from ages 10 to 14 years, and peak bone mass is usually attained between the ages of 20 and 30 years. It is especially important to recognize inadequate intake in young athletes during these critical periods of bone development.[86]

The World Health Organization bases the diagnoses of osteopenia (low BMD) and osteoporosis in postmenopausal women on T-scores that compare individuals to average peak adult BMD values.[87] Criteria for the assessment of bone health among premenopausal women and children have been established by the International Society for Clinical Densitometry (ISCD). The ISCD recommends that BMD be expressed as *z* scores, comparing individuals to age- and sex-matched controls. In premenopausal females and children, a *z* score less than or equal to 2.0 is defined as "below the expected range for age." Among children and adolescents, the ISCD recommends the term *low BMD* when BMD *z* scores are less than or equal to −2.0. Furthermore, the ISCD recommends that the term *osteoporosis* be used only when there is a history of vertebral compression fracture or a history of clinically significant fracture in addition to low BMD.[86]

The American College of Sports Medicine (ACSM) recommends addressing low BMD in athletes with BMD *z* scores of less than −1.0, even if they do not have a history of fracture. The ACSM recommends identifying athletes with BMD *z* scores between −1.0 and −2.0 who also have a history of nutritional deficiencies, hypoestrogenism, or stress fracture as having *low BMD.* The ACSM defines athletes with BMD *z* scores less than or equal to −2.0 and a history of nutritional deficiencies, hypoestrogenism, or stress fracture as having *osteoporosis.*[86]

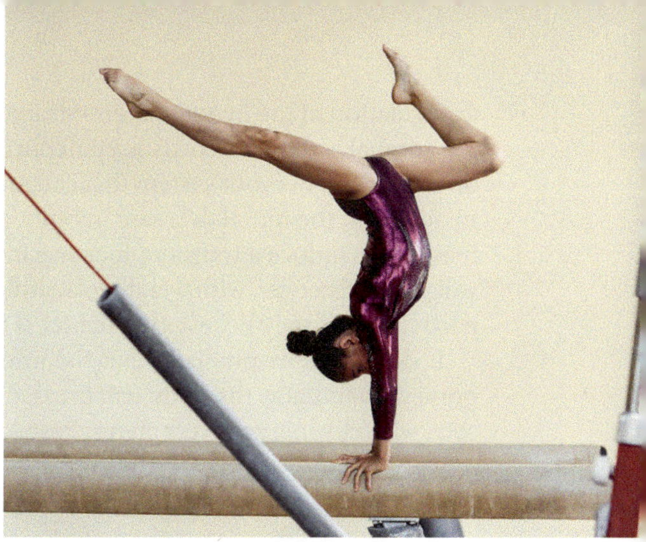

Reproductive Function

Reproductive function may be affected by an ED. It is common for menstruation to be interrupted, especially among those living with AN. Leptin is secreted from adipocytes; a deficiency in leptin triggers an adaptive metabolic response to energy distribution, including disruption of the hypothalamic-gonadal axis. Dysregulation of the hypothalamic-gonadal axis leads to the suppression of reproductive hormones and menstrual disturbance among females. Use of oral contraceptives or other estrogen replacements has not been shown to benefit individuals who experience menstrual disturbance resulting from chronic insufficient energy intake to meet caloric needs.[75] Restoring nutrition and maintaining body weight within a healthy range is the necessary treatment, although in clinical practice, resumption of menses frequently lags the restoration of weight. To resume normal function, it may be necessary to nudge body weight 5% to 10% above the expected recovery weight or about 5 lb above the weight at which menstruation ceased.

Menstrual dysfunction; hypercortisolemia; and reduced levels of androgens, leptin, and insulin-like growth factor 1 are associated with low BMD. Although the essential nutrients calcium and vitamin D are commonly associated with bone growth and development, once bone loss has occurred, supplementation with these nutrients is insufficient to treat or prevent low BMD. Unfortunately, research has failed to show that full recovery from an ED will completely reverse damage to the skeletal system or to the reproductive system. Long-term fracture risk and future problems with fertility may persist.[75,88] The best medicine at this time is treatment of the ED and nutritional restoration.

Comorbidities

By and large, EDs do not exist in isolation. Both psychological and physical comorbidities are found with EDs. The vast majority of people living with an ED are also experiencing another concurrent psychological disorder, and it is extremely important that medical practitioners perform a comprehensive assessment for comorbidities in the evaluation of anyone showing symptoms of an ED.

Many individuals with an ED display a co-occurring personality disorder, such as obsessive-compulsive disorder, dependent personality disorder, or bipolar disorder. Note that body dysmorphic disorder, characterized by a preoccupation with perceived defects in physical appearance, is described as an obsessive-compulsive disorder in *DSM-5* and not as an ED.[3] These personality disorders may predispose an individual to the development of an ED, or a personality disorder may be a consequence of malnutrition. The famous Keys semistarvation study of conscientious objectors during World War II demonstrated the physical effects of dietary restriction to achieve a 25% weight reduction and also psychological distress, including the development of anxiety, depression, rigidity, obsessions, and irritability.[89] Nutritional rehabilitation improves many of these personality traits, although some linger.[13]

ED behaviors may limit the availability of vitamins and minerals, but clinical micronutrient deficiency does not occur as frequently as expected in the ED population.[90] However, overnutrition (obesity) is a problem for some people. Whereas most people who are obese do not have BED, up to two-thirds of individuals with BED are obese and are at risk of the medical complications of obesity.[91]

Special Considerations for Athletic Performance

Surprisingly, anecdotal evidence suggests that athletes practicing DE behaviors often experience an initial, albeit transient, improvement in performance. The reasons for this temporary increase in performance are not completely understood but are thought to be related to the initial physiological and psychological effects of starvation and purging.[93] Starvation and purging are physiological stressors and, as such, produce an upregulation of the hypothalamic-pituitary-adrenal axis (eg, the fight-or-flight response) and an increase in the adrenal hormones cortisol, epinephrine, and norepinephrine. These hormones have a stimulatory effect on the central nervous system that can mask fatigue and evoke feelings of euphoria in an athlete with an ED. In addition, the initial decrease in body weight (particularly before there is a significant decrease in muscle mass) may induce a transient increase in relative maximal oxygen uptake (VO_2 max) per kilogram of body weight.[94] Moreover, with weight loss, athletes may feel lighter, which may afford them a psychological boost, particularly if they believe that lighter is better in terms of performance.

It should be emphasized that the improvement in performance sometimes seen with DE is only temporary. Eventually, the body will break down, and performance will suffer. The decrement in performance seen with chronic or severe energy restriction is likely due to 1 or more of the following factors: nutrient deficiencies, anemia, fatigue, reduced cardiovascular function, frequent infection, illness, or injuries.[28] As previously described, individuals with BN may purge through self-induced vomiting or otherwise attempt to compensate for bingeing episodes by using diuretics, laxatives, enemas, or excessive exercise. If the purging or compensatory behaviors place the athlete in a state of negative energy balance, then the potential effects on performance are similar to those seen with chronic or severe energy restriction. In addition, GI blood losses that often result from chronic vomiting can contribute to iron losses and increase the risk of iron deficiency anemia. Excessive exercise, especially given inadequate energy and nutrient intakes, invariably leads to overuse injuries such as stress fractures. In addition to the resulting energy and nutrient deficiencies, purging poses some unique problems regarding athletic performance, most notably dehydration and electrolyte abnormalities.[92]

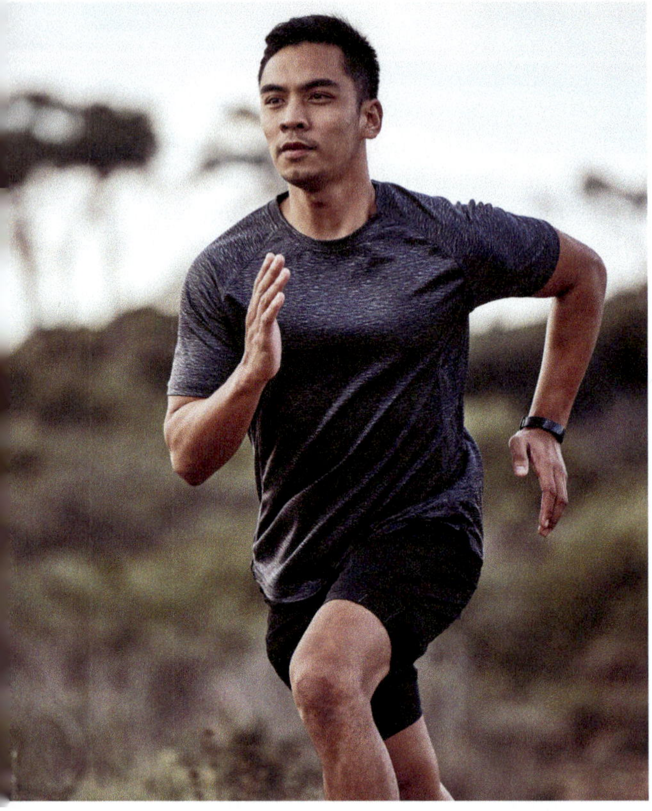

The effects of DE on athletic performance are a function of the severity and duration of the DE behaviors as well as the physiological demands of the sport.[28] Thus, an individual who engages in severe energy restriction or who has been bingeing and purging for a long time will likely experience a greater decrement in performance than one who has engaged in milder weight-control behaviors for a shorter time. Likewise, those who participate in endurance sports and other physical activities with high energy demands (eg, distance running, swimming, cycling, basketball, and field and ice hockey) are likely to be more negatively affected than those in sports with lower energy demands (eg, diving, gymnastics, weightlifting). Finally, athletes who train at a high intensity (eg, elite athletes) are likely to have greater performance decrements than those who engage in lower-intensity exercise (eg, recreational athletes).

ETIOLOGY AND RISK FACTORS FOR THE DEVELOPMENT OF DISORDERED EATING AND EATING DISORDERS

Why do some people develop EDs whereas others do not? An understanding of why one may develop an ED is important in reducing stigma, providing effective treatment, and preventing EDs. Among the most prevalent reasons individuals engage in behaviors that they know are harmful and costly to them physically, psychologically, socially, or in terms of performance and do not seek treatment are shame and fear of being misunderstood or blamed for their ED.[93] Risk factors include biological characteristics (eg, genetic differences) and environmental events (eg, teasing or bullying) or experiences (eg, cultural ideals of thinness). A variety of environmental factors may influence the development of an ED. Examples include the family environment, the sociocultural environment, and environmental experiences of stress and trauma.

Family of Origin

Thinking about how the family contributes to the development of an ED has changed over time. Whereas early research focused on family dysfunction, the family is now considered as part of the larger sociocultural environment. The following types of family dysfunction play a relatively small role in the etiology of eating disturbances and the development of EDs: (1) high-conflict home environment, (2) lack of familial cohesion, (3) poor communication, (4) deficient problem-solving skills, (5) high levels of emotional expression (general criticism, hostility) or low levels of emotional expression, and (6) modeling of dieting or negative body comments.[94]

Culture

Eating plays an important role in the lives of people in most cultures around the globe, and habits that are considered acceptable vary widely among groups. Thus, EDs have been conceptualized as culture-bound syndromes, implying that they occur uniquely in certain cultures or that they represent a culturally shaped expression of an underlying disease.[93-95] The data on the prevalence and risk of EDs suggest that variation, both within and among groups, is largely determined by socioeconomic status; religious affiliation; cultural ideals for body weight, shape, or size; media exposure; local environment (suburban vs urban settings); and the influence of other people who play a significant role in an individual's life.[96] Socioeconomic status has long been held to be a factor in the development of an EDs based on the observation that higher-status individuals are thinner than those of lower status. However, research does not support a direct association between socioeconomic status and the onset of an ED.[93]

According to Striegel-Moore and Bulik,[93] epidemiologic studies on demographics, such as race, ethnicity, and sexual orientation (including homosexuality), are lacking, and thus, it is not possible to draw valid conclusions and offer reliable insight regarding risk associated with cross-cultural differences. EDs occur around the world and may reflect changes in body ideals. Media messages parallel the sociocultural ideal. Researchers reported that the mass media send many types of messages, in both form and content, that "present, elaborate, and reinforce, in a salient fashion, the schematic ingredients, that is, the 'nervosa,' of severely disordered eating" and that those messages include "unattainable for most . . . to dichotomous, contradictory, and mystifying messages about passion, abandon, and indulgence vs control of hunger, sexuality, and other desires."[96] Evidence suggests that media exposure increases body-image concerns, at least in the short run.[93]

Subculture of the Athlete

Culturally based value for a specific body weight, shape, or size and exposure or social pressure to conform to the norm play a significant role in body-image concerns, such as the overvaluation of thinness, weight, shape, or body composition.[93] Both aesthetic (appearance) sports and nonaesthetic sports often involve revealing attire, focusing attention on the body and leading to body consciousness.[97] Excessive exercise to control body shape and weight has been observed among 40.3% to 54.5% of persons with an ED.[67] Although athletic participation may play a role in appreciation of one's body, thereby serving as a protective factor, traditionally, sports participation has been stereotyped as more masculine than feminine.[98,99]

Attention on the body and sexualization of athletes may adversely affect both males and females. Females have been mainly targeted, from subtle suggestions to revealing attire on the cover of mainstream magazines,[99] whereas males are under pressure to conform to the perception of the male athlete as unbreakable, stoic, and self-sacrificing.[100] On a more positive note, both the frequency and serious tone of coverage for female athletes in mainstream media have increased over time. Focus on females as serious competitors has grown, emphasizing their psychological and emotional strengths and athletic performance rather than their physical appearance and personal relationships.[101] More widespread representation of females in athletics may prompt others to value their physical abilities over how their bodies look and serve as a point of reference for athletic females of all ages in the development of their own self-concept.[99]

Whereas all athletes should be considered at risk for the development of an ED, those who seem to have the highest prevalence of EDs are athletes involved in sports that emphasize a low body weight and low body fat, combined with regulations in some weight-sensitive sports.[102] Higher levels of pressure to perform generally predict more EDs; however, the evidence is inconsistent. On the basis of questionnaire results from German high school students, Rosendahl et al[46] reported a higher risk of EDs among nonathlete females (36.1%) and nonathlete males (12.3%) than among female athletes (12.3%) and male athletes (10.4%). In contrast, Martinsen and Sundgot-Borgen[42] used a 2-stage approach (a survey followed by a clinical interview) with male and female Norwegian adolescents and found the rates of EDs to be higher among elite athletes than among age-matched nonathlete controls.

Age and Sex

Age and sex are the two characteristics that are most indicative of risk for an ED. The age of adolescence has long been recognized as the period of greatest vulnerability in terms of developing AN or BN; BED, on the other hand, has an onset well into adulthood.[93] In every study of the prevalence of EDs, females outnumber males. However, sex appears to be less of a factor for BED and OSFED than for AN or BN. Males and females with EDs often engage in similar behaviors but with different goals. For example, females are more likely to focus on weight-control behaviors, whereas males often focus on loss of fat and increasing muscularity. Estimates of male athletes with an ED or DE vary among studies, but prevalence rates are higher among athletes than among the general population.[93,100]

Sex and identity as an athlete confound the risk of having an ED among males, as disordered food-related behaviors may be missed as a problem or even encouraged. Male athletes may also be less likely to seek or accept help as they may be feeling general shame about their symptoms or the stereotype of EDs as a female issue, may fear the stigma around mental health, and may experience emotional conflict around complying with the identity of the male athlete.[100]

People who identify among sexual minorities appear to be at greater risk for disordered eating, unhealthy weight-control behaviors, over- or under-estimation of their body weight, and body dissatisfaction.[103] Individuals in minority sexual and gender populations are at risk for limited access to quality health care, discrimination from a host of people (including coaching staff, teammates, health care practitioners), and violence.[2,103]

Trauma

The association between trauma, both emotional (eg, feelings of failure, loss, disconnection, loss of control) and physical (eg, abuse, injury), and the development of an ED is well established. Many individuals with EDs reveal a history of trauma during the course of treatment and may be diagnosed with posttraumatic stress disorder. Although the specific mechanism that leads to ED development is not understood, psychobiological dysregulation may put some people at greater risk than others.[13] The United Nations and the International Olympic Committee (IOC) describe harm experienced by athletes related to an abuse of actual or perceived differentials in power, based on a cultural context of discrimination as "nonaccidental violence." Whereas nonaccidental violence occurs in all sports and at all levels, athletes at the elite level, child athletes, athletes with a disability, and athletes with diverse sexual identities and gender expressions (eg, lesbian, gay, bisexual, transgender, questioning, and others) are at greater risk.[2]

EATING DISORDER IDENTIFICATION, DIAGNOSIS, AND TREATMENT

Identification

Individuals with EDs may be identified through the use of screening questionnaires. Ideally, practitioners should employ a 2-stage approach, as recommended by Jacobi and colleagues,[104] that uses a broad screen for those at risk, followed by a more specific assessment, such as the clinical interview employed by Martinsen and Sundgot-Borgen,[42] which would more accurately identify individuals with an ED. In research, questionnaires are the most common method of screening, perhaps because self-reporting questionnaires are easy to administer, efficient, and economical. Furthermore, anonymity likely enhances the participants' ease or honesty in response, compared with a face-to-face interview.

The EAT exists in both the original 40-item version and the shorter 26-item version. The EDI and the Eating Disorder Examination Questionnaire (EDE-Q) are among the most widely used screening tools for EDs. The EDE-Q is the self-report version of the Eating Disorder Examination interview (EDE), recognized as one of the gold-standard instruments used in the validation of screening tools.[105] The EDE is reportedly the most commonly used interview tool in clinical studies, but it may not be practical in many situations because of the time and training required for the interviewers.[13]

The health care practitioner should be cautious in using these tools among populations in which they have not been validated, such as in the athletic population where individuals are thought to be 2 to 3 times more at risk compared with nonathletes.[13,105] A variety of tools may be used to identify EDs among athletes, including the SEDA, the FAST, the BULIT-R, the Brief Eating Disorder in Athletes Questionnaire (BEDA-Q), the AMDQ,[29] the EDSA, and the DESA-6.[30] The 2019 IOC consensus statement on mental health in elite athletes suggested use of the AMDQ, version 2; the BEDA-Q, version 2; and the Physiologic Screening Test to Detect Eating Disorders Among Female Athletes.[2] In addition, Lease and Bond[106] compared tools designed to identify maladaptive exercise—namely, the Obligatory Exercise Questionnaire (OEQ), the Exercise Dependence Scale (EDS), and the Frequency, Intensity, Time (FIT) Index—and their associations with DE symptomology. Research supports the personal interview as the preferred method for diagnosis of an ED.[2] Overall, the field needs better identification of athletes at risk. In addition to the RDN, others involved in the health and performance of athletes, including certified athletic trainers, health care practitioners, and coaches, also need to be skilled in observing the behaviors of athletes as a means of detecting DE and EDs.[107]

Diagnosis

The very people who serve as first responders in terms of ED recognition and referral for treatment (coaches, primary care doctors, RDNs) have relatively little formal preparation to do so according to a study from Mahr et al.[108] It is not uncommon for professionals to miss the symptoms of EDs in a culture that idolizes the thin and fit and, in fact, even inadvertently promote DE and EDs through comments or body measurements. The diagnosis of an ED is based on specific criteria and may include physical, behavioral, and cognitive domains. Although the RDN may be among the first to recognize the signs and symptoms of an ED, it is considered outside the scope of the RDN's role to make a conclusive diagnosis. It is essential that individuals exhibiting such symptoms be referred to a physician who is familiar with EDs for a thorough physical and psychological examination to rule out other diseases.

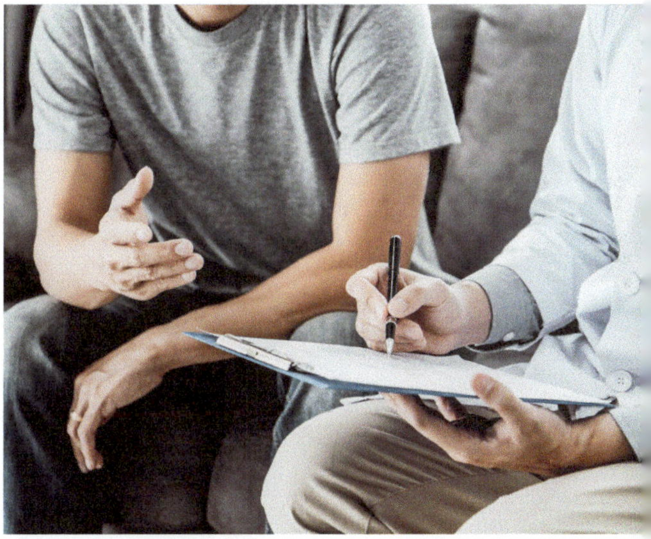

Treatment

THE TREATMENT TEAM

Eating disorders are becoming more commonly recognized, yet statistically speaking, EDs remain relatively rare conditions in the general population and need to be addressed by people who are experienced in treating them. Treatment of EDs through the use of multiple health disciplines has long been advocated.[1,2,109] Effective treatment usually involves clinicians from various health disciplines, including mental health professionals, physicians, RDNs, and nurses knowledgeable about EDs. Inclusion of a physical therapist experienced with EDs is gaining support. Although not all treatment teams include all members for the duration of treatment, thorough assessment and treatment are warranted. Clinical decisions will be deferred to the individual who holds the highest level of responsibility and liability (eg, the physician).

LEVELS OF CARE

A fundamental goal of ED treatment is to work with the individual at the lowest effective level of care. The outpatient setting is less disruptive and less costly than higher levels of care, which are not necessary for the treatment of most people.[110] However, a subset of individuals with an ED will require the safety, structure, and support offered by inpatient or day treatment programs.[111] The APA publishes guidelines for the care of individuals with EDs. Overall physical condition, psychological state, behaviors, and social circumstances all play roles in the decision-making process regarding the appropriate level of care. Adults who weigh less than approximately 85% of their individually estimated healthy body weight are known to have difficulty gaining weight outside of a highly structured, supervised program. Even those who have weights of at least 85% of their expected body weight may also require higher levels of care on account of medical or psychiatric necessity. Levels of care include 24-hour inpatient hospital-based programs for those needing medical stabilization; residential care, which offers a more home-like setting for individuals needing 24-hour supervision and support; partial hospital programs, which entail being at the hospital for part of every day; intensive outpatient programs, which individuals attend for part of most days of the week; outpatient programs, which can have variable settings, practitioners, supports, and schedules; and support groups.

At all levels of care, transition planning is important. When an individual is served by a hospital program, experts recommend that they stay until consistency in food intake and a healthy body weight are achieved and maintained to reduce the chances of relapse. The APA recommends that a specific clinician be identified as the primary care coordinator to ensure continuity and attention to important aspects of treatment.[113]

THE REGISTERED DIETITIAN NUTRITIONIST WITHIN AN INTERDISCIPLINARY TREATMENT TEAM

Collaboration among health care practitioners is essential to high-quality, person-centered care. An interdisciplinary treatment team is composed of professionals across disciplines who communicate, reinforce, and build on the work of one another. Coordination of care for individuals who are living with chronic and complex EDs takes additional time, energy, and effort that is often not reimbursable by insurance. A high-performing team shares patient responsibility and treatment goals, mutual respect, good communication through coordination of care, and a sense of mutual support. Although practitioners may encounter "turf wars" and questions around scope of practice—who knows what, who decides what, and who can do what—it is imperative that all members of the team are reinforcing and building on the work of one another.

Positive interprofessional interactions are protective against burnout; ensure practitioner mental health and improved patient safety; and enhance quality of care, patient health, and patient satisfaction.[113,114] Without having regular communication with other practitioners, a relationship with a patient alone does not constitute collaborative interprofessional care, but rather denotes "care as usual" by separate professions practicing within the silos of their disciplines.[114]

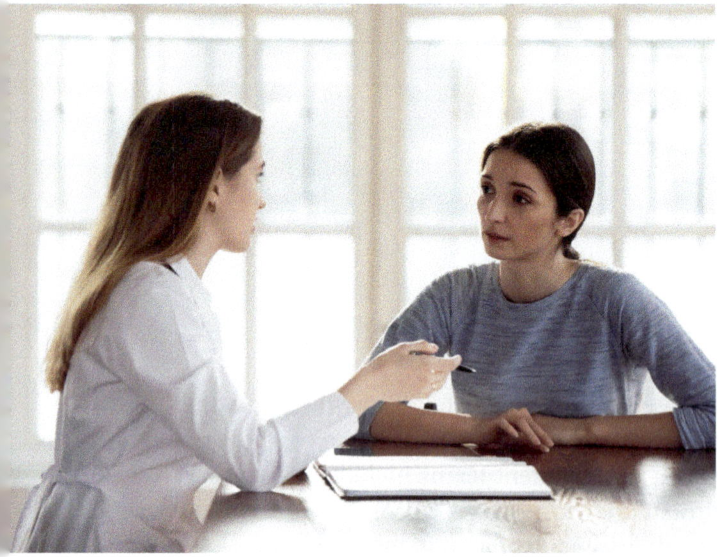

Roles of the Registered Dietitian Nutritionist

Medical nutrition therapy (MNT) for EDs is the evidence-based application of the nutrition care process provided by an RDN. Essential components of MNT include assessment, psychoeducation, reassessment, and monitoring with modification of interventions through ongoing follow-up to support long-term change, evaluation of outcomes, and referral to higher levels of care as needed. An RDN treating individuals who are living with EDs uses a variety of skills, with the primary goal of changing eating behaviors. The interventions combine strategies drawn from different fields (eg, medicine, psychology, and physical therapy) to be applied in a multidisciplinary or interdisciplinary approach. These terms generally refer to treatment that combines disciplines; however, theoretically they are not the same. Multidisciplinary refers to "the addition of the competencies of multiple professionals who stay within the boundaries of their fields, whereas interdisciplinary denotes that the various disciplines are coordinated toward a common and coherent approach."[115] Whereas many of the sources cited within this overview use the term multidisciplinary, the authors believe that the most effective treatment team addressing a complex disorder, such as an ED, is interdisciplinary in contrast to multidisciplinary.

Skills and Competencies of the Registered Dietitian Nutritionist Working With Eating Disorders

RDNs who work with athletes *will, without doubt,* encounter individuals living with DE and EDs; thus, it is imperative to develop the skills and qualifications to treat these serious disorders. One must demonstrate proficiency in the delivery of MNT for individuals with EDs, contributing both technical and collaborative expertise within the treatment team.[116] RDNs who treat athletes with EDs will best serve this population by having a solid foundation in both sports nutrition and EDs. The Board Certified Specialist in Sports Dietetics (CSSD) certification,[117] offered through the Commission on Dietetic Registration, and the Certified Eating Disorders Specialist (CEDS) certification,[118] offered through the International Association of Eating Disorders Professionals, verify foundational knowledge in these areas.

The therapeutic delivery of nutrition care demands that the RDN have the aptitude to combine technical skill with the development and delivery of nutrition care plans. Sports dietitians educate athletes to meet their nutrient needs and play a central role in helping individuals who overexercise set limits and recognize the adverse effects of their actions on their sports performance, as well as on their physical, emotional, and social health.

Depending on the phase of recovery, nutritional counseling and health and wellness coaching skills may be used together to support the individual in making difficult thinking and behavioral changes. In a coaching role, the RDN listens empathetically to the patient's story, engages in a spirit of curiosity, reflects to the patient what has been heard, respects the patient's values, and creatively assists in identifying goals and strategies that will restore the patient's health. Helpful coaching strategies include the modeling of authenticity, affirmation, courage, calm, warmth, appropriate humor, and playfulness. The RDN may take on a more prescriptive role regarding nutrition care and work with family members, guiding them in taking a supervisory role during mealtimes that demonstrates a caring and compassionate attitude, as well as consistency in expectations about meals in terms of amount eaten, time to completion, and acceptable behaviors. Taken together, these skills enable RDNs to build and sustain a close therapeutic relationship with the patient or client and a strong partnership with the treatment team, including family members, coaches, and trainers.

Although MNT is widely endorsed by professional organizations in the treatment of EDs, no standard exists for the delivery of nutrition therapy among the DE or ED population.[119] Research across disciplines and among patients suggests that there is a lack of agreement regarding when, what, and how nutrition therapy for those recovering from an ED should be provided.[120,121] A Delphi study of Australian ED clinicians and consumers revealed disagreement related to whether a nutrition expert should be included at all. Furthermore, the same study reported dissent regarding the specific components of nutritional therapy and whether RDNs involved in such care remained consistent in the provision of evidence-based treatment or drifted from their scope of practice.[120] Mittnacht and Bulik[121] investigated the best nutrition counseling practices for AN among RDNs identified as recognized experts in the treatment of EDs. Consensus (>85% agreement) regarding nutrition treatment among these experts was reached on only 35% (47 of 133) of the questions and statements delivered by the Delphi method, indicating that, although some nutrition counseling approaches are widely applicable to all individuals with EDs, customization for the specific needs of the individual is also necessary. It is clear that all members of the treatment team benefit from being acquainted with the core competencies and skill set of the RDN who specializes in the treatment of EDs. Ideally, the treatment team members should reinforce messages across disciplines, providing consistency for the patient that reinforces trust in the recovery process.

The *Guidebook for Nutrition Treatment of Eating Disorders*,[109] authored by the Nutrition Working Group of the Academy for Eating Disorders, a team of nutrition experts across the spectrum of care, clarifies the role and responsibilities of the RDN in ED care for all treatment team members.

Nutrition Therapy for Eating Disorders

Nutrition therapy includes psychoeducation regarding the disease and nutritional needs, the development and modification of food plans, the supervision of food and beverage intake, and overall accountability for meeting nutritional needs.[109] The sports RDN who has an existing relationship with an athlete who is living with an ED may be well positioned to help them but may also benefit from networking or coordinating care with another RDN who has expertise in the treatment of EDs.

Eating disorders are diseases wherein doubt frequently surfaces: doubt about the seriousness of the ED behaviors, doubt about what recovery will look like, and doubt in both one's treatment team and one's ability to recover. Thus, it is imperative that practitioners who treat individuals with EDs be specifically prepared for and have the experience and confidence to work with this population.

Nonconforming gender subgroups likely have their own unique risk factors,[122] with both physical and psychosocial implications related to diet. The health risks associated with hormonal therapy warrant nutritional consideration among the transgender population.[103] Moreover, it is important that the RDN working with this population engage in a gender-affirming practice, including using the individual's preferred pronouns, engaging in regular cultural competence training, facilitating access to gender-affirming interventions,[122] and staying abreast of emerging research and recommendations in applying the nutrition care process.[103]

All members of the treatment team must also recognize that the patient or client is the one who determines if or when they ultimately choose to recover, partially or fully. It is the practitioner's responsibility to bring forward the best effort and support individuals where they are, recognizing what they are willing and able to do with regard to keeping themselves safe and avoiding further harm. At times, this may result in involuntary treatment. In the world of sports nutrition, those supporting athletes often practice harm reduction (eg, when athletes insist on using supplements without evidence to support any benefit), recognizing the limits of their ability to effect change in another person. In treating an individual who is living with a life-threatening ED, an individualized harm-reduction approach allows a person to maintain their EDs in as healthful a way as possible for them and may be applicable when a patient is unable or unwilling to progress in treatment.[123]

Working with individuals who have these dysfunctions is demanding, and those who serve their patient or client best will be equally committed to self-care. An individual's circumstances may be painful for the RDN to hear, leaving them at risk for compassion fatigue or secondary trauma. Individuals who are living with DE or an ED may have experienced tragedy or trauma and abuse that no human being should have to endure. As a result, patients may engage in self-harm or suicidality. The RDN working with individuals who have DE or EDs needs to have their own coping skills and strategies to prevent burnout. To that end, regular collaboration among treatment team members as a source of support and as a mechanism for setting therapeutic boundaries is recommended. Finally, all members of the treatment team must recognize and respect their own limits. Inadequate or harmful care puts individuals with EDs at even greater risk for abandoning or avoiding treatment and for loss of faith in the medical system.[65]

Phases of Nutrition Therapy

Graves and Scribner[119] have described 3 phases of nutrition therapy with which an athlete familiar with recovery from physical injury may be likely to identify. The phases move from high levels of structure that keep the athlete safe from further injury to lower levels of structure that allow eating with flexibility and for optimal performance; the 3 phases are described in Box 18.4.[119]

Throughout the phases, the role of the RDN shifts from "expert mode" in

BOX 18.4 Three Phases of Nutrition Therapy[119]

Phase	Name	Description
Phase 1	Foundation	The provision of structure is the foundation for healing. The approach is similar to the casting of a broken bone. The registered dietitian nutritionist (RDN) plays a prescriptive role.
Phase 2	Rehabilitation	Change may be difficult and painful. The process is similar to the progression from a cast to physical therapy in the restoration of flexibility and strength.
Phase 3	Synergy	The athlete is striving to achieve their full potential. The RDN serves as an ally to patient-driven progress.

prescribing specific food plans and nutritional supplements to a "nutrition coach" role. This model supports the athlete in holding a vision of recovery as an injured athlete returning to their full potential in the sport according to their readiness as determined by their progress in healing.

The Nutrition Assessment

A thorough assessment of nutritional status requires an investment of time and coordination of care. The goal of the nutrition assessment is to identify nutrition-related problems, their causes, and their consequences. The RDN engages in an ongoing process of reassessing nutritional status compared to accepted standards, recommendations, and/or goals throughout the delivery of MNT.[124] The assessment of risk related to body weight is further confounded by the use of BMI categories that may not appropriately indicate health risk. Flegal and colleagues[125] reported that the health risks associated with underweight are understated, whereas the health risks associated with overweight BMI classes are overstated. Furthermore, weight within a healthy range does not necessarily indicate adequate nutrition because of the body's ability to maintain homeostasis.

Data from other medical practitioners, recent laboratory results or imaging, intake documents, a nutrition focused physical exam, and interviews with the patient and caregivers are fundamental to understanding the patient's condition. The nutrition assessment includes environmental limitations and resources, a physical evaluation, a physical activity assessment, food- and body-related attitudes and beliefs, a summary of past and current reliance on alternate modes of nourishment (eg, supplements, meal replacements, tube feedings), and an assessment of nutritional needs compared with dietary intake. A more thorough explanation of the nutrition assessment for EDs is available in the *Guidebook for Nutrition Treatment of Eating Disorders* from the Academy for Eating Disorders.[109] This resource is listed in Box 18.5, along with others available from various professional organizations.

BOX 18.5 Professional Resources for Eating Disorders

Academy for Eating Disorders

www.aedweb.org

Guidebook for Nutrition Treatment of Eating Disorders

Eating Disorders: A Guide to Medical Care

Information about eating disorders and treatment options

Malnutrition resources: pediatric and adult diagnostic criteria

Professional listserv

International conferences and meetings

Webinar library for members and the public

Continuing education

Academy of Nutrition and Dietetics

www.eatrightpro.org

Academy of Nutrition and Dietetics Pocket Guide to Eating Disorders, 3rd edition

Position of the American Dietetic Association: Nutrition Intervention in the Treatment of Eating Disorders

Position of the American Dietetic Association, Dietitians of Canada, and the American College of Sports Medicine: Nutrition and Athletic Performance

Continued on next page

BOX 18.5 Professional Resources for Eating Disorders (CONTINUED)

Revised 2020 Standards of Practice and Standards of Professional Performance for Registered Dietitians (Competent, Proficient, and Expert) in Eating Disorders

Revised 2021 Standards of Practice and Standards of Professional Performance for Registered Dietitian Nutritionists (Competent, Proficient, and Expert) in Sports and Human Performance Nutrition

Revised 2022 Standards of Practice and Standards of Professional Performance for Registered Dietitian Nutritionists (Competent, Proficient, and Expert) in Pediatric Nutrition

Treatment of Pediatric Overweight and Obesity: Position of the Academy of Nutrition and Dietetics Based on an Umbrella Review of Systematic Reviews

Position of the Academy of Nutrition and Dietetics: Malnutrition (Undernutrition) Screening Tools for All Adults

Sports Nutrition Care Manual

Nutrition Focused Physical Exam Pocket Guide, 3rd edition

Continuing professional education

International Association of Eating Disorders Professionals Foundation

https://iaedpfoundation.com

Conferences and local chapters

Certification as a specialist in eating disorders

National Eating Disorder Association

www.nationaleatingdisorders.org

Conferences

Hotline

Workshops and symposia

International Olympic Committee

https://olympics.com

Information relevant to eating disorders, disordered eating, and mental health in sports

IOC Mental Health in Elite Athletes Toolkit

Stories from athletes who have faced issues with body image, eating disorders, and disordered eating to share with patients

Professionals in Nutrition for Exercise and Sport

https://pinesnutrition.org

Educational resources

Conferences

International Olympic Committee Diploma in Sports Nutrition

Australian Institute of Sport Female Performance & Health Initiative

www.ausport.gov.au/ais/fphi

Free education resources

Royal College of Psychiatrists (UK)

www.rcpsych.ac.uk

Full report: Medical Emergencies in Eating Disorders (MEED): Guidance on Recognition and Management, College Report CR233 (published May 2022, updated October 2023)

Summary sheets for assessing and managing patients with severe eating disorders

Nutrition-Related Treatment Goals

The goals of nutrition therapy for EDs are individualized and holistic. The following are examples of treatment goals[109]:

- » Achieve a regular pattern of intake through a diet that meets nutritional needs and is sustainable.
- » Develop coping and distraction techniques to manage urges to restrict, binge, purge, or engage in excessive exercise.
- » Improve obsessive thoughts, preoccupations, and attitudes about food.
- » Enhance appreciation of the functions of the body and acceptance of genetic determinants of body shape and weight.
- » Restore and maintain a natural, biologically appropriate weight range, emphasizing a healthy state over focus on weight.
- » Restore/maintain normal physiological functions (eg, menstruation, hormone levels, body temperature).
- » Resolve fear of adverse consequences of eating and improve tolerance of the sensory characteristics of food.
- » Improve interest in and enjoyment of eating.

Assessment of short-term weight change is complicated by numerous factors. Body weight fluctuates day to day by about 5 to 6 lb depending on one's hydration status, the contents of the gut and bladder, the time of day, and the presence of menses for menstruating females. Consider the following factors when interpreting weight change[109]:

- » Full bladder and colon: 1 to 2 lb
- » Time of day: weight increases by up to 5 lb over the course of the day
- » Clothes: 2 to 4 lb
- » Menses: 3 to 5 lb

A biologically appropriate weight range[109] is:

- » easily maintained without the need for dieting or inappropriate food and exercise behaviors and reflects premorbid weight, normal physical and psychological function, genetic predisposition, ethnicity, gender, and family history;
- » associated with normal historical development (eg, growth trajectory in children and teenagers);
- » where weight settles when enough food is consumed to attain required nutrients and the individual is physically and emotionally satisfied; and
- » capable of reflecting the individual's weight prior to the onset of the ED.

Weight restoration in restrictive EDs is typically defined as 95% of the median BMI for age and is associated with a reduced risk of long-term medical complications.[126]

Medical Monitoring and Coordination

It is critical that the RDN be prepared to recognize and treat poor nutrition (undernutrition or clinical malnutrition). The RDN's assessment of nutrition parameters of poor nutrition assist the physician or advanced practice practitioner in making an accurate diagnosis and may impact the patient's speed of recovery. Application of the appropriate *ICD* code indicating the severity of undernutrition or malnutrition may influence insurance reimbursement. Evidence-based guidelines that facilitate the nutrition diagnosis among adults include the joint expert panels of the Academy of Nutrition and Dietetics and the American Society for Parenteral and Enteral Nutrition (ASPEN), as well as the Global Leadership Initiative on Malnutrition (GLIM). Whereas the Academy of Nutrition and Dietetics/ASPEN criteria were specifically delineated for the North American population, some insurance companies may adopt the GLIM criteria in making reimbursement decisions. The American Academy of Pediatrics joined the Academy of Nutrition and Dietetics and ASPEN for diagnostic criteria among children (ages 1 month to 18 years) in the United States.[127]

When properly trained and working closely with a physician, the RDN may further contribute to physiological monitoring of the individual with an ED by assessing vital signs, along with providing psychoeducation around the signs of malnutrition and nutritional recovery. RDNs may assess hydration status through urine color, urine frequency, and urine specific gravity. Some individuals with EDs restrict fluid intake, and others may load up on fluids, typically in an attempt to either misguide the treatment team regarding their body weight or quiet hunger signals. Some people consume caffeine in the hopes of suppressing appetite, stimulating metabolism, or both. Table 18.2 identifies some of the physiological monitoring the RDN may contribute in the comprehensive nutritional care of athletes with DE/EDs.[77-79,128-130] It is imperative that the RDN has certifications, as applicable, and documents timely communication with a primary care physician who oversees medical care to reduce the risk of legal issues if adverse medical problems occur. Although physiological screening by the RDN is helpful, the interpretation of vitals and laboratory values requires expertise beyond the RDN credential.

Traditionally, the strategy toward restoring nutrition was to "start low, go slow" in terms of caloric intake. However, research suggests that a more rapid restoration of weight predicts long-term recovery.[126,131] The optimal route, speed, and composition of the diet for refeeding a malnourished patient have not been defined.[126] The generally agreed-upon approach to the restoration of energy intake is to incrementally increase according to the currently recommended ranges (25%–35% of calories from fat, 15%–20% from protein, and 50%–60% from carbohydrate)[131] by approximately 100 kcal per day or by up to approximately 400 kcal every 3 to 4 days with close medical supervision.[109] A reduced-sodium diet may diminish undesirable fluid shifts.[119,126] The physician may prescribe supplemental vitamins or minerals or electrolytes (eg, thiamin, folate, potassium, phosphorus) as needed.

The energy needs for a person who is severely energy-restricted defy typical calculations and may be upward of 3,000 to 4,000 kcal/d, even with low physical activity and with concurrent indicators of the downregulation of metabolism. Research suggests that the thermic effect of food may be elevated by between 14% and 30% among those with AN because of the individual's psychological state (eg, anxiety and depression related to eating) and hormonal response to stress.[132,133] Furthermore, metabolizable energy intake is complicated by diets that are high in fiber and individual differences in absorption. More research is needed to understand the metabolic changes and needs of individuals with EDs.

Therapeutic Nutrition Approaches

It is imperative that practitioners recognize the unpredictability of EDs and maintain vigilance in treatment. For example, it is important to check vital signs and laboratory tests and to proceed with the awareness that individuals with EDs seem to "wear a mask," frequently reporting that they are fine, based on an obscured view of their condition. Individuals with EDs frequently do not feel that they are sick enough to warrant treatment or that they deserve care. Furthermore, they are typically ambivalent about the desire for a change in their food selection or body weight. Stereotypes abound regarding EDs, and individuals who do not fit the image of having an ED may either disregard the symptoms or feel unworthy of medical attention. In their book *Eating Disorders in Sport*, Thompson and Sherman[97] described the phenomenon of "presumption of health," in which people often automatically associate

TABLE 18.2 Physiological Monitoring by the Registered Dietitian Nutritionist[a,77-79,128-130]

Parameter	Description	At risk	Symptomatic for
Heart rate	Change in the normal sequence of electrical impulses, causing an abnormal heartbeat rhythm	Bradycardia: <60 bpm (adults)[77,78] Tachycardia: >100 bpm (adults)[77,78]	Nutritional deficiency/LEA, electrolyte imbalance, dehydration, risk for fainting Tachycardia may reflect nervousness or serious cardiovascular problems or organ damage
Blood pressure	Change in pressure exerted by blood on the blood vessel walls Measured with a validated meter[b]	Hypotension (adults): • Systolic < 90 mm Hg[77,78] • Diastolic < 50 mm Hg[77,78] Hypertension (adults): • Systolic > 140 mm Hg[128] • Diastolic > 90 mm Hg[128]	Low blood pressure may reflect LEA Blood pressure may rise in refeeding syndrome Blood pressure may be elevated with stimulant use
Minimum exertion blood pressure	Change in blood pressure and pulse within 10 s from resting to standing	May be at risk when > 20 mm Hg[77]	Malnutrition/LEA
Orthostatic blood pressure	Change in blood pressure within 2-5 min from supine to standing	Systolic drop > 20 mm Hg[79] Diastolic drop > 10 mm Hg[79]	Malnutrition/LEA
Capillary refill time	Assessment of peripheral perfusion Measure time for blood color to return to an external capillary bed and restore color after pressure is applied by pressing the extremity (nail or fingers) with the thumb and forefinger for 5-10 s Capillary refill time increases as the body conserves energy for circulation to the vital organs and sends less blood to the peripheral tissues	>3 s[129]	Dehydration, inadequate energy

Continued on next page

TABLE 18.2 Physiological Monitoring by the Registered Dietitian Nutritionist[a,77-79,128-130] (CONTINUED)

Parameter	Description	At risk	Symptomatic for
Menstrual tracking	Record of menstrual cycles	Individuals with menstrual irregularities[128]	Menstrual irregularities may indicate inadequate energy intake
Urinalysis[c]	Reagent-coated test strips are used to diagnose, screen, or monitor health issues Urine is a marker of body functioning[128]	Urine SG >1.020 suggests dehydration when accompanied by inadequate fluid intake Urine SG <1.010 suggests overhydration when accompanied by excess fluid intake Can also monitor ketones, pH, blood, nitrites, and leukocytes	Intentional or unintentional over- or underhydration Diuretic or laxative use High ketones may indicate extended fasting High pH may reflect a catabolic state Presence of blood, nitrites, and leukocytes may reflect urinary tract infection Malnutrition may affect kidney functioning
Peripheral edema	Fluid swelling of the extremities[128]	Pressure produces dents in the skin, especially in anorexia nervosa	Malnutrition, purging, cardiac abnormalities, refeeding

[a] The RDN coordinates care with the interdisciplinary team to interpret physiological monitoring. Table 18.2 is not comprehensive. Many caveats apply to the interpretation of vital signs and laboratory tests for people who are living with an ED. In addition to screening for abnormal values, normal or even slightly abnormal values, when taken in the context of an individual patient, may signal trouble.

[b] Blood pressure monitor validation can be checked at the website US Blood Pressure Validated Device Listing (https://validatebp.org).

[c] Under the Clinical Laboratory Improvement Amendments (CLIA) program, health care practitioners who screen for or monitor specific diseases or conditions are required to have the appropriate certificate before they can accept human samples for testing. Analysis of urine within a private practice generally requires a CLIA waiver.[130] Normal values for urine specific gravity span a wide range.

Abbreviations: bpm, beats per minute; LEA, low energy availability; SG, specific gravity (the density of urine as compared to the density of water, where urine contains more solutes than water and so has a slightly higher density)

competition in sport as a reflection of health. Lack of awareness and/or training or a desire to avoid recognizing DE or an ED may result in coaches, family members, and medical practitioners missing clues that indicate a serious problem.

An RDN working with individuals with DE may draw from a variety of domains, including compassionate communication (also known as nonviolent communication), motivational interviewing, and appreciative inquiry, as well as several psychological therapy practices. Box 18.6 presents some of the more common therapeutic approaches and modalities that RDNs may use in providing MNT to those who have an ED.[112,119,134-143]

BOX 18.6 Therapeutic Approaches to Nutrition Therapy[112,119,134-143]

Cognitive behavior therapy (CBT)

CBT is regarded as the leading evidence-based treatment for adults with eating disorders (EDs); it is generally considered more effective for treating bulimia nervosa (BN) and binge-eating disorder (BED) than anorexia nervosa (AN).[120,135]

Therapists provide psychoeducation about the disease and its treatment. Patients recognize thought patterns, the power of those patterns, and the triggers that lead to symptomatic behavior.

Recovery is focused on managing self-defeating thought patterns and engaging in planned strategies that lead to healthful, recovery-oriented behavioral patterns.[112]

Dialectical behavior therapy (DBT)

Developed by Marsha Linehan, DBT uses elements from CBT, with the additions of mindfulness, distress tolerance, and acceptance.[135]

Treatment can be modified for the treatment of patients with complex, multidiagnostic EDs.[136,137]

Individuals learn rational thinking and decision-making skills that allow them to move beyond black-and-white thinking to develop coping strategies for perceived crises.[138]

Acceptance and commitment therapy (ACT)

ACT was developed by Steven Hayes, Kelly Wilson, and Kirk Strosahl and focuses on accepting thoughts.[139]

ACT differs from CBT in that, rather than striving to change or control thoughts, people learn that thoughts may be uncontrollable.

ACT teaches recognition and tolerance of negative thoughts and feelings in an effort to live a better life in the face of distress, accepting pain as a normal part of living.[140]

ACT embodies the belief that everyone will have pain and suffering. Patients with EDs are viewed as attempting to avoid the pain of life through their behaviors.

ACT is based on the following founding principles[140]:

- Accept your thoughts and feelings and be present.
- Choose a valued direction.
- Take action.

Family-based treatment (FBT)

FBT emerged from the family-based, home-based treatment practiced at Maudsley Hospital in London. Parents are an integral part of the recovery.

The treatment model is brief (15–20 outpatient sessions over 6–12 months).

Continued on next page

BOX 18.6 *Therapeutic Approaches to Nutrition Therapy*[112,119,134-143]

Family-based treatment (FBT) (continued)

FBT uses 3 phases:

- Uniting parents to take temporary control of all food-related decisions and restore a healthful weight range
- Transitioning control back to the adolescent
- Establishing normal adolescent development and identity.

The treatment provides a manualized approach with guides for the treatment of AN and BN among adolescents.[141]

FBT does not specifically use the expertise of an RDN.[142]

The principles of FBT may also be used with older patients or clients by enlisting the support of those who play the supportive roles of the family.

Motivational interviewing (MI)

MI emphasizes 4 general principles:

- Expressing empathy
- Developing discrepancy
- Rolling with resistance
- Supporting self-efficacy

RDNs who are trained in MI use these principles to help patients and clients become increasingly aware of thoughts and feelings that lead to behaviors. Awareness of precipitating thoughts and feelings facilitates the resolution of resistance to change.[143]

Exposure treatment

Exposure treatment with response prevention is considered an adjunct therapeutic technique.[144]

RDNs may engage in therapeutic meals and snacks with patients, as well as help parents and other practitioners expose patients to foods that are fearful for them to gain familiarity and confidence in adding those foods back into the diet.

A progressive twist on the concept of exposure therapy is to change one's relationship with food through involvement in growing, cooking, and preparing food.

Psychoeducation and Dietary Manipulation

No clear protocol exists for manipulating macronutrients or micronutrients among the ED population. The RDN explores and addresses beliefs held by the individual with an ED about the benefits and risks of energy-producing nutrients, vitamins, and minerals and about the use of supplements, including ergogenic agents. Although it is beyond the scope of this chapter to describe the details of dietary manipulation, food or meal plans are key behavioral interventions. Food plans generally progress from specific (prescribing or dosing of food as medicine based on the amount and timing) to more general as the individual makes progress, with the end goal of establishing an adequate energy and nutrient intake with balance among food groups and a variety of foods. The type of food plan recommended depends on the type and severity of the disorder, as well as the individual's needs and preference. The *Guidebook for Nutrition Treatment of Eating Disorders* provides a description of food plan approaches.[109] Individuals with inadequate energy intake are more likely to experience symptoms of gastroparesis.[83] Gastrointestinal pain and bloating make increased food intake more difficult. Engaging in small, frequent eating episodes; using foods that are soft and can be mashed into smaller particle size; limiting high-fiber foods; and replacing solid foods with liquids to meet nutritional needs are strategies that may be helpful.[144]

Most individuals with DE or an ED express a desire to return to normal eating, characterized by mindfulness and intuition. Retraining a patient to eat in response to internal cues, using mindfulness or an approach termed intuitive eating, would generally follow weight restoration and requires that the patient be in a frame of mind such that they are able to integrate interoceptive awareness (ability to perceive physical, bodily sensations) with emotional regulation and respond to their own needs in a timely manner. One principle of intuitive eating is unconditional permission to eat. According to food addiction theory, implementation of all of the principles of mindful or intuitive eating may need to be delayed or may never be effective or appropriate.[145]

As previously described, the role of the RDN is determined by training and certification. An advanced practitioner who is a certified eating disorder specialist (CEDS) may have the knowledge and skill to apply an assortment of physiological monitoring, behavior change strategies, and psychological therapy techniques within the scope of an interdisciplinary team as part of MNT. It is critical that the RDN communicate the results of physiological monitoring to the physician and coordinate the use of psychological approaches with mental health providers. An RDN who holds expertise in sports nutrition (eg, Board Certified Specialist in Sports Dietetics, CSSD) provides education to assist the patient or client in fueling athletic activity. Athletes generally understand, at least cognitively, the need for carbohydrate-rich foods as fuel for the brain, power for the muscles, and a vehicle for fiber and phytochemicals. They also relate to the necessity of adequate protein as a bridge supporting satiety signals, as well as a connector for building muscle and producing neurotransmitters.[119] Although fears of eating may apply to any of the macronutrients, fear of body fat often translates into a fear of dietary fat.

Athletes are not immune to nutrition myths, and they are aware that weight loss may result in an initial performance improvement. What many athletes have a difficult time understanding is the transience of this benefit. The first impression is lasting, and even after continued efforts to lose weight through dietary restriction that result in nutritional deficits, fatigue, loss of strength, impaired immunity, and illness, the initial success may propel the athlete and, through contagion, teammates and others to move along the same path toward developing a clinical ED, including purging by vomiting, use of diuretics or laxatives, or excessive exercise.[13] The devastation of a poor performance due to injury or illness pales in comparison to the potential for a life-threatening cardiac event due to hypoglycemia, dehydration, or an electrolyte imbalance. RDNs are uniquely qualified to educate athletes and coaches on the critical role of nutrition in health and performance.

When someone displays symptoms of an ED, a thorough nutritional and medical assessment, with ongoing monitoring, is warranted. Fast-paced restoration of nutrition, especially among adults, can be life threatening when it results in a rapid shift of phosphorus from the serum into the cells. Low serum phosphorus can cause muscle breakdown (eg, rhabdomyolysis), blood cell dysfunction, respiratory failure, seizure, and cardiac arrest.[65]

The term *refeeding* may refer to either (1) the process of restoring nutrition or (2) the potentially life-threatening condition that results from improved energy intake (especially from carbohydrate), known as refeeding syndrome. It is important for the RDN and other health care practitioners to know that, theoretically, any patient could experience refeeding syndrome in the process of increasing nutritional intake. Refeeding syndrome, like other aspects of ED treatment, is ideally treated at the lowest effective level of care. Consider the needed support and availability of medical monitoring alongside the patient's resources and circumstances, including the personal, educational, and social needs of the patient. Medical complications and serum phosphorus and electrolytes should be monitored every 1 to 2 days for the first 1 to 2 weeks of refeeding at any level of care.[109]

Whereas no single indicator exists to precisely identify who will develop refeeding syndrome, the Clinical Guidelines of the National Institute for Health and Care Excellence provide criteria for identifying those at higher risk (Box 18.7 on page 480).[146]

BOX 18.7 Criteria for Determining Individuals at High Risk of Developing Refeeding Syndrome[146]

Patient has 1 or more of the following	OR	Patient has 2 or more of the following
BMI of less than 16		BMI of less than 18.5
Unintentional weight loss greater than 15% within the previous 3 to 6 months		Unintentional weight loss greater than 10% within the previous 3 to 6 months
Little or no nutritional intake for more than 10 days		Little or no nutritional intake for more than 5 days
Low levels of potassium, phosphate, or magnesium prior to feeding		A history of alcohol or drug use or abuse including insulin, chemotherapy, antacids, or diuretics

RETURNING TO COMPETITION

Determining appropriate levels of physical activity based on both nutritional status and emotional readiness can be a responsibility of the RDN, especially if the athlete does not have an interdisciplinary sports medicine team. When a patient or client wishes to increase physical activity, it is important to explore their intention, as well as potential benefits and risks. In general, a gradual return to training is recommended. However, because some athletes have an addictive nature regarding physical activity, they may never be able to safely return to physical activity at the competitive level.

Return-to-Play Guidelines

Athletes who present with an ED or otherwise have signs or symptoms of dysfunction (energy deficiency relative to energy intake or exercise dependence) should undergo a thorough medical examination for safe participation. Screening tools should be used to identify and guide management of LEA with the goal of maintaining the athlete's safety, identifying athletes who should refrain from participation and require further medical attention, and monitoring such athletes before they return to play.[147]

The female athlete triad and the male athlete triad indicate the health of the athlete based on 3 interrelated spectrums that exist on a continuum from optimal health to disease: energy deficiency/LEA, suppression of the hypothalamic-pituitary-gonadal axis, and impaired bone health. The male athlete triad was adapted from the female athlete triad based on evidence that adolescent and young adult male athletes in certain sports (eg, lean-sport, endurance, and weight-class) are at greater risk. Both triads evaluate health based on a point system using similar criteria[148] known as the Triad Cumulative Risk Assessment (Triad CRA) (refer to Figures 18.1[149] and 18.2[148]). The assessment assigns the risk of an athlete as high (restricted from training and competition), moderate (provisional or limited clearance), or low (full clearance). The clearance level can be modified at the practitioner's discretion.[147]

The International Olympic Committee (IOC) introduced the term *relative energy deficiency in sport* (RED-S) in 2014, provided an update on the condition in 2018 and a further update in 2023 (now abbreviated as REDs). REDs extends and emphasizes the risks described in the female athlete triad to include males and persons from various ethnic groups, expanding on the many global health and performance consequences of LEA.[147,150,151] The *British Journal of Sports Medicine* dedicated its entire September 2023 issue to REDs, providing an updated consensus statement, a thorough review of the potential mental and physiological health outcomes of exposure to LEA, and clinical guidance for the prevention and management of REDs in athletes. The update also features a "traffic-light" continuum depicting 4 levels of

Risk Factors	Magnitude of Risk Low Risk = 0 points each	 Moderate Risk = 1 point each	 High Risk = 2 points each
Low EA with or without DE/ED	☐ No dietary restriction	☐ Some dietary restriction‡; current/past history of DE;	☐ Meets DSM-V criteria for ED*
Low BMI	☐ BMI ≥ 18.5 **or** ≥ 90% EW** or weight stable	☐ BMI 17.5 < 18.5 **or** < 90% EW **or** 5 to < 10% weight loss/month	☐ BMI ≤17.5 **or** < 85% EW **or** ≥ 10% weight loss/month
Delayed Menarche	☐ Menarche < 15 years	☐ Menarche 15 to < 16 years	☐ Menarche ≥16 years
Oligomenorrhea and/or Amenorrhea	☐ > 9 menses in 12 months*	☐ 6-9 menses in 12 months*	☐ < 6 menses in 12 months*
Low BMD	☐ Z-score ≥ -1.0	☐ Z-score -1.0*** < - 2.0	☐ Z-score ≤ -2.0
Stress Reaction/Fracture	☐ None	☐ 1	☐ ≥ 2; ≥ 1 high risk or of trabecular bone sites†
Cumulative Risk (total each column, then add for total score)	**____ points +**	**____ points +**	**____ points = ____ Total Score**

FIGURE 18.1 Female Athlete Triad cumulative risk assessment tool[149]

‡ Some dietary restriction as evidenced by self-report or low/inadequate energy intake on diet logs.

* Current or past history.

** ≥90% EW; absolute BMI cut-offs should not be used for adolescents.

*** Weight-bearing sport.

† High-risk skeletal sites associated with low BMD and delay in return to play in athletes with 1 or more components of the Triad include stress reaction/fracture of trabecular sites (femoral neck, sacrum, pelvis).

Abbreviations: BMD, bone mineral density; BMI, body mass index; DE, disordered eating; EA, energy availability; ED, eating disorder; EW, expected weight

Reproduced with permission from reference 149: De Souza MJ, Nattiv A, Joy E, et al. 2014 Female Athlete Triad Coalition consensus statement on treatment and return to play of the female athlete triad: 1st International Conference held in San Francisco, California, May 2012 and 2nd International Conference held in Indianapolis, Indiana, May 2013. *Br J Sports Med.* 2014;48(4):289. doi:10.1136/bjsports-2013-093218

Risk Factor	Low Risk = 0 points each	Moderate Risk = 1 point each	High Risk = 2 points each
Low EA with or without ED/DE	☐ No dietary restriction	☐ Some dietary restriction*; current or past DE	☐ Meets DSM-5 criteria for ED
Low BMI	☐ BMI ≥ 18.5 in adults, OR % Median BMI** ≥ 90% in adolescents/children, OR weight stable	☐ BMI 17.5 < 18.5 in adults, OR % Median BMI 86-89% in adolescents, OR 5<10% weight loss/12mo†	☐ BMI ≤ 17.5 in adults, OR % Median BMI ≤ 85% in adolescents, OR ≥ 10% weight loss/past 12mo
Low BMD	☐ Z-score ≥ -1.0	☐ Z-score -1.0*** < -2.0	☐ Z-score ≤ -2.0
Stress Reaction/Fracture	☐ None	☐ 1	☐ ≥ 2; OR ≥ 1 high risk‡ or trabecular bone site
Cumulative Risk (total each column, then add together for total score)	____ points +	____ points +	____ points = ____ total

FIGURE 18.2 Male Athlete Triad cumulative risk assessment tool[148]

* Some dietary restriction as evidenced by self-report or energy deficiency/low EA on diet logs or validated surveys. In adolescents, absolute BMI cut-offs should not be used, and clinicians should rely on age-adjusted and gender-adjusted BMI percentiles (**% median BMI, CDC BMI-for-age growth charts, or BMI Z-scores) or † % change in weight in the past 12 months.

*** Weight-bearing sport.

‡ High-risk skeletal sites associated with low BMD and delay in return-to-play include stress reaction/fracture of trabecular sites (femoral neck, sacrum, and pelvis).

Abbreviations: BMD, bone mineral density; BMI, body mass index; CDC, Centers for Disease Control and Prevention; DE, disordered eating; EA, energy availability; ED, eating disorder

Reproduced with permission from reference 148: Fredericson M, Kussman A, Misra M, et al. The male athlete triad—A consensus statement from the Female and Male Athlete Triad Coalition Part II: Diagnosis, treatment, and return-to-play. *Clin J Sport Med.* 2021;31(4):349-366. doi:10.1097/JSM.0000000000000948 progressing risk (green, yellow, orange, red) related to guidelines for participation in sports activity.[152]

The 2023 IOC REDs Clinical Assessment Tool (CAT2)[151,152] replaces the prior version. REDs is a clinical diagnosis made by a multidisciplinary athlete health and performance team based on a 3-step model that guides clinicians in the diagnosis, treatment, and prevention of REDs[153]:

- **Step 1**: Screen for REDs using a population-specific, REDs-related questionnaire or clinical interview. Screening may be part of an annual periodic health examination, and/or it may be done when an athlete presents with changes in mood, habits, or behaviors or health and performance concerns. A variety of potential screening tools were presented earlier in this chapter.
- **Step 2**: Conduct an in-depth assessment using the REDs Severity/Risk Assessment Table (refer to Box 18.8). Based on the results, athletes are then stratified according to the REDs Stratification and Sports Participation Guidelines (refer to Figure 18.3 on page 485) Athletes using sex hormone–altering medications are not scored for menstrual cycle. Additional information, including a scoring assistance tool, can be found in the article by Heikura et al (available online at https://stillmed.olympics.com/media/Documents/Athletes/Medical-Scientific/Consensus-Statements/REDs/IOC-REDs-CAT-Version-2.pdf).
- **Step 3**: The collective results from Step 1 and Step 2 are intended to be used by a physician (ideally a sports medicine physician) for final diagnosis. Athletes in the red, orange, or yellow zones need medical evaluation and treatment. Treatment of REDs should be undertaken by a team of health professionals versed in sports medicine, including a physician, sports RDN, exercise physiologist, athletic therapist or trainer, and sports psychologist/psychiatrist as needed. Although it is imperative that patient confidentiality is honored, it is equally important that the athlete's coach, and when appropriate, parents/guardians are aware of the diagnosis and supportive of the treatment plan.

Box 18.9 lists the global effects of LEA on physical and mental health as well as athletic performance.[153]

The Triad CRA scoring system is easy to use, aside from the requirement of BMD measurement. REDs CAT uses available health data to assign risk but lacks precision for some criteria (eg, low body fat, "severe" ED, and bradycardia).[152] Many athletic training programs employ their own specific return-to-play protocols, and protocols may vary from program to program. Both athletes and the practitioners who work with them need a greater understanding of both physical and psychological recovery from REDs and optimum readiness to return to play.[2]

BOX 18.8 Relative Energy Deficiency in Sport Severity/Risk Assessment[153]

Indicator	Description
Severe primary indicators (2 points)	
Primary amenorrhea (females)	Failure to reach menarche by the age of 15 years, when the development of secondary sexual characteristics is evident or by the age of 14 years when no secondary sexual characteristics are present
Prolonged secondary amenorrhea due to functional hypothalamic amenorrhea (FHA)	Absence of 12 or more consecutive menstrual cycles
Clinically low free or total testosterone (males)	
Primary indicators (1 point)	
Secondary amenorrhea caused by FHA (females)	Absence of 3 to 11 consecutive menstrual cycles

Indicator	Description
Subclinically low free or total testosterone (males)	Testosterone within the lowest quartile of the laboratory and age-specific reference range
Subclinically or clinically low total or free triiodothyronine (T3)	Within or below the lowest quartile of the laboratory and age-specific reference range
History of bone stress injury (BSI)	1 or more high-risk BSI (femoral neck or total hip, sacrum, pelvis) **OR** 2 or more low-risk BSI (all other BSI locations) within the previous 2 years **OR** absence of 6 months or more from training due to BSI in the previous 2 years
History of low bone mineral density (BMD)	Adults/adolescents (aged ≥15 years): BMD z score assessed by dual-energy x-ray absorptiometry (DXA) within the past 6 months of less than −1 at the lumbar spine, total hip, or femoral neck **OR** decrease in BMD z score from prior testing using pediatric norms and software for individuals aged less than 20 years
	Child/adolescent (aged <15 years): BMD z score assessed by DXA within the past 6 months of less than −1 at the spine or in total-body-less-head scan **OR** decrease in BMD z score from prior testing
A deviation of a pediatric or adolescent athlete's previous growth trajectory (height and/or weight)	
An elevated score for the Eating Disorder Examination Questionnaire (EDE-Q) global **AND/OR** clinically diagnosed *Diagnostic and Statistical Manual of Mental Disorders, 5th ed, Text Revision*-defined eating disorder	EDE-Q global score of more than 2.30 in females or more than 1.68 in males Only 1 primary indicator for either or both outcomes
Secondary indicators	
History of 1 low-risk BSI within the previous 2 years and absence of less than 6 months from training due to BSI in the previous 2 years	Refer to high- vs low-risk definition earlier in this table

Continued on next page

BOX 18.8 Relative Energy Deficiency in Sport Severity/Risk Assessment[153] (CONTINUED)

Indicator	Description
Secondary indicators (continued)	
Oligomenorrhea caused by FHA	More than 35 days between periods for a maximum of 8 periods per year
Clinically diagnosed depression and/or anxiety	Only 1 secondary indicator for either or both outcomes
Elevated total or low-density lipoprotein (LDL) cholesterol	Total or LDL cholesterol above reference range
Potential indicators[a] (0 points)	
Subclinically or clinically low insulin-like growth factor-1 (IGF-1)	Within or below the lowest quartile of the reference range
Clinically low blood glucose	Below the reference range
Clinically low blood insulin	Below the reference range
Chronically poor or sudden decline in iron studies	Ferritin, iron, transferrin, and/or hemoglobin
Lack of ovulation	Via urinary ovulation detection
Elevated resting or 24-h urine cortisol	Above the reference range or significant change for the individual
Urinary incontinence (females)	
Gastrointestinal or liver dysfunction or adverse gastrintestinal symptoms at rest and during exercise	
Reduced or low resting metabolic rate (RMR) **OR** intake of less than 30 kcal per kilogram of fat-free mass per day **OR** RMR ratio of less than 0.90	
Reduced or low libido/sex drive (especially in males) and decreased morning erections (males)	
Symptomatic orthostatic hypotension	
Sleep disturbances	

[a] These indicators are pending further research to quantify parameters and cut-offs more accurately.

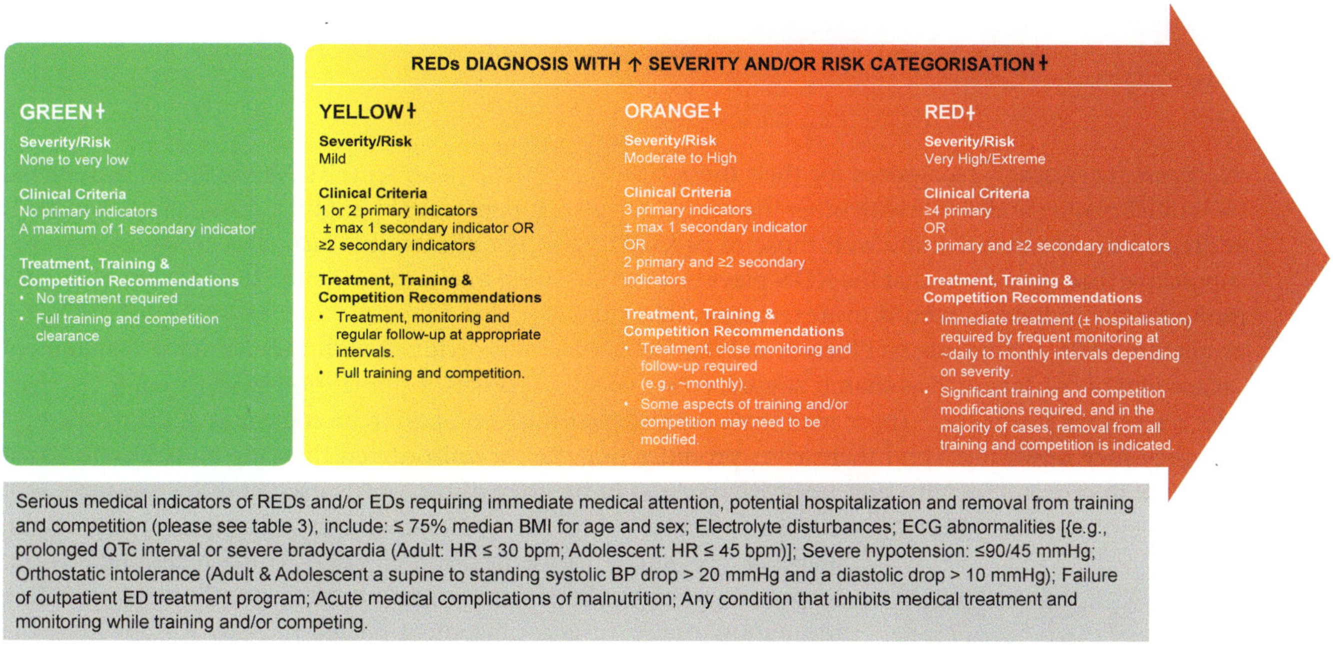

Disclaimer: The IOC REDs CAT2 Severity/Risk Assessment and Stratification and Sport Participation Guidelines is not to be used in isolation and is not to be used solely for diagnosis. Furthermore, this tool is less reliable in situations where it is not possible to assess all indicators in theREDs Severity/Risk Assessment Table. The IOC REDs CAT2 Severity/Risk Assessment and Sport Participation Guidelines is not a substitute for professional clinical diagnosis, advice and/or treatment from a team of REDs health and performance experts led by a sports medicine physician. Along with the evaluation of health status presented here, sport participation decisions also need to be made in the context of various decision modifiers, such as level of the athlete, sport type, participation risk, conflict of interest, athlete/coach pressures, timing, and season etc.[13]

FIGURE 18.3 **Relative energy deficiency in sport traffic-light continuum of severity and/or risk**[153] Adapted with permission from reference 153: Heikura IA, Mountjoy ML, Ackerman K, et al. IOC REDs CAT2. International Olympic Committee (IOC) relative energy deficiency in sport (REDs) clinical assessment tool version 2 (CAT2). Accessed August 20, 2023. https://stillmed.olympics.com/media/Documents/Athletes/Medical-Scientific/Consensus-Statements/REDs/IOC-REDs-CAT-Version-2.pdf

BOX 18.9 Effects of Low Energy Availability on Health and Performance[153]

The effects of low energy availability exist on a spectrum. Effects may be mild, while stronger symptoms may lead to adverse REDs (relative energy deficiency in sport) outcomes.

Effects on health	Effects on performance
Impaired growth and development	Decreased athlete availability
Reduced immunity	Decreased training response
Impaired reproductive function	Decreased recovery
Impaired bone health	Decreased cognitive performance/skill
Impaired gastrointestinal function	Decreased motivation
Impaired energy metabolism/regulation	Decreased muscle strength
Impaired hematological function	Decreased endurance performance
Urinary incontinence	Decreased power performance
Impaired glucose and lipid metabolism	
Mental health issues	
Impaired neurocognitive function	

PREVENTING DISORDERED EATING AND EATING DISORDERS IN ATHLETES

RDNs are increasingly recognized for their therapeutic role in ED treatment. RDNs trained in therapeutic modalities play a parallel role with other therapists on the treatment team by aligning the language and goals addressed in nutrition therapy with those of psychotherapy. For clients, this facilitates recognition of the supportive therapeutic role that the RDN plays beyond imposing intake of unwanted food or setting activity limits for the individual who is overexercising. Remain aware that EDs carry one of the highest risks for premature death among mental illnesses and that because most individuals with EDs do not seek treatment on account of barriers such as shame, stigma, economics, or accessibility, practitioners must not focus their efforts solely on treatment.[12] Those who work in this field are called upon to be cognizant of the many ways that they may unwittingly find themselves promulgating the very disordered thinking and behaviors that they seek to prevent, identify, and treat. RDNs need to be wary of the words used and the messages sent regarding the physical and emotional environment provided. Be cautious about associating any body weight, shape, or size with a disease or disorder. *DSM-5* recognizes that AN can occur at any weight; therefore, it is imperative to strictly avoid providing admiration, praise, or encouragement related to body weight. Keep the conversation about health, strength, performance, and being connected in ways that are important to the athlete; overall, the less health care practitioners talk about bodies and body image, the better people seem to do.

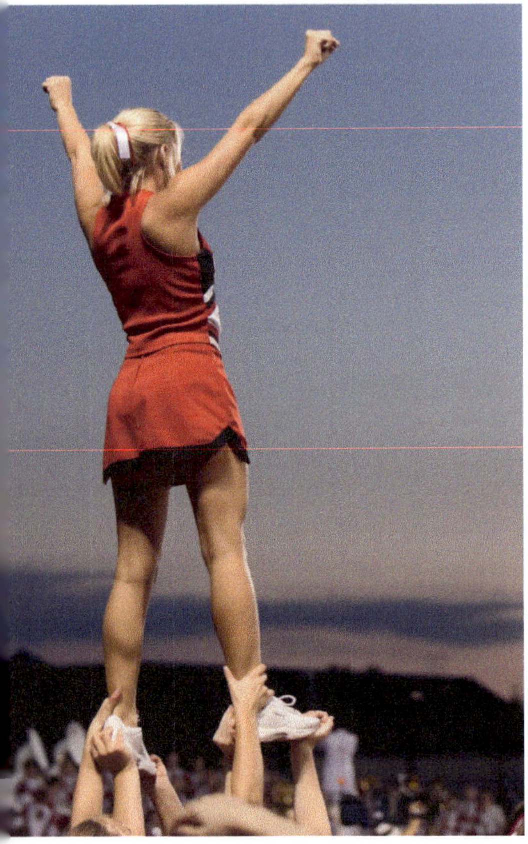

Prevention programs are generally divided into 3 categories as defined by the Caplan model: primary, secondary, and tertiary. Primary (also known as universal) prevention aims to reduce the number of cases in a population by targeting people who do not have signs or symptoms. Secondary prevention seeks to reduce the prevalence by selectively targeting high-risk individuals and those who may be showing early signs or symptoms of disorder. Tertiary prevention is directed toward minimizing the damaging effects among those who have been diagnosed with a disorder. It is often difficult to discriminate between populations that are targets for primary or secondary interventions because differentiation between healthy individuals and those with a subclinical condition may be difficult. Reactive prevention efforts are directed at creating resistance to potential risk factors, whereas proactive prevention seeks to reduce or eliminate exposure to known risk factors.[12] Little empirical evidence exists regarding the prevention of DE and EDs among athletes. Peer-led and practitioner-led programs have been modified to address some of the unique needs and circumstances of the culture of the athlete.

At any level, prevention begins with an awareness of risks, signs, and symptoms. Often, dietary restriction, which results in relative energy deficiency, is the first sign of an ED.[13] Unfortunately, relatively little is actually known about the diets of individual athletes. This calls for greater attention to the dietary and weight-management practices of athletes.[12] The RDN who works with athletes should be aware of the importance of building a trusting interpersonal relationship in which athletes view the sports dietitian as a safe resource and are willing to share the details of their dietary practices. For many people, what they eat, what they put into their body, is a very intimate topic of conversation.

Some additional factors that place an athlete at risk for REDs include injuries and illness (injured athletes fear unwanted weight gain during recovery); a decline in the quality of performance as a result of the loss of lean body mass and strength; the sharing of nutrition myths or pressure to lose weight by misinformed training staff; fear of eating when traveling, perhaps especially in fast-food restaurants; lack of nutrition knowledge or skills to choose or prepare nutritious food; and personality traits of a good athlete (eg, perfectionism, competitiveness, willingness to train through pain).[97,102,153]

Additional efforts toward prevention include the following:

- Develop mandatory educational programs for coaches, trainers, and athletes across all sports regarding the risk factors, signs, and symptoms of DE and EDs.[13]
- Educate male and female athletes about the athlete triads and REDs so they recognize the nutrition and health requirements necessary for safe participation in sport.
- Adopt a protocol to identify EDs and appropriate actions to take. Consider the IOC REDs CAT2, the Female Athlete Triad Cumulative Risk Assessment Tool, and a sample athlete contract for clearance and ready-to-play decisions.
- Monitor the modeling of beliefs and behaviors to reduce contagion between athletes and influential others.
- Deemphasize body weight and composition.
- Promote healthful eating behaviors.
- Destigmatize EDs.
- Foster individuality among and within athletes.

FUTURE NEEDS

Formal ED curricula for RDNs include various programs; brief training workshops; specialized ED conferences; web-based courses; and collaborative learning, teaching, and supervision.[110] Despite these programs, more training is needed, specifically for RDNs on therapeutic modalities for the ED population.

Although education for athletes and coaches does not directly translate into changes in attitudes or behavior, education does contribute to awareness. Educational programs that emphasize the central role of nutrition in both physical and mental health, in addition to weight as a factor in performance, increase awareness of the potential detriment of critical comments about body size, weight, and/or shape and support the creation of safe and trusting relationships to encourage open communication about eating problems.

Although the determinants of mental health are complex, the emerging and compelling evidence for nutrition as a crucial factor in the high prevalence and incidence of mental disorders suggests that diet is as important to psychiatry as it is to cardiology, endocrinology, and gastroenterology. Evidence is steadily growing for the relationship between dietary quality (and potential nutritional deficiencies) and mental health and for the select use of nutrient-based supplements to address deficiencies or to provide monotherapies or augmentation therapies.

SUMMARY

This chapter discusses EDs, especially among the athletic population. Although the data suggest individual risk factors, it is important to view every athlete as being at risk. If the health care and sports communities address the entire culture of sport, it is more likely that substantial strides will be made toward the prevention and early identification of EDs on a large scale, positively affecting countless at-risk athletes. It is also important that the health care community dispel the commonly held belief that those with DE or OSFED are not as at risk as those diagnosed with other EDs. Similarly, it is a mistake to assume that a person is healthy based on performance or simple observation. It is imperative that those who work with athletic populations recognize their own attitudes and gaps in knowledge and seek to improve their skills. RDNs should look for opportunities to increase their knowledge about EDs by seeking out formal education opportunities. Finally, it is necessary to overcome stigma among athletes so that all "members of this population come to understand that the 'mental toughness' required for success in sport is compatible with mental health help seeking."[2]

KEY TAKEAWAYS

Disordered eating behaviors exist on a spectrum.

Athletes in any and every sport may be at risk for DE/EDs.

The health and performance consequences of DE/EDs are significant and can be severe.

RDNs who treat athletes with DE/EDs require specialized training and experience.

The treatment of DE/EDs requires an interdisciplinary team including at the very least a physician, a mental health professional, and an RDN.

REFERENCES

1. Wells KR, Jeacocke NA, Appaneal R, et al. The Australian Institute of Sport (AIS) and National Eating Disorders Collaboration (NEDC) position statement on disordered eating in high performance sport. *Br Sports Med.* 2020;54(21):1247-1258. doi:10.1136/bjsports-2019-101813
2. Reardon CL, Hainline B, Aron CM, et al. Mental health in elite athletes: International Olympic Committee consensus statement (2019). *Br Sports Med.* 2019;53:667-699. doi:10.1136/bjsports-2019-100715
3. American Psychiatric Association. From Planning to Publication: Developing DSM-5-TR. Accessed January 22, 2023. www.psychiatry.org/File%20Library/Psychiatrists/Practice/DSM/DSM-5-TR/APA-DSM5TR-FromPlanningtoPublication.pdf
4. American Psychiatric Association. Attention to Culture, Racism, and Discrimination in DSM-5-TR. Accessed January 22, 2023. www.psychiatry.org/File%20Library/Psychiatrists/Practice/DSM/DSM-5-TR/APA-DSM5TR-AttentiontoCultureRacismandDiscrimination.pdf
5. American Psychiatric Association. Coding and Recording Procedures. Accessed January 22, 2023. www.psychiatry.org/File%20Library/Psychiatrists/Practice/DSM/DSM-5-TR/APA-DSM5TR-Coding.pdf
6. World Health Organization. ICD-11 Implementation. Accessed January 23, 2023. www.who.int/standards/classifications/frequently-asked-questions/icd-11-implementation
7. World Health Organization. ICD-11 Implementation or Transition Guide. Accessed January 23, 2023. https://icd.who.int/en/docs/ICD-11%20Implementation%20or%20Transition%20Guide_v105.pdf
8. American Psychiatric Association. *Diagnostic and Statistical Manual of Mental Disorders, Fifth Edition, Text Revision (DSM-5-TR).* Accessed January 23, 2023. https://dsm.psychiatryonline.org/doi/book/10.1176/appi.books.9780890425787
9. American Psychiatric Association. *Diagnostic and Statistical Manual of Mental Disorders, Fifth Edition (DSM-5).* American Psychiatric Association; 2013.
10. World Health Organization. International Statistical Classification of Diseases and Related Health Problems, 10th Revision. Accessed January 23, 2023. https://icd.who.int/browse10/2019/en
11. World Health Organization. ICD-11 Coding Tool: Mortality and Morbidity Statistics (MMS). Accessed January 23, 2023. https://icd.who.int/ct11/icd11_mms/en/release
12. Filion AJ, Haines J. Why prevention? The case for upstream strategies. In: Smolak L, Levine MP, eds. *The Wiley Handbook of Eating Disorders.* John Wiley & Sons, Ltd; 2015:555-568.
13. de Oliveira Coelho GM, da Silva Gomes AI, Ribeiro BG, de Abreu Soares E. Prevention of eating disorders in female athletes. *Open Access Sports Med.* 2014;5:105-113. doi:10.2147/OAJSM.S36528
14. Hay P, Girosi F, Mond J. Prevalence and sociodemographic correlates of DSM-5 eating disorders in the Australian population. *Eat Disord.* 2015;3:19. doi:10.1186/s40337-015-0056-0
15. National Eating Disorders Association. Statistics. Accessed January 23, 2023. www.nationaleatingdisorders.org/statistics-research-eating-disorders
16. Von Essen E, *Mårtensson* F. Young adults' use of food as a self-therapeutic intervention. *Int Qual Stud Health Well-being.* 2014;9:23000. doi:10.3402/qhw.v9.23000
17. Bratman S, Knight D. *Health Food Junkies: Orthorexia Nervosa: Overcoming the Obsession with Healthful Eating.* Broadway Books; 2000.
18. Moroze RM, Dunn TM, Holland CJ, Yager J, Weintraub P. Microthinking about micronutrients: a case of transition from obsessions about healthy eating to near-fatal "orthorexia nervosa" and proposed diagnostic criteria. *Psychosomatics.* 2015;56(4):397-403. doi:10.1016/j.psym.2014.03.003
19. Uher R, Rutter M. Classification of feeding and eating disorders: review of evidence and proposals for ICD-11. *World Psychiatry.* 2012;11(2):80-92. doi:10.1016/j.wpsyc.2012.05.005
20. Elgaddal N, Kramarow EA, Reuben C. Physical Activity Among Adults Aged 18 and Over: United States, 2020. NCHS Data Brief, no 443. National Center for Health Statistics, Center for Disease Control and Prevention. Last Reviewed: August 30, 2022. Accessed January 23, 2023. www.cdc.gov/nchs/products/databriefs/db443.htm
21. O'Keefe JO, Patil HR, Lavie CJ, Magalski A, Vogel RA, McCullough PA. Potential adverse cardiovascular effects from excessive endurance exercise. *Mayo Clin Proc.* 2012;87(6):587-595. doi:10.1016/j.mayocp.2012.04.005
22. Lichtenstein MB, Melin AK, Szabo A, et al. The prevalence of exercise addiction symptoms in a sample of national level elite athletes. *Front Sports Act Living.* 2021;3:635418. doi:10.3389/fspor.2021.635418
23. National Health Interview Survey. Glossary. National Center for Health Statistics, Center for Disease Control and Prevention. Last Reviewed: February 17, 2017. Accessed January 20, 2023. www.cdc.gov/nchs/nhis/physical_activity/pa_glossary.htm
24. Landolfi E. Exercise addiction. *Sports Med.* 2013;43(2):111-119. doi:10.1007/s40279-012-0013-x
25. Cook BJ, Hausenblas HA. The role of exercise dependence for the relationship between exercise behavior and eating pathology: mediator or moderator? *Health Psychol.* 2008;13(4):495-502. doi:10.1177/1359105308088520
26. Szabo A, Pinto A, Griffiths MD, Kovácsik R, Demetrovics Z. The psychometric evaluation of the Revised Exercise Addiction Inventory: Improved psychometric properties by changing item response rating. *Behav Addict.* 2019;8(1):157-161. doi:10.1556/2006.8.2019.06
27. Mari-Sanchis A, Burgos-Balmaseda J, Hidalgo-Borrajo R. Eating disorders in sport. Update and proposal for an integrated approach. *Endocrinol Diabetes Nutr (Engl Ed).* 2022;69(2):131-143. doi:10.1016/j.endien.2022.02.016

28. Beals K. *Disordered Eating Among Athletes: A Comprehensive Guide for Health Professionals*. Human Kinetics; 2004.

29. Knapp J, Aerni G, Anderson J. Eating disorders in female athletes: use of screening tools. *Curr Sports Med Rep*. 2014;13(4):214-218. doi:10.1249/JSR.0000000000000074

30. Schaefer LM, Crosby RD, Machado PPP. A systematic review of instruments for the assessment of eating disorders among adults. *Curr Opin Psychiatry*. 2021;34(6):543-562. doi:10.1097/YCO.0000000000000746

31. Schaal K, Tafflet M, Nassif H, et al. Psychological balance in high level athletes: gender-based differences and sport-specific patterns. *PLoS One*. 2011;6(5):e19007. doi:10.1371/journal.pone.0019007

32. Berg S, Pritchett, K, Ogan D, Larson A. Self-reported history of eating disorders, training, weight-control methods and body satisfaction in elite female runners competing at the 2020 US Olympic marathon trials. *Int Exerc Sci*. 2022;15(2):721-732.

33. Smith AB, Gay JL, Monsma EV, et al. Investigation of eating disorder risk and body image dissatisfaction among female competitive cheerleaders. *Int Environ Res Public Health*. 2022;19(4):2196. doi:10.3390/ijerph19042196

34. Borgelt S, Burmeister JM. Disordered eating in collegiate English equestrian athletes in aesthetic and nonaesthetic disciplines. *Eat Behav*. 2022;46:101661. doi:10.1016/j.eatbeh.2022.101661

35. Martínez-Rodríguez A, Vicente-Martínez M, Sánchez-Sánchez J, Miralles-Amorós L, Martínez-Olcina M, Sánchez-Sáez JA. Eating disorders in top elite beach handball players: cross sectional study. *Children (Basel)*. 2021;8(3):245. doi:10.3390/children8030245

36. Joubert LM, Gonzalez GB, Larson A. Prevalence of disordered eating among international sport lead rock climbers. *Front Sports Act Living*. 2020;2:86. doi:10.3389/fspor.2020.00086

37. Prather H, Hunt D, McKeon K, et al. Are elite female soccer athletes at risk for disordered eating attitudes, menstrual dysfunction and stress fractures? *PM R*. 2016;8(3):208-213. doi:10.1016/j.pmrj.2015.07.003

38. Thiemann P, Legenbauer T, Vocks S, Platen P, Auyeung B, Herpertz S. Eating disorders and their putative risk factors among female German professional athletes. *Eur Eat Disord Rev*. 2015;23:269-276. doi:10.1002/erv.2360

39. Fortes LS, Kakeshita I, Almeida S, Gomes A, Ferreira M. Eating behaviours in youths: a comparison between female and male athletes and non-athletes. *Scand Med Sci Sports*. 2014;24:e62-e68. doi:10.1111/sms.12098

40. Chatterton J, Petrie TA. Prevalence of disordered eating and pathogenic weight control behaviors among male collegiate athletes. *Eat Disord*. 2013;21(4):328-341. doi:10.1080/10640266.2013.797822

41. Goltz F, Stenzel L, Schneider C. Disordered eating behaviors and body image in male athletes. *Rev Bras Psiquiatr*. 2013;35(3):237-242. doi:10.1590/1516-4446-2012-0840

42. Martinsen M, Sundgot-Borgen J. Higher prevalence of eating disorders among adolescent elite athletes than controls. *Med Sci Sports Exerc*. 2013;45(6):1188-1197. doi:10.1249/MSS.0b013e318281a939

43. Thein-Nissenbaum JM, Rauh MJ, Carr KE, Loud KJ, McGuine TA. Associations between disordered eating, menstrual dysfunction, and musculoskeletal injury among high school athletes. *Orthop Sports Phys Ther*. 2011;41(2):60-69. doi:10.2519/jospt.2011.3312

44. Martinsen M, Bratland-Sanda S, Eriksson AK, Sundgot-Borgen J. Dieting to win or to be thin? A study of dieting and disordered eating among adolescent elite athletes and non-athlete controls. *Br Sports Med*. 2010;44(1):70-76. doi:10.1136/bjsm.2009.068668

45. Greenleaf C, Petrie TA, Carter J, Reel JJ. Female collegiate athletes: prevalence of eating disorders and disordered eating behaviors. *Amer Coll Health*. 2009;57(5):489-495. doi:10.3200/JACH.57.5.489-496

46. Rosendahl J, Bormann B, Aschenbrenner K, Aschenbrenner F, Strauss B. Dieting and disordered eating in German high school athletes and non-athletes. *Scand Med Sci Sports*. 2009;19(5):731-739. doi:10.1111/j.1600-0838.2008.00821.x

47. Petrie TA, Greenleaf C, Reel J, Carter J. Prevalence of eating disorders and disordered eating behaviors among male collegiate athletes. *Psychol Men Masc*. 2008;9:267-277. doi:10.1037/a0013178

48. Torstveit MK, Rosenvinge JH, Sundgot-Borgen J. Prevalence of ED and the predictive power of risk models in female elite athletes: a controlled study. *Scand Med Sci Sports*. 2008;18(1):108-118. doi:10.1111/j.1600-0838.2007.00657.x

49. Nichols JF, Rauh MJ, Barrack MT, Barkai H-S, Pernick Y. Disordered eating and menstrual irregularity in high school athletes in lean-build and nonlean-build sports. *Int Sport Nutr Exerc Metab*. 2007;17(4):364-377. doi:10.1123/ijsnem.17.4.364

50. Nichols JF, Rauh MJ, Lawson MJ, Ji M, Barkai H-S. Prevalence of the female athlete triad syndrome among high school athletes. *Arch Pediatr Adolesc Med*. 2006;160(2):137-142. doi:10.1001/archpedi.160.2.137

51. Beals KA, Hill AK. The prevalence of disordered eating, menstrual dysfunction, and low bone mineral density among US collegiate athletes. *Int Sport Nutr Exerc Metab*. 2006;16(1):1-23. doi:10.1123/ijsnem.16.1.1

52. Toro J, Gailiea B, Martinez-Mallén E, et al. Eating disorders in Spanish female athletes. *Int Sports Med*. 2005;26(8):679-700. doi:10.1055/s-2004-830378

53. Sundgot-Borgen J, Torstveit MK. Prevalence of eating disorders in elite athletes is higher than in the general population. *Clin Sport Med*. 2004;14(1):25-32. doi:10.1097/00042752-200401000-00005

54. Byrne S, McLean N. Elite athletes: effects of the pressure to be thin. *Sci Med Spor*. 2002;5(2):80-94. doi:10.1016/s1440-2440(02)80029-9

55. Beals KA, Manore MM. Disorders of the female athlete triad among collegiate athletes. *Int Sport Nutr Exerc Metab*. 2002;12(3):281-293. doi:10.1123/ijsnem.12.3.281

56. Johnson C, Powers P, Dick R. Athletes and eating disorders: the National Collegiate Athletic Association study. *Int Eat Disord*. 1999;26(2):179-188. doi:10.1002/(sici)1098-108x(199909)26:2<179::aid-eat7>3.0.co;2-z

57. Sundgot-Borgen J. Prevalence of eating disorders in elite female athletes. *Int Sport Nutr*. 1993;3(1):29-40. doi:10.1123/ijsn.3.1.29

58. Kosmiski L, Schmiege S, Mascolo M, Gaudiani J, Mehler P. Chronic starvation secondary to anorexia nervosa is associated with an adaptive suppression of resting energy expenditure. *Clin Endocrinol Metab.* 2014;99(3):908-914. doi:10.1210/jc.2013-1694
59. Keeler JL, Konyn CY, Treasure J, et al. "Your mind doesn't have room for anything else": a qualitative study of perceptions of cognitive functioning during and after recovery from anorexia nervosa. *Eat Disord.* 2022;10(1):201. doi:10.1186/s40337-022-00723-6
60. Burke LM, Lundy B, Fahrenholtz IL, Melin AK. Pitfalls of conducting and interpreting estimates of energy availability in free-living athletes. *Int Sport Nutr Exerc Metab.* 2018;28(4):350-363. doi:10.1123/ijsnem.2018-0142
61. Taguchi M, Manore MM. Reexamining the calculations of exercise energy expenditure in the energy availability equation of free-living athletes. *Front Sports Act Living.* 2022;4:885631. doi:10.3389/fspor.2022.885631
62. O'Hara CB, Keyes A, Renwick B, Leyton M, Campbell IC, Schmidt U. The effects of acute dopamine precursor depletion on the reinforcing value of exercise in anorexia nervosa. *PLoS One.* 2016;11(1):e0145894. doi:10.1371/journal.pone.0145894
63. Watford M. Starvation: metabolic changes. Wiley Online Library, 2015. Accessed February 15, 2023. https://doi.org/10.1002/9780470015902.a0000642.pub2
64. Physical status: the use and interpretation of anthropometry. Report of a WHO expert committee. Technical Report Series No. 854. 1995. World Health Organization website. Accessed May 5, 2016. www.who.int/childgrowth/publications/physical_status/en
65. Gaudiani JL, Mehler PS. Rare medical manifestations of severe restricting and purging: "Zebras," missed diagnoses, and best practices. *Int Eat Disord.* 2016;49(3):331-344. doi:10.1002/eat.22475
66. Mehler PS, Krantz MJ, Sachs KV. Treatments of medical complications of anorexia nervosa and bulimia nervosa. *Eat Disord.* 2015;3:15. doi:10.1186/s40337-015-0041-7
67. Fisher BA, Schenkman M. Functional recovery of a patient with anorexia nervosa: physical therapist management in the acute care hospital setting. *Phys Ther.* 2012;92(4):595-604. doi:10.2522/ptj.20110187
68. Campbell K, Peebles R. Eating disorders in children and adolescents: state of the art review. *Pediatrics.* 2014;134(3):582-592. doi:10.1542/peds.2014-0194
69. Sidiropoulos M. Anorexia nervosa: the physiological consequences of starvation and the need for primary prevention efforts. *McGill Med.* 2007;10(1):20-25.
70. Definition & Facts for Binge Eating Disorder. National Institute of Diabetes and Digestive and Kidney Diseases website. Accessed February 9, 2023. www.niddk.nih.gov/health-information/weight-management/binge-eating-disorder/definition-facts
71. Tewksbury C, Nwankwo R, Peterson J. Academy of Nutrition and Dietetics: Revised 2022 Standards of Practice and Standards of Professional Performance for Registered Dietitian Nutritionists (Competent, Proficient, and Expert) in Adult Weight Management. *Acad Nutr Diet.* 2022;122(10):1940-1954.e45. doi:10.1016/j.jand.2022.06.008
72. Kirk S, Ogata B, Wichert E, Handu D, Rozga M. Treatment of pediatric overweight and obesity: position of the Academy of Nutrition and Dietetics based on an umbrella review of systematic reviews. *Acad Nutr Diet.* 2022;122(4):848-861. doi:10.1016/j.jand.2022.01.008
73. Spodick DH. Normal sinus heart rate; appropriate rate thresholds for sinus tachycardia and bradycardia. *South Med J.* 1996;89(7):666-667. doi:10.1097/00007611-199607000-00003
74. Chiu SN, Lin LY, Wang JK, et al. Long-term outcomes of pediatric sinus bradycardia. *Pediatr.* 2013;163(3):885-889.e1. doi:10.1016/j.jpeds.2013.03.054
75. Mehler PS, Brown C. Anorexia nervosa medical complications. *Eat Disord.* 2015;3:11. doi:10.1186/s40337-015-0040-8
76. Yahalom M, Spitz M, Sandler L, Heno N, Roguin N, Turgeman Y. The significance of bradycardia in anorexia nervosa. *Int Angiol.* 2013;22(2):83-94. doi:10.1055/s-0033-1334138
77. ACUTE Center for Eating Disorders & Severe Malnutrition. Low heart rate (bradycardia) and anorexia. Updated February 25, 2021. Accessed October 7, 2023. www.acute.org/resource/bradycardia-anorexia
78. Mehler P. Anorexia nervosa in adults and adolescents: Medical complications and their management. In: Yager J, Solomon D, eds. *UpToDate.* Wolters Kluwer; July 29, 2022. Accessed October 20, 2023. www.uptodate.com/contents/14705#!
79. Wertli MM, Ruchti KB, Steurer J, Held U. Diagnostic indicators of non-cardiovascular chest pain: a systematic review and meta-analysis. *BMC Med.* 2013;11:239. doi:10.1186/1741-7015-11-239
80. Birmingham CL. Medical complications and diagnosing eating disorders. In: Smolak L, Levine MP, eds. *The Wiley Handbook of Eating Disorders.* John Wiley & Sons, Ltd; 2015:170-182.
81. Fisher B, Schenkman M. Functional recovery of a patient with anorexia nervosa: physical therapist management in the acute care hospital setting. *Phys Ther.* 2012;92(4):595-604. doi:10.2522/ptj.20110187
82. D'Souza AD, Bucchi A, Johnsen AB, et al. Exercise training reduces resting heart rate via downregulation of the funny channel HCN_4. *Nat Commun.* 2014;5:3775. doi:10.1038/ncomms4775
83. Zheng T, Camilleri M. Management of gastroparesis. *Gastroenterol Hepatol (N Y).* 2021;17(11):515-525.
84. Lacy BE, Gabbard SL, Crowell MD. Pathophysiology, evaluation, and treatment of bloating: hope, hype, or hot air? *Gastroenterol Hepatol (NY).* 2011;7(11):729-739.
85. Kleiman SC, Carroll IM, Tarantino LM, Bulik CM. Gut feelings: a role for the intestinal microbiota in anorexia nervosa? *Int Eat Disord.* 2015;48(5):449-451. doi:10.1002/eat.22394
86. Weiss Kelly A, Hecht S. The female athlete triad. *Ann Joint.* 2022;7:6. doi:10.21037/aoj-2020-03
87. Nattiv A, Loucks AB, Manore MM, Sanborn CF, Sundgot-Borgen J, Warren MP; American College of Sports Medicine. American College of Sports Medicine position stand. The female athlete triad. *Med Sci Sports Exerc.* 2007;39(10):1867-1882. doi:10.1249/mss.0b013e318149f111

88. Faje AT, Fazeli PK, Miller KK, et al. Fracture risk and areal bone mineral density in adolescent females with anorexia nervosa. *Int Eat Disord.* 2014;47(5):458-466. doi:10.1002/eat.22248
89. Kalm LM, Semba RD. They starved so that others be better fed: remembering Ancel Keys and the Minnesota Experiment. *Nutr.* 2005;135(6):1347-1352. doi:10.1093/jn/135.6.1347
90. Hadigan CM, Anderson EJ, Miller KK, et al. Assessment of macronutrient and micronutrient intake in women with anorexia nervosa. *Int Eat Disord.* 2000;28(3):284-292. doi:10.1002/1098-108x(200011)28:3<284::aid-eat5>3.0.co;2-g
91. Statistics. National Eating Disorders Association website. Accessed January 23, 2023. www.nationaleatingdisorders.org/statistics
92. Otis CL, Goldingay R. *The Athletic Woman's Survival Guide: How to Win the Battle Against Eating Disorders, Amenorrhea, and Osteoporosis.* Human Kinetics Publishers; 2000.
93. Striegel-Moore RH, Bulik CM. Risk factors for eating disorders. *Am Psychol.* 2007;62(3):181-198. doi:10.1037/0003-066X.62.3.181
94. Crowther J, Smith KE, Williams GA. Familial risk factors and eating disorders. In: Smolak L, Levine MP, eds. *The Wiley Handbook of Eating Disorders.* John Wiley & Sons, Ltd; 2015:338-351.
95. Uher R, Rutter M. Classification of feeding and eating disorders: review of evidence and proposals for ICD-11. *World Psychiatry.* 2012;11(2):80-92. doi:10.1016/j.wpsyc.2012.05.005
96. Wildes JE, Forbush KT. Ethnicity as a risk factor for eating disorders. In: Smolak L, Levine MP, eds. *The Wiley Handbook of Eating Disorders.* John Wiley & Sons, Ltd; 2015:324-337.
97. Thompson RA, Sherman RT. *Eating Disorders in Sport.* Routledge; 2010.
98. Smolak L, Murnen SK, Ruble AE. Female athletes and eating problems: a meta-analysis. *Int Eat Disord.* 2000;27(4):371-380. doi:10.1002/(sici)1098-108x(200005)27:4<371::aid-eat1>3.0.co;2-y
99. Daniels EA. Sex objects, athletes, and sexy athletes: how media representations of women athletes can impact adolescent girls and college women. *Adolesc Res.* 2009;24(4):399-422. doi:10.1177/0743558409336748
100. Eichstadt M, Luzier J, Cho D, Weisenmuller C. Eating disorders in male athletes. *Sports Health.* 2020;12(4):327-333. doi:10.1177/1941738120928991
101. Wolter S. A quantitative analysis of photographs and articles on espnW: positive progress for female athletes. *Commun Sport.* 2015;3(2):168-195. doi:10.1177/2167479513509368
102. Sundgot-Borgen J, Meyer NL, Lohman TG, et al. How to minimise the health risks to athletes who compete in weight-sensitive sports review and position statement on behalf of the Ad Hoc Research Working Group on Body Composition, Health and Performance, under the auspices of the IOC Medical Commission. *Br Sports Med.* 2013;47(16):1012-1022. doi:10.1136/bjsports-2013-092966
103. Rahman R, Linsenmeyer WR. Caring for transgender patients and clients: nutrition-related clinical and psychosocial considerations. *Acad Nutr Diet.* 2019;119(5):727-732. doi:10.1016/j.jand.2018.03.006
104. Jacobi C, Abascal L, Taylor CB. Screening for eating disorders and high-risk behavior: caution. *Int Eat Disord.* 2004;36(3):280-295. doi:10.1002/eat.20048
105. Rodgers RF, Franko DL. Screening for eating disorders: An updated guide. In: Smolak L, Levine MP, eds. *The Wiley Handbook of Eating Disorders.* John Wiley & Sons, Ltd; 2015:507-523.
106. Lease H, Bond M. Correspondence between alternate measures of maladaptive exercise, and their associations with disordered eating symptomatology. *Behav Addict.* 2013;2(3):153-159. doi:10.1556/JBA.2.2013.012
107. Bonci CM, Bonci LJ, Granger LR, et al. National Athletic Trainers' Association position statement: preventing, detecting, and managing disordered eating in athletes. *Athl Train.* 2008;43(1):80-108. doi:10.4085/1062-6050-43.1.80
108. Mahr F, Farahmand P, Bixler E, et al. A national survey of eating disorder training. *Int Eat Disord.* 2015;48(4):443-445. doi:10.1002/eat.22335
109. Academy for Eating Disorders (AED), Nutrition Working Group. *Guidebook for Nutrition Treatment of Eating Disorders.* 2021. Accessed October 10, 2023. https://higherlogicdownload.s3.amazonaws.com/AEDWEB/27a3b69a-8aae-45b2-a04c-2a078d02145d/UploadedImages/Publications_Slider/FINAL_AED_Purple_Nutrition_Book.pdf
110. National Collaborating Centre for Mental Health, National Institute for Clinical Excellence (NICE). *Eating Disorders: Core Interventions in the Treatment and Management of Anorexia Nervosa, Bulimia Nervosa and Related Eating Disorders.* National Clinical Guideline Number CG9. The British Psychological Society and The Royal College of Psychiatrists; 2004.
111. Dalle Grave R, Calugi S, Conti M, Doll H, Fairburn CG. Inpatient cognitive behaviour therapy for anorexia nervosa: a randomized controlled trial. *Psychother Psychosom.* 2013;82(6):390-398. doi:10.1159/000350058
112. Yager J, Devlin MJ, Halmi KA, et al. *Practice Guideline for the Treatment of Patients with Eating Disorders.* 3rd ed. American Psychiatric Association; 2006. Accessed October 30, 2015. http://psychiatryonline.org/pb/assets/raw/sitewide/practice_guidelines/guidelines/eatingdisorders.pdf
113. Dow AW, Baernholdt M, Santen SA, Baker K, Sessler CN. Practitioner wellbeing as an interprofessional imperative. *Interprof Care.* 2019;33(6):603-607. doi:10.1080/13561820.2019.1673705
114. Morgan KH, Barroso CS, Bateman S, Dixson M, Brown KC. Patients' experiences of interprofessional collaborative practice in primary care: a scoping review of the literature. *Patient Exp.* 2020;7(6):1466-1475. doi:10.1177/2374373520925725
115. Choi BCK, Pak AWP. Multidisciplinarity, interdisciplinarity and transdisciplinarity in health research, services, education and policy: 1. Definitions, objectives, and evidence of effectiveness. *Clin Invest Med.* 2006;29(6):351-364.

116. Tholking MM, Mellowspring AC, Eberle SG, et al. American Dietetic Association: standards of practice and standards of professional performance for registered dietitians (competent, proficient, and expert) in disordered eating and eating disorders (DE and ED). *Am Diet Assoc.* 2011;111(8):1242-1249.e37. doi:10.1016/j.jada.2011.05.021
117. Commission on Dietetic Registration. CSSD Eligibility Requirements. Accessed February 14, 2023. www.cdrnet.org/cssd-eligibility-requirements
118. International Association of Eating Disorders Professionals. Certification for Eating Disorder Professionals. Accessed February 14, 2023. https://iaedpfoundation.com/certification
119. Graves LL, Scribner C. Medical nutrition therapy for eating disorders. In: Smolak L, Levine MP, eds. *The Wiley Handbook of Eating Disorders.* John Wiley & Sons, Ltd; 2015:843-858.
120. McMaster CM, Wade T, Franklin J, Hart S. Discrepancies between Australian eating disorder clinicians and consumers regarding essential components of dietetic treatment. *Acad Nutr Diet.* 2022;122(8):1543-1557. doi:10.1016/j.jand.2021.12.006
121. Mittnacht AM, Bulik C. Best nutrition counseling practices for the treatment of anorexia nervosa: a Delphi study. *Int Eat Disord.* 2015;48(1):111-122. doi:10.1002/eat.22319
122. Parker LL, Harriger JA. Eating disorders and disordered eating behaviors in the LGBT population: a review of the literature. *Eat Disord.* 2020;8:51. doi:10.1186/s40337-020-00327-y
123. Janse van Rensburg M. COVID19, the pandemic which may exemplify a need for harm-reduction approaches to eating disorders: a reflection from a person living with an eating disorder. *Eat Disord.* 2020;8:26. doi:10.1186/s40337-020-00306-3
124. Swan WI, Vivanti A, Hakel-Smith NA, et al. Nutrition Care Process and Model update: toward realizing people-centered care and outcomes management. *Acad Nutr Diet.* 2017;117(12):2003-2014. doi:10.1016/j.jand.2017.07.015
125. Flegal KM, Graubard BI, Williamson DF, Gail MH. Excess deaths associated with underweight, overweight, and obesity: an evaluation of potential bias. *Vital Health Stat 3.* 2018;(42):1-21.
126. Bargiacchi A, Clarke J, Paulsen A, Leger J. Refeeding in anorexia nervosa. *Eur Pediatr.* 2019;178(3):413-422. doi:10.1007/s00431-018-3295-7
127. Phillips W, Doley J, Boi K. Malnutrition definitions in clinical practice: To be E43 or not to be? *Health Inf Manag.* 2020;49(1):74-79. doi:10.1177/1833358319852304
128. Quesnel DA, Cooper M, Fernandez-Del-Valle M, Reilly A, Calogero RM. Medical and physiological complications of exercise for individuals with an eating disorder: A narrative review. *Eat Disord.* 2023;11(1):3. doi:10.1186/s40337-022-00685-9
129. *Emergency Triage Assessment and Treatment (ETAT): Manual for Participants.* Department of Child and Adolescent Health and Development, World Health Organization, 2005. https://apps.who.int/iris/bitstream/handle/10665/43386/9241546875_eng.pdf?sequence=1
130. US Food & Drug Administration. Clinical Laboratory Improvement Amendments (CLIA). Updated July 17, 2023. Accessed August 8, 2023. www.fda.gov/medical-devices/ivd-regulatory-assistance/clinical-laboratory-improvement-amendments-clia
131. Garber AK, Sawyer SM, Golden NH, et al. A systematic review of approaches to refeeding in patients with anorexia nervosa. *Int Eat Disord.* 2016;49(3):293-310. doi:10.1002/eat.22482
132. Rigaud D, Verges B, Colas-Linhart N, et al. Hormonal and psychological factors linked to the increased thermic effect of food in malnourished fasting anorexia nervosa. *Clin Endocrinol Metab.* 2007;92(5):1623-1629. doi:10.1210/jc.2006-1319
133. Castellini G, Castellani W, Lelli L, et al. Association between resting energy expenditure, psychopathology and HPA-axis in eating disorders. *World Clin Cases.* 2014;2(7):257-264. doi:10.12998/wjcc.v2.i7.257
134. Anderson AE, Yager J. Eating disorders. In: Sadock BJ, Sadock VA, Ruiz P, eds. *Kaplan and Sadock's Comprehensive Textbook of Psychiatry.* Vol 1. 9th ed. Lippincott Williams and Wilkins; 2009:2128-2149.
135. Federici A, Wisniewski L. An intensive DBT program for patients with multidiagnostic eating disorder presentations: a case series analysis. *Int Eat Disord.* 2013;46(4):322-331. doi:10.1002/eat.22112
136. Federici A, Wisniewski L, Ben-Porath DD. Development and feasibility of an intensive DBT outpatient program for multi-diagnostic clients with eating disorders. *Couns Dev.* 2012;90:330-338. doi:10.1002/j.1556-6676.2012.00041.x
137. Rathaus JH, Miller AL. *DBT Skills Manual for Adolescents.* Guilford Press; 2014.
138. Juarascio A, Shaw J, Forman E, et al. Acceptance and commitment therapy as a novel treatment for eating disorders: an initial test of efficacy and mediation. *Behav Modif.* 2013;37(4):459-489. doi:10.1177/0145445513478633
139. Gorham E. The use of acceptance and commitment therapy (ACT) in the treatment of eating disorders. Paper presented at: 3rd annual Rocky Mountain Eating Disorders Conference; August 19-20, 2011; Denver, CO.
140. Ciao AC, Anderson K, Le Grange D. Family approaches to treatment. In: Smolak L, Levine MP, eds. *The Wiley Handbook of Eating Disorders.* John Wiley & Sons, Ltd; 2015:828-842.
141. Lock J, Le Grange D, Agras WS, Dare C. *Treatment Manual for Anorexia Nervosa: A Family-Based Approach.* Guildford Press; 2013.
142. Miller WR, Rollnick S. *Motivational Interviewing: Preparing People for Change.* 2nd ed. Guilford; 2002.
143. Brauhardt A, de Zwaan M, Hilbert A. The therapeutic process in psychological treatments for eating disorders: a systematic review. *Int Eat Disord.* 2014;47:565-584. doi:10.1002/eat.22287
144. Abell TL, Bernstein RK, Cutts T, et al. Treatment of gastroparesis: a multidisciplinary clinical review. *Neurogastroenterol Motil.* 2006;18(4):263-283. doi:10.1111/j.1365-2982.2006.00760.x

145. Schulte EM, Joyner MA, Potenza MN, Grilo CM, Gearhardt AN. Current considerations regarding food addiction. *Curr Psychiatry Rep*. 2015;17(4):563. doi:10.1007/s11920-015-0563-3
146. National Institute for Health and Care Excellence. Nutrition support for adults: oral nutrition support, enteral tube feeding and parenteral nutrition. Clinical Guideline 32. Published February 22, 2006. Accessed August 28, 2016. www.nice.org.uk/guidance/cg32/chapter/Introduction
147. Holtzman B, Tenforde AS, Parziale AL, Ackerman KE. Characterization of risk quantification differences using Female Athlete Triad Cumulative Risk Assessment and Relative Energy Deficiency in Sport Clinical Assessment Tool. *Int Sport Nutr Exerc Metab.* 2019;29(6):569-575. doi:10.1123/ijsnem.2019-0002
148. Fredericson M, Kussman A, Misra M, et al. The male athlete triad—a consensus statement from the Female and Male Athlete Triad Coalition Part II: Diagnosis, treatment, and return-to-play. *Clin Sport Med.* 2021;31(4):349-366. doi:10.1097/JSM.0000000000000948
149. De Souza MJ, Nattiv A, Joy E, et al. 2014 Female Athlete Triad Coalition consensus statement on treatment and return to play of the female athlete triad: 1st International Conference held in San Francisco, California, May 2012 and 2nd International Conference held in Indianapolis, Indiana, May 2013. *Br Sports Med.* 2014;48(4):289. doi:10.1136/bjsports-2013-093218
150. Mountjoy M, Sundgot-Borgen J, Burke L, et al. The IOC consensus statement: beyond the Female Athlete Triad—Relative Energy Deficiency in Sport (RED-S). *Br Sports Med.* 2014;48(7):491-497. doi:10.1136/bjsports-2014-093502
151. Nattiv A, Loucks AB, Manore MM, Sanborn CF, Sundgot-Borgen J, Warren MP; American College of Sports Medicine. American College of Sports Medicine position stand. The female athlete triad. *Med Sci Sports Exerc.* 2007;39(10):1867-1882. doi:10.1249/mss.0b013e318149f111
152. Mountjoy M, Ackerman KE, Bailey DM, et al. Avoiding the 'REDs Card'. We all have a role in the mitigation of REDs in athletes. *Br Sports Med.* 2023;57:1063-1064. doi:10.1136/bjsports-2023-106749
153. Heikura IA, Mountjoy ML, Ackerman KE, et al. IOC REDs CAT2. International Olympic Committee (IOC) Relative Energy Deficiency in Sport (REDs) Clinical Assessment Tool Version 2 (IOC REDs CAT2). Accessed August 20, 2023. https://stillmed.olympics.com/media/Documents/Athletes/Medical-Scientific/Consensus-Statements/REDs/IOC-REDs-CAT-Version-2.pdf

CHAPTER 19

Athletes With Diabetes

Charlotte Hayes, MMSc, MS, RDN, CSSD, CDCES, ACSM-CEP, and Melissa L. Brown, PhD, RD, CSSD, LD

LEARNING OBJECTIVES

- Summarize the interplay between diabetes pharmacology and exercise physiology.
- Describe the alterations in the endocrine system's response to exercise in athletes with diabetes.
- Examine the multitude of factors that impact glycemic management in athletes with diabetes.
- Develop an athlete-centered nutrition care plan that simultaneously supports glycemic management and athletic performance.

INTRODUCTION

Regular physical activity is a cornerstone of diabetes prevention and management because of the advantages it provides, including improvements in cardiometabolic health, cognitive functioning, and musculoskeletal health, as well as enhanced psychosocial outcomes.[1] These same benefits apply to athletes who have diabetes.[2] Athletes with diabetes are involved in a wide variety of sports and training regimens, each presenting its own unique set of challenges. The number of athletes who have diabetes continues to increase, ranging from youth and recreational athletes to professional, collegiate, and Olympic athletes.[2-7] Expanding knowledge of the biochemical regulation of muscle metabolism, the endocrinology of exercise, the pathophysiology of diabetes, and the practice of prescribing exercise and nutrition allows for better decision making for athletes with diabetes. This expanding knowledge has also made it possible for individuals with diabetes to safely participate in nearly all levels and types of sports.[2-8]

Balancing blood glucose management and athletic performance is challenging, so having the support of knowledgeable practitioners is critical. A sports registered dietitian nutritionist (RDN) who understands the needs of athletes with diabetes can be a valuable part of the athlete's support team, which typically also includes a certified diabetes care and education specialist (CDCES) and an endocrinologist. The desired outcome of nutrition intervention is the achievement of optimal glucose management with exercise so that the athlete with diabetes can realize the many health benefits of an active lifestyle and can achieve performance goals. However, managing diabetes in athletes goes beyond simply encouraging physical activity for the purpose of improving blood glucose management and overall health.[2-7] Athletes with diabetes have 2 important goals: manage blood glucose and optimize sports performance. Health care practitioners working with this population must be aware of both goals and must place maintaining the athlete's overall health as a third, equally important goal. It is common for athletes with diabetes and health care practitioners to become so focused on blood glucose management that they lose sight of the need to fuel for performance. Moreover, as with many athletes, there is a tendency to become so focused on meeting their performance goals that they lose sight of the general nutritional needs for good health.

When developing a quality sports nutrition plan for athletes with diabetes, it is necessary for the sports RDN to consider all 3 of the aforementioned goals. To do so, the sports RDN must have a good understanding of sports nutrition, energy metabolism, exercise physiology, and exercise endocrinology, as well as diabetes pharmacology and the pathophysiology of the various types of diabetes. Fully understanding the variables to be assessed and how they affect one another will enable sports RDNs to design nutrition plans that address the needs of athletes with diabetes. The most common type of diabetes among competitive athletes is type 1 diabetes (T1D),[2,9] however, type 2 diabetes (T2D) also exists among athletes, especially within the masters age group of 50 years or older.[2] (Refer to Chapter 14 for more information on masters athletes. Individuals may move into the masters category as early as the age of 35 years in some sports.) This chapter discusses the needs of and recommendations for athletes with diabetes and also introduces the concept of blood glucose management as a performance-enhancing strategy for athletes without diabetes.

TYPES OF DIABETES AND CONTRAINDICATIONS TO EXERCISE

The term *diabetes* encompasses a group of heterogenous diseases in which there is considerable variation in the clinical presentation and the progression of the disease. Multiple classifications exist under the umbrella diagnosis of diabetes, and the classification is what determines the appropriate treatment and medication; however, in some instances, it may be difficult to classify an individual at the time of diagnosis. Historically, it was rather simple to classify an individual as having either T1D or T2D based on the age of onset: onset in early childhood indicated T1D, whereas onset in adulthood indicated T2D. Currently, diagnosis is no longer that clear cut. Box 19.1 summarizes the classification and diagnosis of diabetes as noted in the American Diabetes Association's *Standards of Care in Diabetes—2023*. Box 19.2 provides a description of the conditions for which exercise is contraindicated for individuals with diabetes.[10]

BOX 19.1 Classification and Diagnosis of Diabetes[10]

Type 1 diabetes	Caused by autoimmune β-cell destruction, usually leading to absolute insulin deficiency, including latent autoimmune diabetes of adulthood
Type 2 diabetes	Caused by a nonautoimmune progressive loss of adequate β-cell insulin secretion frequently on the background of insulin resistance and metabolic syndrome
Gestational diabetes mellitus	Diagnosed in the second or third trimester of pregnancy that was not clearly overt diabetes prior to gestation
Specific types of diabetes due to other causes, such as monogenic diabetes syndromes (eg, neonatal diabetes and maturity-onset diabetes of the young)	Diseases of the exocrine pancreas (such as cystic fibrosis and pancreatitis) and drug- or chemical-induced diabetes (such as with glucocorticoid use, in the treatment of HIV/AIDS, or after organ transplantation)

DIABETES PHARMACOLOGY

Insulin Management

Since its discovery more than 100 years ago, insulin has been a life-sustaining medication for many millions of people living with diabetes.[11] Recent improvements in insulin formulations[12] and in diabetes technology[8] have resulted in increasingly more physiologic replacement therapies. Examples of advances in technology include continuous subcutaneous insulin infusion (CSII, or insulin pump) therapy, continuous glucose

BOX 19.2 Conditions for Which Exercise Is Contraindicated for Individuals With Diabetes[10]

Retinopathy	In individuals with type 1 diabetes or type 2 diabetes who have proliferative diabetic retinopathy, vigorous-intensity aerobic or resistance exercise can increase the risk of vitreous hemorrhage or retinal detachment.
Peripheral neuropathy	Individuals with peripheral neuropathy may have decreased pain sensation that can alter kinesthetic or proprioceptive sensation during physical activity. Peripheral neuropathy can increase the risk of skin breakdown, infection, and Charcot joint destruction. Proper footwear and daily self-examination of feet can help to detect early skin breakdown.
Autonomic neuropathy	Individuals with autonomic neuropathy can be at an increased risk of exercise-induced injury as a result of lowered cardiac responsiveness, postural hypotension, impaired thermoregulation, impaired night vision due to decreased papillary reaction, and greater risk of hypoglycemia. These individuals should be monitored by a cardiologist prior to training.
Albuminuria and nephropathy	Exercise can increase urinary protein excretion. There is no evidence that vigorous-intensity exercise increases the rate of progression of diabetic kidney disease.

monitoring systems (CGM) systems, and automated insulin delivery (AID) systems. AID systems use sophisticated algorithms to pair CGM systems with insulin pumps to automate insulin delivery and have the potential to increase an individual's time in range and reduce their diabetes burden.[8] Time in range is the amount of time spent with blood glucose levels in the target range (ie, 70–180 mg/dL). Individuals can preestablish insulin profiles in pump settings with an AID system to accommodate different types of training, competition, and recovery. Even so, an athlete with T1D or T2D who requires insulin must make numerous decisions when managing insulin to keep glucose in a safe and performance-enhancing range before, during, and after any exercise session.

Insulin therapy entails administering exogenous insulin in both fasting and postprandial states (refer to Table 19.1 on page 498),[12] as follows:

» Rapid- and short-acting insulins have an onset between 1 and 30 minutes and are used before meals to cover the postmeal rise in blood glucose. In addition, rapid-acting insulins are dosed to "correct" above-range glucose levels that may occur throughout the day. These insulins are the sole type of insulin used in insulin pump therapy.

» Long-acting insulin formulations generally have an onset time of 1 to 2 hours and a duration of 24 to 42 hours. They are used to mimic insulin released from the pancreatic β-cells at a low, basal level corresponding to a fasted state.

» Premixed and intermediate-acting insulin formulations include both postprandial and basal components. They are primarily prescribed to individuals with T2D who do not require dosing flexibility or desire the complex task of making multiple insulin dosing decisions throughout the day.

Glucose management for the athlete with diabetes is a dynamic process that requires close attention to blood glucose, fuel availability, circulating insulin on board (IOB), exercise energy systems, and hormonal interplay. Given this complexity, intensive insulin therapy using either multiple daily injections (MDIs) of rapid- and long-acting insulin or CSII is generally the therapy of choice.

INSULIN ON BOARD

The duration of insulin action refers to the length of time during which a dose of rapid-acting insulin will continue to lower blood glucose (refer to Table 19.1). IOB is the calculated amount of active insulin remaining in the bloodstream for a period of time postbolus or postinjection. It typically takes at least 4 to

TABLE 19.1 Insulin Types and Action Profiles[12]

Insulin type[a]	Insulin name[a] (brand name)	Insulin action profile		
		Onset	Peak	Duration
Rapid-acting analogue (U-100)	Glulisine (Apidra)	15 min	1 h	2-4 h
	Lispro (Humalog)	0-15 min	30-90 min	3-5 h
	Aspart (NovoLog)	10-20 min	60-120 min	3-5 h
	Faster-acting aspart (Fiasp)	2.5 min	30-90 min	3-5 h
	Insulin human (Afrezza[b])	1-12 min	35-45 min	1.5-3 h
Short-acting analogue (regular)	Humulin R Novolin R	30 min	2-5 h	5-8 h
Concentrated human (regular)	Humulin R U-500	0.5-1 h	2-8 h	up to 24 h
Intermediate-acting (neutral protamine Hagedorn [NPH])	Humulin N Novolin N	1.5-4 h	4-12 h	10-16 h
Long-acting	Biosimilar glargine (Basaglar)	1-2 h	Flat	24 h
	Glargine (Lantus)	1-2 h	Flat	24 h
	Detemir (Levemir)	0.8-2 h	3-9 h (dose dependent)	up to 24 h
	Degludec (Tresiba)	1 h	9 h (peak concentration)	42 h
Concentrated long-acting	Glargine U-300 (Toujeo) Degludec U-200 (Tresiba)	Not applicable	Not applicable	Not applicable
Premixed insulin[c]	Humulin 70/30 Novolin 70/30 Humalog 50/50 Humalog 75/25 NovoLog 70/30	Dual onset	Dual peaks	10-16 h
Premixed insulin/glucagon-like peptide-1 receptor agonists	Glargine/lixisenatide (Soliqua 100/33) Degludec/liraglutide (Xultrophy 100/3.6)	Not applicable	Not applicable	Not applicable

[a] U-100, 100 units per milliliter; U-200, 200 units per milliliter; U-300, 300 units per milliliter; U-500, 500 units per milliliter.
[b] Ultra-rapid acting, inhaled.
[c] Combination insulins represented by (percentage NPH)/(percentage regular insulin).

6 hours for all of the insulin action from a rapid-acting dose to stop lowering blood glucose. Taking additional insulin when there is still active IOB has an additive effect referred to as *stacking insulin doses*. This is one of the most common causes of hypoglycemia.[13,14] When programming insulin pumps, a CDCES must take into consideration peak insulin action and duration of action to minimize low blood glucose levels caused by stacking. Additional factors considered when programming insulin pumps include individual differences in cellular insulin sensitivity, insulin clearance, and gastric emptying.

Estimating active IOB can be more difficult for individuals on MDI therapy than for those using CSII/insulin pump therapy. Recently, programmable Bluetooth-enabled "smart" insulin pens paired with apps have been developed to improve dosing accuracy and tracking for those who prefer to take insulin by injection.

CONTINUOUS SUBCUTANEOUS INSULIN INFUSION/INSULIN PUMP

Insulin pumps are small computerized devices that infuse insulin subcutaneously through a tiny catheter, allowing for precise management of insulin dosing and thereby increasing the likelihood of achieving goals for time in range.[8,12] These devices are primarily used by individuals with T1D, but they can also be used by those with insulin-requiring T2D. To optimize blood glucose management, insulin pumps must be uniquely programmed and adjusted for individual needs. An athlete's physiological insulin requirements are often altered as their demands of training, level of conditioning, and body weight change. Female athletes may also find variations in insulin needs relative to menstrual cycle phases, especially during the luteal (premenstrual) phase when there is often increased insulin resistance and subsequent hyperglycemia.[15,16]

Insulin pumps are helpful because they allow for tailored basal and bolus insulin coverage.[17] Accurate infusion management formulas are used to initially calculate basal insulin rates, insulin-to-carbohydrate ratios (ICRs), and insulin sensitivity factors (ISFs).[18] A standard pump automatically delivers basal insulin for a period of 24 hours at precalculated rate(s) in units per hour (eg, 0.8 units/h). If an individual is switching from MDI to CSII, the diabetes care team should also consider the dose of long-acting insulin that the individual has been injecting in the determination of their basal insulin settings. A pump is typically programmed with 75% of the current long-acting insulin amount because infused rapid-acting insulin is absorbed more efficiently in hourly increments than single-dose, injected, long-acting insulin. For example, if an individual's dose of long-acting insulin is 24 units/d, the hourly infusion rate of rapid-acting insulin delivered by the pump would be (24 units × 0.75)/24 h = 0.75 unit/h. Insulin pumps can be programmed with multiple basal rates throughout the day to accommodate variations in insulin sensitivity. For example, people who are consistently more insulin resistant in the early morning (called the dawn phenomenon) are able to program a higher basal insulin rate for the early morning hours to prevent elevated blood glucose.[12]

In addition to basal rates, settings for bolus insulin, which is manually delivered when a standard pump is being used, must be programmed into the pump settings. The determination of bolus settings includes both the ICR and the ISF.[12] These are highly individualized calculations that are determined by the diabetes care team in collaboration with the pump wearer. The ICR is used to estimate the number of units of insulin that are needed to cover a set number of grams of carbohydrate; for example, a ratio of 1 unit for every 15 g of carbohydrate may be used to keep postprandial glucose within a goal range. The ISF is used to estimate the amount by which 1 unit of insulin will lower blood glucose (in units of milligrams per deciliter [or millimoles per liter]) if the glucose level is above range. For individuals using AID systems, the pump automates all insulin delivery unless the wearer switches the device into manual mode.

Note that all of the calculated factors can be variable for athletes because insulin sensitivity and insulin-independent uptake of glucose are affected by exercise and stress (in the short term) and by adaptations of training. Thus, these values need to be reevaluated throughout the year as cycles of training, competition, and recovery change.

INSULIN ADJUSTMENT STRATEGIES

The sports RDN is typically adept at adjusting carbohydrates for exercise, but it is beyond the scope of practice for most sports RDNs to advise about insulin adjustments. Thus, it is appropriate for the sports RDN to consult with the athlete's diabetes care team before making recommendations for insulin adjustments. Athletes with T1D will often need to decrease their basal rates during training or competition, especially for endurance sports. This allows for improved glucose management and athletic performance by reducing the risk of hypoglycemia and increasing the percentage of time in range.

In addition to lowering basal rates, athletes using pumps may disconnect from their pump (or untether) for up to 1 hour. For events requiring that an athlete spend a longer time without wearing a pump, the athlete can, with the support of their diabetes team, develop strategies for taking small doses of rapid-acting insulin by pen to replace insulin "gaps" and keep glucose in range. Disconnecting for longer than 1 hour without an insulin replacement strategy puts the athlete at increased risk for hyperglycemia and elevated ketone levels because of the missed basal insulin dose.

Because insulin sensitivity and responsiveness change with exercise, sizable blood glucose fluctuations can occur, especially if the active IOB is too low or too high. Use of CGM alone or alongside frequent self-monitoring of capillary blood glucose before, during, and after exercise is the foundation to making data-driven insulin adjustment decisions. Figure 19.1 illustrates exercise-related insulin adjustment strategies that can be used to maximize IOB.[2,5-7,9,19-26]

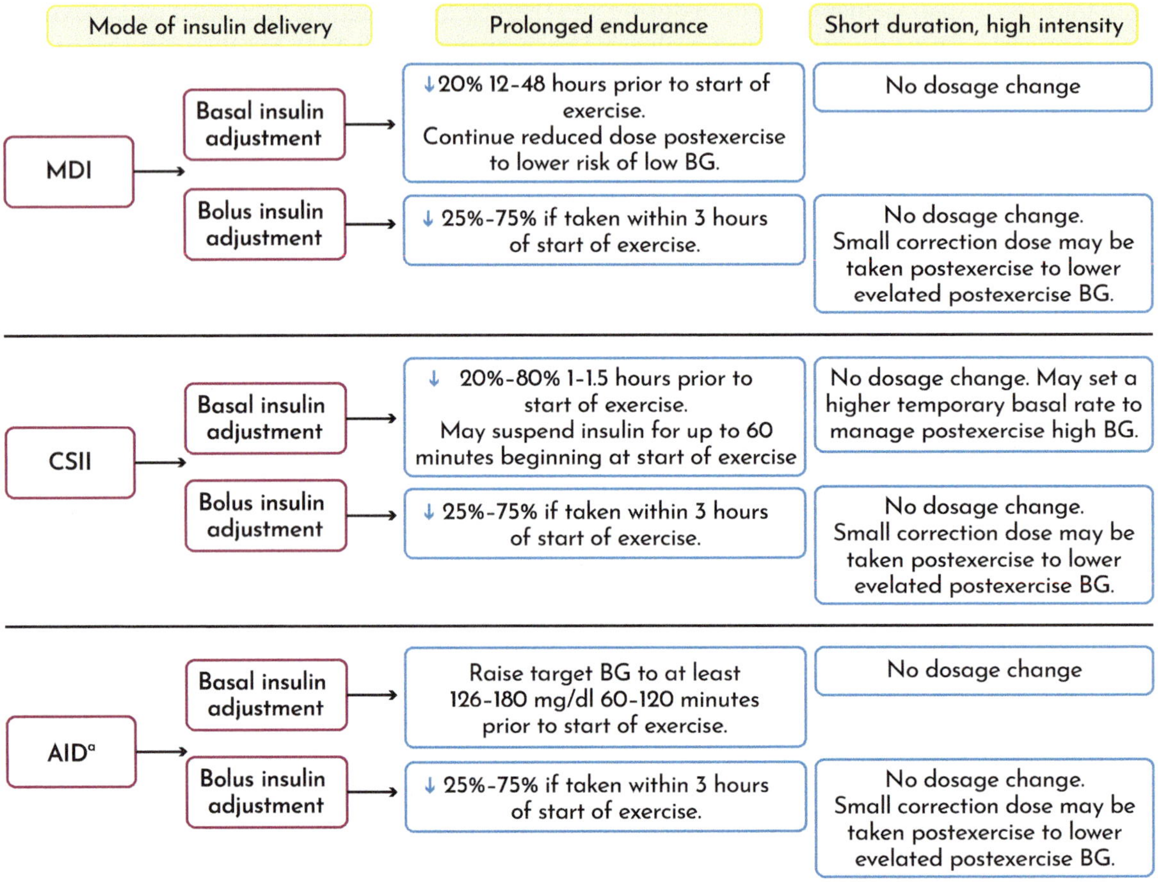

FIGURE 19.1 Exercise-related insulin adjustment strategies for maximizing insulin on board[2,5-7,9,19-26]

[a] Preestablish insulin profiles in the pump settings to accommodate different types of training, competition, and recovery. Turn on the temporary exercise activity feature 1 to 2 hours before the start of exercise or transfer to manual mode. Automatic insulin delivery systems can be transitioned to manual mode during exercise if automated features do not adequately keep glucose in range. An extended lag in continuous glucose monitoring (interstitial glucose) data of 12 to 20 minutes relative to plasma glucose can occur when the glucose level is changing rapidly and can affect the response of automatic insulin delivery systems. A typical protocol would be to raise BG levels to 150 mg/dL at least 1 hour before exercise for those using AID.

Abbreviations: AID, automatic insulin delivery; BG, blood glucose; CSII, continuous subcutaneous insulin infusion; MDI, multiple daily injections

BASAL INSULIN ADJUSTMENTS

Reductions in basal or long-acting insulin dose preceding exercise are typically recommended when an individual plans to do more exercise than usual; reductions are generally necessary for athletes participating in long-duration, high-intensity competitive events lasting longer than 90 minutes when energy demand is high.[1,6,8,20-22] Dosages of basal insulin may also need to be gradually reduced during blocks of increased training. Alternatively, increases in basal insulin become necessary in some scenarios. This is especially true during periods of reduced training, times of physical stress including during illness and postinjury recovery, when inflammatory markers are elevated, at times of heightened emotional stress, and during extended travel. Considering basal insulin adjustments is critical when a pattern of out-of-range morning fasting glucose or overnight glucose is identified. In addition, basal insulin adjustments should be considered if late postprandial glucose (>4 hours since last food intake) is out of range. Approaches for adjusting basal insulin are based on the insulin delivery method and the type of insulin employed (refer to Figure 19.1). Basal adjustments for MDI therapy generally must be made at least 12 hours (and even as much as 48 hours or longer for ultra–long-acting insulin) prior to planned exercise. CSII offers greater flexibility in insulin adjustments than MDI.[8,12] With CSII, basal insulin rates can be set 60 to 90 minutes before exercise, and the current glucose level and dynamics can be more readily weighed in decision making.[21,22]

MEALTIME/RAPID-ACTING INSULIN ADJUSTMENTS

Decisions about mealtime insulin adjustments require that multiple factors be weighed, including insulin program, meal nutrient composition, and timing in relation to the exercise start time, as well as the nature of the exercise session itself.[1,6,8,20-22] Reductions in bolus insulin dosages are advised when the exercise session will occur within 3 hours of a prior rapid-acting insulin injection and the planned exercise duration is longer than 30 to 60 minutes (refer to Figure 19.1). The goal is to reduce the active IOB at a time when the rapid-acting insulin action is high and, thereby, to reduce the risk of hypoglycemia during and after exercise. The degree of dose reduction is relative to the anticipated intensity, duration, and energy demands of the exercise, especially as the duration extends beyond 60 minutes.[6,20]

Travel and Storage

Many types of insulin are stable at room temperature for up to 28 days, after which they must be discarded; however, experts recommend that insulin be refrigerated (at 36 °F to 46 °F) until needed.[27] Insulin should not be frozen; this will decrease its effectiveness.[27] Athletes in cold-weather sports who carry insulin with them should keep it in an inside pocket to insulate it from potentially freezing temperatures. In general, insulin exposed to extreme temperatures may lose its effectiveness. A diabetes management plan should include specific strategies for storing insulin at appropriate temperatures.[27,28] This can be done by storing it in an insulated bag; a special insulin storage container with freezer packs; or a convenient type of lightweight carrying case, which, when soaked in water, keeps insulin cool for up to 48 hours. To avoid exposure to extreme temperatures, insulin and other medications should be kept with the person for whom they are prescribed and not in a cargo hold when traveling. It is also advisable that athletes carry a written copy of all prescriptions, extra diabetes supplies, and food that can be used to treat hypoglycemia or used as a small meal should the need arise.[28]

Oral Hypoglycemic Agents and Glucagon Formulations

Noninsulin pharmacologic diabetes therapies are used primarily to treat T2D, although some are also used to treat polycystic ovary syndrome, gestational diabetes, and other types of diabetes. Although the majority of these are oral medications, a few are noninsulin injectables. Advancements in intensive insulin therapy have been shown to improve time in range and decrease hemoglobin A1c (HbA1c) levels; however, insulin-related weight gain is also recognized as a potential challenging outcome of intensive therapy. In recent years, researchers have paid increasing attention to the co-occurrence of T1D and features of metabolic syndrome, coined *double diabetes*.[29,30] A growing number of randomized control trials and clinical trials have shown evidence of the cardiometabolic and weight benefits of noninsulin glucose-lowering medications as add-on therapy in T1D care. However, this approach is not without potential adverse effects including diabetic ketoacidosis (DKA) in the presence of either hyperglycemia or normoglycemia.[29-31] Close coordination with an individual's diabetes health care team is warranted when add-on therapy is initiated. The additional education, glucose and ketone monitoring, assessment of hydration status, and adjustment of insulin dosages required for add-on treatment necessitate frequent follow-up.[30]

A complete list of noninsulin glucose-lowering medications can be found in Table 19.2 on page 502, along with the mechanism of action, risk of hypoglycemia, administration information, and other considerations for athletes.[12] Table 19.3 on page 504 describes the glucagon formulations available for use in urgent hypoglycemic events in which the blood glucose is severely low and needs to be increased rapidly.[32]

TABLE 19.2 Glucose-Lowering Medications and Considerations for Athletes With Diabetes[12]

Drug class	Medication name(s)	Mechanism(s) of action	Hypoglycemia risk?	Administration	Other considerations
Biguanides	Metformin	Suppresses endogenous glucose production; inhibits intestinal polysaccaridase; increases insulin sensitivity	No[a]	Oral	GI intolerance, as diarrhea or nausea may impede exercise; potential for vitamin B12 deficiency contributing to anemia, muscle weakness, fatigue, and reduced performance; can increase plasma lactate levels (MALA); some weight loss possible
Sodium-glucose cotransporter 2 inhibitors	Canagliflozin Dapagliflozin Empagliflozin Ertugliflozin	Blocks renal glucose reabsorption, leading to increased urinary excretion	No[a]	Oral	Increased diabetic ketoacidosis risk with or without glucose elevation; risk of dehydration or volume depletion could be worsened during exercise, especially in hot or dry environments; risk of genitourinary infections; risk of bone fractures; some weight loss is possible
Glucagon-like peptide 1 receptor agonists and mimetics	Dulaglutide Liraglutide Semaglutide Exenatide Exenatide XR Lixisenatide	Stimulates satiety and insulin secretion	No[a]	Injection	GI side effects, such as nausea, vomiting, or diarrhea, may impede exercise performance; mild to significant weight loss
Glucose-dependent insulinotropic polypeptide/glucagon-like peptide 1 receptor agonist	Tirzepatide	Stimulates satiety and insulin secretion	No[a]	Injection	GI side effects, such as nausea, vomiting, or diarrhea, may impede exercise performance; mild to significant weight loss
Dipeptidyl peptidase IV inhibitor	Alogliptin Saxagliptin Linagliptin Sitagliptin	Inhibits glucagon release	No[a]	Oral	Joint pain could limit exercise tolerance

Thiazolidinediones	Pioglitazone	Increases insulin sensitivity	No	Oral	Fluid retention, heart failure risk, bone fracture risk, potential for weight gain
Sulfonylureas	Glimepiride Glipizide Glyburide	Stimulates insulin secretion	Yes	Oral	Associated with increased cardiovascular mortality risk; potential for weight gain
Meglitinides	Nateglinide Repaglinide	Stimulates insulin secretion	Yes	Oral	Potential for weight gain
α-Glucosidase inhibitors	Acarbose Miglitol	Prevents digestion of carbohydrates	Yes[a,b]	Oral	Adverse GI effects; reduced carbohydrate absorption; potential for weight loss
Bile acid sequestrant	Colesevelam	Improves glucose tolerance (mechanism unknown)	No	Oral	
Dopamine-2 agonist	Bromocriptine	Decreases postprandial blood glucose; decreases endogenous glucose production	No	Oral	Hypotension; dizziness
Amylin mimetic	Pramlintide	Modulates gastric emptying rate; prevents postprandial glucagon rise; promotes satiety	Yes[a]	Injection	Reduced appetite, early satiety, delayed stomach emptying and nutrient delivery, suppressed glucagon response, potential for weight loss

[a] Can contribute to hypoglycemia when used in combination with insulin or sulfonylureas.
[b] α-Glucosidase inhibitors prevent the conversion of sucrose to metabolically available sugars. Glucose must be used for the treatment of hypoglycemia
Abbreviations: GI, gastrointestinal; MALA, metformin-associated lactic acidosis

TABLE 19.3 Glucagon Formulations[32]			
Drug	**Formulation**	**Administration**	**Requires reconstitution?**
Baqsimi	Nasal glucagon	Nasal	No
Gvoke	Liquid-stable glucagon	SC; lower abdomen, outer thigh, outer upper arm	No
Zegalogue (Dasiglucagon)	Glucagon receptor agonist	SC; abdomen, thigh, buttocks, outer upper arm	No
GlucaGen	Lyophilized glucagon powder	SC or IM; upper arm, thigh, buttocks	Yes

Abbreviations: IM, intramuscular; SC, subcutaneous

Newer intranasal and ready-to-inject glucagon preparations are beneficial in terms of ease of use, safety, and efficacy. An individual does not need to be a health care practitioner to safely administer glucagon.[28] Like an epinephrine autoinjector (commonly known by the brand name EpiPen), a ready-to-use glucagon autoinjector is used in emergency situations. Sports RDNs, along with coaches, trainers, and other staff of sports teams with athletes who have diabetes, should be trained to administer glucagon.

THE PHYSIOLOGIC RESPONSE TO EXERCISE

Energy Metabolism

As described in Chapter 1, the amount and type of fuel an athlete should consume during exercise is dependent on the type, intensity, and duration of the activity, as well as the available fuel mix and the athlete's degree of physical fitness.[33-37] This section provides a brief summary of normal metabolism to help illustrate the alterations that occur with diabetes.

Contraction of skeletal muscle triggers the need for energy from adenosine triphosphate (ATP), which is then rapidly replenished by phosphocreatine (PCr). After only a few seconds, the PCr stores are depleted, and alternative fuel sources are needed to provide sustained energy. ATP and PCr levels in individuals with diabetes appear to be similar to those in individuals without diabetes when blood glucose is tightly regulated. When blood glucose levels are not tightly regulated, delayed replenishment of PCr and impairments in mitochondrial function can occur, which can contribute to diminished energy for activity.[38,39]

Anaerobic exercise depends almost exclusively on glucose as a fuel source.[33,37] To help meet the high demand for glucose during anaerobic exercise, the body augments the glucose supply through glycolysis and gluconeogenesis. Thus, anaerobic activities can potentially increase the blood glucose level in athletes with diabetes. This rise in blood glucose may be sustained for prolonged periods in some athletes and short-lived in others. When glycogen stores begin to deplete, however, there may be a rapid drop in blood glucose, resulting in hypoglycemia.

Aerobic exercise is highly dependent on glucose in the early stages but shifts to a greater dependence on fat as a fuel source as its duration increases. Aerobic exercise is less likely to cause sustained elevated blood glucose because the need for glucose as a fuel source is significantly lower; thus, the liver is not inclined to supplement the glucose supply. A typical blood glucose pattern for endurance athletes who do not have diabetes includes a short initial spike in blood glucose followed by a steady state and then a gradual reduction as glycogen stores are depleted if they are not supplemented with exogenous sources of carbohydrate during exercise.[33,37] Although most endurance athletes with diabetes also experience the initial rise in blood glucose with the onset of exercise, the pattern that follows will vary depending on the type of diabetes, medications on board, type and duration of activity, and individual differences unique to each athlete.[2,6,22,34,35]

Exercise Endocrinology

The energy pathways used during exercise are mediated by hormonal responses to exercise. An understanding of exercise endocrinology and hormonal control of carbohydrate metabolism is essential to accurately predict blood glucose patterns in athletes with diabetes. At the onset of exercise, counterregulatory hormones such as epinephrine are released. These, in turn, trigger the secretion of other metabolic hormones including glucagon, growth hormone, and cortisol. A summary of these counterregulatory or stress hormones, their actions, and adaptations to exercise can be found in Table 19.4. In general, these hormones facilitate the mobilization of metabolic fuels from storage to working muscles. Insulin, by contrast, is a storage hormone that facilitates the transport of fuel into cells. A primary function of insulin is to facilitate the transport of glucose into cells where it is either used as an immediate fuel source or stored as glycogen (in liver and muscle cells). Insulin also facilitates the uptake of circulating amino acids and free fatty acids into cells and stimulates glycogen synthesis, protein synthesis, and lipogenesis, thus promoting fuel storage. Insulin inhibits the actions of counterregulatory hormones that promote the mobilization of fuels out of storage through lipolysis, proteolysis, and gluconeogenesis processes. Conversely, counterregulatory hormones inhibit insulin production, thus allowing for the mobilization of glucose, amino acids, and free fatty acids to be available to fuel the muscles and brain.[33,37,40]

TABLE 19.4 Normal Endocrine Response to Exercise[33,37,40]

Hormone	Hormone effects	Hormone response at onset of exercise	Hormone response during recovery	Adaptation to exercise
Glucagon	Stimulates hepatic glucose production via glycogenolysis and gluconeogenesis Stimulates lipolysis Facilitates uptake of FFAs Inhibits insulin production	Increase	Increase	Smaller increase in glucose levels during exercise at both absolute and relative workloads
Epinephrine	Stimulates muscle and some hepatic glycolysis Mobilizes FFAs from adipose tissue Stimulates hepatic gluconeogenesis Inhibits insulin production	Increase	Increase	Decreased secretion at rest
Growth hormone	Stimulates hepatic glucose production via glycolysis and gluconeogenesis Stimulates lipolysis Facilitates uptake of FFAs Inhibits insulin	Increase	Nominal change	Less dramatic rise during exercise
Norepinephrine	Directly stimulates lipolysis Indirectly suppresses glucose utilization Stimulates AA storage	Increase	Nominal change	Nominal change

Continued on next page

TABLE 19.4 Normal Endocrine Response to Exercise[33,37,40] (CONTINUED)				
Hormone	**Hormone effects**	**Hormone response at onset of exercise**	**Hormone response during recovery**	**Adaptation to exercise**
Cortisol	Mobilizes AAs and glycerol as substrates for hepatic gluconeogenesis Mobilizes FFAs as fuel source for muscles Blocks glucose uptake into adipocytes and muscles	Increase during heavy exercise only	Nominal change	Slight elevations during exercise
Insulin	Increases glycogen synthesis Increases lipogenesis Increases AA uptake Increases potassium uptake Decreases proteolysis Decreases gluconeogenesis Decreases renal sodium excretion	Decrease	Increase	Increased sensitivity to insulin Decrease in insulin during exercise

Abbreviations: AA, amino acid; FFA, free fatty acid

The rate-limiting step in the regulation of blood glucose involves 2 cellular transportation mechanisms: an insulin-dependent mechanism and an insulin-independent mechanism.[41,42] In the insulin-dependent mechanism, when insulin binds to receptors on the surface of cells, the intracellular glucose transporter type 4 (GLUT4) is activated and migrates to the interior surface of the cell membrane, where GLUT4 moves glucose into the cell. In the second mechanism, muscle contractions activate GLUT4 independent of insulin. Thus, during exercise, insulin is not needed to transport glucose into cells of working muscles, and insulin production is necessarily inhibited to allow the cells to switch from a fuel storage mode to a fuel utilization mode. In addition, exercising muscles have increased insulin sensitivity, making them more responsive to any insulin that is present.[6,23,43-45]

Glucagon remains high for approximately 1 hour after exercise. At the cessation of exercise, high concentrations of glucagon and catecholamine are retained, the insulin sensitivity of muscles increases, the intestinal absorption of glucose increases, and insulin production rebounds. During the hour following exercise, the body is primed to store glycogen. Insulin sensitivity and insulin production remain high for several hours, allowing the body to transport glucose into muscles 3 to 5 times faster than normal. The elevated glucagon level encourages hepatic glucose production, which is used to replenish muscle glycogen. Even though fuel storage is most efficient during this phase, completely replenishing glycogen stores can take up to 48 hours postexercise.[6,23,43-45]

For athletes with T1D, all insulin is exogenously supplied, so the body does not have the ability to downregulate insulin during exercise.[2,6,27-29,33,43-45] These athletes are, therefore, at greater risk of hypoglycemia secondary to exercise than those who produce their own insulin because some amount of baseline circulating insulin (from the injection of long-acting insulin or an insulin pump's basal rate) remains present even after exercise has activated GLUT4 receptors independent of insulin.[24,25,46-49] This results in both glucose transport mechanisms occurring simultaneously, allowing for the rapid depletion of blood glucose.[24,25,41,42,46-49] Postexercise, athletes with T1D often experience an initial rise in blood glucose, followed by a decrease in blood glucose.[2,6,24,25,46-49]

Health care practitioners must understand that each athlete with T1D has a unique pattern of postexercise glucose response. This pattern varies with regard to the timing and magnitude of the glucose response. Some athletes with T1D will experience a dramatic spike in blood glucose immediately after exercise, whereas others may have a delayed rise in blood glucose that can occur up to several hours later.[2,6,24,25,46-49] The rise is a result of continued hepatic glucose output without the compensatory insulin response that people without diabetes experience. The eventual decrease in blood glucose corresponds to the decreased concentration of stress hormones in conjunction with increased insulin sensitivity.

The timing and extent of the postexercise rise in blood glucose is also dependent on the type of exercise and can vary during different types or intensities of activity for a single athlete.[2,6,24,25,46-49] Knowledge of an athlete's patterns helps determine how to tailor insulin recommendations and the ideal timing of recovery nutrition. This pattern is most easily determined by CGM, although it can be roughly estimated by performing multiple finger-stick glucose checks postexercise.

In athletes with T2D, insulin sensitivity and insulin secretion will typically be elevated postexercise, as with athletes who do not have diabetes. These athletes typically have a net decrease in blood glucose postexercise. Athletes who have T2D and take insulin will benefit from additional monitoring around exercise and may need to consider reducing their insulin dose if their postexercise blood glucose is consistently low.[2]

Training Adaptations

In addition to the acute responses to exercise, training adaptations occur that affect energy metabolism. As an athlete's level of fitness improves, insulin sensitivity increases, and exercise-induced insulin secretion decreases. A reduction occurs in the secretion of epinephrine and in the response of growth hormone to exercise, which subsequently decreases exercise-induced hepatic glucose production.[40]

These adaptations in a person with T2D may result in decreased insulin secretion in response to ingested carbohydrate, decreased levels of circulating insulin between feedings, and a subsequent decreased tendency to store fat. Given that 2 hallmarks of T2D are insulin resistance and increased hepatic glucose production, regular exercise, especially aerobic exercise that involves large muscle groups, can be an effective tool for managing blood glucose. As training intensity increases and fitness improves, the athlete and their diabetes care team are strongly advised to monitor blood glucose trends and adjust doses of diabetes medications as appropriate. This is especially important for athletes with T2D who take insulin or oral hypoglycemic agents, such as sulfonylureas, which put them at an increased risk of hypoglycemia. Athletes with T2D may be able to successfully decrease their dose or discontinue their diabetes medications as their fitness improves.[1] This may require working with the prescribing medical practitioner to decrease the dose in a stepwise progression, bearing in mind that most diabetes specialists lack experience with athletes.

For athletes with T1D, the primary implications of adaptation to exercise include an increased risk of hypoglycemia secondary to increased insulin sensitivity and decreased hepatic glucose production.[2,6,23,43]

GLUCOSE MANAGEMENT AND SPORT PERFORMANCE

Glucose and Ketone Monitoring

The management plan for athletes with diabetes needs to anticipate the blood glucose response to training and competition.[28] Thus, the self-monitoring of blood glucose (SMBG) is essential. The data from SMBG can be used to determine how to adjust food, medication, and other parameters that may affect blood glucose. SMBG and pattern management are critical skills for all athletes with diabetes. Athletes should understand how insulin, exercise, and carbohydrate intake affect their glucose values and performance. Frequent monitoring helps identify hypoglycemia or hyperglycemia and allows the individual to treat each situation.

Ideally, blood glucose should be in the range from 126 to 180 mg/dL (7.0–10.0 mmol/L) preexercise to reduce hypoglycemia risk and support performance. Some athletes may prefer to maintain their glucose levels above this range when competition and safety are at stake.[2,6,39,40,43-48] The frequency of an individual's glucose monitoring depends on the type of diabetes; type of medication(s); type, frequency, and intensity of exercise; and individual needs. Although most individuals who require insulin are advised to check their blood glucose before each meal and at bedtime, practitioners should individualize recommendations.

Athletes typically need to monitor more frequently, especially before, during, and after a bout of exercise. An athlete with diabetes benefits from knowing their initial blood glucose concentration, as well as its direction and rate of change around any exercise session (refer to Figures 19.2 and 19.3).[2,5-7,10,11,20-26] This is most efficiently determined by CGM but can also be done with SMBG by taking at least 3 blood glucose readings at 20- to 30-minute intervals before, during, and after the exercise session. The slope of the line created by SMBG data points will indicate the rate and direction of blood glucose change and enable the athlete to make preemptive adjustments to prevent hypoglycemia and hyperglycemia.

PROS AND CONS OF CONTINUOUS GLUCOSE MONITORS

A CGM is a small medical device that uses a subcutaneous sensor to measure the glucose in interstitial fluid. Because interstitial glucose differs slightly from blood glucose, a CGM system uses an algorithm to predict the blood glucose value from sensor-measured values. It transmits a glucose value every 1 to 5 minutes to a receiver or smart phone app. CGM systems can be programmed for target ranges and will signal an alarm if glucose is above or below range. To prevent alarm fatigue, it is not uncommon for alarms to be set outside the target glucose range so that, when the alarm sounds, the individual is more likely to respond to it. The receiver or app shows both a predicted glucose value and a glucose trend arrow. A standard blood glucose meter gives a single blood glucose value but no predicted direction or rate-of-change information.[8] Manufacturers suggest that a CGM sensor can be worn for up to 14 days, although the precise amount of time varies by CGM manufacturer.

The use of a CGM system does not completely negate the need for capillary blood glucose monitoring. SMBG should be performed when diabetes treatment decisions are being made, when sensor readings or alerts do not match symptoms, and when a CGM system does not display glucose data or displays data that are inconsistent. Although the accuracy of CGM technology has continually improved, the data can be inaccurate, especially when rate of change in blood glucose is high. There is a lag time of 5 to 20 minutes between the equilibration of interstitial and capillary glucose. When glucose is rapidly rising or falling, as can occur during exercise, the lag time is increased. This can create a significant obstacle to obtaining accurate CGM readings at critical times.[20] As such, if there is a question about sensor readings, glucose values measured on a CGM system should be verified by SMBG, especially when insulin dosing decisions are being made.

The added value of a CGM system is its usefulness in tracking near-real-time glucose trends. This gives the user the ability to identify the direction and rate of glucose change, and to adjust insulin dosing and carbohydrate intake accordingly before blood glucose is significantly out of range. The athlete with diabetes is advised to check blood glucose every 30 to 60 minutes during prolonged exercise, within 30 minutes after exercise ends, and then every 2 to 4 hours postexercise. If preexercise blood glucose is between 90 and 250 mg/dL, it is generally safe to begin training. CGM is much more convenient and preferred if a sensor can be safely positioned on the body and a receiver or smart phone is accessible to receive and view the data during training and sports competition. Most CGM systems are now water resistant, and sensors can be covered with protective waterproof patches that make their use in water sports possible. Even so, use of CGM may not be possible or practical in all situations. In these cases, alternative monitoring strategies, primarily using fingerstick BG monitoring, may need to be employed.[20-24]

KETONE MONITORING

Athletes who take insulin should check for ketones when blood glucose is greater than 250 mg/dL and the presence of hyperglycemia is unexplained. Blood ketone levels can be checked with a handheld meter (similar to a glucose meter). If blood ketones are moderately elevated (up to 1.4 mmol/L), the athlete should limit activity to moderate intensity for a maximum duration of 30 minutes and focus on hydration, as there is an increased risk of dehydration when ketones are elevated. A small dose of correction insulin may be needed to clear blood ketones before exercise is initiated, especially if the blood glucose level is greater than 350 mg/dL. With a significantly elevated glucose level (>350 mg/dL, even if blood ketones are less than 0.5 mmol/L), the athlete should correct with a 10% to 20% reduced dosage of insulin calculated from their ISF and then proceed with caution. If ketones are elevated (≥1.5 mmol/L), exercise is contraindicated. If the athlete does not have a blood ketone meter, the athlete can use a urine test strip instead. The athlete should follow the directions provided with the product to interpret the results. Aggressive glucose and ketone management is necessary in this situation, and the individual's diabetes care team should immediately be contacted to assist with management decisions.

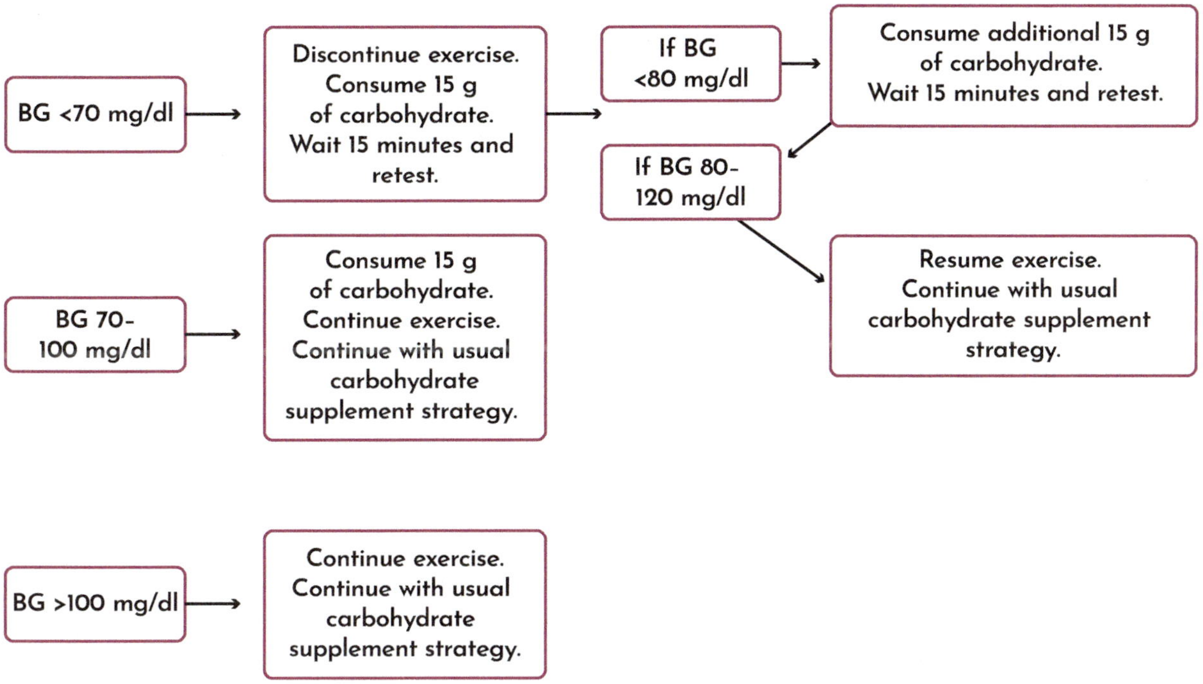

FIGURE 19.2 During-exercise decision tree for athletes with diabetes using self-monitoring of blood glucose[2,5-7,10,11,20-26] Abbreviation: BG, blood glucose

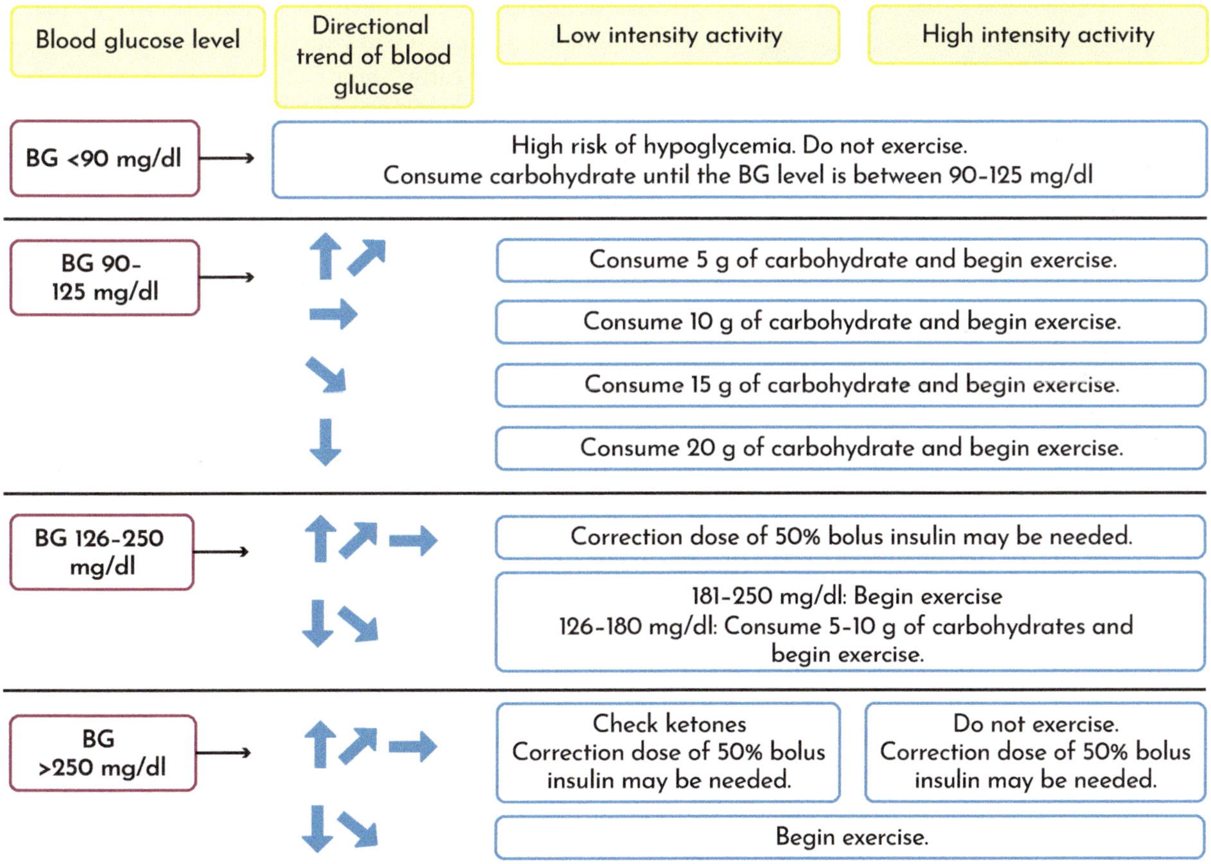

FIGURE 19.3 Preexercise management of blood glucose for athletes with type 1 diabetes using continuous glucose monitoring[6,10,20-22,24,25] Abbreviation: BG, blood glucose

Glucose Response to Different Types of Exercise

A primary concern for managing athletes with diabetes is preventing acute complications of hypoglycemia and hyperglycemia.[1,2,6] There is no single means to do this. The type of diabetes; duration, intensity, and type of exercise; and type of medication can each affect glycemic control. Figures 19.1, 19.2, and 19.3 provide recommendations to aid in appropriate decision making for athletes with T1D and insulin-requiring T2D.

Preventing and Managing Hypoglycemia

As mentioned previously, exercise may increase the risk of hypoglycemia in individuals who take insulin or insulin secretagogues. This is due to the insulin-independent ability of exercise to lower blood glucose. Consumption of carbohydrate is advised before, during, and/or after exercise if the blood glucose value is below 90 mg/dL. Some athletes who have a known pattern of significant blood glucose reductions during exercise often find it necessary to start exercise with a blood glucose level that is above their normally recommended range, especially if they are participating in sports during which they will be unable to ingest carbohydrate. Athletes who take insulin secretagogues may need to adjust their dose on days when they exercise in order to avoid hypoglycemic episodes. Any changes to the medication dose and/or timing should be made in conjunction with their health care practitioner. For athletes who take insulin, knowing how much active insulin is on board helps to accurately predict additional carbohydrate needs.[14] If an athlete has a clear pattern of hypoglycemic tendencies during or after exercise, it is prudent to decrease insulin accordingly to proactively prevent hypoglycemic events. Athletes who use CSII/insulin pumps often achieve this by temporarily decreasing the basal insulin. The degree to which athletes need to decrease basal insulin varies greatly. Some will reduce the basal rate by 20%; others may reduce it by up to 80%. The extent and timing of the temporary adjustment will depend on the individual athlete's typical blood glucose patterns, which give an indication of changes in the ISF around exercise. Many athletes find it helpful to decrease basal and bolus insulin before prolonged endurance exercise to effectively limit active IOB and to increase back to a normal basal rate near the cessation of exercise, based on their historical blood glucose trends around exercise.[2,6,14,24] Examples of recommended starting points for insulin adjustments can be found in Figure 19.1 on page 500.

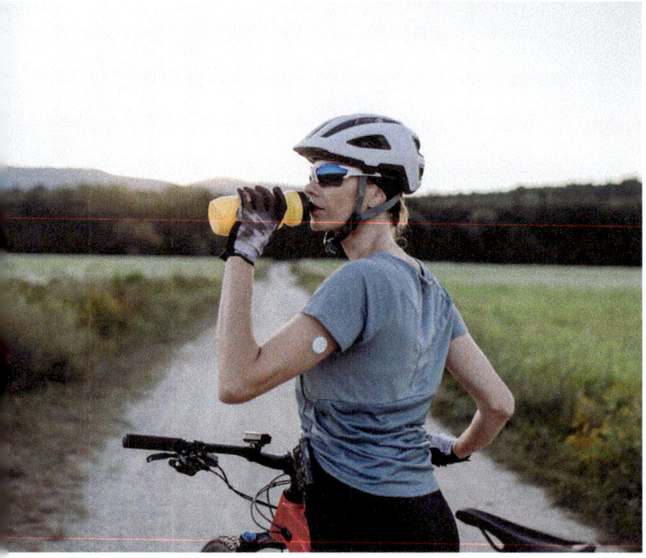

Following exercise, athletes on insulin therapy often experience hypoglycemia soon after completion, within a few hours, or as delayed-onset hypoglycemia.[2,6,25,26,49-52] The postexercise recovery period is crucial for achieving maximum training adaptations, but this can be hampered by these episodes of hypoglycemia. Doses of insulin may need to be modified for an extended time after extreme or prolonged activity, when insulin sensitivity and muscle glycogen repletion are increased. The period of heightened sensitivity to insulin can last for up to 36 hours after extreme exercise. Delayed-onset hypoglycemia may occur overnight and sometimes even the following day. This pattern is common in endurance athletes with T1D after an event such as a triathlon, marathon, or century cycle. CGM can be extremely useful for detecting delayed hypoglycemia and alerting the wearer in time to treat it. Postexercise recovery guidelines addressing delayed-onset hypoglycemia are lacking in the published literature. Therefore, to reap the benefits of the postexercise phase while avoiding delayed-onset hypoglycemia, each athlete with T1D must work with their health care practitioners to develop a personalized strategy that works for them. Frequent SMBG, including monitoring during the night (eg, at 3:00 AM), is an advisable precautionary measure.[50]

Symptoms of mild hypoglycemia may include an urgency to eat, nervousness, shakiness, and excessive perspiration. If blood glucose continues to drop, neurologic symptoms of moderate hypoglycemia will arise. These symptoms typically correspond to blood glucose levels of less than 55 mg/dL and may include changes in mood such as irritability, anxiety, restlessness, or anger; confusion; difficulty concentrating; blurred vision; dizziness; headache; low energy; poor coordination; slurred speech; and decreased communication.[51] Because not all individuals have the same signs and symptoms, it is advisable to ask athletes with diabetes how they personally react when their blood glucose is low and how they would like teammates and coaching staff to respond when symptoms are noticed. This is an important part of the diabetes care plan because it is possible for individuals with diabetes to have hypoglycemic unawareness, in which case they do not experience the physical symptoms of hypoglycemia and may not recognize it.[28]

Suspected hypoglycemia should be confirmed with measured blood glucose values before treatment. In most cases of mild and moderate hypoglycemia, individuals are able to self-treat hypoglycemic events using the "rule of 15" (also known as the "15:15 rule").[52] This simple protocol suggests consuming 15 g of a quick-acting carbohydrate source, such as glucose tablets, gel, or juice, and then rechecking blood glucose after 15 minutes. If blood glucose has not responded to treatment, the protocol is repeated until blood glucose is within acceptable limits. The 15-minute checks verify that blood glucose is indeed returning to acceptable limits. The second check helps ensure that the individual did not overcorrect and end up with rebounded high blood glucose. In anticipation of such events, an athlete's diabetes management plan should stipulate having a source of quick-acting carbohydrate readily available at all times.

Severe hypoglycemia typically occurs when blood glucose falls below 54 mg/dL and the individual is nonresponsive or too debilitated to self-treat with oral carbohydrate. Symptoms of severe hypoglycemia may include an altered state of consciousness, coma, seizure, or hypothermia.[51] Severe hypoglycemia is a medical emergency demanding immediate attention. In some cases, it can be treated orally with assistance from others, but if the patient cannot safely swallow or is unable to cooperate, a glucagon injection may be necessary. Athletes with diabetes who take insulin should have a glucagon kit readily available during training and competition, and their diabetes plan should include designated individuals who are trained to prepare and administer glucagon if needed.[26,28] Older versions of the glucagon kit consist of a syringe of saline that must be freshly mixed into a small vial of dry glucagon powder before injection. Newer versions, such as Gvoke, do not require reconstitution, and in the case of Baqsimi, the glucagon is delivered as a nasal spray. Injectable glucagon is administered into the buttocks, thigh, or deltoid and works immediately to increase blood glucose by stimulating production and release of glucose from the liver.[32] Table 19.3 on page 504 summarizes the various options for glucagon formulations.

Preventing and Managing Hyperglycemia

Whereas transient hyperglycemia is not uncommon, prolonged or extreme hyperglycemia is a cause for concern. Chronic high blood glucose (ie, blood glucose >250 mg/dL) can result in long-term complications, including damage to the nerves, eyes, kidneys, and blood vessels. Common symptoms of chronic hyperglycemia include fatigue, thirst, frequent urination, and possible urinary tract or genital yeast infections. Individuals with chronic hyperglycemia may not feel well but can continue their usual daily activities. By contrast, episodes of acute hyperglycemia can be life threatening. Signs and symptoms of progressing hyperglycemia may include nausea, dehydration, reduced cognition, slowed visual reaction times, and fatigue. Severe hyperglycemia may result in DKA, with possible additional symptoms that include rapid breathing, fruity odor of the breath, extreme fatigue or sleepiness, inattentiveness, decreased appetite, increased thirst, and frequent urination.[51] DKA is most commonly associated with T1D, although it is also possible with other types of diabetes. It is due to insufficient insulin to transport glucose into cells and results in metabolic acidosis, severe dehydration, and electrolyte imbalance. Any action that increases blood glucose and decreases insulin action can contribute to the development of DKA. Athletes with T1D are advised to have urine ketone strips or a ketone meter available to test for ketoacidosis when blood glucose is excessively high.[26]

In athletes with T2D, hyperosmolar hyperglycemic state (HHS) is the most common form of acute hyperglycemic illness. HHS is the result of high blood glucose (>600 mg/dL) compounded by profound dehydration (plasma osmolality > 320 mOsm/kg).[51] An associated loss of 12% or more of body weight may also occur. Symptoms of HHS are similar to those of DKA but with the notable absence of ketones.[48] Like DKA, HHS is a life-threatening condition and requires immediate treatment. The goals of treatment include rehydration, the restoration of electrolyte balance, and the provision of insulin to normalize blood glucose. Prevention of severe hyperglycemia includes attention to hydration. Exercising with ketones is dangerous and can lead to DKA.[10] Athletes with blood glucose levels greater than 250 mg/dL without ketones should hydrate (and may also require a corrective dose of insulin) to help bring blood glucose into a desired range. If athletes have glucose levels greater than 250 mg/dL and ketone levels greater than 0.6 mmol/L, they should treat with insulin and hydration and should not exercise until ketones are cleared.

Exercise-induced hyperglycemia is most often associated with short-duration, high-intensity exercise that stimulates endogenous production of glucose in the liver. Blood glucose elevation in this situation is usually transient, and use of supplemental insulin as a corrective measure is typically not indicated. Any type of physiological or psychological stress can also contribute to elevated blood glucose through the action of stress hormones.[2,6] Thus, an illness, injury, inflammation, pain, or even preevent anxiety can influence blood glucose. In most cases, blood glucose will decrease without intervention after the cessation of exercise, so caution should be used when considering treating hyperglycemia with insulin because this may result in subsequent hypoglycemia.[2,6,9,26,36] Hyperglycemia can also occur if an insulin pump fails, if the insulin is expired or spoiled from exposure to extreme temperatures, or if the injection site is unusable because of excessive scar tissue. In these instances, it is entirely appropriate to provide the missing insulin to correct the hyperglycemia. The diabetes management plan should include protocols for treating hyperglycemia using a sliding scale for insulin based on the insulin sensitivity of the individual athlete.[28]

SPECIAL CONSIDERATIONS FOR ATHLETES WITH TYPE 1 DIABETES

T1D is a complex autoimmune disease that has many associated risks and complications. Health care practitioners who work with athletes with T1D benefit from being informed about adjunct concerns that may affect these athletes and will be better prepared to address these issues if needed.

Circadian Rhythms

Circadian rhythms refer to naturally occurring biological rhythms that follow a daily pattern. Of particular relevance to those with diabetes are the diurnal variations in glucose metabolism. These are primarily mediated by direct autonomic innervations that target organs from the hypothalamus and are independent of insulin or glucagon levels.[53,54] Secretion of glucocorticoid typically increases before dawn and targets the liver to stimulate hepatic glucose production. Other actions tied to circadian rhythms include reduced skeletal muscle blood flow and increased insulin resistance, which occur in anticipation of a need for energy for the day.[53] This is often referred to as the dawn phenomenon and helps explain why blood glucose is often highest in the morning, despite coming after an overnight fast.[12] This pattern is important to keep in mind for athletes who may train and compete at different times of day.

Sleep

College athletes may sacrifice sleep in favor of studying to meet academic demands. Professional athletes frequently lose sleep when they travel between time zones. Endurance athletes and outdoor adventurists often begin the day before dawn. What effect does sleep deprivation have on glycemic control? In 1 study, participants who went without sleep for 1 to 5 days developed insulin resistance and β-cell dysfunction, resulting in increased fasting and postprandial glucose levels. In another study, participants who restricted sleep to 4 to 5 hours per night exhibited a reduction in glucose tolerance, decreased muscle glucose uptake, increased hepatic glucose output, and pancreatic β-cell dysfunction.[55]

Altitude and Ambient Temperature

Athletes often perform in extraordinary conditions that include high altitude and extreme temperatures. Although obvious examples include mountain climbers, skiers, rock climbers, and endurance trail runners, teams who travel from sea level to destinations several thousand feet higher also experience radical climate changes. Altitude exposure can increase levels of epinephrine, norepinephrine, and cortisol, causing a subsequent rise in blood glucose.[3,56,57] Temperature extremes (heat and cold), humidity, and high altitude can cause physiological stress that results in elevated counterregulatory hormones and subsequent hyperglycemia despite exercise.[56] Frequent glucose monitoring is warranted, but the glucometer and CGM readings may be inaccurate at high altitude and in extreme heat or cold. Additionally, heat and cold can destroy insulin, so efforts must be made to insulate it from the elements.[27] Dehydration is also common under such extreme conditions and contributes to increased blood glucose.[56,57]

Autoimmune Comorbidities

Health care practitioners working with athletes with T1D should be aware of the increased risk for other autoimmune diseases, such as celiac disease, autoimmune thyroid disease, and rheumatoid arthritis because of the common genetic predisposition and the interplay between environmental and immunologic factors.[58-60] Celiac disease is one of the most common coexisting autoimmune diseases for people with T1D.[58,59] Celiac disease is characterized by damaged intestinal villi that appear flattened and atrophied. Classic symptoms of celiac disease include diarrhea, gastrointestinal bloating, possible weight loss, and failure to thrive and delayed puberty in children. Nonclassic symptoms may include constipation, neuropathy, ataxia, and heartburn. Not everyone with celiac disease experiences gastrointestinal symptoms. In fact, the majority of people with T1D who have celiac disease do *not* present with classic symptoms or may have only very mild gastrointestinal symptoms, which can be overlooked.[58] Other possible indicators of celiac disease are iron deficiency anemia and low bone density.[58] These clinical signs are a result of poor micronutrient absorption secondary to inflamed and damaged intestinal villi. Because anemia and low bone density (often identified as a result of stress fractures) are not uncommon in athletes, sports RDNs must be aware of this possible non–sports-related etiology of these conditions, especially in populations at high risk for celiac disease. Iron-deficiency anemia that does not respond to iron supplementation may warrant screening for celiac disease. In addition, undiagnosed and untreated celiac disease can be an underlying cause of glycemic variations despite the individual's adherence to a strict diabetes management plan. Treatment of celiac disease in athletes with T1D is the same as for those without T1D: adherence to a gluten-free diet (excluding wheat, barley, and rye).

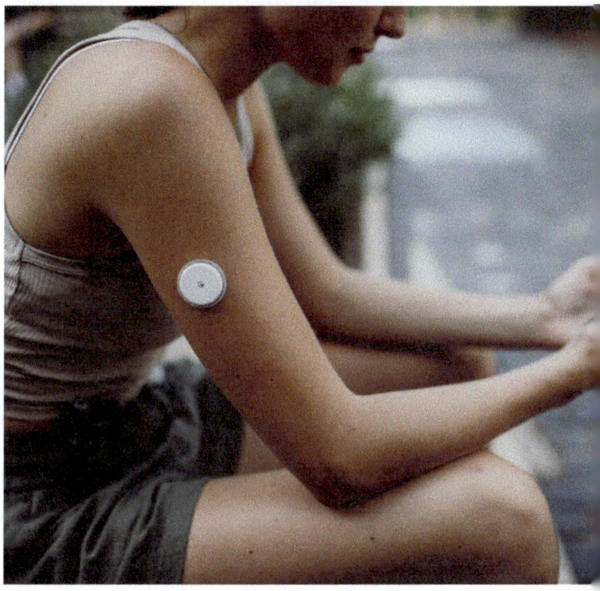

"Diabulimia" and Other Eating Disorders

Because disordered eating is prevalent in many sports, it is always wise to screen for such disorders in athletes. It is particularly important to do so for athletes who have T1D because they have an additional and dangerous component to add to their weight-loss arsenal. Withholding insulin can be a very effective means of inducing weight loss, but it is extremely dangerous for athletes with T1D because it results in hyperglycemia and often ketosis.[61] See Chapter 18 for information on eating disorders in athletes.

ATHLETE-CENTERED CARE AND THE PERFORMANCE NUTRITION CARE PLAN

Evidence-based performance nutrition standards have been established for athletes,[62] and evidence-based medical nutrition therapy (MNT) standards have been established for individuals with diabetes.[1,63] The challenge for sports RDNs working with athletes with diabetes is to develop a nutrition care plan that incorporates both sets of standards. The performance nutrition standards are the same for athletes with diabetes as for those without, and the MNT standards for nonathletic individuals with diabetes also apply to athletes with diabetes. Essentially, athletes with diabetes have the same basic nutritional needs as any athlete, which means that their carbohydrate and energy requirements are higher than those of nonathletes. Sports nutrition plans need to be athlete-centered and must be tailored to meet individual goals and needs.

Nutrition Assessment

The initial assessment of an athlete with diabetes should follow a standard approach as described in Chapter 8, with the consideration of additional factors. These factors include the type of diabetes; the length of time since diagnosis; the progression of the disease; the presence of complications and comorbidities; the type, intensity, and duration of training; the athlete's level of fitness; the type of diabetes medications and their mode of delivery; the individual blood glucose patterns; and the habits of each individual athlete. An example of questions to ask during the initial assessment can be found in Box 19.3. Assessing the athlete's understanding of diabetes and readiness to manage it are top priorities. For example, if an athlete is newly diagnosed, the entire focus should be on stabilizing the blood glucose levels first; training may need to be put on the back burner until that occurs. Commitment to a diabetes management plan that maintains adequate glycemic control is necessary for safe athletic participation.[28] The preparticipation medical exam should ensure that the athlete is up to date on recommended routine diabetes screenings for cardiovascular disease, renal function, retinopathy, and neuropathy (including a diabetic foot exam). Laboratory tests should include fasting blood glucose, HbA1c, blood lipids, and glomerular filtration rate. If a medical professional suspects prediabetes or T2D, the practitioner should perform additional tests for glucose tolerance, hyperinsulinemia, and insulin resistance (by the hyperinsulinemic-euglycemic clamp technique). Additionally, athletes can be screened for skin alterations related to insulin resistance such as acanthosis nigricans. Athletes who take metformin should also be screened for vitamin B12 deficiency.[64] Additional key assessment tools for sports RDNs working with athletes with diabetes include training logs, food and beverage logs, blood glucose logs, and CGM data.

BOX 19.3 Examples of Questions to Ask When Caring for an Athlete With Diabetes

What type of diabetes does the athlete have?

When was the athlete diagnosed with diabetes?

What has the progression of the disease looked like for the athlete and are there any complications and/or comorbidities?

What is the athlete's training schedule including type of training, intensity, and duration?

Does the athlete know the medications they are taking and understand how they work?

How often does the athlete check their blood glucose and/or continuous glucose monitoring system data?

What challenges does the athlete encounter in checking blood glucose?

Can the athlete sense when their blood glucose is too high or too low?

Does the athlete know how to effectively treat hyperglycemia and hypoglycemia?

Does the athlete follow a particular eating pattern, such as consistent carbohydrates, or use advanced carbohydrate counting with an insulin-to-carbohydrate ratio?

Does the athlete understand how diet affects blood glucose and know how to appropriately adjust diet and/or insulin as dictated by pattern management of blood glucose readings?

Does the athlete understand how various types of exercise can affect blood glucose patterns and whether or not different blood glucose levels may lead to changes in performance?

Does the athlete understand how stress (psychological or physiological) can affect blood glucose?

Does the athlete have an emergency plan, and if so, what does it look like?

Is the athlete comfortable letting others know that they have diabetes?

Are the athlete's teammates and coaches willing to assist them if needed, and are they educated in basic diabetes management?

The Performance Nutrition Plan

An athlete-centered nutrition care plan should be developed to support the athlete's body composition and performance goals with careful consideration given to the athlete's medication regimen. Athletes with diabetes will need to adjust carbohydrate intake to manage blood glucose; however, carbohydrate recommendations should be kept as close as possible to the recommendations for those without diabetes to help meet performance needs. Strategies that maximize carbohydrate intake and control blood glucose focus on distributing carbohydrates throughout the day. This often means encouraging larger carbohydrate intake at the times of day when insulin sensitivity is highest, such as evening and postexercise. Because there may be a need to limit but not overrestrict carbohydrate in T2D, athletes with T2D and their diabetes care teams often place more emphasis on "just-in-time fueling." This means that individuals with T2D may need to intentionally fuel just before and during exercise to provide fuel for optimal performance. This strategy is suggested because they are not able to efficiently process relatively large doses of carbohydrate, so their glycogen stores are likely to be smaller than those of athletes who do not have diabetes.[65]

For athletes with T1D, the 2 most critical components of the nutrition performance plan are the amount of carbohydrates and the available insulin. The preferred approach is to determine the athlete's carbohydrate needs for optimal performance and to then adjust the insulin to fit the recommended plan. Note, however, that insulin is a prescription medication, and only providers who are qualified to prescribe it can legally make adjustments to an athlete's insulin prescription. Therefore, the athlete with diabetes should consult with a CDCES or endocrinologist when insulin adjustments are deemed necessary. That said, most CDCESs and endocrinologists are not well acquainted with exercise endocrinology and the nutritional needs of athletes, so they will likely benefit from the expertise and guidance of a health care practitioner who is skilled in sports nutrition, such as a sports RDN.

The most common mistake made by athletes with diabetes is excessive restriction of carbohydrates. Carbohydrate is the macronutrient with the most immediate effect on blood glucose levels, and many athletes with diabetes have been taught that limiting carbohydrate is necessary for managing blood glucose. However, by doing so, they often compromise athletic performance in favor of well-controlled blood glucose. A better approach is to titrate carbohydrate up to the estimated amount needed to optimize performance, making corresponding incremental adjustments in insulin in the process.

Carbohydrate supplements are useful when activity is spontaneous or unplanned and is typically necessary during long-duration training or competitive events when energy expenditure is high.[10,37,43] Carbohydrate can be consumed before, during, and/or after such exercise. As a general rule, preexercise intake of supplemental carbohydrate is indicated when the blood glucose is less than 90 mg/dL prior to the start of activity (refer to Figures 19.2 and 19.3). Individuals who participate in long-duration or competitive events that last longer than 60 minutes will likely need to consume carbohydrate during exercise to maintain optimal blood glucose control and to delay fatigue.

Muscle efficiency and performance seem to be best when blood glucose values are maintained between 80 and 180 mg/dL—or as near normal as possible—during exercise.[26] However, as more athletes use CGM technology, refinement of the current understanding of optimal glucose levels for competitive performance is possible. Enough carbohydrate should be consumed during exercise to keep the blood glucose in this optimal range. Intake of 15 to 30 g of carbohydrate every 30 to 60 minutes of exercise is a general, safe starting guideline for supplementing carbohydrate.[62] Sport drinks and diluted juices (<8% carbohydrate) replace fluid as well as carbohydrate and are certainly appropriate for individuals with diabetes. Energy gels or sport bars are easy-to-carry, portion-controlled, carbohydrate-controlled supplement options and are convenient to use during training and competition. Taking additional insulin to cover carbohydrate consumed for the purpose of maintaining target-range blood glucose levels during exercise is generally not advised. Because numerous variables can influence blood glucose response to exercise, strategies for supplementing carbohydrate must be highly individualized. Glucose monitoring and pattern management allow the individual to draw on prior exercise experience, fine-tune carbohydrate supplementation strategies, and achieve optimal blood glucose levels for peak performance. Further, recent evidence suggests that carbohydrate is not the only macronutrient that impacts blood glucose levels. Some individuals with diabetes will have a delayed rise in blood glucose after consuming protein and/or fat (2–5 hours after a meal).[66,67] Therefore, athletes with diabetes should determine their own individual responses to all 3 macronutrients.

Endurance athletes with T1D typically should not employ carbohydrate loading in the traditional sense, but when done with care, they may use similar strategies for manipulating carbohydrate intake to optimize glycogen stores prior to long events.[26] If an athlete with T1D attempted to significantly increase carbohydrate intake in the days preceding a sporting event (ie, carbohydrate loading), the athlete would have to significantly alter their insulin dosing to accommodate the change in intake. Doing so would risk compromising blood glucose control and training. The better approach for athletes with diabetes is to find a macronutrient balance and energy level that meets their training needs and focus more on keeping their glycogen stores topped off rather than maximized. This will mean that just-in-time fueling strategies must be built into their nutrition plans and that the timing and distribution of foods—especially carbohydrate food sources—may be more important than for nonathletes with diabetes.

For many athletes with T1D, their greatest fear is exercise-induced hypoglycemia, and they will intentionally begin exercise in a hyperglycemic state to prevent hypoglycemia. It is usually more appropriate to decrease basal or long-acting insulin to prevent hypoglycemia. Athletes who use an insulin pump can set a temporary basal rate that is decreased about 90 minutes before exercise and during exercise. For those prone to blood glucose spikes immediately after exercise, turning the basal rate back up about 30 minutes before the end of exercise can help normalize postexercise blood glucose. For those who have a delayed postexercise blood glucose spike, the timing and duration of the temporary basal rate will necessarily differ to accommodate individual blood glucose patterns around exercise. There is no one-size-fits-all recommendation for insulin adjustments.

As mentioned previously, the type, duration, and intensity of exercise will influence blood glucose levels around exercise, as will the amount of stored glycogen, nutrient timing, stress factors surrounding exercise, and individual differences. Athletes with T1D on MDIs sometimes benefit from decreasing their long-acting insulin and adjusting their mealtime insulin as needed to manage blood glucose on exercise days. Recreational athletes on MDIs sometimes choose to take their long-acting insulin in the morning rather than at bedtime so they can be more spontaneous about outdoor activities that may be weather dependent. Optimizing both blood glucose and athletic performance, including fueling to make exercise easier and more enjoyable, requires an understanding of the blood glucose patterns around exercise so that nutrient timing and insulin dosing and timing can be adjusted to best support the unique needs of each athlete. Extra carbohydrate is often necessary after exercise when insulin sensitivity is increased and glycogen synthesis is enhanced.[63] Intake of additional carbohydrate at this time both promotes glycogen storage and reduces the likelihood of hypoglycemia. SMBG should be done every 1 to 2 hours after exercise to assess the blood glucose response and make any necessary adjustments in food intake and insulin doses.[2,6,43,50]

CONTINUOUS GLUCOSE MONITORING FOR THE ATHLETE WITHOUT DIABETES

Continuous glucose monitors were originally designed with the intention for use by individuals with diabetes as a glucose management tool. The interest in CGM systems has now crossed over into the athletic population, and a growing number of athletes without diabetes are using CGM systems with the overall objective of maximizing substrate availability around exercise to perform at optimal levels, essentially creating an energy management system. This strategy depends on interstitial glucose serving as a valid biomarker for carbohydrate availability, which has not yet been tested in rigorous research studies. The complex and multifactorial physiology behind glucose regulation makes it highly challenging to use for the purpose of energy management.[68,69]

The practice of using CGM for energy management involves additional challenges as well as practical and technical issues.[68,69] Practical issues include the need for context knowledge to correctly interpret the large amount of data obtained by CGM, the high cost of the sensor and subscription for the mobile applications used with the sensor, and the regulatory issues regarding use in sport. For example, the Australian Institute of Sport (AIS) bans the use of CGM under the "no needle policy,"[70] and the Union Cycliste Internationale (UCI) bans the use of CGM in competition.[71] The UCI ban is not related to a no-needle policy, but rather is due to the ability of the devices to provide data on metabolic values such as glucose and lactate. The AIS and UCI bans are intended solely for athletes who do not have a legitimate medical reason for use of the devices such as diabetes.

Technical issues may include loss of data due to transmission failures and dislodged sensors during activity. Sensors are attached to the body by an adhesive compound, and although most sensors are quite sturdy and reliable, they may become dislodged under certain conditions. For example, this may occur as a result of friction contact with uniforms or protective equipment, direct contact with another individual (eg, in contact and combat sports), or heavy sweating or immersion in water loosening the sensor adhesive material. The last possibility suggests that those competing in water sports may find CGM to be of little use. Finally, the acquisition of a CGM system is generally challenging. Currently, CGM systems are available for use by individuals without diabetes in only a handful of countries. As of December 2022, the devices available for use include the Abbott FreeStyle 2 (www.abbott.com; paired with the Ultrahuman M1 mobile application for data management, www.ultrahuman.com; available in India) and the Abbott FreeStyle Libre (www.abbott.com; paired with Veri and Levels mobile applications for data management; Veri is available in the Europe, the United States, Switzerland, Ireland, and Norway, www.veri.co; Levels is available in the United States, www.levelshealth.com).[68]

The limited research into the validity of using CGM in the athletic population without diabetes mainly consists of small sample sizes and/or case studies focusing on endurance or ultraendurance events. A literature search reported by Bowler et al[68] yielded 5 studies with a combined sample size of 34 athletes (74% male).[72-76] All 5 studies measured changes in glucose response either during exercise or during exercise and the postexercise recovery period. Ishihara et al[72] and Sengoku et al[73] studied 7 endurance runners (4 males, 3 females) and 2 male ultraendurance runners, respectively. Thomas et al[74] and Doering et al[75] studied 10 cyclists (7 males, 3 females) and 7 cyclists (6 males, 1 female), respectively, and Francois et al[76] studied adventure racers (6 males, 2 females). The overall conclusion from these 5 studies was that the observed changes in glucose response as measured by CGM had no correlation with glycogen restoration or substrate availability. However, in the study by Ishihara et al,[72] runners with carbohydrate intakes of less than 0.8 g/kg/h trended toward lower running speeds with corresponding lower CGM readings. These results should be interpreted with caution given the small sample sizes. Evidence does not yet exist to suggest that hypoglycemia equals low substrate availability, normoglycemia equals adequate substrate availability, and hyperglycemia equals excessive substrate availability. However, the concept is intriguing and warrants further study. The identification of an individual's optimal performance glucose range could have significant implications for training and competition in the sports nutrition world. Studies with larger cohorts should provide the information needed to make evidence-based recommendations in the future.

CASE STUDY

A case study of an elite cyclist with T1D is presented below. The case study walks through the steps of the Nutrition Care Process while illustrating the various challenges involved in the care of an athlete with diabetes.

Athlete History

DH is a 23-year-old male who began competitively cycling when he was 17 years old and is now moving up in the ranks of professional cycling. During the competitive season, he trains from 1 to 5 hours per day, riding approximately 30 km on a recovery day and 157.0 km or more on a long race day. DH was diagnosed with type 1 diabetes (T1D) 8 years ago at age 15 years and has had routine diabetes care since his diagnosis. DH uses an intermittently scanned continuous glucose monitor and a blood glucose (BG) meter for capillary BG monitoring in situations when glucose data measured by continuous glucose monitoring (CGM) are unavailable. DH follows training programs developed by his coaches to optimize race preparation and recovery. He and the coaches use the online application TrainingPeaks to communicate and track training data. DH is preparing for upcoming stage races with mountain stages and requested an appointment with his sports registered dietitian nutritionist (RDN) and certified diabetes care and education specialist (CDCES) to assist with 2 priority areas:

1) DH has experienced high glucose variability during and after races and wants to find strategies for reducing occurrences of above- and below-range glucose at times of competition.
2) He and his coach would like to achieve a gradual and modest weight loss and reduction in body fat percentage without compromising his training and overall health. (Note that, although DH's percent body fat is at the low end of a healthy range for a male his age, further reducing body mass and body fat in cycling improves the power-to-weight ratio and benefits performance.)

CASE STUDY

Step 1: Assessment

The information that follows was collected by the sports RDN.

ANTHROPOMETRICS

Height: 182 cm (5 ft, 11.5 in)

Weight: 73.1 kg (160.8 lb)

Body fat: 8.2%

PAST MEDICAL HISTORY

T1D and hypothyroidism

MEDICATIONS

Multiple daily injections of insulin

- Ultra-long-acting insulin degludec (brand name Tresiba, 14 units at 9 pm)
- Premeal insulin aspart (brand name NovoLog, insulin-to-carbohydrate ratio [ICR] of 1:10)
  - 2 to 5 units before breakfast depending on planned training
  - 2 to 4 units before lunch
  - 5 to 6 units before dinner
  - 1 to 2 units before evening snack
  - If glucose is above range, DH corrects with 1 to 2 units depending on the degree of glucose elevation.

50 mcg of L-thyroxine daily

GLUCOSE MANAGEMENT

DH's day-to-day diabetes self-management skills are sound, and he comprehends the fundamentals of insulin therapy; however, adapting management at times of competition and travel has proven challenging. Using a target glucose range of 70 to 180 mg/dL, DH achieved the following results during a recent block of racing (refer to the Figure 19.c1):

- 66% time in range (goal is to be in range 70% of the time, so this is 4% below goal)
- 10% time below range (goal is to spend no more than 5% of the time below range)
- 24% time above range (meets the goal); however, 6% of the time was spent in the very high range (>250 mg/dL); goal is to be in the very high range <5% of the time
- Glucose variability score (coefficient of variation) is 44.0%.
- Glucose management indicator (estimated HbA1c) is 6.7%.
- The values of the coefficient of variation and glucose management indicator reflect a high amount of glucose variability while achieving a target HbA1c value of <7.0%.

GLUCOSE STATISTICS AND TARGETS

18 March 2023-31 March 2023 — **14 Days**

Time Sensor Active: — **77%**

Ranges and targets for	Type 1 or type 2 diabetes
Glucose ranges	**Targets** % of Readings (Time/Day)
Target Range 70-180 mg/dl	Greater than 70% (16h 48min)
Below 70 mg/dl	Less than 4% (58 min)
Below 54 mg/dl	Less than 1% (14min)
Above 180 mg/dl	Less than 25% (6h)
Above 250 mg/dl	Less than 5% (1h 12min)

Each 5% increase in time range (70-180 mg/dl) is clinically beneficial.

Average Glucose — **140** mg/dl

Glucose Management Indicator (GMI) — **6.7% or 49** mmol/mol

Glucose Variability — **44.0%**

Defined as percent coefficient of variation (%CV)

TIME IN RANGES

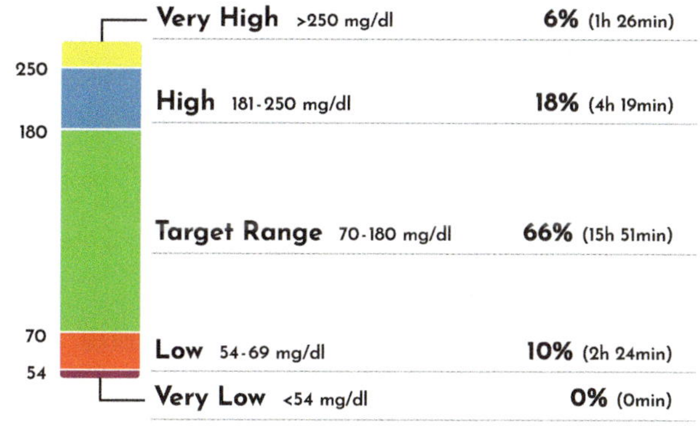

FIGURE 19.c1 Initial ambulatory glucose profile report

GLUCOSE PATTERNS (14 Days)

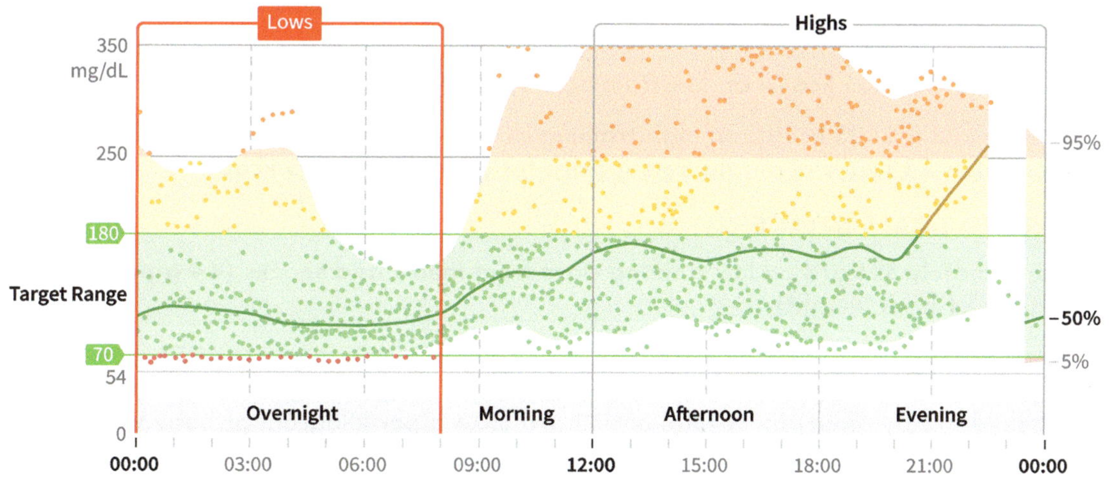

FIGURE 19.c2 Initial glucose patterns

DAILY GLUCOSE PROFILES

Each daily profile represents a midnight to midnight period with the date displayed in the upper left corner.

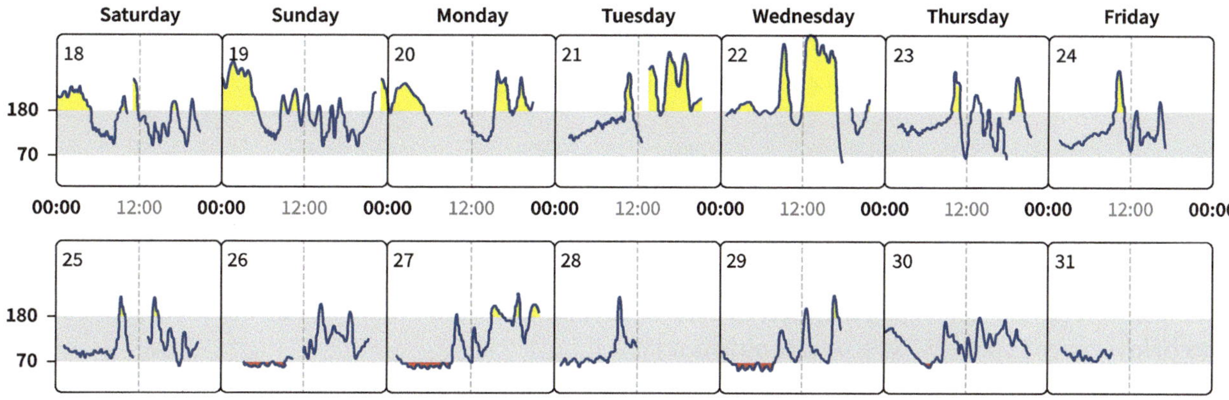

FIGURE 19.c3 Initial daily glucose profiles

CASE STUDY

Glucose patterns showed that the time segment when DH's glucose tended to be most elevated was midday through late afternoon. He also tended to have a high postmeal glucose rise in the late evening, as well as nighttime hypoglycemia during periods of travel and competition. The daily profiles show several instances of significant rises and falls in glucose levels contributing to an elevated glucose variability score (refer to Figures 19.c2 and 19.c3).

ESTIMATED EXERCISE ENERGY EXPENDITURE

- ~500 kcal during recovery rides
- ~4,000 kcal during a 5-hour road race

NUTRITION HISTORY AND USUAL DIETARY INTAKE

When at home, DH follows a consistent nutrition plan, typically eating 3 meals and an evening snack. He consumes higher amounts of carbohydrates on heavy training and race days, primarily from larger portions of pasta and rice in his prerace and recovery meals and from gels, a carbohydrate-containing sports drink mix, bars, and other food he consumes on the bike.

ENERGY INTAKE

Approximately 1,855 kcal/d on low training days from meals and snacks

Approximately 2,505 kcal/d on high training days from meals and snacks plus up to an additional 1,200 kcal during 5-hour rides for a total of ~3,705 kcal/d

CARBOHYDRATE INTAKE

Approximately 324 g/d on low training days from meals and snacks (4.4 g per kilogram of body weight)

Approximately 459 g/d on high training days from meals and snacks (6.3 g per kilogram of body weight) plus up to an additional 300 g during 5-hour rides (60 g of carbohydrate per hour) for a total of 759 g/d (10.4 g per kilogram of body weight)

PROTEIN INTAKE

92 to 108 g/d (1.25-1.5 g per kilogram of body weight)

Breakfast: 615 kcal, 104 g of carbohydrate, 35 g of protein

Lunch and dinner

Low training: ~900 kcal, ~175 g of carbohydrate, ~40 g of protein

High training: ~1,550 kcal, 310 g of carbohydrate, ~56 g of protein

Evening snack: 340 kcal, 45 g of carbohydrate, 17 g of protein

The nutrition-focused interview indicated that DH understands fundamental principles of diabetes and sports nutrition; however, he would benefit from a personalized and more targeted nutrition plan. At times, he was able to consume carbohydrate according to plan if his glucose was above range during racing and recovery, but at other times, he had to consume extra unplanned carbohydrate if his glucose was below range (up to 45–50 g of carbohydrate).

ENERGY NEEDS

Approximately 2,800 to 5,200 kcal/d (based on the Mifflin-St. Jeor equation)

CARBOHYDRATE NEEDS

292 to 584 g/d (based on 4–8 g per kilogram of body weight)

PROTEIN NEEDS

110 to 146 g/d (based on 1.5–2 g per kilogram of body weight)

Step 2: Nutrition Diagnosis

1. Inadequate protein-energy intake
2. Excessive carbohydrate intake
3. Altered nutrition-related laboratory value: *blood glucose*

EXAMPLE PROBLEM, ETIOLOGY, SIGNS AND SYMPTOMS (PES) STATEMENT

Altered nutrition-related blood glucose level related to inappropriate insulin dosing, insulin type, and distribution of carbohydrates as evidenced by only 66% time in the target range of 70 to 180 mg/dL with glucose variability of 44% (coefficient of variation).
Note: Nutrition diagnosis 3 was chosen because correction of the etiology causing the problem of glucose variability will also address diagnoses 1 and 2.

Step 3: Intervention

DH was advised to use his CGM and BG meter for capillary blood glucose monitoring in situations when CGM-measured glucose data are unavailable or inconsistent. In addition, he was informed of the importance of confirming his BG before and after races, when glucose variability can be high and certainty of his glucose number is critical to making decisions about insulin dosing and fueling strategy. His glucose goal range was revised to 90 to 120 mg/dL when not exercising so that he would be alerted to potential hypoglycemia earlier. During training and racing his goal range was set higher at 110 to 200 mg/dL.

Based on his recent pattern of nighttime hypoglycemia, DH was advised by his endocrinologist to reduce his 9 PM insulin degludec dosage to 12 units (15% reduction). He was also referred to his endocrinologist to have his premeal insulin aspart prescription changed to the brand Fiasp, which has a quicker onset, earlier peak time, and shorter duration of action. Based on total daily insulin dosage, the ICR was changed to 1 unit of insulin for every 45 g of carbohydrate (1:45 ratio) at breakfast and 1 unit of insulin for every 50 g of carbohydrate (1:50 ratio) at lunch and dinner. DH's insulin sensitivity factor (ISF) was estimated to be 1:75, so that 1 unit of insulin is expected to lower his BG by 75 mg/dL. His revised premeal insulin dosages based on his ICR are shown on next page.

BREAKFAST

2 units of insulin for 90 g of carbohydrate (reduced by 50% to 1 unit for 90 g on heavy training days); 0 units for fasted training rides

LUNCH (POSTTRAINING)

2 units of insulin for 100 g of carbohydrate or 4 units for 200 g of carbohydrate, depending on recovery nutrition plan

DINNER

2 units of insulin for 100 g of carbohydrate or 4 units for 200 g of carbohydrate

EVENING

Protein snack with minimal carbohydrate covered by 1 unit of insulin for BG greater than 120 mg/dL; no insulin for BG less than 120 mg/dL

To reduce high postmeal glucose spikes, DH was advised to inject his premeal insulin at least 15 minutes before eating unless his glucose is below range, in which case he was advised to take insulin with his first bite of food. He was also advised that eating salads and other low-carbohydrate vegetables and proteins before consuming carbohydrate sources is a strategy that can help delay and reduce postmeal glucose rise.

DH worked closely with his sports RDN to develop a nutrition and fueling plan that strategically guided carbohydrate and protein intake and timing to match his needs based on his training plans. To support recovery from training with moderate energy restriction, his protein intake was increased to 2.0 g/kg and distributed across the day. His in-ride nutrition was also adapted to the demands of training and racing. On recovery days, he was advised to consume 15 g of carbohydrate only if his glucose fell below 90 mg/dL. During endurance training rides, his goal was to consume 45 to 60 g of carbohydrate per hour. During high-effort training and racing, his aim was 60 to 90 g of carbohydrate per hour using a combination of foods including gels and drink mixes with multiple transportable carbohydrates. He was advised to not inject rapid-acting insulin to cover in-ride carbohydrates unless his glucose was greater than 200 mg/dL. In-ride insulin dosing decisions were based on both glucose level and CGM rate-of-change arrow indications and were reduced by 50% or more of the usual calculated dose.

Step 4: Monitoring and Evaluation

By applying a more targeted approach to nutrition and fueling, glucose monitoring, and insulin dosing strategies, DH reduced his body weight to 72.2 kg and his body fat to 7.9% within 2 months, which translated to a 0.5-kg reduction in fat mass. He was also able to reduce his glucose variability and increase his glucose time in range, achieving 84% time in range with only 1% time below range and 15% time above range. In addition, he achieved very acceptable values of a coefficient of variation of 36.2% and a glucose management indicator of 6.4% (refer to the Figure 19.c4). DH will continue to work closely with his sports RDN, CDCES, coaches, and clinical diabetes care team, understanding the complex and dynamic scenarios that can contribute to unique glucose management challenges.

GLUCOSE STATISTICS AND TARGETS

20 May 2023-2 June 2023 **14 Days**
Time Sensor Active: **87%**

Ranges and targets for	Type 1 or type 2 diabetes
Glucose ranges	**Targets** % of Readings (Time/Day)
Target Range 70-180 mg/dl	Greater than 70% (16h 48min)
Below 70 mg/dl	Less than 4% (58 min)
Below 54 mg/dl	Less than 1% (14min)
Above 180 mg/dl	Less than 25% (6h)
Above 250 mg/dl	Less than 5% (1h 12min)
Each 5% increase in time range (70-180 mg/dl) is clinically beneficial.	

Average Glucose **131** mg/dl
Glucose Management Indicator (GMI) **6.4% or 47** mmol/mol
Glucose Variability **36.2%**
Defined as percent coefficient of variation (%CV)

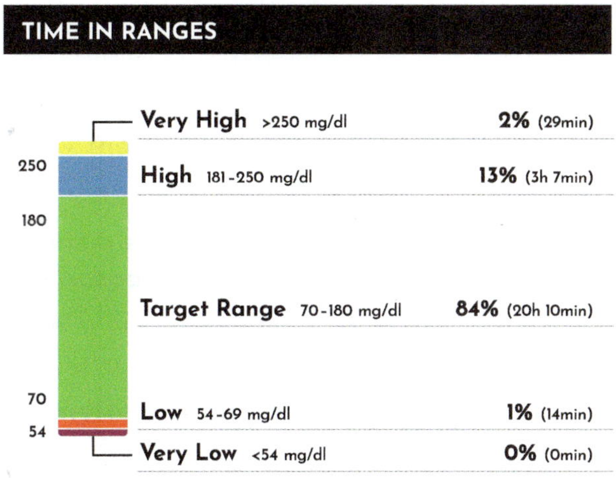

FIGURE 19.c4 **Ambulatory glucose profile report postintervention**

SUMMARY

For individuals with T2D and those with prediabetes, regular physical activity can improve blood glucose control and may even alleviate symptoms of the disease. However, for individuals with T1D, exercise does not have the same tendency to improve glycemic control. Rather, it has the potential to contribute to substantial blood glucose variability and considerable management challenges. Even so, all individuals with diabetes should be encouraged to follow active lifestyles to achieve the many health benefits of physical activity. The athlete with diabetes who is striving for competitive performance should be offered the support and self-management training needed to achieve optimal performance. This chapter provides general guidelines and strategies for adapting diabetes medications and MNT to accommodate exercise. This chapter also introduces the concept of using CGM as a performance tool while acknowledging that there is not yet enough evidence to support widespread use in athletes without diabetes. Strategies must be modified and individualized based on the uniqueness of each individual and each exercise situation. SMBG and pattern management allow successful strategies to be developed and fine-tuned to minimize exercise risk while maximizing performance.

KEY TAKEAWAYS

Athletes with diabetes present with challenges that need to be addressed.

If a determined athlete has a solid plan for training and diabetes management, there is no reason diabetes should prevent them from achieving great feats.

Athletes with diabetes are often more prepared than other athletes on the course or field. By necessity, they have to think through variables and anticipate potential needs more carefully than others.

Preparation and planning are key to the success of athletes with diabetes. Each athlete should have an individual diabetes management plan for training and competition that includes prevention and treatment strategies. Athletes with diabetes are also advised to have a diabetes management kit that includes emergency plans, medications, and items to treat hypoglycemia if needed.

Managing the needs of an athlete with diabetes demands a team approach and necessitates excellent communication between members of the team. The team includes health care practitioners (endocrinologist, CDCES, and others) who are involved in the athlete's diabetes care; pertinent members of the coaching and training staff; the sports RDN; and most importantly, the athlete. The better the communication, the better the outcome.

Every athlete with diabetes has unique needs. Understanding the underlying science will provide valuable insights, but for the best results, there must also be an understanding of each athlete's individual blood glucose response to exercise. Flexible treatment is the key to success!

The interest in CGM has now crossed over into the athletic population, and a growing number of athletes without diabetes are using CGM systems; however, there is not enough evidence yet to support their use for this purpose.

REFERENCES

1. ElSayed N, Aleppo G, Aroda V, et al. Facilitating positive health behaviors and well-being to improve health outcomes: Standards of Care in Diabetes—2023. *Diabetes Care*. 2023;46(suppl 1):S68-S96. doi:10.2337/dc23-S005
2. Trojian T, Colberg S, Harris G, et al. American Medical Society for Sports Medicine Position Statement on the Care of the Athlete and Athletic Person with Diabetes. *Clin Sport Med* 2022;32(1):8-20. doi:10.1097/JSM.0000000000000906
3. Malcolm G, Rilstone S, Sivasubramaniyam S, et al. Managing diabetes at high altitude: personal experience with support from a multidisciplinary physical activity and diabetes clinic. *BM Open Sport Exerc Med*. 2017;3:e000238. doi:10.1136/bmjsem-2017-000238
4. Milewski M. Peak performance. *Diabetes Forecast*. 2006;59:60-63.
5. Colberg SR, Sigal RJ, Yardley JE, et al. Physical activity/exercise and diabetes: a position statement of the American Diabetes Association. *Diabetes Care*. 2016;39(11):2065-2079. doi:10.2337/dc16-1728
6. Riddell MC, Gallen IW, Smart CE, et al. Exercise management in type 1 diabetes: a consensus statement. *Lancet Diabetes Endocrinol*.2017;5(5):377-390. doi:10.1016/S2213-8587(17)30014-1
7. Harris GD, White RD. Diabetes in the competitive athlete. *Curr Sports Med Rep*. 2012;11(6):309-315. doi:10.1249/JSR.0b013e3182751007
8. ElSayed NA, Aleppo G, Aroda VR, et al; American Diabetes Association. 7. Diabetes technology: *Standards of Care in Diabetes—2023. Diabetes Care*. 2023;46(suppl 1):S111-S127. doi:10.2337/dc23-S007
9. Hornsby WG Jr, Chetlin RD. Management of competitive athletes with diabetes. *Diabetes Spectr*. 2005;18(2):102-107. doi:10.1007/s00125-020-05183-8
10. ElSayed NA, Aleppo G, Aroda VR, et al; American Diabetes Association. 2. Classification and diagnosis of diabetes: *Standards of Care in Diabetes—2023. Diabetes Care*. 2023;46(suppl 1):S19-S40. doi:10.2337/dc23-S002
11. Bliss M. History of insulin. *Diabetes Care*. 1993;16(suppl 3):4-7. doi:10.2337/diacare.16.3.4
12. ElSayed NA, Aleppo G, Aroda VR, et al; American Diabetes Association. 9. Pharmacologic approaches to glycemic treatment: *Standards of Care in Diabetes—2023. Diabetes Care*. 2023;46(suppl 1):S140-S157. doi:10.2337/dc23-S009
13. Hirsch I. Insulin analogs. *N Engl Med*. 2005;352(2):174-183. doi:10.1056/NEJMra040832
14. Walsh J, Roberts R. *Pumping Insulin: Everything You Need for Success on a Smart Insulin Pump*. Torrey Pines Press; 2006.
15. Devries MC, Hamadeh MJ, Phillips SM, Tarnopolsky MA. Menstrual cycle phase and sex influence muscle glycogen utilization and glucose turnover during moderate-intensity endurance exercise. *Am Physiol Regul Integr Comp Physiol*. 2006;291(4):R1120-R1128. doi:10.1152/ajpregu.00700.2005
16. Yardley JE, Brockman NK, Bracken RM. Could age, sex and physical fitness affect blood glucose responses to exercise in type 1 diabetes? *Front Endocrinol (Lausanne)*. 2018;9:674. doi:10.3389/fendo.2018.00674
17. Millstein R, Becerra N, Shubrook J. Insulin pumps: beyond basal-bolus. *Clev Clin Med*. 2015;82(12):835-842. doi:10.3949/ccjm.82a.14127
18. Davidson PC, Hebblewhite HR, Steed RD, Bode BW. Analysis of guidelines for basal-bolus insulin dosing: basal insulin, correction factor and carbohydrate-to-insulin ratio. *AACE Endocrine Pract*. 2008;14(9):1095-1101. doi:10.4158/EP.14.9.1095
19. Colberg SR. Nutrition and exercise performance in adults with type 1 diabetes. *Can Diabetes*. 2020;44(8):750-758. doi:10.1016/j.jcjd.2020.05.014
20. Riddell MC, Peters AL. Exercise in adults with type 1 diabetes mellitus. *Nat Rev Endocrinol*. 2023;19(2);98-111. doi:10.1038/s41574-022-00756-6
21. Moser O, Riddell MC, Eckstein ML, et al. Glucose management for exercise using continuous glucose monitoring (CGM) and intermittently scanned CGM (isCGM) systems in type 1 diabetes: a position statement of the European Association for the Study of Diabetes (EASD) and of the International Society for Pediatric and Adolescent Diabetes (ISPAD) endorsed by JDRF and supported by the American Diabetes Association (ADA). *Diabetologia*. 2020;63(12):2501-2520. doi:10.1007/s00125-020-05263-9
22. Riddell MC, Scott SN, Fournier PA, et al. The competitive athlete with type 1 diabetes. *Diabetologia*. 2020;63(8):1475-1490. doi:10.1007/s00125-020-05183-8
23. Lisle D, Trojian T. Managing the athlete with type 1 diabetes. *Curr Sports Med Rep*. 2006;5(2):93-98. doi:10.1097/01.csmr.0000306527.66877.5f
24. Horton W, Subauste J. Care of the athlete with type 1 diabetes mellitus: a clinical review. *Int Endocrinol Metab*. 2016;14(2):e36091. doi:10.5812/ijem.36091
25. Pereira WVC, Vancea DMM, de Andrade Oliveira R, et al. 2022: Position of Brazilian Diabetes Society on exercise recommendations for people with type 1 and type 2 diabetes. *Diabetol Metab Syndr*. 2023;15(1):2. doi:10.1186/s13098-022-00945-3
26. Chetty T, Shetty V, Fournier PA, et al. Exercise management for young people with type 1 diabetes: a structured approach to exercise consultation. *Front Endocrinol (Lausanne)*. 2019;10:326. doi:10.3389/fendo.2019.00326
27. Makoni M. Insulin storage without refrigeration. *Lancet Diabetes Endocrinol*. 2021;9(4):202. doi:10.1016/S2213-8587(21)00057-7
28. Handelsman Y, Bloomgarden ZT, Grunberger G, et al. American Association of Clinical Endocrinologists and American College of Endocrinology clinical practice guidelines for developing a diabetes mellitus comprehensive care plan. *Endocr Pract*. 2015:21(suppl 1):1-87. doi:10.4158/EP15672.GL

29. Aberer F, Bieber TR, Eckstein ML, et al. Glucose-lowering therapy beyond insulin in type 1 diabetes: a narrative review on existing evidence from randomized controlled trials and clinical perspective. *Pharmaceutics.* 2022;14(6):1180. doi:10.3390/pharmaceutics14061180
30. Isaacs D. Non-insulin medications for type 1 diabetes. *On the Cutting Edge.* 2018;39(2):12-18.
31. Evans M, Hicks D, Patel D, Patel V, McEwan P, Dashora U. Optimizing the benefits of SGLT2 inhibitors for type 1 diabetes. *Diabetes Ther.* 2020:11(1);37-52. doi:10.1007/s13300-019-00728-6
32. Warwick K. Hypoglycemia. *On the Cutting Edge.* 2022;43(2):35-37.
33. Kenny WL, Wilmore JH, Costill DL. *Physiology of Sport and Exercise.* 8th ed. Human Kinetics; 2022.
34. Riddell MC, Zaharieva DP, Tansey M, et al. Individual glucose responses to prolonged moderate intensity aerobic exercise in adolescents with type 1 diabetes: the higher they start, the harder they fall. *Pediatr Diabetes.* 2019;20(1):99-106. doi:10.1111/pedi.12799
35. Vartak V, Chepulis L, Driller M, Paul RG. Comparing two treatment approaches for patients with type 1 diabetes during aerobic exercise: a randomised, crossover study. *Sports Med Open.* 2021;7(1):29. doi:10.1186/s40798-021-00319-5
36. García-García F, Kumareswaran K, Hovorka R, Hernando ME. Quantifying the acute changes in glucose with exercise in type 1 diabetes: a systematic review and meta-analysis. *Sports Med.* 2015;45(4):587-599. doi:10.1007/s40279-015-0302-2
37. McArdle WD, Katch FI, Katch VL. *Exercise Physiology: Energy, Nutrition, and Human Performance.* 3rd ed. Lea & Febiger; 1991.
38. Sedivy P, Dezotova M, Drobny M, et al. Differences in muscle metabolism in patients with type I diabetes - influence of gender and nephropathy studied by ^{31}P MR spectroscopy. *Physiol Res.* 2018;67(3):433-441. doi:10.33549/physiolres.933745
39. Monaco CMT, Hughes MC, Ramos SV, et al. Altered mitochondrial bioenergetics and ultrastructure in the skeletal muscle of young adults with type 1 diabetes. *Diabetologia.* 2018;61(6):1411-1423. doi:10.1007/s00125-018-4602-6
40. Borer K. *Exercise Endocrinology.* Human Kinetics; 2003.
41. Kubo K, Foley JE. Rate-limiting steps for insulin-mediated glucose uptake into perfused rat hindlimb. *Am Physiol.* 1986;250(1 pt 1):E100-E102. doi:10.1152/ajpendo.1986.250.1.E100
42. Douen AG, Ramlal T, Rastogi S, et al. Exercise induces recruitment of the "insulin-responsive glucose transporter": evidence for distinct intracellular insulin- and exercise-recruitable transporter pools in skeletal muscle. *Biol Chem.* 1990;265(23):13427-13430.
43. Colberg SR. *Diabetic Athlete's Handbook.* Human Kinetics; 2009.
44. Minuk HL, Vranic M, Marliss EB, Hanna AK, Albisser AM, Zinman B. Glucoregulatory and metabolic response to exercise in obese noninsulin-dependent diabetes. *Am Physiol.* 1981;240(5):E458-E464. doi:10.1152/ajpendo.1981.240.5.E458
45. Pedersen O, Bak JF, Andersen PH, et al. Evidence against altered expression of GLUT1 or GLUT4 in skeletal muscle of patients with obesity for NIDDM. *Diabetes.* 1990;39(7):865-870. doi:10.2337/diab.39.7.865
46. Yardley JE, Zaharieva DP, Jarvis C, Riddell MC. The "ups" and "downs" of a bike race in people with type 1 diabetes: dramatic differences in strategies and blood glucose responses in the Paris-to-Ancaster Spring Classic. *Can Diabetes.* 2015;39(2):105-110. doi:10.1016/j.jcjd.2014.09.003
47. Macknight JM, Mistry DJ, Pastors JG, Holmes V, Rynders CA. The daily management of athletes with diabetes. *Clin Sports Med.* 2009;28(3):479-495. doi:10.1016/j.csm.2009.02.005
48. Gallen IW, Hume C, Lumb A. Fuelling the athlete with type 1 diabetes. *Diabetes Obes Metab.* 2011;13(2):130-136. doi:10.1111/j.1463-1326.2010.01319.x
49. Jensen TE, Richter EA. Regulation of glucose and glycogen metabolism during and after exercise. *Physiol.* 2012;590(5):1069-1076. doi:10.1113/jphysiol.2011.224972
50. Scott SN, Fontana FY, Cocks M, et al. Post-exercise recovery for the endurance athlete with type 1 diabetes: a consensus statement. *Lancet Diabetes Endocrinol.* 2021;9(5):304-317. doi:10.1016/S2213-8587(21)00054-1
51. ElSayed NA, Aleppo G, Aroda VR, et al.; American Diabetes Association. 6. Glycemic targets: *Standards of Care in Diabetes—2023. Diabetes Care.* 2023;46(suppl 1):S97-S110. doi:10.2337/dc23-S006
52. Centers for Disease Control and Prevention. Treatment of low blood sugar (hypoglycemia). December 30, 2022. Accessed April 16, 2023. www.cdc.gov/diabetes/treatment/treatment-low-blood-sugar-hypoglycemia.html
53. Jimenez C, Corcoran M, Crawley J, et al. National Athletic Trainers' Association position statement: management of the athlete with type 1 diabetes mellitus. *J Athl Train.* 2007;42(4):536-545.
54. Challet E. Keeping circadian time with hormones. *Diabetes Obes Metab.* 2015;17(suppl 1):76-83. doi:10.1111/dom.12516
55. Halson SL. Sleep in elite athletes and nutritional interventions to enhance sleep. *Sports Med.* 2014;44(suppl 1):S13-S23. doi:10.1007/s40279-014-0147-0
56. Richards P, Hillebrandt D. The practical aspects of insulin at high altitude. *High Alt Med Biol.* 2013;14(3):197-204. doi:10.1089/ham.2013.1020
57. de Mol P, de Vries ST, de Koning EG, Gans ROB, Bilo HJG, Tack CJ. Physical activity at altitude: challenges for people with diabetes: a review. *Diabetes Care.* 2014;37(8):2404-2413. doi:10.2337/dc13-2302
58. Cohn A, Sofia AM, Kupfer SS. Type 1 diabetes and celiac disease: clinical overlap and new insights into disease pathogenesis. *Curr Diabetes Rep.* 2014;14(8):517. doi:10.1007/s11892-014-0517-x
59. Kurien M, Mollazadegan K, Sanders DS, Ludvigsson JF. Celiac disease increases risk of thyroid disease in patients with type 1 diabetes: a nationwide cohort study. *Diabetes Care.* 2016;39(3):371-375. doi:10.2337/dc15-2117
60. Pham-Short A, Donaghue KC, Ambler G, Phelan H, Twigg S, Craig ME. Screening for celiac disease in type 1 diabetes: a systematic review. *Pediatrics.* 2015;136(1):e170-e176. doi:10.1542/peds.2014-2883

61. Bermudez O, Sommer J. T1D Intel: Learning about the dual diagnosis of an eating disorder and type 1 diabetes. JDRF website. October 15, 2012. Accessed May 21, 2023. www.jdrf.org/blog/2012/10/15/t1d-intel-learning-about-the-dual-diagnosis-of-an-eating-disorder-and-type-1-diabetes
62. Thomas DT, Erdman KA, Burke LM. Position of the American Dietetic Association, Dietitians of Canada, and the American College of Sports Medicine: nutrition and athletic performance. *Acad Nutr Diet.* 2016;116(3):501-528. doi:10.1016/j.jand.2015.12.006
63. Franz M, MacLeod J, Evert A, et al. Academy of Nutrition and Dietetics nutrition practice guidelines for type 1 and type 2 diabetes in adults: systematic review of evidence for medical nutrition therapy effectiveness and recommendations for integration into the nutrition care process. *Acad Nutr Diet.* 2017;117(10):1659-1679. doi:10.1016/j.jand.2017.03.022
64. Aroda VR, Edelstein SL, Goldberg RB, et al. Long-term metformin use and vitamin B12 deficiency in the Diabetes Prevention Program Outcomes Study. *Clin Endocrinol Metab.* 2016;101(4):1754-1761. doi:10.1210/jc.2015-3754
65. Beck-Nielsen H. The role of glycogen synthase in the development of hyperglycemia in type 2 diabetes: "To store or not to store glucose, that's the question". *Diabetes Metab Res Rev.* 2012;28(8):635-644. doi:10.1002/dmrr.2337
66. Bell KJ, Fio CZ, Twigg S, et al. Amount and type of dietary fat, postprandial glycemia, and insulin requirements in type 1 diabetes: A randomized within-subject trial. *Diabetes Care.* 2020;43(1):59-66. doi:10.2337/dc19-0687
67. Bell KJ, Smart CE, Steil GM, et al. Impact of fat, protein, and glycemic index on postprandial glucose control in type 1 diabetes: implications for intensive diabetes management in the continuous glucose monitoring era. *Diabetes Care.* 2015;38(6):1008-1015. doi:10.2337/dc15-0100
68. Bowler A-LM, Whitfield J, Marshall L, Coffey VG, Burke LM, Cox GR. The use of continuous glucose monitors in sport: possible applications and considerations. *Int Sport Nutr Exerc Metab.* 2022;33(2):121-132. doi:10.1123/ijsnem.2022-0139
69. Klonoff DC, Nguyen KT, Xu NY, Gutierrez A, Espinoza JC, Vidmar AP. Use of continuous glucose monitors by people without diabetes: an idea whose time has come? *Diabetes Sci Technol.* 2023;17(6):1686-1697. doi:10.1177/19322968221110830
70. Hughes D. Australian Institute of Sport. No needles policy. October 2018. Accessed November 1, 2023. www.sportaus.gov.au/__data/assets/pdf_file/0006/687624/AIS_No_Needles_Policy_-_November_2018.pdf
71. Union Cycliste Internationale. Clarification guide of the UCI technical regulation. May 10, 2021. Accessed November 1, 2023. https://assets.ctfassets.net/761l7gh5x5an/7s1ma6mVAVlFwi8rRgy0Iw/1bef531d-d9e9f534c34ff016c68e3c72/Clarification_Guide_of_the_UCI_Technical_Regulation_-_20211005_-_ENG.pdf
72. Ishihara K, Uchiyama N, Kizaki S, et al. Application of continuous glucose monitoring for assessment of individual carbohydrate requirement during ultramarathon race. *Nutrients.* 2020;12(4):1121. doi:10.3390/nu12041121
73. Sengoku Y, Nakamura K, Ogata H, Nabekura Y, Nagasaka S, Tokuyama K. Continuous glucose monitoring during a 100-km race: a case study in an elite ultramarathon runner. *Int Sports Physiol Perform.* 2015;10(1):124-127. doi:10.1123/ijspp.2013-0493
74. Thomas F, Pretty CG, Desaive T, Chase JG. Blood glucose levels of subelite athletes during 6 days of free living. *Diabetes Sci Technol.* 2016;10(6):1335-1343. doi:10.1177/1932296816648344
75. Doering TM, Cox GR, Areta JL, Coffey VG. Repeated muscle glycogen supercompensation with four days' recovery between exhaustive exercise. *Sci Med Sport.* 2019;22(8):907-911. doi:10.1016/j.jsams.2019.03.009
76. Francois ME, Cosgrove SD, Walker NM, Lucas SJ, Black KE. Physiological responses to a five-day adventure race: Continuous blood glucose, hemodynamics and metabolites the 2012 GODZone field-study. *Exerc Sci Fit.* 2018;16(3):78-82. doi:10.1016/j.jesf.2018.07.002

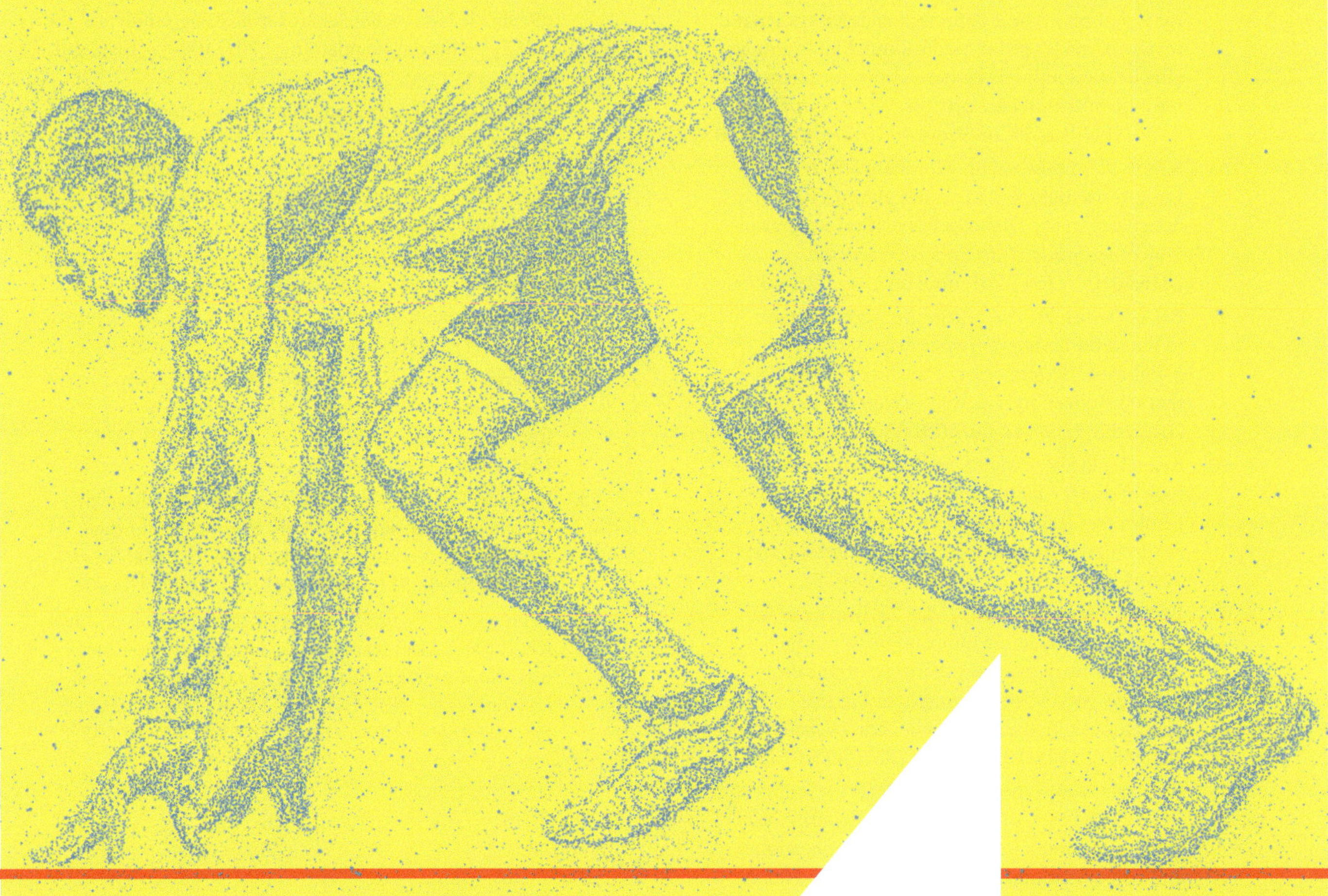

SECTION 4

ACTIVITY-SPECIFIC NUTRITION GUIDELINES

The practice of sports nutrition has come a long way. The chapters in this section synthesize the science of sports nutrition and exercise to provide guidelines for athletes participating in sports ranging from the very high–intensity but short all-out effort (such as the 100-m sprint that crowns the "fastest" athlete in the world) to the ultraendurance events (such as the Run Around Australia, which covers 9,053 miles in 191 days of competition). Athletes have very different nutritional needs depending on their exercise intensity and duration. These chapters pinpoint the nutritional requirements for training and competition for athletes competing in very high–intensity, high-intensity short-duration, and high-intensity intermittent exercise, as well as endurance and ultraendurance events. The science is provided along with practical tips for fueling athletes to help the sports registered dietitian nutritionist (RDN) establish food and fluid goals to help athletes achieve their dreams. This section also explores activity-specific nutrition guidelines from an occupational standpoint and ends with a new chapter that focuses on tactical performance nutrition.

CHAPTER 20

Nutrition for Short-Duration, Very High- and High-Intensity Sports

Christine A. Karpinski, PhD, RD, CSSD, LDN

LEARNING OBJECTIVES

- Discuss the energy pathways and substrate utilization most common for short-duration, very high-intensity and high-intensity sports.
- Identify the macronutrients and micronutrients most at-risk for insufficient intake among athletes who participate in short-duration, very high-intensity and high-intensity sports.
- Understand how the macronutrient, micronutrient, hydration, and body composition demands of training and competition affect dietary recommendations for short-duration, very high-intensity and high-intensity athletes.
- Analyze the risks and benefits of weight-loss practices, weight-gain practices, and dietary supplements as they relate to short-duration, very high-intensity and high-intensity athletes.

INTRODUCTION

Limited research focuses on high-intensity sports compared with endurance and intermittent sports, and even less focuses on what is referred to as short-duration, very high–intensity and high-intensity sports. Events typically included in the very high–intensity category are sports or training that requires all-out effort or near-maximal effort (>90% of the maximum oxygen consumption [VO_2 max] or 1-repetition maximum) and lasts less than 30 seconds. Short-duration, high-intensity sports require near-maximal effort that can last several minutes. These sports are often referred to as *power sports* or *explosive sports* and can include single sprints (eg, run, cycle, swim, skate), middle-distance events (eg, running, rowing), jumping or throwing events (field), or a single move or play during the course of a game or match (eg, football, baseball, basketball, soccer). Olympic and power weightlifting and certain strength-training protocols can also fall into this category. Box 20.1 lists examples of events that involve short-duration, very high–intensity and high-intensity exercise.

Bodybuilding and physique competitions (eg, bikini, figure, fitness) are not included in this chapter because their strength-training programs typically are higher volume, use higher repetition ranges (10–12 repetitions), include more muscle groups, and incorporate little rest between sets compared with most power sports.[1] Another unique aspect of bodybuilding and other aesthetic sports is that the competition is not intended to generate power or speed, as the athlete holds an isometric pose for up to 20 seconds. Finally, the diets of bodybuilders and physique competitors vary greatly during different phases of training, with the ultimate goal of achieving body-fat levels below guidelines recommended for most performance athletes. Although these practices are common among coaches and competitors, they are not supported by the scientific literature. Refer to the At a Glance section for more information on physique sports.

BOX 20.1 Events and Sports That Involve Very High-Intensity or High-Intensity Exercise

Mode	Event (approximate duration)
Very high intensity	
Running sprint	50-m dash (6 s), 100 m dash (10 s), 200 m dash (20 s)
Hurdles	100-m or 110-m hurdle (12–16 s)
Jumping	High jump, long jump, triple jump, pole vault (no set duration)
Cycle sprint	200 m (10 s)
Swimming sprint	50 m (22 s)
Throwing	Shotput, javelin, discus, hammer (several seconds)
Olympic weightlifting	Snatch, clean, and jerk (≤1 s)
Power lifting	Bench press, squat, deadlift (several seconds)
Gymnastics	Multiple events (no set duration)
Team sports with sprints	Multiple, including football and baseball (no set duration)
High intensity	
Running	400 m (50 s), 600 m (1 min 30 s), 800 m (2 min)
Swimming	100 m (1 min), 200 m (2 min)
Skating	1,000 m (1 min 15 s), 1,500 m (2 min)

Because the events discussed in this chapter are extremely short in duration, the importance of nutrition may be minimized by athletes and coaches; however, for these sports, hundredths of seconds can be the difference between first and second place, and nutrition can play an important role in the outcome. Short-duration, very high– and high-intensity athletes face unique nutritional challenges because of the nature of their sports, including demanding training schedules, multiple-event days, travel, and a high level of focus. For example, an elite swim sprinter can train up to 3 or 4 hours per day, yet their event lasts less than 2 minutes. It is common for track-and-field athletes and gymnasts to have several events in 1 day with limited recovery time between events. This chapter reviews the energy systems and substrate utilization involved in these types of sports; typical dietary intake; energy, macronutrient, and micronutrient needs; nutritional guidelines; and nutritional strategies that address training and competition for athletes involved in short-duration, very high–intensity and high-intensity sports.

ENERGY SYSTEM AND SUBSTRATE UTILIZATION

The ability to perform high-intensity and very high–intensity efforts in sport depends on many factors, including reaction time, muscle power, skill, muscle fiber type, and psychological factors. From a metabolic standpoint, adenosine triphosphate (ATP) availability, rate of ATP breakdown, and rate of ATP resynthesis are critical. The rate of ATP production needed to perform these events is high. For example, the power output during a 30-second sprint is approximately twice that achieved at VO_2 max, and the energy need for a 1,500-m running race may be approximately 115% of VO_2 max.[2] A substantial amount of the ATP required to fuel these events is produced anaerobically; the shorter the duration of maximal effort, the higher the percentage of ATP generated from anaerobic sources. For example, ATP used in a 30-second sprint is approximately 80% anaerobically generated, whereas that used in a 10-second sprint is approximately 97% anaerobically fueled.[3] Although the specific crossover point varies by individual, in general, events of effort longer than 2 minutes obtain a majority of ATP from the aerobic system, and the contribution from anaerobic pathways diminishes.

The briefest, highest-intensity efforts are fueled by ATP produced anaerobically by the breakdown of phosphocreatine (PCr) within the muscle. The rate of ATP production (in micromoles per second per kilogram) is estimated at[4]:

- 6.0 for PCr (maximal rate of production),
- 1.5 for anaerobic glycolysis,
- 0.24 for aerobic generation from fat, and
- 0.5 for aerobic generation from carbohydrate.

This means that efforts that require very rapid generation of ATP use will rely heavily on the breakdown of PCr. Because PCr stores are limited and their use is rapid with high-intensity work, it is possible to substantially reduce PCr stores during a brief exercise bout. For example, research shows that a 30-second sprint can decrease PCr by 75%, a 20-second sprint (eg, 200-m run, 50-m swim) can decrease PCr by about 50%, and even a 10-second maximal effort (eg, 100-m run, 200-m cycle) can decrease PCr by 40%.[3,4]

Once PCr donates its phosphate group to adenosine diphosphate (ADP), it must return to the mitochondria to be rephosphorylated, which takes approximately 1 to 2 minutes. Therefore, a limiting factor for performance of these very high–intensity efforts could be initial muscle PCr stores. It is logical to begin the event, game, or match with high muscle PCr. Sprint training can increase PCr stores. Another way to boost muscle creatine stores is through supplementation with oral creatine (discussed later in this chapter and in Chapter 7). The rate of recovery for muscular PCr depends on many factors, including the magnitude of reduction, oxygen availability, pH, and substrate level, but it can take up to 1 minute to regain the initial levels. Although PCr is resynthesized rapidly, replenishment may not be complete if a second very high–intensity bout occurs close to the first.

In addition to PCr, the fuel that provides ATP anaerobically for high- and very high–intensity efforts is glucose generated through glycolysis. The use of glycolysis for ATP generation rather than PCr increases with the duration of a sprint. A 10-second sprint depends on glycolysis for approximately 44% of the ATP used, whereas a 30-second sprint will likely get more than 50% of the ATP from this system.[3] However, because muscles have much more glycogen than PCr, these brief, very high–intensity efforts do not substantially reduce muscle glycogen. The magnitude of reduction in muscle glycogen depends on the intensity and duration of an exercise bout, as well as the type of activity (Figure 20.1).[4-6] The magnitude of glycogen depletion during resistance exercise is related to the intensity of the lift and the amount of work performed. Most of the studies available to date use a high-volume resistance exercise workout; little research has been done on glycogen use with low-volume, high-intensity workouts.

Although it is unlikely that modestly reduced glycogen stores will influence the performance of a single very high–intensity effort, it could impair high-intensity efforts interspersed within a game that involves substantial aerobic exercise (eg, basketball or soccer) if it is concurrent with a lower-carbohydrate diet (eg, less than 3–4 g per kilogram of body weight).

Acidosis that occurs secondary to lactate production during anaerobic glycolysis is a limiting factor for performance during brief, high-intensity events.[7] Some research suggests that acidosis directly impairs muscle force development, whereas other research suggests that it may have an indirect effect through the impairment of enzyme activity critical for ATP generation. Other metabolic factors, such as the accumulation of intracellular phosphate with the subsequent disruption of calcium release from the sarcoplasmic reticulum, could play a role in fatigue for middle-distance events.[8]

In summary, brief, very high–intensity efforts are primarily fueled by PCr stores, with increasing reliance on glycogen stores occurring with longer sprints or middle-distance events, such as the 800-m sprint. This results in substantial use of the PCr stores but typically use of less than one-third of the muscle glycogen stores. Accumulation of such metabolites as hydrogen ions and inorganic phosphates can contribute to fatigue that lasts for several minutes during high-intensity events.

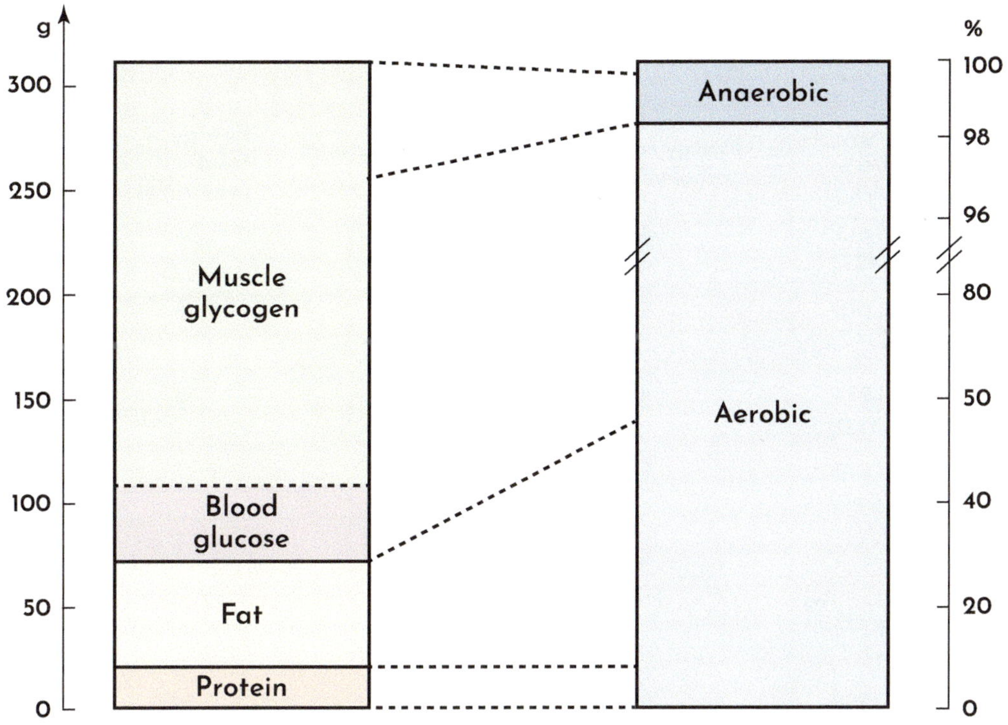

FIGURE 20.1 Percentage muscle glycogen reduction for sprints and resistance-exercise workouts[4-6] The left-hand scale represents the grams of substrate being used. The right-hand scale represents the percentage of adenosine triphosphate produced from aerobic vs anaerobic energy pathways.

NUTRITIONAL INTAKE

There is a distinct lack of current studies focusing on the nutritional intake of athletes participating in short-duration, very high–intensity and high-intensity sports. Data from 2 studies included in the last edition of this book have been included here because they were conducted after 2010.[9,10] A search of the literature for studies assessing the nutritional intake of athletes between 2014 and 2022 revealed that most have focused on athletes participating in endurance or team sports. A few studies on young children involved in short-duration, very high– and high-intensity sports exist,[11,12] but they are not discussed here. In addition, some of these data were collected on athletes from different countries, adding variations due to cultural differences and levels of competition. It should be emphasized again that although the competitive events of many of these athletes may last less than a few minutes, their training regimens are high volume, often lasting several hours per day, and thus, their everyday diets may not reflect their competition needs. The data obtained in some studies that evaluated the diets of high-intensity or very high–intensity athletes using dietary records are reported in Tables 20.1 and 20.2 on page 534.[9,10,13-17]

Data on the micronutrient intake of power and strength athletes is also sparse. Of the studies that collected macronutrient data listed in Tables 20.1 and 20.2, 4 also collected data on some key micronutrients[10,13,15,16]; calcium and iron were common to all 4 studies. A few studies have focused on just the micronutrient intake of athletes participating in short-duration, very high–intensity and high-intensity sports.[18-20] Results for mean calcium intake were mixed, with young Indonesian gymnasts and female Slovenian swimmers below the recommended intake (at 1,157 ± 516 mg and 899 ± 347 mg, respectively).[13,15] Lovell[18] assessed the vitamin D levels of elite female gymnasts and found calcium intakes similar to those of the Slovenian swimmers (mean = 823 mg). On the other hand, the mean calcium intake of male Slovenian swimmers and female swimmers in the United States exceeded recommendations (1,716 ± 353 mg and 1,579 mg, respectively).[15,16] Only the Indonesian gymnasts did not meet the Recommended Dietary Allowance for iron intake (8.4 ± 2.7 mg).[13] Specifically, Pouramir et al[19] found that the training regimen of the Bulgarian male gymnasts was associated with a reduction in body iron stores, although they did not discuss their study participants' dietary intake.

TABLE 20.1 Reported Diet Quality and Quantity for Female Athletes Involved in Short-Duration, High-Intensity Exercise[9,10,13-16]

Type of athlete	Energy, kcal/d (kcal/kg)	Energy from carbohydrate, %	Carbohydrate, g/kg	Energy from protein, %	Energy from fat, %
Gymnasts[13]	1,613 (42.7)	48	5.1	14	36
Sprinters[9]	2,007 (54.7)	55	5.1	16	30
Jumpers[10]	1,984 (34.0)	41	3.5	16	42
Swimmers[14] (combined male and female)	4,048 (63.0)	55	8.0	17	27
Swimmers[15] (national junior)	34 kcal/kg of FFM	N/A	6.9	1.7 g/kg	26
Swimmers[16] (collegiate)	3,229 (N/A)	54	N/A	14	31

Abbreviations: N/A, not available; FFM, fat-free mass

TABLE 20.2 Reported Diet Quality and Quantity for Male Athletes Involved in Short-Duration, High-Intensity Exercise[9,10,14,15,17]

Type of athlete	Energy, kcal/d (kcal/kg)	Energy from carbohydrate, %	Carbohydrate, g/kg	Energy from protein, %	Energy from fat, %
Sprinters[9]	3,117 (50.9)	56	6.0	14	30
Jumpers[10]	2,673 (35.0)	40	3.6	20	40
Swimmers[14] (combined male and female)	4,048 (63.0)	55	8.0	17	27
Swimmers[15] (national junior)	43 kca/kg of FFM	N/A	8.8	2.7 g/kg	26
Weight lifters[17]	3,564 (52)	61	7.8	17	29

Abbreviations: N/A, not available; FFM, fat-free mass

Simič and Mohorko[15] assessed vitamin D intake out of concern that Slovenian swimmers might be lacking the internal synthesis of vitamin D because of their lower exposure to sun as a result of the country's geographic location. The authors recognized that they could not compare the reported low estimated intake values to the recommended intake level of 20 mcg because they could not account for internal synthesis, but they concluded that the swimmers were most likely at risk. In fact, Geiker et al[20] reported that 45% of the 29 swimmers residing at latitude 55 °N to 56 °N had 25-hydroxyvitamin D levels lower than

50 nmol/L in the early spring months. Lovell[18] reported that 15 of 18 female gymnasts aged 10 to 17 years had levels below recommended guidelines for optimal bone growth (<75 nmol/L), with 6 having vitamin D levels less than 50 nmol/L.

Bogdanis et al[10] completed a comprehensive assessment of the micronutrient intakes of Greek elite high jumpers and found that the male athletes consumed less than the Dietary Reference Intake (DRI) for 4 of 12 vitamins and 4 of 6 minerals. The female athletes consumed less than the DRI for 7 of 12 vitamins and 5 of 6 minerals. Both sexes consumed less than the recommended levels of vitamin D, pantothenic acid, biotin, folate, calcium, magnesium, zinc, and selenium. Interestingly, the male athletes (but not the female athletes) had inadequate vitamin C intake. The female athletes had inadequate intakes of several B vitamins and iron compared with the males. Clearly, there is a need for more consistent research in this area, but the data suggest that these athletes may be at risk for insufficient intake of some key micronutrients for health and performance.

MACRONUTRIENT AND MICRONUTRIENT DEMANDS

The effects of nutritional quality or quantity on performance for high-intensity and very high–intensity efforts are not as well researched as the effects on performance for endurance events. The nutrition recommendations that follow are based on the theoretical limitations to performance discussed earlier in this chapter, as well as the limited research that has been done.

Carbohydrate

MUSCLE STRENGTH AND POWER

Glycogen levels can be depleted by 16% to 41% in a single resistance-training session, depending on the intensity and duration.[21] This wide range in glycogen utilization is based on several factors, including the lower energy expenditure of eccentric contractions,[22] the amount of rest between sets,[23] and the ability to use the PCr system.[24] Glycogen depletion starts affecting neuromuscular functioning only when levels are reduced by approximately 40% from baseline, depending on the preexercise levels. Thus, high-intensity, resistance-training workouts are not likely to deplete enough glycogen to impair performance.[25]

A 2022 systematic review and meta-analysis compared 49 studies that manipulated carbohydrate intake (19 acute, 17 long-term, and 4 abstracts).[21] This analysis closely aligns with short-duration, high-intensity or very high–intensity exercise because the authors included only resistance workouts with up to 10 sets per muscle group, which are unlikely to deplete glycogen stores. The review concluded that the literature showed no significant difference in strength-training performance or strength development between acute and long-term high-carbohydrate and low-carbohydrate intakes if the diets were isocaloric. One question addressed the acute effects of carbohydrate on strength-training performance. Eleven of the 19 studies found no significant effects of acute carbohydrate intake on strength-training performance. The 11 studies that saw no significant effects included low-volume workouts, whereas acute carbohydrate intake may benefit higher-volume workouts or athletes who have a short recovery period between workouts.[21]

Although the literature does not indicate that carbohydrate has much of a mechanistic effect on strength development, other nonmetabolic factors may be worth considering, such as the satiating effect of low-carbohydrate and ketogenic diets that may result in lower energy intakes and greater exercise effort.[21,26] Both of these factors could theoretically lead to lower gains in lean body mass over time.

ANAEROBIC PERFORMANCE

The increased focus on ketogenic diets during the past 10 years has provided a substantial amount of data on the effects of low-carbohydrate diets on endurance performance, yet only a few studies have examined the effects of low-carbohydrate diets on anaerobic performance.[27-30] Additionally, these studies used different levels and durations of carbohydrate restriction and a wide range of performance measures.

Two studies examining the ketogenic diet and its effect on high-intensity exercise involved study participants who were moderately trained, recreational athletes; therefore, the application of the results of these studies to elite athletes is limited.[27,28] These parallel group design studies were similar in many ways, with both test protocols involving graded exercise tests and a high-intensity test with a 2:1 recovery theme. Cipryan et al[27] applied the ketogenic diet for 4 weeks with 18 participants, whereas Dostal et al[28] extended the ketogenic diet to 12 weeks for 24 participants. Both studies reported no significant differences between the very low-carbohydrate, high-fat diet (VLCHFD; maximum of 50 g of carbohydrate per day) and the habitual diet (HD) for time to exhaustion or VO_2 max.

Michalczyk et al[29] had 15 competitive basketball players complete the Wingate test (a test that requires the participant to exercise at maximal effort for 30 seconds) before and after a 7-day low-carbohydrate diet (in which carbohydrate comprises 10% of total calories) and then again after a subsequent 7-day carbohydrate-loading diet (75% of total calories). Neither the low-carbohydrate diet nor the carbohydrate-loading diet was found to affect peak power. However, after the low-carbohydrate diet, the athletes' total work, blood pH, bicarbonate, and lactate were all found to have decreased significantly. In addition, a small crossover study on 8 elite male gymnasts compared the body-composition and performance measures of the athletes after they had followed a modified ketogenic diet for 30 days. No significant differences were seen in any performance measures after the VLCHFD or the HD, although the VLCHFD group did exhibit significant decreases in body weight and body fat compared to the HD group.[30] Both of these studies pose important questions regarding what the priorities should be when considering extreme dietary manipulation for short-duration, high-intensity or very high–intensity athletes.

Millard-Stafford et al[31] investigated anaerobic performance and carbohydrate timing by assessing the blood lactate response to a pretrial carbohydrate feeding for 23 highly trained swimmers (12 male and 11 female). The study participants completed five 200-m freestyle swims at increasing intensity from approximately 75% to 100% maximum at 5-minute intervals. Although the primary purpose of the study focused on the lactate response, the secondary findings of relevance showed that there were no significant differences in swim velocity, heart rate, or rating of perceived exertion regardless of whether the athlete drank the carbohydrate drink or the placebo after an overnight fast.

RECOVERY

Some power and strength athletes perform in repeated events or games during a single day, so they need to recover as quickly as possible. Consumption of carbohydrate after exercise will accelerate glycogen replenishment. For example, Pascoe et al[32] showed that muscle glycogen decreased to approximately 70% of resting values after a multiset resistance exercise bout, but consumption of a carbohydrate beverage (1.5 g/kg body weight) after exercise increased muscle glycogen to 75% of baseline after 2 hours and to 91% of baseline after 6 hours. On the other hand, no restoration of muscle glycogen occurred even after 6 hours when a water placebo was ingested after exercise instead.

The evidence is not conclusive that consuming a high-carbohydrate diet between 2 high-intensity exercise bouts enhances subsequent performance. Two studies using similar methodologies but different participant populations yielded completely different conclusions regarding the importance of high carbohydrate intake between bouts. Haub et al[33] reported that 6 moderately trained men were able to maintain their maximal exercise performance of a 100-kJ cycle ergometer test compared to an initial test when they consumed carbohydrate (0.7 g/kg body weight) during the 60 minutes between the 2 tests; in contrast, the time to complete the 100-kJ test was longer when participants consumed a placebo during the recovery period. Although these results suggest a benefit of high-carbohydrate ingestion on recovery from high-intensity performance, a subsequent study with the same protocol involving 7 competitive cyclists found no benefit on performance after high-carbohydrate consumption between bouts.[34] Because training, especially sport-specific training, is such an important variable, it is difficult to compare the 2 studies. The differences between these studies emphasize the importance of employing athletes specific to the event of interest in dietary intervention studies.

More recently, attention has focused on the *type* of carbohydrate and the ability to replenish glycogen during recovery. Although the coingestion of glucose and fructose provides higher rates of carbohydrate absorption, the research has not shown that it further enhances muscle glycogen repletion rates beyond that of glucose polymer ingestion alone. However, liver glycogen repletion rates are almost doubled with the glucose-fructose combination, and gastrointestinal distress is significantly alleviated as the maximum absorption rate of 1.2 g/min is approached.[35] The sports RDN should consider these effects when making postworkout recommendations, especially when athletes have less than 24 hours between trainings or competitions.

INTAKE RECOMMENDATIONS

Dietary carbohydrate can ensure that glycogen stores are adequate and that blood glucose is maintained. As discussed earlier, very high–intensity exercise drains some muscle glycogen, but not to the extent that it causes impaired performance as may occur in longer events or events involving repeated sprints. Therefore, the value of high initial muscle glycogen content on a single, short, maximal effort is debatable. However, many of these athletes perform multiple events in competitions, which could lead to depleted glycogen stores over the course of the day. Additionally, these athletes often participate in high-volume training, including weightlifting sessions, in which glycogen depletion may become a concern, so maintaining adequate glycogen stores remains crucial.

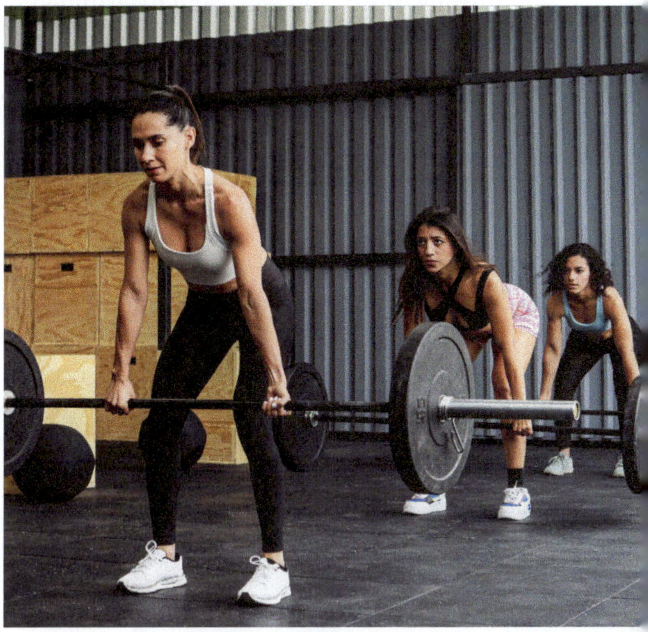

This complex situation makes carbohydrate intake recommendations for short-duration, high-intensity or very high–intensity athletes difficult. There is no consensus that a high-carbohydrate diet is superior to a moderate-carbohydrate diet for anaerobic performance or muscular strength and power. The carbohydrate content of the diet may come into play for athletes competing in multiple events over the course of a day or for those doing substantial aerobic activity in addition to sprints (eg, basketball). Furthermore, athletes who do high-volume aerobic training but compete in brief, very high–intensity events (eg, sprint swimmers) will need to consume substantial amounts of carbohydrate to replenish the glycogen used during training. In most cases, athletes involved in very high–intensity sports or events are advised to consume approximately 5 to 7 g of carbohydrate per kilogram of body weight, with the lower end of the range recommended for athletes with lower energy needs and little aerobic training and the higher end is recommended for those participating in modest amounts of aerobic training in addition to the high-intensity work. The consumption of carbohydrate foods shortly after an event will enhance the rate of glycogen replacement, which becomes more important if athletes are training or competing again within 24 hours.[36]

Protein

Ideal muscle protein synthesis depends on the provision of substrate (amino acids), as well as the appropriate hormonal environment (eg, insulin) to enhance protein synthesis. Most studies are consistent in concluding that the consumption of protein before or after a bout of resistance exercise is beneficial for protein retention and superior to the consumption of the same energy as carbohydrate alone.[37-40] Research on protein intake in the immediate postexercise period or the "window of anabolic opportunity" has been confirmed by several researchers, although recent research has clarified that the tight postexercise time (<1 hour) may be extended when discussing anabolic gains.[41]

In fact, the postexercise window can last up to 24 hours, but most researchers agree that early feeding is more advantageous because earlier in the window is when muscle protein synthesis is greatest.[42,43] Recently, the focus of research has clearly shifted from the total amount of protein consumed in a day to evaluating the timing and type of protein consumed to maximize metabolic adaptations initiated by the training stimulus.[38,44] The intake recommendation is 0.3 g of protein per kilogram of body weight after key exercise sessions and then again every 3 to 5 hours over multiple meals.[45,46] Longitudinal training studies have verified that increases in strength and muscle mass are greatest with the immediate postexercise provision of protein.[47] The International Olympic Committee Consensus Statement on Sports Nutrition encourages protein consumption in the postexercise period to aid in the long-term maintenance of muscle and bone and to repair tissues damaged by acute exercise.[48]

The type of dietary protein that is best for muscle protein gains is controversial; earlier studies reported either no difference in the response of muscle protein synthesis to the ingestion of different types of protein or a superior response to one type of protein compared to the others.[49-52] However, more recent studies comparing isonitrogenous quantities of soy, casein, and whey proteins and the stimulation of muscle protein both at rest and following resistance exercise have demonstrated an advantage for whey protein.[51] The reasons for the superiority of milk proteins are not clear, but it appears that the amino acid leucine, which is abundant in milk protein, could be critically important, possibly along with the other branched-chain amino acids. Leucine has an ability to activate key signaling proteins in the protein kinase B-mammalian target of rapamycin (mTOR) pathway that are responsible for translation initiation in muscle protein synthesis and resultant hypertrophy.[53] Phillips et al[54] examined the amino acid composition of high-quality protein foods (milk, meat, and eggs) and determined that 10 g of essential amino acids (EAAs) can be found in about 25 g of each of these proteins. Most complete proteins are approximately 40% EAAs, hence the recommendation to consume 20 to 25 g of intact, high-quality protein after exercise. Current recommendations that are appropriate for strength athletes include consuming 10 g of EAAs (0.25 to 0.3 g per kilogram of body weight) or 15 to 25 g of protein postexercise, with more than 40 g showing no additional benefit.[36,40,44,55] Refer to Chapter 3 for a complete review of protein.

INTAKE RECOMMENDATIONS

Because most athletes performing brief, maximal-effort movements depend on high muscularity and function, nutritional strategies that enhance fat-free mass (FFM) are often employed throughout the year. Current data suggest that dietary protein intake necessary to support metabolic adaptation, repair, remodeling, and protein turnover generally ranges from 1.2 to 2.0 g per kilogram of body weight per day.[36,38,56] Two meta-analyses separately analyzing 49 and 82 articles concluded that consuming protein in amounts greater than 1.6 and 1.5 g per kilogram of body weight per day, respectively, does not further contribute to gains in FFM.[57,58] Exceeding the recommended protein intake appears to provide no additional benefit for athletes desiring to increase their FFM, as long as they are consuming adequate total calories.[45] Although the research is limited, higher intakes of protein (1.8–2.0 g per kilogram of body weight per day) are typically recommended for short periods during intensified training or when energy intake is reduced.[38,59] For a more individualized recommendation, using a calculation based on kilograms of FFM may be more accurate. The range of 2.3 to 3.1 g per kilogram of FFM has been recommended to minimize loss of lean tissue, with athletes having a lower percentage of body fat tending toward the higher end of this range.[60]

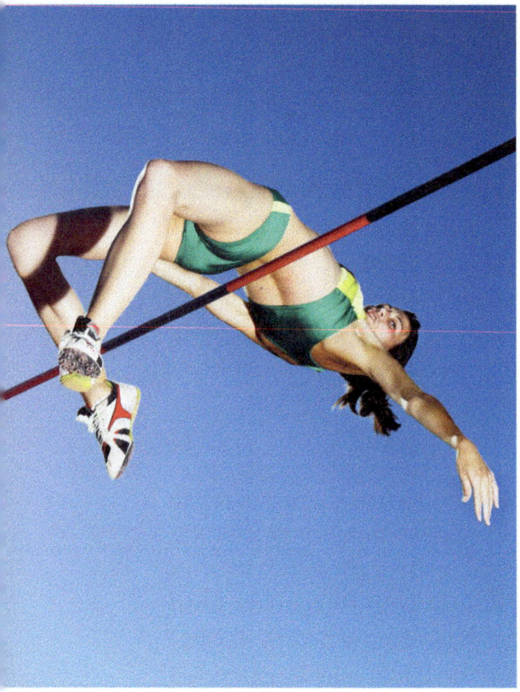

Fat

Intake of dietary fat and its direct effect on performance are of little concern for power athletes. Dietary fat intake is likely to be most relevant for power athletes as a means to achieve adequate energy intake and to support cardiometabolic health. Many of these athletes would find it difficult to achieve their high energy requirements if they followed a very low-fat diet, as dietary fat is 2 times more energy dense than carbohydrate or protein. Obviously, dietary fat and overall calories need to be limited for athletes who are trying to decrease weight. In addition, although the quality of dietary fat has minimal effect on performance, practitioners should take fat into consideration as part of the athlete's overall diet and long-term health.

As previously mentioned, research into ketogenic diets and fat adaptation has increased during the past 10 years, mostly in the context of endurance exercise. The scant literature discussing ketogenic diets and power athletes is the same as discussed earlier in this chapter regarding low-carbohydrate diets and anerobic performance.[27-30] More information on dietary fat is provided in Chapter 4.

INTAKE RECOMMENDATIONS

The only evidence-based recommendation for dietary fat that currently exists, from a joint position statement issued by the Academy of Nutrition and Dietetics, Dietitians of Canada, and the American College of Sports Medicine, states that fat is a necessary component of the diet and should not comprise less than 20% of total calories in the diet.[36] Any reduction beyond this level would put the athlete at risk for inadequate intake of fat-soluble vitamins and essential fatty acids, especially omega-3 fatty acids.

Micronutrients

The micronutrient demands of athletes performing short-duration, very high–intensity or high-intensity sports correlate to energy intake. Most athletes will meet the DRI for micronutrients as long as they are meeting their energy needs and consuming a wide variety of foods.[61,62] Athletes following low-energy diets (those with relative energy deficiency in sport, REDs), limiting the intake of certain food groups (eg, dairy, meat), training at altitude, or receiving limited sun exposure may be at risk for certain micronutrient deficiencies that require supplementation. A blood test is recommended to confirm certain deficiencies, such as deficiencies of iron and vitamin D.[62]

Two specific considerations for power athletes are oxidative stress and joint health. More than 150 articles have been published on the association between antioxidants and exercise-induced skeletal muscle damage and impaired muscle function. Although these mostly small-scale, low-quality studies have shown that antioxidant supplementation attenuates exercise-induced oxidative stress, most have not shown an effect on muscle damage and performance.[62,63] It is widely known that nutrition can play an important role in joint health, but the necessity of dietary supplementation is not supported. Micronutrients that support joint health include calcium, phosphorus, and zinc, as well as vitamins C, D, and E.[62,64] Refer to Chapter 5 for a detailed discussion of micronutrients.

HYDRATION

The risk of dehydration is highly variable among athletes participating in short-duration, high-intensity and very high–intensity sports because of both individual differences and the diverse nature of their training regimens and events.[65] Whereas the influence of dehydration on the performance of endurance athletes has been studied extensively, the literature on power and strength athletes is lacking.[66]

- A 2014 review by Cheuvront and Kenefick[67] suggested that dehydration of 2% or greater could lead to a decrease in endurance exercise performance. Interestingly, the authors also found that impaired strength and power were associated with dehydration, but the threshold and mechanism could not be established.
- Judelson et al[68] reviewed the research for findings on the effects of dehydration on performance of muscle strength, power, and high-intensity endurance. They determined that dehydration of 3% to 4% caused a reduction in muscle strength of approximately 2%, a reduction in muscle power of approximately 3%, and a reduction in muscle high-intensity endurance of approximately 10%.
- A meta-analysis assessing the impact of hypohydration on non–bodyweight-dependent muscle performance found that muscle strength (−5.5% ± 1.0%) and anerobic power (−5.8% ± 2.3%) decreased significantly with hypohydration, but overall anaerobic capacity (−3.5% ± 2.3%) and vertical jumping ability (0.9% ± 0.7%) were not significantly different.[69]
- Jones et al[70] used the Wingate test to explore the effects of active dehydration on anaerobic performance. They found that peak power was significantly decreased by 14.48% in the upper body and by 18.36% in the lower body, but there were no significant differences between the euhydrated and dehydrated conditions for power output.

An interesting 2021 study assessed the knowledge, attitudes, and behaviors of collegiate track-and-field athletes with regard to hydration. The Rehydration and Refueling in Collegiate Track and Field Throwers Survey was completed by athletes at all division levels. Ninety-four of the 284 athletes (93.9%) indicated that dehydration would decrease athletic performance, and half (50.5%) believed that thirst was the best indicator of dehydration.[71] Although the best manner to acutely determine hydration is equivocal, experts including including the National Athletic Trainers' Association often recommend that a combination of measures such as thirst, urine color, body weight change, and urine osmolality be used.[72] Although not necessarily related to hydration, another finding from the collegiate hydration study is that only 1.4% of the athletes recognized that consuming sports drinks would also aid in restoring glycogen.[71] Thus, although the athletes were found to be fairly knowledgeable on the topic of hydration, they may need more education on the overall purpose of sports drinks.

Acute dehydration is modestly harmful to sport performance involving maximal muscle strength and power. Dehydration becomes more detrimental when the high-intensity effort in a sport or exercise is longer or when sprints are interspersed within prolonged aerobic exercise,[66] as is the case for runners, team sports athletes, and CrossFit athletes. Although each athlete can respond differently to dehydration, a strong body of evidence demonstrates that hypohydration can negatively affect strength and anaerobic power, with the magnitude of dehydration resulting in a proportionate negative effect on performance.[67] Clearly, the effect of hypohydration on power and strength athletes requires further research. Specific recommendations for individual athletes depend on body mass, sweating rate, the environment, training status, and tolerance.[72,73] Refer to Chapter 6 for more information on hydration.

BODY WEIGHT AND BODY COMPOSITION

Body composition has been identified as one of the key factors influencing the health and performance of athletes,[74,75] and one can assume that these factors can be directly applied to most power and strength athletes. Increased muscle mass has the advantage of enhanced force generation, but any extra body fat can be a disadvantage for performance.

Few current data are available on the effects of body composition on power and strength athletes. Attempting to extrapolate data gathered prior to 2000 to data from today's athletes is difficult, as power and strength athletes have become much more specialized, stronger, and leaner. The authors of a 2020 cross-sectional study on adolescent gymnasts (5 male and 15 female, 10–18 years of age) provided the participants with a 30-item questionnaire used to determine their level of nutrition knowledge. The researchers reported the mean body-fat percentages for the "good" nutrition-knowledge group and the "poor" nutrition-knowledge group to be 17.9% ± 3.0% and 13.9% ± 6.1%, respectively.[13] Although a difference was detected between the 2 groups, it was not statistically significant. The body-fat percentages of these athletes were higher than those of the gymnasts observed in a 2016 study done by Silva and Paiva,[75] in which the mean body fat of the rhythmic gymnasts (aged 18.7 ± 2.9 years) was 9.2% ± 2.2% (6%–16%) for the highest-scoring performance group and 8.9% ± 2.0% (6%–15%) for the lowest-scoring performance groups. A study with the primary goal of assessing the dietary intake of elite Japanese male and female swimmers (aged 21.9 ± 2.3 years) also measured their body fat. The mean body fat for the males was 12.5% ± 3.4% and that for the females was 17.7% ± 4%.[14] The body compositions of 60 collegiate track-and-field athletes (aged 19.2 ± 1.4 years) were assessed after the athletes had been stratified into 6 event groups.[76] Table 20.3 lists the absolute body composition results from the study. Overall, the throwers had greater values for body weight, fat mass, and percent body fat than the runners and jumpers. This is not surprising, considering the importance of mass in the success of throwing events.[77] The sprinters and jumpers were relatively similar in all measures, which is also not surprising, as many of these athletes often overlap in these events.

Although the values in Table 20.3 help to provide some context, many other important factors determine performance. Some of these factors have the potential unintended consequence of encouraging rapid weight loss as athletes try to comply with rigid minimum-body-fat standards. Evidence indicates that because of these unrealistic standards, weight loss is common in short-duration, high-intensity athletes as a result of efforts to maximize their power-to-weight ratio. Some researchers have reported no effect of short-term weight loss on performance in high-intensity exercise, whereas others have reported decrements. In general, rapid or substantial weight loss is more likely to impair performance than gradual or modest weight loss.[78] A 2011 study compared the effects of a slower weekly weight-loss goal of 0.7% vs a faster weekly weight loss goal of 1.4% on a 1-repetition maximum-strength test for 36 elite male and female athletes. The group engaging in slower weight loss significantly increased their lean body mass and improved all 3 of their 1-repetition maximum tests compared to the rapid-weight-loss group.[79]

A 2022 systematic review and meta-analysis investigated whether a ketogenic diet without energy restriction generates increases in FFM in resistance-trained study participants. The researchers analyzed 5 studies that included 111 resistance-trained participants (87 male and 24 female). The results of the meta-analysis did not show significant differences in FFM between the control group and the ketogenic diet group, although the differences between the means were favorable to the ketogenic diet group. An interesting con-

TABLE 20.3 Anthropometric Measures of Various Track-and-Field Positions[76]

	Sprints	MidD	Multis	Jumps	PV/Jav	Throws	Men	Women
Weight (kg)	67.1 ± 8.8[a,b]	70.9 ± 8.0[a]	77.0 ± 14.3[a]	67.6 ± 9.1[a]	68.1 ± 11.9[a]	90.4 ± 18.3	78.4 ± 11.6	67.0 ± 14.2[c]
FM (kg)	10.1 ± 2.0[a]	10.8 ± 5.1[a]	13.7 ± 3.0[a]	10.5 ± 1.4[a]	11.7 ± 1.6[a]	21.6 ± 11.0	10.5 ± 3.1	15.1 ± 7.7[c]
LBM (kg)	53.3 ± 9.0	56.3 ± 7.7	59.1 ± 13.3	53.4 ± 9.3	53.0 ± 11.6	64.2 ± 11.7	63.5 ± 8.4	48.5 ± 6.8[c]
BF (%)	15.6 ± 4.1[a]	15.4 ± 6.7[a]	18.5 ± 4.8[a]	16.1 ± 3.7[a]	17.8 ± 4.1[a]	23.6 ± 7.8	13.5 ± 2.1	22.0 ± 5.3[c]
BMC (kg)	2.7 ± 0.5[a,b]	2.9 ± 0.5	3.1 ± 0.6	2.7 ± 0.5[a]	2.5 ± 0.4[a,b]	3.3 ± 0.5	3.2 ± 0.5	2.5 ± 0.4[c]

Abbreviations: BF, body fat; BMC, bone mineral content; FM, fat mass; Jav, javelin; LBM, lean body mass; MidD, middle distance; Multis, heptathletes and decathletes; PV, pole vault

[a] Significantly different from throwers.

[b] Significantly different from multis.

[c] Significantly differently from men.

Adapted with permission from reference 76: Hirsch KR, Smith-Ryan AE, Trexler ET, Roelofs EJ. Body composition and muscle characteristics of division i track and field athletes. *J Strength Cond Res*. 2016;30(5):1231-1238. doi:10.1519/JSC.0000000000001203

clusion by the authors was that the ketogenic diet does not seem to be an optimal diet strategy for more than 8 weeks because of its satiating nature and adherence challenges.[26]

The evidence for higher protein intakes during weight loss among strength athletes is supported for maintaining lean body mass; however, evidence for its effect on athletic performance is lacking.[59] Because energy restriction could negatively affect sports performance, body composition recommendations should be flexible and individualized for athletes with different body types and weight histories. There is no guarantee that any individual athlete will improve performance as a result of weight loss. In fact, as discussed, performance may be impaired during the weight-loss phase. Other potential consequences of rapid weight loss include decreases in muscle mass and possible effects on linear growth, hormonal changes, and nutrient deficiencies.[37] There is a need for further research into the optimal macronutrient mix for both weight-loss and mass-building diets for power and strength athletes.

Female athletes dieting for weight loss are particularly susceptible to the female athlete triad or REDs. These conditions include disruption of reproductive hormones, reduced bone strength concurrent with disordered eating, and low energy availability (Chapter 18). Athletes who need to lose weight should be encouraged to lose weight gradually and during the offseason to minimize any detrimental effects on performance and specifically to minimize loss of lean body mass. It is standard practice to monitor weight loss through the accurate assessment and reassessment of body composition. Working closely with a sports RDN is crucial to avoid negative effects on training. Athletes interested in gains in muscle mass should also work closely with a sports RDN to ensure that they consume adequate energy to support their resting metabolic rate, ingest adequate protein based on lean body mass, and participate in strenuous resistance training.[37] Protein for gains in lean mass is discussed in Chapter 3.

SPORTS FOODS AND ERGOGENIC AIDS

Many athletes may be tempted by various claims from supplement companies. Sports RDNs should find out what supplements athletes may be taking or are considering taking and be open to having a conversation with them about this topic. Supplements that have no evidence of benefit, that have evidence of potential to be harmful, and that are banned by sports governing bodies should be strongly discouraged. Additionally, athletes need to understand that there is little regulation of the dietary supplement industry, and the risk of contamination or banned substances is very real. However, the use of sports foods and dietary supplements can be considered with an evidence-based approach that takes into consideration the specific scenario, goals, and commitment of the athelete.[80]

Sports foods are specially formulated food products designed for a specific nutritional function. The 4 main physiologic goals are adequate fueling, optimal hydration, increased anabolism, and maintenance of osmolality. All 4 of these may be important goals for power and strength athletes. Sports foods often contain many of the same ingredients or nutrient densities of whole foods, but they may offer the practical advantage of combining all of the nutrients needed for a specific goal in a single source. In addition, sports foods are often easier to transport, store, prepare, and consume, especially before, during, and after/between competition events and training sessions.[80]

Dietary supplements are defined as manufactured products intended to supplement one's diet in the form of a pill, capsule, tablet, powder, or liquid. Dietary supplements that are attractive to athletes involved in power and strength sports are those that may increase the availability of PCr, increase lean body mass, enhance recovery time, and/or improve reaction time or focus. Enhancement of lactic acid buffering capacity may be helpful for high-intensity events lasting up to several minutes. The dietary supplement that is primarily used to maximize the PCr system is creatine monohydrate. Dietary supplements that are commonly used to enhance lactic acid buffering capacity are sodium bicarbonate and β-alanine. Dietary supplements that are commonly used to improve reaction time and focus include caffeine and β-alanine. Although dietary nitrate/beetroot originally showed benefits for aerobic endurance, recent studies suggest that dietary nitrate supplementation may also enhance the performance of muscle power, sprint, multiple-sprint, and high-intensity intermittent exercise.[81] Creatine, branched-chain amino acids, leucine, and protein powders are dietary supplements commonly used for increasing lean body mass. During periods of heavy training, supplements such as collagen and *N*-acetylcysteine and increased dietary intake of food polyphenols and other antioxidants might be warranted.[82] The efficacy and safety of dietary supplements are discussed in Chapter 7.

NUTRITIONAL STRATEGIES FOR TRAINING AND COMPETITION

Providing nutritional support to short-duration, very high– and high-intensity athletes encompasses 2 distinct situations: training and competition. As mentioned previously, the training protocols of these athletes can be very different from their competitions. Additionally, most athletes practice some level of training periodization throughout the year, which correspondingly changes their nutritional requirements. Thus, nutritional support needs to be adjusted accordingly. In addition to performance concerns, the diets of these athletes should remain healthy, which means consuming a balanced, varied diet with approximately 55% of energy from carbohydrate and at least 1.2 g of protein per kilogram of body weight, with an abundant intake of whole grains, fruits, and vegetables.

High-priority considerations for training include the following:

- maintaining energy and glycogen levels,
- maintaining adequate hydration,
- promoting maximal recovery,
- supporting training adaptations, and
- achieving an ideal power-to-weight ratio.

High-priority considerations for competition include the following:

- maintaining focus and concentration,
- maximizing reaction time, and
- managing fueling around events.

It would be prudent for the athlete to plan what to eat before, during, and after training or competition. To avoid gastrointestinal distress during the event, athletes should consume a balanced preevent meal at least 90 minutes prior, with only liquids closer to the event. A low-fiber, low-fat meal is recommended because

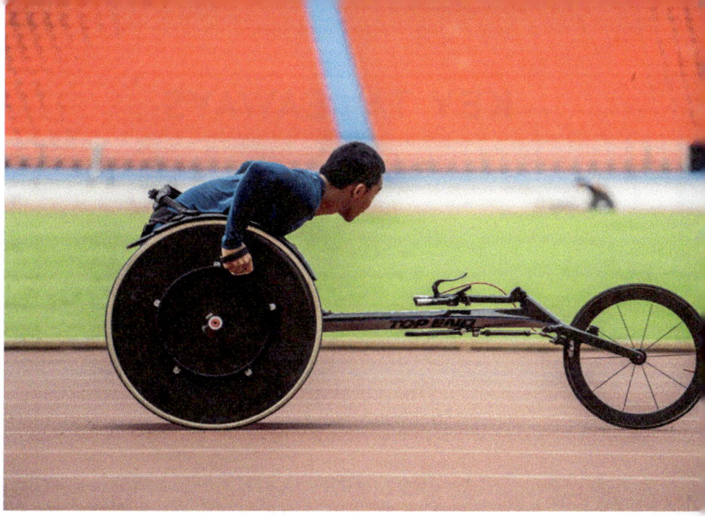

it will leave the stomach and intestines more quickly. Inclusion of protein with carbohydrate in the meal will make it more likely that blood glucose will be at a normal concentration before the event. Experts recommend that the athlete consume 1 to 4 g of carbohydrate per kilogram of body weight 1 to 4 hours before exercise, along with a small to moderate amount of protein (7–21 g).[36]

Immediately after a high-volume training session, the athlete can maximize muscle glycogen replacement and protein synthesis by consuming 0.75 to 1.5 g of carbohydrate per kilogram of body weight, as well as 20 to 30 g of high-quality protein within the first 2 hours.[36] If the athlete will not be training or competing for 24 hours, the urgency of nutritional intake immediately after exercise decreases, as long as the athlete consumes adequate calories and macronutrients over the course of the next 24 hours.

Athletes should consume fluids at each meal, between meals, and during workouts to maintain hydration. Athletes can use measurement of body weight before and after a workout or monitoring of the color of urine as an index of dehydration, and they should make an effort to rehydrate before the next workout or competition. If a training session or competition lasts less than 60 minutes, consumption of water is recommended. However, if an intense training session lasts longer than 60 minutes, the athlete may benefit from consuming the high-glycemic-index carbohydrates found in sports drinks.

Athletes competing in several events or matches during a single day have a special challenge in deciding what they can tolerate that will also help their performance. A light snack, such as yogurt with fruit, a small sandwich (without high-fat sauces or cheeses), cereal with milk, regular or dried fruit, a commercial liquid meal, granola bars, fruit bars (eg, fig), or muffins, along with sport drinks or water, are appropriate between events. The choice and size of snack, including protein and carbohydrate contents, will vary based on the time available between events, the event type, and the appropriateness of preevent nutritional strategies to optimize performance. Because the food provided at the concession stands at most sporting events often does not fit this profile, it is best if athletes or their trainers pack snacks for the day.

All athletes, including those who compete in very high–intensity sports, should be discouraged from consuming a very low-carbohydrate diet. Such a diet may impair performance and is often less healthful because of its low vitamin, mineral, and fiber contents.

Some athletes may know that there is less evidence for an effect of diet on performance in very high–intensity events and may therefore believe that they can eat whatever they want. Practitioners making dietary recommendations for these athletes must consider the same health issues as for any other individual. Therefore, it is important that the sports RDN assess the overall diet and provide education about making changes to improve the quality and healthfulness of the diet, as well as to improve performance.

SUMMARY

For most short-duration, very high–intensity events, specific nutritional strategies will have less of an impact on performance than genetics, training, and motivational factors. Only very low-carbohydrate diets or moderately low-carbohydrate diets paired with low energy intake have been found to have a detrimental effect on performance in single, maximal efforts. The benefits of nutrition for high-intensity exercise performance are most often observed when high-intensity efforts are interspersed with substantial amounts of other aerobic exercise. The training practices of athletes engaged in such sports are often different from those of their actual competition, and the sports RDN should take this factor into consideration when discussing nutritional strategies. Dehydration in the range of 1% to 2% can reduce muscle strength and power slightly and can substantially reduce muscle high-intensity endurance. By consuming more total energy as well as protein before or after each resistance exercise bout, an athlete can improve their muscle protein balance and long-term gain. Although not without controversy, most evidence suggests that supplements such as creatine, caffeine, and bicarbonate may benefit athletes performing high-intensity exercise. Cost, efficacy, and safety should always be considered before an athlete uses any supplement.

KEY TAKEAWAYS

Short-duration, very high- and high-intensity athletes predominantly utilize the phosphagen and anaerobic energy pathways.

Nutritional strategies have minimal impact on performance for most power and strength events, but they have a substantial impact on training and multiple events.

The athlete should use fueling strategies for before, during, and after exercise.

These athletes should consume a balanced diet with approximately 55% of energy from carbohydrate and at least 1.2 g of protein per kilogram of body weight, with an abundance of whole grains, fruits, and vegetables.

Athletes should ingest 0.3 g of protein per kilogram of body weight, or approximately 20 g, after key exercise sessions and every 3 to 5 hours over multiple meals.

Dietary supplements worth consideration include caffeine, creatine, dietary nitrate/beetroot, sodium bicarbonate, β-alanine, and sports foods, under certain circumstances.

REFERENCES

1. Lambert CP, Flynn MG. Fatigue during high-intensity intermittent exercise: application to bodybuilding. *Sports Med.* 2002;32(8):511-522. doi:10.2165/00007256-200232080-00003
2. Stellingwerff T, Boit MK, Res PT; International Association of Athletics Federations. Nutritional strategies to optimize training and racing in middle-distance athletes. *J Sports Sci.* 2007;25(suppl 1):S17-S28. doi:10.1080/02640410701607213
3. Spriet LL, Perry CGR, Talanian JL. Legal pre-event nutritional supplements to assist energy metabolism. *Essays Biochem.* 2008;44:27-43. doi:10.1042/BSE0440027
4. Lamb DR. *Physiology of Exercise: Responses and Adaptations.* 2nd ed. Macmillan; 1984.
5. Gaitanos GC, Williams C, Boobis LH, Brooks S. Human muscle metabolism during intermittent maximal exercise. *J Appl Physiol (1985).* 1993;75(2):712-719. doi:10.1152/jappl.1993.75.2.712
6. Esbjörnsson-Liljedahl M, Bodin K, Jansson E. Smaller muscle ATP reduction in women than in men by repeated bouts of sprint exercise. *J Appl Physiol (1985).* 2002;93(3):1075-1083. doi:10.1152/japplphysiol.00732.1999
7. Haff GG, Lehmkuhl MJ, McCoy LB, Stone MH. Carbohydrate supplementation and resistance training. *J Strength Cond Res.* 2003;17(1):187-196. doi:10.1519/1533-4287(2003)017<0187:csart>2.0.co;2
8. Ament W, Verkerke GJ. Exercise and fatigue. *Sports Med.* 2009;39(5):389-422. doi:10.2165/00007256-200939050-00005
9. Aerenhouts D, Deriemaeker P, Hebbelinck M, Clarys P. Dietary acid-base balance in adolescent sprint athletes: a follow-up study. *Nutrients.* 2011;3(2):200-211. doi:10.3390/nu3020200
10. Bogdanis G, Veligekas P, Selima E, Christofi E, Pafili Z. Elite high jumpers exhibit inadequate nutrient intakes. *J Phys Educ Sport.* 2013;13(3):330-337. doi:10.7752/jpes.2013.03054
11. Kolimechkov S, Yanev I, Kiuchukov I, et al. Nutritional status and body composition of young artistic gymnasts from Bulgaria. *J Appl Sports Sci.* 2019;1:39-52. doi:10.37393/jass.2019.01.4
12. Karabudak E, Köksal E, Ertaş Öztürk Y, Kucukerdonmez O. Dietary intake of Turkish gymnast and non-gymnast children. *Nutr Diet.* 2016;73(2):184-189. doi:10.1111/1747-0080.12191
13. Gifari N, Nuzrina R, Kuswari M, Hutami N, Ghalda A. Relationship between nutrition knowledge and aerobic fitness in young gymnasts. *Sci Gymnast J.* 2020;12(2):195-202. doi:10.52165/sgj.12.2.195-202
14. Mizugaki A, Kato H, Suzuki H, Kurihara H, Ogita F. Nutritional practice and nitrogen balance in elite Japanese swimmers during a training camp. *Sports (Basel).* 2021;9(2):17. doi:10.3390/sports9020017
15. Simič V, Mohorko N. Nutritional strategies of Slovenian national junior swimming team. *Ann Kinesiol.* 2018;9(1):15-34. doi:10.35469/ak.2018.158
16. Hoogenboom BJ, Morris J, Morris C, Schaefer K. Nutritional knowledge and eating behaviors of female, collegiate swimmers. *N Am J Sports Phys Ther.* 2009;4(3):139-148.
17. Nazni P, Vimala S. Nutrition knowledge, attitude and practice of college sportsmen. *Asian J Sports Med.* 2010;1(2):93-100. doi:10.5812/asjsm.34866
18. Lovell G. Vitamin D status of females in an elite gymnastics program. *Clin J Sport Med.* 2008;18(2):159-161. doi:10.1097/JSM.0b013e3181650eee
19. Pouramir M, Haghshenas O, Sorkhi H. Effects of gymnastic exercise on the body iron status and hematologic profile. *Iranian J Med Sci.* 2004;29(3):140-141.
20. Geiker NRW, Hansen M, Jakobsen J, et al. Vitamin D status and muscle function among adolescent and young swimmers. *Int J Sport Nutr Exerc Metab.* 2017;27(5):399-407. doi:10.1123/ijsnem.2016-0248
21. Henselmans M, Bjørnsen T, Hedderman R, Vårvik FT. The effect of carbohydrate intake on strength and resistance training performance: a systematic review. *Nutrients.* 2022;14(4):856. doi:10.3390/nu14040856
22. Herzog W. Why are muscles strong, and why do they require little energy in eccentric action? *J Sport Health Sci.* 2018;7(3):255-264. doi:10.1016/j.jshs.2018.05.005
23. Grgic J, Schoenfeld BJ, Skrepnik M, Davies TB, Mikulic P. Effects of rest interval duration in resistance training on measures of muscular strength: a systematic review. *Sports Med.* 2018;48(1):137-151. doi:10.1007/s40279-017-0788-x
24. Baker JS, McCormick MC, Robergs RA. Interaction among skeletal muscle metabolic energy systems during intense exercise. *J Nutr Metab.* 2010;2010:905612. doi:10.1155/2010/905612
25. Ørtenblad N, Nielsen J, Saltin B, Holmberg H-C. Role of glycogen availability in sarcoplasmic reticulum Ca^{2+} kinetics in human skeletal muscle. *J Physiol.* 2011;589(Pt 3):711-725. doi:10.1113/jphysiol.2010.195982
26. Vargas-Molina S, Gómez-Urquiza JL, García-Romero J, Benítez-Porres J. Effects of the ketogenic diet on muscle hypertrophy in resistance-trained men and women: a systematic review and meta-analysis. *Int J Environ Res Public Health.* 2022;19(19):12529. doi:10.3390/ijerph191912629
27. Cipryan L, Plews DJ, Ferretti A, Maffetone PB, Laursen PB. Effects of a 4-week very low-carbohydrate diet on high-intensity interval training responses. *J Sports Sci Med.* 2018;17(2):259-268.
28. Dostal T, Plews DJ, Hofmann P, Laursen PB, Cipryan L. Effects of a 12-week very-low carbohydrate high-fat diet on maximal aerobic capacity, high-intensity intermittent exercise, and cardiac autonomic regulation: non-randomized parallel-group study. *Front Physiol.* 2019;10:912. doi:10.3389/fphys.2019.00912

29. Michalczyk MM, Chycki J, Zajac A, Maszczyk A, Zydek G, Langfort J. Anaerobic performance after a low-carbohydrate diet (LCD) followed by 7 days of carbohydrate loading in male basketball players. *Nutrients*. 2019;11(4):778. doi:10.3390/nu11040778

30. Paoli A, Grimaldi K, D'Agostino D, et al. Ketogenic diet does not affect strength performance in elite artistic gymnasts. *J Int Soc Sports Nutr*. 2012;9(1):34. doi:10.1186/1550-2783-9-34

31. Millard-Stafford ML, Brown MB, Snow TK. Acute carbohydrate ingestion affects lactate response in highly trained swimmers. *Int J Sports Physiol Perform*. 2010;5(1):42-54. doi:10.1123/ijspp.5.1.42

32. Pascoe DD, Costill DL, Fink WJ, Robergs RA, Zachwieja JJ. Glycogen resynthesis in skeletal muscle following resistive exercise. *Med Sci Sports Exerc*. 1993;25(3):349-354.

33. Haub MD, Potteiger JA, Jacobsen DJ, Nau KL, Magee LA, Comeau MJ. Glycogen replenishment and repeated maximal effort exercise: effect of liquid carbohydrate. *Int J Sport Nutr*. 1999;9(4):406-415. doi:10.1123/ijsn.9.4.406

34. Haub MD, Haff GG, Potteiger JA. The effect of liquid carbohydrate ingestion on repeated maximal effort exercise in competitive cyclists. *J Strength Cond Res*. 2003;17(1):20-25. doi:10.1519/1533-4287(2003)017<0020:teolci>2.0.co;2

35. Gonzalez JT, Fuchs CJ, Betts JA, van Loon LJ. Glucose plus fructose ingestion for post-exercise recovery-greater than the sum of its parts? *Nutrients*. 2017;9(4):344. doi:10.3390/nu9040344

36. Thomas DT, Erdman KA, Burke LM. Position of the Academy of Nutrition and Dietetics, Dietitians of Canada, and the American College of Sports Medicine: nutrition and athletic performance. *J Acad Nutr Diet*. 2016;116(3):501-528. doi:10.1016/j.jand.2015.12.006

37. Koopman R, Saris WHM, Wagenmakers AJM, van Loon LJC. Nutritional interventions to promote post-exercise muscle protein synthesis. *Sports Med*. 2007;37(10):895-906. doi:10.2165/00007256-200737100-00005

38. Phillips SM, Van Loon LJC. Dietary protein for athletes: from requirements to optimum adaptation. *J Sports Sci*. 2011;29(suppl 1):S29-S38. doi:10.1080/02640414.2011.619204

39. Tipton KD, Jeukendrup AE, Hespel P; International Association of Athletics Federations. Nutrition for the sprinter. *J Sports Sci*. 2007;25(suppl 1):S5-S15. doi:10.1080/02640410701607205

40. Areta JL, Burke LM, Ross ML, et al. Timing and distribution of protein ingestion during prolonged recovery from resistance exercise alters myofibrillar protein synthesis. *J Physiol*. 2013;591(9):2319-2331. doi:10.1113/jphysiol.2012.244897

41. Cermak NM, Res PT, de Groot LCPGM, Saris WHM, van Loon LJC. Protein supplementation augments the adaptive response of skeletal muscle to resistance-type exercise training: a meta-analysis. *Am J Clin Nutr*. 2012;96(6):1454-1464. doi:10.3945/ajcn.112.037556

42. Burd NA, Tang JE, Moore DR, Phillips SM. Exercise training and protein metabolism: influences of contraction, protein intake, and sex-based differences. *J Appl Physiol (1985)*. 2009;106(5):1692-1701. doi:10.3945/ajcn.112.037556

43. Schoenfeld BJ, Aragon AA, Krieger JW. The effect of protein timing on muscle strength and hypertrophy: a meta-analysis. *J Int Soc Sports Nutr*. 2013;10(1):53. doi:10.1186/1550-2783-10-53

44. Phillips SM. Dietary protein requirements and adaptive advantages in athletes. *Br J Nutr*. 2012;108(suppl 2):S158-S167. doi:10.1017/S0007114512002516

45. Moore DR, Robinson MJ, Fry JL, et al. Ingested protein dose response of muscle and albumin protein synthesis after resistance exercise in young men. *Am J Clin Nutr*. 2009;89(1):161-168. doi:10.3945/ajcn.2008.26401

46. Phillips SM. A brief review of higher dietary protein diets in weight loss: a focus on athletes. *Sports Med*. 2014;44(suppl 2):S149-S153. doi:10.1007/s40279-014-0254-y

47. Josse AR, Atkinson SA, Tarnopolsky MA, Phillips SM. Diets higher in dairy foods and dietary protein support bone health during diet- and exercise-induced weight loss in overweight and obese premenopausal women. *J Clin Endocrinol Metab*. 2012;97(1):251-260. doi:10.1210/jc.2011-2165

48. IOC consensus statement on sports nutrition 2010. *J Sports Sci*. 2011;29(suppl 1):S3-S4. doi:10.1080/02640414.2011.619349

49. Tipton KD, Elliott TA, Cree MG, Wolf SE, Sanford AP, Wolfe RR. Ingestion of casein and whey proteins result in muscle anabolism after resistance exercise. *Med Sci Sports Exerc*. 2004;36(12):2073-2081. doi:10.1249/01.mss.0000147582.99810.c5

50. Anthony TG, McDaniel BJ, Knoll P, Bunpo P, Paul GL, McNurlan MA. Feeding meals containing soy or whey protein after exercise stimulates protein synthesis and translation initiation in the skeletal muscle of male rats. *J Nutr*. 2007;137(2):357-362. doi:10.1093/jn/137.2.357

51. Tang JE, Moore DR, Kujbida GW, Tarnopolsky MA, Phillips SM. Ingestion of whey hydrolysate, casein, or soy protein isolate: effects on mixed muscle protein synthesis at rest and following resistance exercise in young men. *J Appl Physiol (1985)*. 2009;107(3):987-992. doi:10.1152/japplphysiol.00076.2009

52. Wilkinson SB, Tarnopolsky MA, Macdonald MJ, Macdonald JR, Armstrong D, Phillips SM. Consumption of fluid skim milk promotes greater muscle protein accretion after resistance exercise than does consumption of an isonitrogenous and isoenergetic soy-protein beverage. *Am J Clin Nutr*. 2007;85(4):1031-1040. doi:10.1093/ajcn/85.4.1031

53. Phillips SM, Tang JE, Moore DR. The role of milk- and soy-based protein in support of muscle protein synthesis and muscle protein accretion in young and elderly persons. *J Am Coll Nutr*. 2009;28(4):343-354. doi:10.1080/07315724.2009.10718096

54. Phillips SM, Moore DR, Tang JE. A critical examination of dietary protein requirements, benefits, and excesses in athletes. *Int J Sport Nutr Exerc Metab*. 2007;17(suppl):S58-S76. doi:10.1123/ijsnem.17.s1.s58

55. Beelen M, Burke LM, Gibala MJ, van Loon JCL. Nutritional strategies to promote postexercise recovery. *Int J Sport Nutr Exerc Metab*. 2010;20(6):515-532. doi:10.1123/ijsnem.20.6.515

56. Houtkooper L, Abbot JM, Nimmo M; International Association of Athletics Federations. Nutrition for throwers, jumpers, and combined events athletes. *J Sports Sci*. 2007;25(suppl 1):S39-S47. doi:10.1080/02640410701607262

57. Tagawa R, Watanabe D, Ito K, et al. Synergistic effect of increased total protein intake and strength training on muscle strength: a dose-response meta-analysis of randomized controlled trials. *Sports Med Open*. 2022;8(1):110. doi:10.1186/s40798-022-00508-w

58. Morton RW, Murphy KT, McKellar SR, et al. A systematic review, meta-analysis and meta-regression of the effect of protein supplementation on resistance training-induced gains in muscle mass and strength in healthy adults. *Br J Sports Med*. 2018;52(6):376-384. doi:10.1136/bjsports-2017-097608

59. Mettler S, Mitchell N, Tipton KD. Increased protein intake reduces lean body mass loss during weight loss in athletes. *Med Sci Sports Exerc*. 2010;42(2):326-337. doi:10.1249/MSS.0b013e3181b2ef8e

60. Helms ER, Zinn C, Rowlands DS, Brown SR. A systematic review of dietary protein during caloric restriction in resistance trained lean athletes: a case for higher intakes. *Int J Sport Nutr Exerc Metab*. 2014;24(2):127-138. doi:10.1123/ijsnem.2013-0054

61. Volpe SL. Micronutrient requirements for athletes. *Clin Sports Med*. 2007;26(1):119-130. doi:10.1016/j.csm.2006.11.009

62. Beck KL, von Hurst PR, O'Brien WJ, Badenhorst CE. Micronutrients and athletic performance: A review. *Food Chem Toxicol*. 2021;158:112618. doi:10.1016/j.fct.2021.112618

63. Peternelj TT, Coombes JS. Antioxidant supplementation during exercise training: beneficial or detrimental? *Sports Med*. 2011;41(12):1043-1069. doi:10.2165/11594400-000000000-00000

64. Clark KL. Nutritional considerations in joint health. *Clin Sports Med*. 2007;26(1):101-118. doi:10.1016/j.csm.2006.11.006

65. Casa DJ, Cheuvront SN, Galloway SD, Shirreffs SM. Fluid needs for training, competition, and recovery in track-and-field athletes. *Int J Sport Nutr Exerc Metab*. 2019;29(2):175-180. doi:10.1123/ijsnem.2018-0374

66. Maughan RJ, Shirreffs SM. Development of hydration strategies to optimize performance for athletes in high-intensity sports and in sports with repeated intense efforts. *Scand J Med Sci Sports*. 2010;20(suppl 2):59-69. doi:10.1111/j.1600-0838.2010.01191.x

67. Cheuvront SN, Kenefick RW. Dehydration: physiology, assessment, and performance effects. *Compr Physiol*. 2014;4(1):257-285. doi:10.1002/cphy.c130017

68. Judelson DA, Maresh CM, Anderson JM, et al. Hydration and muscular performance: does fluid balance affect strength, power and high-intensity endurance? *Sports Med*. 2007;37(10):907-921. doi:10.2165/00007256-200737100-00006

69. Savoie FA, Kenefick RW, Ely BR, Cheuvront SN, Goulet ED. Effect of hypohydration on muscle endurance, strength, anaerobic power and capacity and vertical jumping ability: a meta-analysis. *Sports Med*. 2015;45(8):1207-1227. doi:10.1007/s40279-015-0349-0

70. Jones LC, Cleary MA, Lopez RM, Zuri RE, Lopez R. Active dehydration impairs upper and lower body anaerobic muscular power. *J Strength Cond Res*. 2008;22(2):455-463. doi:10.1519/JSC.0b013e3181635ba5

71. Judge LW, Bellar DM, Popp JK, et al. Hydration to maximize performance and recovery: knowledge, attitudes, and behaviors among collegiate track and field throwers. *J Hum Kinet*. 2021;79:111-122. doi:10.2478/hukin-2021-0065

72. Casa DJ, Armstrong LE, Hillman SK, et al. National Athletic Trainers' Association position statement: fluid replacement for athletes. *J Athl Train*. 2000;35(2):212-224.

73. American College of Sports Medicine; Sawka MN, Burke LM, Eichner ER, Maughan RJ, Montain SJ, Stachenfeld NS. American College of Sports Medicine position stand. Exercise and fluid replacement. *Med Sci Sports Exerc*. 2007;39(2):377-390. doi:10.1249/mss.0b013e31802ca597

74. Malina R, Geithner C. Body composition of young athletes. *Am J Lifestyle Med*. 05/17 2011;5:262-278. doi:10.1177/1559827610392493

75. Silva MR, Paiva T. Poor precompetitive sleep habits, nutrients' deficiencies, inappropriate body composition and athletic performance in elite gymnasts. *Eur J Sport Sci*. 2016;16(6):726-735. doi:10.1080/17461391.2015.1103316

76. Hirsch KR, Smith-Ryan AE, Trexler ET, Roelofs EJ. Body composition and muscle characteristics of Division I track and field athletes. *J Strength Cond Res*. 2016;30(5):1231-1238. doi:10.1519/jsc.0000000000001203

77. O'Connor H, Olds T, Maughan RJ; International Association of Athletics Federations. Physique and performance for track and field events. *J Sports Sci*. 2007;25(suppl 1):S49-S60. doi:10.1080/02640410701607296

78. Rankin JW. Weight loss and gain in athletes. *Curr Sports Med Rep*. 2002;1(4):208-213. doi:10.1249/00149619-200208000-00004

79. Garthe I, Raastad T, Refsnes PE, Koivisto A, Sundgot-Borgen J. Effect of two different weight-loss rates on body composition and strength and power-related performance in elite athletes. *Int J Sport Nutr Exer Metab*. 2011;21(2):97-104. doi:10.1123/ijsnem.21.2.97

80. Peeling P, Castell LM, Derave W, de Hon O, Burke LM. Sports foods and dietary supplements for optimal function and performance enhancement in track-and-field athletes. *Int J Sport Nutr Exerc Metab*. 2019;29(2):198-209. doi:10.1123/ijsnem.2018-0271

81. Thompson C, Vanhatalo A, Jell H, et al. Dietary nitrate supplementation improves sprint and high-intensity intermittent running performance. *Nitric Oxide*. 2016;61:55-61. doi:10.1016/j.niox.2016.10.006

82. The Australian Sports Commission, Australian Institute of Sport. Supplements: Benefits and risks of using supplements and sports foods. Accessed November 20, 2022. www.ais.gov.au/nutrition/supplements

CHAPTER 21

Nutrition for High-Intensity, Intermittent Sports

Isaac Hicks III, RDN, CSSD, LDN, CSCS, and Kayla Lawson, MS, RD, LDN

LEARNING OBJECTIVES

- Differentiate sports and training regimens that fit the profile of high-intensity, intermittent sports.
- Discuss the energy systems that are used during high-intensity, intermittent sports.
- Describe nutritional strategies for high-intensity, intermittent sports.
- Discuss the hydration requirements and strategies of athletes participating in high-intensity, intermittent sports.

INTRODUCTION

The term *high-intensity, intermittent exercise* (HIIE) refers to activities that require short periods of all-out effort (eg, sprints of up to 2–7 seconds), punctuated by periods of less-intense effort (eg, jogging sustained over 5–10 minutes) and low-intensity effort (eg, walking and standing still). Examples of HIIE sports include team sports such as soccer, football, basketball, lacrosse, field hockey, ice hockey, rugby, and volleyball and individual sports such as tennis and squash.[1] HIIE sports can vary from competition to competition or per sport based on in-game play (eg, rest periods, substitutions, style of play, game length). All of these sports, however, commonly require bursts of intense effort mixed with periods of lower effort; examples of these bursts include running bases in baseball, driving to the rim in basketball, accelerating in ice hockey, or sprinting to a ball in soccer.

Intermittent sports are classified as endurance-based field sports (eg, soccer, field hockey, lacrosse), arena or court sports (eg, basketball, ice hockey, volleyball, tennis), batting sports (eg, baseball, softball, cricket), and strength- and power-based field sports (eg, American football, rugby). Success in HIIE sports is largely dependent on an athlete's ability to sustain skill execution while minimizing fatigue. In addition, aspects of cognitive function such as attention, decision-making, and response time can affect performance. The stop-and-go nature of these sports often results in impaired performance after periods of intense effort and near the end of the competition.[2] In a study examining muscle metabolism and fatigue during a simulated ice hockey game, muscle glycogen decreased by more than 50% during the match, leading to depletion of glycogen in both fast- and slow-twitch muscle fibers and an impaired ability to maintain sprint performance in the latter stages of competition.[3] Taken as a whole, HIIE sports require a range of exercise intensities from low to very high in varying durations during which all of the major energy systems are tapped. Box 21.1 lists examples of intermittent high-intensity team sports.[1,4]

Soccer has been studied extensively and can provide a good base for understanding the physiological demands and nutritional implications of HIIE.[5] Other HIIE sports have also been studied, but to a lesser degree.[6] Soccer is mainly aerobic in nature because of the large distances covered during competition (estimated as 8–13 km or 5–8 miles). However, the tempo during matches varies, potentially involving more than

BOX 21.1 Categories of Intermittent High-Intensity Team Sports[1,4]

Classification	Sport	Sport distinctions	Physiological burden
Endurance-based field sports	Soccer, field hockey, lacrosse	Large playing area, longer distances covered at high speed, change of direction, continuous activity at variable speeds	Glycogen repletion, hydration status
Strength and power field sports	American football, rugby	Cover less running distance; frequent bursts of short sprints with bouts of contact, scrimmage, and tackling	Carbohydrate intake to match training goals an support performance and recovery, hydration status, possibly lower carbohydrate needs for rugby union
Batting sports	Baseball, softball, cricket	Lower overall energy demands, many hours in the sun, greater rest duration between efforts, increased focus needs and quick decision-making	Maintaining blood glucose during game, hydration status
Arena or court sports	Basketball, volleyball, tennis, badminton, team handball, racquetball, squash, ice hockey	Smaller playing area, shorter-duration games, frequent substitution, often several games per day or over several days, much time spent traveling	Training period requires high energy and fluid demands, potential for suboptimal glycogen repletion due to schedule

700 different movements including dynamic changes in direction and high-intensity sprinting bouts and turns, of which most, if not all, are anaerobic in nature during a 90-minute match. As a result, energy and nutrient demands also vary greatly. Needs may also vary by team and individual role because of potentially large differences that occur on the field, including actual distance covered, gameplay limitations (running clock, breaks, limited substitutions), and the specific individual or team playing style.[2,7-10] During competition, both anaerobic and aerobic body systems are stressed, and players may experience cognitive strain to execute sport-specific skills (high-speed decision making, ball handling), placing further importance on optimizing nutrition strategies that can support training and competition performance.[2-5,11]

By comparison, a professional ice hockey game has 60 minutes of regulation play but usually lasts approximately 150 minutes because of intermissions and time-outs. An ice hockey game is characterized by intense bouts of play lasting 45 to 60 seconds, seldom exceeding 90 seconds. The average ice time is less than 16 minutes for most ice hockey players, although some players may receive as much as 35 minutes of ice time.[12] Studies on fatigue development in professional male ice hockey athletes suggest that both the anaerobic and aerobic systems are commonly stressed during competitions, with heart rate values at approximately 85% of an athlete's maximal heart rate. Almost half of a player's time on the ice is classified as high intensity.[13] These distinguishing features of each sport create various physiological challenges and focus areas for addressing the nutritional needs of HIIE athletes.

The nutrient needs of athletes performing HIIE can be high. The goal is to focus on a diet that provides sufficient energy to meet the demands of training and competition, along with strategic food and fluid selection (eg, nutrient timing) to meet additional nutrient demands. Observations of the dietary practices of athletes engaged in HIIE sports suggest that many athletes have an inadequate diet, increasing the need for assistance in managing these needs.[14-25]

PHYSIOLOGICAL DEMANDS OF HIGH-INTENSITY, INTERMITTENT EXERCISE

Energy Systems Used Depend on the Sport and Movements Required

Anaerobic and aerobic energy production are both equally important to the HIIE athlete.[7,12,26-29] Anaerobic energy production is essential for high-intensity exercise when the demand for adenosine triphosphate (ATP) exceeds the body's ability to produce it aerobically. At the onset of high-intensity exercise, anaerobically produced ATP provides the majority of the energy used because of the short supply of oxygen, and it continues to play a role in sustained high-intensity exercise[5,12,30-36] (Refer to Table 21.1.[37])

TABLE 21.1 Approximate Relative Energy Contributions During Selected Periods of High-Intensity Exercise[37]

Duration, seconds	Anaerobic, %	Aerobic, %
30	80	20
60-90	45	55
120-180	30	70

Both the intensity and duration of exercise increase energy demands during vigorous, stop-and-go exercise that lasts for 60 minutes or more.[32] The ability to perform sprints and short-duration recovery is an important element of performance in intermittent sports.[12,26,36,38] Given that HIIE sports have been identified as glycogen-depleting because of their unique physiological demands, any decrease in running or repeated sprint performance observed in later stages of competition may be due to fatigue. This can occur at different times throughout training and competition and result from different physiological mechanisms. Players experience temporary fatigue during the game after bouts of high-intensity effort and longer-lasting fatigue toward the end of the game.[39-41] Transient fatigue is associated with repeated high-intensity efforts and insufficient recovery (<30 s), but researchers have not clearly identified the factors contributing to transient fatigue and its effect on subsequent running performance.[42-44]

Unique variations in the type of intermittent sport (eg, strength- or endurance-based), the sex of the athlete, the level of play (recreational, elite domestic, and international), the location, and other environmental factors make it challenging to determine the exact demands of a game, but performance is often dependent on nutritional factors. Ongoing considerations include achieving and maintaining optimal body mass and composition as well as meeting the nutrient demands of the training program. Acute issues in training or competition include keeping athletes adequately hydrated and fueled throughout activity. Recovery between events (whether training or competition) is a major priority and should always address rehydration, refueling, and repair.

Unique to endurance-type intermittent sports is their reliance on aerobic metabolism because of the duration of the games. Aerobic pathways support increasing the availability of oxygen for the resynthesis of phosphocreatine stores that can help compensate for the lowered capabilities of the anaerobic system to provide energy because of the intermittent nature of HIIE.[3] During a 90-minute soccer match, the average work intensity, measured by heart rate, is close to the anaerobic threshold, with mean and peak heart rates reaching approximately 85% and 98%, respectively, of the maximum heart rate.[31,33,45,46] Total energy expended is directly related to the distance covered during the 90 minutes of the game, typically in the range from 8 to 13 km (5–8 miles).[5,27,31,36] Although the greatest percentage of distance covered is done at lower speeds, elite soccer players can perform 150 to 250 brief intense actions during a game, indicating that they also experience periods of high anaerobic energy turnover. Consider that athletes are required to sprint, jog, stride, walk, and move sideways and backward while tackling, jumping, accelerating, and turning.

In addition to the general physiological demands on soccer athletes, elite soccer players also display differences in match performance based on sex and level of play, adding to the need for individualization. Males cover more total distance at higher speed thresholds and during the most intense period of a match. Females tend to cover their match distances at a lower average speed threshold of less than 12 km/h vs a standard of more than 15 km/h for males.[47] Major differences in the physical demands have been observed because of the level of play, with a greater amount of high-intensity exercise in top-class players compared with those of a lower standard.[48] Although measurements of high-intensity running, mean recovery time, and maximal running speed are similar in elite domestic and international soccer players, they vary markedly among playing positions. Midfielders, fullbacks, and attackers tend to cover greater distances at higher intensities than defenders.[43]

Ice hockey is metabolically unique in that it requires finely trained aerobic and anaerobic energy pathways. Bursts of intense muscular activity demand exceptional aerobic power and endurance along with intense glycolytic activity. Vigh-Larsen et al[3] found that, of the approximately 6,000 m covered in a simulated ice hockey match, nearly half that distance was covered through high-speed skating, with 95 to 123 explosive efforts noted during the competition. The involvement of the anaerobic system may depend on the efficiency of the aerobic system. Using sport-specific testing methods, Peterson et al[49] investigated the relationship between maximal oxygen uptake (VO_2 peak) and repeated on-ice sprint ability in 45 male college hockey players. The results of the study suggest that an athlete's ability to complete repeated on-ice sprints is associated with their VO_2 peak value and the final stage they completed during the graded exercise test, pointing to the association of aerobic metabolism and fatigue in ice hockey players. A comparison of position-specific energy demands indicated that defensemen experienced a larger physical burden than forwards, highlighting the need for individualization when explaining nutritional needs to hockey athletes.[13]

Duration of play and relative exercise intensity are major factors in determining the fuel mixture needed during exercise. Exercise intensity is expressed as a percentage of maximum oxygen consumption (VO_2 max), which is influenced by age, sex, genetic makeup, and level of aerobic training.[50,51] Muscles' primary fuel, glycogen, is an essential fuel during prolonged vigorous exercise and is required by athletes who engage in HIIE sports, as evidenced by increased glycogen metabolism at the cellular level during high-intensity efforts. A strong link between glycogen storage and associated depletion rates based on activity and HIIE performance has been established. Both impairments in performance and the onset of fatigue are strongly tied to glycogen depletion. Glycogen is heterogeneously stored within the muscle tissue to be readily available for the contraction of various muscle fibers, type I (slow twitch) and type II (fast twitch), as needed to perform a particular exercise or activity.[52] The nature of the activity in stop-and-go team sports requires use of both types of fibers.[53,54] Type II fibers exhibit the greatest degree of glycogen depletion after sprint-type activities.[55] Costill et al[56] showed that, in distance running, glycogen was selectively depleted in type I fibers but type II fibers also bore some of the load. From these studies, it seems that type I fibers are activated at lower workloads and that type II fibers are used during 2 conditions: when type I fibers are depleted of glycogen and during high-intensity output.[55,57,58] Table 21.2 lists muscle energy pathways used during activities of varying intensity.[50,51]

TABLE 21.2 Muscle Energy Pathways Used During Activities of Varying Intensity[50,51]

	Type of activity (% MHR)	Duration of activity	Muscle energy pathway(s)
Immediate	Surges and sprints (≥80-90)	1-6 s	ATP in muscles
		7-20 s	ATP + PCr
		20-45 s	ATP + PCr + muscle glycogen
Short term	Moderate-intensity running (70-80)	45-120 s	Muscle glycogen
		120-180 s	Muscle glycogen + lactic acid
Long term	Low- to moderate-intensity running (<69)	>30 min, limited by oxygen	Muscle glycogen + free fatty acids

Abbreviations: ATP, adenosine triphosphate; MHR, maximum heart rate; PCr, phosphocreatine

Green examined glycogen utilization in the muscle fibers of ice hockey players and found that muscle glycogen depletion averaged 60%. This depletion indicates the utilization of both type I and type II fibers, with the greatest decline occurring in type I fibers. No apparent differences were detected in the amount and pattern of glycogen depletion between forwards and defensemen.[59] Krustrup et al[60] found that muscle glycogen was reduced to 150 to 350 mmol/kg by the end of a soccer match, with half of the fibers of both types being depleted or almost depleted. The authors theorized that the pattern of glycogen depletion in some fibers may limit an athlete's maximal sprint effort.

Effects of High-Intensity, Intermittent Exercise on Substrate Utilization

The relative contributions of fat and carbohydrate as fuel depend on the intensity and duration of exercise, with an increasingly greater total and relative contribution from carbohydrate as the exercise intensity increases above approximately 60% of VO_2 max.[58,61] Endurance exercise training triggers metabolic adaptations that lead to a marked sparing of carbohydrate as a result of a slower utilization of glucose and muscle and liver glycogen during sustained exercise of the same intensity.[62,63] Consequently, endurance training leads to a relatively smaller reliance on carbohydrates than on fatty acids during prolonged steady-state exercise. The reduced reliance on blood glucose and muscle glycogen during exercise in a trained state is one of the mechanisms by which exercise enhances endurance.

In addition to a relative shift in substrate, the absolute amount of fat used decreases as work rate increases.[50,64] Plasma glucose and muscle glycogen utilization both increase in response to an increase in exercise intensity (Figure 21.1).[50] Plasma glucose contributes approximately 10% to 15% of total energy at all work rates, whereas muscle glycogen supplies approximately 60% of the energy requirement during strenuous exercise at approximately 80% of VO_2 max.[50,51]

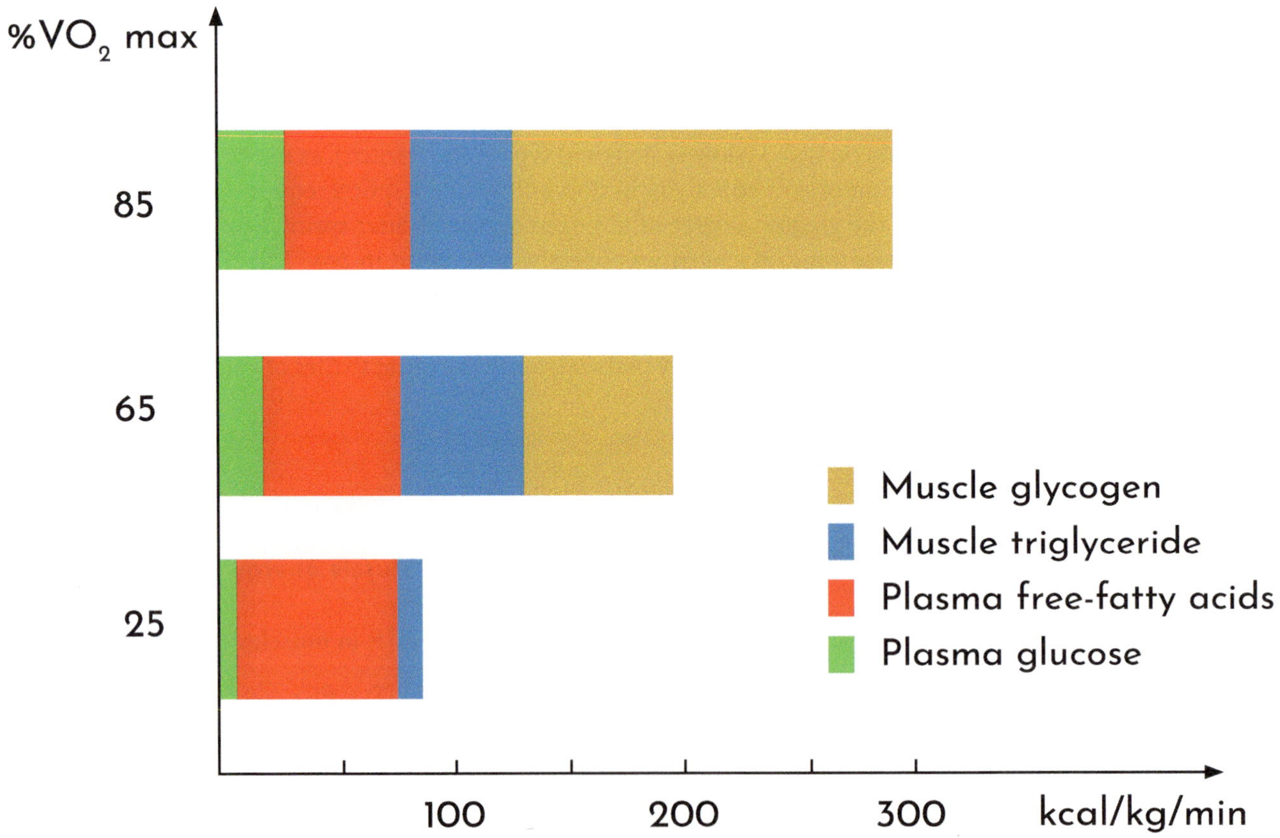

FIGURE 21.1 Muscle energy pathways used during activities of varying intensity Abbreviation: VO_2 max, maximum oxygen consumption

Adapted with permission from reference 50: Romijn JA, Coyle EF, Sidossis LS, et al. Regulation of endogenous fat and carbohydrate metabolism in relation to exercise intensity and duration. *Am J Physiol.* 1993;265(3 pt 1):E380-E391. doi:10.1152/ajpendo.1993.265.3.E380

Whereas the following sections focus on the body's utilization of carbohydrate and fat as substrates to support HIIE, practitioners should note that studies indicate that in a glycogen-depleted state, athletes may experience increased utilization of protein as a substrate because of the high aerobic nature of HIIE. Depending on the duration of the HIIE and related rest periods supporting the fluctuation of substrate utilization throughout the activity, protein utilization seems to depend on preexercise glycogen levels. As in short-term starvation, when both muscle and liver glycogen stores are depleted, prolonged exercise at higher intensities may increase protein catabolism as a result of the decreased ability to synthesize ATP from the body's primary substrates of carbohydrate and fat.[65] Furthermore, researchers understood that during aerobic exercise of longer duration, amino acid oxidation increases with decreased glycogen availability.[66]

Aerobic Energy System

Intermittent exercise has an effect on oxygen consumption similar to that of submaximal continuous running.[33] HIIE activity at moderate intensity levels of 65% to 85% of VO_2 max relies heavily on fat oxidation, with plasma free fatty acids and intramuscular triglycerides contributing more than half of the required energy for activity (refer to Figure 21.1 on page 552).[67] Aerobic metabolism of glucose and lipids at submaximal levels spares muscle glycogen use (primarily used at intensities greater than 85% of VO_2 max), delaying the onset of fatigue and impaired high-intensity exercise.[52,62,63] For example, anaerobic activity is an important component of soccer, but the majority of the time in matches is spent in a submaximal state (less than 85% VO_2 max) with relative work rates estimated at between 70% and 80% of VO_2 max, demonstrating that the greater demand is on aerobic metabolism,[31-33,36] Studies on soccer players suggest an average estimate of VO_2 max of 60 mL/kg/min.[54] Soccer matches are 90 minutes in length, with a 2:1 ratio of low-intensity to high-intensity activity and a 7:1 ratio of relative time spent at low intensity vs high intensity.[33] Sprinting occurs no more than 1.5% of total playing time.[8,68]

Researchers have attempted to determine the contribution of aerobic energy during HIIE performance in soccer by measuring oxygen uptake (VO_2); however, the procedure interferes with normal play, and the results are most likely imprecise. Heart rate is used to estimate oxygen uptake, but heart rate does not always provide an accurate reflection of oxygen uptake. Factors such as dehydration, hyperthermia, and mental stress elevate heart rate without affecting oxygen uptake. In addition to its use in predicting oxygen uptake, heart rate provides a useful index of the overall physiological demands of soccer.[32]

During a match, soccer players spend a considerable amount of time working at heart rates estimated to be more than 160 beats per minute, with mean and peak heart rates at approximately 85% and 98%, respectively, of the maximal value and heart rates rarely lower than 65% of maximum values.[31,36,69] Heart rates of ice hockey players have been reported at between 79.0% and 89.5% of maximum heart rate, with oxygen uptakes of as much as 82.5% of VO_2 max.[12,70,71] Physiological profiles of players in other HIIE team sports, such as basketball, field hockey, ice hockey, and tennis, have shown similar patterns, pointing to the importance of the aerobic energy pathway in HIIE sports.[26,28,72,73] Table 21.3 provides a summary of heart rate patterns among HIIE athletes.[26,31,32,36,38,74-79]

TABLE 21.3 Heart Rate Patterns of Athletes in High-Intensity, Intermittent Sports[26,31,32,36,38,74-79]

Sport	Maximum heart rate, %
Basketball	>85
Ice hockey	85-90
Racquet sports, including squash and badminton	80-85
Rugby	>85
Soccer	80-100
Tennis	80-85

Fat as a Substrate During High-Intensity Intermittent Exercise

Studies on soccer players have shown that blood free fatty acid (FFA) concentration increases during a soccer match, with greater increase in the second half vs the first half or after the game.[60] The blood FFA concentration during a soccer match is the net result of the uptake of FFAs in various tissues and the release of FFAs from adipose tissue. Hormonal responses during HIIE also exert a significant influence on metabolism,[33] which impacts the availability of FFAs and glycerol during HIIE. Bracken et al[80] studied the catecholamine response in 12 nonspecifically trained men who completed ten 6-second cycle ergometer sprints, with a 30-second recovery period after each sprint. Plasma epinephrine increased 6.3-fold from baseline, whereas norepinephrine increased 14.5-fold at the end of sprinting. Trapp et al[81] examined the metabolic response to 2 forms of HIIE—short sprint and long sprint—in 16 trained and untrained women. The observed increase in glycerol concentration suggested an increased reliance on fats for fuel despite increased lactate concentrations and was attributed to periods of rest and a slower pace during the second half of the exercise, allowing more blood flow to adipose tissue and possibly promoting higher FFA release. This process, when coupled with hormonal changes (specifically, decreased insulin), increases catecholamines and stimulates lipolysis and the release of FFAs into the blood. These changes lead to a greater uptake of FFAs and utilization of triglycerides by contracting muscles. Such adaptations favor high blood glucose concentrations and may be compensatory mechanisms for progressively decreasing muscle glycogen levels. A high uptake of glycerol in various tissues (primarily the liver) is assumed, indicating that glycerol might be an important gluconeogenic precursor. Ketone bodies may also function as a minor fat source during exercise.

As low-carbohydrate diets and the subsequent use of very high–fat diets are becoming more popular, especially among endurance athletes, more support is still needed for such dietary strategies to be fully recommended for athletes engaged in HIIE team sports. Dostal et al[82] examined the effects of a very low-carbohydrate, high-fat (VLCHF) diet on aerobic capacity and HIIE. Similarly to other studies on fat adaptation and aerobic performance, they found that the VLCHF diet did not negatively affect HIIE or cardiorespiratory performance in fat-adapted individuals. The study examined a 12-week protocol in which the experimental group ingested a maximum intake of 50 g of carbohydrate per day with protein and fat intakes ad libitum and was compared with a control group that consumed the habitual diet, including a higher carbohydrate intake. The results of this study are contrary to those of another literature report[52] stating that a limiting factor in HIIE performance is adequate glycogen stores directly correlated with carbohydrate ingestion. However, specific conclusions cannot be drawn from this study, as 2 significant variables prevent this study from having a direct application for team athletes who participate in HIIE sports. First, the results from the Dostal et al study can be applied only to intermittent exercises lasting up to 25 minutes in duration, whereas the duration of HIIE in team sports is often triple that value and likely exhausts glycogen stores to a greater extent than was demonstrated in the study. Second, athletes will need to be disciplined enough to become adapted to a fat-rich diet to achieve similar results in performance. For fat adaptation to occur, a fat-rich diet would need to be followed for longer than 4 weeks to improve the body's efficiency in its use of lipids in HIIE and endurance activities. Fat adaptation is crucial for the ability to maintain high-intensity activity on a VLCHF diet.

Although the data suggest promising results for fat-adapted HIIE athletes, more studies are needed to validate additional benefits to VLCHF diets over the current mixed-diet recommendations. Moderate- to high-carbohydrate dietary approaches have stronger support in the current literature for maintaining adequate glycogen stores and improving aerobic performance throughout the full duration of HIIE team-sport activities.

Carbohydrate as a Substrate During High-Intensity, Intermittent Exercise

As exercise intensity increases, the percentage of carbohydrate used as an energy substrate increases to meet most of the energy demands of muscle contraction at an intensity near an individual's VO_2 max. The relative contribution of fat decreases with a concomitant increase in carbohydrate oxidation from 40% to 85% of VO_2 max. For moderate- and high-intensity exercise (50% to 85% of VO_2 max), plasma fatty acids and muscle triglycerides supply the fats that are oxidized.[50,64,83,84]

During vigorous exercise in trained athletes, there is an initial burst of glycogenolysis and a resulting production of lactic acid, followed by a decrease in the rate of glycogenolysis and a reduction in muscle and blood lactate levels. Glycogen, an essential fuel during prolonged vigorous exercise, is required by athletes engaged in HIIE sports, especially when completing high-intensity efforts. The contraction of skeletal muscle and the function of the central nervous system depend on carbohydrate as a fuel substrate, but the body's stores of carbohydrate are limited, and often, the fuel requirements of training and competition for HIIE team sports substantially exceed carbohydrate availability. In a simulated soccer match, the rate of muscle glycogen use decreased from the first to the second half, with the rate reaching its highest value (4.0 ± 1.2 mmol/kg/min) during the warm-up and first 15 minutes of play and becoming progressively lower during intervals from 15 to 60 minutes (1.8 ± 0.5 mmol/kg/min) and 60 to 90 minutes (0.9 ± 1.2 mmol/kg/min).[85] When muscle glycogen stores are depleted, fatigue—both physical and mental—sets in, and performance is compromised.[86-88]

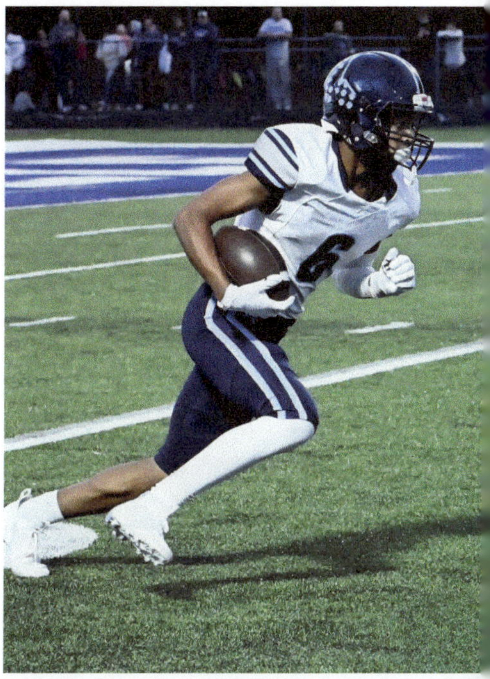

A study involving 20 male and female college students with experience playing team sports consisted of experimental trials of varying intensity to examine the effects of a 6% carbohydrate solution on performance and central nervous system function. Compared with a placebo, carbohydrate feedings resulted in fourth-quarter improvements, including faster sprint times, higher average jump heights, enhanced motor skills, and improved mood, suggesting that carbohydrate feedings during HIIE benefit the function of both the peripheral and central nervous systems.[89]

Anaerobic Energy System

Considerable energy fluctuations occur when a person is performing HIIE sports. Although the majority of work is done at submaximal intensities, high-intensity exercise plays a crucial role, and the athlete's ability to successfully carry out these high-intensity activities affects the results of the game.

ADENOSINE TRIPHOSPHATE AND PHOSPHOCREATINE

Phosphocreatine concentrations fluctuate throughout HIIE sports competitions because of the intermittent nature of the games, and they may decrease below resting values if a number of intense bouts of exercise are accompanied by a short recovery time.[60] Despite a small net utilization, phosphocreatine plays an important role as an energy buffer, providing phosphate for the resynthesis of ATP during rapid increases in exercise intensity.[27,33] Aerobic fitness enhances recovery from HIIE through increased aerobic response, improved lactate removal, and enhanced phosphocreatine regeneration.[90]

BLOOD LACTATE

Glycolysis is activated and lactate is formed almost immediately once exercise starts.[33] Because lactate is produced at a high rate during intense activity, blood lactate concentrations have been used as indicators of anaerobic energy production in soccer players.[31,33] The concentration of blood lactate fluctuates throughout a soccer match. Lactate is metabolized within the active muscle after high-intensity exercise. When high-intensity exercise is coupled with low-intensity exercise, lactate metabolism increases. Evidence suggests that lactate is an important metabolic intermediate as a substrate for oxidative metabolism in cardiac and skeletal muscle and as a precursor for gluconeogenesis.[91] Thus, measurements of blood lactate concentrations represent the balance of lactate released by muscle and taken up by blood and do not fully reflect lactate production during a soccer match.

During HIIE, blood lactate may be high, whereas muscle lactate may be relatively low.[36] Blood lactate concentrations are used to estimate the contribution of anaerobic glycolysis to metabolism during team sports, with mean values reported to lie between 3.0 and 9.0 mmol/L in soccer, between 6.5 and 8.5 mmol/L in rugby, between 4.94 and 6.05 mmol/L in male basketball players, and between 3.7 and 5.2 mmol/L in female basketball players.[26,28,36,92,93] Note that blood lactate represents the balance of the production, release, and removal of lactate. Lactate is metabolized by active muscles after high-intensity activity and varies according to the intensity of play. However, not all of the lactate produced is reflected in the blood. Lactate released from active muscles into the blood is taken up by different tissues, such as the heart, liver, kidney, and inactive muscles. Lactate production may be very high at points during a soccer game, with mean blood lactate concentrations ranging from 2 to 10 mmol/L during a match.[31,33,60] Similarly, blood lactate levels of male tennis players were found to increase during a singles tennis match by 50% to near, but not beyond, the anabolic threshold.[77] The authors attributed this finding to several factors, including the athletes' highly trained aerobic systems and variations in play that allowed their blood lactate levels to clear. In a separate, smaller study on elite male basketball players, McInnes et al[75] reported blood lactate levels averaging 6.8 ± 2.8 mmol/L during competition to support the high involvement of glycolysis in energy production in HIIE athletes.

ENERGY AND MACRONUTRIENT NEEDS

Energy Needs and Summary of Current Intakes

The specific nutritional needs of HIIE athletes are hard to quantify collectively, as each sport has its own physiological demands, length of training and competition, level of gameplay, and style of play. In addition, each athlete is unique in their level of fitness and conditioning, age, daily activity, body composition, and weight, among other factors. The estimation of an athlete's energy requirements starts with an estimation of their energy expenditure and is then based on their goals and training calendar. It is helpful for athletes to work with an experienced sports dietitian to help periodize energy, macronutrient, and micronutrient intake. The intakes of energy and carbohydrate are 2 areas on which an athlete should largely focus to optimize energy and glycogen levels, which foundationally support HIIE performance. Energy availability (EA) can be used as a starting point to assess whether an athlete is meeting their basic metabolic needs while factoring in expenditures in activity. Maintaining an EA of 30 to 45 kcal per kilogram of fat-free mass per day while adding in calories expended during activity can help provide an estimate for caloric needs and energy balance for each athlete.[94,95] Specific macronutrient and micronutrient recommendations to assist in optimizing the athlete's whole diet are discussed in later sections of this chapter.

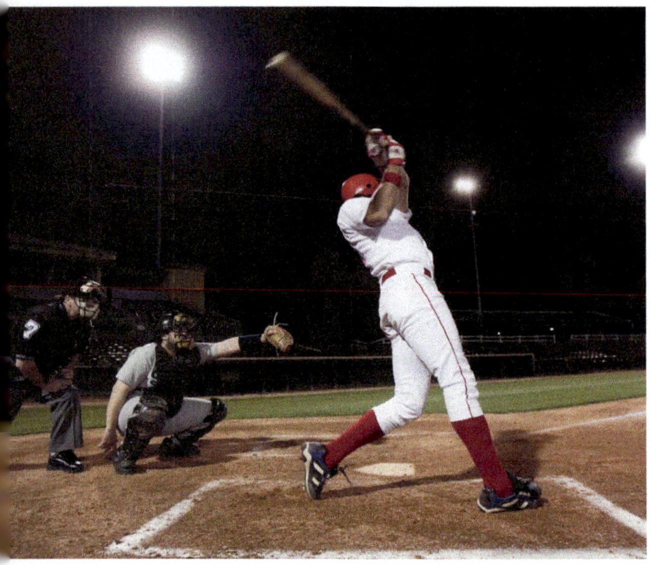

The energy demands of HIIE athletes are high because of the intermittent nature of stop-and-go sports, and the energy intake of an HIIE athlete must be adequate to support training and competition.[96] Researchers have attempted to determine the energy expended during HIIE sports, but to date, none of these attempts have resulted in accurate and valid data. Values that have been measured by oxygen uptake are likely underestimated, and the equipment needed to accurately measure such values can often interfere with gameplay or training, leading to inaccurate results. Establishing a relationship between heart rate and oxygen uptake may allow for an accurate indirect assessment of oxygen uptake during HIIE, as regression equations from treadmill running show a linear connection between heart rate and VO_2 and may allow for oxygen consumption to be estimated for team sports. As mentioned earlier in this chapter, however, it should be noted that, even though this may be an accepted method for estimating VO_2 in HIIE, other factors such as stress and dehydration can elevate the heart rate without affecting oxygen uptake, so the accuracy of these estimations may be affected.[97] In 1 study on elite soccer athletes, energy expenditure was estimated at approximately 1,360 kcal over the course of a match on the basis of heart rate data (at an estimated 70% of VO_2 max) for a 75 kg player with a maximum oxygen uptake of 60 mL/kg/min.[27] Additional studies have yielded the following results:

- Stølen et al[98] estimated an average exercise intensity of 85% of the maximum heart rate, corresponding to approximately 75% of VO_2 max during a soccer match. This corresponds to average oxygen uptakes of 45.0, 48.8, and 52.5 mL/kg/min for a player performing at 60%, 65%, and 70% of VO_2 max, respectively. For a player who weighs 75 kg, these estimates correspond to energy expenditures of 1,519, 1,645, and 1,772 kcal, respectively, over the course of a 90-minute match (at 5 kcal per liter of oxygen per minute).
- Bangsbo et al[36] estimated that elite soccer players, despite spending more than half their time playing at a lower intensity, expended 1,608 kcal on average during each training session in the 2 weeks leading

up to the men's World Cup. This corresponded to an average exercise intensity of approximately 73% of their maximum heart rate at an average of 70% of VO_2 max. Practitioners should note that although female soccer athletes experience similar exercise intensities during a match, they often expend less energy than males because of their typically lower body masses.

Despite the high energy expenditures experienced by soccer players during both training and competition, several studies have suggested that the majority of soccer athletes may not be meeting optimal energy and nutrient intakes.[10,96,99-102] This finding was also corroborated by M Macedonio in a summary report on the nutrition management of the Cleveland Force soccer team (unpublished data, 1987). More recent data examining the diets of athletes involved in intermittent sports support these findings and indicate that the nutritional intakes of both male and female athletes participating in various HIIE sports may be inadequate.[15,17,19-21,24,100-109] In a 2022 literature review by Danielik et al,[10] the intakes of male soccer players were assessed in terms of whether they met the recommendations of a Union of European Football Associations (UEFA) expert group on applied sports nutrition. The researchers estimated the athletes' average energy intake as 2,813 ± 446 kcal/d, whereas the energy recommendations from the UEFA expert group were between 2,900 and 3,500 kcal/d. Caloric averages from this study ranged from 2,164 ± 498 to 3,789 ± 532 kcal/d. In addition:

- In a study of 75 National Collegiate Athletic Association Division III soccer players, intakes of total energy, carbohydrates, and dietary fiber were reported to be lower than recommendations. Significant differences were found between the target intakes for total energy (2,789.9 ± 352.3 kcal vs 2,470 ± 522.8 kcal), total carbohydrate (420.1 ± 55.9 g vs 318.2 ± 82.7 g), and dietary fiber (39.1 ± 4.9 g vs 20.9 ± 8.6 g).[110]
- An examination of the dietary intakes of 24 female college athletes (field hockey, cross country, tennis, and golf) revealed that the intakes of carbohydrate and energy were less than the recommended values (1,513 ± 406 kcal/d), with iron and calcium intakes that were 30% below the corresponding Recommended Dietary Allowances (RDAs). Practitioners should note that 14 of the 24 athletes participating in this study were attempting to lose weight.[111] The author concluded that nutrition counseling is necessary to advise female players on ways to balance energy and nutrient intake with attempts to achieve a desired performance weight.

Additional studies have provided a variety of information on the dietary intakes of HIIE athletes:

- Data reported in 2003 on female collegiate soccer players indicated that they met the Dietary Reference Intakes (DRIs) for total energy (37 kcal per kilogram of body weight), protein, and fat during the preseason and that their intakes were substantially higher than the DRIs during the playing season. Although the athletes' protein and fat intakes during the preseason were higher than the minimum recommendations, their carbohydrate intakes were not sufficient to promote glycogen repletion. In this study, although protein and fat helped supply the energy requirements during preseason training, they displaced carbohydrate-rich, nutrient-dense foods, which caused the athletes to fail at meeting the appropriate energy, carbohydrate, and micronutrient recommendations and potentially compromised their performance.[102]
- Papadopoulous et al[112] assessed the macronutrient and micronutrient intakes of 2 Greek teams of adolescent female volleyball players (the Junior National Team and the Junior National Championship Team) and found that, although the protein intakes were satisfactory (approximately 16% of total kilocalories), fat intakes were generally higher than desired (approximately 37.5% of total kilocalories) at the expense of carbohydrate consumption (45.9% of total kilocalories), with mean energy intakes at less-than-optimal levels (2,013 and 1,529 kcal, respectively). As a whole, the volleyball players fell short of meeting the RDA values for calcium (935 ± 497 mg, RDA 1,200 mg), iron (7.9 ± 4.0 mg, RDA 15.0 mg), folic acid (163 ± 98 mcg, RDA 400 mcg), magnesium (207 ± 130 mg, RDA 300 mg), zinc (7 ± 5 mg, RDA 12 mg), and vitamins A (554 ± 495 retinol equivalents, RDA 800 retinol equivalents), B1 (0.9 ± 0.5 mg, RDA 1.1 mg), B2 (1.2 ± 0.6 mg, RDA 1.2 mg), and B6 (0.8 ± 0.7 mg, RDA 1.5 mg). The mean daily energy intake (1,648 kcal/d) was lower than the RDA (by 44 kcal/d) for very active females.[112]
- Holway and Spriet[1] summarized 30 years of published reports on the energy and macronutrient intakes of team-sport athletes. The mean carbohydrate, protein, and fat intakes were 49%, 17%, and 34%, respectively, for male athletes and 50%, 15%, and 35%, respectively, for female athletes, with male athletes

reaching an average carbohydrate consumption of 5.6 ± 1.3 g per kilogram of body weight per day and female athletes consuming 4.0 ± 0.7 g per kilogram of body weight per day. Generally, the preseason intakes were found to be greater than the in-season intakes; larger athletes consumed more energy; and the average carbohydrate intake, at 49%, was lower than some past recommendations of 55% to 65%.

- Gravina et al[16] studied the effects of macronutrient and micronutrient intake on markers of oxidative stress, muscle damage, and inflammatory and immune response in 28 female soccer players, aged 21 ± 6 years. All players engaged in training plus 1 match per weekend. An 8-day diet record and blood samples collected both immediately after and 18 hours after 4 official soccer matches were analyzed. The mean reported energy intake was 2,271 ± 578 kcal/d with a macronutrient distribution that was higher in protein (15% ± 2%); lower in carbohydrate (44.3% ± 6%); and higher in total fat (37% ± 7%), saturated fat (12.4% ± 3%), and cholesterol (340 mg/d) than recommendations (protein, 10% to 12%; carbohydrate, 50% to 60%; fat, 35%; cholesterol, <300 mg). The fiber intake was lower (20 ± 7 g/d) than the recommended level of 25 to 26 g/d. The intakes of folic acid (230 ± 100 mcg/d), vitamin D (3.3 ± 2 mcg/d), magnesium (315 ± 97 mg/d), and potassium (2,973 ± 971 mg/d) were also suboptimal and lower than the DRI. Players who followed the guidelines for the recommended intakes had higher levels of total antioxidant status and lower levels of creatine kinase and lactate dehydrogenase, both of which are markers of oxidative stress. The authors concluded that their data revealed an association between nutritional intake and muscle damage, oxidative stress, immunity, and inflammation markers and that adequate intakes of specific nutrients may help prevent undesirable physiological effects related to HIIE.
- Briggs et al[113] investigated energy intake and expenditure (using a triaxial accelerometer) of adolescent male academy-level soccer players aged 15.4 ± 0.3 years during a competitive 7-day period. The mean energy intake (2,245 ± 321 kcal) was significantly lower than the mean energy expenditure (2,552 ± 321 kcal), resulting in a daily deficit of 311 ± 397 kcal. Significant differences were observed between energy intake and energy expenditure on heavy training days (−505 ± 539 kcal) and match days (−544 ± 551 kcal). Only on rest days was a mean positive energy balance (153 ± 286 kcal) observed. Carbohydrate intake (5.6 ± 0.4 g/kg/d), mainly from starchy foods, was suboptimal, especially during training and on match days. Protein intake (1.5 ± 0.2 g per kilogram of body weight per day), mainly from poultry and dairy foods, was within an optimal range to support growth and development. The mean fat intake (29% ± 2%) was at the upper limit, with saturated fat values of 26 ± 3 g/d (12% of total kcal). This suggests that having athletes reduce their intakes of saturated fat rather than total fat may be advisable. Researchers have observed energy deficits among young athletes in similar populations and indicate a need for nutrition education and intervention to support optimal growth, development, and performance of adolescent athletes.

Research suggests that nutrition education can be correlated with better food selection with respect to carbohydrate, fruit, and vegetable intakes, suggesting that knowledge of sports nutrition concepts can help mitigate inadequate food and energy consumption. In a study investigating the effects of low energy availability on female Australian rules football players, inadequate carbohydrate, iron, and calcium intake levels were found compared to the suggested recommendations for athletes. Thirty percent of the players were at risk for low energy availability. This study looked at nutrition knowledge scores and found that the average score (percent of correct answers) was 54.5%. Sections on general nutrition concepts, fluids, recovery, weight control, and supplements were presented. Although this study focused on knowledge within the female population, similar comparisons of the level of sports nutrition knowledge were also found in male Australian football players. It is suggested that team-sport athletes, overall, would benefit from education that may lead to better performance outcomes.[114] In addition, periodic dietary evaluations from a sports dietitian can detect early trouble signs, help prevent serious nutritional deficiencies, and screen for possible disordered eating.

Carbohydrate

The abundant aerobic energy production in HIIE sports and the substantial anaerobic energy turnover are associated with the extensive consumption of substrates, predominantly carbohydrate and fat. The body's carbohydrate is stored as glycogen in the liver (~100 g) and skeletal muscle (~300–700 g). These endogenous carbohydrate stores are relatively small, supplying less than 5% of the body's total energy storage. When carbohydrate requirements of training or competition exceed endogenous carbohydrate stores, carbohydrate availability is compromised. In a review of studies of cyclists, Maughan et al[115] compared the effects of low-carbohydrate diets vs high-carbohydrate diets on high-intensity exercise. A low-carbohydrate diet (<10% of total energy from carbohydrate) was found to result in reduced endurance time. Conversely, diets that provided 65% to 84% of calories from carbohydrate were associated with increased performance, more consistently so with carbohydrate intakes at the higher end. Also noted was that a high-protein diet, particularly in conjunction with a low-carbohydrate diet, resulted in metabolic acidosis, which is associated with fatigue. Although many questions about the causal mechanisms remain unanswered, the authors concluded the review with 2 distinct messages. The first is that it is possible to improve the performance of short-duration, high-intensity exercise with a high-carbohydrate, low-protein diet for a few days before competition. Second, performance of this type may be impaired by a high-protein diet with insufficient carbohydrate or an energy-restricted diet in the precompetition period.

Based on the effects of nutrition interventions on molecular and cellular processes during exercise and recovery, Hawley et al[116] recommended that the diet of athletes performing HIIE approach 7 g of carbohydrate per kilogram of body mass during intense training to maintain adequate muscle glycogen stores to meet the periods of strenuous demands during competition.

MUSCLE GLYCOGEN

The demands on muscle glycogen are considerable, and early researchers almost unanimously agreed that performance improves when carbohydrate is supplied before and during HIIE. Carbohydrate used during HIIE is primarily supplied by the glycogen stored within exercising muscle, although muscles may also use glucose circulating in blood. Although most of the early studies supported the use of a carbohydrate-electrolyte solution during HIIE, they were subject to methodological limitations. Of particular concern was the use of exercise protocols that employed a constant exercise intensity, lacked work at high or maximal intensity, and included long periods of seated recovery, thus clearly failing to replicate the activity patterns and physiological demands of exercise during team sports and limiting their applicability to actual team sports.[117]

Bangsbo et al[118] reported that, by increasing the carbohydrate content of the diet from 39% to 65% before a soccer match, muscle glycogen levels increased and resulted in a higher work rate and improved intermittent endurance. In a study of Swedish elite ice hockey players, Akermark et al[76] compared the performance of ice hockey players given a carbohydrate-enriched diet to that of players given a mixed diet. During a 3-day period between 2 games, players were fed a mixed diet of approximately 40% carbohydrate or a diet of approximately 60% carbohydrate. Distance skated, number of shifts skated, amount of time skated within shifts, and skating speed were all found to improve with the higher carbohydrate intake, leading the researchers to conclude that these differences may be related to muscle glycogen metabolism.

Glycogen depletion can seriously limit players' ability to maintain high-intensity work output, distance covered, and sprinting frequency, particularly during the later stages of a game. The glycogen utilization in leg muscle is markedly increased during bouts of intense exercise. During periods of rest and low-intensity play, glycogen is resynthesized.[119] In 2 studies, researchers found low levels of muscle glycogen at the end of a soccer match and reported higher glycogen use in the first half compared with the second half.[53,120] The muscle glycogen concentration was only 50% of the prematch values 2 days after the match.[51] The difference in muscle glycogen measured before and after a match represents the net glycogen utilization and does not fully reflect the total glycogen turnover during play.[27,33] Toward the end of a match, players were found to experience fatigue and a decrease in perfor-

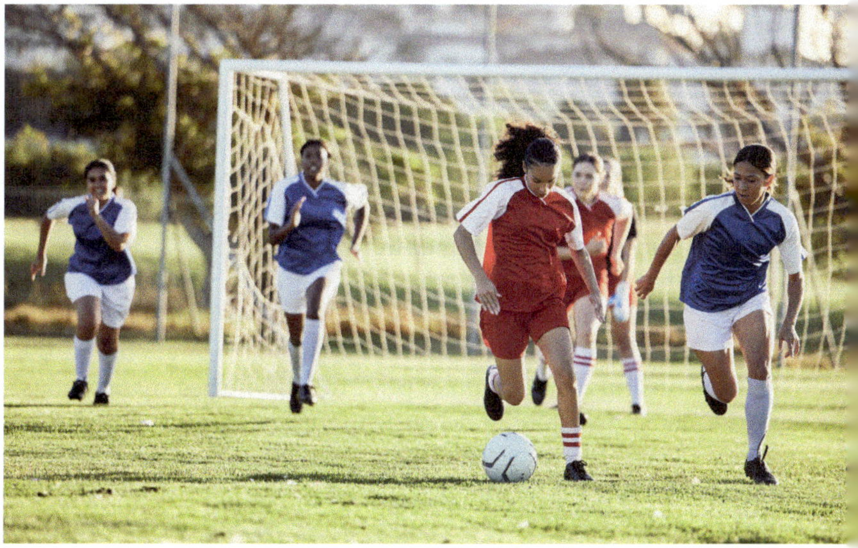

mance. Although an exact mechanism for this phenomenon has not been identified, low levels of muscle glycogen may be a factor. Saltin[120] observed that players with low levels of glycogen covered 24% less distance, 50% of which was covered at a walk. Without sufficient muscle glycogen, exercise is fueled by fat, and the intensity of that exercise is typically less than 50% of capacity.[50,121] Krustrup et al[60] measured a decrease in muscle glycogen of 150 to 350 mmol per kilogram of dry weight (42% ± 6%) as a result of repeated sprinting: Postgame measures at rest were 225 ± 22 mmol per kilogram of dry weight (compared with 449 mmol per kilogram of dry weight). Sprint performance was reduced both temporarily after intense exercise and at the end of the match. Half of the glycogen in individual muscle fibers of both types were either depleted or almost depleted, possibly preventing maximal sprint effort.

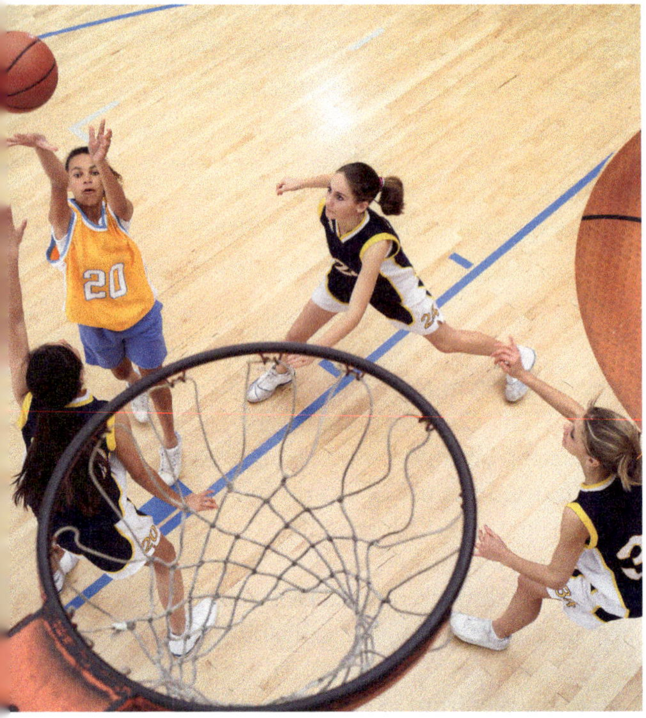

The effect of low muscle glycogen is more likely to have greater consequence in intermittent sports where endogenous stores of glycogen are insufficient to meet energy demands for the full duration of play, during overtime, or during tournament competition. It is, therefore, important that athletes begin exercise with full glycogen stores and replenish glycogen stores as soon as possible after glycogen-depleting exercise. In the absence of severe muscle damage, an adequate carbohydrate intake can restore muscle glycogen stores within 24 hours of reduced exercise.[122]

BLOOD GLUCOSE

The role of liver glycogen is to regulate blood glucose to meet the needs of the whole organism, including the central nervous system. The stored glycogen in skeletal muscle provides a major portion of carbohydrate used during a soccer match, but blood glucose may also be used by exercising muscles and may, in fact, spare muscle glycogen.[33,123] Muscle contraction causes an increase in the uptake of glucose from the blood. As exercise duration increases, the carbohydrate from muscle glycogen decreases, whereas that from blood glucose increases.[50] Blood glucose concentrations increase during HIIE, as long as there are sufficient liver glycogen and glucose precursors.[31,33,123]

Hypoglycemia and glycogen depletion are associated with fatigue and reduced performance. Ferrauti et al[124] assessed the incidence of hypoglycemia in tennis players during repeated tournament and practice matches by examining the change in glucose concentrations during the test period. The results indicated that glucose homeostasis is disrupted several times during tennis tournaments, leading to a decrease in glucose concentration and an increased risk of hypoglycemia, especially after a long match with only short breaks. In the absence of carbohydrate supplementation during extended play, the blood glucose concentration can decrease. To reduce the risk of hypoglycemia, a continuous intake of carbohydrates with a low glycemic index is recommended beginning with the third set through the end of the match and during changeovers.

CARBOHYDRATE RECOMMENDATIONS

A 1994 review by Hargreaves[125] presented an overview of the early research on the role of carbohydrates in the performance of soccer players before, during, and after games and intensive training. Hargreaves concluded that a prematch diet of at least 55% of total energy as carbohydrate, accompanied by additional carbohydrate consumed during and after a match, maximized liver and muscle glycogen stores and enhanced the performance of athletes.

The effects of consuming carbohydrate during HIIE have been investigated in multiple studies.[126,127] Davison et al[128] demonstrated that consumption of a 6% carbohydrate-electrolyte solution in the amount of 8 mL/kg 15 minutes prior to HIIE helped maintain higher blood glucose compared with a placebo or no fluid, resulting in delayed fatigue and improved performance. More recently, Phillips et al[129] demonstrated that ingesting a 6% carbohydrate-electrolyte solution significantly improves the endurance capacity but not the sprint performance of adolescents during intermittent, high-intensity exercise. Sporting skills have been shown to decline during or following exercise.[86,130] In an earlier work, Phillips et al[117] performed a literature review on the effects of carbohydrate intake on team-sport performance. On the basis of studies mimicking the demands of team sports and using appropriate methodologies, the authors concluded that carbohydrate supplementation resulted in an increase in the blood glucose concentration, significantly higher carbohydrate oxidation rates, and attenuated fat oxidation rates and FFA levels in soccer, rugby, and field hockey players.

Russell et al[131] reported that a 6% sucrose-electrolyte beverage administered during a soccer match simulation attenuated the athletes' declining shooting performance through improved shot speed and overall shooting performance at the end of the simulation but did not improve their precision, success, ball speed, or performance in passing and dribbling. The carbohydrate beverage did not prevent an exercise-induced glycemic response when exercise was resumed after halftime. Another study by Russell et al[132] documented a transient reduction in blood glucose when players consumed a carbohydrate-electrolyte beverage during team play. Despite evidence that blood glucose concentrations can be maintained beyond 90 minutes and during more than 30 minutes of extra time, researchers recommended that team-sport athletes ingest carbohydrate during exercise to preserve their endogenous glycogen and maintain running performance late in exercise.[133]

Jeukendrup[134] noted that carbohydrates can be oxidized at different rates during exercise because of differences in absorption rates and the need to convert specific carbohydrates into substrates that can be used by skeletal muscle. In another study, Jeukendrup[135] compared glucose, fructose, galactose, sucrose, and maltose polymers, finding that fructose was oxidized at slightly lower rates than glucose and that the rate of oxidation of galactose was 50% lower than that of glucose. Recommendations for specific types and overall amount of carbohydrates should largely depend on the duration of the activity. Consequently, athletes are advised to consume carbohydrates at a rate no higher than 1 g/min (30 to 60 g/h) for events less than 2.5 hours in length. For events lasting longer than 2.5 hours, the consumption of up to 90 g/h may be beneficial only if multiple transportable carbohydrates are being used. Recent research has demonstrated that ingesting multiple transportable carbohydrates that use different intestinal transporters increases carbohydrate delivery and that such combinations of carbohydrates can be oxidized at rates exceeding 1 g/min.

A 2015 literature review on the effects of ingesting 30 to 60 g of carbohydrate per hour on performance in intermittent sports showed mixed results for sprinting, sport-specific skills, and change-of-direction speed. Carbohydrate ingestion was minimally effective for jumping and cognitive function; however, carbohydrate ingestion seemed to have the greatest impact on the development of permanent fatigue and hypoglycemia, such as toward the end of a long match.[136] The available research suggests that intake of 30 to 60 g of carbohydrate per hour consistently enhances high-intensity, intermittent performance with longer time to exhaustion and greater distance covered, and it may be more important to performance when carbohydrate is consumed before or during a high-intensity event than a lower-intensity session.[129,137] Solid (bar form) or semisolid (gel or chew form) carbohydrates are oxidized at the same rate as carbohydrate solution as long as sufficient water is consumed. Research has shown that carbohydrate gels can improve endurance capacity in HIIE.[137] The exact amount and timing of the carbohydrate intake should be determined according to the individual's needs and a number of factors specific to the sport. For a detailed discussion and recommended guidelines for determining individual recommendations, refer to the review by Baker et al.[136]

Carbohydrate recommendations are more precisely expressed on a gram per kilogram basis.[126,138,139] The current recommendations for athletes engaged in HIIE are summarized in Table 21.4 on page 562.[122,139,140] Specific recommendations should be tailored to the needs of the individual athlete. The recommendations of Burke et al[122] for carbohydrate intake according to total energy needs, specific training needs, and feedback from training performance provide guidelines for achieving high carbohydrate availability to promote optimal performance in competition or key training sessions. These guidelines became the foundation for the carbohydrate recommendations in the 2016 joint position statement on Nutrition and Athletic Performance by the Academy of Nutrition and Dietetics, Dietitians of Canada, and the American College of Sports Medicine.[122,135,141]

Although more research is needed, practitioners should give additional consideration to carbohydrate utilization for females during the different phases of menstruation. The utilization and storage of carbohydrates varies throughout the menstrual cycle, thus affecting the benefits of carbohydrate loading. In a study observing both male and female cyclists, Tarnopolsky et al[142] found that female participants who were in the follicular phase of their menstrual cycle did not experience any significant changes in performance or muscle glycogen content even after an increase to 70% carbohydrate intake. In contrast, the male participants in the study exhibited improvements in both areas after increasing carbohydrates to 70% of daily intake. Therefore, it may be more beneficial to give carbohydrate loading recommendations for females in terms of grams of carbohydrate per kilogram of body weight.

TABLE 21.4 Carbohydrate Guidelines for High-Intensity, Intermittent Exercise[122,139,140]

Training or competition	Carbohydrate intake to promote high carbohydrate availability	Additional considerations
Fueling for moderate exercise of 30-90 min	5-7 g/kg/24 h spread throughout the day	Once adequate energy intake is met, timing can be determined by individual or sport-specific needs.
Fueling for events involving <90 min exercise	7-12 g/kg/24 h	Once adequate energy intake is met, timing can be determined by individual or sport-specific needs.
Fueling for events involving >90 minutes of sustained intermittent exercise	10-12 g/kg/24 h for 36-48 h	Once adequate energy intake is met, timing can be determined by individual or sport-specific needs.
Preevent fueling for events lasting >60 min	1-4 g/kg approximately 1-4 h before competition, or >200 g	Solid carbohydrate with a low glycemic index may be beneficial.
Fueling during exercise of 1.0-2.5 h	30-60 g/h	Ingest a 6%-8% carbohydrate beverage or carbohydrate gel.
Speedy refueling: <8 h recovery between 2 fuel-demanding sessions	1.0-1.2 g/kg/h for the first 4 h, then resume daily fuel needs; 0.8 g of carbohydrate per kilogram per hour plus 0.2-0.4 g of protein per kilogram per hour	Consider the fat and fiber contents as well as the glycemic index for athletes with lower gastrointestinal thresholds for carbohydrate ingestion immediately postexercise.

A 2018 study found that carbohydrate rinsing can be ergogenic to performance. This is especially evident when preexercise carbohydrate intake is insufficient and athletes have lower muscle glycogen stores.[143] A quick mouth rinse is an alternative to carbohydrate ingestion and can immediately increase maximal force production. In a study in which carbohydrate mouth rinsing was employed during intermittent sprinting, Beaven et al[144] predicted a better power output when there were longer breaks between periods of exertion or only a single sprint was required. Researchers have suggested that athletes use mouth rinsing for activities of 30 to 75 minutes in duration alongside smaller, additional amounts of carbohydrates if needed.[135]

Before adopting any new eating and drinking strategies for use immediately before or during a match, players should be cautioned to experiment on training days to establish a comfortable routine and to avoid any untoward consequences.

GLYCOGEN REPLETION

In spite of measures to minimize glycogen losses, match play sharply reduces glycogen stores. Glycogen depletion is associated with fatigue and a decrease in exercise intensity. Resynthesis of depleted glycogen stores is both an important consideration and a challenge in postexercise recovery. When enough carbohydrate is supplemented immediately after exercise with sufficient recovery time, the rate of glycogen synthesis and the amount stored are optimal, increasing muscle glycogen up to 7-fold.[145-147] Several studies have suggested that the consumption of foods with a moderate to high glycemic index after exercise may be beneficial.[147-150] A large body of research supports the need for dietary carbohydrate before, during, and after exercise to fuel muscle glycogen stores and replenish liver glycogen content to help delay fatigue and maximize performance. Refer to Chapter 2 for more information on carbohydrates and exercise.

Protein

Studies have shown that amino acids can be oxidized for energy during endurance exercise and that amino acid oxidation is inversely related to muscle glycogen availability.[151,152] During team sports of intermittent exercise, muscle glycogen can be depleted, depending on the pregame glycogen stores and the intensity and duration of exercise. The higher the intensity of exercise, the greater the glycogen utilization and amino acid oxidation. If the amino acids are not replaced through the diet, a net loss in amino acids can occur over time, with losses in muscle strength and possibly performance.

Protein recommendations for soccer players are based on research that shows the strength component of soccer and the use of protein as an energy source. Lemon[153] concluded that soccer players need more dietary protein than sedentary individuals and suggested a protein intake of 1.4 to 1.7 g per kilogram of body weight per day for competitive soccer players. In a study of eleven 15-year-old soccer players by Boisseau et al[103] in which the mean daily energy intake of the athletes (2,345 kcal or 38.9 kcal/kg body weight) was less than the RDA for nonactive 15-year-olds, a protein intake of 1.57 g/kg body weight was necessary to achieve nitrogen balance. A later study of 14-year-old male soccer players demonstrated that both protein intake and energy balance were important determinants of nitrogen balance, and the authors recommended a protein intake of 1.4 g per kilogram of body weight per day for adolescent boys.[104] Current data suggest that the dietary protein intake necessary for metabolic adaptations, repair, and remodeling, as well as for protein turnover, ranges from 1.2 to 2.0 g per kilogram of body weight and that higher intakes may be necessary for short periods of intense training or when overall energy intake is being reduced.[141]

Researchers have paid attention to the possible benefits of combining protein with carbohydrate during exercise to delay fatigue and immediately after exercise to maximize muscle glycogen synthesis.[154-158] The results of such strategies have been mixed, with inconclusive evidence to support the addition of protein in the presence of adequate carbohydrate intake. However, for glycogen repletion when energy intake does not provide sufficient carbohydrate, the addition of protein to carbohydrate during recovery may enhance overall glycogen recovery, as well as assist in muscle repair.

Fat

Fat is certainly an important component of a balanced diet, but the absolute quantity and percentage of energy distribution contributed by fat should be limited. It is generally recommended that fat should contribute no more than 35% of total energy. However, no performance benefits for any sports have been associated with diets providing less than 20% of total energy from fat.[141]

To achieve energy intake levels that support weight and weight-training goals, athletes often consume diets that are high in fat. In a review of the role of dietary macronutrients in optimizing performance, Stellingwerff et al[158] observed reduced glycogenolysis during a sprint exercise after 5 days of a high-fat diet followed by 1 day of carbohydrate restoration and postulated that the muscle glycogen sparing observed in studies of high-fat diets followed by carbohydrate restoration might be an impairment of glycogenolysis. In a review of the training adaptations occurring through nutritional interventions, Hawley et al[116] cautioned against high-fat, low-carbohydrate diets as a strategy for HIIE. In 2019, Michalczyk et al[159] conducted a study involving well-trained male basketball players to investigate the effects of a 4-week high-fat, low-carbohydrate diet followed by up to 7 days of carbohydrate loading. The researchers found that, although the low-carbohydrate diet phase decreased the athletes' total work capacity, neither intervention affected their peak power. Therefore, the explosive activities and short repeated bursts characterized by basketball training did not trigger adaptive changes from either the low- or high-carbohydrate intervention.

Athletes benefit from nutrition education on the most beneficial food choices that support both their training and performance goals and their long-term health. Factors that may contribute to less-than-optimal dietary intake include competition travel, access to food, time limitations, ability to cook, and insufficient nutrition knowledge. Dietitians working with athletes who participate in HIIE can make the following recommendations with regard to fat intake:

- Determine carbohydrate and protein intakes and then aim for 20% to 35% of energy from fat.
- Limit saturated fat to less than 10% of energy.
- Emphasize heart-healthy fats, including rich sources of essential fatty acids, especially omega-3 fatty acids.
- Give practical guidelines for food selections that will control the contribution from fat, especially sources of hidden fats, such as full-fat dairy products, meats, processed foods, and foods prepared with fat, including restaurant and fast foods.
- Focus on selecting lean protein sources.
- Include tips for choosing foods away from home.

MICRONUTRIENT NEEDS

The demands of HIIE training and competition are considerable and include the need for adequate intakes of all nutrients involved in energy production. There are no known micronutrient needs specific to athletes engaged in HIIE, so the DRIs are appropriate goals for micronutrient intakes.[160-163] Fogelholm[164] presented data on micronutrient status and the effects of micronutrient supplementation on exercise performance related to soccer and other team sports. In an effort to understand the micronutrient needs and intakes of athletes and to determine whether any performance benefit can be gained from micronutrient supplementation, data were reported from 9 studies examining dietary the intakes of athletes involved in soccer, football, basketball, hockey, volleyball, and handball, as well as 3 studies assessing the effects of micronutrient supplementation. The data from these studies suggest that, overall, micronutrient intakes correlate with energy intake. The micronutrient intakes of male athletes were mostly in line with the DRIs. Female athletes with energy intakes of less than 2,400 kcal/d were more likely to have lower intakes than the DRIs for minerals and trace elements, such as calcium, magnesium, iron, and zinc. The data also suggest that the vitamin B6 intake was less than the DRIs for all groups studied, but this may be due to incomplete data from vitamin B6 nutrient databases.[165]

With regard to supplementation, no clear evidence that micronutrient supplementation can improve the performance of well-nourished athletes has been reported, and the number of study participants was small.[164] There are 2 exceptions to this conclusion. First, female athletes with infrequent or irregular menstruation may benefit from calcium and vitamin D supplementation to help stem the loss of bone density. In the presence of estrogen deficiency, calcium and vitamin D supplementation alone will not improve bone density. Second, iron-depleted female athletes (those with serum ferritin levels of <12 mcg/L) may benefit from daily supplementation with 100 mg of elemental iron for 3 months or longer. The iron status of female athletes should be assessed annually. Those who are symptomatic (serum ferritin <35 mcg/L) or at high risk for iron deficiency should be rescreened 3 to 4 months after the initial assessment.[166]

More recently, research has shown a prevalence of low vitamin D levels in athletes across a wide variety of sports. Vitamin D concentrations lower than 20 ng/mL are apparent especially during the winter months.[167]

In an effort to understand the impact of magnesium on strength, Santos et al[168] analyzed 7 days of 24-hour diet records from 26 male team athletes (basketball, handball, and volleyball) aged 21.1 ± 4.9 years and compared the intakes with the results of a series of strength tests. The magnesium intakes were significantly lower than recommendations, and the calcium-to-magnesium ratios were higher than recommendations. A regression analysis showed a direct association between magnesium intake and trunk flexion, trunk rotation, and handgrip maximal strength, as well as jumping performance tests. The effect of magnesium on muscle strength seems to be independent of total dietary intake, illustrating the importance of magnesium in muscle performance and suggesting that performance could be improved with adequate magnesium intakes.

FLUID REQUIREMENTS

The major causes of fatigue in endurance sports are depletion of muscle glycogen and problems associated with thermoregulation and fluid loss. HIIE requires that players exercise at high intensities for a prolonged period, often at elevated ambient temperatures and high humidity. The added factor of clothing and equipment make heat dissipation, and thus thermoregulation, more difficult, as exemplified in the sports of American football and ice hockey.[169] Palmer and Spriet[170] studied the hydration status and habits of elite ice hockey players and found that more than 50% of players arrived at practice in various degrees of hypohydration. In general, among players who drank sports drinks before practice and replaced 60% of lost fluid with water during practice, 30% still had a greater than 1% loss of body mass. All players had high sweat rates during practice, with substantial loss of sodium in sweat that was not replaced by either the sports drinks consumed before practice or the water consumed during practice.

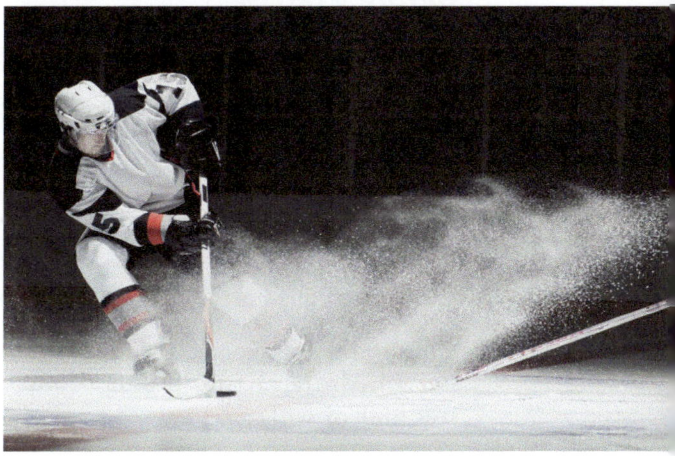

In a study by Arnaoutis et al,[171] the hydration statuses of 107 young soccer players were evaluated on the first day of soccer camp. Seventy-two of the athletes agreed to undergo testing on 2 additional days. Hydration assessments showed that 88.7% (95 of 107) of the youth were hypohydrated based on the urine specific gravity tests conducted on the first morning. Evaluation based on a urine color chart classified 93.7% (100 of 107) as hypohydrated. Measurements taken before training on the third and fifth days of camp showed that 8.4% and 12.5%, respectively, were euhydrated. After training, 95.8% and 97.2%, respectively, were dehydrated. A majority of young players were hypohydrated and remained hypohydrated throughout camp.

The energy demands of stop-and-go sports greatly reduce muscle glycogen stores and fluid reserves, which must be replenished before the next competition. Repletion of muscle glycogen depends not only on carbohydrate intake but also on fluid intake because each gram of muscle glycogen is stored with 2.7 g of water.

Studies examining the effects of carbohydrate-electrolyte solutions on performance during HIIE found that muscle glycogen utilization was reduced, endurance running capacity was improved, time to fatigue was delayed, and mental function was improved when a carbohydrate-electrolyte solution was consumed.[86,89,172,173] At moderate temperatures (10 °C [50 °F]), the sweat losses of soccer players during a match may be as much as 2 L, and at high temperatures, they can reach a mean loss of 3 L or more.[32,150] When the ambient temperature is higher than skin temperature, the body builds up additional heat, and this reduces the capacity to perform prolonged exercise. Players who sweat profusely are likely to become dehydrated and fatigued toward the end of an exercise session. Players working in the heat should focus on fluid ingestion along with maintenance of their hydration status. Tennis players have been shown to sweat more than 2.5 L/h and replace fluids at a lower rate during competition than during practice. In warm and hot environments, researchers recommend that tennis players consume a carbohydrate-electrolyte beverage in amounts greater than 200 mL per changeover and ideally closer to 400 mL per changeover to maintain physiological homeostasis and performance.[174]

Full rehydration after exercise requires replacement of both fluid and electrolytes, primarily sodium, lost in sweat. A study by Shirreffs et al[175] suggested that full rehydration after intense exercise is best achieved when the replacement fluid contains sufficient sodium and is consumed as 150% of the fluid lost through exercise.

The majority of studies evaluating internal body temperature in relation to dehydration have included male participants. Therefore, more research is needed to determine the impacts that sex differences may have on hydration status. During the luteal phase of the menstrual cycle, the internal body temperature increases. This increase in body temperature may put individuals in the luteal phase of menstruation at a higher risk of heat illness. In addition, females may be more prone to dehydration as progesterone increases, causing less fluid retention.[176]

More information on hydration and fluids can be found in Chapter 6. Box 21.2 on page 566 summarizes hydration strategies for HIIE.[175,177-182]

Special Considerations for Young Athletes

Special consideration and care should be given to the fluid needs of young athletes, particularly prepubescent youth.[183] During exercise, children produce a smaller amount of heat than adults yet have a greater surface area-to-body mass ratio (~20% higher than that of adults). When skin temperature is hotter than the environment, the direction of heat flux is from the body outward. However, when ambient temperatures are

BOX 21.2 Hydration Goals in High-Intensity, Intermittent Exercise[a,181,183-188]

Before exercise

Maximize fluid intake during the 24 h preceding training or competition.

Drink extra fluid during the last 10 to 15 min before the game begins.

A carbohydrate-electrolyte solution consumed 15 min before exercise improves endurance.

During exercise

Consume fluid early and at regular intervals during exercise.

Choose cool, flavored beverages that are more palatable and contain 4% to 8% carbohydrate (30-60 g of carbohydrate per hour) and electrolytes (0.5-0.7 g of sodium per liter of water).

After exercise

Achieve rapid and complete repletion of fluid, electrolytes, and carbohydrates lost during training and exercise. Each pound lost is equivalent to approximately 480 mL (~16 oz) of fluid.

Drink at least 150% or 2.5 cups of fluid for every pound lost through exercise to cover obligatory urine loss.

[a] General precaution: Alcohol is dehydrating. Avoid alcohol within 72 hours before or after training.

greater than skin temperature, children's greater surface area becomes a liability. An influx of heat results in greater heat absorption from the environment. In addition, children have less capacity for sweating, relying on dry means to dissipate heat, and they take longer to acclimatize to warm weather.[183-185] The difference in sweating rate widens with increasing exercise intensity or heat stress. These factors increase young athletes' risk for dehydration and heat illness. When children become dehydrated, their core temperatures increase faster than they do in dehydrated adults, underscoring the need for strict enforcement of hydration practices. Given the heightened risk of hyperthermia in children, the following precautions and practical measures should be taken:

- At 2 to 4 hours before exercise, young athletes should consume a fluid volume of 5 to 10 mL per kilogram of body weight to achieve urine that is pale yellow. Allow sufficient time for voiding.[141]
- For most athletes, an intake of 0.4 to 0.8 L/h will supply sufficient fluids to replace sweat losses to limit total body fluid losses to less than 2% of body weight. Approximately 3.5 to 6.75 oz of fluid should be consumed at least every 15 to 20 minutes during training and exercise in the heat, with fluid needs customized to the athlete's tolerance and experience.[141]
- Fluids should be cool and palatable to encourage drinking. In 1 study, grape was the preferred flavor and the flavor that encouraged the greatest rehydration following mild dehydration.[186]
- Overdrinking fluids in excess of sweat and urinary losses is the prime cause of hyponatremia (blood sodium <135 mmol/L), also known as water intoxication.
- When large sweat losses occur (>1.2 L/h), sodium should be ingested.
- In warm weather, individuals should avoid unnecessary layers of clothing. For example, soccer goalkeepers should remove the team jersey when wearing the goalkeeper shirt.
- Clothing should be made of wicking material. Sweat-drenched clothing should be replaced with dry clothing when possible.
- Athletes should reduce the intensity of exercise when the relative humidity and ambient temperature are high.

- Coaches should allow frequent breaks.
- Teams should provide shelter from direct sunlight during hot weather when players are on the sidelines.
- After exercise, effective rehydration requires a fluid intake 125% to 150% for every kilogram of body weight lost.[141]

SUPPLEMENTATION: ERGOGENIC AIDS IN HIGH INTENSITY, INTERMITTENT EXERCISE

Although the primary focus is on macronutrients and the use of whole foods to meet the energy demands of athletes engaged in HIIE, micronutrient supplementation and other ergogenic aids may offer potential benefits to such athletes. Caffeine, dietary nitrate, creatine monohydrate, β-alanine, and sodium bicarbonate each have potential roles in improving performance outcomes through increasing substrate availability, minimizing fatigue development, and/or improving aerobic efficiency. In summarizing the emerging literature in this "food first, but not food only" approach, Stecker et al[187] provided guidelines considering the timing and impact on exercise performance these aids may have, which are summarized in Table 21.5 on page 568. Calcium and iron and their potential benefits are also summarized alongside recommended dosing protocols. Practitioners should note that not every athlete will benefit from specific supplementation because of their current nutrient status, individualized issues related to digestive tolerance, and true physiological and genetic response (such as with CYP1A2, an enzyme that impacts caffeine metabolism, affecting individual ergogenic response). Athletes are encouraged to seek out a registered dietitian nutritionist (RDN) specializing in sports performance or a Board-Certified Specialist in Sports Dietetics (CSSD) to discuss whether and how they should appropriately incorporate these performance aids into their training and competition routines.

SUMMARY

HIIE athletes place significant strain on both the aerobic and anaerobic metabolic pathways to support the physiological demands of their sports. Although such athletes may spend a considerable amount of time engaged aerobically in low to moderate activity, the remaining activity can be spent near their anabolic threshold. This presents challenges in estimating energy demands for each athlete, as their level of training, level and timing of competition, aerobic fitness, age, sex, and other factors will impact their energy, fluid, and macronutrient requirements. Using energy availability equations and individualized assessment measures such as VO_2 max and heart rate data, if available, HIIE athletes and sports dietitians can get closer to identifying exact needs throughout the athlete's training calendar to optimize training and performance.

Carbohydrates continue to be a limiting factor in maintaining consistent performance outcomes in HIIE activity, especially for athletes who may not be fat-adapted. Increasing carbohydrate intake both before and during HIIE activities of longer duration delays the onset of fatigue and improves overall endurance in performance. Educating athletes on foundational nutrition concepts as well as the benefits of a carbohydrate-rich and balanced diet has been shown to benefit performance outcomes and prevent low energy availability and associated symptoms of fatigue resulting from poor dietary choices. Beyond dietary intervention through education on energy, macronutrient, fluid, and micronutrient targets, several performance aids may also be used to additionally support and enhance HIIE performance. Before employing such aids, however, an athlete should discuss individual considerations related to dosing, timing, and overall use within the athlete's current diet with a qualified nutrition professional.

TABLE 21.5 Timing Implications of Acute Supplement Administration

Nutrient/ dietary supplement	Mechanism of action	Purported benefit	Recommended dosing protocol
Documented evidence of timing benefit			
Caffeine	Adenosine receptor antagonist	↑ fat utilization ↑ mental drive ↑ performance ↓ perceptions of fatigue ↑ force production ↑ muscular endurance	*Time:* 2-0 h prior *Absolute dose:* 100-300 mg *Relative dose:* 3-6 mg per kilogram of body mass
Nitrates	↑ nitric oxide ↑ blood flow ↑ muscular contractility ↓ O_2 cost during aerobic exercise	↑ endurance ↑ intermittent exercise	*Time:* 2-3 h prior *Dose:* >5 mmol/serving
Creatine monohydrate	↑ PCr ↑ ATP	↑ high-intensity exercise capacity ↑ muscle mass ↑ strength	*Time:* 10-12 weeks *Absolute dose:* 5 g *Relative dose:* 0.1 g per kilogram of body mass
Iron	Oxygen transportation DNA synthesis Electron transportation	↑ aerobic performance ↑ oxygen carrying capacity	*Time:* 3-6 weeks *Dose:* 100 mg/d
Unexplored, but potential timing effect			
β-alanine	↑ production of carnosine	↑ high intensity exercise ↑ resistance training volume ↓ neuromuscular fatigue	*Time:* 4×/d *Dose:* 1.3-1.6 g (6-7 g/d)
Calcium	Muscular contraction Blunt ↑ levels of PTH	↑ bone density ↓ PTH levels	*Time:* 60 min prior to exercise for up to 12 months *Dose:* 1,000 mg/d
Sodium bicarbonate	↓ metabolic acidosis	↑ repeated sprints ↑ high intensity exercise	*Time:* 1-3 h prior *Relative dose:* 0.3 g per kilogram of body mass

Abbreviations: ATP, adenosine triphosphate, DNA, deoxyribonucleic acid; O_2, oxygen; PCr, phosphocreatine; PTH, parathyroid hormone
Adapted under CC BY 4.0 from reference 187: Stecker RA, Harty PS, Jagim AR, Candow DG, Kerksick CM. Timing of ergogenic aids and micronutrients on muscle and exercise performance. *J Int Soc Sports Nutr.* 2019:16(1):37. doi:10.1186/s12970-019-0304-9

KEY TAKEAWAYS

The stop-and-go nature of HIIE sports places great physiological and metabolic demands on the body and involves all 3 energy systems. These sports require bursts of all-out effort interspersed with periods of moderate- and low-intensity effort.

The primary goal of nutrition in HIIE sports is to support peak performance by ensuring adequate amounts of energy and nutrients, the right blend of fuel for a given effort, adequate hydration, and a plan for the rapid replacement of fluids and muscle glycogen. Coaches and trainers must take precautions to avoid or minimize the pitfalls of HIIE, such as fatigue, hypoglycemia, impaired performance, and dehydration and its consequences.

Carbohydrate is the preferred fuel for much of the work in stop-and-go sports. It is crucial to supply sufficient intakes of carbohydrate before, during, and after exercise to ensure adequate energy availability to support training, performance, and recovery. The general carbohydrate recommendation is 7 g per kilogram of body weight per day, with a range from 7 to 12 g per kilogram of body weight per day during training and competition. Both the timing of ingestion and the amount of carbohydrate help fuel the athlete and enhance their endurance and power.

The recommended daily protein intake is 1.2 to 2.0 g per kilogram of body weight per day. Higher intakes may be indicated during periods of intense training, reduced energy intake, or a prolonged period until the next feeding. Protein intake after exercise should be individualized to optimize muscle protein synthesis. Excessive protein intake, generally above 2 g per kilogram of body weight per day, has not been shown to provide additional benefits and may limit carbohydrate intake.

The percentage of total energy consumed as fat is best set within the guideline of 20% to 35% and should be determined after carbohydrate and protein needs are established. Heart-healthy fats should be stressed to limit saturated fats to less than 10% of total energy.

Sports nutritionists should educate HIIE athletes to carefully choose nutrient-rich foods that also provide ample vitamins and minerals essential for health and fuel production and to support training adaptations and recovery.

Fluid intake is critical, especially because many HIIE sports are played in hot and humid conditions. Hydration strategies should be planned to replace fluid and sodium lost in sweat as soon after exercise as possible.

REFERENCES

1. Holway FE, Spriet LL. Sport-specific nutrition: practical strategies for team sports. *J Sports Sci.* 2011;29(suppl 1):S115-S125. doi:10.1080/02640414.2011.605459
2. Rampinini E, Impellizzeri FM, Castagna C, Coutts AJ, Wisløff U. Technical performance during soccer matches of the Italian Serie A league: effect of fatigue and competitive level. *J Sci Med Sport.* 2009;12(1):227-233. doi:10.1016/j.jsams.2007.10.002
3. Vigh-Larsen JF, Ermidis G, Rago V, et al. Muscle metabolism and fatigue during simulated ice hockey match-play in elite players. *Med Sci Sports Exerc.* 2020;52(10):2162-2171. doi:10.1249/MSS.0000000000002370
4. Bradley WJ, Cavanagh B, Douglas W, et al. Energy intake and expenditure assessed 'in-season' in an elite European rugby union squad. *Eur J Sport Sci.* 2015;15(6):469-479. doi:10.1080/17461391.2015.1042528
5. Reilly T, Thomas V. A motion analysis of work rate in different positional roles in professional football match play. *J Hum Mov Stud.* 1976;2(2):87-97.
6. Pincivero DM, Bompa TO. A physiological review of American football. *Sports Med.* 1997;23(4):247-260. doi:10.2165/00007256-199723040-00004
7. Mujika I, Burke LM. Nutrition in team sports. *Ann Nutr Metab.* 2010;57(suppl 2):26-35. doi:10.1159/000322700
8. Bangsbo J, Nørregaard L, Thorsø F. Activity profile of competition soccer. *Can J Sport Sci.* 1991;16(2):110-116.
9. Carling C, Dupont G. Are declines in physical performance associated with a reduction in skill-related performance during professional soccer match-play? *J Sports Sci.* 2011;29(1):63-71. doi:10.1080/02640414.2010.521945
10. Danielik K, Książek A, Zagrodna A, Słowińska-Lisowska M. How do male football players meet dietary recommendations? A systematic literature review. *Int J Environ Res Public Health.* 2022;19(15):9561. doi:10.3390/ijerph19159561
11. Macuh M, Levec J, Kojić N, Knap B. Dietary intake, body composition and performance of professional football athletes in Slovenia. *Nutrients.* 2023;15(1):82. doi:10.3390/nu15010082
12. Cox MH, Miles DS, Verde TJ, Rhodes EC. Applied physiology of ice hockey. *Sports Med.* 1995;19(3):184-201. doi:10.2165/00007256-199519030-00004
13. Rago V, Muschinsky A, Deylami K, Vigh-Larsen JF, Mohr M. Game demands of a professional ice hockey team with special emphasis on fatigue development and playing position. *J Hum Kinet.* 2022;84:195-205. doi:10.2478/hukin-2022-000078
14. García-Rovés PM, García-Zapico P, Patterson AM, Iglesias-Gutiérrez E. Nutrient intake and food habits of soccer players: analyzing the correlates of eating practice. *Nutrients.* 2014;6(7):2697-2717. doi:10.3390/nu6072697
15. Gibson JC, Stuart-Hill L, Martin S, Gaul C. Nutrition status of junior elite Canadian female soccer athletes. *Int J Sport Nutr Exerc Metab.* 2011;21(6):507-514. doi:10.1123/ijsnem.21.6.507
16. Gravina L, Ruiz F, Diaz E, et al. Influence of nutrient intake on antioxidant capacity, muscle damage and white blood cell count in female soccer players. *J Int Soc Sports Nutr.* 2012;9(1):32. doi:10.1186/1550-2783-9-32
17. Iglesias-Gutiérrez E, García A, García-Zapico P, et al. Is there a relationship between the playing position of soccer players and their food and macronutrient intake? *Appl Physiol Nutr Metab.* 2012;37(2):225-232. doi:10.1139/h11-152
18. Maroon JC, Mathyssek CM, Bost JW, et al. Vitamin D profile in National Football League players. *Am J Sports Med.* 2015;43(5):1241-1245. doi:10.1177/0363546514567297
19. Martínez Reñón C, Sánchez Collado P. Nutritional study of a third division soccer team. Article in Spanish. *Nutr Hosp.* 2013;28(2):319-324. doi:10.3305/nh.2013.28.2.6304
20. Ono M, Kennedy E, Reeves S, Cronin L. Nutrition and culture in professional football. A mixed method approach. *Appetite.* 2012;58(1):98-104. doi:10.1016/j.appet.2011.10.007
21. Russell M, Pennock A. Dietary analysis of young professional soccer players for 1 week during the competitive season. *J Strength Cond Res.* 2011;25(7):1816-1823. doi:10.1519/JSC.0b013e3181e7fbdd
22. Santos DA, Matias CN, Monteiro CP, et al. Magnesium intake is associated with strength performance in elite basketball, handball and volleyball players. *Magnes Res.* 2011;24(4):215-219. doi:10.1684/mrh.2011.0290
23. Shriver LH, Betts NM, Wollenberg G. Dietary intakes and eating habits of college athletes: are female college athletes following the current sports nutrition standards? *J Am Coll Health.* 2013;61(1):10-16. doi:10.1080/07448481.2012.747526
24. Valliant MW, Emplaincourt HP, Wenzel RK, Garner BH. Nutrition education by a registered dietitian improves dietary intake and nutrition knowledge of a NCAA female volleyball team. *Nutrients.* 2012;4(6):506-516. doi:10.3390/nu4060506
25. Zapolska J, Witczak K, Mańczuk A, Ostrowska L. Assessment of nutrition, supplementation and body composition parameters on the example of professional volleyball players. *Rocz Panstw Zakl Hig.* 2014;65(3):235-242.
26. Gabbett T, King T, Jenkins D. Applied physiology of rugby league. *Sports Med.* 2008;38(2):119-138. doi:10.2165/00007256-200838020-00003
27. Bangsbo J. Energy demands in competitive soccer. *J Sports Sci.* 1994;12(spec no):S5-S12.
28. Ben Abdelkrim N, El Fazaa S, El Ati J. Time-motion analysis and physiological data of elite under-19-year-old basketball players during competition. *Br J Sports Med.* 2007;41(2):69-75. doi:10.1136/bjsm.2006.032318
29. Sheppard JM, Gabbett TJ, Stanganelli LC. An analysis of playing positions in elite men's volleyball: considerations for competition demands and physiologic characteristics. *J Strength Cond Res.* 2009;23(6):1858-1866. doi:10.1519/JSC.0b013e3181b45c6a
30. Withers RT, Maricic Z, Wasilewski S, Kelly L. Match analyses of Australian professional soccer players. *J Hum Mov Stud.* 1982;8(4):159-176.

31. Ekblom B. Applied physiology of soccer. *Sports Med.* 1986;3(1):50-60. doi:10.2165/00007256-198603010-00005

32. Reilly T. Energetics of high-intensity exercise (soccer) with particular reference to fatigue. *J Sports Sci.* 1997;15(3):257-263. doi:10.1080/026404197367263

33. Bangsbo J. The physiology of soccer—with special reference to intense intermittent exercise. *Acta Physiol Scand Suppl.* 1994;619:1-155.

34. Drust B, Reilly T, Rienzi E. Analysis of work rate in soccer. *Sports Exerc Inj.* 1988;4(4):151-155.

35. Shephard RJ. Biology and medicine of soccer: an update. *J Sport Sci.* 1999;17(10):757-786. doi:10.1080/026404199365498

36. Bangsbo J, Mohr M, Krustrup P. Physical and metabolic demands of training and match-play in the elite football player. *J Sports Sci.* 2006;24(7):665-674. doi:10.1080/02640410500482529

37. McArdle WD, Katch VL. *Exercise Physiology: Nutrition, Energy, and Human Performance.* 6th ed. Lippincott Williams & Wilkins; 200

38. Ben Abdelkrim N, Chaouachi A, Chamari K, Chtara M, Castagna C. Positional role and competitive-level differences in elite-level men's basketball players. *J Strength Cond Res.* 2010;24(5):1346-1355. doi:10.1519/JSC.0b013e3181cf7510

39. Mohr M, Krustrup P, Bangsbo J. Fatigue in soccer: a brief review. *J Sports Sci.* 2005;23(6):593-599. doi:10.1080/02640410400021286

40. Mohr M, Krustrup P, Andersson H, Kirkendal D, Bangsbo J. Match activities of elite women soccer players at different performance levels. *J Strength Cond Res.* 2008;22(2):341-349. doi:10.1519/JSC.0b013e318165fef6

41. Krustrup P, Zebis M, Jensen JM, Mohr M. Game-induced fatigue patterns in elite female soccer. *J Strength Cond Res.* 2010;24(2):437-441. doi:10.1519/JSC.0b013e3181c09b79

42. Bangsbo J, Iaia FM, Krustrup P. Metabolic response and fatigue in soccer. *Int J Sports Physiol Perform.* 2007;2(2):111-127. doi:10.1123/ijspp.2.2.111

43. Bradley PS, Di Mascio M, Peart D, Olsen P, Sheldon B. High-intensity activity profiles of elite soccer players at different performance levels. *J Strength Cond Res.* 2010;24(9):2343-2351. doi:10.1519/JSC.0b013e3181aeb1b3

44. Abt G, Siegler JC, Akubat I, Castagna C. The effects of a constant sprint-to-rest ratio and recovery mode on repeated sprint performance. *J Strength Cond Res.* 2011;25(6):1695-1702. doi:10.1519/JSC.0b013e3181dbdc06

45. Krustrup P, Mohr M, Ellingsgaard H, Bangsbo J. Physical demands during an elite female soccer game: importance of training status. *Med Sci Sports Exerc.* 2005;37(7):1242-1248. doi:10.1249/01.mss.0000170062.73981.94

46. Reilly T, Thomas V. Estimated daily energy expenditures of professional association footballers. *Ergonomics.* 1979;22(5):541-548. doi:10.1080/00140137908924638

47. Bradley PS, Dellal A, Mohr M, Castellano J, Wilkie A. Gender differences in match performance characteristics of soccer players competing in the UEFA Champions League. *Hum Mov Sci.* 2014;33:159-171. doi:10.1016/j.humov.2013.07.024

48. Mohr M, Krustrup P, Bangsbo J. Match performance of high-standard soccer players with special reference to development of fatigue. *J Sports Sci.* 2003;21(7):519-528. doi:10.1080/0264041031000071182

49. Peterson BJ, Fitzgerald JS, Dietz CC, et al. Aerobic capacity is associated with improved repeated shift performance in hockey. *J Strength Cond Res.* 2015;29(6):1465-1472. doi:10.1519/JSC.0000000000000786

50. Romijn JA, Coyle EF, Sidossis LS, et al. Regulation of endogenous fat and carbohydrate metabolism in relation to exercise intensity and duration. *Am J Physiol.* 1993;265(3 pt 1):E380-E391. doi:10.1152/ajpendo.1993.265.3.E380

51. Roberts TJ, Weber JM, Hoppeler H, Weibel ER, Taylor CR. Design of the oxygen and substrate pathways. II. Defining the upper limits of carbohydrate and fat oxidation. *J Exp Biol.* 1996;199(pt 8):1651-1658. doi:10.1242/jeb.199.8.1651

52. Vigh-Larsen JF, Ørtenblad N, Spriet LL, Overgaard K, Mohr M. Muscle glycogen metabolism and high-intensity exercise performance: a narrative review. *Sports Med.* 2021;51(9):1855-1874. doi:10.1007/s40279-021-01475-0

53. Jacobs I, Westin N, Karlsson J, Rasmusson M, Houghton B. Muscle glycogen and diet in elite soccer players. *Eur J Appl Physiol.* 1982;48(3):297-302. doi:10.1007/BF00430219

54. Tumilty D. Physiological characteristics of elite soccer players. *Sports Med.* 1993;16(2):80-96. doi:10.2165/00007256-199316020-00002

55. Gollnick PD, Armstrong RB, Sembrowich WL, Shepherd RE, Saltin B. Glycogen depletion pattern in human skeletal muscle fibers after heavy exercise. *J Appl Physiol.* 1973;34(5):615-618. doi:10.1152/jappl.1973.34.5.615

56. Costill D, Gollnick PD, Jansson ED, Saltin B, Stein EM. Glycogen depletion pattern in human muscle fibers during distance running. *Acta Physiol Scand.* 1973;89(3):374-383. doi:10.1111/j.1748-1716.1973.tb05532.x

57. Gollnick PD, Piehl K, Saubert CW IV, Armstrong RB, Saltin B. Diet, exercise, and glycogen changes in human muscle fibers. *J Appl Physiol.* 1972;33(4):421-425. doi:10.1152/jappl.1972.33.4.421

58. Brooks G, Mercier J. Balance of carbohydrate and lipid utilization during exercise: the "crossover" concept. *J Appl Physiol (1985).* 1994;76(6):2253-2261. doi:10.1152/jappl.1994.76.6.2253

59. Green HJ. Glycogen depletion patterns during continuous and intermittent ice skating. *Med Sci Sports.* 1978;10(3):183-187.

60. Krustrup P, Mohr M, Steensberg A, Bencke J, Kjaer M, Bangsbo J. Muscle and blood metabolites during a soccer game: implications for sprint performance. *Med Sci Sports Exerc.* 2006;38(6):1165-1174. doi:10.1249/01.mss.0000222845.89262.cd

61. Brooks GA. Importance of the "crossover" concept in exercise metabolism. *Clin Exp Pharmacol Physiol.* 1997; 24(11):889-895. doi:10.1111/j.1440-1681.1997.tb02712.x

62. Coggan AR, Kohrt WM, Spina RJ, Bier DM, Holloszy JO. Endurance training decreases plasma glucose turnover and oxidation during moderate-intensity exercise in men. *J Appl Physiol (1985).* 1990;68(3):990-996. doi:10.1152/jappl.1990.68.3.990

63. Hurley BF, Nemeth PM, Martin WH III, Hagberg JM, Dalsky GP, Holloszy JO. Muscle triglyceride utilization during exercise: effect of training. *J Appl Physiol (1985).* 1986;60(2):562-567. doi:10.1152/jappl.1986.60.2.562

64. Sidossis LS, Gastaldelli A, Klein S, Wolfe RR. Regulation of plasma fatty acid oxidation during low- and high-intensity exercise. *Am J Physiol.* 1997;272(6 pt 1):E1065-E1070. doi:10.1152/ajpendo.1997.272.6.E1065

65. Lemon PW, Mullin JP. Effect of initial muscle glycogen levels on protein catabolism during exercise. *J Appl Physiol Respir Environ Exerc Physiol.* 1980;48(4):624-629. doi:10.1152/jappl.1980.48.4.624
66. Packer JE, Wooding DJ, Kato H, Courtney-Martin G, Pencharz PB, Moore DR. Variable-intensity simulated team-sport exercise increases daily protein requirements in active males. *Front Nutr.* 2017;4:64. doi:10.3389/fnut.2017.00064
67. Ramadoss R, Stanzione JR, Volpe SL. A comparison of substrate utilization profiles during maximal and submaximal exercise tests in athletes. *Front Psychol.* 2022;13:854451. doi:10.3389/fpsyg.2022.854451
68. Orendurff MS, Walker JD, Jovanovic M, Tulchin KL, Levy M, Hoffmann DK. Intensity and duration of intermittent exercise and recovery during a soccer match. *J Strength Cond Res.* 2010;24(10):2683-2692. doi:10.1519/JSC.0b013e3181bac463
69. Smodlaka VN. Cardiovascular aspects of soccer. *Phys Sportsmed.* 1978;6(7):66-70. doi:10.1080/00913847.1978.11948391
70. Montgomery DL. Physiology of ice hockey. *Sports Med.* 1988;5(2):99-126. doi:10.2165/00007256-198805020-00003
71. Stanula AJ, Gabryś TT, Roczniok RK, Szmatlan-Gabryś UB, Ozimek MJ, Mostowik AJ. Quantification of the demands during an ice-hockey game based on intensity zones determined from the incremental test outcomes. *J Strength Cond Res.* 2016;30(1):176-183. doi:10.1519/JSC.0000000000001081
72. Smekal G, von Duvillard SP, Rihacek C, et al. A physiological profile of tennis match play. *Med Sci Sports Exerc.* 2001;33(6):999-1005. doi:10.1097/00005768-200106000-00020
73. Yagüe PL, Del Valle ME, Egocheaga J, Linnamo V, Fernández A. The competitive demands of elite male rink hockey. *Biol Sport.* 2013;30(3):195-199. doi:10.5604/20831862.1059211
74. Sirotic AC, Coutts AJ, Knowles H, Catterick C. A comparison of match demands between elite and semi-elite rugby league competition. *J Sports Sci.* 2009;27(3):203-211. doi:10.1080/02640410802520802
75. McInnes SE, Carlson JS, Jones CJ, McKenna MJ. The physiological load imposed on basketball players during competition. *J Sports Sci.* 1995;13(5):387-397. doi:10.1080/02640419508732254
76. Akermark C, Jacobs I, Rasmusson M, Karlsson J. Diet and muscle glycogen concentration in relation to physical performance in Swedish elite ice hockey players. *Int J Sport Nutr.* 1996;6(3):272-284. doi:10.1123/ijsn.6.3.272
77. Bergeron MF, Maresh CM, Kraemer WJ, Abraham A, Conroy B, Gabaree C. Tennis: a physiological profile during match play. *Int J Sports Med.* 1991;12(5):474-479. doi:10.1055/s-2007-1024716
78. Therminarias A, Dansou P, Chirpaz-Oddou MF, Gharib C, Quirion A. Hormonal and metabolic changes during a strenuous match: effect of ageing. *Int J Sports Med.* 1991;12(1):10-16. doi:10.1055/s-2007-1024647
79. Docherty D. A comparison of heart rate responses in racquet games. *Br J Sports Med.* 1982;16(2):96-100. doi:10.1136/bjsm.16.2.96
80. Bracken RM, Linnane DM, Brooks S. Plasma catecholamine and nephrine responses to brief intermittent maximal intensity exercise. *Amino Acids.* 2009;36(2):209-217. doi:10.1007/s00726-008-0049-2
81. Trapp EG, Chisholm DJ, Boutcher SH. Metabolic response of trained and untrained women during high-intensity intermittent cycle exercise. *Am J Physiol Regul Integr Comp Physiol.* 2007;293(6):R2370-R2375. doi:10.1152/ajpregu.00780.2006
82. Dostal T, Plews DJ, Hofmann P, Laursen PB, Cipryan L. Effects of a 12-week very-low carbohydrate high-fat diet on maximal aerobic capacity, high-intensity intermittent exercise, and cardiac autonomic regulation: non-randomized parallel-group study. *Front Physiol.* 2019;10:912. doi:10.3389/fphys.2019.00912
83. Martin WH III, Dalsky GP, Hurley BF, et al. Effect of endurance training on plasma free fatty acid turnover and oxidation during exercise. *Am J Physiol.* 1993;265(5 pt 1):E708-E714. doi:10.1152/ajpendo.1993.265.5.E708
84. Weber J, Brichon G, Zwingelstein G, et al. Design of the oxygen and substrate pathways. IV. Partitioning energy provision from fatty acids. *J Exp Biol.* 1996;199(pt 8):1667-1674. doi:10.1242/jeb.199.8.1667
85. Bendiksen M, Bischoff R, Randers MB, et al. The Copenhagen Soccer Test: physiological response and fatigue development. *Med Sci Sports Exerc.* 2012;44(8):1595-1603. doi:10.1249/MSS.0b013e31824cc23b
86. Welsh RS, Davis JM, Burke JR, Williams HG. Carbohydrates and physical/mental performance during intermittent exercise to fatigue. *Med Sci Sports Exerc.* 2002;34(4):723-731. doi:10.1097/00005768-200204000-00025
87. Newsholme EA, Blomstrand E, Ekblom B. Physical and mental fatigue: metabolic mechanisms and importance of plasma amino acids. *Br Med Bull.* 1992;48(3):477-495. doi:10.1093/oxfordjournals.bmb.a072558
88. Bergström J, Hermansen L, Hultman E, Saltin B. Diet, muscle glycogen and physical performance. *Acta Physiol Scand.* 1967;71(2):140-150. doi:10.1111/j.1748-1716.1967.tb03720.x
89. Winnick JJ, Davis JM, Welsh RS, Carmichael MD, Murphy EA, Blackmon JA. Carbohydrate feedings during team sport exercise preserve physical and CNS function. *Med Sci Sports Exerc.* 2005;37(2):306-315. doi:10.1249/01.mss.0000152803.35130.a4
90. Tomlin DL, Wenger HA. The relationship between aerobic fitness and recovery from high-intensity intermittent exercise. *Sports Med.* 2001;31(1):1-11. doi:10.2165/00007256-200131010-00001
91. Brooks GA. Current concepts in lactate exchange. *Med Sci Sports Exerc.* 1991;2(8):895-906.
92. Matthew D, Delextrat A. Heart rate, blood lactate concentration, and time-motion analysis of female basketball players during competition. *J Sports Sci.* 2009;27(8):813-821. doi:10.1080/02640410902926420
93. Scanlan AT, Dascombe BJ, Reaburn P, Dalbo VJ. The physiological and activity demands experienced by Australian female basketball players during competition. *J Sci Med Sport.* 2012;15(4):341-347. doi:10.1016/j.jsams.2011.12.008

94. Mota JA, Nuckols G, Smith-Ryan AE. Nutritional periodization: applications for the strength athlete. *Strength Cond J.* 2019;41(5):69-78. doi:10.1519/ssc.0000000000000488
95. Dobrowolski H, Karczemna A, Włodarek D. Nutrition for female soccer players—recommendations. *Medicina (Kaunas).* 2020;56(1):28. doi:10.3390/medicina56010028
96. Williams C, Nicholas CW. Nutrition needs for team sport. *Sport Sci Exch.* 1998;11(3):70.
97. da Silva HS, Nakamura FY, Papoti M, da Silva AS, Dos-Santos JW. Relationship between heart rate, oxygen consumption, and energy expenditure in futsal. *Front Psychol.* 2021;12:698622. doi:10.3389/fpsyg.2021.698622
98. Stølen T, Chamari K, Castagna C, Wisløff U. Physiology of soccer: an update. *Sports Med.* 2005;35(6):501-536. doi:10.2165/00007256-200535060-00004
99. Clark K. Nutritional guidance to soccer players for training and competition. *J Sports Sci.* 1994;12(spec no):S43-S50.
100. Brewer J. Nutritional aspects of women's soccer. *J Sports Sci.* 1994;12(spec no):S35-S38.
101. Economos CD, Bortz SS, Nelson ME. Nutritional practices of elite athletes. Practical recommendations. *Sports Med.* 1993;16(6):381-399. doi:10.2165/00007256-199316060-00004
102. Clark M, Reed DB, Crouse SF, Armstrong RB. Pre- and post-season dietary intake, body composition, and performance indices of NCAA division I female soccer players. *Int J Sport Nutr Exerc Metab.* 2003;13(3):303-319. doi:10.1123/ijsnem.13.3.303
103. Boisseau N, Le Creff C, Loyens M, Poortmans JR. Protein intake and nitrogen balance in male non-active adolescents and soccer players. *Eur J Appl Physiol.* 2002;88(3):288-293. doi:10.1007/s00421-002-0726-x
104. Boisseau N, Vermorel M, Rance M, Duché P, Patureau-Mirand P. Protein requirements in male adolescent soccer players. *Eur J Appl Physiol.* 2007;100(1):27-33. doi:10.1007/s00421-007-0400-4
105. Iglesias-Gutiérrez E, Garcıa-Rovés P, García A, Patterson AM. Food preferences do not influence adolescent high-level athletes' dietary intake. *Appetite.* 2008;50(2-3):536-543. doi:10.1016/j.appet.2007.11.003
106. Noda Y, Iide K, Masuda R, et al. Nutrient intake and blood iron status of male collegiate soccer players. *Asia Pac J Clin Nutr.* 2009;18(3):344-350.
107. Mielgo-Ayuso J, Zourdos MC, Calleja-Gonzalez J, Urdampilleta A, Ostojic SM. Dietary intake habits and controlled training on body composition and strength in elite female volleyball players during the season. *Appl Physiol Nutr Metab.* 2015;40(8):827-834. doi:10.1139/apnm-2015-0100
108. Papadopoulou SK, Papadopoulou SD. Nutritional status of top team-sport athletes according to body fat. *Nutr Food Sci.* 2010;40(1):64-73. doi:10.1108/00346651011015935
109. Nikic M, Pedišic Z, Šatalic Z, Jakovljevic S, Venus D. Adequacy of nutrient intakes in elite junior basketball players. *Int J Sport Nutr Exerc Metab.* 2014;24(5):516-523. doi:10.1123/ijsnem.2013-0186
110. Gomez-Hixson K, Biagioni E, Brown ML. Significant differences in dietary intake of NCAA Division III soccer players compared to recommended levels. *J Am Coll Health.* 2022;70(1):150-157. doi:10.1080/07448481.2020.1728279
111. Nutter J. Seasonal changes in female athletes' diets. *Int J Sport Nutr.* 1991;1(4):395-407. doi:10.1123/ijsn.1.4.395
112. Papadopoulou SK, Papadopoulou SD, Gallos GK. Macro- and micro-nutrient intake of adolescent Greek female volleyball players. *Int J Sport Nutr Exerc Metab.* 2002;12(1):73-80. doi:10.1123/ijsnem.12.1.73
113. Briggs MA, Cockburn E, Rumbold PL, Rae G, Stevenson EJ, Russell M. Assessment of energy intake and energy expenditure of male adolescent academy-level soccer players during a competitive week. *Nutrients.* 2015;7(10):8392-8401. doi:10.3390/nu7105400
114. Condo D, Lohman R, Kelly M, Carr A. Nutritional intake, sports nutrition knowledge and energy availability in female Australian rules football players. *Nutrients.* 2019;11(5):971. doi:10.3390/nu11050971
115. Maughan RJ, Greenhaff PL, Leiper JB, Ball D, Lambert CP, Gleeson M. Diet composition and the performance of high-intensity exercise. *J Sports Sci.* 1997;15(3):265-275. doi:10.1080/026404197367272
116. Hawley JA, Tipton KD, Millard-Stafford ML. Promoting training adaptations through nutritional interventions. *J Sports Sci.* 2006;24(7):709-721. doi:10.1080/02640410500482727
117. Phillips SM, Sproule J, Turner AP. Carbohydrate ingestion during team games exercise: current knowledge and areas for future investigation. *Sports Med.* 2011;41(7):559-585. doi:10.2165/11589150-000000000-00000
118. Bangsbo J, Nørregaard L, Thorsø F. The effect of carbohydrate diet on intermittent exercise performance. *Int J Sports Med.* 1992;13(2):152-157. doi:10.1055/s-2007-1021247
119. Nordheim K, Vollestad NK. Glycogen and lactate metabolism during low-intensity exercise in man. *Acta Physiol Scand.* 1990;139(3):475-484. doi:10.1111/j.1748-1716.1990.tb08949.x
120. Saltin B. Metabolic fundamentals in exercise. *Med Sci Sports Exerc.* 1973;5(3):137-146.
121. Kirkendall DT. Effects of nutrition on performance in soccer. *Med Sci Sports Exerc.* 1993;25(12):1370-1374.
122. Burke LM, Hawley JA, Wong SH, Jeukendrup AE. Carbohydrates for training and competition. *J Sports Sci.* 2011;29(suppl 1):S17-S27. doi:10.1080/02640414.2011.585473
123. Coyle EF. Substrate utilization during exercise in active people. *Am J Clin Nutr.* 1995;61(suppl 4):968S-979S. doi:10.1093/ajcn/61.4.968S
124. Ferrauti A, Pluim BM, Busch T, Weber K. Blood glucose responses and incidence of hypoglycaemia in elite tennis under practice and tournament conditions. *J Sci Med Sport.* 2003;6(1):28-39. doi:10.1016/s1440-2440(03)80006-3
125. Hargreaves M. Carbohydrate and lipid requirements of soccer. *J Sports Sci.* 1994;12(spec no):S13-S16.
126. Ali A, Williams C, Nicholas C, Foskett A. The influence of carbohydrate-electrolyte ingestion on soccer skill performance. *Med Sci Sports Exerc.* 2007;39(11):1969-1976. doi:10.1249/mss.0b013e31814fb3e3
127. Kingsley M, Penas-Ruiz C, Terry C, Russell M. Effects of carbohydrate-hydration strategies on glucose metabolism, sprint performance and hydration during a soccer match simulation in recreational players. *J Sci Med Sport.* 2014;17(2):239-243. doi:10.1016/j.jsams.2013.04.010

128. Davison GW, McClean C, Brown J, et al. The effects of ingesting a carbohydrate-electrolyte beverage 15 minutes prior to high-intensity exercise performance. *Res Sports Med.* 2008;16(3):155-166. doi:10.1080/15438620802103155
129. Phillips SM, Turner AP, Gray S, Sanderson MF, Sproule J. Ingesting a 6% carbohydrate-electrolyte solution improves endurance capacity, but not sprint performance, during intermittent, high-intensity shuttle running in adolescent team games players aged 12-14 years. *Eur J Appl Physiol.* 2010;109(5):811-821. doi:10.1007/s00421-010-1404-z
130. Russell M, Benton D, Kingsley M. The effects of fatigue on soccer skills performed during a soccer match simulation. *Int J Sports Physiol Perform.* 2011;6(2):221-233. doi:10.1123/ijspp.6.2.221
131. Russell M, Benton D, Kingsley M. Influence of carbohydrate supplementation on skill performance during a soccer match simulation. *J Sci Med Sport.* 2012;15(4):348-354. doi:10.1016/j.jsams.2011.12.006
132. Russell M, Benton D, Kingsley M. Carbohydrate ingestion before and during soccer match play and blood glucose and lactate concentrations. *J Athl Train.* 2014;49(4):447-453. doi:10.4085/1062-6050-49.3.12
133. Harper LD, Briggs MA, McNamee G, et al. Physiological and performance effects of carbohydrate gels consumed prior to the extra-time period of prolonged simulated soccer match-play. *J Sci Med Sport.* 2015;19(6):509-514. doi:10.1016/j.jsams.2015.06.009
134. Jeukendrup AE. Carbohydrate and exercise performance: the role of multiple transportable carbohydrates. *Curr Opin Clin Nutr Metab Care.* 2010;13(4):452-457. doi:10.1097/MCO.0b013e328339de9f
135. Jeukendrup A. A step towards personalized sports nutrition: carbohydrate intake during exercise. *Sports Med.* 2014;44(suppl 1):S25-S33. doi:10.1007/s40279-014-0148-z
136. Baker LB, Rollo I, Stein KW, Jeukendrup AE. Acute effects of carbohydrate supplementation on intermittent sports performance. *Nutrients.* 2015;7(7):5733-5763. doi:10.3390/nu7075249
137. Phillips SM. Carbohydrate supplementation and prolonged intermittent high-intensity exercise in adolescents: research findings, ethical issues and suggestions for the future. *Sports Med.* 2012;42(10):817-828. doi:10.1007/BF03262296
138. Burke LM, Cox GR, Cummings NK, Desbrow B. Guidelines for daily carbohydrate intake: do athletes achieve them? *Sports Med.* 2001;31(4):267-299. doi:10.2165/00007256-200131040-00003
139. Burke LM. Fueling strategies to optimize performance: training high or training low? *Scand J Med Sci Sports.* 2010;20(suppl 2):48-58. doi:10.1111/j.1600-0838.2010.01185.x
140. Cermak NM, van Loon LJC. The use of carbohydrates during exercise as an ergogenic aid. *Sports Med.* 2013;43(11):1139-1155. doi:10.1007/s40279-013-0079-0
141. Thomas DT, Erdman KA, Burke LM. Position of the Academy of Nutrition and Dietetics, Dietitians of Canada, and the American College of Sports Medicine: nutrition and athletic performance. *J Acad Nutr Diet.* 2016;116(3):501-528. doi:10.1016/j.jand.2015.12.006
142. Tarnopolsky MA, Atkinson SA, Phillips SM, MacDougall JD. Carbohydrate loading and metabolism during exercise in men and women. *J Appl Physiol (1985).* 1995;78(4):1360-1368. doi:10.1152/jappl.1995.78.4.1360
143. Hearris M, Hammond K, Fell J, Morton J. Regulation of muscle glycogen metabolism during exercise: implications for endurance performance and training adaptations. *Nutrients.* 2018;10(3):298. doi:10.3390/nu10030298
144. Beaven CM, Maulder P, Pooley A, Kilduff L, Cook C. Effects of caffeine and carbohydrate mouth rinses on repeated sprint performance. *Appl Physiol Nutr Metab.* 2013;38(6):633-637. doi:10.1139/apnm-2012-0333
145. Ivy JL. Optimization of glycogen stores. In: Maughan RJ, ed. *Nutrition in Sport.* Blackwell Science; 2000:97-111.
146. Mondazzi L, Arcelli E. Glycemic index in sport nutrition. *J Am Coll Nutr.* 2009;28(suppl):455S-463S. doi:10.1080/07315724.2009.10718112
147. Burke LM, Collier GR, Davis PG, Fricker PA, Sanigorski AJ, Hargreaves M. Muscle glycogen storage after prolonged exercise: effect of the frequency of carbohydrate feedings. *Am J Clin Nutr.* 1996;64(1):115-119. doi:10.1093/ajcn/64.1.115
148. Rankin J. Glycemic index and exercise metabolism. *Sports Sci Exch.* 1997;10(1):64.
149. Burke LM, Hargreaves M, Collier GR. Muscle glycogen storage after prolonged exercise: effect of the glycemic index of carbohydrate feedings. *J Appl Physiol (1985).* 1993;75(2):1019-1023. doi:10.1152/jappl.1993.75.2.1019
150. Coyle EE. Timing and method of increased carbohydrate intake to cope with heavy training, competition and recovery. *J Sports Sci.* 1991;9(spec no):29-51; discussion 51-52. doi:10.1080/02640419108729865
151. Evans WJ, Fisher EC, Hoerr RA, Young VR. Protein metabolism and endurance exercise. *Phys Sports Med.* 1983;11(7):63-162. doi:10.1080/00913847.1983.11708585
152. Lemon PW, Mullin JP. Effect of initial muscle glycogen levels on protein catabolism during exercise. *J Appl Physiol Respir Environ Exerc Physiol.* 1980;48(4):624-629. doi:10.1152/jappl.1980.48.4.624
153. Lemon PW. Protein requirements of soccer. *J Sports Sci.* 1994;12(spec no):S17-S22.
154. Ivy JL, Goforth HW Jr, Damon BM, McCauley TR, Parsons EC, Price TB. Early postexercise muscle glycogen recovery is enhanced with a carbohydrate-protein supplement. *J Appl Physiol (1985).* 2002;93(4):1337-1344. doi:10.1152/japplphysiol.00394.2002
155. Davis JM, Welsh RS, De Volve KA, Alderson NL. Effects of branched-chain amino acids and carbohydrate on fatigue during intermittent, high-intensity running. *Int J Sports Med.* 1999;20(5):309-314. doi:10.1055/s-2007-971136
156. Lemon PW. Beyond the zone: protein needs of active individuals. *J Am Coll Nutr.* 2000;19(5 suppl):513S-521S. doi:10.1080/07315724.2000.10718974
157. Gunnarsson TP, Bendiksen M, Bischoff R, et al. Effect of whey protein- and carbohydrate-enriched diet on glycogen resynthesis during the first 48 h after a soccer game. *Scand J Med Sci Sports.* 2013;23(4):508-515. doi:10.1111/j.1600-0838.2011.01418.x
158. Stellingwerff T, Spriet LL, Watt MJ, et al. Decreased PDH activation and glycogenolysis during exercise following fat adaptation with carbohydrate restoration. *Am J Physiol Endocrinol Metab.* 2006;290(2):E380-E388. doi:10.1152/ajpendo.00268.2005

159. Michalczyk M, Chycki J, Zajac A, Maszczyk A, Zydek G, Langfort J. Anaerobic performance after a low-carbohydrate diet (LCD) followed by 7 days of carbohydrate loading in male basketball players. *Nutrients*. 2019;11(4):778. doi:10.3390/nu11040778

160. Standing Committee on the Scientific Evaluation of Dietary Reference Intakes; Panel on Calcium and Related Nutrients; Subcommittee on Upper Reference Levels of Nutrients; Food and Nutrition Board, Institute of Medicine. *Dietary Reference Intakes for Calcium, Phosphorus, Magnesium, Vitamin D, and Fluoride*. National Academies Press; 1997. doi:10.17226/5776

161. Institute of Medicine. *Dietary Reference Intakes for Calcium, Phosphorus, Magnesium, Vitamin D, and Fluoride*. National Academies Press; 2010.

162. Standing Committee on the Scientific Evaluation of Dietary Reference Intakes and its Panel on Folate, Other B Vitamins, and Choline; Subcommittee on Upper Reference Levels of Nutrients; Food and Nutrition Board, Institute of Medicine. *Dietary Reference Intakes for Thiamin, Riboflavin, Niacin, Vitamin B_6, Folate, Vitamin B_{12}, Pantothenic Acid, Biotin, and Choline*. National Academies Press; 1998. doi:10.17226/6015

163. Panel on Dietary Antioxidants and Related Compounds; Subcommittees on Upper Reference Levels of Nutrients and Interpretation and Uses of Dietary Reference Intakes; Standing Committee on the Scientific Evaluation of Dietary Reference Intakes; Food and Nutrition Board, Institute of Medicine. *Dietary Reference Intakes for Vitamin C, Vitamin E, Selenium, and Carotenoids*. National Academies Press; 2000. doi:10.17226/9810

164. Fogelholm M. Vitamins, minerals and supplementation in soccer. *J Sports Sci*. 1994;12(spec no):S23-S27.

165. Reynolds RD. Determination of dietary vitamin B-6 intake: is it accurate? *J Am Diet Assoc*. 1990;90(6):799-801.

166. Nielsen P, Nachtigall D. Iron supplementation in athletes. Current recommendations. *Sports Med*. 1998;26(4):207-216. doi:10.2165/00007256-199826040-00001

167. de la Puente Yagüe M, Collado Yurrita L, Ciudad Cabañas MJ, Cuadrado Cenzual MA. Role of vitamin D in athletes and their performance: current concepts and new trends. *Nutrients*. 2020;12(2):579. doi:10.3390/nu12020579

168. Santos DA, Dawson JA, Matias CN, et al. Reference values for body composition and anthropometric measurements in athletes. *PLoS One*. 2014;9(5):e97846. doi:10.1371/journal.pone.0097846

169. Kulka TJ, Kenney WL. Heat balance limits in football uniforms: how different uniform ensembles alter the equation. *Phys Sportsmed*. 2002;30(7):29-39. doi:10.3810/psm.2002.07.377

170. Palmer MS, Spriet LL. Sweat rate, salt loss, and fluid intake during an intense on-ice practice in elite Canadian male junior hockey players. *Appl Physiol Nutr Metab*. 2008;33(2):263-271. doi:10.1139/H08-011

171. Arnaoutis G, Kavouras SA, Kotsis YP, Tsekouras YE, Makrillos M, Bardis CN. Ad libitum fluid intake does not prevent dehydration in suboptimally hydrated young soccer players during a training session of a summer camp. *Int J Sport Nutr Exerc Metab*. 2013;23(3):245-251. doi:10.1123/ijsnem.23.3.245

172. Nicholas CW, Tsintzas K, Boobis L, Williams C. Carbohydrate-electrolyte ingestion during intermittent high-intensity running. *Med Sci Sports Exerc*. 1999;31(9):1280-1286. doi:10.1097/00005768-199909000-00008

173. Nicholas CW, Williams C, Lakomy H, Phillips G, Nowitz A. Influence of ingesting a carbohydrate-electrolyte solution on endurance capacity during intermittent, high-intensity shuttle running. *J Sports Sci*. 1995;13(4):283-290. doi:10.1080/02640419508732241

174. Kovacs M. A review of fluid and hydration in competitive tennis. *Int J Sports Physiol Perform*. 2008;3(4):413-423. doi:10.1123/ijspp.3.4.413

175. Shirreffs SM, Taylor AJ, Leiper JB, Maughan RJ. Post-exercise rehydration in man: effects of volume consumed and drink sodium content. *Med Sci Sports Exerc*. 1996;28(10):1260-1271. doi:10.1097/00005768-199610000-00009

176. Giersch GEW, Charkoudian N, Stearns RL, Casa DJ. Fluid balance and hydration considerations for women: review and future directions. *Sports Med*. 2019;50(2):253-261. doi:10.1007/s40279-019-01206-6

177. Convertino VA, Armstrong LE, Coyle EF, et al. American College of Sports Medicine position stand. Exercise and fluid replacement. *Med Sci Sports Exerc*. 1996;28(1):i-vii. doi:10.1097/00005768-199610000-00045

178. Greenleaf JE, Castle BL. Exercise temperature regulation in man during hypohydration and hyperthermia. *J Appl Physiol*. 1971;30(6):847-853. doi:10.1152/jappl.1971.30.6.847

179. Maughan RJ, Leiper JB. Fluid replacement requirements in soccer. *J Sports Sci*. 1994;12(spec no):S29-S34.

180. Shi X, Gisolfi CV. Fluid and carbohydrate replacement during intermittent exercise. *Sports Med*. 1998;25(3):157-172. doi:10.2165/00007256-199825030-00003

181. Horswill CA. Effective fluid replacement. *Int J Sport Nutr Exerc Metab*. 1998;8(2):175-195. doi:10.1123/ijsn.8.2.175

182. Burke LM, Hawley JA. Fluid balance in team sports. Guidelines for optimal practices. *Sports Med*. 1997;24(1):38-54. doi:10.2165/00007256-199724010-00004

183. Petrie HJ, Stover EA, Horswill CA. Nutritional concerns for the child and adolescent competitor. *Nutrition*. 2004;20(7-8):620-631. doi:10.1016/j.nut.2004.04.002

184. American Academy of Pediatrics. Committee on Sports Medicine and Fitness. Climatic heat stress and the exercising child and adolescent. *Pediatrics*. 2000;106(1 pt 1):158-159.

185. Falk B, Dotan R. Children's thermoregulation during exercise in the heat: a revisit. *Appl Physiol Nutr Metab*. 2008;33(2):420-427. doi:10.1139/H07-185

186. Meyer F, Bar-Or O, Salsberg A, Passe D. Hypohydration during exercise in children: effect of thirst, drink preferences, and rehydration. *Int J Sport Nutr Exerc Metab*. 1994;4(1):22-35. doi:10.1123/ijsn.4.1.22

187. Stecker RA, Harty PS, Jagim AR, Candow DG, Kerksick CM. Timing of ergogenic aids and micronutrients on muscle and exercise performance. *J Int Soc Sports Nutr*. 2019;16(1):37. doi:10.1186/s12970-019-0304-9

CHAPTER 22

Nutrition for Endurance and Ultraendurance Sports

Eve Pearson, MBA, RDN

LEARNING OBJECTIVES

- Identify current sports nutrition information as it specifically relates to endurance athletes.
- Learn how to prescribe nutrition and hydration needs for the endurance athlete before, during, and after training and races.
- Recognize when micronutrient deficiencies are a concern in endurance athletes.
- Understand the varying types of endurance events and how they differ.

INTRODUCTION

Endurance events encompass a wide range of competitions, including half-marathon and marathon runs, 20k and 50k race walking events, Olympic distance triathlons, cross-country ski races, adventure races, obstacle course races, road and mountain cycling events, and short-course swimrun events. Ultraendurance events involve races that last from 4 to 24 hours and include marathon rowing, running 31 to 100 miles, cycling 100 miles or more, the longest obstacle course races (eg, Toughest Mudder and Spartan Beast), triathlons ranging from Half Ironman events to the Ultraman distance, and long-course swimrun events. Multistage or multiday ultraendurance events entail competing over consecutive days, such as the Tour de France bicycle race (~2,200 miles over 21 days), the Race Across America (RAAM) cycling event (3,000 miles), the Barkley Marathons (one of the toughest 100-mile run courses with a 60-hour time cutoff), the self-supported mountain bike race Tour Divide (2,745 miles), and some adventure races.

Endurance racing has become very popular, even among nonelite athletes, many of whom participate in these races for fun and to finish rather than to vie for the title. These recreational athletes also need individualized nutrition and hydration plans. Although much of the existing research discussed in this chapter involves elite athletes, an increasing number of studies have included amateur and female athletes. The results of these studies provide a starting point from which adjustments can be made for the individual needs of recreational athletes as well.

ENERGY SYSTEMS AND FUEL USAGE

Endurance athletes have unique nutrient demands because of their high energy expenditures, and they must cope with a variety of challenges to achieve their fuel and fluid replacement goals. The predominant energy system for endurance athletes is the aerobic energy system, with brief, intermittent involvement of the anaerobic energy systems. During prolonged exercise, the oxidative metabolism of carbohydrate (muscle glycogen and plasma glucose) and fat (intramuscular triglycerides and plasma fatty acids) provides the vast majority of adenosine triphosphate for muscle contraction. Although amino acid oxidation occurs to a limited extent during endurance exercise, carbohydrate and fat are the most important oxidative substrates.[1,2]

During high-intensity endurance events, the exercise intensity is often 85% of the maximum rate of oxygen consumption (VO_2 max) or more, and carbohydrate (primarily muscle glycogen) is the primary fuel source. An endurance athlete can sustain exercise at 85% of VO_2 max for approximately 90 minutes without exogenous fuel. During ultraendurance events, the exercise intensity averages 65% of VO_2 max, where fat oxidation reaches its peak for male athletes. An ultraendurance athlete can sustain exercise at 65% of VO_2 max for approximately 8 hours with exogenous fuel.[2] The length of time at a certain percentage of VO_2 max will vary with modality, training, sex, and environmental conditions; it varies widely among athletes.[3] Refer to Chapter 4 for more on fat utilization during exercise at different intensities and durations.

GENERAL NUTRITION REQUIREMENTS

Energy needs among endurance athletes vary based on a variety of factors, making it important to fully assess the athlete and create an individualized plan. Fueling strategies should be fine-tuned based on exercise intensity, duration, mode, and environmental conditions. General nutrition requirements and recommendations are discussed here, and those specific to training and competition are discussed later in this chapter.

Energy Needs

Endurance athletes should consume adequate daily energy, especially carbohydrate, during various phases of training to maintain a desirable training intensity and, thus, maximize training adaptations. As shown in Table 22.1 on page 578, these athletes have high energy requirements.[4-14] In a study by Frączek et al,[15] different methods of assessing energy expenditure were found to produce different results. Female endurance athletes' daily energy expenditure was assessed as 2,654 to 3,432 kcal using a chronometric-tabular method compared to 2,022 to 2,440 kcal using a kinematic method. Similarly, male endurance athletes' daily energy expenditures were determined to be 3,121 to 4,435 kcal and 3,505 to 4,569 kcal, respectively.

To meet energy demands, endurance athletes often need to eat meals and snacks continuously throughout the day, especially surrounding their training sessions. Testing specific foods and fluids before, during, and after training sessions allows the athlete to determine effective fueling strategies for competition.[16-18] Prioritizing adequate fueling is recommended to optimize endurance athletes' health. Failure to match energy intake to energy expenditure during training impairs endurance performance, most likely because of the depletion of muscle and liver glycogen. Therefore, changes in body weight or composition that limit energy intake should be reserved for the offseason or early in the training cycle when training volume is lower.[19] See Chapter 18 for more information on the repercussions of disordered eating practices that result in low energy availability.

Experts previously thought that compared to male endurance athletes, female endurance athletes were more likely to consume insufficient energy.[20] In reality, endurance athletes may severely underestimate their caloric intake, thereby making it difficult to assess energy balance.[21] A few studies have reported the maintenance of body weight even when energy intake falls short of energy expenditure, indicating underreporting.[22,23] Even with chronic underreporting in research studies, a more recent systematic review by Heydenreich et al[24] found an apparent negative energy balance among male and female endurance athletes. This is also demonstrated in additional studies including women who report menstrual irregularities and amenorrhea.[20]

However, Martin et al[8] and Sjöden et al,[11] in studies on elite female cyclists and female cross-country skiers, respectively, reported that most of the cyclists and some of the skiers modulated their energy intakes based on energy expenditure. In addition, a review by Burke et al[20] showed that male elite cyclists consumed approximately 51 to 63 kcal per kilogram of body weight per day and female elite cyclists consumed approximately 39 to 50 kcal per kilogram of body weight per day.

Heydenreich et al[24] also found that many endurance athletes experience a higher total energy expenditure during their competition phase than during other training phases. Therefore, sports dietitians should consider the unique energetic needs of each training phase when making recommendations. Table 22.2 on page 579 lists examples of athlete macronutrient intakes during training and competition phases.[4,5,7-9,12,25-31] The competition phase varies tremendously among different types of endurance athletes; it could consist of a single competition day or a multiday event, or it could involve weeks of back-to-back competition days.

TABLE 22.1 Daily Energy Expenditures and Intakes of Endurance and Ultraendurance Athletes During the Training/Preparation Phase[4-14]

Type of athlete	Daily energy expenditure for training	Daily energy intake for training
Male elite ultraendurance triathletes[a,4]	Data not available	3,287-4,903 kcal/d
Male marathon runners[b,4]	Data not available	2,905-4,235 kcal/d
Male elite Kenyan distance runners[c,5]	3,243-3,742 kcal/d	2,847-3,483 kcal/d
Male Japanese distance runners[6]	3,775-5,253 kcal/d	3,693-3,875 kcal/d
Male elite road cyclists[d,7,13]	2,867-3,584 kcal/d	4,948-5,760 kcal/d
Female elite road cyclists[8]	Data not available	2,868-3,585 kcal/d
Female elite lightweight rowers[e,10]	2,738-5,176 kcal/d	1,901-2,527 kcal/d
Female cross-country skiers[f,11]	3,609-4,828 kcal/d	3,752-4,876 kcal/d
Male cross-country skiers[g,11]	6,071-8,341 kcal/d	6,142-7,027 kcal/d
Female elite runners[h,12,14]	2,514-3,138 kcal/d	2,575-3,405 kcal/d
Male adventure racer[i,9]	Data not available	44.6 ± 8.0 kcal/kg/d
Female adventure racer[j,9]	Data not available	48.1 ± 19.8 kcal/kg/d

[a] 8.1 miles swimming, 202 miles cycling, 47 miles running per week.
[b] 91.6 miles per week.
[c] 117 miles or more per week.
[d] 405 miles per month.
[e] 90-300 minutes per day plus 2 strength workouts per week.
[f] 153-187 minutes per day.
[g] 196-228 minutes per day.
[h] 7-13 miles per day.
[i] 10.4-15.8 hours per week (running, cycling, rowing, and strength exercises).
[j] 9.1-15.9 hours per week (running, cycling, rowing, and strength exercises).

Because recreational athletes typically train around their professional jobs and personal responsibilities, finding time for eating and food preparation adds a layer of difficulty to their schedule. Often, their meal and snack times are dictated by work and personal demands, meetings, or other commitments. All of this makes it increasingly important to educate such athletes on the importance of pretraining and posttraining fueling to meet daily energy demands.

Macronutrients

As for their energy needs, the carbohydrate, protein, and fat needs of the endurance athlete also vary based on exercise intensity, duration, mode, and environmental conditions. When counseling athletes, the sports dietitian can calculate protein and carbohydrate needs based on body weight and then adjust fat accordingly using the guidelines that follow.

TABLE 22.2 Average Daily Macronutrient Intakes for Endurance and Ultraendurance Athletes[4,5,7-9,12,25-31]

Type of athlete	Carbohydrate, g per kg of body weight	Protein, g per kg of body weight	Fat, g per kg of body weight (percentage of energy intake)
Male elite ultraendurance triathletes, training[4]	9.0	2.0	1.8 (27%)
Male amateur ultraendurance triathletes, racing[a,31]	Cycling: 0.8 Running: 4.7	Cycling: 0.6 Running: 0.1	Cycling: 0.9 (10.5%) Running: 0.1 (2.2%)
Male marathon runners[4]	8.0	2.0	2.0 (32%)
Male elite Kenyan distance runners[5]	9.8	2.2	1.0 (17%)
Female elite runners, training[b,12]	6.3	1.4	1.3 (27%)
Male ultraendurance runners, racing[c,25]	12.0	1.1	1.5 (22%)
Female ultraendurance runners, racing[c,25]	8	1.1	1.5 (22%)
Male elite road cyclists[7]	Training: 11.0 Racing: 12.0	Training: 2.9 Racing: 2.6	Training: 2.8 (30%) Racing: 2.2 (25%)
Female elite road cyclists[8]	Training: 9.0 Racing: 9.9	Training: 2.6 Racing: 2	Training and racing: 1.0 (17%)
Male Tour de France cyclists[26]	12.0	3.1	2.1 (23%)
Male Pony Express Trail cyclists,[d] racing[27]	18.0	2.7	3.5 (27%)
Male Tour de Spain cyclists, racing[28]	12.6	3.0	2.3 (26)
Male Sydney to Melbourne runner,[e] racing[29]	17.0	2.9	3.2 (27%)
Male Race Across America cyclist,[f] racing[30]	22.6	3.6	1.0 (9%)
Male Race Across America cyclist (4th-place finish),[g] racing[31]	24.8	2.8	2.3 (16%)
Male Adventure racers[h,9]	5.7	1.9	1.5 (30%)
Female Adventure racers[h,9]	6.9	2.0	1.5 (28%)

[a] 2.4-mile swim, 112-mile bike, 26.2-mile run.
[b] 7-13-miles per week.
[c] 24-hour trail race.
[d] 2,050 miles in 10 days.
[e] 628 miles in 8.5 days.
[f] 10 days, 7 hours, and 53 minutes.
[g] 9 days, 16 hours, and 45 minutes.
[h] 149 hours, 33 minutes.

CARBOHYDRATE

Adequate carbohydrate stores (muscle, liver glycogen, and blood glucose) are critical for optimum endurance performance. Fatigue during endurance exercise is often associated with muscle glycogen depletion or hypoglycemia. Thus, nutritional strategies that optimize carbohydrate availability before, during, and after exercise are recommended to improve endurance performance.[1] Nutrient-rich carbohydrate foods and fluids should be emphasized because they contain other nutrients, such as vitamins and minerals, that are important for the overall diet as well as exercise recovery.[18]

The athlete's carbohydrate and energy intakes should be adjusted or periodized (possibly on a daily basis) to meet the requirements of the particular training cycle or phase of their sport. (Carbohydrate loading is discussed later in this chapter and in more detail in Chapter 2.) Excessive energy intake, including excessive carbohydrate intake, during light training can cause an increase in body fat, which may have a negative effect on performance. Conversely, inadequate carbohydrate and energy intake during heavy training can cause a loss of lean tissue, depleted carbohydrate stores, and impaired performance. The recommendations for daily carbohydrate intake for endurance athletes are listed in Box 22.1.

Examples of average daily macronutrient intakes for endurance and ultraendurance athletes can be found in Table 22.2.[4,5,7-9,12,25-31]

BOX 22.1 Daily Carbohydrate Intake Recommendations for Endurance and Ultraendurance Athletes

Daily carbohydrate intake should be in the range of 5 to 12 g per kilogram of body weight. Adjust intake goals based on the athlete's total energy needs, specific training needs, and feedback from training performance.

Carbohydrate intake should be spread over the day (before, during, and after exercise) to promote fuel availability for key training sessions.

The amount of carbohydrate per day can vary daily if the athlete's training varies in length and intensity (eg, in 1 week, an athlete may have 2 days of 4- to 5-hour training sessions, 2 days of 1-hour training sessions, and 3 days of 1- to 3-hour training sessions, making the athlete's carbohydrate requirements vary daily).

The following are examples of daily guidelines for various activity levels:

- 5 to 7 g/kg body weight: moderate-intensity training programs for 1 h/d
- 6 to 10 g/kg body weight: moderate- to high-intensity endurance exercise for 1 to 3 h/d
- 8 to 12 g/kg body weight: moderate- to high-intensity exercise for 4 to 5 h/d

Several studies have reported that male runners and male and female cyclists consume adequate carbohydrate (9, 11, and 9 g/kg body weight, respectively) during training.[5,7,8,12,25,31,32] However, 1 study suggested that both male and female adventure racers and female runners are likely consuming inadequate amounts of carbohydrate (5.7, 6.9, and 6.3 g/kg body weight, respectively).[9] Training for endurance events involves hours of prolonged exercise that may include multiple daily training sessions. The stress of such rigorous training can decrease appetite, resulting in reduced consumption of energy and carbohydrate.[18,33] As discussed in Chapter 2, athletes who train heavily and have difficulty eating enough can consume a high-carbohydrate liquid supplement to meet energy and carbohydrate needs. To demonstrate this, Brouns et al[33] evaluated the effect of a simulated Tour de France on food and fluid intake, energy balance, and substrate oxidation. Although the cyclists consumed 630 g of carbohydrate (8.6 g per kilogram of body weight per day), they oxidized 850 g of carbohydrate per day (11.6 g per kilogram of body weight per day). Despite ad libitum intake of conventional foods, the cyclists were unable to ingest sufficient carbohydrate and calories to compensate for their increased energy expenditure. When the diet was supplemented with a 20% carbohydrate beverage, carbohydrate intake increased to 16 g per kilogram of body weight, and carbohydrate oxidation rose to 13 g per kilogram of body weight per day. In addition, Lindeman[30] reported that a male cyclist who competed in the RAAM obtained most of his total energy intake from a high-carbohydrate liquid supplement (23% carbohydrate). Saris et al[26] reported that approximately 30% of the total carbohydrate consumed by Tour de France cyclists came from high-carbohydrate beverages (eg, sports drinks, soft drinks, and liquid meals).

Athletes who have extremely high carbohydrate requirements and suppressed appetites as a result of heavy endurance training or competition should include compact, low-fiber forms of carbohydrate, such as pasta, white rice, sports nutrition bars and gels, baked goods (cake, tarts, biscuits), cereal, granola bars, and sugar-rich foods (eg, candy) in their diets. Carbohydrate-rich fluids, such as sports drinks, juices, low-fat chocolate milk, high-carbohydrate liquid supplements, soft drinks, commercial liquid meals, milk shakes, yogurt drinks, and fruit smoothies, may also be appealing to athletes who are very tired and dehydrated.[18,34]

Practitioners can recommend a large range of carbohydrate foods for endurance and ultraendurance athletes, provided that the foods are easy to consume, portable, and easy to store, ensuring athlete compliance. Daily carbohydrate intake can be in liquid, semisolid, or solid form and will depend on each athlete's preference and tolerance. Additional carbohydrate foods used by Tour de France cyclists and 1 ultraendurance runner include sweet cakes, bread, muesli, yogurt, pancakes, toast, porridge, sandwiches with protein fillings, instant noodle meals, muffins, fruit, sweets, and pastries.[26,29]

PROTEIN

Although acute endurance exercise results in the oxidation of several amino acids, the total amount of amino acid oxidation amounts to only 1% to 6% of the total energy cost of exercise. A low-energy and low-carbohydrate intake will increase amino acid oxidation and total protein requirements.[34,35] During low- to moderate-intensity endurance activity, protein intake of 1.2 g per kilogram of body weight per day is sufficient when energy and carbohydrate intakes are adequate.[36] Elite male endurance athletes may require 1.5 to 1.8 g of protein per kilogram of body weight per day to maintain their nitrogen balance.[33,36-38] Several studies suggest that higher protein intake of up to 2.0 g per kilogram of body weight per day may be necessary when energy is restricted[22,39,40] or when male endurance athletes are in heavy training blocks.[33]

Research has shown that because of its high oxidation rate, the amino acid leucine is of great importance to endurance athletes, more so in male athletes than their female counterparts.[41,42] Foods containing the highest amounts of leucine include eggs, soy protein, seaweed, elk, tuna, chicken and turkey breast meat, cod, buffalo, and haddock.

Protein timing and dose are of particular importance, with intake of a quality protein source in the amount of 0.25 to 0.3 g/kg body weight recommended within 2 hours postexercise.[42-45] Meal doses above 0.3 g/kg body weight have not been shown to have any additional benefit. Protein doses are most useful when consumed at 3- to 5-hour increments.[42]

Studies of male endurance athletes suggest that they are consuming appropriate amounts of protein. The data on female endurance athletes continues to be limited, as shown in Table 22.2. The athlete's sex affects protein metabolism. During endurance exercise, females oxidize more lipids and less carbohydrate and protein compared with equally trained and nourished males. Because of sex-based hormonal responses that promote fat metabolism in females and carbohydrate and protein metabolism in males, female endurance athletes may have a 10% to 20% lower protein requirement than their male counterparts.[35] Furthermore, during the follicular phase of the menstrual cycle, the protein needs of female endurance athletes may increase to 1.63 g/kg/d to maintain their nitrogen balance or when energy or carbohydrate intake is low.[22]

Although most endurance athletes consume sufficient protein (including leucine), those with low-energy or reduced-carbohydrate intakes and those who are vegetarians or vegans could benefit from nutrition counseling to optimize and increase their dietary protein intake.[35]

FAT

The Food and Nutrition Board of the Institute of Medicine established an acceptable macronutrient distribution range for fat at 20% to 35% of total energy intake.[40] Research indicates that this range is also acceptable for endurance athletes. Studies of male endurance athletes suggest that they are consuming an appropriate amount of fat. The data on female endurance athletes are extremely limited, as shown in Table 22.2.

The relevance of fat adaptation remains a question among endurance athletes and their coaches. Although researchers continue to conduct studies in this area, it is clear that a low-carbohydrate, high-fat diet (also referred to as keto-adaptation) coupled with training does improve fat oxidation and reduce carbohydrate oxidation.[46] In a review article, Yeo et al[47] found that some well-trained athletes have responded positively when attempting to increase fat metabolism during training and races, whereas others have not. Some instances of gastrointestinal distress have been reported when athletes have tried to use medium-chain triglyceride oils for improved fat metabolism.[41] In several studies, eating a high-fat, low-carbohydrate diet was found to affect performance outcomes negatively[42,48,49] and to make it difficult to train and race at higher intensities.[42]

As previously mentioned, some athletes participate in endurance events not to win but rather to finish; therefore, if they are training at low intensities, fat adaptation might be on option for these individuals. This concept of fat adaptation is practiced among coaches and athletes alike, thereby making it important to assess each athlete individually and determine the best approach. This topic is discussed in more detail in Chapter 4.

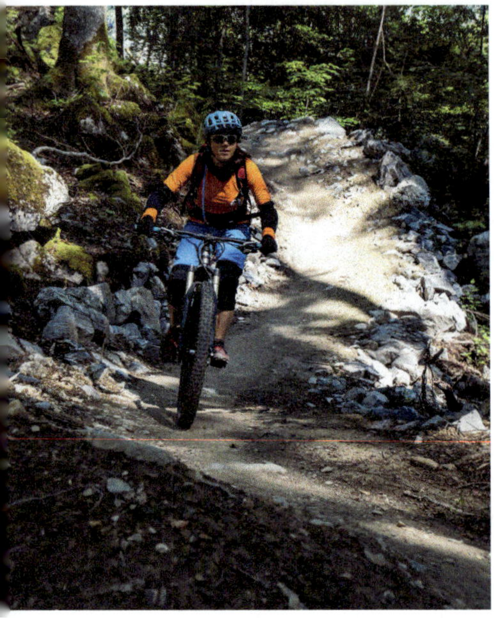

Fluid

In 2004, the Institute of Medicine established the Dietary Reference Intake (DRI) for water as 16 cups for males and 12 cups for females.[50] These recommendations are meant for sedentary individuals. As noted in Chapter 6, there is no one fluid recommendation that will suffice for everyone, especially for the wide variety of endurance athletes. When working with endurance athletes, the sports dietitian should begin with the DRI and add more daily fluids based on the sweat rate, which is discussed later in this chapter. Each athlete needs a specific daily hydration plan based on their training plan. Also of concern is hyponatremia, which may occur in endurance athletes who are heavier and slower, and which can be fatal.

Athletes can easily monitor their daily hydration status by checking the color of their urine, observing daily changes in their body weight, and comparing their pre- and post-training weights. Darkly colored urine is an indication of dehydration, whereas light-colored urine generally represents a euhydrated state, making this a simple discussion with athletes. When considering daily weight changes, especially before and after training sessions, having multiple days of data are helpful. When athletes participate in multiple sports within an event (eg, triathlon), they should collect weight-change data for each event (eg, swim, bike, run).

Another subjective, inexpensive measurement of hydration status in the recent literature is urine specific gravity (USG). Although USG has not been recognized as a valid measure of hydration status on its own, collecting and monitoring the data regularly can serve as an additional tool if athletes are not severely dehydrated. A USG value of less than 1.020 indicates that an athlete is hydrated, and a measurement greater than 1.030 indicates dehydration.[51,52]

Using data from 3 simple field tests (weight change, urine, and thirst) in a Venn diagram decision tool may be the best approach to assess hydration.[53] A combination of any 2 markers means that dehydration is likely, and the presence of all 3 markers means that dehydration is very likely. Additional information on hydration can be found in Chapter 6.

Micronutrients

Although limited data are available on the micronutrient intakes of endurance athletes, those who consume adequate total energy usually meet or exceed population reference values such as the DRIs for vitamins and minerals.[20,28,31,34,54] Experts found that intakes of thiamin and riboflavin might be inadequate[26,27,29]; however, when athletes are consuming supplements, whether as pills or injections, deficiency is not a concern.[26]

Endurance athletes who regularly restrict energy or eat a limited variety of foods may be at risk for suboptimal micronutrient intakes. As discussed in Chapter 16, vegan and vegetarian athletes may have suboptimal intakes of specific nutrients. Some endurance and ultraendurance athletes may have increased requirements because of excessive losses in sweat or urine. Sodium is of highest concern, followed by magnesium and calcium. Consuming a nutrient-dense diet containing fruits, vegetables, whole grains, legumes, lean meats, and dairy foods during training helps to ensure adequate micronutrient intake.

Supplementation with single micronutrients is not recommended unless there is a medical necessity (eg, iron to treat iron deficiency anemia).[55] When supplementing micronutrients, athletes should not exceed the DRI Tolerable Upper Intake Level for any nutrient to prevent possible adverse effects on health and performance.

SODIUM

Because of the nature of endurance training, endurance athletes may have greater sodium needs than the general population or even other athletes. Sodium requirements vary widely depending on intensity and time of training sessions, sodium concentration in sweat, and sweat rate. As for water intake, the daily sodium intake can be addressed by starting with typical recommendations of no more than 2,300 mg/d.[50] When devising a plan, the athlete and their sports nutritionist should consider the athlete's sweat rate. Sweat sodium losses in athletes have been shown to average 800 mg of sodium per liter of sweat lost, with the range of sodium losses extending from 10 to 70 mEq/L. Heat acclimatization improves the ability to reabsorb sodium and chloride; thus, individuals who are heat acclimatized usually have lower sweat sodium concentrations for any given sweating rate. Considering these multiple factors, daily sodium requirements for endurance athletes may exceed normal sodium dietary guidelines, especially during days involving multiple hours of training and during competition. The athlete's current eating habits should be considered with respect to sodium, as most people far exceed the recommended 2,300 mg/d, making it likely that there will be no need to increase an athlete's daily sodium intake on low to moderate training days.[56]

IRON

Endurance training can increase iron requirements (because of increases in hemoglobin, myoglobin, and iron-containing proteins involved in aerobic metabolism), iron losses (through sweating, gastrointestinal bleeding, mechanical trauma such as foot-strike hemolysis), and upregulated hepcidin postexercise.[57-59] Iron depletion can progress to iron deficiency anemia if untreated. The debilitating effects of iron deficiency anemia on endurance performance are well established. Anemia impairs erythropoiesis (red blood cell formation), thereby limiting oxygen delivery to the muscles and decreasing VO_2 max and endurance performance.[60-62]

Endurance and ultraendurance athletes, especially female athletes and runners of both sexes, are at risk for depleting their iron stores.[61] Although depleted iron stores should not affect VO_2 max because hemoglobin levels are not compromised, inadequate tissue iron stores may reduce oxidative metabolism in the muscle and impair endurance performance.[63,64] One indicator of tissue iron deficiency, known as serum transferrin receptor, suggests that even stage 1 iron deficiency (depleted iron stores) may compromise aerobic and endurance capacity. Hinton et al[63] found that iron supplementation in iron-depleted, nonanemic women significantly improved endurance capacity, serum ferritin, and serum transferrin receptor concentrations, but the supplementation did not affect hemoglobin concentrations. Further analysis of these data showed that tissue iron deficiency impaired adaptations to endurance training.[64] DellaValle and Haas[65] found improved energy efficiency with iron supplementation regardless of menstrual status. Individuals with the most tissue iron depletion also showed the greatest improvement in endurance capacity after supplementation.[66] An increase in plasma and storage iron increases the synthesis of hepcidin; therefore, a decrease in hepcidin may be an early marker of iron deficiency.[67]

Athletes at risk for iron deficiency should have routine checks of their iron status. A low plasma ferritin level (<20 mcg/L) or serum hepcidin levels of less than 20 ng/mL indicate tissue iron deficiency, which can impair endurance.[68] An athlete's iron stores can be increased through diet and iron supplementation to prevent the negative consequences of iron deficiency.[60]

CALCIUM AND VITAMIN D

Inadequate intakes of dietary calcium and vitamin D increase the risk of low bone mineral density and stress fractures. Female endurance and ultraendurance athletes who have low energy intakes or menstrual dysfunction or who eliminate dairy products are at high risk for low bone mineral density. One study on female cyclists showed that a calcium-rich (1,352 mg) meal within the 2 hours before a training session did not improve or hinder performance, but it did decrease exercise-induced bone resorption markers during the follicular and luteal phases of the menstrual cycle.[69] Vitamin D status can be easily checked through a routine blood draw by the athlete's physician or sports medicine team. Supplementation with calcium and vitamin D should be determined after a nutrition assessment.[62]

MAGNESIUM

Although the direct correlation between performance and magnesium status is still unclear, a deficient magnesium status in endurance athletes may result in cellular damage.[70] Magnesium losses through sweat and urine in prolonged endurance exercise could lead to a deficit, weakening muscles and affecting neuromuscular function, as indicated by changes in the amount of magnesium in red blood cells.[67] Because assessing magnesium status is invasive, it is difficult to measure in practice, and assessing intake could prove beneficial. This has led some researchers to report that a magnesium intake 10% to 20% higher than the average sedentary person may be necessary for endurance athletes, especially those with high sweat rates.[70]

ANTIOXIDANTS

The dietary antioxidants vitamins C and E play an important role in protecting cell membranes from oxidative damage. Although endurance exercise is associated with increased oxidative stress, it also increases the body's enzymatic and nonenzymatic antioxidant defenses as an adaptation to training.[71] In fact, the routine consumption of antioxidant supplements during endurance training may have negative effects. Several studies have found that the suppression of free-radical generation during exercise can attenuate some of the signals for endogenous adaptation to endurance training.[72,73] Until research suggests otherwise, it is prudent to recommend that endurance and ultraendurance athletes consume an antioxidant-rich diet, rather than supplements, to protect against oxidative damage.[71-73]

TRAINING AND COMPETITION DAY NUTRITION RECOMMENDATIONS

Although recommendations for training and competition are combined in this section, several important differences should be noted. First, energy requirements for competition days are often higher than those for training days, especially for ultraendurance events (eg, Ironman triathlon, 100-mile runs) and multiday events, as demonstrated in Table 22.3.[25-32,74-79] It is neither necessary nor practical to replace 100% of calories burned during ultraendurance events. However, during multiday events (eg, Tour de France, RAAM), energy intake should match energy expenditure as much as possible to promote glycogen restoration, preservation of lean tissue, an adequate intake of macronutrients and micronutrients, and optimal continued performance.[6] Second, endurance athletes should try different products to see what works best for them during training; the athlete should never try anything new on race day. Therefore, the race-day plan comes together during training, and the athlete can practice the plan to implement on race day. Typically, a weekly endurance training schedule will include 1 or 2 long training sessions of 3 hours or more. These are the perfect days to replicate race-day nutrition.

Although endurance athletes are reported to have a calorie deficit during events and training lasting less than 24 hours, it is important to note that, during training, energy will be replaced before or after the training session. The athlete should develop and refine a fueling and hydration plan months ahead of the priority race by experi-

TABLE 22.3 Energy Intake and Energy Expenditure of Endurance and Ultraendurance Athletes During Competition[25-32,74-79]

Type of athlete	Energy intake and expenditure during competition, kcal/d
Male New Zealand Ironman triathletes[74]	Intake: 3,940 Expenditure: 10,036
Female New Zealand Ironman triathletes[74]	Intake: 3,115 Expenditure: 8,570

Type of athlete	Energy intake and expenditure during competition, kcal/d
Nonprofessional male triathletes[a,32]	Intake: 3,643 Expenditure: 11,009
Male ultrarunners[b,75]	Intake: 6,047 Expenditure: 13,560
Male and female ultrarunners[c,76]	Intake: 7,022 Expenditure: 9,538
Male amateur ultrarunners[d,25]	Intake: 5,497 Expenditure: 13,862
Female amateur ultrarunners[d,25]	Intake: 3,107 Expenditure: 10,755
Male Race Around Australia runners[e,75,79]	Intake: ~6,000[79] Expenditure: 6,321[74]
Male Sydney to Melbourne runner[e,29]	Intake: 5,952 Expenditure: Not reported
Male Tour de France cyclists[26]	Intake: 5,785 Expenditure: 6,069
Male Pony Express Trail cyclists[g,27]	Intake: 7,125 Expenditure: Not reported
Male Tour de Spain cyclists[28]	Intake: 5,595 Expenditure: Not reported
Male Race Across America cyclist[h,30]	Intake: 8,429 Expenditure: Not reported
Male Race Across America cyclist (4th-place finish)[i,31]	Intake: 9,612 Expenditure: Not reported
Female Race Across America cyclist (1st-place finish)[j,31]	Intake: 7,950 Expenditure: Not reported
Male elite road cyclists[k,76]	Intake: 4,918 Expenditure: 6,420
Male elite road cyclists[l,77]	Intake: 6,525 Expenditure: 6,549
Male amateur road cyclists[m,78]	Intake: 5,449 Expenditure: 10,253

[a] 3.8-km swim, 180-km bike, 42.2-km swim.
[b] 100-mile run, 24.3 hours.
[c] 100-mile run, 26.2 hours.
[d] 24-hour trail run, looped course.
[e] 2,050 miles in 10 days.
[f] 9,053 miles in 191 days.
[g] 628 miles in 8.5 days.
[h] 10 days, 7 hours, and 53 minutes.
[i] 9 days, 16 hours, and 45 minutes.
[j] 12 days, 6 hours, and 21 minutes.
[k] Race Across America, 4-person team completed in 6 days, 10 hours, 51 minutes, relay style.
[l] 6 days, 10 stages.
[m] 24-hour cycle race, closed circuit.

menting during training and in lower-priority races. As previously mentioned, experts do not suggest attempting weight loss during the preparation phase. The fueling plan should be tested while the athlete is training at race pace and in environmental conditions that simulate the race conditions for best results.[17] Athletes should not consume untested foods or fluids during the race because this may result in severe gastrointestinal distress and poor performance. Endurance athletes should consume liquid, semisolid, or solid fuel before feeling hungry or tired, usually within the first hour of training, depending on the timing of the last meal before the training session. Consuming small amounts at frequent intervals (every 15–20 minutes) helps prevent gastrointestinal upset, maintain blood glucose levels, and promote hydration.[17,29] The athlete's foods and fluids should be easily digestible, familiar (tested in training), and enjoyable (to encourage eating and drinking).[17,28,29,34]

Kimber et al[74] determined that the average energy expenditures of triathletes in the New Zealand Ironman triathlon was much greater than their average energy intake, creating a substantial energy deficit for both men (5,973 kcal) and women (5,213 kcal). This finding indicates that the triathletes obtained a large amount (59%) of their energy during the Ironman from endogenous fuel stores. The authors noted that total energy expenditure was similar between the sexes when adjusted for fat-free mass. Another study of male triathletes showed a race-day energy deficit ranging from 6,070 to 8,651 kcal.[32] Glace et al[75] found that male ultrarunners incurred an energy deficit of 7,513 kcal in 24.3 hours during a 100-mile run. In another study, Glace et al[80] found that male and female ultrarunners incurred an energy deficit of 2,516 kcal in 26.2 hours during a 100-mile run.

For multiday events, Saris et al[26] found that mean daily energy intake of 5 male cyclists competing in the Tour de France (5,785 kcal) closely matched their average daily energy expenditure (6,069 kcal), so that they maintained their body weights and compositions during the race. Two case studies, 1 involving a runner and the other involving 2 cyclists, found that the athletes maintained their body weights and compositions over 9 to 10 days of ultraendurance exercise, suggesting that their energy intakes were adequate to meet their energy demands.[27,29] Remarkably, an athlete who ran around Australia lost only about 5 kg after averaging approximately 47 miles/d for 191 days. O'Connor and Cox[34] noted that a typical day's intake for this athlete provided about 100 g of protein, more than 1,000 g of carbohydrate, and 120 g of fat.

Carbohydrate Loading

An additional point to consider when devising a race nutrition strategy is that male and female athletes differ with respect to carbohydrate loading before racing. Female athletes oxidize more fat and less carbohydrate during endurance training compared with their male counterparts.[79] According to a review by Burke et al,[81] carbohydrate loading appears to be most effective in men running more than 30 km. The research available regarding women and carbohydrate loading is scarce and inconclusive, likely because of small sample sizes; however, a few studies have demonstrated improvements in performance for carbohydrate loading by female endurance athletes. In addition, carbohydrate loading is only effective if the athlete is consuming adequate energy and carbohydrate leading into the race. The regimen can be viewed as an extended period of fueling up to prepare for competition. Carbohydrate loading guidelines are provided in Chapter 2.

Intake Before Training and Competition

Consuming carbohydrate before an endurance event helps to maintain blood glucose levels during prolonged exercise. The athlete should consume 1 to 4 g of carbohydrate per kilogram of body weight 1 to 4 hours before exercise. García-Rovés et al[28] noted that the Tour de Spain cyclists consumed carbohydrate in the amount of 4.5 g/kg approximately 3 hours before competition. Foods typically consumed prior to endurance and ultraendurance events include liquid meals, muesli, porridge, milk, yogurt, fruit and fruit juice, toast, jam, pancakes, waffles, bagels and biscuits, and jam or honey.[26,28,29,34]

Intake During Training and Competition

Consuming carbohydrate is neither practical nor necessary during endurance exercise lasting less than 60 minutes.[82] Small amounts of carbohydrate from sports drinks or foods or a carbohydrate mouth rinse may enhance performance during sustained high-intensity endurance exercise lasting 45 to 75 minutes. In a systematic review by Silva et al, carbohydrate rinsing with a 6.4% to 10% carbohydrate beverage every 5 to 10 minutes improved performance by approximately 2% to 3%. This technique could be used by athletes who experience gastrointestinal distress at high intensities.[83] Athletes should consume 30 to 60 g of carbohydrate per hour from carbohydrate-rich fluids or foods during endurance sports and exercise lasting 1 to 2.5 hours.[82] As the duration of the event increases, so does the amount of carbohydrate required to enhance performance. During endurance and ultraendurance exercise lasting 2.5 to 3 hours and longer, athletes should consume 80 to 90 g of carbohydrate per hour from products that provide multiple transportable carbohydrates.[82] Based on Jeukendrup's 2010 review, [4] it appears that a glucose-fructose or maltodextrin-fructose mixture provides the most benefit, allowing for carbohydrate oxidation at a rate of 1.75 g/min.

Consuming carbohydrate during training enables the athlete to maintain a desirable training pace (and therefore maximize training adaptations), in addition to practicing fueling strategies for competition. Athletes should individually determine a fueling plan that meets their nutritional goals (including hydration) and minimizes gastrointestinal distress by consuming familiar foods or fluids in 10- to 20-minute intervals. Table 22.4 lists the carbohydrate intakes of athletes during specific ultraendurance events.

Kimber et al[74] found that New Zealand Ironman triathletes consumed substantially more energy during the bike segment (2,233 kcal for women; 2,896 kcal for men) than during the run segment of the race (883 kcal for women; 1,049 kcal for men). Energy intake during cycling provided 73% of the total energy intake throughout the race. This is not surprising because foods and fluid are easier to consume and digest when a person is on a bike, and the cycling portion is approximately 54% of the total race time. The bike portion of an Ironman also provides the opportunity to obtain energy and fluid in preparation for the marathon run.

Saris et al[26] found that male Tour de France cyclists consumed nearly half of their daily energy during the race and that about 30% of the total carbohydrate consumed came from high-carbohydrate beverages. Gabel et al[27] found that 2 male cyclists consumed about 24% of their total energy intake from high-carbohydrate beverages (eg, sports drinks, fruit juices) during a 10-day, 2,050-mile ride. Eden and Abernathy[29] reported that a male ultradistance runner in the Sydney to Melbourne race used a combination of high-carbohydrate solid foods and a sports drink during running to meet his energy requirements.

Although high-carbohydrate beverages help increase carbohydrate and energy intakes during endurance and ultraendurance events, they can also cause gastrointestinal distress when consumed in large volumes. Lindeman[30] noted that a male RAAM cyclist's reliance on a 23% carbohydrate solution to meet the majority of his energy needs contributed to gastrointestinal distress during the race despite consistent dilution. Gastrointestinal distress during training or racing is attributable to the types of carbohydrate being consumed in addition to the osmotic pressure exerted in the small intestine when particular drinks and products are

TABLE 22.4 Carbohydrate Intakes During Ultraendurance Events[26-29,34,74-76]

Type of athlete	Carbohydrate intake, g/h
Male and female New Zealand Ironman triathletes[74]	Males: 82 Females: 62
Male ultrarunners[a,75]	44
Male and female ultrarunners[b,76]	54
Male Tour de France cyclists[26]	94
Male Pony Express Trail cyclists[c,27]	60-75
Male Tour de Spain cyclists[28]	25
Male Sydney to Melbourne runner[d,29]	39
Male 24-hour mountain bike racer[34]	75

[a] 100-mile run, 24.3 hours.
[b] 100-mile run, 26.2 hours.
[c] 2,050 miles in 10 days.
[d] 628 miles in 8.5 days.

ingested.[85-87] The perfect sports drink or product for every athlete in every condition does not exist. Thus, the goal for the sports nutritionist is to help formulate the best nutrition plan for each individual athlete and their personal preferences while avoiding gastrointestinal distress and maximizing performance.

It is essential for a variety of carbohydrate-rich foods and fluids to be available during ultraendurance and multiday events to prevent flavor fatigue and an associated decrease in energy intake. Alternating between sweet choices (eg, gels, sodas, candy) and savory and/or salty choices (eg, vegetable soup or broth, pretzels, baked chips) helps to maintain the athlete's desire to eat. Consuming solid foods with small amounts of protein and fat (eg, a turkey, cheese, or peanut butter sandwich) also helps provide satiety and variety.[34]

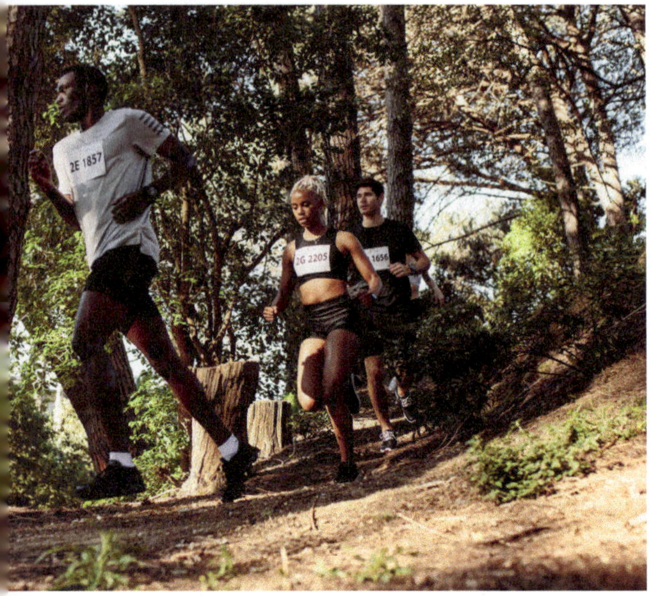

Consuming a small amount of protein during prolonged exercise improves the athlete's protein balance. Koopman et al[88] found that the combined ingestion of protein (0.25 g/kg body weight per hour) and carbohydrate (0.7 g/kg body weight per hour) before, during, and after prolonged moderate-intensity exercise (6 hours at 50% of VO_2 max) improved the net protein balance at rest, during exercise, and during subsequent recovery in endurance athletes; however, this did not necessarily equate to better performance. For more information on protein, refer for Chapter 3.

Gabel et al[27] reported that 2 men who cycled 2,050 miles in 10 days achieved an optimal intake because of the variety and palatability of foods that were available during the event. The cyclists consumed sports drinks, fruit juices, sodas, potato chips, crackers, fruit, cookies, sandwiches, and candy. Eden and Abernathy[29] noted that the foods eaten by a male runner during the Sydney to Melbourne race were based on what he had enjoyed eating during training and what he could tolerate while competing. The runner consumed a sports drink, pasta with meat sauce, rice, bread, biscuits, cheese, vegetable soup, a muffin with egg and cheese, fruit, and fruit juice. O'Connor and Cox[34] noted that an athlete who completed the Race Around Australia consumed sports drinks, fruit juice, soft drinks, high-carbohydrate supplements, milk shakes, and liquid meals during the run.

High-fiber foods should be limited during competition to avoid gut distress such as abdominal bloating, cramping, and diarrhea.[17] Lindeman[30] noted that a male RAAM cyclist's high fiber intake (57 g/d) from consuming fiber-rich sports bars and fruit may have contributed to his gastrointestinal distress during the race. When an athlete's blood flow to the gut is low (eg, during intense cycling or running), the athlete should emphasize carbohydrate-rich fluids (sports drinks, liquid meals, high-carbohydrate liquid supplements, fruit juices, and carbohydrate gels) to promote rapid gastric emptying and intestinal absorption. When the athlete's blood flow to the gut is moderate (eg, during moderate-paced cycling or slow running), the athlete may be able to consume easily digested carbohydrate-rich foods such as sports bars, fruit, and grain products (fig bars, bagels, graham crackers) in addition to liquid foods and fluids.[89] Because endurance athletes training and racing for longer than 2 hours will need to rely on exogenous carbohydrates, it is important to note that the gastrointestinal tract is highly adaptable and can be "trained," as explained by Jeukendrup.[90]

Recreational athletes often travel away from their home training base for races, which can create uncertainty in their results. They may train in a hot, humid environment and travel to race in a cooler, drier part of the country or world. They may train at low elevation in an area with little elevation change but race in the mountains. This makes it extremely important to gather data (eg, average heart rates, sweat tests) year-round, not only during the time of year the race will occur. This might also dictate the type of fueling and hydration plan the athlete should practice at home. For example, if a large amount of elevation change is expected during the race, liquid nutrition might be easier for an athlete to consume while climbing than solid food. If the athlete will race at altitude, they may require a higher energy intake compared to what they would consume where they normally train. These are just some of the reasons that an athlete and their support team must be knowledgeable about the environmental conditions where the race will occur, the time of year when the race will occur, and some details about the race course.

Intake After Training and Competition

Restoring muscle and liver glycogen stores, replacing fluid and electrolyte losses, and promoting muscle repair are important for recovery after strenuous endurance training and multiday events. When the time period between workouts or competitions that deplete muscle glycogen stores is less than 8 hours, the athlete should start consuming carbohydrate immediately after the first exercise session to maximize the effective recovery time between sessions. Specifically, the athlete should consume carbohydrate at a rate of 1 to 1.2 g per kilogram of body weight per hour for the first 4 hours after glycogen-depleting exercise. Consuming small amounts of carbohydrate frequently (every 15 to 30 minutes) further enhances muscle glycogen synthesis. During longer periods of recovery (eg, 24 hours), it does not matter how carbohydrate intake is spaced throughout the day as long as the athlete consumes adequate carbohydrate and energy.[82] Liquid forms of carbohydrate may be desirable when athletes have decreased appetites as a result of fatigue or dehydration.

In addition to carbohydrate, the athlete's initial recovery snack or meal should include high-quality protein in the amount of 15 to 25 g[82] or 0.25 to 0.3 g per kilogram of body weight.[42,43,45,91] Protein can be consumed through liquids, such as a recovery drink, or through solid food, such as a meal or snack. Consuming protein with recovery snacks and meals helps to increase the net muscle protein balance, promote muscle tissue repair, and enhance adaptations involving the synthesis of new proteins.[92] Adding a small amount of protein (~0.3 g per kilogram of body weight per hour) to a suboptimal carbohydrate intake (<1 g per kilogram of body weight per hour) also accelerates muscle glycogen restoration.[93] Recovery meals and snacks contribute to an athlete's daily protein and carbohydrate requirements. In consideration of multiday events, García-Rovés et al[28] noted that Tour of Spain cyclists consumed carbohydrate at a rate of 1.1 g per kilogram of body weight per hour and protein at a rate of 0.35 g per kilogram of body weight per hour for the first 6 hours after the race. This combined dose of carbohydrate and protein helped promote muscle glycogen restoration and muscle tissue repair.

The foods consumed during recovery meals and snacks should contribute to the athlete's overall nutrient intake. Nutritious carbohydrate-rich foods and lean sources of protein and dairy also contain vitamins and minerals that are essential for health and performance. These micronutrients are important for postexercise recovery processes. Athletes should avoid consuming large amounts of foods high in fat or protein when total energy requirements or gastrointestinal distress limits food intake during recovery. These foods can displace carbohydrate-rich foods and reduce muscle glycogen storage.[18] It is common for endurance athletes to not feel hungry after long training sessions, especially in hot weather. Working with athletes to try a liquid recovery option could be important for a sports nutritionist to improve compliance and ensure that the athlete consumes an adequate amount of recovery calories and macronutrients.

TRAINING AND COMPETITION DAY FLUID AND SODIUM RECOMMENDATIONS

The research on fluid and sodium intakes on body weight changes during endurance events and their effects on performance is limited. Endurance athletes can experience both hyperhydration and hypohydration, especially during ultraendurance events. As illustrated in the "General Nutrition Requirements" section of this chapter, the fluid and sodium requirements for endurance athletes exhibit large degrees of variability. The same holds true during training and racing, thereby making it necessary to consider each athlete's needs individually. In addition, sweat rates during training may not closely reflect sweat rates on race day of an endurance event as a result of many factors.[94] It is not possible to develop a one-size-fits-all fluid and electrolyte replacement schedule because of the multiple factors that influence the sweating rate and sweat electrolyte concentration.[56] Endurance and ultraendurance athletes who have high sweat rates and high sodium concentrations in their sweat ("salty sweat") can sustain substantial losses of sodium.[95] However, high sodium sweat losses could also be due to a high daily sodium intake, and it remains unclear if this factor affects all athletes in the same way.[96]

Symptomatic exercise-associated hyponatremia (plasma sodium concentration <135 mmol/L) can occur in prolonged endurance exercise lasting more than 4 hours. Factors that contribute to exercise-associated hyponatremia include drinking an amount of fluid that exceeds sweat and urinary water losses, as well as excessive loss of total body sodium.[67] According to the 2015 Third International Exercise-Associated Hyponatremia Consensus Statement, those at higher risk include smaller persons and possibly those who regularly use nonsteroidal anti-inflammatory drugs (NSAIDs), although more research is needed on NSAID use.[97] In addition, several studies have indicated that female athletes are at higher risk for exercise-induced hyponatremia than their male counterparts.[95,96]

In events that last less than 4 hours, hyponatremia is primarily caused by overdrinking before, during, and after the event.[95,98] During a marathon, symptomatic hyponatremia is more likely to occur in smaller and less lean participants who run slowly, sweat less, and drink excessively before, during, and after the race, as well as female athletes.[96,98-100]

Endurance athletes can experience health problems from both dehydration and overdrinking. Dehydration is more common and can impair exercise performance and contribute to serious heat illness. However, symptomatic hyponatremia is more dangerous and can cause grave illness or death. Because of the considerable variability among individuals in the rates and electrolyte contents of sweat, athletes should customize their fluid replacement plans.[56]

Intake Before Training and Competition

Endurance athletes should begin exercise with normal hydration and plasma electrolyte levels. Prior to exercise, an athlete should drink approximately 5 to 7 mL of fluid per hour per kilogram of body weight about 4 hours before exercise. At the top of this range, 7 mL per kilogram of body weight is equivalent to approximately 1 oz for every 10 lb of body weight. Drinking several hours before exercise allows adequate time for the urine output to return toward normal.[64]

The Sports Dietitians Australia position statement on nutrition for exercise in hot environments notes that glycerol has been removed from the World Anti-Doping Agency Prohibited List and that it is an effective osmolyte that enhances fluid retention.[101] One study by Goulet et al[102] supported adding glycerol to the sodium and fluid requirements preceding exercise in hot environments to encourage additional fluid retention. In addition, Sims et al[103] found that an acute sodium-fluid load (20–40 mg of sodium with 10 mL of fluid per kilogram of body weight) before training can improve physiological tolerance to warmer temperatures, even when no fluid is ingested during exercise. Athletes should experiment with different preexercise foods and fluids during training. Before competition, the athlete should choose familiar, well-tolerated, and palatable foods and fluids.[16]

Intake During Training and Competition

During prolonged ultraendurance exercise (eg, Ironman triathlon), total sodium losses can induce symptomatic hyponatremia if the athlete is drinking either not enough or too much fluid.[56] Previously, researchers thought that high sweat rates and a high concentration of sodium in sweat confer a greater risk of developing hyponatremia because less fluid intake is required to produce dangerously low blood sodium levels. However, more recent information suggests that low blood sodium levels are due to overdrinking.[94,95,97]

Hydration during endurance exercise is necessary to prevent the detrimental effects of excessive dehydration (>2% body weight loss) and electrolyte loss on exercise performance and health. A loss of 1% to 2% of body weight is likely to occur from factors unrelated to sweat losses (eg, substrate oxidation) and is acceptable.[17] Dehydration increases physiological stress as measured by core temperature, heart rate, and perceived exertion, and these effects are accentuated during exercise in warm to hot and humid weather. The greater the shortage of body water, the greater the physiological strain and the greater the impairment of endurance performance.[56] However, in a 2013 meta-analysis of field research, Goulet et al[102] demonstrated that body mass losses of 4% or less of body weight in outdoor, real-world, time-trial exercise are unlikely to impair performance. In addition, a weight loss of up to 3% may be tolerable and may not impair performance in cool weather.[56] Glace et al[75] estimated that the loss of body fat (according to skinfold measurements) accounted for about 1.13 kg of the average of 1.6 kg lost (2% of body weight) by study participants during a 100-mile run. In a second study, Glace et al[80] found that high fluid intakes during a 100-mile run were associated with decreased serum sodium levels and increased risk of mental status change, suggesting possible fluid overload.

To prevent hyponatremia, endurance athletes should avoid overconsumption of fluids and associated weight gain.[56] Some studies suggest that consuming a sodium-containing sports drink helps to maintain plasma sodium levels and may reduce the risk of hyponatremia during prolonged exercise,[84] whereas other studies have demonstrated that sodium supplementation does not affect endurance performance during cycling time trials[104] and that it is not required to maintain serum sodium levels during Ironman triathlon.[105] For the time being, experts recommend that the fluid consumed for rehydration contain 20 to 50 mmol of sodium per liter.[106] This is equivalent to 460 to 1,150 mg/L. This practice is especially important for heavy or salty sweaters as well as for training sessions exceeding 3 hours.

Athletes participating in endurance exercise lasting longer than 3 hours should be particularly meticulous about establishing their fluid replacement schedule. As the exercise duration increases, the cumulative effects of slight disparities between fluid intake and fluid loss can cause extreme dehydration or hyponatremia.[56] Athletes training for 1 hour or less may not need hydration during training, depending on the environment and the prehydration and posthydration plan.

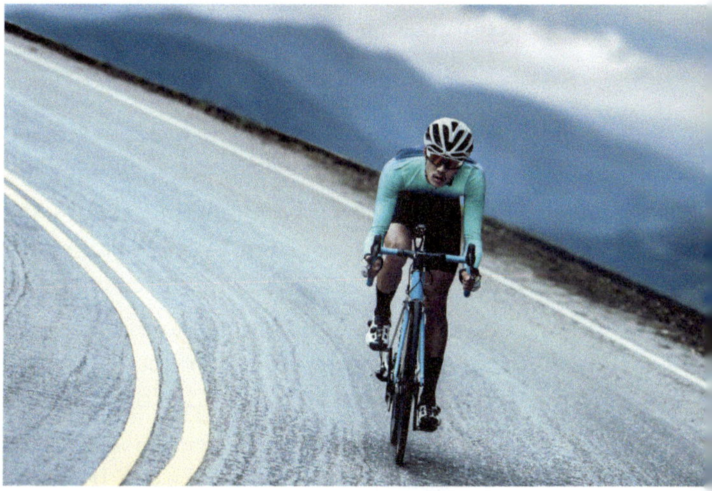

During training, athletes should experiment with different fluid replacement drinks and adjust their drinking strategies based on the workout intensity, duration, and environmental conditions. Drinking appropriately during workouts enables the athlete to maintain a desirable training pace (and maximize training adaptations), protects the athlete against heat illness, and allows the athlete to practice proper drinking strategies for competition.[56] The athlete may also choose water as the hydration source, employing gels, gummies, or other sports nutrition products to provide the electrolytes and carbohydrates. The sports nutritionist should use caution when recommending that an athlete use a fluid replacement drink to also meet their carbohydrate needs. Because of changes in fluid needs related to seasonal changes in temperatures, this could severely affect glycogen replacement. Worse, it could cause the athlete to overhydrate when trying to meet their carbohydrate needs during cooler temperatures.

Intake After Training and Competition

Ideally, the athlete should fully restore fluid and electrolyte losses between exercise sessions.[56] Consuming sodium during recovery promotes fluid retention and stimulates thirst.[107] Precise sodium losses are harder to determine than water losses because each athlete has vastly different rates of electrolyte losses in sweat. Although drinks containing sodium (eg, sports drinks) may be beneficial, many foods can supply the needed electrolytes. Extra salt can be added only when necessary to meals and recovery fluids when sweat sodium losses are high, as ½ tsp (2.5 g) of salt supplies 1,000 mg of sodium.[56] Keep in mind that this may not be an issue that needs to be addressed for many recreational athletes. Practitioners should consider the athlete's individual needs for the best nutrition and hydration plan.

Athletes should drink 24 oz of fluid for each pound lost to achieve rapid and total recovery from dehydration.[108] The additional volume (150% of sweat losses) is required to compensate for the increased urine production that goes along with the rapid intake of large volumes of fluid.[56,108] Additional information on fluid and sodium needs is provided in Chapter 6.

SPORT- AND RACE-SPECIFIC INFORMATION

Several overarching similarities exist among all endurance events that sports dietitians should consider when working with endurance athletes:

- An elite athlete's time to finish an event can differ tremendously from a recreational athlete's time. For many recreational athletes, finish times are double that of their elite counterparts.
- More often than not, an elite athlete has the opportunity to acclimatize in the race environment before event day. This is rarely the case for a recreational athlete. It is important to know the details of the race location and weather for the race; some races have extreme temperature shifts throughout the race day(s), making it necessary to make adjustments throughout the race.

- For most endurance races, professional athletes or those competing at the elite level have a special feed zone, and their exact nutrition bottle or food is handed to them by volunteers or teammates, depending on the sport. This makes it easy to plan for this level of athlete. Recreational athletes have to bring their own nutrition, rely on products provided on the course, or have a club teammate who is not racing hand them nutrition in designated feed zones. In many races, disqualification occurs if aid is not received in the designated feed zones.
- Each type of athlete and group of athletes has their own rituals, desires, and beliefs, making it important for athlete education to become a priority. Sports dietitians should encourage practice and application during long training sessions. The sports dietitian should get to know the sport culture to be able to build a rapport with each athlete individually. It is worth noting that recreational athletes are consumers that may fall prey to media hype of different diets, supplements, and practices, making it important to help them understand the research available in these areas affecting sports performance and health.
- One unique consideration with regard to sports nutrition products is the weather. If it is very cold, gummies and gels will solidify, making them difficult to chew or swallow. Solid food will also feel dry and tough to consume in cold weather. Body heat can keep the product warm if it is near the athlete's body, as opposed to being stored in their equipment (eg, bike or pack).
- At endurance and ultraendurance events, it is not uncommon for athletes to unknowingly drop their nutrition on the ground or not be able to find it easily for various reasons. Having extra fuel or salt tabs at feed stations or in a pocket or pack is always a good idea.
- Finally, for endurance events, it is crucial that the athlete practice their race nutrition and hydration plan many times before race day. If the athlete is wearing a heart rate monitor, a timer can be set to remind the athlete to eat and drink in the same way as was practiced.

For practical applications of nutrition, the following sections present specific details that are unique to different sports. The discussion of each sport is divided into endurance and ultraendurance events, and if there is a multiday event for that sport, this is addressed as well.

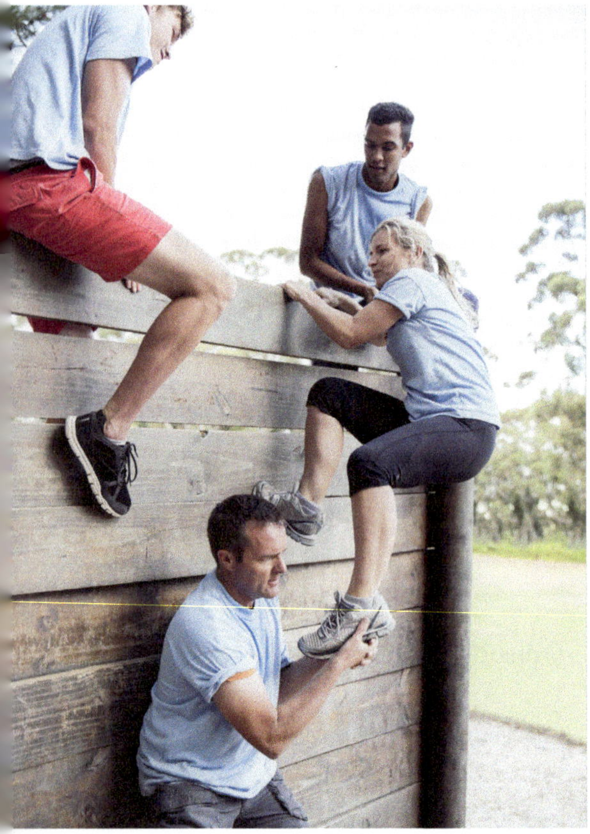

Adventure Racing

Adventure racing, also called expedition racing, is typically a team sport involving different distances, times, and disciplines (eg, trekking, mountain biking, paddling, and climbing).

ENDURANCE RACING

Shorter sprint adventure races can last 3 to 6 hours, making this an endurance sport. Athletes are responsible for nutrition and hydration because there are no aid stations on the course. A light-weight pack is necessary to carry hydration, and the shorter distance lends itself to a faster pace and higher heart rate. What the athlete chooses to consume depends on their preferences and what they practiced in training. One easy nutrition plan is to combine energy with hydration in the pack because the course is short enough for this possibility. If this method is not possible because of athlete preference, quick, low-fiber carbohydrates are easy and light to carry.

ULTRAENDURANCE RACING

The next level of endurance adventure race lasts 12 or 24 hours. These races typically have a checklist of gear that all athletes must carry in their pack, making it heavy at times. At this level, athletes compete in teams of 2 to 4 racers. There is a transition area between sections of the course where the athletes can leave their nutrition and hydration of choice to keep their packs as light as possible. This allows the athletes to add additional fuel and hydration for each section of the race.

Obstacle Course Racing

Obstacle course racing involves foot racing with various physical challenges in the form of obstacles. The most popular obstacle course races in the United States to date are Tough Mudder (www.toughmudder.com), Spartan Trail (www.spartan.com), and Savage Race (www.savagerace.com).

ENDURANCE OBSTACLE COURSE RACING

The Spartan Super and Spartan Beast, Tough Mudder, and Savage races fall into the endurance category.

The Spartan Super race covers 10K and has 25 obstacles; the Spartan Beats covers 21K and includes 30 obstacles. Finish times for Spartan races depend on the location and terrain of the race. Some Spartan Beast races are won in approximately 2 hours, and others take up nearly 4 hours to win. Because of the wide variety of Spartan race terrain (eg, some flat and some mountainous), the availability of aid stations at each race is not consistent, which makes it difficult to depend on course nutrition and hydration support. There is no time limit on Spartan Super or Beast races.

The Tough Mudder races are typically more consistent; all endurance courses are 10K or 15K and have 20 to 25 obstacles. Racers can often carry sports drinks and water throughout the course. Winners typically finish in less than 2 hours, but any competitors who have not reached a specific time limit at the designated halfway point are given a modified course route that allows them to cross the finish line. Tough Mudder is more conducive to athletes using course nutrition and hydration support.

The Savage Race is a 5- to 7-mile course with 27 or more obstacles. One or 2 aid stations are usually positioned along the course that athletes can use if they do not carry their own nutrition and hydration. However, it is difficult to know what products will be available, which makes it difficult to practice race nutrition ahead of time.

One last consideration in nutrition planning for this type of race is the wave start times. Groups of athletes are released at 15- to 30-minute time increments to put space between participants. Additionally, start times run in waves between 8 AM and 3 PM.

ULTRAENDURANCE OBSTACLE COURSE RACING

Spartan's longest race, called the Ultra, takes place over 50K, includes 60 or more obstacles, and has an average finish time of approximately 12 hours. Race start times vary and can be morning or night. Athletes are allowed to access a drop bin, a box of goods created prior to the race in which athletes can store extra clothing, food, drinks, and so on. If they choose to carry their own nutrition and hydration while racing, athletes can also refuel during the loops as they need to. Some aid stations are available on the course. To date, the race has been held in hot and cold environments with rugged to moderate terrain.

The World's Toughest Mudder consists of a 5-mile course; the winner is the athlete who finishes the most laps in 24 hours. Depending on the location and the terrain, this could be as much as 100 miles or as little as 55 miles. Because this course is a loop, it is easy for athletes to control their nutrition and hydration schedules. The race location changes every year and could be international. This event has a mass start instead of wave start times.

Cross-Country Skiing

Although cross-country skiing is widely practiced as a recreational activity, cross-country ski competitions involve a variety of formats for races over courses of varying lengths, including marathons.

ENDURANCE SKIING

The sheer nature of the cross-country ski gear and the need for gloves during a race make it difficult for the cross-country ski athlete to open certain types of nutrition packages. It is possible to carry a waist pack with a water bottle and access it regularly. The bottle could contain most of the calories the athlete needs, as well as their hydration. In this case, liquid nutrition may be the most viable option. Keep in mind that, depending on the temperature, liquids can also freeze and become unusable.

Cycling

Road bicycle racing involves both team and individual competitions and, by nature, is significantly longer than running events.

ENDURANCE CYCLING

Endurance cycling events are fast and furious in the elite field, making it very difficult for the athlete to consume nutrition, especially when a volunteer is responsible for handing out the nutrition products. These events are typically 75 to 125 miles, and teams usually work together in a draft legal race structure (cyclists rotate through a *peloton* [the main field or group of cyclists in a race], taking turns riding up front "pulling" the rest of the group before peeling off and latching onto the back). A team member or a volunteer at designated feed zones can hand nutrition and hydration to the cyclist, or there may be a caravan where teammates can hand the athlete nutrition and hydration. For nonelite cyclists, endurance cycling events range from 100k (approximately 62 miles) to 160K (approximately 100 miles). Athletes typically carry their own nutrition and hydration or take only water or sports drinks at aid stations, choosing to finish the race faster than they would if they stopped at aid stations for nutrition. For the athlete's safety, if the nutrition plan includes solid food choices, it is important to have packages open and accessible.

Gravel cycling is an event newer to the endurance cycling world, and it is gaining interest very quickly. The endurance distances and nutrition challenges are similar to those of the road cycling events just described.

ULTRAENDURANCE CYCLING

Many types of ultraendurance cycling events exist. Some consist of a specific number of hours of a time trial, such as 6, 12, or 24 hours. These races consist of a loop course, and the winner is the person who completes the most loops in the set amount of time. Some races are draft legal (riding directly behind someone without being penalized) and some are not, which sometimes affects the athlete's ability to reach for and implement the nutrition on their bike. Elite athletes do not participate in these types of races, but they are very popular among recreational athletes.

Other ultraendurance cycling races total a set number of miles, such as 100, 200, 400, or 500 miles, with a maximum of 250 miles for a single-day event. Although an elite racer can finish 100 miles in approximately 3 hours 30 minutes, it may take a recreational athlete as long as 8 hours to finish. This ultimately dictates the type of nutrition plan that each athlete would follow. Most courses have aid stations containing some or all of the following items: sports drinks, salt tablets, pickle juice, baked goods, salty snacks, soft drinks, candy, peanut butter sandwiches, and boiled potatoes. The elite athletes receive their planned nutrition handed to them at designated feed zones as they are riding through, whereas the recreational athletes occasionally stop at aid stations to rest, refuel, and rehydrate for a long day.

A hydration pack may be necessary, depending on the spacing of aid stations and individual sweat losses. Riders can fit 2 to 4 bottles on their bikes and can carry 1 or 2 bottles in their race jerseys. However, for every bottle of fluid, the athlete is adding weight to the bike, which can make carrying too many bottles a hard sell. Asking the right questions can help the sports dietitian develop a better plan for the athlete. As a reminder, recreational athletes are most at risk for fluid and electrolyte imbalances and hyponatremia because of the time spent on the course.

Ultraendurance gravel racing is gaining popularity, similarly to endurance gravel racing. Distances include 142 to 200 miles in a single day. The nutrition availability and challenges that exist are like those of ultraendurance road cycling events. Popular US events include Steamboat Gravel (www.sbtgrvl.com), Unbound Gravel (www.unboundgravel.com), and Big Sugar (www.bigsugarclassic.com).

Running

Endurance running, also called long-distance running, can include track running, road running, and cross-country running. It is primarily an individual sport.

ENDURANCE RUNNING

Endurance running consists of road and trail races ranging in distance from a half-marathon (13.1 miles) to full marathon (26.2 miles). The finish times for these distances vary widely depending on each athlete's experience and goals. The largest attended road races now have corrals with wave starts.

For road races, there are typically aid stations on the course at designated spaces throughout the race. Some aid stations are sponsored, especially in large races. Information on what is offered at the aid stations is generally available on the race website. This helps the sports dietitian plan ahead for how the athlete should use the nutrition and hydration provided on the course. Otherwise, many different fuel belts and bottles and hydration packs are available for carrying nutrition and hydration to ensure that the athletes have what they need and what they used during training.

The availability of water is typically reliable on a race course, and only occasionally does the event run out when temperatures reach unusual highs. The availability of sports drinks may not be as reliable because of the way they are mixed (concentrations are usually either diluted or strong), and races tend to run out of sports drinks before water. One other issue with on-course nutrition is that the flavors of the sports drinks, gummies, or gels the race distributes may not be the same flavor the athlete used during training, which may make them difficult to consume.

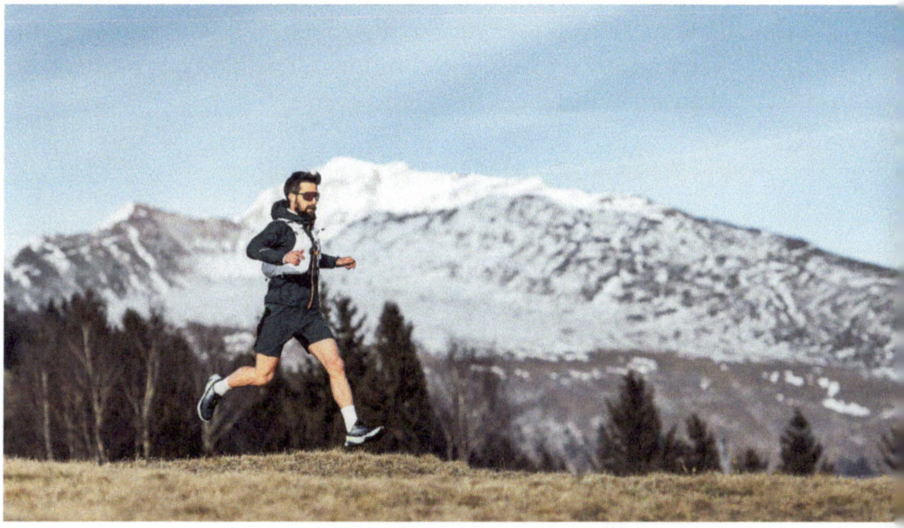

Most trail runs have a mass start. For trail races, the aid stations are spaced farther apart because of trail access points. Athletes can choose from many more fueling options, including solid, liquid, sugary, and salty snacks. The limited number of stations, however, makes it easier for the athlete to potentially eat too much at one time and not properly space out nutrition, as discussed previously in this chapter. This is especially true for slower runners. To improve the athlete's trail running plan for those using on-course nutrition, educate them to take small amounts of aid from each aid station, allowing them to spread out their energy intake over time. The sports dietitian should encourage athletes to carry a handheld bottle or race hydration pack for the best hydration plan.

ULTRAENDURANCE RUNNING

Ultraendurance running distance is typically no more than 135 miles for a single-day event. Examples include the Badwater Ultramarathon road race (www.badwater.com) and the Western States Endurance Run trail race (www.wser.org). Many of these races are held in the United States and throughout the world. The elite field is small, making many of the entrants recreational. Even though these distances involve constant running, many participants will not finish in a 24-hour time frame. The fastest times at Badwater are just shy of 24 hours for men. Although a 100-mile trail run, such as Western States, is won in under 15 hours, the slowest runner may finish in twice that time.

For some ultraendurance trail races, the course is set up in a loop structure, making it easy for the athlete to access their own nutrition and hydration products of choice and not have to rely on the course support. This is important for athletes with certain constraints (eg, celiac disease, past gastrointestinal distress). During a 100K-trail race, it is not uncommon for a runner to have a pacer, usually a friend or multiple friends who can help remind the runner to eat and drink in the event their motor skills are declining.

Many ultraendurance runners carry 2 handheld race bottles or wear a hydration backpack or waist pack. With a hydration pack, it is difficult for athletes to know how much they are drinking because the pack is not clear. Discussing their hydration plan in terms of swallows or sips per 10 minutes, or similar measure, is helpful. The athlete can better gauge their fluid intake when using handheld bottles or waist packs with individual bottles.

Marathon Rowing

Rowing, also referred to as crew in the United States, involves propelling a boat (racing shell) on water using oars. Athletes compete in a number of boat classes, ranging from an individual shell to an 8-person shell.

ENDURANCE ROWING

Finishing times for rowing races can range from just over 3 hours to up to 6 hours. It is somewhat easy for a rower to put nutrition and hydration in the boat. If the nutrition plan includes solid food choices, it is important to have packages open and easy to access. This is another sport in which the athlete's hands are being used, so the quicker the athlete can consume nutrition the better, especially when racing as a single. One final consideration is wind. Some races can be extremely windy, making consuming nutrition and hydration even more difficult, in addition to increasing the athlete's workload and energy output.

Triathlon

A triathlon is a multiple-stage competition that includes the completion of 3 endurance disciplines in immediate succession over various distances. Although several combinations exist, the most popular combination is swimming, cycling, and running. A triathlon can be an on-road or off-road event, with the off-road events differing in distances from road events.

ENDURANCE TRIATHLON

Olympic distance triathlons are considered endurance events. Average age-group times range from approximately 2 hours 30 minutes to 3 hours 10 minutes depending on the course, with the last athletes coming in at approximately 4 hours. The course has aid stations on the bike and run portions, and some races are sponsored, so specific products may be available at aid stations. This information is typically available on the race website. Volunteers are responsible for handing out hydration and nutrition, but they are not always experienced. Getting hydration on the bike can be difficult as is, especially when the athlete is also inexperienced.

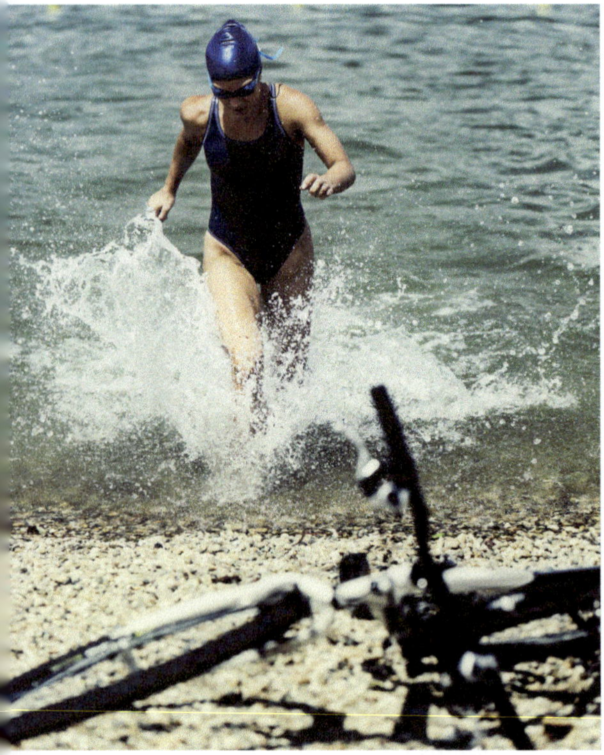

Unlike ultraendurance triathlons, in endurance triathlons, each split is longer than 1 hour, making it difficult to follow an hourly plan. It is much easier to discuss nutrition in terms of "on the bike," "in transition," or "on the run," instead of following a plan based on an hourly clock. This still allows for nutrition and hydration every 10 to 20 minutes, but the athlete will not have to think about time as much during the race. For example, the sports dietitian could advise the athlete to "consume *X* calories of *X* product at the beginning, middle, and end of the bike portion of the race."

ULTRAENDURANCE TRIATHLON

Ultraendurance triathlon events take more than 4 hours to finish and could be a Half Ironman (1.2-mile swim, 56-mile bike, 13.1-mile run) or Ironman (2.4-mile swim, 112-mile bike, 26.22-mile run) (www.ironman.com). In these races, it is important to consider the differences in nutrition tolerance during the bike and run phases of the race. Athletes can generally consume more calories per hour cycling than running.[18] Ironman triathlon competitors often decrease their calorie intake toward the end of the bike segment so they can start the run with a fairly empty gut. During the run segment of a triathlon, the athletes usually consume only sports drinks, gels, gummies, broth, and water to reduce the risk of gut distress.

Many races have implemented a wave start. It is important for the athlete to find out in which wave they will begin because it could be as much as an hour after the official race start, and this dictates the prerace meal. Additionally, there are course cutoff times when athletes are removed from the course if they do not make it to a specified point by a certain time.

The aid stations in these races are similar to those in Olympic distance courses. On an Ironman course, the bike and run portions have special needs stations at the halfway point, and athletes are allowed to put any nutrition or hydration products of choice in their numbered bag. The numbering makes it easy for a volunteer to quickly identify the correct bag when an athlete enters the special needs area. Athletes are not required to stop to get their bags, but it sometimes helps to have extra nutrition and hydration available in case something unexpected occurs.

Most ultraendurance nutrition plans should be discussed with the athlete in terms of "per hour on the bike" and "per hour on the run" for best compliance. The sports dietitian should be aware of the hydration system that is available on the athlete's bike. Some athletes have hydration systems between the handlebars that make it very easy to drink. Others have cages for water bottles on the bike frame, and others store hydration behind the seat. Knowing this information will help with planning.

It is not uncommon for some athletes to wear fuel belts or to carry a handheld water bottle on the run portion of the course, which enables them to use their product of choice instead of relying on the on-course nutrition. This also improves fluid consumption because the athletes do not have to wait until they arrive at aid stations to drink.

Mountain Biking

Mountain biking events are off-road and are grouped into 2 main categories: cross-country and downhill. Cross-country mountain biking is considered an endurance sport.

ENDURANCE AND ULTRAENDURANCE BIKING

In mountain biking, a marathon can range from 37 to 99 miles, as defined by Union Cycliste Internationale. However, there are many single-day mountain bike races that are longer than 99 miles. Mountain bike races can also be 6-, 12-, or 24-hour events; the winner is the rider who completes the most loops of a course within that time frame. Times can vary wildly for distance races because of differences in terrain; for example, the most recent Leadville Trail 100 (a 100-mile race, www.leadvilleraceseries.com/mtb/leadvilletrail100mtb) was won in just under 6 hours, whereas the Wilderness 101 (www.mtntouring.com) was most recently won in just under 7 hours. Marathon races are usually cross-country races that usually have a mass start. However, some events are moving to a wave start because of the increasing numbers of participants. There are typically course cutoff times: If cyclists do not make it to certain points by certain times, they are removed from the course. Aid stations are available throughout the course for athletes to refuel and rehydrate. These aid stations are similar to trail-running aid stations and have many different options to choose from.

In such events, the recreational athlete will typically carry a hydration pack. Even with a hydration pack, it is difficult for the athlete to know how much they are drinking because the pack is not clear. Therefore, sports dietitians will find it helpful to discuss the hydration plan with athletes in terms of swallows or sips per 10 minutes or some similar metric.

Knowledge of the course is crucial to help the athlete be compliant with a nutrition plan. For example, if there are long periods of climbing in the mountains, it is unrealistic for the athlete to eat solid food during that time. In this case, compliance can be improved if the sports dietitian recommends that the athlete consume liquids during that portion of the race. In some longer mountain bike races, the athlete will dismount their bike at aid stations to refuel and rehydrate before continuing.

Swimrun

In swimrun events (www.swimrun.com), athletes alternate between swimming and running various distances. The terrain generally includes elevation, and the water temperatures are cold, requiring a wetsuit. Athletes keep their clothing of choice, including shoes, on during both the run and swim portions. Swimming might be done in the ocean or lakes. These athletes swim from island to island and run across the islands, with each distance between islands unknown unless the athlete has completed that exact course before. A few events allow athletes to race solo, but the majority of athletes race with a partner, requiring a tether on every swim portion. Athletes carry all equipment, and nutrition and hydration are generally tucked away in their wetsuits when not in use. All of these elements make following a set nutrition plan difficult. The dietitian can help the athlete understand their overarching nutrition and hydration needs, but the timing may need to be flexible. Aid stations are available on the course, with water and electrolyte replacement drinks that athletes can use to refill a collapsible cup that they are given.

ENDURANCE SWIMRUN

Short-course swimrun events range from 10.5 to 14.75 miles in total, with an average of 84% of the miles from running.

ULTRAENDURANCE SWIMRUN

Long-course swimrun events range from 18.75 to 28.5 miles in total, with an average of 82% of the miles from running.

Multiday Events

Cycling is the most common multiday sport, with professional stage races such as the Tour de France (www.letour.fr/en) and recreational races such as the Register's Annual Great Bicycle Ride Across Iowa (www.ragbrai.com) and RAAM (www.raceacrossamerica.org). For mountain biking, a race such as the Tour Divide (http://tourdivide.org) falls into this category. Adventure races take place over multiple days, and occasionally, endurance run events are held over multiple days (eg, Mount Rainier Circumnavigation on the Wonderland Trail).

The importance of proper fueling and hydration during ultraendurance and multiday events cannot be overemphasized. The athlete's fueling and fluid replacement strategies can be the difference between completing the event and dropping out of the race. During the event, the athlete's primary nutritional requirements are water, carbohydrate, and sodium.[18,34] Athletes should limit foods that are high in fat, protein, and fiber during the race to decrease the risk of gastrointestinal distress. The following pointers are also helpful:

- The food plan should be built around the athlete's food preferences and should include a variety of foods (savory, salty, and sweet) rather than a restricted assortment.
- Intakes of food and fluid should be closely monitored during multiday events. The crew should be prepared to enforce an eating and drinking schedule. If necessary, separate timers can be set for both liquid and solid feedings.[81]
- Food records and body weight should be assessed daily during multiday events. By tracking the athlete's food and fluid intakes and body weight, the crew can take immediate corrective action, without overfeeding or causing gastrointestinal distress, if the athlete starts to fall behind on fluid or energy intake.[27,81]
- Solid food should be easy to handle, chew, and digest. Beverages should promote rapid absorption of fluids and nutrients. Concentrated nutrition, such as high-carbohydrate supplements or liquid meals, may be offered immediately before scheduled rest.

The advice of a sports dietitian is recommended to determine the multiday athlete's nutritional requirements and develop an individualized dietary plan. The sports dietitian can also help monitor the athlete's nutrition during multiday events and help enforce food and fluid intake plans when necessary.

SUMMARY

Endurance athletes should consume adequate energy and carbohydrate (5 to 12 g per kilogram of body weight per day) during training to maintain a desirable training intensity and thus maximize training adaptations. They have increased protein requirements (~1.2 to 1.6 g per kilogram of body weight per day) and should consume 20% to 35% of calories from fat.

Endurance athletes who consume adequate total energy usually meet or exceed population reference values, such as the DRI for vitamins and minerals. Consuming a nutrient-dense diet containing fruits, vegetables, whole grains, legumes, lean meat, and dairy foods during training and competition also helps to ensure adequate micronutrient intakes. However, many groups of endurance athletes have an apparent negative energy balance. Endurance training can increase the need for certain micronutrients, such as iron and magnesium. Therefore, it is prudent to encourage energy balance and variety, to check for nutrient deficiencies, and to supplement as needed to improve menstrual dysfunction and performance.

Drinking during endurance exercise is necessary to prevent the detrimental effects of excessive dehydration (>2% body weight loss) and electrolyte loss on exercise performance and health. Athletes should have customized fluid replacement plans because of the considerable variability in sweating rates and sweat electrolyte content among individuals.

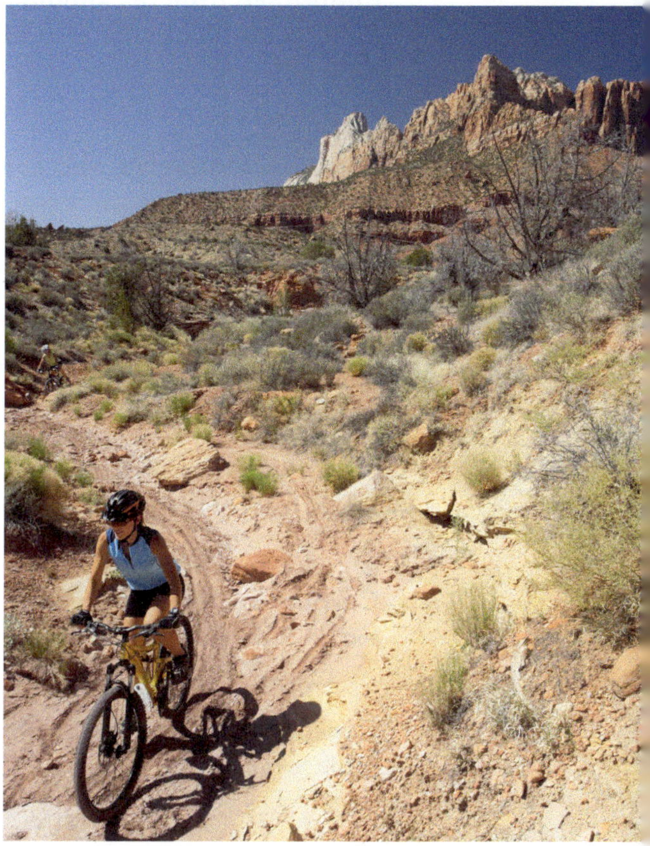

Carbohydrate loading can improve an athlete's performance in endurance events exceeding 90 minutes. For most athletes, a carbohydrate loading regimen will involve 2 to 3 days of a high-carbohydrate intake (10 to 12 g of carbohydrate per kilogram of body weight) and tapered training. Consuming carbohydrate before exercise can help performance by topping off muscle and liver glycogen stores. The preexercise meal should contain approximately 1 to 4 g of carbohydrate per kilogram of body weight, consumed 1 to 4 hours before exercise. The athlete should also slowly consume fluid at a rate of approximately 5 to 7 mL/kg/hr at least 4 hours before activity.

Consuming carbohydrate during exercise can improve performance by maintaining blood glucose levels and carbohydrate oxidation. A carbohydrate mouth rinse may enhance performance during sustained high-intensity endurance exercise lasting 45 to 75 minutes. Athletes should consume 30 to 60 g of carbohydrate per hour during endurance sports and exercise lasting 1 to 2.5 hours. During endurance and ultraendurance exercise lasting 2.5 to 3 hours and longer, athletes should consume up to 80 to 90 g of carbohydrate per hour from multiple transportable carbohydrates.

Consuming carbohydrate following exercise facilitates rapid refilling of one's carbohydrate stores. During the early period of recovery (0 to 4 hours), the endurance athlete should consume 1 to 1.2 g per kilogram of body weight per hour. The athlete's initial recovery snack or meal should also include 15 to 25 g of high-quality protein to promote muscle tissue repair. Endurance athletes should drink 24 oz of fluid for each pound lost and should consume adequate sodium to achieve rapid and total recovery from dehydration.

Endurance athletes should practice adjusting their fueling strategies based on workout intensity, workout duration, and environmental conditions. Testing specific foods and fluids before, during, and after training sessions also allows the athlete to determine effective fueling strategies for competition.

KEY TAKEAWAYS

Endurance athletes should consume adequate energy and carbohydrate (5-12 g per kilogram of body weight per day) during training to maintain a desirable training intensity and thus maximize training adaptations.

Endurance athletes who consume adequate total energy usually meet or exceed population reference values, such as the DRI for vitamins and minerals; however, it is hypothesized that many groups of endurance athletes are in negative energy balance.

Drinking during endurance exercise is necessary to prevent the detrimental effects of excessive dehydration and electrolyte loss on exercise performance and health. The best start is to minimize body weight loss to <2% and adjust from there. For ultraendurance events, body weight loss of 3% to 4% appears to be tolerated.

Carbohydrate loading can improve performance in endurance events exceeding 90 minutes.

Consuming carbohydrate during exercise can improve performance by maintaining blood glucose levels and carbohydrate oxidation.

Endurance athletes should practice adjusting their fueling strategies based on workout intensity, workout duration, and environmental conditions.

REFERENCES

1. Hargreaves M. Exercise physiology and metabolism. In: Burke L, Deakin V, eds. *Clinical Sports Nutrition*. 3rd ed. McGraw-Hill; 2006:1-20.
2. Coyle EF. Substrate utilization during exercise in active people. *Am J Clin Nutr*. 1995;61(4 suppl):968S-979S. doi:10.1093/ajcn/61.4.968S
3. Achten J, Jeukendrup AE. Maximal fat oxidation during exercise in trained men. *Int J Sports Med*. 2003;24(8):603-608. doi:10.1055/s-2003-43265
4. Burke LM, Gollan RA, Read RS. Dietary intakes and food use of groups of elite Australian male athletes. *Int J Sport Nutr*. 1991;1(4):378-394. doi:10.1123/ijsn.1.4.378
5. Fudge BW, Westerterp KR, Kiplamai FK, et al. Evidence of negative energy balance using doubly labelled water in elite Kenyan endurance runners prior to competition. *Br J Nutr*. 2006;95(1):59-66. doi:10.1079/bjn20051608
6. Motonaga K, Yoshida S, Yamagami F, Kawano T, Takeda E. Estimation of total daily energy expenditure and its components by monitoring the heart rate of Japanese endurance athletes. *J Nutr Sci Vitaminol (Tokyo)*. 2006;52(5):360-367. doi:10.3177/jnsv.52.360
7. García-Rovés PM, Terrados N, Fernández S, Patterson AM. Comparison of dietary intake and eating behavior of professional road cyclists during training and competition. *Int J Sport Nutr Exerc Metab*. 2000;10(1):82-98. doi:10.1123/ijsnem.10.1.82
8. Martin MK, Martin DT, Collier GR, Burke LM. Voluntary food intake by elite female cyclists during training and racing: influence of daily energy expenditure and body composition. *Int J Sport Nutr Exerc Metab*. 2002;12(3):249-267. doi:10.1123/ijsnem.12.3.249
9. Zalcman I, Guarita HV, Juzwiak CR, et al. Nutritional status of adventure racers. *Nutrition*. 2007;23(5):404-411. doi:10.1016/j.nut.2007.01.001
10. Hill RJ, Davies PS. Energy intake and energy expenditure in elite lightweight female rowers. *Med Sci Sports Exerc*. 2002;34(11):1823-1829. doi:10.1097/00005768-200211000-00020
11. Sjödin AM, Andersson AB, Högberg JM, Westerterp KR. Energy balance in cross-country skiers: a study using doubly labeled water. *Med Sci Sports Exerc*. 1994;26(6):720-724. doi:10 .1249/00005768-199406000-00011
12. Schulz LO, Alger S, Harper I, Wilmore JH, Ravussin E. Energy expenditure of elite female runners measured by respiratory chamber and doubly labeled water. *J Appl Physiol (1985)*. 1992;72(1):23-28. doi:10.1152/jappl.1992.72.1.23
13. Vogt S, Heinrich L, Schumacher YO, et al. Energy intake and energy expenditure of elite cyclists during preseason training. *Int J Sports Med*. 2005;26(8):701-706. doi:10.1055/s-2004-830438
14. Edwards JE, Lindeman AK, Mikesky AE, Stager JM. Energy balance in highly trained female endurance runners. *Med Sci Sports Exerc*. 1993;25(12):1398-1404.
15. Frączek B, Grzelak A, Klimek AT. Analysis of daily energy expenditure of elite athletes in relation to their sport, the measurement method and energy requirement norms. *J Hum Kinet*. 2019;70:81-92. doi:10.2478/hukin-2019-0049
16. Burke L. Preparation for competition. In: Burke L, Deakin V, eds. *Clinical Sports Nutrition*. 3rd ed. McGraw-Hill; 2006:355-384.
17. Maughan RJ. Fluid and carbohydrate intake during exercise. In: Burke L, Deakin V, eds. *Clinical Sports Nutrition*. 3rd ed. McGraw-Hill; 2006:385-414.
18. Burke L. Nutrition for recovery after training and competition. In: Burke L, Deakin V, eds. *Clinical Sports Nutrition*. 3rd ed. McGraw-Hill; 2006:415-453.
19. O'Connor H, Caterson I. Weight loss and the athlete. In: Burke L, Deakin V, eds. *Clinical Sports Nutrition*. 3rd ed. McGraw-Hill; 2006:135-173.
20. Burke LM. Nutritional practices of male and female endurance cyclists. *Sports Med*. 2001;31(7):521-532. doi:10.2165/00007256-200131070-00007
21. Magkos F, Yannakoulia M. Methodology of dietary assessment in athletes: concepts and pitfalls. *Curr Opin Clin Nutr Metab Care*. 2003;6(5):539-549. doi:10.1097/00075197-200309000-00007
22. Houltham SD, Rowlands DS. A snapshot of nitrogen balance in endurance-trained women. *Appl Physiol Nutr Metab*. 2014;39(2):219-225. doi:10.1139/apnm-2013-0182
23. Jonnalagadda SS, Benardot D, Dill MN. Assessment of under-reporting of energy intake by elite female gymnast. *Int J Sport Nutr Exerc Metab*. 2000;10(3):315-325. doi:10.1123/ijsnem.10.3.315
24. Heydenreich J, Kayser B, Schutz Y, Melzer K. Total energy expenditure, energy intake, and body composition in endurance athletes across the training season: a systematic review. *Sports Med Open*. 2017;3(1):8. doi:10.1186/s40798-017-0076-1
25. Costa RJS, Gill SK, Hankey J, Wright A, Marczak S. Perturbed energy balance and hydration status in ultra-endurance runners during a 24 h ultra-marathon. *Br J Nutr*. 2014;112(3):428-437. doi:10.1017/S0007114514000907
26. Saris WH, van Erp-Baart MA, Brouns F, Westerterp KR, ten Hoor F. Study on food intake and energy expenditure during extreme sustained exercise: the Tour de France. *Int J Sports Med*. 1989;10(suppl 1):S26-S31. doi:10.1055/s-2007-1024951
27. Gabel KA, Aldous A, Edgington C. Dietary intake of two elite male cyclists during 10-day, 2,050-mile ride. *Int J Sport Nutr*. 1995;5(1):56-61. doi:10.1123/ijsn.5.1.56
28. García-Rovés PM, Terrados N, Fernández SF, Patterson AM. Macronutrients intake of top level cyclists during continuous competition—change in the feeding pattern. *Int J Sports Med*. 1998;19(1):61-67. doi:10.1055/s-2007-971882
29. Eden BD, Abernethy PJ. Nutritional intake during an ultraendurance running race. *Int J Sport Nutr*. 1994;4(2):166-174. doi:10.1123/ijsn.4.2.166

30. Lindeman AK. Nutrient intake of an ultraendurance cyclist. *Int J Sport Nutr.* 1991;1(1):79-85. doi:10.1123/ijsn.1.1.79
31. Knechtle B, Enggist A, Jehle T. Energy turnover at the Race Across AMerica (RAAM) - a case report. *Int J Sports Med.* 2005;26(6):499-503. doi:10.1055/s-2004-821136
32. Barrero A, Erola P, Bescós R. Energy balance of triathletes during an ultra-endurance event. *Nutrients.* 2014;7(1):209-222. doi:10.3390/nu7010209
33. Brouns F, Saris WH, Stroecken J, et al. Eating, drinking, and cycling. A controlled Tour de France simulation study, Part II. Effect of diet manipulation. *Int J Sports Med.* 1989;10(suppl 1):S41-S48. doi:10.1055/s-2007-1024953
34. O'Connor H, Cox G. Feeding ultra-endurance athletes: an interview with Dr. Helen O'Connor and Gregory Cox. Interview by Louise M. Burke. *Int J Sport Nutr Exerc Metab.* 2002;12(4):490-494.
35. Tarnopolsky M. Protein and amino acid needs for bulking up. In: Burke L, Deakin V, eds. *Clinical Sports Nutrition.* 3rd ed. McGraw-Hill; 2006:73–111.
36. Tarnopolsky M. Protein requirements for endurance athletes. *Nutrition.* 2004;20(7-8):662-668. doi:10.1016/j.nut.2004.04.008
37. Tarnopolsky MA, MacDougall JD, Atkinson SA. Influence of protein intake and training status on nitrogen balance and lean body mass. *J Appl Physiol (1985).* 1988;64(1):187-193. doi:10.1152/jappl.1988.64.1.187
38. Friedman JE, Lemon PW. Effect of chronic endurance exercise on retention of dietary protein. *Int J Sports Med.* 1989;10(2):118-123. doi:10.1055/s-2007-1024886
39. Phillips SM. Dietary protein requirements and adaptive advantages in athletes. *Br J Nutr.* 2012;108(suppl 2):S158-S167. doi:10.1017/S0007114512002516
40. Panel on Macronutrients; Panel on the Definition of Dietary Fiber; Subcommittee on Upper Reference Levels of Nutrients; Subcommittee on Interpretation and Uses of Dietary Reference Intakes; Standing Committee on the Scientific Evaluation of Dietary Reference Intakes; Food and Nutrition Board, Institute of Medicine. *Dietary Reference Intakes for Energy, Carbohydrate, Fiber, Fat, Fatty Acids, Cholesterol, Protein, and Amino Acids.* National Academies Press; 2005. doi:10.17226/10490
41. Burke LM, Hawley JA. Fat and carbohydrate for exercise. *Curr Opin Clin Nutr Metab Care.* 2006;9(4):476-481. doi:10.1097/01.mco.0000232911.69236.3b
42. Jäger R, Kerksick CM, Campbell BI, et al. International Society of Sports Nutrition position stand: protein and exercise. *J Int Soc Sports Nutr.* 2017;14:20. doi:10.1186/s12970-017-0177-8
43. Thomas DT, Erdman KA, Burke LM. Position of the Academy of Nutrition and Dietetics, Dietitians of Canada, and the American College of Sports Medicine: nutrition and athletic performance. *J Acad Nutr Diet.* 2016;116(3):501-528. doi:10.1016/j.jand.2015.12.006
44. Cox GR, Clark SA, Cox AJ, et al. Daily training with high carbohydrate availability increases exogenous carbohydrate oxidation during endurance cycling. *J Appl Physiol (1985).* 2010;109(1):126-134. doi:10.1152/japplphysiol.00950.2009
45. Kerksick CM, Arent S, Schoenfeld BJ, et al. International Society of Sports Nutrition position stand: nutrient timing. *J Int Soc Sports Nutr.* 2017;14:33. doi:10.1186/s12970-017-0189-4
46. Burke LM, Whitfield J, Heikura IA, et al. Adaptation to a low carbohydrate high fat diet is rapid but impairs endurance exercise metabolism and performance despite enhanced glycogen availability. *J Physiol.* 2021;599(3):771-790. doi:10.1113/JP280221
47. Yeo WK, Carey AL, Burke L, Spriet LL, Hawley JA. Fat adaptation in well-trained athletes: effects on cell metabolism. *Appl Physiol Nutr Metab.* 2011;36(1):12-22. doi:10.1139/H10-089
48. Getzin AR, Milner C, Harkins M. Fueling the triathlete: evidence-based practical advice for athletes of all levels. *Curr Sports Med Rep.* 2017;16(4):240-246. doi:10.1249/JSR.0000000000000386
49. Getzin AR, Milner C, LaFace KM. Nutrition update for the ultraendurance athlete. *Curr Sports Med Rep.* 2011;10(6):330-339. doi:10.1249/JSR.0b013e318237fcdf
50. Panel on Dietary Reference Intakes for Electrolytes and Water; Standing Committee on the Scientific Evaluation of Dietary Reference Intakes; Food and Nutrition Board, Institute of Medicine. *Dietary Reference Intakes for Water, Potassium, Sodium, Chloride, and Sulfate.* National Academies Press; 2004. doi:10.17226/10925
51. Armstrong LE. Assessing hydration status: the elusive gold standard. *J Am Coll Nutr.* 2007;26(5 suppl):575S-584S. doi:10.1080/07315724.2007.10719661
52. Fernández-Elías VE, Martínez-Abellán A, López-Gullón JM, et al. Validity of hydration non-invasive indices during the weightcutting and official weigh-in for Olympic combat sports. *PLoS One.* 2014;9(4):e95336. doi:10.1371/journal.pone.0095336
53. Cheuvront SN, Sawka MN. Hydration assessment of athletes. *Sports Sci Exch.* 2005;18(2):1-6.
54. Singh A, Evans P, Gallagher KL, Deuster PA. Dietary intakes and biochemical profiles of nutritional status of ultramarathoners. *Med Sci Sports Exerc.* 1993;25(3):328-334.
55. Fogelholm M. Vitamin, mineral, and antioxidant needs of athletes. In: Burke L, Deakin V, eds. *Clinical Sports Nutrition.* 3rd ed. McGraw-Hill; 2006:313-342.
56. American College of Sports Medicine, Sawka MN, Burke LM, et al. American College of Sports Medicine position stand. Exercise and fluid replacement. *Med Sci Sports Exerc.* 2007;39(2):377-390. doi:10.1249/mss.0b013e31802ca597
57. Peeling P. Exercise as a mediator of hepcidin activity in athletes. *Eur J Appl Physiol.* 2010;110(5):877-883. doi:10.1007/s00421-010-1594-4
58. Peeling P, Dawson B, Goodman C, et al. Cumulative effects of consecutive running sessions on hemolysis, inflammation and hepcidin activity. *Eur J Appl Physiol.* 2009;106(1):51-59. doi:10.1007/s00421-009-0988-7
59. Peeling P, Sim M, Badenhorst CE, et al. Iron status and the acute post-exercise hepcidin response in athletes. *PLoS One.* 2014;9(3):e93002. doi:10.1371/journal.pone.0093002
60. Deakin V. Iron depletion in athletes. In: Burke L, Deakin V, eds. *Clinical Sports Nutrition.* 3rd ed. McGraw-Hill; 2006:263-312.

61. Schumacher YO, Schmid A, Grathwohl D, Bültermann D, Berg A. Hematological indices and iron status in athletes of various sports and performances. *Med Sci Sports Exerc.* 2002;34(5):869-875. doi:10.1097/00005768-200205000-00022
62. American Dietetic Association; Dietitians of Canada; American College of Sports Medicine, Rodriguez NR, Di Marco NM, Langley S. American College of Sports Medicine position stand. Nutrition and athletic performance. *Med Sci Sports Exerc.* 2009;41(3):709-731. doi:10.1249/MSS.0b013e31890eb86
63. Hinton PS, Giordano C, Brownlie T, Haas JD. Iron supplementation improves endurance after training in iron-depleted, nonanemic women. *J Appl Physiol (1985).* 2000;88(3):1103-1111. doi:10.1152/jappl.2000.88.3.1103
64. Brownlie T 4th, Utermohlen V, Hinton PS, Giordano C, Haas JD. Marginal iron deficiency without anemia impairs aerobic adaptation among previously untrained women. *Am J Clin Nutr.* 2002;75(4):734-742. doi:10.1093/ajcn/75.4.734
65. DellaValle DM, Haas JD. Iron supplementation improves energetic efficiency in iron-depleted female rowers. *Med Sci Sports Exerc.* 2014;46(6):1204-1215. doi:10.1249/MSS.0000000000000208
66. Brownlie T 4th, Utermohlen V, Hinton PS, Haas JD. Tissue iron deficiency without anemia impairs adaptation in endurance capacity after aerobic training in previously untrained women. *Am J Clin Nutr.* 2004;79(3):437-443. doi:10.1093/ajcn/79.3.437
67. Resina A, Gatteschi L, Castellani W, Galvan P, Panise G, Rubenni MG. Effects of aerobic training and exercise on plasma and erythrocyte magnesium concentration. In: Kies CV, Driskell JA, eds. *Sports Nutrition: Minerals and Electrolytes.* CRC Press; 1995:189-203.
68. Ziemann E, Kasprowicz K, Kasperska A, Zembroń-Lacny A, Antosiewicz J, Laskowski R. Do high blood hepcidin concentrations contribute to low ferritin levels in young tennis players at the end of tournament season? *J Sports Sci Med.* 2013;12(2):249-258.
69. Haakonssen EC, Ross ML, Knight EJ, et al. The effects of a calcium-rich pre-exercise meal on biomarkers of calcium homeostasis in competitive female cyclists: a randomised crossover trial. *PLoS One.* 2015;10(5):e0123302. doi:10.1371/journal.pone.0123302
70. Laires MJ, Monteiro CP, Matias CN, Santos DA, Silva AM, Bicho M. Magnesium status and exercise performance in athletes. *J Trace Elem Electrolytes.* 2014;31(1):13-20.
71. Watson T. The science of anti-oxidants and exercise performance. In: Burke L, Deakin V, eds. *Clinical Sports Nutrition.* 3rd ed. McGraw-Hill; 2006:343-353.
72. Gomez-Cabrera MC, Domenech E, Romagnoli M, et al. Oral administration of vitamin C decreases muscle mitochondrial biogenesis and hampers training-induced adaptations in endurance performance. *Am J Clin Nutr.* 2008;87(1):142-149. doi:10.1093/ajcn/87.1.142
73. Ristow M, Zarse K, Oberbach A, et al. Antioxidants prevent health-promoting effects of physical exercise in humans. *Proc Natl Acad Sci U S A.* 2009;106(21):8665-8670. doi:10.1073/pnas.0903485106
74. Kimber NE, Ross JJ, Mason SL, Speedy DB. Energy balance during an Ironman triathlon in male and female triathletes. *Int J Sport Nutr Exerc Metab.* 2002;12(1):47-62. doi:10.1123/ijsnem.12.1.47
75. Glace B, Murphy C, McHugh M. Food and fluid intake and disturbances in gastrointestinal and mental function during an ultramarathon. *Int J Sport Nutr Exerc Metab.* 2002;12(4):414-427. doi:10.1123/ijsnem.12.4.414
76. Hulton AT, Lahart I, Williams KL, et al. Energy expenditure in the Race Across America (RAAM). *Int J Sports Med.* 2010;31(7):463-467. doi:10.1055/s-0030-1251992
77. Rehrer NJ, Hellemans IJ, Rolleston AK, Rush E, Miller BF. Energy intake and expenditure during a 6-day cycling stage race. *Scand J Med Sci Sports.* 2010;20(4):609-618. doi:10.1111/j.1600-0838.2009.00974.x
78. Bescós R, Rodríguez FA, Iglesias X, et al. Nutritional behavior of cyclists during a 24-hour team relay race: a field study report. *J Int Soc Sports Nutr.* 2012;9(1):3. doi:10.1186/1550-2783-9-3
79. Tarnopolsky MA. Gender differences in substrate metabolism during endurance exercise. *Can J Appl Physiol.* 2000;25(4):312-327. doi:10.1139/h00-024
80. Glace BW, Murphy CA, McHugh MP. Food intake and electrolyte status of ultramarathoners competing in extreme heat. *J Am Coll Nutr.* 2002;21(6):553-559. doi:10.1080/07315724.2002.10719254
81. Burke LM, Millet G, Tarnopolsky MA; International Association of Athletics Federations. Nutrition for distance events. *J Sports Sci.* 2007;25(suppl 1):S29-S38. doi:10.1080/02640410701607239
82. Burke LM, Hawley JA, Wong SH, Jeukendrup AE. Carbohydrates for training and competition. *J Sports Sci.* 2011;29(suppl 1):S17-S27. doi:10.1080/02640414.2011.585473
83. de Ataide e Silva T, Di Cavalcanti Alves de Souza ME, de Amorim JF, Stathis CG, Leandro CG, Lima-Silva AE. Can carbohydrate mouth rinse improve performance during exercise? A systematic review. *Nutrients.* 2013;6(1):1-10. doi:10.3390/nu6010001
84. Jeukendrup AE. Carbohydrate and exercise performance: the role of multiple transportable carbohydrates. *Curr Opin Clin Nutr Metab Care.* 2010;13(4):452-457. doi:10.1097/MCO.0b013e328339de9f
85. Gisolfi CV, Lambert GP, Summers RW. Intestinal fluid absorption during exercise: role of sport drink osmolality and [Na^+]. *Med Sci Sports Exerc.* 2001;33(6):907-915. doi:10.1097/00005768-200106000-00009
86. Gisolfi CV, Summers RW, Lambert GP, Xia T. Effect of beverage osmolality on intestinal fluid absorption during exercise. *J Appl Physiol (1985).* 1998;85(5):1941-1948. doi:10.1152/jappl.1998.85.5.1941
87. Hunt JB, Elliott EJ, Fairclough PD, Clark ML, Farthing MJ. Water and solute absorption from hypotonic glucose-electrolyte solutions in human jejunum. *Gut.* 1992;33(4):479-483. doi:10.1136/gut.33.4.479
88. Koopman R, Pannemans DL, Jeukendrup AE, et al. Combined ingestion of protein and carbohydrate improves protein balance during ultra-endurance exercise. *Am J Physiol Endocrinol Metab.* 2004;287(4):E712-E720. doi:10.1152/ajpendo.00543.2003

89. Laursen PB, Rhodes EC, Buchanan JM. Physiological analysis of a high intensity ultraendurance event. *Strength Cond J.* 1999;21(1):26-38. doi:10.1519/00126548-199902000-00006

90. Jeukendrup AE. Training the gut for athletes. *Sports Med.* 2017;47(suppl 1):101-110. doi:10.1007/s40279-017-0690-6

91. Burd NA, West DWD, Moore DR, et al. Enhanced amino acid sensitivity of myofibrillar protein synthesis persists for up to 24 h after resistance exercise in young men. *J Nutr.* 2011;141(4):568-573. doi:10.3945/jn.110.135038

92. Phillips SM, Moore DR, Tang JE. A critical examination of dietary protein requirements, benefits, and excesses in athletes. *Int J Sport Nutr Exerc Metab.* 2007;17(suppl):S58-S76. doi:10.1123/ijsnem.17.s1.s58

93. Betts JA, Williams C. Short-term recovery from prolonged exercise: exploring the potential for protein ingestion to accentuate the benefits of carbohydrate supplements. *Sports Med.* 2010;40(11):941-959. doi:10.2165/11536900-000000000-00000

94. Maughan RJ, Shirreffs SM, Leiper JB. Errors in the estimation of hydration status from changes in body mass. *J Sports Sci.* 2007;25(7):797-804. doi:10.1080/02640410600875143

95. Montain SJ, Cheuvront SN, Sawka MN. Exercise associated hyponatraemia: quantitative analysis to understand the aetiology. *Br J Sports Med.* 2006;40(2):98-105. doi:10.1136/bjsm.2005.018481

96. Allsopp AJ, Sutherland R, Wood P, Wootton SA. The effect of sodium balance on sweat sodium secretion and plasma aldosterone concentration. *Eur J Appl Physiol Occup Physiol.* 1998;78(6):516-521. doi:10.1007/s004210050454

97. Hew-Butler T, Rosner MH, Fowkes-Godek S, et al. Statement of the Third International Exercise-Associated Hyponatremia Consensus Development Conference, Carlsbad, California, 2015. *Clin J Sport Med.* 2015;25(4):303-320. doi:10.1097/JSM.0000000000000221

98. Wagner S, Knechtle B, Knechtle P, Rüst CA, Rosemann T. Higher prevalence of exercise-associated hyponatremia in female than in male open-water ultra-endurance swimmers: the 'Marathon-Swim' in Lake Zurich. *Eur J Appl Physiol.* 2012;112(3):1095-1106. doi:10.1007/s00421-011-2070-5

99. Eijsvogels TM, Scholten RR, van Duijnhoven NT, Thijssen DH, Hopman MT. Sex difference in fluid balance responses during prolonged exercise. *Scand J Med Sci Sports.* 2013;23(2):198-206. doi:10.1111/j.1600-0838.2011.01371.x

100. Hew TD, Chorley JN, Cianca JC, Divine JG. The incidence, risk factors, and clinical manifestations of hyponatremia in marathon runners. *Clin J Sport Med.* 2003;13(1):41-47. doi:10.1097/00042752-200301000-00008

101. McCubbin AJ, Allanson BA, Caldwell Odgers JN, et al. Sports Dietitians Australia position statement: nutrition for exercise in hot environments. *Int J Sport Nutr Exerc Metab.* 2020;30(1):83-98. doi:10.1123/ijsnem.2019-0300

102. Goulet ED, Aubertin-Leheudre M, Plante GE, Dionne IJ. A meta-analysis of the effects of glycerol-induced hyperhydration on fluid retention and endurance performance. *Int J Sport Nutr Exerc Metab.* 2007;17(4):391-410. doi:10.1123/ijsnem.17.4.391

103. Sims ST, van Vliet L, Cotter JD, Rehrer NJ. Sodium loading aids fluid balance and reduces physiological strain of trained men exercising in the heat. *Med Sci Sports Exerc.* 2007;39(1):123-130. doi:10.1249/01.mss.0000241639.97972.4a

104. Cosgrove SD, Black KE. Sodium supplementation has no effect on endurance performance during a cycling time-trial in cool conditions: a randomised cross-over trial. *J Int Soc Sports Nutr.* 2013;10:30. doi:10.1186/1550-2783-10-30

105. Hew-Butler TD, Sharwood K, Collins M, Speedy D, Noakes T. Sodium supplementation is not required to maintain serum sodium concentrations during an Ironman triathlon. *Br J Sports Med.* 2006;40(3):255-259. doi:10.1136/bjsm.2005.022418

106. Sharp RL. Role of sodium in fluid homeostasis with exercise. *J Am Coll Nutr.* 2006;25(3 suppl):231S-239S. doi:10.1080/07315724.2006.10719572

107. Nose H, Mack GW, Shi XR, Nadel ER. Involvement of sodium retention hormones during rehydration in humans. *J Appl Physiol (1985).* 1988;65(1):332-336. doi:10.1152/jappl.1988.65.1.332

108. Shirreffs SM, Maughan RJ. Volume repletion after exercise-induced volume depletion in humans: replacement of water and sodium losses. *Am J Physiol.* 1998;274(5 pt 2):F868-F875.

CHAPTER 23

Tactical Performance Nutrition

Drew E. Gonzalez, PhD, SCCC, CISSN, CSCS,*D, TSAC-F,*D, EP-C, Sarah Johnson, MS, Jillian M. Joyce, PhD, RD, Nicholas Barringer, PhD, RDN, CSSD, CSCS, Douglas S. Kalman, PhD, RD, FACN, FISSN, and Richard B. Kreider, PhD, FACSM, FASEP, FISSN, FACN, FNAK

LEARNING OBJECTIVES

- Understand the occupation-specific demands and issues that influence energy expenditure and subsequent nutritional needs for the tactical athlete.
- Determine the best individualized "food first, but not food only" approach for the tactical athlete.
- Understand that the incorporation of enriched or fortified foods or those that are labeled as "functional foods" also includes supplemental nutrition.
- Identify supplements to augment the tactical athlete's diet during high-stress conditions.
- Understand the social determinants of health as related to the tactical athlete in an effort to meet each tactical athlete where they are in their overall health and fitness status.

INTRODUCTION

The term *tactical athlete* refers to military personnel, law enforcement officers, and firefighters,[1] all of whom can have some of the most physically demanding and stressful occupations.[2-5] For example, essential occupational tasks may include lifting and carrying heavy objects or maneuvering rapidly to gain a tactical advantage or maintain safety. Typically, an individual performs these tasks while wearing personal protective equipment and carrying other occupation-specific articles, which may collectively add additional weight that can range from approximately 10 to 70 kg (22–155 lb) depending on the operator and their respective occupational needs or task-specific demands.[6,7] Considering the various occupational demands and burdens faced, it is clear the tactical athlete has a strong need for nutritional guidance and intervention to promote optimal health and performance, as well as operational readiness (ie, the ability to be prepared and to perform occupational demands or missions). In 2022, the International Society of Sports Nutrition (ISSN) published the first academic position stand on nutrition for tactical athletes.[8] The ISSN position paper on tactical athlete nutrition summarizes the current evidence-based nutritional strategies specific to the tactical athlete. This chapter reviews these and other strategies related to the tactical athlete's health, performance, and operational readiness. In addition, the chapter summarizes the ISSN recommendations, while emphasizing the need for a "food first, but not food only" approach to best fuel the tactical athlete.

Note that there are several other public service members who might be classified as "tactical athletes," including (but not limited to) wildland firefighters, border patrol agents, Special Weapons and Tactics

(SWAT) team members, rescue personnel, emergency medical technicians, national guard members, and coast guard members. Although this chapter focuses primarily on the 3 main categories of tactical athlete (military personnel, firefighters, and law enforcement officers), practitioners working with these various service members should consider the nutritional and supplementation recommendations provided here, as well as the occupation-specific nature of the individual(s) with whom they work.

UNDERSTANDING THE DEMANDS OF THE TACTICAL ATHLETE

The tactical athlete often experiences high physical and mental stress coupled with poor dietary habits and sleep patterns.[8] The provision and timing of adequate energy, macronutrients, micronutrients, and fluids to meet daily needs can vary dramatically depending on the specific job status (eg, deployed vs nondeployed military personnel, sedentary desk jobs vs in-the-field jobs). There is no one-size-fits-all approach to nutrition for these occupational groups. In addition, the high allostatic load and even overload often experienced by these groups has been implicated in poor health outcomes.[9] Allostatic load refers to the cumulation of various chronic stressors and life events experienced by the individual. In particular to the service member, allostatic load may lead to *operator syndrome*, which refers to the interrelated health and functional impairments resulting from the accumulation of chronic stressors and adverse patterns or factors, such as traumatic brain injuries (TBIs), suicidal ideation, depression, posttraumatic stress disorder (PTSD), obstructed sleep and sleep deprivation, chronic joint pain, community dysfunction, and cognitive impairment (to name a few). Whereas an extensive discussion of operator syndrome and allostatic load is beyond the scope of this chapter, the practitioner should be aware of these tactical-specific stressors that, over time, can wear down the individual's health and manifest in increased impairments and disease risk.[10] It is critical for registered dietitians and other supportive health care practitioners who may work with this group (eg, certified sports nutritionist of the ISSN, certified nutrition specialist, certified strength and conditioning specialist, tactical strength and conditioning facilitator) to understand the occupational demands (including physical training loads), common stressors, and health burdens within this population. These factors are summarized in Figure 23.1.[8]

Considerations Based on Physical Exertion

Tactical athletes are subject to a barrage of occupational challenges, which are usually influenced by geography, weather, and operational start time and duration, as well as the specifics of the occupational code (eg, submariner, pilot) or job title or status (eg, assistant fire chief vs structural or wildland firefighter).

MILITARY PERSONNEL

For modern-day military personnel, some common intense physical exertion challenges faced in typical assignments include load carriage and heavy lifting requirements, offensive and defensive combative maneuvers, and running or sprinting. Soldiers are often required to carry heavy loads that can exceed 45 kg (99 lb). The physiological costs and biomechanical responses to these loads, though varying with the contexts in which they are carried, have led to soldier injuries. These injuries can range from musculoskeletal injuries (eg, joint or ligamentous injuries and stress fractures) to neurological injuries (eg, paresthesia) and can impact both the soldier and the military force in which they serve. The loads carried by the soldier may reduce their physiological capabilities, mobility, attention to task, marksmanship, and grenade-throwing ability.[11]

The physiological, biomechanical, and clinical implications of load carrying have been studied, but the effects of load carriage on cognition have received less attention. Several critical military tasks involve a cognitive component, including maintaining vigilance through attentional processes, perceiving and processing verbal communications, and using executive processes to respond to threats and stimuli in the environment. The evolving demands of future warfare indicate that there is likely to be an increased requirement for high levels of cognitive performance in the field. For example, the requirement to integrate warfighter-worn technology to support situation awareness continues. It is essential to consider both the physical and cognitive aspects of military tasks when assessing soldier performance in order to understand any resulting decrements and consider how to train personnel to optimize performance under dualtasking and multitasking conditions.[12]

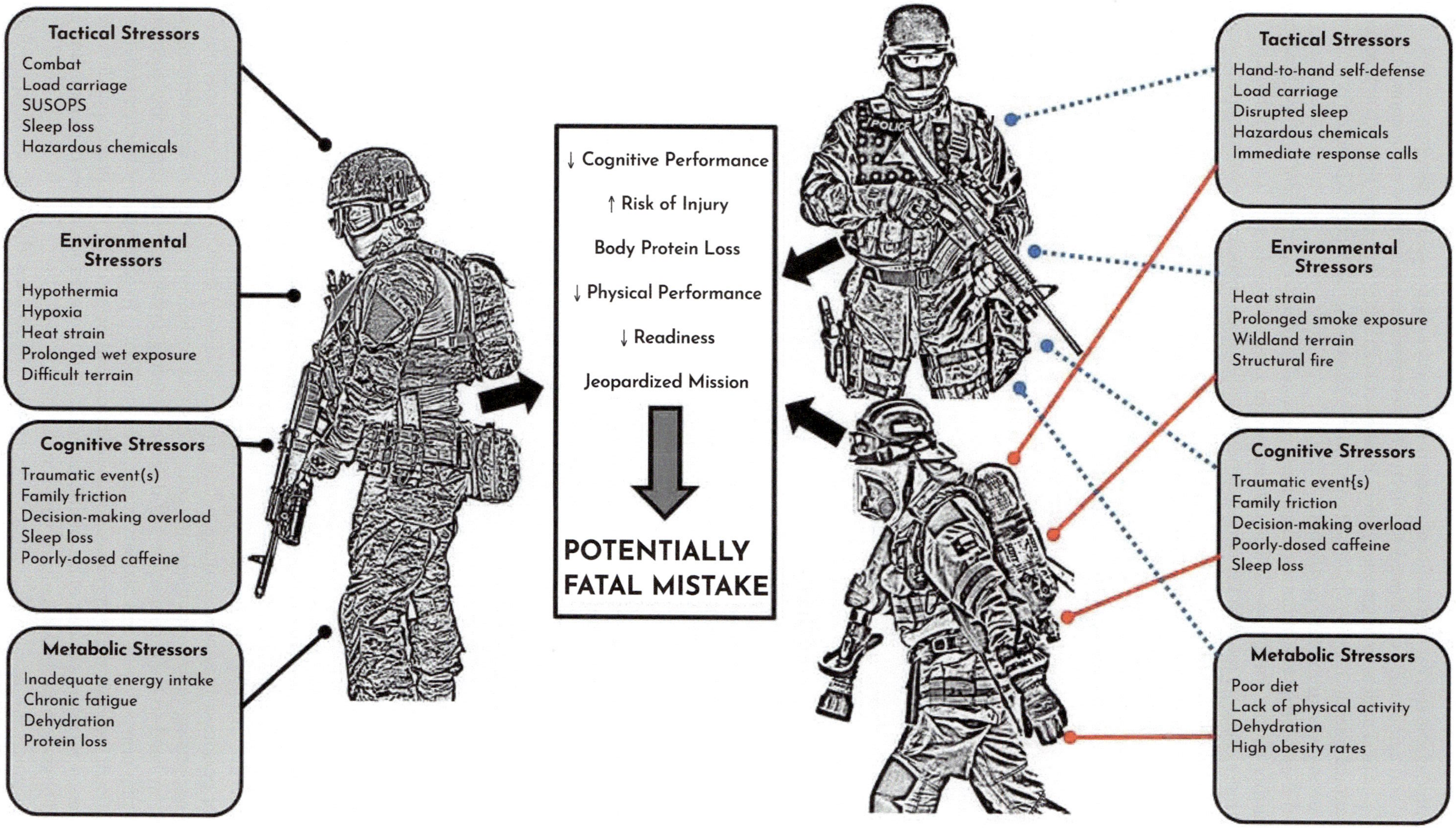

FIGURE 23.1 Common stressors faced by tactical athletes The left side depicts common military stressors, whereas the right side depicts common first-responder stressors. Abbreviations: SUSOPS, sustained operations

Adapted under CC BY 4.0 from reference 8: Gonzalez DE, McAllister MJ, Waldman HS, et al. International society of sports nutrition position stand: tactical athlete nutrition. *J Int Soc Sports Nutr.* 2022;19(1):267-315. doi:10.1080/15502783.2022.2086017

Given the unpredictable and varying nature of modern-day warfare challenges, military personnel should be anaerobically and aerobically conditioned to effectively meet the demands of the occupation. It is not uncommon for a tactical athlete to require an energy intake between 2,000 and more than 6,000 kcal daily based on occupational roles and responsibilities. Table 23.1[13-20] lists a range of energy expenditures that have been estimated among various military personnel.

In addition to these energy expenditure estimations, personal protective equipment and load carriage requirements further elevate energy needs. The carried weight is an added drag or load that requires the body to expend more energy to move in the same manner. Another major concern for military personnel is being subject to a prolonged period of energy deficit, which can negatively impact physical performance[21] and make the operator susceptible to direct enemy threats or actions. This undernutrition can impair an individual's ability to respond quickly to dynamic situations. Taken together, this information on energy expenditure can help dietitians and other support practitioners plan appropriate feeding and nutrient strategies to meet occupational demands and better support the health of military personnel.

TABLE 23.1 Estimated Energy Expenditure of Military Personnel[13-20]

Occupational role	Energy expenditure (kcal/d)
Combat support personnel (female)[13]	~2,500
Military personnel during sustained periods of training or combat operations[14,15]	~2,500-4,500
Marine Corps Forces Special Operations Command[16]	~6,500[a]
Ranger Assessment and Selection Program[16]	~4,200[a]
US Army Special Forces Small Unit Tactics Training groups[16]	~5,200[a]
Army Ranger School and US Army Special Forces Assessment and Selection[17,18]	~4,100-5,200
Special Operations Forces[19]	~2,500-6,300
Marines (male, strenuous, cold weather)[20]	~7,000

[a] Estimates are based on the following predictive equations: model A (kcal/d) = [47.97 × BM (kg)] + [706.33 × PAF] – 467.22 and model B (kcal/d) = [61.99 × FFM (kg)] + [716.49 × PAF] – 721.30. Refer to reference 16 for more information.
Abbreviations: BM, body mass; FFM, fat-free mass; PAF, physical activity factor

FIRST RESPONDERS

The physiological demands on first responders (eg, law enforcement personnel and firefighters) vary considerably and are quite different from those of military personnel. First responders engage in a wide range of occupation-specific tasks that can be relatively mundane or immediately life-threatening. For instance, law enforcement personnel may need to quickly shift from a sedentary state to one of maximal physical exertion when responding to various emergency calls.[3] This may include pursuing and apprehending suspects, engaging in hand-to-hand combat or self-defense, entering unfamiliar and unfriendly scenarios, lifting and carrying heavy objects, and maneuvering quickly on foot.[22] In addition, the burden of personal protective equipment increases the energy needs of law enforcement personnel.[6,23] All first responders are at risk for musculoskeletal injury because of the biomechanical (eg, postural issues, ranges of motion, and gait kinematics) and physiological challenges faced while on the job.[24,25]

Similarly, firefighters are faced with high-stress occupational scenarios that may occur sporadically throughout an on-duty shift. For the structural firefighter, routine occupational tasks may include lifting, carrying, and dragging heavy and odd objects or tools; advancing charged hose lines; climbing multiple flights of stairs with equipment; dragging and carrying victims; and conducting search-and-rescue operations.[26] In contrast, wildland firefighters face very different occupational demands and challenges, and common tasks may include building fire lines, operating chainsaws, and hiking with external loads over wildland terrain to conduct fire suppression activities.[27] All of this can be metabolically taxing, especially for the undertrained, undernourished individual. An individual must wear fire-resistant personal protective equipment when engaged in emergency response, and this adds an additional load of approximately 26 kg (57 lb) for structural firefighters and 6 to 20 kg (13–44 lb) for wildland firefighters. The added weight and its distribution on the human body add to the metabolic stressors that can impact physical and occupational performance (eg, increasing metabolic demands and cardiovascular strain).[28-31]

Unlike for military personnel, fewer data are available regarding estimated or known energy expenditures for first responders. For one sample of law enforcement personnel (Polish police), daily energy expenditure was estimated at approximately 1,800 to 3,000 kcal/d.[32] Among structural firefighters, a 2021 study noted that those participating in 2 days of occupation-specific training experienced an average energy expenditure of approximately 3,600 kcal/d.[33] To date, 2 studies have been published regarding the total daily energy expenditure for wildland firefighters, which was estimated to be between 2,800 and 6,200 kcal/d depending on the occupational demands.[34,35] Based on the limited data, it is advisable for nutrition and other support practitioners to take into consideration all occupational demands and any individual health and fitness goals of the first responder. This includes nutrition beyond simply needed calories, such as the relative amounts of macronutrients and any impacts on vitamin or mineral needs. (Note that, in the remainder of this chapter, the discussion of firefighters focuses primarily on structural, rather than wildland, firefighters.)

Current Health Status and Burdens of the Tactical Athlete

The tactical athlete is susceptible to the same conditions and diseases as the general public, such as obesity, cancer, and cardiovascular disease. The risk of cardiometabolic or other disease exists across all stages of their career (recruit/candidate, rookie, professional).[36-40] Prior to making energy, nutrient, and/or supplementation recommendations, it is paramount for nutrition and other health care practitioners to gather information on the individual's current health status (current and past medical history, medication usage, etc), dietary and lifestyle habits, and other determinants of health and behaviors (including socioeconomic factors). Lifestyle approaches for health and wellness as part of longevity and health promotion are encouraged as part of continuing education in this population.

MILITARY PERSONNEL: DUTY-SPECIFIC HEALTH BURDENS

Military personnel are faced with an increased prevalence of overweight and obesity,[41] which is associated with several chronic conditions, such as cardiovascular disease (eg, hyperlipidemia, hypertension) and type 2 diabetes, as well as mental health challenges (eg, mood state changes, varying levels of depression and anxiety). Although fitness standards are in place to determine employability and occupational specialty, data indicate that 20% of military personnel are classified as obese.[42] This prevalence of obesity in the military can create issues related to warfighter readiness, health status, economic costs, and more. Historically as measured by BMI standards, the military had a better "healthy profile" than the civilian US population; however, this status has been shifting and is a concern for military leaders.[43]

The use of BMI as a method of estimating health status and body composition is controversial among scientists and other groups. A recently published systematic review examined the relationship between BMI and health and occupational performance of all tactical groups, including military personnel. The review indicated a J-shaped curve between BMI and both health and occupational performance for all tactical groups, such that individuals who have a "healthy" or "normal" weight classification are at the lowest risk for chronic disease (eg, cardiovascular disease and type 2 diabetes) and injury and have the highest levels of performance across speed and endurance activities.[44,45] Thus, whereas military personnel are expected to exhibit high levels of physical fitness to meet occupational demands, it is likely that operational readiness is compromised by the high prevalence of overweight and/or obesity currently observed in the military and across other first-responder groups. In addition, chronic sleep restriction and sleep loss are common among military personnel and are associated with obesity as well as adverse health outcomes (eg, insulin resistance, impaired glucose tolerance) and increased risk of cardiovascular disease and musculoskeletal injury (related to obesity and overuse).[46-52]

Body composition and fitness are also associated with success in passing courses, such as the Special Forces Assessment and Selection course. Interestingly, higher BMI and body mass have been associated with better road march performance; however, among other fitness testing parameters (2-mile run, pull-ups, push-ups, etc), having a lower BMI and a lower body mass or percent body fat is favorable for performance. This observation that higher BMI and body mass are related to better road march performance is likely due to the necessary muscular strength and power requirements of load carriage during a marching task; therefore, those with a high BMI and body mass (ideally due to lean tissue) may have greater strength and power compared to individuals a lower BMI and body mass. This finding further demonstrates the need to maintain appropriate body composition (fat mass vs lean mass) and fitness for combat readiness.[53] Thus, despite common yet anecdotal perceptions that military personnel are in peak fitness and health, they are experiencing an increased prevalence of members who are overweight or obese, and as such, the potential burden of added injuries and chronic disease are matters worthy of addressing through nutrition counseling.

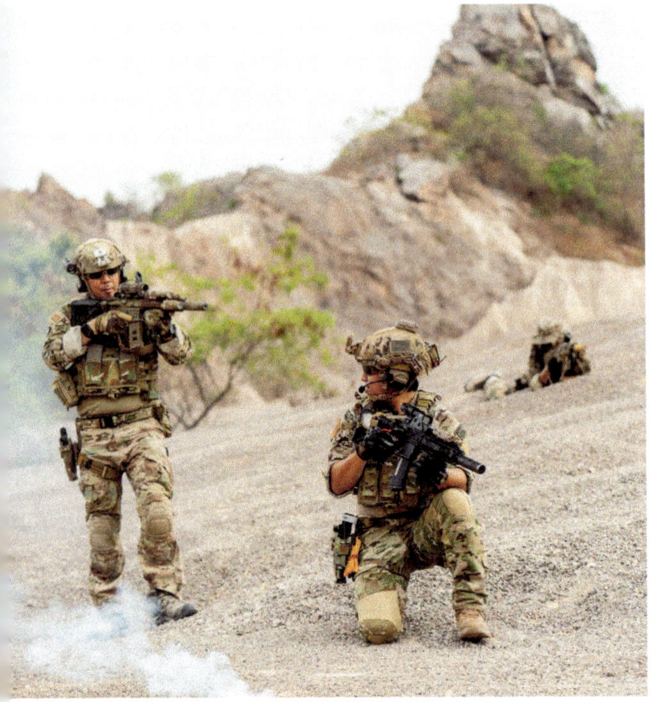

Beyond these challenges, TBI in military populations is an additional area in which enhanced nutrient delivery may afford positive outcomes.[54] Head injuries resulting from shock waves from explosives, violent impact, and/or bullet penetration are some of the main causes of TBIs.[55] Blunt impacts to the head (eg, deceleration injuries) and whiplash are common mechanisms of concussion among military personnel.[56] Unfortunately, TBIs are associated with various psychiatric and neurobehavioral issues, such as suicidality, major depressive disorder, and PTSD.[57] It is also important to note that suicide rates among US military personnel have increased,[58] and there is a need for the assessment and subsequent treatment of PTSD as a means of attenuating the risk of completed suicide.[59,60] Scientists have a growing interest in understanding and optimizing the potential benefits of various forms of nutritional supplementation with regard to cognitive function, mental health, and brain health. Although much more research is needed, 3 ingredients are briefly discussed later in this chapter because of their potential to positively impact cognitive performance and brain health: omega-3 fatty acids, β-alanine, and L-tyrosine.

LAW ENFORCEMENT PERSONNEL: DUTY-SPECIFIC HEALTH BURDENS

Law enforcement personnel appear to exhibit trends for obesity and cardiovascular disease risk that are similar to those of firefighters.[40,61,62] Reports suggest that approximately 40.5% of US law enforcement personnel are classified as obese,[63] and data indicate that the risk for metabolic syndrome is increased by 6.8- and 10.9-fold for personnel who are overweight and obese, respectively.[64] This shift in law enforcement weight and obesity status mirrors changes observed over recent years in the US population. In addition, compared to the general public, law enforcement personnel appear to have a greater risk for cardiovascular disease.[65,66] In fact, the stressful conditions of occupation-specific duties are associated with an increased risk of suffering a significant cardiac event on-duty. More specifically, nonroutine tasks result in a sudden increase in cardiovascular strain and heightened psychological stress, which appears to be responsible for approximately 77% of all significant cardiac events among law enforcement personnel.[61] Unfortunately, law enforcement personnel, like other populations within the United States, may adopt sedentary physical activity patterns and poor dietary habits, which, along with lower fitness levels, can further exacerbate the risk for obesity, obesity-related conditions, and on-duty cardiac events.[62,67] Moreover, law enforcement personnel with higher body fat percentages tend to have lower aerobic capacity and muscular endurance and, thus, a greater risk for cardiometabolic disease.[64,68] Therefore, there is a critical need for dietary and physical training interventions that can (1) prevent body fat accrual and improve lean mass, (2) mitigate the deleterious effects of higher percent body fat relative to lean mass on physical and occupational performance, (3) improve overall health and performance outcomes for the law enforcement officer, and (4) provide individualized nutrition assessments and plans to support the physical and health goals.

FIREFIGHTERS: DUTY-SPECIFIC HEALTH BURDENS

The second leading cause of mortality among firefighters (after exposure) is sudden cardiac death on-duty.[69,70] Data suggest that firefighters have a high prevalence of cardiovascular disease risk factors, such as being classified as overweight or obese (~75% for both career and volunteer firefighters).[39,69] Compared to firefighters who are at a healthy weight, those who are obese generally present with higher total cholesterol, lower high-density lipoprotein cholesterol, and higher triglycerides, as well as higher blood pressure and lower fitness levels.[39,71] In addition, firefighters are exposed to high-stress conditions that are often followed by extended periods of physical inactivity. These inactive periods may give rise to poor nutritional choices.[72] The firehouse is rooted in tradition and may be resistant to change, which could pose an issue for fostering a favorable food environment.[73] Therefore, practitioners should consider implementing health and wellness policies and a supportive food environment, as well as encouraging healthy eating and the use of evidence-based nutritional practices.[8]

Fire suppression activities increase the risk of cardiovascular disease and significant cardiac events on-duty. Significant cardiac events appear to be related to underlying cardiovascular disease, and data suggest that mortality from cardiovascular disease is related to poor lifestyle habits. Stressful conditions increase free-radical damage from reactive oxygen species, lead to elevations in stress hormones, and increase markers of inflammation, all of which contribute to the development and progression of cardiovascular disease.[74,75] Beyond cardiovascular disease, firefighters are also at increased risk for numerous types of cancer (including melanoma and lung, colorectal, and prostate cancers) relative to the general population.[76,77] Thus, in addition to considering performance nutrition needs for occupational demands, dietitians and other nutrition practitioners should also consider lifestyle interventions for health longevity beyond the job.

Considerations Based on Environment

The tactical athlete is commonly faced with extreme environmental factors, such as extreme hot or cold weather; increased elevation; and exposure to smoke, fire, or chemicals and other toxins. The tactical athlete needs to be prepared for all conditions; thus, all possibilities must be contemplated in advance for effective preparation. Tactical athletes who are deployed in the field or in a field-based training environment may also need to rely on dietary supplementation if they do not have access to adequate food supplies or the ability to cook or to store foods properly. Being a first responder presents unique situations. It is important that health care practitioners evaluate all environmental factors when creating a comprehensive nutrition intervention for the first responder.

ENERGY AND MACRONUTRIENT GUIDELINES FOR THE TACTICAL ATHLETE

Military Personnel: Macronutrient and Micronutrient Guidance

The military established a nutritional standard, termed military dietary reference intakes (MDRIs), which are codified in Army Regulation 40-25 (AR 40-25) and reflect the energy and nutrient needs of military personnel.[78] It is critical for practitioners to account for the physical activity levels and environmental factors specific to military personnel as these may cause energy and nutrient needs to increase. AR 40-25 outlines the MDRIs for carbohydrate, protein, and fat, as well as dietary fiber, iron, and electrolytes. Recommendations for carbohydrate intake are based on the 2016 position stand from the Academy of Nutrition and Dietetics, Dietitians of Canada, and American College of Sports Medicine.[79] The joint guidance indicates that military personnel should aim to consume carbohydrate in the range of 340 to 680 g/d for males and 276 to 552 g/d for females (~50%–55% of total energy intake). During prolonged operations, carbohydrate requirements may need to be increased to offset increases in energy expenditure. It is important for dietitians and other nutrition practitioners to consider the barriers to healthy eating and the constraints that may be present when military personnel are deployed (including limited storage of military rations on one's person, environmental barriers to food and water, cost and access to healthy options, and the additional load carried when factoring in ammunition and food rations).[80] To this end, a "food first, but not food only" approach is warranted, especially during prolonged missions in which access to food or storage of rations is limited and the soldier is subject to a catabolic or energy-deficit state.

During prolonged operations, military personnel may be subject to severe energy deficits that can result in weight loss, mostly due to muscle loss. To combat the adverse impacts of these catabolic or energy-deficit states, researchers have tested and advise the delivery of essential amino acids (EAAs) through whole food or free-form EAA supplementation, as discussed in a later section of this chapter. To meet the EAA needs, in AR 40-25 experts recommend that military personnel, both male and female, consume protein within the range of 0.8 to 1.6 g per kilogram of body weight per day[78]; however, the practitioner should consider increasing protein intake to 1.4 to 2.0 per kilogram of body weight per day for a more robust delivery of protein and subsequent favorable body composition, enhanced exercise/training recovery, and lean tissue accretion response.[8] Refer to Box 23.1 for more information.[81]

Experts recommended in AR 40-25 that military personnel consume 30% of total energy intake from fat, which should consist of linoleic acid (17 g/d for males and 12 g/d for females) and α-linolenic acid (1.6 g/d for males and 1.1 g/d for females), while limiting the consumption of saturated fats, *trans* fatty acids, and dietary cholesterol. AR 40-25 also contains recommendations for fiber, iron, and fluids. Experts recommend that male and female military personnel consume fiber in the amounts of 34 and 24 g/d, respectively.[78] It is important that the dietitian or other nutrition practitioner working with military personnel who are deployed consider the utility of the Meal, Ready-To-Eat (MRE) and help the soldier identify suitable substitutes should that be preferred.

The recommendations for iron intake by male and female military personnel are 8 and 18 mg/d, respectively. Female military personnel are likely to benefit from at least 15 mg of iron daily to maintain physical and cognitive performance. Finally, to avoid dehydration, military personnel are advised to consume carbohydrate-containing beverages that contain 82 to 163 mg of sodium and 18 to 46 mg of potassium per 8 fl oz when actively training or engaged in physically demanding conditions.[78] More specifics regarding hydration are discussed in a later section.

First Responders: Macronutrient and Micronutrient Guidance

No energy and macronutrient guidelines have been established specifically for first responders because of the lack of data regarding the nutrient intakes of both law enforcement personnel and firefighters. However, it is plausible that first responders can benefit from energy, macronutrient, and micronutrient recommendations similar to those set for the general public and for athletes.

A 2020 study noted that firefighters consume inadequate amounts of total calories; fiber; linolenic and α-linolenic fatty acids; vitamins D, E, and K; potassium; zinc; magnesium; and carbohydrates when compared to the MDRIs and the Dietary Reference Intakes (DRIs).[82] In addition, a 2021 systematic review highlighted that law enforcement personnel consumed below the MDRI values for total energy and carbohydrate intake.[83] Although these 2 studies offer potential insight to the dietary intake patterns and habits of first-responder populations, practitioners should note that the MDRIs were established for military personnel, whereas first responders often have dramatically different demands and needs based on their occupation. It is also important to note that these dietary data were obtained from self-reported food records. Self-reports may serve as a limitation of these studies, as the first responders may have underreported their total daily energy intakes. It is not atypical for individuals to underestimate their food intake; this often occurs on food diaries and recall analysis.[84] Therefore, although the data offer some insights, they should be interpreted with caution, as more research is needed to better understand these dietary differences and potential shortcomings.

The dietitian or other nutritional practitioner should use the Mifflin-St. Jeor equation or the Harris-Benedict equation[85-87] coupled with the appropriate activity factor to estimate energy needs. If objective indirect metabolic testing is available, use of a portable metabolic rate testing device (ie, one that has been cleared by the US Food and Drug Administration in accordance with the 510[k] premarket review process) is recommended. First responders can also benefit from the nutritional guidance put forth in the ISSN position stands on nutrition for the tactical athlete, sport nutrition, protein, and caffeine, as well as the ISSN's updated review of research and recommendations related to the optimization of training and performance

BOX 23.1 International Society of Sports Nutrition Position Statement: Protein and Exercise

The International Society of Sports Nutrition provides an objective and critical review related to the intake of protein for healthy, exercising individuals. Based on the current available literature, the position of the Society is as follows:

1. An acute exercise stimulus, particularly resistance exercise, and protein ingestion both stimulate muscle protein synthesis (MPS) and are synergistic when protein consumption occurs before or after resistance exercise.
2. For building muscle mass and for maintaining muscle mass through a positive muscle protein balance, an overall daily protein intake in the range of 1.4 to 2.0 g of protein per kilogram of body weight per day (g/kg/d) is sufficient for most exercising individuals, a value that falls in line within the acceptable macronutrient distribution range published by the Institute of Medicine for protein.
3. Higher protein intakes (2.3–3.1 g/kg/d) may be needed to maximize the retention of lean body mass in resistance-trained subjects during hypocaloric periods.
4. Novel evidence suggests higher protein intakes (>3.0 g/kg/d) may have positive effects on body composition in resistance-trained individuals (ie, promote loss of fat mass).
5. Recommendations regarding the optimal protein intake per serving for athletes to maximize MPS are mixed and are dependent on age and recent resistance exercise stimuli. General recommendations are 0.25 g of a high-quality protein per kilogram of body weight, or an absolute dose of 20 to 40 g.
6. Acute protein doses should strive to contain 700 to 3,000 mg of leucine and/or a higher relative leucine content, in addition to a balanced array of the essential amino acids (EAAs).
7. These protein doses should ideally be evenly distributed, every 3 to 4 hours, across the day.
8. The optimal time period during which to ingest protein is likely a matter of individual tolerance, as benefits are derived from pre- or postworkout ingestion; however, the anabolic effect of exercise is long-lasting (at least 24 hours) but likely diminishes with increasing time postexercise.
9. Although it is possible for physically active individuals to obtain their daily protein requirements through the consumption of whole foods, supplementation is a practical way of ensuring the intake of adequate protein quality and quantity while minimizing caloric intake, particularly for athletes who typically complete high volumes of training.
10. Rapidly digested proteins that contain high proportions of EAAs and adequate leucine are most effective in stimulating MPS.
11. Different types and quality of protein can affect amino acid bioavailability following protein supplementation.
12. Athletes should consider focusing on whole food sources of protein that contain all of the EAAs (ie, it is the EAAs that are required to stimulate MPS).
13. Endurance athletes should focus on achieving adequate carbohydrate intake to promote optimal performance; the addition of protein may help to offset muscle damage and promote recovery.
14. Presleep intake of casein protein (30–40 g) provides increases in overnight MPS and metabolic rate without influencing lipolysis.

Adapted under CC BY 4.0 from reference 81: Jäger R, Kerksick CM, Campbell BI, et al. International Society of Sports Nutrition position stand: protein and exercise. *J Int Soc Sports Nutr.* 2017;14:20. doi:10.1186/s12970-017-0177-8 enhancement through exercise training and nutrition.[8,88-91] With regard to macronutrients, the goals of the first responder will dictate the ratio of macronutrients recommended.

HYDRATION CONSIDERATIONS FOR THE TACTICAL ATHLETE

Several vital physiological processes rely on optimal hydration (digestion/hydrolysis, thermoregulation, joint lubrication, metabolic waste removal). However, hypohydration and dehydration pose real and serious implications for performance, as well as the overall health of the individual.[92] The same is true for a tactical athlete. Ideally, the tactical athlete should practice daily hydration strategies to prevent dehydration and most certainly to limit any hypohydration leading toward dehydration. Hydration losses beyond approximately 2% loss in body weight should be avoided, as significant impairments to physical and cognitive performance can occur beyond this threshold.[93] However, it is quite difficult to pinpoint precise recommendations for the tactical athlete because of the various job duties, levels of physical activity on the job, and environmental conditions of tactical athletes. Cheuvront and Sawka[94] suggested a 3-step approach to assess and correct potential hypohydration through the (1) evaluation of thirst, (2) monitoring of urine color,[95,96] and (3) monitoring of weight. In addition, the Institute of Medicine recommends spreading water intake evenly throughout the day, and it advises females to aim for a fluid intake of 2.7 L/d and males to aim for 3.7 L/d.[97] In practice, it appears that the recommendation of ingesting 0.5 to 1 L/h after exercise to aid in hydration balance is typical. The ability for the tactical athlete to achieve this recommended approach will be limited by operational demands and access to resources.

Under hot and humid conditions and during prolonged activities (>2 h), electrolyte-containing beverages are advised.[79,98] Specific to the firefighter community, during any structural or wildland active-duty fire suppression, firefighters wear personal protective equipment that is encapsulating, significantly limits heat dissipation, and subsequently increases cardiovascular strain and risk for dehydration.[99,100] Research has clearly established that dehydration decreases physical performance, compromises thermoregulation, and impairs key cardiovascular responses during exercise.[101-106] Limited data are available with respect to firefighter-specific hydration needs, but it is recommended that firefighters be made aware of the dangers of their equipment and the environmental conditions in which they conduct active fire suppression activities. It is ideal for the firefighter to follow the 3-step approach of Cheuvront and Sawka[94] and to spread hydration evenly throughout the day; they should also consider consuming electrolyte-containing beverages after responding to a fire. All fluids, excluding alcohol, contribute toward hydration (water, sport drinks, protein-carbohydrate shakes, juices, etc). Foods also contain fluids, with fruit and vegetables providing more than protein foods, grains, breads, and the like. Limiting food intake also impacts hydration status. Refer to Chapter 6 for more information on electrolytes and hydration.

NUTRITIONAL SUPPLEMENTATION FOR THE TACTICAL ATHLETE

Although it is advisable to follow a food-first approach, this might not always be feasible for the tactical athlete. Therefore, dietary supplementation may help to improve or optimize nutrient intake and to provide the individual with an opportunity for nutritional adequacy in challenging feeding scenarios. In addition, supplementation may present the tactical athlete with a competitive edge that could mean the difference between life and death (eg, the ability to evade deadly fire in combat for military personnel or the ability to stave off detrimental effects of heat stress for a firefighter).

The aim of this section is to aid the dietitian in understanding the potential or real practices of tactical athletes with respect to dietary supplements and to identify those that are both common and evidence-based. This section reviews recommendations of the ISSN as stated in its position papers for such, with a primary emphasis on data from military personnel. The data evaluating dietary supplements for performance maintenance or improvement in the tactical athlete are somewhat limited, but growing.[107-112] Perhaps the most appropriate approach is to compare and contrast the tactical athlete with what is known about sports performance nutrition (as nutrition for acute performance is about the immediate task and not necessarily long-term health). In contrast, lifestyle education aids in a better understanding and application of nutrition for health as opposed to performance.

β-Alanine, caffeine, and creatine monohydrate offer ergogenic benefits that have utility for the tactical athlete. Other dietary ingredients that offer benefit through their mechanism of action and through structure/function effects include omega-3 fatty acids (eg, eicosapentaenoic acid [EPA], docosahexaenoic acid [DHA] and β-hydroxy-β-methylbutyrate [HMB]).[88,113] For greater metabolic and physiological support, along with other goals, a "food first, but not food only" approach is most appropriate. Dietary ingredient supplementation practices are a means to augment dietary intake in order to achieve optimal health and performance outcomes, as well as increasing occupational readiness. Table 23.2 outlines some of the more commonly used nutritional supplements that may confer health and performance benefits to the tactical athlete.[88,90,91,114-118]

TABLE 23.2 Commonly Used Supplements Consumed by Tactical Athletes[88,90,91,114-118]

Ingredient[a]	Dosage	Function	Potential benefit	Evidence[b]
EAAs	6-12 g/d[88,90]	Increase protein synthesis/ turnover	Increase or help better maintain fat-free mass and strength during training or caloric insufficiency; may increase recovery	Strong
Arginine	2-9 g/d (UL = 20 g/d)[114]	Increase blood flow, increase nitric oxide	Increase exercise performance, increase growth hormone production, support immune function, promote accretion of fat-free mass	Little to none
Citrulline	3-6 g/d[88]	Increase nitric oxide production	Increase aerobic and anaerobic performance	Mixed or limited
Beetroot juice or sodium nitrate	2-3 h preexercise; 300-600 mg or 0.1 mmol/kg/d[88]	Increase blood flow	Improve work efficiently, reduce phosphocreatine degradation, improve time-trial performance, decrease blood pressure	Mixed or limited
β-Alanine	4-6 g/d for 2-4 wk[115] or 0.8 to 1.6 g × 4 doses[88]	Increase carnosine, buffer acidity, and increase pH	Increase high-intensity exercise capacity, primarily in events lasting 30 s to 4 min	Strong
HMB	1 g, 3 times daily (3 g/d)[88]	Decrease protein breakdown, increase protein synthesis	Promote improvements in fat-free mass, peak isometric force, isokinetic torque production, and decreases in fat mass; improve aerobic performance; improve muscular strength; attenuate muscle damage	Mixed or limited
BCAAs	6-14 g/d in 3:1:1 leucine-to-valine-to-isoleucine ratio[88]	Increase exercise capacity, increase recovery	Improve psychological perception of fatigue (central fatigue), promote recovery, mitigate soreness, mitigate loss of force production	Mixed or limited
Caffeine	3-6 mg/kg/d[91]	Increase energy, improve mood, increase endurance	Spare carbohydrate, improve endurance exercise capacity, improve alertness, improve cognitive function	Strong

Continued on next page

TABLE 23.2 Commonly Used Supplements Consumed by Tactical Athletes[88,90,91,114-118] (CONTINUED)

Ingredient[a]	Dosage	Function	Potential benefit	Evidence[b]
Creatine	Load 4-5 g/d for 7 days; 3-5 g daily thereafter[89,116]	Increase energy/ATP, neuroprotection	Increase explosive sprint capacity, recovery from sprints, muscle endurance, and fat-free mass gains during training	Strong
Omega-3 fatty acids	1-3 g/d	Regulation of blood pressure and vascular function	Cardioprotective benefits[117] and improved cognition	Strong
Glutamine	5 g or 0.3 g/kg/d[88]	Increase recovery, immune function	Tolerate stress, enhance strength and muscle mass, improve glycogen stores, improve recovery	Little to none
Melatonin	0.5-3 mg (starting with a lower dose is recommended)[114]	Regulate internal timing of biological rhythms to promote sleep	Improve sleep and optimize sleep quality[118]	Little to none
Multivitamin	Once daily	Supplements nutrients that are in a state of deficiency	Improve vitamin status, support immune system	Strong health benefits
Protein (eg, whey)	Variable, 20-40 g post-workout[88,90]	Increase protein turnover/synthesis	Promote retention of lean body mass, positive effects on body composition, improved strength, reduced risk of injury	Strong
Glucosamine	1,500 mg/d spread out over 3 doses	Reduce osteoarthritis pain	Slow cartilage degeneration, reduced degree of joint pain, may postpone or prevent joint problems[88]	Little to none
Chondroitin	1,200 mg/d in split doses	Reduce osteoarthritis pain	Slow cartilage degeneration, reduced degree of joint pain, may postpone or prevent joint problems[88]	Little to none

[a] Listing of an ingredient does not indicate an endorsement of such.
[b] Indicates strength of evidence to support efficacy and safety.
Abbreviations: ATP, adenosine triphosphate; BCAA, branched-chain amino acid; DHA, docosahexaenoic acid; EAA, essential amino acid; EPA, eicosapentaenoic acid; HMB, β-hydroxy-β-methyl butyrate; UL, upper limit

Ergogenic Aids for the Tactical Athlete

β-ALANINE

β-Alanine, a nonproteinogenic amino acid, is the rate-limiting precursor to carnosine synthesis. Carnosine is a powerful physiological buffer linked to focus, alertness, and cognitive function during stressful and fatigued conditions. Research has established that β-alanine can confer an ergogenic benefit during brief, high-intensity activities (ie, 60–300 s).[115,119,120] In general, the literature suggests that one must consume daily doses of 4 to 6 g of β-alanine (dividing the total of 4–6 g into doses of 2 g or less is advised) for approximately

4 weeks to significantly augment muscle carnosine concentrations and gain the subsequent ergogenic benefits (refer to Box 23.2).[115]

To date, only a handful of studies have examined β-alanine supplementation among military personnel. Hoffman et al[121] assessed the impacts of β-alanine supplementation at 6 g/d for 4 weeks on both physical and cognitive performance outcomes among Israeli military personnel. The researchers had 20 military service members perform a battery of physically demanding tasks and then conduct shooting tasks and cognitive assessments in which shooting accuracy, marksmanship, and target engagement speed were observed. Following the 4 weeks of supplementation, shooting accuracy, marksmanship, and target engagement speed improved, but no improvements were noted for cognitive function. A separate study by Hoffman et al[122] demonstrated that 30 days of β-alanine supplementation significantly elevated skeletal muscle carnosine concentrations in addition to improving military-specific performance, which was assessed by a 50-m casualty carry task. In contrast to Hoffman et al,[121] Hoffman et al[122] found significant improvements for cognitive performance in a 2-minute serial subtraction test that was performed simultaneously while shooting at nearby targets. This finding is critically important to the military, as well as law enforcement personnel, as it demonstrates the ability of an individual to maintain improved focus under stressful, anxiety-inducing conditions along with the ability to maintain proficiency at task switching (multitasking) after β-alanine supplementation. These findings are promising for both physical and cognitive performance enhancements, especially under stressful conditions.

CAFFEINE

Caffeine is arguably one of the most popular naturally occurring food ingredients in the world, and its popularity is noted among tactical athletes.[112,123,124] Caffeine is widely accepted as a central nervous system stimulant that can enhance performance through increased myofibrillar calcium availability, optimize energy metabolism, and reduce perceptual and physical fatigue.[125-128] The 2021 ISSN position stand on caffeine provides a comprehensive review of its ergogenic effects, as well as its mechanism of action and recommendations for supplementation practices (refer to Box 23.3 on page 618).[91] Although the general

BOX 23.2 International Society of Sports Nutrition Position Statement: β-Alanine

The International Society of Sports Nutrition (ISSN) provides an objective and critical review of the mechanisms and use of β-alanine supplementation. Based on the current available literature, the conclusions of the ISSN are as follows:

1. Four weeks of β-alanine supplementation (4-6 g daily) significantly augments muscle carnosine concentrations, thereby acting as an intracellular pH buffer.
2. β-Alanine supplementation currently appears to be safe in healthy populations at recommended doses.
3. The only reported adverse effect is paresthesia (tingling), but studies indicate this can be attenuated by using divided lower doses (1.6 g) or using a sustained-release formula.
4. Daily supplementation with 4 to 6 g of β-alanine for at least 2 to 4 weeks has been shown to improve exercise performance, with more pronounced effects in open end-point tasks/time trials lasting 1 to 4 min in duration.
5. β-Alanine attenuates neuromuscular fatigue, particularly in older subjects, and preliminary evidence indicates that β-alanine may improve tactical performance.
6. Combining β-alanine with other single or multi-ingredient supplements may be advantageous when supplementation of β-alanine is high enough (4-6 g daily) and long enough (minimum 4 weeks).
7. More research is needed to determine the effects of β-alanine on strength, endurance performance beyond 25 minutes in duration, and other health-related benefits associated with carnosine.

BOX 23.3 International Society of Sports Nutrition Position Stand: Caffeine and Exercise Performance

Following critical evaluation of the available literature, the International Society of Sports Nutrition position regarding caffeine intake is as follows:

1. Supplementation with caffeine has been shown to acutely enhance various aspects of exercise performance in many but not all studies. Small to moderate benefits of caffeine use include, but are not limited to, muscular endurance, movement velocity and muscular strength, sprinting, jumping, and throwing performance, as well as a wide range of aerobic and anaerobic sport-specific actions.
2. Aerobic endurance appears to be the form of exercise with the most consistent moderate-to-large benefits from caffeine use, although the magnitude of its effects differs between individuals.
3. Caffeine has consistently been shown to improve exercise performance when consumed in doses of 3 to 6 mg/kg of body mass. Minimal effective doses of caffeine currently remain unclear, but they may be as low as 2 mg/kg of body mass. Very high doses of caffeine (eg, 9 mg/kg) are associated with a high incidence of adverse effects and do not seem to be required to elicit an ergogenic effect.
4. The most commonly used timing of caffeine supplementation is 60 minutes preexercise. Optimal timing of caffeine ingestion likely depends on the source of caffeine. For example, as compared to caffeine capsules, caffeine chewing gums may require a shorter waiting time from consumption to the start of the exercise session.
5. Caffeine appears to improve physical performance in both trained and untrained individuals.
6. Interindividual differences in sport and exercise performance as well as adverse effects on sleep or feelings of anxiety following caffeine ingestion may be attributed to genetic variation associated with caffeine metabolism, and physical and psychological response. Other factors such as habitual caffeine intake also may play a role in between-individual response variation.
7. Caffeine has been shown to be ergogenic for cognitive function, including attention and vigilance, in most individuals.
8. Caffeine may improve cognitive and physical performance in some individuals under conditions of sleep deprivation.
9. The use of caffeine in conjunction with endurance exercise in the heat and at altitude is well supported when dosages range from 3 to 6 mg/kg and 4 to 6 mg/kg, respectively.
10. Alternative sources of caffeine such as caffeinated chewing gum, mouth rinses, energy gels and chews have been shown to improve performance, primarily in aerobic exercise.
11. Energy drinks and pre-workout supplements containing caffeine have been demonstrated to enhance both anaerobic and aerobic performance.

Adapted under CC BY 4.0 from reference 91: Guest NS, VanDusseldorp TA, Nelson MT, et al. International Society of Sports Nutrition position stand: caffeine and exercise performance. *J Int Soc Sports Nutr.* 2021;18(1):1. doi:10.1186/s12970-020-00383-4

recommendation in AR 40-25 is to consume caffeine in the amount of 100 to 200 mg (100 mg per 2 hours or 200 mg per 4 hours) throughout a 24-hour period (while aiming to abstain from caffeine consumption for 6 hours prior to bedtime),[78] researchers have reported that the daily average consumption of caffeine among military personnel is roughly between 200 and 300 mg/d.[124] This is equal to 1 to 2 premium coffees per day (Starbucks grande, Dunkin' Donuts medium, etc).

Caffeine use can potentially improve time to exhaustion during tactical-specific tasks following periods of sleep loss among military personnel. Sleep deprivation is common in the military. Caffeine administered in varying doses over the course of 3 days of sleep loss (using caffeinated gum at specific time intervals) resulted in improved 6.3-km run times under sleep-deprived conditions.[129] Kamimori et al[130] also demonstrated that a total daily dose of 800 mg of caffeine was effective in overcoming the adverse effects of successive sleep loss among Special Forces personnel. Practitioners should note that the US Food and Drug Administration recommends that an individual consume no more than 400 mg of caffeine per day to reduce their chances of an adverse event (eg, tremor, palpitations, restlessness, irritability, nausea, paresthesia, headache).[131] These findings of enhanced multitasking and improved physical performance, among others, are critical to military personnel and potentially also to first responders who are faced with periods of extended wakefulness when optimal sleep is not feasible.[130,132,133]

Beyond the ergogenic benefits, caffeine is also known to enhance cognitive performance and mood states when appropriate doses (3–6 mg/kg of body weight) are consumed.[134-136] Improved attention, vigilance, reaction time, ability to perform complex activities, problem-solving, and reasoning are several critical cognitive benefits to military personnel. In addition, several studies have illustrated the ability of caffeine to improve marksmanship under conditions of sleep deprivation.[133,137,138] Total caffeine doses of 200 to 300 mg have been reported to augment correct responses on a 4-choice visual reaction time assessment (by 73% and 81%, respectively) and premature errors (by 98% and 88%, respectively) compared to placebo during Navy SEAL candidates' "Hell Week" training.[138] Moreover, intake of 200 mg of caffeine improved marksmanship as noted by reduced distance from center of mass (23%), reduced misses (44%), increased precision (47%), and faster sighting time (23%) compared to placebo.[133,138] Outcomes of life or death for the military and first responders are very real; therefore, any nutritional strategy that may enhance the skills of the operator may prove to be beneficial beyond performance alone.

CREATINE MONOHYDRATE

Creatine monohydrate has been extensively researched for its ergogenic effects, which include performance outcomes such as increases in high-intensity exercise capacity, peak power output, maximal muscular strength, number of repetitions completed before fatigue, and fat-free mass (refer to Box 23.4 on page 620).[116,139] Although data are limited among tactical athletes, the observed ergogenic outcomes from supplementation with creatine monohydrate in athletic populations are relevant. First, research has demonstrated that creatine monohydrate supplementation improves recovery and attenuates skeletal muscle tissue damage following an intense bout of exercise,[140] which could benefit tactical athletes responding to emergencies or during intense training. In addition, researchers found that collegiate-level athletes using creatine monohydrate demonstrated a lower incidence of skeletal muscle–related injuries and/or other diagnoses, such as strains and pulls, cramping and heat illness, and total injuries, which are also experienced by tactical athletes.[141] In terms of the thermoregulatory benefits of creatine monohydrate, data indicate that supplementation can increase intracellular water (positively impacting cellular hydration) in addition to reducing heart rate, rectal temperature, and sweat rates during prolonged exercise under hot environmental conditions,[142] which could benefit tactical athletes working in extreme environments.

Creatine monohydrate has also been shown to confer cognitive benefits.[143] Emerging data have demonstrated the ability for creatine monohydrate to increase brain creatine concentrations by approximately 5% to 10%,[143,144] which may explain why there is some published evidence supporting neuroprotective properties for creatine monohydrate.[143,145,146] Although experts do not yet know specifics on optimal dosage, it appears that higher daily doses given for longer durations (ie, 10–20 g/d for 2 weeks or longer) might be needed to enhance brain creatine concentrations.[144,147] These cognitive and neuroprotective properties of creatine monohydrate could confer critical benefits to the tactical athlete; however, more research is needed, specifically in these populations.

With regard to safety, clinical studies on creatine monohydrate using dosages of up to 30 g/d for 5 years have shown safety and no untoward effects. Overall, creatine monohydrate is a safe and efficacious dietary supplement.[88,116,139,148] It is important to note that the amount of creatine provided in whole foods is approximately a net yield of 1 g/d and varies depending on the source (eg, 11 g/kg in raw and dried herring fillet, and 0 for any plant-based foods).[149] Therefore, consideration of supplementation is recommended to optimize creatine provision.

BOX 23.4 International Society of Sports Nutrition Position Stand: Safety and Efficacy of Creatine Supplementation in Exercise, Sport, and Medicine

The purpose of this review was to provide an update to the current literature regarding the role and safety of creatine supplementation in exercise, sport, and medicine and to update the position stand of International Society of Sports Nutrition.

1. Creatine is one of the most popular nutritional ergogenic aids for athletes.
2. Studies have consistently shown that creatine supplementation increases intramuscular creatine concentrations, which may help explain the observed improvements in high-intensity exercise performance leading to greater training adaptations.
3. In addition to athletic and exercise improvement, research has shown that creatine supplementation may enhance post-exercise recovery, injury prevention, thermoregulation, rehabilitation, and concussion and/or spinal cord neuroprotection.
4. Additionally, a number of clinical applications of creatine supplementation have been studied involving neurodegenerative diseases (eg, muscular dystrophy, Parkinsons, Huntingtons disease), diabetes, osteoarthritis, fibromyalgia, aging, brain and heart ischemia, adolescent depression, and pregnancy. These studies provide a large body of evidence that creatine can not only improve exercise performance but can play a role in preventing and/or reducing the severity of injury, enhancing rehabilitation from injuries, and helping athletes tolerate heavy training loads.
5. Additionally, researchers have identified a number of potentially beneficial clinical uses of creatine supplementation. These studies show that short- and long-term supplementation (up to 30 g/d for 5 years) is safe and well tolerated in healthy individuals and in a number of patient populations ranging from infants to the elderly.
6. Moreover, significant health benefits may be provided by ensuring habitual low dietary creatine ingestion (eg, 3 g/d) throughout the lifespan.

Adapted under CC BY 4.0 from reference 116: Kreider RB, Kalman DS, Antonio J, et al. International Society of Sports Nutrition position stand: safety and efficacy of creatine supplementation in exercise, sport, and medicine. *J Int Soc Sports Nutr.* 2017;14:18. doi:10.1186/s12970-017-0173-z

Limiting Catabolism in Military Personnel

ESSENTIAL AMINO ACIDS

Military personnel perform highly physical tasks over long periods of time with little rest and less-than-optimal feeding conditions. This may occur in training or in deployment to a combat zone. In this scenario, providing adequate nutrition for fueling and, consequently, muscle protein maintenance is exceedingly difficult. Because of the physical demands of the job and the need to maintain lean mass for occupational performance and life preservation in combat, preserving whole-body muscle protein becomes a major priority. To date, approximately 70 clinical trials have been completed among the general public, and these studies indicate the benefits of ingestion of and/or supplementation with EAAs. Seminal work regarding muscle protein synthesis has demonstrated the critical role of EAAs in maximally stimulating muscle protein synthesis.[150-152] Several studies have demonstrated the benefits of EAA supplementation and intake regarding skeletal muscle anabolism, lean mass, and functional outcomes, as well as rehabilitative mitigation of skeletal muscle loss postsurgery.[153-158] Moreover, free-form EAA supplementation, in combination with exercise training, confers a strong anabolic effect on skeletal muscle.[159] Other factors, such as the dose ingested, can also augment the response in skeletal muscle protein synthesis rates.[160-162] It is important for the tactical athlete, especially military personnel, to increase EAA intake during periods of energy deficit for the maintenance of body protein.[8]

The inclusion of free-form EAAs in the rations of military personnel may be an important pragmatic consideration when they are in garrison (military outpost where military personnel are stationed to provide protection to surrounding area) and subject to prolonged periods of a caloric deficit. In fact, there are commercially available, free-form EAA products that are highly palatable, water-soluble, and packaged into compact and lightweight delivery formats. The consumption of 3 to 6 g of EAAs appears to be efficacious from an anabolic standpoint when taken postexercise (1 and 2 hours post),[163] whereas a maximal response can be leveraged from 10 to 15 g taken before and after exercise bouts.[150,164] However, one does not need to supplement both before and after to achieve an added impact on muscle protein synthesis. Moreover, Tipton et al[164] demonstrated that 10- to 15-g doses of EAAs could promote high protein accretion even over a 24-hour period. These findings are consistent with studies assessing the efficacy of the ingestion of 25 to 30 g of protein per serving, combined with exercise, on maximal stimulation of skeletal muscle protein synthesis.[165] Interestingly, the ingestion of free-form EAAs appears to result in greater skeletal muscle protein synthesis than the equivalent given in a high-quality protein bolus.[151] The recommended efficacious dose of EAAs is between 10 and 15 g.[166] Based on these data, the tactical athlete is advised to consume a daily diet consisting of the optimal EAA dose at each meal (ingesting intact protein sources as part of meals may aid in this goal).[8]

The research mentioned in this section has thus far summarized the effects of EAAs under optimally fed conditions, which is not always the case for military personnel, especially when in forward deployment. Research by Gwin et al[166] demonstrated that 5 days of a 30% energy deficit increased the body's need for EAAs to maintain the whole-body protein balance. In this study, 2 EAA doses of 0.10 g/kg (ie, ~8 g/dose) or 0.30 g/kg were administered immediately postexercise, and whole-body protein homeostasis was achieved with both doses. Moreover, the higher dose resulted in greater rates of whole-body protein synthesis, which resulted in a 2-fold greater response compared to that observed with the lower dose. Gwin et al[167] conducted additional work assessing 3 different postexercise ingestion delivery formats of 35-g protein doses (a free-form EAA plus whey protein formula, whey protein alone, or a mixed macronutrient meal) while individuals were subjected to 5 days of a 30% energy deficit. The results demonstrated that the whole-body protein synthesis and net protein balance were greater in response to the free-form EAA/whey combination. Finally, other studies in both civilian and military contexts have demonstrated that adding protein to the diet optimizes EAA delivery while also mitigating the loss of lean tissue and optimizing the loss of fat tissue in the face of energy deficits of 30% to 40%.[168,169] Taken together, these data indicate that efficient delivery of EAAs can be beneficial to the tactical athlete, especially when exposed to energy-deficit conditions. The major challenge for the tactical athlete is the necessity of carrying large amounts of provisions when personal load carriage is already very high and when there is an unpredictability in terms of logistics downrange. For this reason, among others, the use of free-form EAAs may be a suitable method for withstanding periods in which the tactical athlete is subject to a catabolic state (eg, deployed military personnel).

Additional Nutritional Supplementation Considerations

L-TYROSINE

L-Tyrosine, a proteogenic amino acid, is the precursor to the synthesis of dopamine, norepinephrine, and epinephrine. Although tyrosine is not considered an EAA, data indicate the potential neuroprotective impacts of L-tyrosine supplementation. The body can synthesize tyrosine through transamination and other processes; one precursor to the production of tyrosine is phenylalanine. However, the brain does not convert enough tyrosine from phenylalanine to meet its demands, which may have potential occupational performance and readiness implications when considering the need for the tactical athlete to have optimal cognitive function. In fact, the tactical athlete is likely to be vulnerable during stressful conditions and sleep loss, when neural catecholamine activity can increase and become more precursor sensitive.[170] L-Tyrosine supplementation affects cognitive processes largely through activity in the prefrontal cortex. Dopamine activity in the prefrontal cortex is particularly critical for working memory, decision making, task switching, attention, and general executive control functions.[171] These cognitive processes are vital to the life-preserving activities of tactical athletes. Several studies have reported that L-tyrosine supplementation during stressful conditions can preserve cognitive processing. Mahoney et al[172] reported that L-tyrosine supplementation in the amount of 150 mg/kg improved information processing speed and accuracy prior to two 90-minute cold-water immersions among military personnel. In addition, Shurtleff et al[173] demonstrated that an identical dose of l-tyrosine improved matching accuracy after 30 minutes of cold exposure. Finally, supplementation with 300 mg of L-tyrosine per kilogram of body mass has been shown to improve vigilance (9% increase) among soccer players training in a hot environment when administered 5 hours and 1 hour prior to the training.[174] Tactical athletes may face both hot and cold environmental conditions that could impact physical and cognitive performance; therefore, these findings may provide important implications for the consideration of L-tyrosine supplementation in tactical athletes.

OMEGA-3 FATTY ACIDS

Omega-3 fatty acids, consisting of the fatty acids eicosapentaenoic acid (EPA) and docosahexaenoic acid (DHA), have been referred to as "nutritional armor" in terms of cognitive health and performance.[175] Within the brain, DHA is a primary structural component for the neuronal cell membrane, accounting for 10% and 97% of total lipid and omega-3 fatty acid contents, respectively.[176,177] TBIs reduce DHA brain content, and the tactical athlete is commonly exposed to combat and training environments that increase the risk of head trauma and mild to severe TBIs, as well as associated negative effects. Therefore, it is plausible that the tactical athlete may benefit from prophylactic DHA supplementation, as well as omega-3 fatty acid supplementation in general, to boost resilience to TBIs and head trauma.[8] Limited data on such as approach exist, especially among tactical athletes; however, recent studies conducted with athletic populations exposed to repetitive head trauma could provide useful insight regarding the nutritional factors available to reduce the prevalence and severity of TBIs.

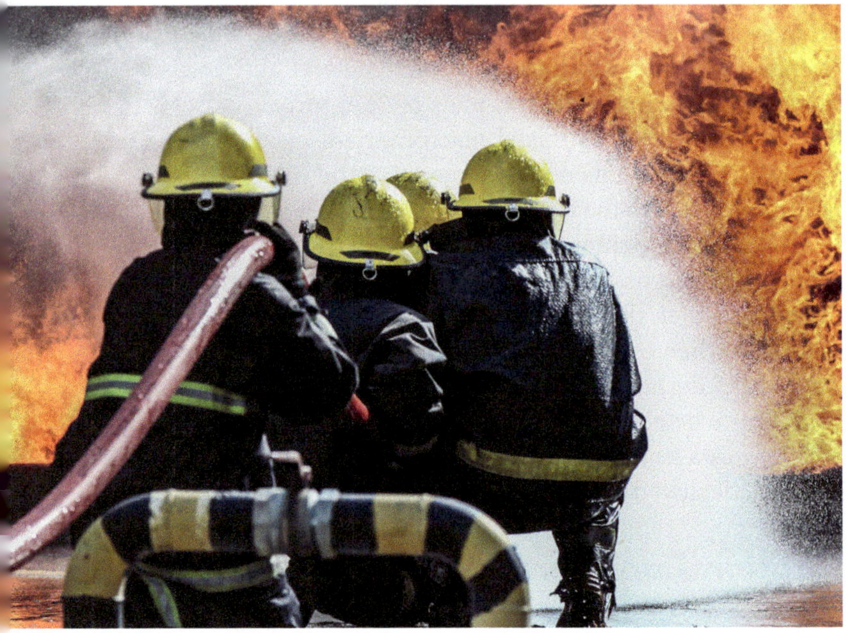

DHA supplementation at a dosage of 2 g/d or greater (delivered as either 2, 4, or 6 g/d) has been shown to favorably improve reliable markers of head trauma, such as the serum levels of neurofilament light chain among American football players who were subjected to repetitive head impacts during training and competition.[178] Heileson et al[179] demonstrated similar reductions in neurofilament light chain levels among collegiate football players who supplemented with multiple omega-3 fatty acids (2 g of DHA, 0.56 g of EPA, and 0.32 g of docosapentaenoic acid). Apart from the neuroprotective benefits, omega-3 fatty acids have also been shown to improve cognitive outcomes, such as sleep quality, mood, episodic memory, and reaction time.[180-182]

Data also suggest a link between insufficiencies or deficiencies in omega-3 fatty acids and elevated deployment-induced stress that can manifest as depression and completed suicide.[183] Importantly, supplementation with both EPA and DHA at 2 g/d for 12 weeks has been shown to reduce suicidal ideation by 45% and depression by 30% among athletic populations.[184-186] Warfighters with low DHA levels are 62% more likely to have committed suicide.[183] Hallahan et al reported a 45% reduction in suicidal ideation and a 30% reduction in depression for individuals who consumed 2 g of EPA and DHA per day for at least 12 weeks.[186] Finally, these data were thoroughly summarized in a review by Hibbeln and Gow[184] that advocated for increases in EPA and DHA in warfighters' diets to reduce military psychiatric distress and increase force sustainability. These recommendations were also firmly supported by a military expert panel who concluded that it would be unethical to *not* attempt to increase the omega-3 status among US military personnel.[186,187]

In addition, omega-3 fatty acids have been shown to improve recovery from rigorous exercise and exercise-induced muscle damage, in addition to reducing delayed-onset muscle soreness among athletic populations.[180,185,187-189] Given that the tactical athlete endures a high degree of physiological and psychological stress, as well as exposure to dangerous environments with increased risk of suffering from head trauma, prophylactic omega-3 fatty acid supplementation is a pragmatic nutritional practice to enhance cognitive performance and combat the detrimental impacts of overexertion among tactical athletes.

VITAMIN D

A high prevalence of vitamin D insufficiency and deficiency has been noted among tactical athletes, and northerly stationed service members may be at an increased risk for vitamin D deficiency.[190-192] Maintaining adequate levels of vitamin D is necessary for supporting skeletal and bone health, and research indicates blood vitamin D concentrations are associated with muscle mass, muscular strength and power, mental health, aerobic endurance, Army Combat Fitness Test parameters, and testosterone.[191-198] Healthy individuals ages 1 to 70 years are advised to consume 600 IU/d (15 mcg/d) to maintain nutrient adequacy, whereas consumption of 1,500 to 2,000 IU/d (37.5 to 50 mcg/d) may be necessary to consistently maintain sufficient levels. Serum 25-hydroxyvitamin D levels of at least 30 ng/mL are considered sufficient, whereas the ranges of 20 to 29 ng/mL and less than 20 ng/mL are considered insufficient and deficient, respectively.[199] Importantly, poor vitamin D status has been noted as an important modifiable risk factor for the development of stress fractures, and the risk among military personnel, especially among trainees and females, is high.[200,201]

Firefighters have also been identified as a group who has inadequate amounts of vitamin D in their diets,[202] and there is a likelihood that the wear and tear of the occupational demands of firefighting could lead to the risk of stress fractures. In fact, other first-responder personnel, such as law enforcement officers, also have a risk of stress fractures that can be attributed to the occupational demands and likely inadequate vitamin D status.[8,203] In addition, tactical athletes deficient in vitamin D may also be at risk for being diagnosed with depression.[192] Therefore, tactical athletes should generally be encouraged to consume a minimum of 600 IU of vitamin D per day.

Combating Traumatic Brain Injuries and Concussions

Tactical athletes, especially military personnel, are susceptible to suffering mild TBIs and concussions because of the nature of their occupation[55]; therefore, nutritional interventions that can aid brain function and improve recovery post-TBI are of particular interest. In general, fueling strategies to treat and aid recovery from TBIs are targeted at (1) restoring cellular energetics/metabolism, (2) reducing oxidative stress and inflammation, and (3) supporting repair and recovery.[204] Early feeding strategies (within the first 24 hours) that focus on adequate energy and protein intakes post-TBI can improve mortality and neurological outcomes.[205,206] Data from the Brain Trauma Foundation suggest that mortality improves significantly by each 10 kcal increase in energy intake per kilogram of body weight.[207] Moreover, a recent narrative review on nutrition management among patients with TBIs noted that energy requirements may increase by 100% to 200% of baseline resting energy expenditure values and that these increased requirements can persist for weeks to months depending on the severity of the injury. Experts recommend that the practitioner use either indirect calorimetry or predication equations (eg, the Harris-Benedict, Ireton-Jones, or Penn State predictive equations) to measure energy needs post-TBI and to combat the risk of death postinjury.[208] In addition, protein intakes are recommended to account for 15% to 20% of one's total daily caloric goal, which may translate into total protein requirements of approximately 2 g/kg/d.[209]

Several dietary supplements including omega-3 fatty acids; isolated antioxidants (eg, curcumin, resveratrol) and polyphenols; creatine monohydrate; melatonin; and vitamins C, D, and E have shown promising results in animal studies in mitigating the symptoms of concussion, combating oxidative stress and inflammation, and aiding in the repair and recovery of TBI.[204,210,211] Briefly, supplementation with omega-3 fatty acids before an individual has sustained a concussion has been shown to protect against reduced plasticity of neurons and impaired learning by normalizing the levels of proteins associated with normal neural function.[212] Research has shown that omega-3 fatty acid supplementation before a concussion can reduce the biological markers of brain injury and cellular apoptosis.[213] Omega-3 fatty acids may also provide resistance to oxidative stress induced by a concussion and help maintain genomic stability and cellular homeostasis, in addition to decreasing the amount of injury the brain sustains.[214-216]

With regard to antioxidants, curcumin supplementation before an individual has sustained a concussion has been shown to result in improved balance as well as transduction and monitoring of cellular energy compared to a control group.[217] Supplementation with curcumin after a concussion has been shown to improve membrane function, the restoration of homeostasis, neuronal plasticity, synaptic plasticity, and neuronal signaling, in addition to significantly reducing neural inflammation by decreasing the levels of microglia and macrophages that aid in neuronal apoptosis.[217,218]

Finally, creatine monohydrate could theoretically decrease hyperglycolysis and oxidative damage. The use of proton magnetic resonance spectroscopy to measure the levels of creatine preconcussion and postconcussion has revealed that creatine levels in the brain decrease after an individual has sustained a concussion.[219] Two human-based randomized prospective studies have investigated the use of creatine supplementation in children after they had sustained a moderate to severe TBI. These open-label studies showed that, compared with the control group, the children who were supplemented with creatine had significantly improved cognition, communication, self-care, personality, and behavior, as well as significantly decreased headaches, dizziness, and fatigue.[220,221] Judging from these studies, creatine shows promise for the treatment of concussions; however, given that these studies were evaluating patients with TBIs with a longer time to recovery, experts are not certain whether creatine would improve outcomes in patients with concussions whose symptoms have generally resolved in a shorter time frame. Furthermore, there is a critical need for more research with respect to these nutrients among military personnel. Presently, the approach of increasing energy and protein intakes to meet the higher energy needs of individuals post-TBI, as well as providing supplementation with omega-3 and other isolate dietary supplements to combat oxidative stress and inflammation and aid the recovery process, appears to hold promise.

Nutritional Supplementation Specific to the First Responder

Few studies have been published regarding the use of dietary supplements among first responders. First responders are guided to place an emphasis on lifestyle changes necessary to reduce their risk for obesity, cardiovascular disease, and other associated comorbidities. However, the use of dietary supplements may help first responders achieve these goals. Supplements such as caffeine, creatine, protein, β-alanine, and EAAs are safe and efficacious and can be recommended for these personnel. The ISSN position stands on caffeine,[91] creatine,[116] and protein,[81] as well as the updated review of research and recommendations related to the optimization of training and performance enhancement through exercise training and nutrition,[88] can help the practitioner better understand how to incorporate these supplements into a first responder's regimen.

Given the heighted risk for cardiovascular disease and cancer among first responders, natural antioxidants and anti-inflammatory ingredients have gained interest. Isolated ingredients with antioxidant properties, such as curcumin and astaxanthin, have been investigated for their antioxidative and anti-inflammatory benefits.[222,223] These benefits may improve the cardiometabolic health profiles of individuals, including the tactical athlete.[224,225] In addition, these ingredients may reduce biological inflammatory or oxidative stress markers and also improve recovery from muscle-damaging exercise or movements.[226,227] At the time of this writing, only 1 study has been published regarding curcumin supplementation among a cohort of firefighters.[108] More research is warranted to generate firm recommendations regarding antioxidants and other dietary ingredients for first responders. Practitioners may consider recommending supplementation with natural antioxidants and anti-inflammatory ingredients in addition to recommending a diet high in these nutrients.

DIETARY PATTERN CONSIDERATIONS

Of major concern among tactical athletes, specifically first responders, are the challenges resulting from poor dietary patterns and habits (eg, hypercaloric diets, frequent snacking); physical inactivity; and an increased prevalence of obesity, cardiovascular disease, and other associated comorbidities. Dietary intakes are influenced by busy schedules, shift work, long hours, inconsistent and infrequent mealtimes, tiredness and sleep loss, motivation, and convenience.[228-230] In general, first responders should modify their dietary habits to meet appropriate energy, macronutrient, micronutrient, and dietary fiber needs to maintain and improve their overall health and fitness status.[8] Dietary programs should target a reduction of fat mass, an increase in lean mass, and improvements in both health and fitness outcomes while employing a "food first, but not food only" approach. No one dietary pattern is best to practice for all tactical athletes; however, the Mediterranean diet or a diet that combines the Mediterranean diet with the DASH (dietary approaches to stop hypertension) diet called the MIND (Mediterranean-DASH intervention for neurodegenerative delay) diet could be beneficial given the associated favorable cardiometabolic and cognitive health outcomes of these dietary approaches.[231-234] Discussing the efficacy of every dietary strategy is outside the scope of this chapter; however, approaches focused on portion control, limited intake of energy-dense foods, and increased intake of nutrient-dense foods and dietary fiber are likely to provide the greatest benefit for the tactical athlete.[8]

Time-Restricted Feeding or Intermittent Fasting

A small number of investigations have been completed using time-restricted feeding (similar to intermittent fasting), low-carbohydrate diets, and the Mediterranean diet, and these studies have been conducted primarily within the firefighting community. Time-restricted feeding (also known as time-restricted eating) has gained popularity within the past decade because of its potential health benefits, such as improved blood lipids and markers of inflammation in active, trained, and overweight populations.[235-237] In addition, some data suggest that the benefits of time-restricted feeding are not entirely linked to caloric restriction.[238] Specifically, McAllister et al[239] demonstrated significant reductions in blood pressure and percent body fat, as well as increased high-density lipoprotein cholesterol and adiponectin concentrations, following a 16:8 (fasting hours to feeding hours) time-restricted feeding protocol among healthy college-aged individuals. In firefighters, a protocol involving a 14:10 ratio of fasting hours to feeding hours resulted in reduced inflammation and oxidative stress, as well as reductions in inflammation after simulated fire suppression activities (ie, ladder carry, hose deployment, victim removal, and forced-entry tasks).[239,240] In terms of physical performance, it appears that 7 weeks of time-restricted feeding does not negatively affect fitness outcomes, such as the 1-repetition maximums for barbell back squat and bench press, vertical jump height, and number of repetitions for push-ups and sit-ups.[241]

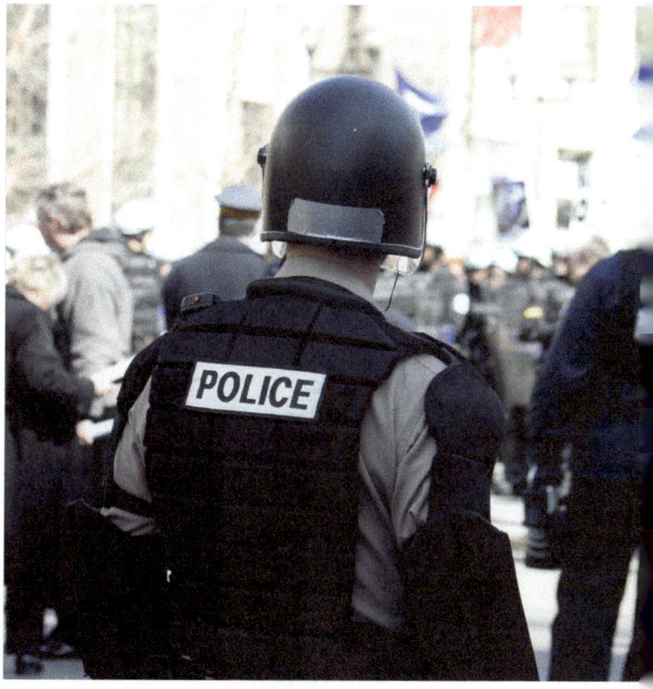

Low-Carbohydrate Diets

In addition to time-restricted feeding, low-carbohydrate diets have garnered interest among tactical athletes for producing similar outcomes, such as reducing body weight and body fat and improving metabolic health and physical performance. To date, 1 study has been completed that examined the effects of 28 days of carbohydrate-restricted dieting among a cohort of firefighters. This study noted improvements in fat mass (~2.4-kg reduction, specifically around the abdominal section), decreases in both the systolic and diastolic blood pressure readings (by 6.0 and 5.0 mm Hg, respectively), and increased fat oxidation rates, as well as improvements in various cardiometabolic health markers (malondialdehyde, advanced oxidation protein products, high-density lipoprotein cholesterol, and triglycerides) following the intervention. In terms of physical performance, the firefighters improved their 2.41-km run times (~3% faster times) and increased the maximum number of push-ups performed (~15% increase).[242] Although these data are limited, it appears that time-restricted feeding and low-carbohydrate diets may be useful tools for first responders; however, caution is warranted, as more research is needed on the dietary quality and nutrient adequacy of these diets within these populations.

Mediterranean Diet

The Mediterranean diet has gained continued interest and popularity because of its less restrictive approach to food choices,[232,243] as well as evidence demonstrating its potential benefits in terms of cardiovascular health (ie, favorable blood lipid and weight changes).[244,245] For example, Yang et al[231] reported that, among a cohort of firefighters, the Mediterranean diet was inversely associated with weight gain (odds ratio, 0.57; 95% confidence interval, 0.39–0.84) and favorably improved both high-density lipoprotein cholesterol and low-density lipoprotein cholesterol. Almeida et al[246] demonstrated that the Mediterranean diet coupled with exercise training was effective in improving cardiometabolic health profiles among a cohort of firefighters. However, the civilian control group of this study demonstrated higher overall adherence to the diet intervention.

Although the Mediterranean diet appears to be of interest to first responders,[231] there is no one-size-fits-all dietary approach, and the best strategy to achieve health and performance outcomes is one that can be followed. More research is needed to examine the impact of potential modulators toward health, performance, and occupational readiness. The results from these investigations can best inform researchers and practitioners regarding the potential efficacy of a combination of various diet and exercise training strategies to improve the health and performance of first-responder populations.

SOCIAL DETERMINANTS OF HEALTH FOR TACTICAL POPULATIONS

The tactical athlete is unique from the general population in terms of social determinants of health, which should be taken into consideration when finding fueling solutions for this group that are feasible, realistic, and sustainable. According to Healthy People 2030,[247] the Centers for Disease Control and Prevention,[248] and the World Health Organization,[249] *social determinants of health* are conditions or environments in which people are born, grow up, and age; live; learn; work; play; and worship that affect or shape health, functioning, and quality of life. Social determinants of health are classified into the following 5 domains: economic stability, built environment, health care, social and community context, and education (refer to Figure 23.2).[247] For tactical athletes, social determinants of health have a greater influence on health behaviors than health care or individual lifestyle choices, create unique health inequities, and may explain as much as 30% to 55% of health outcomes.[249]

Economic Stability

Economic stability factors for the tactical athlete include employment, food security, and access to safe housing.[247-249] Jobs within the tactical field range widely in their impact on economic stability, depending on the following factors:

- branch of service (career, volunteer, or contractual [wildland] fire; municipal, university, county, state, or special operations law enforcement; active duty, National Guard, or Reserves military),
- rank (varies by service; examples include lieutenant, captain, major, colonel, etc),
- time in service (typically leads to time-based or rank-based pay raises with longer time in service), and
- living arrangements (some military members may be required to live in barracks, and some first responders may sleep at their place of duty during extended shifts or time on call).

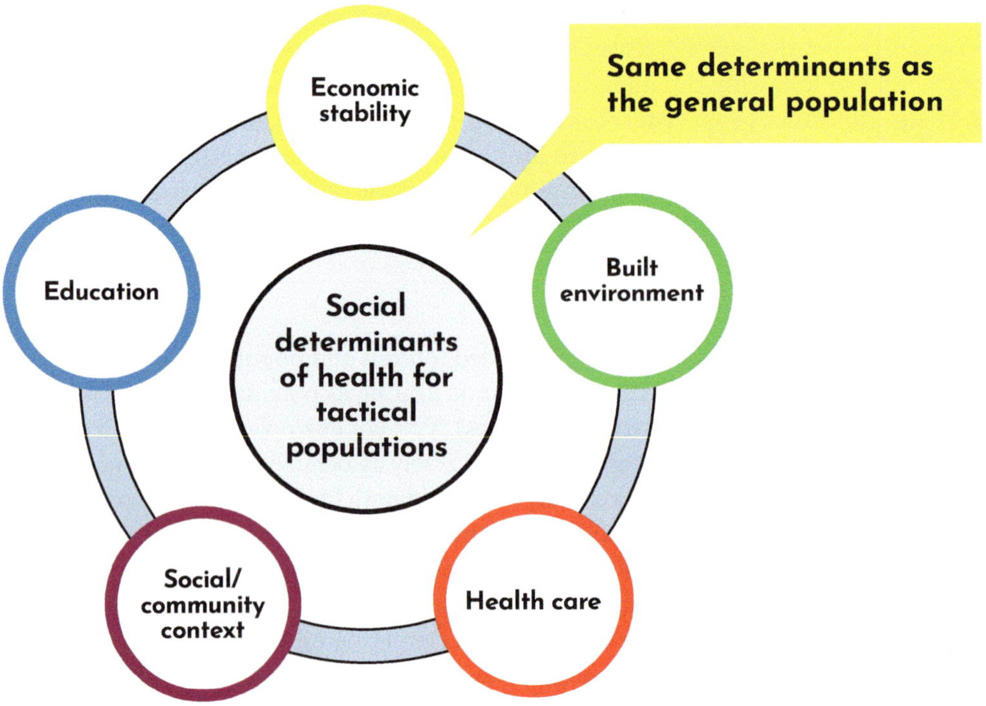

FIGURE 23.2 **Social determinants of health for tactical populations**[247]

For individuals serving in multiple occupations simultaneously, numerous combinations could exist. For example, a law enforcement officer may also serve in the National Guard. Additionally, seasonal or part-time tactical groups (eg, wildland firefighters) often experience instability and low pay without benefits, which is even reportedly leading to homelessness.[250-252] Moreover, average annual income varies widely and is often lower than the general population perceives. According to popular employment websites, as of 2024, the average annual income of a career firefighter in the midwestern and southern United States was about $34,000 per year, which was about $4,000 above the then-current federal poverty limit for a 4-person household.[253,254] Firefighters in the 25th percentile for the same region earn just below $25,000 per year.[253] Another factor contributing to potential financial stress, as found in a systematic review by Blakely et al,[255] is that it is difficult for spouses of tactical athletes to be employed because of frequent moves and the need to manage the household in unpredictable and extremely stressful conditions. Thus, it is important that dietitians and other nutrition practitioners ask questions about economic stability when developing fueling solutions for tactical populations, as financial conditions vary widely.

Built Environment

Built environmental factors to consider include access to healthy food, environmental conditions, and safety.[247-249] When working with tactical populations, health care practitioners should consider several environmental factors, including:

- access to cooking equipment and safe food storage, which is often limited or even nonexistent (eg, working an 8-hour shift in a patrol car with no refrigerator or microwave)[65,256,257];
- access to vending machines, which is often excessive and does not generally include healthy options[65,73,256-258];
- location of the duty station, which may exist in a food desert (limited access to nutrient-dense food) or food swamp (excessive access to energy-dense, nutrient-poor food)[65,73,256-258];
- stations or working conditions that lack opportunities for physical activity or training (eg, old fire stations with no room for a gym, patrol cars), leading to high levels of inactivity and lower energy needs[72,259]; and
- hazardous occupational exposure, including the following:
  - Firefighters may be exposed to aldehydes, benzene, carbon monoxide, dichlorofluoromethane, hydrogen chloride, hydrogen cyanide, sulfur dioxide, and particulates.[260] Exposure depends on building materials, building contents, and fire conditions.[261]
  - Law enforcement officers may be exposed to oleoresin capsicum sprays (mace), lead from gunshot residue, and toxic materials used in illicit drug-making laboratories, to name a few.[262-264]
  - Military personnel may be exposed to hazardous occupational exposures that are combat- or noncombat-related and fall into 5 categories according to the Department of Veterans Affairs: chemicals (eg, contaminated drinking water and Agent Orange), radiation (eg, nuclear weapons and x-rays), air pollutants (eg, dust and smoke from burn pits), occupational hazards (eg, lead from gunshot residue), and chemical or biological weapons.[265]

Overall, tactical populations often report that their food and physical activity environments are not conducive to starting or maintaining healthy behaviors. These environments vary widely, and unique feeding conditions should be considered by health care practitioners when providing fueling solutions for these populations.

Health Care

Health care factors to consider with tactical athletes include health literacy and access to a primary care physician and other health care services.[247-249] The general population often assumes that tactical populations have stable and high-quality access to health care services, but that is not always the case. Instability and the part-time nature of contractual work for groups such as wildland firefighters result in a lack of benefits from their fire service job and difficulty holding a full-time (ie, benefit-providing) job outside the fire service.[250-252]

Health care practitioners such as physicians, nurses, registered dietitians, and others should be mindful of their weight perceptions (biases) when working with tactical populations. A study by Wilkinson et al[266] reported that fewer than half of firefighters with obesity received weight counseling from their primary care physicians. Additionally, the study found that most fire and law enforcement departments did not require annual physicals. Tactical athletes also often perceive themselves to be healthier than they truly are.[73,267] Another topic of interest to researchers is whether tactical populations have fatalistic mindsets surrounding health because of the fact that risk is a normal element of their everyday lives,[268-270] which could make changing fueling behaviors more difficult.

Social and Community Context

Social and community factors to consider with tactical athletes include discrimination, social cohesion, and norms.[247-249] Practitioners in the tactical field often find this to be one of the strongest factors influencing fueling behaviors because of the tight-knit team nature of tactical groups, which is invaluable to success on the job. When considering cultural food norms, tactical populations often have a strong traditional workplace food culture in which energy-dense, nutrient-poor foods are the norm.[75] Historically, there has been a strong family-like nature to meals among tactical groups; therefore, one may be influenced to go along with the norms of the group when eating in a group (as is common for first responders).[73,258] Risky behavior is another social norm that can make changing fueling behaviors difficult.[268-270] Finally, tactical populations work fast-paced, unpredictable jobs, which can make having a plan for healthy fueling difficult.[73,258]

However, as registered dietitians and other health professionals are being increasingly employed by tactical populations (especially by the Army's Holistic Health and Fitness system [H2F] and by military contractors), this indicates a greater interest in not only the performance but also the health of employees and members. Initial analysis of the H2F system indicates that nutrition knowledge is significantly improving among service members.[271] A related avenue of research involves identifying individuals who serve as leading influences on the tactical athlete's off-duty and on-duty eating behaviors, such as spouses or significant others. Nutritional education can then be provided to these individuals as well, in an effort to offer additional social support to the tactical athlete in making positive changes in their fueling behavior.

Education

Educational factors to consider with tactical athletes include literacy rates, access to early childhood education, and high school graduation rates.[247-249] This social determinant of health is often not a major factor, in that the majority of tactical professions require the same base level of education, which is at least a high school diploma or GED or higher.[272-274] Within the first-responder community, an immense need exists for education regarding dietary and other lifestyle habits to support or improve work performance and to enhance health throughout the life cycle. In addition, considering that many tactical professions require cardiopulmonary resuscitation and emergency medical technician training, basic health and medical knowledge is sometimes higher than that of the general population.[272]

SUMMARY

The tactical athlete has highly variable nutrition needs depending on their roles and responsibilities, physiological demands, environmental factors, and chronic disease risk. Using an individualized assessment is crucial in formulating a strategic nutrition plan, as well as meeting the tactical athlete where they are (emotionally and intellectually) in terms of their health, fitness, and readiness to perform occupational tasks. Registered dietitians and other nutrition practitioners should always take a "food first, but not food only" approach. It is critical for the nutrition practitioner to know when to rely more on supplements for tactical athletes, such as during deployment or field simulation events when food-based meals are not as accessible or realistic and energy and nutrient demands are high. Tactical performance nutrition is a growing and exciting area, and the literature is increasing exponentially. As more information becomes available, practitioners working with tactical athletes should continually consider the occupation-specific demands, energy expenditure, physical fitness requirements or recommendations, and job-related health burdens of the tactical athlete to effectively implement recommendations and guidelines that are practical and will promote optimal health, performance, and operational readiness within this population.

KEY TAKEAWAYS

The physiological demands faced by the tactical athlete vary considerably depending on their intended mission or job tasks.

Load carriage, chronic sleep loss, and environmental stressors impact the health and performance of tactical athletes and should be considered when developing fueling regimens to optimize occupational success.

Army Regulation 40-25 provides general nutrition guidance for military personnel.

No nutrient guidelines specific to first responders currently exist, so it is advisable for these personnel to follow the ISSN recommendations or those for the general public.

Supplements to consider for the tactical population include caffeine, creatine monohydrate, omega-3 fatty acids, vitamin D, β-alanine, L-tyrosine, antioxidants, EAAs, and protein.

Early fueling strategies should be employed to lower the risk of death post-TBI. These strategies include increasing total energy and protein intakes. Supplementation with certain nutrients (ie, creatine monohydrate, omega-3 fatty acids) could be beneficial as well in the repair and recovery process post-TBI.

The tactical athlete is challenged with irregular and often hypercaloric dietary habits, as well as low physical activity behaviors that can lead to various diseases. Therefore, dietary modifications should focus on fostering healthy eating habits that promote favorable changes in health and fitness profiles.

When providing nutritional strategies to tactical populations, the dietitian or other health care practitioner should ask questions about financial status, daily schedules, food environments on the job, sleep habits, hydration habits, access to health care services, health knowledge and perceptions, and family and workplace community context to provide solutions that are feasible and sustainable.

REFERENCES

1. Scofield DE, Kardouni JR. The tactical athlete: a product of 21st century strength and conditioning. *Strength Cond J*. 2015;37(4):2-7. doi:10.1519/ssc.0000000000000149
2. Davis MR, Easter RL, Carlock JM, et al. Self-reported physical tasks and exercise training in special weapons and tactics (SWAT) teams. *J Strength Cond Res*. 2016;30(11):3242-3248. doi:10.1519/jsc.0000000000001411
3. Dawes JJ, Kornhauser CL, Crespo D, Elder CL, Lindsay KG, Holmes RJ. Does body mass index influence the physiological and perceptual demands associated with defensive tactics training in state patrol officers? *Int J Exerc Sci*. 2018;11(6):319-330.
4. Johnson QR, Goatcher JD, Diehl C, et al. Heart rate responses during simulated fire ground scenarios among full-time firefighters. *Int J Exerc Sci*. 2020;13(2):374-382.
5. Knapik JJ, Reynolds KL, Harman E. Soldier load carriage: historical, physiological, biomechanical, and medical aspects. *Mil Med*. 2004;169(1):45-56. doi:10.7205/milmed.169.1.45
6. Baran K, Dulla J, Orr R, Dawes JJ, Pope R. Duty loads carried by the Los Angeles Sheriff's Department deputies. *J Aust Strength Cond*. 2018;26(5):34-38.
7. Knapik J, Reynolds K. Load carriage in military operations: a review of historical, physiological, biomechanical, and medical aspects. In: Santee WR, Friedl KE, eds. *Military Quantitative Physiology: Problems and Concepts in Military Operational Medicine*. Borden Institute; 2012:303-337.
8. Gonzalez DE, McAllister MJ, Waldman HS, et al. International society of sports nutrition position stand: tactical athlete nutrition. *J Int Soc Sports Nutr*. 2022;19(1):267-315. doi:10.1080/15502783.2022.2086017
9. Guidi J, Lucente M, Sonino N, Fava GA. Allostatic load and its impact on health: a systematic review. *Psychother Psychosom*. 2020;90(1):11-27. doi:10.1159/000510696
10. Frueh BC, Madan A, Fowler JC, et al. "Operator syndrome": A unique constellation of medical and behavioral health-care needs of military special operation forces. *Int J Psychiatry Med*. 2020;55(4):281-295. doi:10.1177/0091217420906659
11. Orr R, Pope R, Lopes TJA, et al. Soldier load carriage, injuries, rehabilitation and physical conditioning: an international approach. *Int J Environ Res Public Health*. 2021;18(8):4010. doi:10.3390/ijerph18084010
12. Armstrong NC, Smith SJR, Risius D, et al. Cognitive performance of military men and women during prolonged load carriage. *BMJ Mil Health*. 2023;169(1):37-45. doi:10.1136/bmjmilitary-2021-002000
13. Baker-Fulco CJ, Kramer FM, Lesher LL, Merrill E, Johnson J. Dietary intakes of female and male combat support hospital personnel subsisting on meal-focused or standard versions of the meal, ready-to-eat. USARIEM Technical Report T-02/23. US Army Research Institute of Environmental Medicine; September 2002. https://apps.dtic.mil/sti/pdfs/ADA406726.pdf
14. Nindl BC, Barnes BR, Alemany JA, Frykman PN, Shippee RL, Friedl KE. Physiological consequences of U.S. Army Ranger training. *Med Sci Sports Exerc*. 2007;39(8):1380-1387. doi:10.1249/MSS.0b013e318067e2f7
15. Sepowitz JJ, Armstrong NJ, Pasiakos SM. Energy balance and diet quality during the US Marine Corps Forces Special Operations Command Individual Training Course. *J Spec Oper Med*. 2017;17(4):109-113. doi:10.55460/RKM3-KDFU
16. Barringer ND, Pasiakos SM, McClung HL, Crombie AP, Margolis LM. Prediction equation for estimating total daily energy requirements of special operations personnel. *J Int Soc Sports Nutr*. 2018;15:15. doi:10.1186/s12970-018-0219-x
17. Fairbrother B, Shippee R, Kramer T, Askew W, Mays M. Nutritional and Immunological Assessment of Soldiers During the Special Forces Assessment and Selection Course. Technical Report T95-22. US Army Research Institute of Environmental Medicine; August 11, 1995. https://apps.dtic.mil/sti/pdfs/ADA299556.pdf
18. Nindl BC, Leone CD, Tharion WJ, et al. Physical performance responses during 72 h of military operational stress. *Med Sci Sports Exerc*. 2002;34(11):1814-1822. doi:10.1249/01.MSS.0000037093.39080.3E
19. Shippee R, Askew E, Bernton E, Martinez-Lopez L, Kramer M. Nutritional and immunological assessment of ranger students with increased caloric intake. Technical Report T95-5. US Army Research Institute of Environmental Medicine; December 1994. https://apps.dtic.mil/sti/pdfs/ADA290252.pdf
20. Hoyt R, Jones T, Stein T, et al. Doubly labeled water measurement of human energy expenditure during strenuous exercise. *J Appl Physiol (1985)*. 1991;71(1):16-22. doi:10.1152/jappl.1991.71.1.16
21. Murphy NE, Carrigan CT, Karl JP, Pasiakos SM, Margolis LM. Threshold of energy deficit and lower-body performance declines in military personnel: a meta-regression. *Sports Med*. 2018;48(9):2169-2178. doi:10.1007/s40279-018-0945-x
22. Bissett D, Bissett J, Snell C. Physical agility tests and fitness standards: Perceptions of law enforcement officers. *Police Pract Res*. 2012;13(3):208-223. doi:10.1080/15614263.2011.616142
23. Carlton SD, Carbone PD, Stierli M, Orr RM. The impact of occupational load carriage on the mobility of the tactical police officer. *J Aust Strength Cond*. 2014;22(1):32-37.
24. Marins EF, Cabistany L, Farias C, Dawes J, Del Vecchio FB. Effects of personal protective equipment on metabolism and performance during an occupational physical ability test for Federal Highway Police officers. *J Strength Cond Res*. 2020;34(4):1093-1102. doi:10.1519/jsc.0000000000002892
25. Keeler JM, Pohl MB, Bergstrom HC, Thomas JM, Abel MG. The effect of tactical tasks and gear on muscle activation of SWAT officers. *J Strength Cond Res*. 2022;36(1):238-244. doi:10.1519/JSC.0000000000003396

26. Abel MG, Palmer TG, Trubee N. Exercise program design for structural firefighters. *Strength Cond J.* 2015;37(4):8-19. doi:10.1519/ssc.0000000000000123
27. Rodríguez-Marroyo JA, López-Satue J, Pernía R, et al. Physiological work demands of Spanish wildland firefighters during wildfire suppression. *Int Arch Occup Environ Health.* 2012;85(2):221-228. doi:10.1007/s00420-011-0661-4
28. Eves ND, Jones RL, Petersen SR. The influence of the self-contained breathing apparatus (SCBA) on ventilatory function and maximal exercise. *Can J Appl Physiol.* 2005;30(5):507-519. doi:10.1139/h05-137
29. Punakallio A, Lusa S, Luukkonen R. Protective equipment affects balance abilities differently in younger and older firefighters. *Aviat Space Environ Med.* 2003;74(11):1151-1156.
30. Park K, Rosengren KS, Horn GP, Smith DL, Hsiao-Wecksler ET. Assessing gait changes in firefighters due to fatigue and protective clothing. *Saf Sci.* 2011;49(5):719-726. doi:10.1016/j.ssci.2011.01.012
31. Lesniak AY, Bergstrom HC, Clasey JL, Stromberg AJ, Abel MG. The effect of personal protective equipment on firefighter occupational performance. *J Strength Cond Res.* 2020;34(8):2165-2172. doi:10.1519/jsc.0000000000003384
32. Bertrandt J, Anyżewska A, Łakomy R, et al. Assessment of energy expenditure of police officers trained in polish police schools and police training centers. *Int J Environ Res Public Health.* 2022;19(11):6828. doi:10.3390/ijerph19116828
33. Koizumi N, Negishi Y, Ogata H, Rakwal R, Omi N. Estimating total energy expenditure for fire-fighters during large scale disaster response training using a tri-axial accelerometer. *Nutrients.* 2021;13(8):2789. doi:10.3390/nu13082789
34. Cuddy JS, Sol JA, Hailes WS, Ruby BC. Work patterns dictate energy demands and thermal strain during wildland firefighting. *Wilderness Environ Med.* 2015;26(2):221-226. doi:10.1016/j.wem.2014.12.010
35. Ruby BC, Shriver TC, Zderic TW, Sharkey BJ, Burks C, Tysk S. Total energy expenditure during arduous wildfire suppression. *Med Sci Sports Exerc.* 2002;34(6):1048-1054. doi:10.1097/00005768-200206000-00023
36. Shrestha A, Ho TE, Vie LL, et al. Comparison of cardiovascular health between US army and civilians. *J Am Heart Assoc.* 2019;8(12):e009056. doi:10.1161/JAHA.118.009056
37. McGraw LK, Turner BS, Stotts NA, Dracup KA. A review of cardiovascular risk factors in US military personnel. *J Cardiovasc Nurs.* 2008;23(4):338-344. doi:10.1097/01.JCN.0000317437.75081.e7
38. Smith DL, Fehling PC, Frisch A, Haller JM, Winke M, Dailey MW. The prevalence of cardiovascular disease risk factors and obesity in firefighters. *J Obes.* 2012;2012:908267. doi:10.1155/2012/908267
39. Tsismenakis AJ, Christophi CA, Burress JW, Kinney AM, Kim M, Kales SN. The obesity epidemic and future emergency responders. *Obesity (Silver Spring).* 2009;17(8):1648-1650. doi:10.1038/oby.2009.63
40. Zimmerman FH. Cardiovascular disease and risk factors in law enforcement personnel: a comprehensive review. *Cardiol Rev.* 2012;20(4):159-166. doi:10.1097/CRD.0b013e318248d631
41. Almond N, Kahwati L, Kinsinger L, Porterfield D. The prevalence of overweight and obesity among U.S. military veterans. *Mil Med.* 2008;173(6):544-549. doi:10.7205/milmed.173.6.544
42. *2022 Health of the Force Report.* Defense Centers for Public Health-Aberdeen; May 10, 2023. Accessed March 14, 2024. https://ph.health.mil/Periodical%20Library/2022-hof-report-web.pdf
43. Centers for Disease Control and Prevention. Unfit to Serve: Obesity and physical activity are impacting national security. Last Reviewed June 20, 2023. Accessed June 23, 2023. www.cdc.gov/physicalactivity/resources/unfit-to-serve/index.html
44. Sergi TE, Bode KB, Hildebrand DA, Dawes JJ, Joyce JM. Relationship between body mass index and health and occupational performance among law enforcement officers, firefighters, and military personnel: a systematic review. *Curr Dev Nutr.* 2023;7(1):100020. doi:10.1016/j.cdnut.2022.100020
45. Clerc PG, Mayer SB, Graybill S. Overweight BMI (25-29) in active duty military: excess fat or more lean mass? A look at the evidence. *Mil Med.* 2021;187(7-8):201-203. doi:10.1093/milmed/usab447
46. Capaldi VF, Balkin TJ, Mysliwiec V. Optimizing sleep in the military: challenges and opportunities. *Chest.* 2019;155(1):215-226. doi:10.1016/j.chest.2018.08.1061
47. Patel S. Reduced sleep as an obesity risk factor. *Obes Rev.* 2009;10(suppl 2):61-68. doi:10.1111/j.1467-789X.2009.00664
48. Spiegal K, Tasali E, Penev P, Van Cauter E. Sleep curtailment in healthy young men is associated with decreased leptin levels, elevated ghrelin levels and increased hunger and appetite. *Ann Int Med.* 2004;141(11):846-850. doi:10.7326/0003-4819-141-11-200412070-00008
49. Spiegel K, Leproult R, Van Cauter E. Impact of sleep debt on metabolic and endocrine function. *Lancet.* 1999;354(9188):1435-1439. doi:10.1016/S0140-6736(99)01376-8
50. Grier T, Dinkeloo E, Reynolds M, Jones BH. Sleep duration and musculoskeletal injury incidence in physically active men and women: a study of U.S. Army Special Operation Forces soldiers. *Sleep Health.* 2020;6(3):344-349. doi:10.1016/j.sleh.2020.01.004
51. Ulmer CS, Bosworth HB, Germain A, et al. Associations between sleep difficulties and risk factors for cardiovascular disease in veterans and active duty military personnel of the Iraq and Afghanistan conflicts. *J Behav Med.* 2015;38(3):544-555. doi:10.1007/s10865-015-9627-4
52. Sammito S, Hadzic V, Karakolis T, et al. Risk factors for musculoskeletal injuries in the military: a qualitative systematic review of the literature from the past two decades and a new prioritizing injury model. *Mil Med Res.* 2021;8(1):66. doi:10.1186/s40779-021-00357-w
53. Farina EK, Thompson LA, Knapik JJ, Pasiakos SM, McClung JP, Lieberman HR. Anthropometrics and body composition predict physical performance and selection to attend special forces training in United States army soldiers. *Mil Med.* 2021;187(11-12):1381-1388. doi:10.1093/milmed/usab315

54. Vincent AS, Roebuck-Spencer T, Lopez MS, et al. Effects of military deployment on cognitive functioning. *Mil Med.* 2012;177(3):248-255. doi:10.7205/milmed-d-11-00156

55. Kong LZ, Zhang RL, Hu SH, Lai JB. Military traumatic brain injury: a challenge straddling neurology and psychiatry. *Mil Med Res.* 2022;9(1):2. doi:10.1186/s40779-021-00363-y

56. Tschiffely AE, Haque A, Haran FJ, et al. Recovery from mild traumatic brain injury following uncomplicated mounted and dismounted blast: a natural history approach. *Mil Med.* 2018;183(3-4):e140-e147. doi:10.1093/milmed/usx036

57. Howlett JR, Nelson LD, Stein MB. Mental health consequences of traumatic brain injury. *Biol Psychiatry.* 2022;91(5):413-420. doi:10.1016/j.biopsych.2021.09.024

58. Stanley IH, Rogers ML, Hanson JE, Gutierrez PM, Joiner TE. PTSD symptom clusters and suicide attempts among high-risk military service members: a three-month prospective investigation. *J Consult Clin Psychol.* 2019;87(1):67-78. doi:10.1037/ccp0000350

59. Helmkamp JC, Kennedy RD. Causes of death among U.S. military personnel: a 14-year summary, 1980-1993. *Mil Med.* 1996;161(6):311-317.

60. Castro CA, Kintzle S. Suicides in the military: the post-modern combat veteran and the Hemingway effect. *Curr Psychiatry Rep.* 2014;16(8):460. doi:10.1007/s11920-014-0460-1

61. Varvarigou V, Farioli A, Korre M, Sato S, Dahabreh IJ, Kales SN. Law enforcement duties and sudden cardiac death among police officers in United States: case distribution study. *BMJ.* 2014;349:g6534. doi:10.1136/bmj.g6534

62. Sörensen L, Smolander J, Louhevaara V, Korhonen O, Oja P. Physical activity, fitness and body composition of Finnish police officers: a 15-year follow-up study. *Occup Med (Lond).* 2000;50(1):3-10. doi:10.1093/occmed/50.1.3

63. Can SH, Hendy HM. Behavioral variables associated with obesity in police officers. *Ind Health.* 2014;52(3):240-247. doi:10.2486/indhealth.2013-0237

64. Anderson AA, Yoo H, Franke WD. Associations of physical activity and obesity with the risk of developing the metabolic syndrome in law enforcement officers. *J Occup Environ Med.* 2016;58(9):946-951. doi:10.1097/jom.0000000000000833

65. Ramey SL, Downing NR, Franke WD. Milwaukee police department retirees: cardiovascular disease risk and morbidity among aging law enforcement officers. *AAOHN J.* 2009;57(11):448-453. doi:10.3928/08910162-20091019-02

66. Kales SN, Tsismenakis AJ, Zhang C, Soteriades ES. Blood pressure in firefighters, police officers, and other emergency responders. *Am J Hypertens.* 2009;22(1):11-20. doi:10.1038/ajh.2008.296

67. Violanti JM, Ma CC, Fekedulegn D, et al. Associations between body fat percentage and fitness among police officers: a statewide study. *Saf Health Work.* 2017;8(1):36-41. doi:10.1016/j.shaw.2016.07.004

68. Dawes JJ, Orr RM, Elder CL, Rockwell C. Association between body fatness and measures of muscular endurance among part-time SWAT officers. *J Aust Strength Cond.* 2014;22(4):33-36.

69. Poston WSC, Haddock CK, Jahnke SA, Jitnarin N, Tuley BC, Kales SN. The prevalence of overweight, obesity, and substandard fitness in a population-based firefighter cohort. *J Occup Environ Med.* 2011;53(3):266-273. doi:10.1097/JOM.0b013e31820af362

70. US Department of Homeland Security, Federal Emergency Management Agency, US Fire Administration, National Fire Data Center, National Fallen Firefighters Foundation. Firefighter Fatalities in the United States in 2021. July 2023. Accessed March 14, 2024. www.usfa.fema.gov/downloads/pdf/publications/firefighter-fatalities-2021.pdf

71. McAllister MJ, Gonzalez DE, Leonard M, et al. Firefighters with higher cardiorespiratory fitness demonstrate lower markers of cardiovascular disease risk. *J Occup Environ Med.* 2022;64(12):1036-1040. doi:10.1097/JOM.0000000000002632

72. Eastlake AC, Knipper BS, He X, Alexander BM, Davis KG. Lifestyle and safety practices of firefighters and their relation to cardiovascular risk factors. *Work.* 2015;50(2):285-294. doi:10.3233/wor-131796

73. Jahnke SA, Poston WS, Jitnarin N, Haddock CK. Health concerns of the US fire service: perspectives from the firehouse. *Am J Health Promot.* 2012;27(2):111-118. doi:10.4278/ajhp.110311-QUAL-109

74. Webb HE, Garten RS, McMinn DR, Beckman JL, Kamimori GH, Acevedo EO. Stress hormones and vascular function in firefighters during concurrent challenges. *Biol Psychol.* 2011;87(1):152-160. doi:10.1016/j.biopsycho.2011.02.024

75. Huang C-J, Webb HE, Garten RS, Kamimori GH, Evans RK, Acevedo EO. Stress hormones and immunological responses to a dual challenge in professional firefighters. *Int J Psychophysiol.* 2010;75(3):312-318. doi:10.1016/j.ijpsycho.2009.12.013

76. Sritharan J, Kirkham TL, MacLeod J, et al. Cancer risk among firefighters and police in the Ontario workforce. *Occup Environ Med.* 2022;79(8):533-539. doi:10.1136/oemed-2021-108146

77. Jalilian H, Ziaei M, Weiderpass E, Rueegg CS, Khosravi Y, Kjaerheim K. Cancer incidence and mortality among firefighters. *Int J Cancer.* 2019;145(10):2639-2646. doi:10.1002/ijc.32199

78. Departments of the Army, the Navy, and the Air Force. Army Regulation 40-25. Nutrition and Menu Standards for Human Performance Nutrition. January 3, 2017. Accessed March 24, 2024. www.armyresilience.army.mil/ard/images/pdf/Policy/AR%2040-25%20Nutrition%20and%20Menu%20Standards%20for%20Human%20Performance%20Optimization.pdf

79. Thomas DT, Erdman KA, Burke LM. Position of the Academy of Nutrition and Dietetics, Dietitians of Canada, and the American College of Sports Medicine: nutrition and athletic performance. *J Acad Nutr Diet.* 2016;116(3):501-528. doi:10.1016/j.jand.2015.12.006

80. Chukwura CL, Santo TJ, Waters CN, Andrews A. 'Nutrition is out of our control': soldiers' perceptions of their local food environment. *Public Health Nutr.* 2019;22(15):2766-2776. doi:10.1017/s1368980019001381

81. Jäger R, Kerksick CM, Campbell BI, et al. International Society of Sports Nutrition position stand: protein and exercise. *J Int Soc Sports Nutr.* 2017;14:20. doi:10.1186/s12970-017-0177-8
82. Johnson BVB, Mayer JM. Evaluating nutrient intake of career firefighters compared to Military Dietary Reference Intakes. *Nutrients.* 2020;12(6):1876. doi:10.3390/nu12061876
83. MacKenzie-Shalders KL, Tsoi AV, Lee KW, Wright C, Cox GR, Orr RM. Free-living dietary intake in tactical personnel and implications for nutrition practice: a systematic review. *Nutrients.* 2021;13(10):3502. doi:10.3390/nu13103502
84. Graber E. Dietary Assessment: Do We Really Know What People Are Eating? American Society for Nutrition. July 20, 2022. Accessed June 24, 2023. https://nutrition.org/dietary-assessment-do-we-really-know-what-people-are-eating
85. Roza AM, Shizgal HM. The Harris Benedict equation reevaluated: resting energy requirements and the body cell mass. *Am J Clin Nutr.* 1984;40(1):168-182. doi:10.1093/ajcn/40.1.168
86. Harris JA, Benedict FG. A biometric study of human basal metabolism. *Proc Natl Acad Sci U S A.* 1918;4(12):370-373. doi:10.1073/pnas.4.12.370
87. Mifflin MD, St. Jeor ST, Hill LA, Scott BJ, Daugherty SA, Koh YO. A new predictive equation for resting energy expenditure in healthy individuals. *Am J Clin Nutr.* 1990;51(2):241-247. doi:10.1093/ajcn/51.2.241
88. Kerksick CM, Wilborn CD, Roberts MD, et al. ISSN exercise & sports nutrition review update: research & recommendations. *J Int Soc Sports Nutr.* 2018;15(1):38. doi:10.1186/s12970-018-0242-y
89. Kreider RB, Wilborn CD, Taylor L, et al. ISSN exercise & sports nutrition review: research & recommendations. *J Int Soc Sports Nutr.* 2010;7(1):7. doi:10.1186/1550-2783-7-7
90. Jäger R, Kerksick CM, Campbell BI, et al. International Society of Sports Nutrition position stand: protein and exercise. *J Int Soc Sports Nutr.* 2017;14(1):20. doi:10.1186/s12970-017-0177-8
91. Guest NS, VanDusseldorp TA, Nelson MT, et al. International society of sports nutrition position stand: caffeine and exercise performance. *J Int Soc Sports Nutr.* 2021;18(1):1. doi:10.1186/s12970-020-00383-4
92. Popkin BM, D'Anci KE, Rosenberg IH. Water, hydration, and health. *Nutr Rev.* 2010;68(8):439-458. doi:10.1111/j.1753-4887.2010.00304.x
93. Peacock OJ, Stokes K, Thompson D. Initial hydration status, fluid balance, and psychological affect during recreational exercise in adults. *J Sports Sci.* 2011;29(9):897-904. doi:10.1080/02640414.2011.568511
94. Cheuvront SN, Sawka MN. Hydration assessment of athletes. *Sports Sci Exch.* 2005;18(2):1-6.
95. Armstrong LE, Maresh CM, Castellani JW, et al. Urinary indices of hydration status. *Int J Sport Nutr.* 1994;4(3):265-279. doi:10.1123/ijsn.4.3.265
96. Armstrong LE, Soto JA, Hacker FT Jr, Casa DJ, Kavouras SA, Maresh CM. Urinary indices during dehydration, exercise, and rehydration. *Int J Sport Nutr.* 1998;8(4):345-355. doi:10.1123/ijsn.8.4.345
97. Committee to Review Dietary Reference Intakes for Vitamin D and Calcium, Food and Nutrition Board, Institute of Medicine. Ross AC, Taylor CL, Yaktine AL, Del Valle HB, eds. *Dietary Reference Intakes for Calcium and Vitamin D.* National Academies Press; 2011: Summary Table 4. Accessed March 14, 2024. www.ncbi.nlm.nih.gov/books/NBK56068/table/summarytables.t4/?report=objectonly
98. Kalman DS, Lepeley A. A Review of Hydration. *Strength Cond J.* 2010;32(2):56-63. doi:10.1519/SSC.0b013e3181c21172
99. Larsen B, Snow R, Williams-Bell M, Aisbett B. Simulated firefighting task performance and physiology under very hot conditions. *Front Physiol.* 2015;6:322. doi:10.3389/fphys.2015.00322
100. Cheung SS, McLellan TM, Tenaglia S. The thermophysiology of uncompensable heat stress. Physiological manipulations and individual characteristics. *Sports Med.* 2000;29(5):329-359. doi:10.2165/00007256-200029050-00004
101. Cheuvront SN, Kenefick RW. Dehydration: physiology, assessment, and performance effects. *Compr Physiol.* 2014;4(1):257-285. doi:10.1002/cphy.c130017
102. Baker LB, Conroy DE, Kenney WL. Dehydration impairs vigilance-related attention in male basketball players. *Med Sci Sports Exerc.* 2007;39(6):976-983. doi:10.1097/mss.0b013e3180471ff2
103. Casa DJ, Armstrong LE, Hillman SK, et al. National athletic trainers' association position statement: fluid replacement for athletes. *J Athl Train.* 2000;35(2):212-224.
104. Wendt D, van Loon LJC, Lichtenbelt WD. Thermoregulation during exercise in the heat: strategies for maintaining health and performance. *Sports Med.* 2007;37(8):669-682. doi:10.2165/00007256-200737080-00002
105. González-Alonso J. Human thermoregulation and the cardiovascular system. *Exp Physiol.* 2012;97(3):340-346. doi:10.1113/expphysiol.2011.058701
106. González-Alonso J, Crandall CG, Johnson JM. The cardiovascular challenge of exercising in the heat. *J Physiol.* 2008;586(1):45-53. doi:10.1113/jphysiol.2007.142158
107. McAllister MJ, Holland AM, Chander H, Waldman HS, William Smith J, Basham SA. Impact of ketone salt containing supplement on cardiorespiratory and oxidative stress response in firefighters exercising in personal protective equipment. *Asian J Sports Med.* 2019;10(1):e82404. doi:10.5812/asjsm.82404
108. McAllister MJ, Basham SA, Smith JW, et al. Effects of environmental heat and antioxidant ingestion on blood markers of oxidative stress in professional firefighters performing structural fire exercises. *J Occup Environ Med.* 2018;60(11):e595-e601. doi:10.1097/jom.0000000000001452
109. Knapik JJ, Trone DW, Steelman RA, Farina EK, Lieberman HR. Dietary supplement and prescription medication use among US military service members with clinically diagnosed medical conditions: The US Military Dietary Supplement Use Study. *J Acad Nutr Diet.* 2022;122(10):1841-1850. doi:10.1016/j.jand.2022.05.007

110. Knapik JJ, Trone DW, Steelman RA, Farina EK, Lieberman HR. Prevalence of and factors associated with dietary supplement use in a stratified, random sample of US military personnel: The US Military Dietary Supplement Use Study. *J Nutr.* 2021;151(11):3495-3506. doi:10.1093/jn/nxab239

111. Knapik JJ, Trone DW, Steelman RA, Farina EK, Lieberman HR. Adverse effects associated with multiple categories of dietary supplements: The Military Dietary Supplement Use Study. *J Acad Nutr Diet.* 2022;122(10):1851-1863. doi:10.1016/j.jand.2022.01.014

112. Knapik JJ, Austin KG, McGraw SM, Leahy GD, Lieberman HR. Caffeine consumption among active duty United States Air Force personnel. *Food Chem Toxicol.* 2017;105:377-386. doi:10.1016/j.fct.2017.04.050

113. Wilson JM, Fitschen PJ, Campbell B, et al. International Society of Sports Nutrition Position Stand: beta-hydroxy-beta-methylbutyrate (HMB). *J Int Soc Sports Nutr.* 2013;10(1):6. doi:10.1186/1550-2783-10-6

114. Alver BA, Sell K, Deuster PA, eds. *NSCA's Essentials of Tactical Strength and Conditioning.* Human Kinetics; 2017.

115. Trexler ET, Smith-Ryan AE, Stout JR, et al. International society of sports nutrition position stand: beta-alanine. *J Int Soc Sports Nutr.* 2015;12:30. doi:10.1186/s12970-015-0090-y

116. Kreider RB, Kalman DS, Antonio J, et al. International Society of Sports Nutrition position stand: safety and efficacy of creatine supplementation in exercise, sport, and medicine. *J Int Soc Sports Nutr.* 2017;14:18. doi:10.1186/s12970-017-0173-z

117. Kris-Etherton PM, Harris WS, Appel LJ. Fish consumption, fish oil, omega-3 fatty acids, and cardiovascular disease. *Circulation.* 2002;106(21):2747-2757. doi:10.1161/01.CIR.0000038493.65177.94

118. Costello RB, Lentino CV, Boyd CC, et al. The effectiveness of melatonin for promoting healthy sleep: a rapid evidence assessment of the literature. *Nutr J.* 2014;13(1):106. doi:10.1186/1475-2891-13-106

119. Artioli GG, Gualano B, Smith A, Stout J, Lancha AH Jr. Role of β-alanine supplementation on muscle carnosine and exercise performance. *Med Sci Sports Exerc.* 2010;42(6):1162-1173. doi:10.1249/MSS.0b013e3181c74e38

120. Hoffman JR, Stout JR, Harris RC, Moran DS. β-Alanine supplementation and military performance. *Amino Acids.* 2015;47(12):2463-2474. doi:10.1007/s00726-015-2051-9

121. Hoffman JR, Landau G, Stout JR, et al. β-alanine supplementation improves tactical performance but not cognitive function in combat soldiers. *J Int Soc Sports Nutr.* 2014;11(1):15. doi:10.1186/1550-2783-11-15

122. Hoffman JR, Landau G, Stout JR, et al. β-Alanine ingestion increases muscle carnosine content and combat specific performance in soldiers. *Amino Acids.* 2015;47(3):627-636. doi:10.1007/s00726-014-1896-7

123. Knapik JJ, Trone DW, McGraw S, Steelman RA, Austin KG, Lieberman HR. Caffeine use among active duty Navy and Marine Corps personnel. *Nutrients.* 2016;8(10):620. doi:10.3390/nu8100620

124. Chaudhary NS, Taylor BV, Grandner MA, Troxel WM, Chakravorty S. The effects of caffeinated products on sleep and functioning in the military population: a focused review. *Pharmacol Biochem Behav.* 2021;206:173206. doi:10.1016/j.pbb.2021.173206

125. Rosser JI, Walsh B, Hogan MC. Effect of physiological levels of caffeine on Ca^{2+} handling and fatigue development in *Xenopus* isolated single myofibers. *Am J Physiol Regul Integr Comp Physiol.* 2009;296(5):R1512-R1517. doi:10.1152/ajpregu.90901.2008

126. Barcelos RP, Lima FD, Carvalho NR, Bresciani G, Royes LFF. Caffeine effects on systemic metabolism, oxidative-inflammatory pathways, and exercise performance. *Nutr Res.* 2020;80:1-17. doi:10.1016/j.nutres.2020.05.005

127. Harpaz E, Tamir S, Weinstein A, Weinstein Y. The effect of caffeine on energy balance. *J Basic Clin Physiol Pharmacol.* 2017;28(1):1-10. doi:10.1515/jbcpp-2016-0090

128. Keisler BD, Armsey TD 2nd. Caffeine as an ergogenic aid. *Curr Sports Med Rep.* 2006;5(4):215-219. doi:10.1097/01.csmr.0000306510.57644.a7

129. McLellan TM, Bell DG, Kamimori GH. Caffeine improves physical performance during 24 h of active wakefulness. *Aviat Space Environ Med.* 2004;75(8):666-672. PMID: 15328782

130. Kamimori GH, McLellan TM, Tate CM, Voss DM, Niro P, Lieberman HR. Caffeine improves reaction time, vigilance and logical reasoning during extended periods with restricted opportunities for sleep. *Psychopharmacology (Berl).* 2015;232(12):2031-2042. doi:10.1007/s00213-014-3834-5

131. Willson C. The clinical toxicology of caffeine: A review and case study. *Toxicol Rep.* 2018;5:1140-1152. doi:10.1016/j.toxrep.2018.11.002

132. McLellan TM, Riviere LA, Williams KW, McGurk D, Lieberman HR. Caffeine and energy drink use by combat arms soldiers in Afghanistan as a countermeasure for sleep loss and high operational demands. *Nutr Neurosci.* 2019;22(11):768-777. doi:10.1080/1028415x.2018.1443996

133. Tharion WJ, Shukitt-Hale B, Lieberman HR. Caffeine effects on marksmanship during high-stress military training with 72 hour sleep deprivation. *Aviat Space Environ Med.* 2003;74(4):309-314.

134. Fine BJ, Kobrick JL, Lieberman HR, Marlowe B, Riley RH, Tharion WJ. Effects of caffeine or diphenhydramine on visual vigilance. *Psychopharmacology (Berl).* 1994;114(2):233-238. doi:10.1007/BF02244842

135. Rees K, Allen D, Lader M. The influences of age and caffeine on psychomotor and cognitive function. *Psychopharmacology (Berl).* 1999;145(2):181-188. doi:10.1007/s002130051047

136. Butt MS, Sultan MT. Coffee and its consumption: benefits and risks. *Crit Rev Food Sci Nutr.* 2011;51(4):363-373. doi:10.1080/10408390903586412

137. Tikuisis P, Keefe AA, McLellan TM, Kamimori G. Caffeine restores engagement speed but not shooting precision following 22 h of active wakefulness. *Aviat Space Environ Med.* 2004;75(9):771-776.

138. Lieberman HR, Tharion WJ, Shukitt-Hale B, Speckman KL, Tulley R. Effects of caffeine, sleep loss, and stress on cognitive performance and mood during U.S. Navy SEAL training. Sea-Air-Land. *Psychopharmacology (Berl).* 2002;164(3):250-261. doi:10.1007/s00213-002-1217-9

139. Wax B, Kerksick CM, Jagim AR, Mayo JJ, Lyons BC, Kreider RB. Creatine for exercise and sports performance, with recovery considerations for healthy populations. *Nutrients*. 2021;13(6):1915. doi:10.3390/nu13061915
140. Cooke MB, Rybalka E, Williams AD, Cribb PJ, Hayes A. Creatine supplementation enhances muscle force recovery after eccentrically-induced muscle damage in healthy individuals. *J Int Soc Sports Nutr*. 2009;6:13. doi:10.1186/1550-2783-6-13
141. Greenwood M, Kreider RB, Greenwood L, Byars A. Cramping and injury incidence in collegiate football players are reduced by creatine supplementation. *J Athl Train*. 2003;38(3):216-219.
142. Kilduff LP, Georgiades E, James N, et al. The effects of creatine supplementation on cardiovascular, metabolic, and thermoregulatory responses during exercise in the heat in endurance-trained humans. *Int J Sport Nutr Exerc Metab*. 2004;14(4):443-460. doi:10.1123/ijsnem.14.4.443
143. Dolan E, Gualano B, Rawson ES. Beyond muscle: the effects of creatine supplementation on brain creatine, cognitive processing, and traumatic brain injury. *Eur J Sport Sci*. 2019;19(1):1-14. doi:10.1080/17461391.2018.1500644
144. Roschel H, Gualano B, Ostojic SM, Rawson ES. Creatine supplementation and brain health. *Nutrients*. 2021;13(2):586. doi:10.3390/nu13020586
145. Kreider RB, Melton C, Rasmussen CJ, et al. Long-term creatine supplementation does not significantly affect clinical markers of health in athletes. *Mol Cell Biochem*. 2003;244(1-2):95-104.
146. Kreider RB, Stout JR. Creatine in health and disease. *Nutrients*. 2021;13(2):447. doi:10.3390/nu13020447
147. Dechent P, Pouwels P, Wilken B, Hanefeld F, Frahm J. Increase of total creatine in human brain after oral supplementation of creatine-monohydrate. *Am J Physiol*. 1999;277(3):R698-R704. doi:10.1152/ajpregu.1999.277.3.R698
148. Kreider RB, Stout JR. Creatine in health and disease. *Nutrients*. 2021;13(2):447.
149. Ostojic SM. Creatine as a food supplement for the general population. *J Funct Foods*. 2021;83:104568. doi:10.1016/j.jff.2021.104568
150. Tipton KD, Gurkin BE, Matin S, Wolfe RR. Nonessential amino acids are not necessary to stimulate net muscle protein synthesis in healthy volunteers. *J Nutr Biochem*. 1999;10(2):89-95. doi:10.1016/s0955-2863(98)00087-4
151. Church DD, Hirsch KR, Park S, et al. Essential amino acids and protein synthesis: insights into maximizing the muscle and whole-body response to feeding. *Nutrients*. 2020;12(12):3717. doi:10.3390/nu12123717
152. Wolfe RR, Baum JI, Starck C, Moughan PJ. Factors contributing to the selection of dietary protein food sources. *Clin Nutr*. 2018;37(1):130-138. doi:10.1016/j.clnu.2017.11.017
153. Cuthbertson DJ, Babraj J, Leese G, Siervo M. Anabolic resistance does not explain sarcopenia in patients with type 2 diabetes mellitus, compared with healthy controls, despite reduced mTOR pathway activity. *Clin Nutr*. 2017;36(6):1716-1719. doi:10.1016/j.clnu.2016.11.012
154. Dillon EL, Sheffield-Moore M, Paddon-Jones D, et al. Amino acid supplementation increases lean body mass, basal muscle protein synthesis, and insulin-like growth factor-I expression in older women. *J Clin Endocrinol Metab*. 2009;94(5):1630-1637. doi:10.1210/jc.2008-1564
155. Ispoglou T, White H, Preston T, McElhone S, McKenna J, Hind K. Double-blind, placebo-controlled pilot trial of l-leucine-enriched amino-acid mixtures on body composition and physical performance in men and women aged 65-75 years. *Eur J Clin Nutr*. 2016;70(2):182-188. doi:10.1038/ejcn.2015.91
156. Negro M, Perna S, Spadaccini D, et al. Effects of 12 weeks of essential amino acids (EAA)-based multi-ingredient nutritional supplementation on muscle mass, muscle strength, muscle power and fatigue in healthy elderly subjects: a randomized controlled double-blind study. *J Nutr Health Aging*. 2019;23(5):414-424. doi:10.1007/s12603-019-1163-4
157. Dreyer HC, Owen EC, Strycker LA, et al. Essential amino acid supplementation mitigates muscle atrophy after total knee arthroplasty: a randomized, double-blind, placebo-controlled trial. *JB JS Open Access*. 2018;3(2):e0006. doi:10.2106/JBJS.OA.18.00006
158. Dreyer HC, Strycker LA, Senesac HA, et al. Essential amino acid supplementation in patients following total knee arthroplasty. *J Clin Invest*. 2013;123(11):4654-4666. doi:10.1172/JCI70160
159. Rasmussen BB, Tipton KD, Miller SL, Wolf SE, Wolfe RR. An oral essential amino acid-carbohydrate supplement enhances muscle protein anabolism after resistance exercise. *J Appl Physiol (1985)*. 2000;88(2):386-392. doi:10.1152/jappl.2000.88.2.386
160. Tipton KD, Ferrando AA, Phillips SM, Doyle D Jr, Wolfe RR. Postexercise net protein synthesis in human muscle from orally administered amino acids. *Am J Physiol*. 1999;276(4 pt 1):E628-E634. doi:10.1152/ajpendo.1999.276.4.E628
161. Tipton KD, Rasmussen BB, Miller SL, et al. Timing of amino acid-carbohydrate ingestion alters anabolic response of muscle to resistance exercise. *Am J Physiol Endocrinol Metab*. 2001;281(2):E197-E206. doi:10.1152/ajpendo.2001.281.2.E197
162. Kerksick CM, Arent S, Schoenfeld BJ, et al. International society of sports nutrition position stand: nutrient timing. *J Int Soc Sports Nutr*. 2017;14:33. doi:10.1186/s12970-017-0189-4
163. Miller SL, Tipton KD, Chinkes DL, Wolf SE, Wolfe RR. Independent and combined effects of amino acids and glucose after resistance exercise. *Med Sci Sports Exerc*. 2003;35(3):449-455. doi:10.1249/01.MSS.0000053910.63105.45
164. Tipton KD, Borsheim E, Wolf SE, Sanford AP, Wolfe RR. Acute response of net muscle protein balance reflects 24-h balance after exercise and amino acid ingestion. *Am J Physiol Endocrinol Metab*. 2003;284(1):E76-E89. doi:10.1152/ajpendo.00234.2002
165. Moore DR, Churchward-Venne TA, Witard O, et al. Protein ingestion to stimulate myofibrillar protein synthesis requires greater relative protein intakes in healthy older versus younger men. *J Gerontol A Biol Sci Med Sci*. 2015;70(1):57-62. doi:10.1093/gerona/glu103

166. Gwin JA, Church DD, Hatch-McChesney A, et al. Effects of high versus standard essential amino acid intakes on whole-body protein turnover and mixed muscle protein synthesis during energy deficit: A randomized, crossover study. *Clin Nutr.* 2021;40(3):767-777. doi:10.1016/j.clnu.2020.07.019

167. Gwin JA, Church DD, Hatch-McChesney A, et al. Essential amino acid-enriched whey enhances post-exercise whole-body protein balance during energy deficit more than iso-nitrogenous whey or a mixed-macronutrient meal: a randomized, crossover study. *J Int Soc Sports Nutr.* 2021;18(1):4. doi:10.1186/s12970-020-00401-5

168. Pasiakos SM, Cao JJ, Margolis LM, et al. Effects of high-protein diets on fat-free mass and muscle protein synthesis following weight loss: a randomized controlled trial. *FASEB J.* 2013;27(9):3837-3847. doi:10.1096/fj.13-230227

169. Longland TM, Oikawa SY, Mitchell CJ, Devries MC, Phillips SM. Higher compared with lower dietary protein during an energy deficit combined with intense exercise promotes greater lean mass gain and fat mass loss: a randomized trial. *Am J Clin Nutr.* 2016;103(3):738-746. doi:10.3945/ajcn.115.119339

170. Lieberman HR. Amino acid and protein requirements: cognitive performance, stress and brain function. In: *The Role of Protein and Amino Acids in Sustaining and Enhancing Performance.* National Academies Press; 1999:289-307.

171. Ott T, Nieder A. Dopamine and cognitive control in prefrontal cortex. *Trends Cogn Sci.* 2019;23(3):213-234. doi:10.1016/j.tics.2018.12.006

172. Mahoney CR, Castellani J, Kramer FM, Young A, Lieberman HR. Tyrosine supplementation mitigates working memory decrements during cold exposure. *Physiol Behav.* 2007;92(4):575-582. doi:10.1016/j.physbeh.2007.05.003

173. Shurtleff D, Thomas JR, Schrot J, Kowalski K, Harford R. Tyrosine reverses a cold-induced working memory deficit in humans. *Pharmacol Biochem Behav.* 1994;47(4):935-941. doi:10.1016/0091-3057(94)90299-2

174. Coull NA, Watkins SL, Aldous JW, et al. Effect of tyrosine ingestion on cognitive and physical performance utilising an intermittent soccer performance test (iSPT) in a warm environment. *Eur J Appl Physiol.* 2015;115(2):373-386. doi:10.1007/s00421-014-3022-7

175. Montain S, Jonas WB. Nutritional armor: omega-3 for the warfighter. *Mil Med.* 2014;179(11 suppl):1. doi:10.7205/milmed-d-14-00452

176. Kitson AP, Metherel AH, Chen CT, et al. Effect of dietary docosahexaenoic acid (DHA) in phospholipids or triglycerides on brain DHA uptake and accretion. *J Nutr Biochem.* 2016;33:91-102. doi:10.1016/j.jnutbio.2016.02.009

177. Bailes JE, Patel V. The potential for DHA to mitigate mild traumatic brain injury. *Mil Med.* 2014;179(11 suppl):112-116. doi:10.7205/milmed-d-14-00139

178. Oliver JM, Jones MT, Kirk KM, et al. Effect of docosahexaenoic acid on a biomarker of head trauma in American football. *Med Sci Sports Exerc.* 2016;48(6):974-982. doi:10.1249/mss.0000000000000875

179. Heileson JL, Anzalone AJ, Carbuhn AF, et al. The effect of omega-3 fatty acids on a biomarker of head trauma in NCAA football athletes: a multi-site, non-randomized study. *J Int Soc Sports Nutr.* 2021;18(1):65. doi:10.1186/s12970-021-00461-1

180. Black KE, Witard OC, Baker D, et al. Adding omega-3 fatty acids to a protein-based supplement during pre-season training results in reduced muscle soreness and the better maintenance of explosive power in professional Rugby Union players. *Eur J Sport Sci.* 2018;18(10):1357-1367. doi:10.1080/17461391.2018.1491626

181. Fontani G, Corradeschi F, Felici A, Alfatti F, Migliorini S, Lodi L. Cognitive and physiological effects of omega-3 polyunsaturated fatty acid supplementation in healthy subjects. *Eur J Clin Invest.* 2005;35(11):691-699. doi:10.1111/j.1365-2362.2005.01570.x

182. Fontani G, Lodi L, Migliorini S, Corradeschi F. Effect of omega-3 and policosanol supplementation on attention and reactivity in athletes. *J Am Coll Nutr.* 2009;28(suppl):473S-481S. doi:10.1080/07315724.2009.10718114

183. Lewis MD, Hibbeln JR, Johnson JE, Lin YH, Hyun DY, Loewke JD. Suicide deaths of active-duty US military and omega-3 fatty-acid status: a case-control comparison. *J Clin Psychiatry.* 2011;72(12):1585-1590. doi:10.4088/JCP.11m06879

184. Hibbeln JR, Gow RV. The potential for military diets to reduce depression, suicide, and impulsive aggression: a review of current evidence for omega-3 and omega-6 fatty acids. *Mil Med.* 2014;179(11 suppl):117-128. doi:10.7205/milmed-d-14-00153

185. Lewis NA, Daniels D, Calder PC, Castell LM, Pedlar CR. Are there benefits from the use of fish oil supplements in athletes? A systematic review. *Adv Nutr.* 2020;11(5):1300-1314. doi:10.1093/advances/nmaa050

186. Hallahan B, Hibbeln JR, Davis JM, Garland MR. Omega-3 fatty acid supplementation in patients with recurrent self-harm. Single-centre double-blind randomised controlled trial. *Br J Psychiatry.* 2007;190:118-122. doi:10.1192/bjp.bp.106.022707

187. Coulter ID. The response of an expert panel to Nutritional armor for the warfighter: can omega-3 fatty acids enhance stress resilience, wellness, and military performance? *Mil Med.* 2014;179(11 suppl):192-198. doi:10.7205/milmed-d-14-00189

188. VanDusseldorp TA, Escobar KA, Johnson KE, et al. Impact of varying dosages of fish oil on recovery and soreness following eccentric exercise. *Nutrients.* 2020;12(8):2246. doi:10.3390/nu12082246

189. Kyriakidou Y, Wood C, Ferrier C, Dolci A, Elliott B. The effect of omega-3 polyunsaturated fatty acid supplementation on exercise-induced muscle damage. *J Int Soc Sports Nutr.* 2021;18(1):9. doi:10.1186/s12970-020-00405-1

190. Funderburk LK, Daigle K, Arsenault JE. Vitamin D status among overweight and obese soldiers. *Mil Med.* 2015;180(2):237-240. doi:10.7205/MILMED-D-14-00041

191. Wentz LM, Eldred JD, Henry MD, Berry-Caban CS. Clinical relevance of optimizing vitamin D status in soldiers to enhance physical and cognitive performance. *J Spec Oper Med.* 2014;14(1):58-66. doi:10.55460/52YL-XU05

192. Schaad KA, Bukhari AS, Brooks DI, Kocher JD, Barringer ND. The relationship between vitamin D status and depression in a tactical athlete population. *J Int Soc Sports Nutr.* 2019;16(1):40. doi:10.1186/s12970-019-0308-5

193. Holick MF. Sunlight and vitamin D for bone health and prevention of autoimmune diseases, cancers, and cardiovascular disease. *Am J Clin Nutr.* 2004;80(6 suppl):1678S-1688S. doi:10.1093/ajcn/80.6.1678S

194. Gilsanz V, Kremer A, Mo AO, Wren TA, Kremer R. Vitamin D status and its relation to muscle mass and muscle fat in young women. *J Clin Endocrinol Metab.* 2010;95(4):1595-1601. doi:10.1210/jc.2009-2309

195. Grimaldi AS, Parker BA, Capizzi JA, et al. 25(OH) vitamin D is associated with greater muscle strength in healthy men and women. *Med Sci Sports Exerc.* 2013;45(1):157-162. doi:10.1249/MSS.0b013e31826c9a78

196. Heileson JL, McGowen JM, Moris JM, et al. Body composition, eicosapentaenoic acid, and vitamin D are associated with army combat fitness test performance. *J Int Soc Sports Nutr.* 2022;19(1):349-365. doi:10.1080/15502783.2022.2094717

197. Barringer ND, Kotwal RS, Lewis MD, et al. Fatty acid blood levels, vitamin D status, physical performance, activity, and resiliency: a novel potential screening tool for depressed mood in active duty soldiers. *Mil Med.* 2016;181(9):1114-1120. doi:10.7205/milmed-d-15-00456

198. Wentz L, Berry-Cabán C, Eldred J, Wu Q. Vitamin D correlation with testosterone concentration in US army special operations personnel. *FASEB J.* 2015;29(S1):733.5. doi:10.1096/fasebj.29.1_supplement.733.5

199. Holick MF, Binkley NC, Bischoff-Ferrari HA, et al. Evaluation, treatment, and prevention of vitamin D deficiency: an Endocrine Society clinical practice guideline. *J Clin Endocrinol Metab.* 2011;96(7):1911-1930. doi:10.1210/jc.2011-0385

200. Lappe J, Cullen D, Haynatzki G, Recker R, Ahlf R, Thompson K. Calcium and vitamin D supplementation decreases incidence of stress fractures in female navy recruits. *J Bone Miner Res.* 2008;23(5):741-749. doi:10.1359/jbmr.080102

201. Fogleman SA, Janney C, Cialdella-Kam L, Flint JH. Vitamin D deficiency in the military: It's time to act! *Mil Med.* 2021;187(5-6):144-148. doi:10.1093/milmed/usab402

202. Johnson BVB, Mayer JM. Evaluating nutrient intake of career firefighters compared to military dietary reference intakes. *Nutrients.* 2020;12(6):1876. doi:10.3390/nu12061876

203. Murphy MC, George HA, Naqi M, Owen PJ, Chivers P, Hart NH. Musculoskeletal injury epidemiology in law enforcement and firefighter recruits during physical training: a systematic review. *BMJ Open Sport Exerc Med.* 2022;8(1):e001289. doi:10.1136/bmjsem-2021-001289

204. Institute of Medicine Committee on Nutrition, Trauma, the Brain. Erdman J, Oria M, Pillsbury L, eds. *Nutrition and Traumatic Brain Injury: Improving Acute and Subacute Health Outcomes in Military Personnel.* National Academies Press; 2011.

205. Perel P, Yanagawa T, Bunn F, Roberts I, Wentz R, Pierro A. Nutritional support for head-injured patients. *Cochrane Database Syst Rev.* 2006;2006(4):CD001530. doi:10.1002/14651858.CD001530.pub2

206. Doig GS, Heighes PT, Simpson F, Sweetman EA, Davies AR. Early enteral nutrition, provided within 24 h of injury or intensive care unit admission, significantly reduces mortality in critically ill patients: a meta-analysis of randomised controlled trials. *Intensive Care Med.* 2009;35(12):2018-2027. doi:10.1007/s00134-009-1664-4

207. Härtl R, Gerber LM, Ni Q, Ghajar J. Effect of early nutrition on deaths due to severe traumatic brain injury. *J Neurosurg.* 2008;109(1):50-56. doi:10.3171/jns/2008/109/7/0050

208. Lee HY, Oh B-M. Nutrition management in patients with traumatic brain injury: a narrative review. *Brain Neurorehabil.* 2022;15(1):e4. doi:10.12786/bn.2022.15.e4

209. Quintard H, Ichai C. Nutritional and metabolic supplementation for the injured brain: an update. *Curr Opin Crit Care.* 2019;25(2):126-131. doi:10.1097/mcc.0000000000000588

210. Ainsley Dean PJ, Arikan G, Opitz B, Sterr A. Potential for use of creatine supplementation following mild traumatic brain injury. *Concussion.* 2017;2(2):CNC34. doi:10.2217/cnc-2016-0016

211. Barringer N, Conkright W. Omega-3 fatty acid ingestion as a TBI prophylactic. *J Spec Oper Med.* 2012;12(3):5-7. doi:10.55460/e1w8-7plc

212. Wu A, Ying Z, Gomez-Pinilla F. Dietary omega-3 fatty acids normalize BDNF levels, reduce oxidative damage, and counteract learning disability after traumatic brain injury in rats. *J Neurotrauma.* 2004;21(10):1457-1467. doi:10.1089/neu.2004.21.1457

213. Mills JD, Bailes JE, Sedney CL, Hutchins H, Sears B. Omega-3 fatty acid supplementation and reduction of traumatic axonal injury in a rodent head injury model. *J Neurosurg.* 2011;114(1):77-84. doi:10.3171/2010.5.Jns08914

214. Wu A, Ying Z, Gomez-Pinilla F. The salutary effects of DHA dietary supplementation on cognition, neuroplasticity, and membrane homeostasis after brain trauma. *J Neurotrauma.* 2011;28(10):2113-2122. doi:10.1089/neu.2011.1872

215. Wu A, Ying Z, Gomez-Pinilla F. Omega-3 fatty acids supplementation restores mechanisms that maintain brain homeostasis in traumatic brain injury. *J Neurotrauma.* Oct 2007;24(10):1587-1595. doi:10.1089/neu.2007.0313

216. Bailes JE, Mills JD. Docosahexaenoic acid reduces traumatic axonal injury in a rodent head injury model. *J Neurotrauma.* 2010;27(9):1617-1624. doi:10.1089/neu.2009.1239

217. Sharma S, Zhuang Y, Ying Z, Wu A, Gomez-Pinilla F. Dietary curcumin supplementation counteracts reduction in levels of molecules involved in energy homeostasis after brain trauma. *Neuroscience.* 2009;161(4):1037-1044. doi:10.1016/j.neuroscience.2009.04.042

218. Wu A, Ying Z, Schubert D, Gomez-Pinilla F. Brain and spinal cord interaction: a dietary curcumin derivative counteracts locomotor and cognitive deficits after brain trauma. *Neurorehabil Neural Repair.* 2011;25(4):332-342. doi:10.1177/1545968310397706

219. Vagnozzi R, Signoretti S, Floris R, et al. Decrease in *N*-acetylaspartate following concussion may be coupled to decrease in creatine. *J Head Trauma Rehabil.* 2013;28(4):284-292. doi:10.1097/HTR.0b013e3182795045

220. Sakellaris G, Kotsiou M, Tamiolaki M, et al. Prevention of complications related to traumatic brain injury in children and adolescents with creatine administration: an open label randomized pilot study. *J Trauma*. 2006;61(2):322-329. doi:10.1097/01.ta.0000230269.46108.d5
221. Sakellaris G, Nasis G, Kotsiou M, Tamiolaki M, Charissis G, Evangeliou A. Prevention of traumatic headache, dizziness and fatigue with creatine administration. A pilot study. *Acta Paediatr*. 2008;97(1):31-34. doi:10.1111/j.1651-2227.2007.00529.x
222. Menon VP, Sudheer AR. Antioxidant and anti-inflammatory properties of curcumin. *Adv Exp Med Biol*. 2007;595:105-125. doi:10.1007/978-0-387-46401-5_3
223. Ambati RR, Phang SM, Ravi S, Aswathanarayana RG. Astaxanthin: sources, extraction, stability, biological activities and its commercial applications--a review. *Mar Drugs*. 2014;12(1):128-152. doi:10.3390/md12010128
224. Cao Y, Yang L, Qiao X, Xue C, Xu J. Dietary astaxanthin: an excellent carotenoid with multiple health benefits. *Crit Rev Food Sci Nutr*. 2023;63(18):3019-3045. doi:10.1080/10408398.2021.1983766
225. Fassett RG, Coombes JS. Astaxanthin in cardiovascular health and disease. *Molecules*. 2012;17(2):2030-2048. doi:10.3390/molecules17022030
226. Choi Y, Tanabe Y, Akazawa N, Zempo-Miyaki A, Maeda S. Curcumin supplementation attenuates the decrease in endothelial function following eccentric exercise. *J Exerc Nutrition Biochem*. 2019;23(2):7-12. doi:10.20463/jenb.2019.0010
227. Mallard AR, Briskey D, Richards BA, Rao A. Curcumin improves delayed onset muscle soreness and postexercise lactate accumulation. *J Diet Suppl*. 2021;18(5):531-542. doi:10.1080/19390211.2020.1796885
228. MacKenzie-Shalders K, Matthews C, Dulla J, Orr R. Law enforcement personnel are willing to change, but report influencing beliefs and barriers to optimised dietary intake. *BMC Public Health*. 2020;20(1):1638. doi:10.1186/s12889-020-09716-z
229. MacKenzie-Shalders KL, Lee KW, Wright C, Dulla J, Tsoi A, Orr RM. Dietary intake in law enforcement personnel: occupation is an additional challenge for changing behavior. *Nutrients*. 2022;14(7):1336. doi:10.3390/nu14071336
230. Bucher Della Torre S, Wild P, Dorribo V, Amati F, Danuser B. Eating habits of professional firefighters: comparison with national guidelines and impact healthy eating promotion program. *J Occup Environ Med*. 2019;61(5):e183-e190. doi:10.1097/jom.0000000000001565
231. Yang J, Farioli A, Korre M, Kales SN. Dietary preferences and nutritional information needs among career firefighters in the United States. *Glob Adv Health Med*. 2015;4(4):16-23. doi:10.7453/gahmj.2015.050
232. Christodoulou A, Christophi CA, Sotos-Prieto M, Moffatt S, Kales SN. Eating habits among US firefighters and association with cardiometabolic outcomes. *Nutrients*. 2022;14(13):2762. doi:10.3390/nu14132762
233. Morris MC, Tangney CC, Wang Y, et al. MIND diet slows cognitive decline with aging. *Alzheimers Dement*. 2015;11(9):1015-1022. doi:10.1016/j.jalz.2015.04.011
234. Ardekani AM, Vahdat S, Hojati A, et al. Evaluating the association between the Mediterranean-DASH intervention for neurodegenerative delay (MIND) diet, mental health, and cardio-metabolic risk factors among individuals with obesity. *BMC Endocr Disord*. 2023;23(1):29. doi:10.1186/s12902-023-01284-8
235. Ravussin E, Beyl RA, Poggiogalle E, Hsia DS, Peterson CM. Early time-restricted feeding reduces appetite and increases fat oxidation but does not affect energy expenditure in humans. *Obesity (Silver Spring)*. 2019;27(8):1244-1254. doi:10.1002/oby.22518
236. Peeke PM, Greenway FL, Billes SK, Zhang D, Fujioka K. Effect of time restricted eating on body weight and fasting glucose in participants with obesity: results of a randomized, controlled, virtual clinical trial. *Nutr Diabetes*. 2021;11(1):6. doi:10.1038/s41387-021-00149-0
237. Patterson RE, Sears DD. Metabolic effects of intermittent fasting. *Annu Rev Nutr*. 2017;37(1):371-393. doi:10.1146/annurev-nutr-071816-064634
238. McAllister MJ, Pigg BL, Renteria LI, Waldman HS. Time-restricted feeding improves markers of cardiometabolic health in physically active college-age men: a 4-week randomized pre-post pilot study. *Nutr Res*. 2020;75:32-43. doi:10.1016/j.nutres.2019.12.001
239. McAllister MJ, Gonzalez AE, Waldman HS. Impact of time restricted feeding on markers of cardiometabolic health and oxidative stress in resistance-trained firefighters. *J Strength Cond Res*. 2022;36(9):2515-2522. doi:10.1519/jsc.0000000000003860
240. McAllister MJ, Gonzalez AE, Waldman HS. Time restricted feeding reduces inflammation and cortisol response to a firegrounds test in professional firefighters. *J Occup Environ Med*. 2021;63(5):441-447. doi:10.1097/JOM.0000000000002169
241. Gonzalez AE, Waldman HS, Abel MG, McCurdy KW, McAllister MJ. Impact of time restricted feeding on fitness variables in professional resistance trained firefighters. *J Occup Environ Med*. 2021;63(4):343-349. doi:10.1097/jom.0000000000002144
242. Waldman HS, Smith JW, Lamberth J, Fountain BJ, McAllister MJ. A 28-day carbohydrate-restricted diet improves markers of cardiometabolic health and performance in professional firefighters. *J Strength Cond Res*. 2019;33(12):3284-3294. doi:10.1519/JSC.0000000000003354
243. Sotos-Prieto M, Cash SB, Christophi CA, et al. Rationale and design of feeding America's bravest: Mediterranean diet-based intervention to change firefighters' eating habits and improve cardiovascular risk profiles. *Contemp Clin Trials*. 2017;61:101-107. doi:10.1016/j.cct.2017.07.010
244. Sofi F, Cesari F, Abbate R, Gensini GF, Casini A. Adherence to Mediterranean diet and health status: meta-analysis. *BMJ*. 2008;337:a1344. doi:10.1136/bmj.a1344
245. Mertens E, Mullie P, Deforche B, et al. Cross-sectional study on the relationship between the Mediterranean diet score and blood lipids. *Nutr J*. 2014;13(1):88. doi:10.1186/1475-2891-13-88
246. Almeida AA, Reeve EH, Dickinson RL, Carty M, Gilpin J, Feairheller DL. Civilians have higher adherence and more improvements in health with a Mediterranean diet and circuit training program compared with firefighters. *J Occup Environ Med*. 2022;64(6):488-494. doi:10.1097/jom.0000000000002478

247. Social Determinants of Health. Healthy People 2030 website. Accessed February 2, 2022. https://health.gov/healthypeople/objectives-and-data/social-determinants-health

248. Social Determinants of Health (SDOH). CDC website. Accessed February 2, 2022. www.cdc.gov/socialdeterminants/index.htm

249. Social determinants of health: Overview. WHO website. Accessed February 2, 2022. www.who.int/health-topics/social-determinants-of-health#tab=tab_1

250. Selby A. The Forest Service should embrace a full-time workforce. *High Country News*. June 15, 2020. Accessed February 2, 2022. www.hcn.org/issues/52.7/south-wildfire-the-forest-service-should-embrace-a-full-time-workforce

251. Farivar C, Lozano AV. Federal wildland firefighters say they're burned out after years of low pay, little job stability. *NBC News*. October 31, 2020. Accessed February 2, 2022. www.nbcnews.com/news/us-news/federal-wildland-firefighters-say-they-re-burned-out-after-years-n1245576

252. Osgood B. Wildland firefighters struggle with homelessness. *High Country News*. October 27, 2021. Accessed February 2, 2022. www.hcn.org/articles/labor-wildland-firefighters-struggle-with-homelessness

253. First Responder Salary in Oklahoma City, OK. ZipRecruiter website. Accessed February 2, 2022. www.ziprecruiter.com/Salaries/First-Responder-Salary-in-Oklahoma-City,OK

254. Poverty Guidelines. US Department of Health and Human Services, Office of the Assistant Secretary for Planning and Evaluation (ASPE) website. Accessed February 2, 2022. https://aspe.hhs.gov/topics/poverty-economic-mobility/poverty-guidelines

255. Blakely G, Hennessy C, Chung MC, Skirton H. A systematic review of the impact of foreign postings on accompanying spouses of military personnel. *Nurs Health Sci*. 2012;14(1):121-132. doi:10.1111/j.1442-2018.2011.00659.x

256. Da Silva FC, Hernandez SSS, Goncalves E, Arancibia BAV, Da Silva Castro TL, Da Silva R. Anthropometric indicators of obesity in policemen: a systematic review of observational studies. *Int J Occup Med Environ Health*. 2014;27(6):891-901. doi:10.2478/s13382-014-0318-0

257. Alasagheirin MH, Clark MK, Ramey SL, Grueskin EF. Body mass index misclassification of obesity among community police officers. *AAOHN J*. 2011;59(11):469-475. doi:10.3928/08910162-20111017-01

258. Frattaroli S, Pollack KM, Bailey M, Schafer H, Cheskin LJ, Holtgrave DR. Working inside the firehouse: developing a participant-driven intervention to enhance health-promoting behaviors. *Health Promot Pract*. 2013;14(3):451-458. doi:10.1177/1524839912461150

259. Staley JA, Weiner B, Linnan L. Firefighter fitness, coronary heart disease, and sudden cardiac death risk. *Am J Health Behavior*. 2011;35(5):603-617. doi:10.5993/ajhb.35.5.9

260. Brandt-Rauf PW, Fallon LF Jr, Tarantini T, Idema C, Andrews L. Health hazards of fire fighters: exposure assessment. *Br J Ind Med*. 1988;45(9):606-612. doi:10.1136/oem.45.9.606

261. Firefighter Resources – Job Hazards. CDC, National Institute for Occupational Safety and Health (NIOSH) website. Last reviewed April 13, 2023. Accessed May 31, 2023. www.cdc.gov/niosh/firefighters/hazard.html

262. Lee RJ, Yolton RL, Yolton DP, Schnider C, Janin ML. Personal defense sprays: effects and management of exposure. *J Am Optom Assoc*. 1996;67(9):548-560. PMID: 8888888

263. Burgess JL, Barnhart S, Checkoway H. Investigating clandestine drug laboratories: adverse medical effects in law enforcement personnel. *Am J Ind Med*. 1996;30(4):488-494. doi:10.1002/(sici)1097-0274(199610)30:4<488::AID-AJIM15>3.0.Co;2-0

264. Sylvain DC. Health Hazard Evaluation Report 96-0218-2623. New Hampshire Police Standards and Training Council. January 1997. Accessed March 14, 2024. www.cdc.gov/niosh/hhe/reports/pdfs/1996-0218-2623.pdf

265. Military Exposures. US Department of Veterans Affairs Public Health website. Accessed May 31, 2023. www.publichealth.va.gov/exposures

266. Wilkinson ML, Brown AL, Poston WS, Haddock CK, Jahnke SA, Day RS. Physician weight recommendations for overweight and obese firefighters, United States, 2011-2012. *Prev Chronic Dis*. 2014;11:E116. doi:10.5888/pcd11.140091

267. Baur DM, Christophi CA, Tsismenakis AJ, Jahnke SA, Kales SN. Weight- perception in male career firefighters and its association with cardiovascular risk factors. *BMC Public Health*. 2012;12(1)::480. doi:10.1186/1471-2458-12-480

268. Roşca AC, Burtăverde V, Dan C-I, et al. The dark triad traits of firefighters and risk-taking at work. the mediating role of altruism, honesty, and courage. *Int J Environ Res Public Health*. 2021;18(11):5983. doi:10.3390/ijerph18115983

269. Kelley AM, Athy JR, Cho TH, Erickson B, King M, Cruz P. Risk propensity and health risk behaviors in US army soldiers with and without psychological disturbances across the deployment cycle. *J Psychiatr Res*. 2012;46(5):582-589. doi:10.1016/j.jpsychires.2012.01.017

270. Meadows SO. U.S. Service Members in Generally Good Health, but Risky Behaviors Persist. News release. RAND. April 28, 2021. Accessed February 2, 2022. www.rand.org/news/press/2021/04/28.html

271. Jayne J. Evaluating the effect of the personnel element of the Army's Holistic Health and Fitness system on health-related behaviors and injury: an interim analysis. *J Acad Nutr Diet*. 2022;122(9 suppl):A61. doi:10.1016/j.jand.2022.06.196

272. Calams S. 11 requirements to become a firefighter. Fire Rescue 1 website. Published March 24, 2017. Accessed February 2, 2022. www.firerescue1.com/firefighter-training/articles/11-requirements-to-become-a-firefighter-FO0ZZpNdggP1GAmq

273. Basic Requirements. International Association of Chiefs of Police (IACP) Discover Policing website. Accessed February 2, 2022. www.discoverpolicing.org/about-policing/basic-requirements

274. Answers to the Top Army Questions. Military.com website. Accessed February 2, 2022. www.military.com/join-armed-forces/army-recruiting-faqs.html

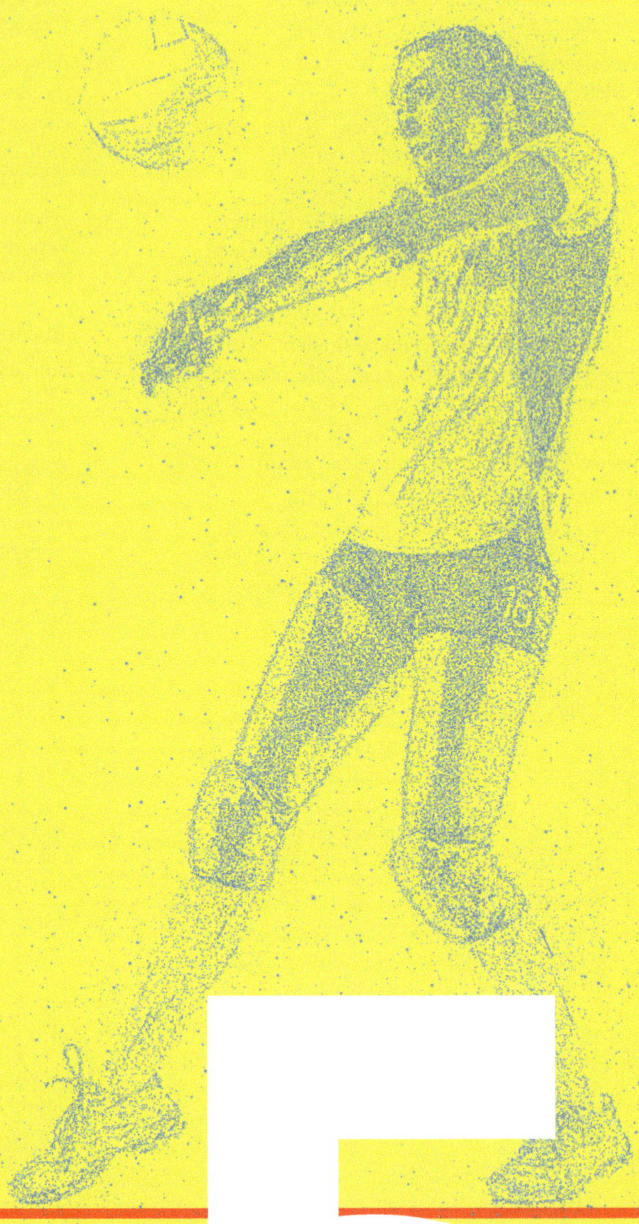

SECTION 5

ADVANCING THE FUTURE

Section 5 is dedicated to advancing not only the future of the performance nutrition field but also the future of the athletes and tactical operators it serves. The section starts with a chapter that explores emerging areas of opportunity for sports dietitians, such as working with CrossFit athletes, obstacle course racers, motorsport drivers, artistic performers (eg, dance, marching arts, musicians, actors), and esports participants. Chapter 24 also demonstrates the commitment of the performance nutrition field to providing inclusive nutrition services to all by summarizing the current knowledge base and best practices for providing evidence-based, compassionate care to transgender and gender-nonconforming athletes. Chapter 25 focuses on dietary patterns and athletes. Energy and macronutrients tend to be the main focus in performance nutrition, and this chapter is a reminder of the importance of overall athlete health both while the athlete is competing and once they have retired from sport. This chapter discusses overall dietary patterns and their role in health promotion and performance. The final chapter in this section, Chapter 26, provides an overview of nutrition operations and management with specific application to athletics and sports nutrition. The role of the sports dietitian has expanded tremendously over the years to truly maximize the training and education that is part of the pathway to becoming a registered dietitian nutritionist, including operations and management. Currently, the available resources specific to nutrition operations and management in athletics and sports nutrition are scarce, and the training and education that sports dietitians typically receive is through a "learn as you go" or an "on the job" approach. The inclusion of this chapter will help to fill this gap in knowledge.

CHAPTER 24

Emerging Opportunities in Sports Nutrition

Elizabeth L. Abbey, PhD, RDN, CDN

LEARNING OBJECTIVES

- Identify athletic populations that have traditionally been underserved in the field of sports nutrition.
- Summarize the physiological and nutritional considerations of athletic populations that have traditionally been underserved in the field of sports nutrition.
- Identify gaps in research and professional practice that a sports registered dietitian nutritionist (RDN) could fill.
- Explain strategies that an RDN could take to expand their professional practice into an emerging arena of sports nutrition.
- Identify best practices for providing evidence-based, compassionate care to transgender and gender-nonconforming athletes.

INTRODUCTION

When he was a swimmer in college, James first became interested in nutrition after working with his university's sports dietitian who helped him to manage a new diagnosis of celiac disease. After completing a dietetics internship and passing the board exam, James became a newly minted registered dietitian nutritionist (RDN) with the goal of earning the certified specialist in sports dietetics (CSSD) credential and pursuing a career in sports nutrition. However, he lives in an area in which there are few opportunities to work with high-level athletes, and he is not in a situation where he can move to a larger market. James has found work as a relief RDN at the local hospital, but he would like a position that would connect him with a more active population so he can start logging CSSD hours. Outside of working with college or professional athletes, James is not sure what opportunities exist for sports dietitians and how to break into the field.

Does James's situation sound familiar? Although the prevalence of RDNs in collegiate and professional athletics continues to grow, in reality, most sports dietitians work with individuals of all skill and activity levels.

When sports dietitians look beyond our traditional athlete populations, there are limitless, untapped opportunities. Several active populations—some that are new and some that have been around for some time—are increasingly seeking out RDNs for their expertise. These include people involved in high-intensity functional training such as CrossFit or boot camp programs, obstacle course races, motorsports, artistic performers, electronic sports (esports), and more. Clearly, there is overlap between some of these groups and those involved in other sports (eg, CrossFitters and participants in short-duration, very high– and high-intensity sports), and the reader is encouraged to refer to the corresponding chapters for more background on the physiological underpinnings of those activities. The purpose of this chapter is not to provide exhaustive detail on each of these sports or populations but to present a general overview of the unique considerations for each of these groups, practical tips from RDNs who currently work with them, and suggestions for how to make inroads into these fields. This chapter also includes a new section on special considerations for transgender athletes, recognizing that their unique needs and circumstances warrant increased attention. Using the information presented in this chapter as an introduction, members of the nutrition and dietetics community are encouraged to explore these and other emerging opportunities in sports nutrition.

CROSSFIT

Description

Since the first CrossFit gym opened in 2000 in Santa Cruz, CA, similar programs have flooded the market.[1] For simplicity's sake, this section focuses on CrossFit, but the same basic principles can apply to other high-intensity functional training (HIFT) and high-intensity interval training (HIIT) programs. CrossFit is a "sport of fitness" that involves "constantly varied, high-intensity, functional movement" with the goal of increasing power.[2] This is achieved by collectively increasing load, distance, and speed. According to Feito et al,[3] CrossFit is a form of HIFT, which is "an exercise modality that emphasizes functional, multi-joint movements that can be modified to any fitness level and elicit greater muscle recruitment than more traditional exercise." The term HIFT is often used interchangeably with HIIT, although the two are distinct. HIIT exercise comprises "short bursts of repeated vigorous activity, interspersed by periods of rest or low-intensity exercise for recovery," whereas HIFT generally involves more varied exercises of different durations that may or may not incorporate rest.

The explosion of CrossFit and CrossFit-like programs may be due to the variety of workouts as well as the camaraderie and competition among participants. To fully engage in the CrossFit community, participants are encouraged to join an affiliate gym staffed by accredited CrossFit trainers. Since the COVID-19 pandemic, options for online programming have taken off. Individuals can also participate without a membership by accessing the *workout of the day* (WOD) online. Top-level CrossFitters can vie for the crown of the Fittest Man and Fittest Woman on Earth at the annual CrossFit Games, a multiday event of back-to-back workouts, each with different movements, equipment, and time domains. Most workout details are unknown until athletes are set to begin the event. Qualifying is a multistage process that begins at local affiliates with the worldwide CrossFit Open, advertised as the "largest participatory sporting event on Earth."[4] The top participants advance to a semifinal round, followed by the finals. The Games also include teenage and masters divisions as well as adaptive categories for athletes with disabilities.

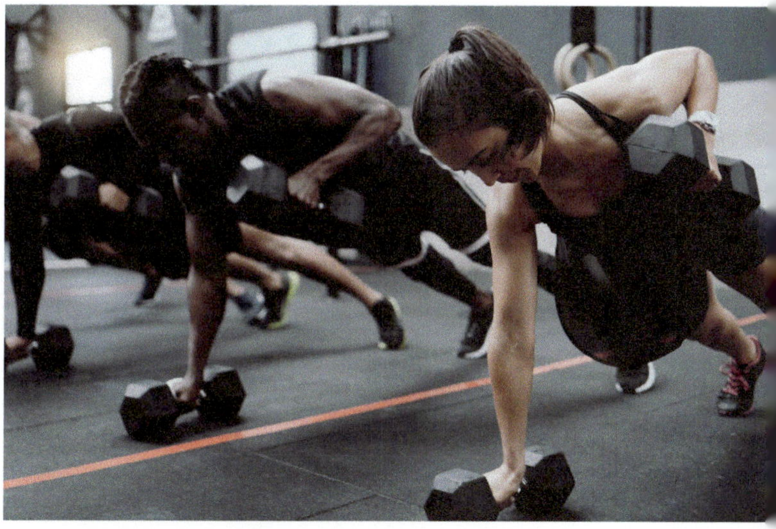

In CrossFit's early years, the image of a typical athlete may have been a chiseled, Special Forces commando. Today, CrossFit attracts individuals from all backgrounds and skill levels. Andrea Givens, MS, RDN, CSSD, (email, September 24, 2022) is a dietitian based in California who has participated in CrossFit since 2013 and has provided 1-on-1 nutrition coaching to CrossFitters, as well as group nutrition education during quarterly 6-week gym challenges. She sees many tactical and military personnel among the CrossFitters with whom she works but notes that the popularity of CrossFit has exploded into the general population, with a growing number of CrossFit affiliate gyms and people doing the workouts at home via online programming. Opportunities to work with CrossFit athletes are not limited to the top-level CrossFitters, as people of all ages and abilities participate in CrossFit to improve their health and fitness and to maintain functional independence. Givens says that most of her clients are 25 to 45 years old and work full-time day jobs, but she has also worked with teenagers and retirees. There is even a CrossFit Kids program with scaled workouts for youth ages 3 to

17 years.[5] According to Givens, the CrossFit Games online leaderboard enables participants to filter scores to see where they place in the world by sex, age, adaptive category, country, and occupation (including RDNs!). Box 24.1[6] explains some common CrossFit terms.

Basic Physiological Demands

CrossFit is unique in that every WOD is different (ie, "constantly varied functional movement"[2]). The average CrossFitter engages in workouts 4.5 days/week, with most classes programmed to be 60 minutes.[7] The typical structure of a 60-minute CrossFit class starts with a warm-up, leading into a strength- or skill-based movement, followed by a metcon. CrossFit is appealing to many because people can get in a good

BOX 24.1 A Selection of Common CrossFit Terms and Abbreviations[a,6]

Affiliate	A local CrossFit gym
Benchmark	A standardized workout that allows a participant to compare their own progress over time and their performance against others (eg, Murph, Fight Gone Bad, CrossFit Total, and "The Girls" workouts)
Box	The traditional name for a CrossFit gym, so-named because they are often in industrial-type warehouses
CrossFit Open	A virtual stage of the CrossFit Games that allows users to register online and compete from anywhere in the world
Hero workout	Several CrossFit benchmark workouts that are named after actual military service members, law enforcement officers, and firefighters who have died in the line of duty; typically very difficult workouts (see Murph)
Macros	Short for macronutrients; tracking or counting macros is a popular diet trend among CrossFitters
Metcon	Short for metabolic conditioning, a type of workout; training with the intent to enhance performance of the 3 metabolic pathways
Murph	A hero workout and one of the most popular and challenging benchmark workouts, named after Navy SEAL and Medal of Honor recipient Michael Murphy, who was killed in Afghanistan in 2005; consists of a 1-mile run followed by 100 pull-ups, 200 push-ups, and 300 bodyweight squats, ending with another 1-mile run, all while wearing a weighted vest
The Girls	Several CrossFit benchmark workouts that are given female names but are not named after actual people, similar to the naming of storms; the workouts are very physically demanding, like a storm just hit you (eg, Fran, Cindy, Karen, Grace, Helen, Jackie)
The Open	Worldwide, 3-week competition in which anyone, regardless of fitness level or ability, can compete at home or an affiliate gym to try to qualify for the CrossFit Games
WOD	Workout of the day; a combination of exercises that changes from day to day

[a] Andrea Givens, MS, RDN, CSSD, (email, September 24, 2022) also contributed to the information provided.

workout relatively quickly. Participants usually take 2 rest days every week. The types of movements and activities vary widely, from Olympic lifting, powerlifting, and body-weight training to sports such as gymnastics, swimming, and running. Although all WODs are performed at a high to very high intensity and therefore rely heavily on anaerobic energy production, aerobic energy production is also important during metcons and longer workouts activities (Givens, email, September 24, 2022). In a systematic review of the physiological and metabolic demands of CrossFit WODs, de Souza et al[8] reported postexercise reductions in cognitive performance and increases in blood lactate (up to 18 mmol/L), markers of muscle damage and inflammation (interleukin-6 [IL-6], interleukin-10 [IL-10], and creatine phosphokinase), sweat rates (21.9–23.8 mL/min), mean heart rates (>90% of the maximum heart rate), oxygen consumption rates (VO_2) (55%–65% of the maximum rate of oxygen consumption [$VO_{2\,max}$]), rates of perceived exertion (7.2–9.8 on 0–10 scale), and muscle fatigue (impaired mean power output, peak power output, countermovement jump, and plank test time). Refer to Chapters 20 and 21 (Nutrition for Short-Duration, Very High- and High-Intensity Sports and Nutrition for High-Intensity, Intermittent Sports, respectively) on sport-specific nutrition guidelines for a more thorough overview of the physiological considerations for these types of activities.

Typical Diets and Lifestyle Trends

Nutrition is a key component of CrossFit and other HIFT programs. CrossFitters are encouraged to observe the following diet recommendations: "Eat meat and vegetables, nuts and seeds, some fruit, little starch, and no sugar. Keep intake to levels that support exercise but not body fat."[9] Even though CrossFit has ridden the wave of popular diet trends, 1 constant has been the promotion of a diet that is low in processed foods and added sugars and high in protein. The Zone diet, developed by Barry Sears, PhD, was commonly promoted during the early years of CrossFit, and more recently, the paleolithic (Paleo) diet has been associated with the sport. In a descriptive study of dietary practices and supplement use among CrossFit participants (N = 2,576), Brisebois et al[7] found that 60.1% of participants reported following a particular diet, with macro counting, intermittent fasting, and Paleo being the most common. The top reasons given for following a specific diet were to improve overall health (45.6%), decrease body fat (29.2%), and improve CrossFit performance (25.2%). These results align with Givens' (email, September 24, 2022) experience: "CrossFitters are probably the first to jump on the train... right now, the most popular is 'tracking macros' or 'macro counting.'" Online calculators for macros are quite popular, and most of these calculators use some version of the 30:30:40 ratio of protein to fat to carbohydrate popularized by the Zone diet, although the specific ratio may not be readily apparent on the website of a given calculator.[10] In terms of a dinner plate, this translates into roughly one-third lean protein, two-thirds nonstarchy fruits and vegetables, and a dash of monounsaturated fat.[11,12] With macros counting, "cheat meals" are less common, as the focus is on well-balanced eating. Givens explained "I like to say, 'eating isn't cheating.'" Givens also mentions that many CrossFitters have a "nutrition coach," who may or may not be a qualified professional such as an RDN. In addition, CrossFit recently launched an 8-hour online, self-paced nutrition course for individuals and coaches that can be taken by anyone who pays the fee.[9]

Other common trends are the use of meal preparation services and, in addition to the counting of macros, the tracking of food intake with smartphone applications such as MyFitnessPal, Cronometer, and LoseIt!. In Givens' (email, September 24, 2022) experience, wearable devices that track recovery and sleep and technology such as continuous glucose monitoring systems have risen in popularity. "CrossFitters are so competitive, they now compete in their recovery scores."

Nutrition Issues

ENERGY AVAILABILITY AND HYDRATION

The high-intensity, muscle-fatiguing nature of CrossFit, with subsequent training sessions sometimes occurring within 24 to 48 hours, makes energy availability, recovery nutrition, and nutrition timing high priorities. Local competitions may be individual or consist of teams of 2 to 4 individuals, and they can have multiple workouts in 1 day. "Each workout may only last 10 to 20 minutes, and there is downtime in between to recover, rehydrate, and refuel" (Givens, email, September 24, 2022). If a CrossFitter consumes anything during a workout, it is likely water, but even that may be difficult because of the sustained intensity of the workout.

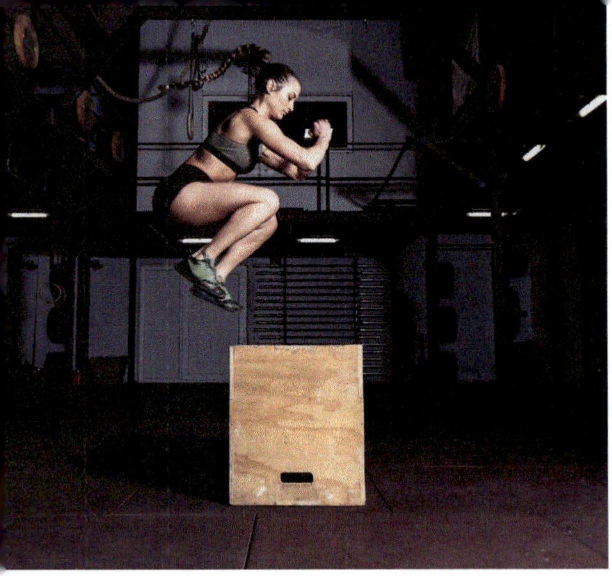

The hot environment of many gyms may also put participants at a higher risk for dehydration and heat illness. Practitioners should emphasize fluid intake preworkout and postworkout in addition to appropriate recovery. See Chapter 6 for fluid guidelines and Chapters 20 and 21 for sport-specific nutrition guidelines.

SUPPLEMENTS AND ERGOGENIC AIDS

According to Brisebois et al,[7] about 82% of surveyed CrossFitters reported taking at least 1 supplement, with the most popular being protein (51.2%), creatine (22.9%), and preworkout or energy supplements (20.7%). Givens (email, September 24, 2022) reports that branched-chain amino acids in carbonated drinks; omega-3 supplements; magnesium; cannabidiol; and unfortunately, performance-enhancing drugs (PEDs) are quite popular. Among the top reasons give for consuming supplements are wanting to improve recovery (52.6%), wanting to improve overall health (51.4%), and wanting to increase muscle mass or strength (41.7%).[7] Whether any of these supplements have a significant impact on CrossFit performance is inconclusive. In a review of the effects of diet interventions, dietary supplements, and performance-enhancing substances on CrossFit performance, Dos Santos Quaresma et al[13] found no clear support for any of the aforementioned measures, except possibly for sodium bicarbonate. CrossFitters' primary sources of supplement information include the internet (53.1%), coaches and trainers (27.0%), and peer-reviewed research (23.0%).[7] Notably absent from this list are RDNs. Givens (email, September 24, 2022) emphasizes that "RDNs working with this population need to be well-versed in supplement safety, including the legality, risks, and dangers of PEDs."

Expert Nutrition Tips

Following are some tips for working with CrossFit athletes:

- CrossFitters tend to be extremely focused, driven individuals who are willing to push their bodies to the limit. They have also often received a great deal of misinformation regarding nutrition and can take that to an extreme. Givens (email, September 24, 2022) advises, "It's common for CrossFitters to want to go full throttle all the time (in workouts, workout schedule 4+ days/week, and year-round), but rest and periodization need to be appreciated and honored. That has not been well-communicated or executed in CrossFit culture."
- As with counseling any athlete, Givens (email, September 24, 2022) says that it is important to "keep an open mind and work from the beginning to build a strong rapport." When an athlete chooses to follow a specific diet, she emphasizes providing guidance on evidence-based sports nutrition and, if necessary, working with the athlete to modify the diet plan to fit their unique needs.

How to Get a Foot in the Door

In a survey of CrossFitters, the top sources for nutrition information were the internet (47.5%); coaches and trainers (28.7%); and lastly, nutritionists and/or dietitians (26.2%).[7] There is clearly room for improvement. Givens (email, September 24, 2022) has observed an increase in nutrition coaching jobs, or "macros coaches," through nutrition coaching companies, but an RDN credential is not always required. She reports that the best opportunity for RDNs to work with CrossFitters is for the RDN to be part of a CrossFit affiliate or training facility. "This is one 'sport' where the athlete may only value your expertise if you are doing this type of workout too, so they feel you truly understand the metabolic demands and the food culture." CrossFit gyms, social media, and online courses are areas where she recommends getting involved. Strong background knowledge in exercise science (eg, a degree or college courses), the Certified Strength and Conditioning Specialist (CSCS) credential, the CSSD credential, comfortableness with evaluating and providing education on supplements, and a passion for educating are all helpful qualities. Signing up for at least an introductory workout series is the best way to become acquainted with the physical demands and jargon of CrossFit.

CrossFitters are a loyal, highly connected group. Because of the lack of credentialed nutrition experts in this arena, a highly engaged RDN can make a significant impact. Fostering connections in the "sport of fitness" may open several doors for a motivated RDN.

OBSTACLE COURSE RACES

Description

Whereas multievent competitions, such as the ancient pentathlon, have been in existence for thousands of years, the earliest contemporary obstacle course race (OCR), the Tough Guy Competition, was held in 1987 in the United Kingdom.[14] Participation in OCR surged in popularity around 2010 at the founding of some of the most well-known OCRs (ie, Spartan Race and Tough Mudder).[15] Participation continued to grow into the mid-2010s, when it started to level off. Between 2009 and 2013, participation in nontraditional running events (eg, theme races and obstacle races) increased 40-fold to more than 4 million participants in the United States annually.[16] According to the World Obstacle Federation (Fédération Internationale de Sports d'Obstacles), the nonprofit sole world governing body for OCR, more than 2,500 OCRs are currently held worldwide annually.[17]

Theme races (eg, mud, color) tend to be short (5 km; typically called "5K") and attract individuals whose main goals are to finish and to have a good time with friends. Obstacle races tend to be more intense and geared toward athletes who are looking for a new challenge that combines endurance with strength and skill. Adventure races are sometimes categorized with OCRs, but they require more orienteering and can last multiple days or weeks.[15] The two most popular OCRs are Spartan Race and Tough Mudder. Both are team-oriented endurance events with obstacle courses throughout. Spartan Race offers the most variety in race types: Sprint (5K with 20 obstacles), Super (10K with 25 obstacles), Beast (20K with 30 obstacles), and Ultra Beast (50K with 60 obstacles).[18] Standard Tough Mudder events range from 5K to 15K with obstacles, and 12- and 24-hour events are offered.[19] The exact obstacles are not disclosed until the day of the event, although signature challenges are usually included (eg, barbed-wire crawl, mud pit, rope climbs, live wires, and fire rings). Race distances and obstacles have become more standardized over the years as the World Obstacle Federation works to make OCRs an Olympic sport.[17] Most OCRs are for-profit events (participants pay for their entry), and typically, some amount of the profit is donated to charity. OCRs attract participants of varied backgrounds, ranging from elite-level participants to beginners. Bob Seebohar, MS, RDN, CSSD, CSCS, (email, October 7, 2022) works in private practice with athletes in many sports including OCRs. Whether athletes are purely recreational or elite, "all can and will use sports nutrition services, but I have found those who really seek out nutrition coaching from a sports RD are doing the longer OCR races." In most Tough Mudder events, times are not recorded.[20] Spartan Races, however, provide an elite racing division (Spartan Series) that has an annual scoring system that culminates in a world championship race with prize money available.[21] This division attracts former Olympic athletes and elite triathletes and runners.

Basic Physiological Demands

Because of the varied nature of OCRs, racers do not fit neatly into one physiological category. Athletes are expected to quickly transition among sprinting, jumping, climbing, crawling, and lifting over the course of many miles through any number of terrain types (usually involving some amount of mud). The physical demands of these events can be equated to those of a marathon or ultramarathon but with additional strength concerns (Amy Culp, RDN, CSSD, email, October 18, 2022). These races primarily require endurance, but nutritional guidance should also consider recommendations for very high–intensity, short-duration sports, as well as high-intensity, intermittent sports (refer to Chapters 20 and 21). For OCRs that require more time to complete than a typical marathon, refer to information on ultraendurance sports in Chapter 22. Because these events last for multiple hours, the daily macronutrient guidelines for an endurance athlete, or an ultraendurance athlete for those competing in longer events, are recommended. One exception to this general guideline is to consider increasing protein intake to a range of at least 1.2 to 2.0 g per kilogram of body weight per day, aiming for the higher end, particularly during difficult training.[22] As discussed in previous chapters, the timing of protein intake before and after exercise is an important consideration to promote training adaptations and to speed recovery.

Corrina Coffin, MS, RDN, CSSD, (email, October 24, 2022) has her own virtual nutrition coaching practice and has competed at the Spartan Race World Championships herself. She shares, "I love the emphasis on both endurance and strength training with OCR athletes. You have to be fast and aerobic, but if you don't have upper body strength, you won't be successful in this sport. Because you need both, you see a lot of different training approaches based on an individual's strengths and weaknesses, which is fun to then plan nutrition around." She says that the unique physiological demands of OCR require a periodized approach depending on where someone is in the racing season. "Most of the championship races [Spartan] are in the fall, but the Series races start in the early spring and go until the fall, so it can be a very long season. Working with an athlete to determine their A-races and peak performance timeline is essential for building an appropriate nutrition plan. The offseason is usually focused on strength building so that the in-season focus can be on speed and endurance." Coffin also highlights that the sport is "constantly evolving as race companies continue to create ways to expand upon this new 'hybrid fitness' trend that requires speed, endurance, and strength."

Nutrition Issues

ENERGY AVAILABILITY AND HYDRATION

Obstacle course races vary in terms of the nutritional products they do and do not provide on the course. Some might not provide any sports drinks or food at all. Even when fluids are available, the unpredictable nature of these events can make adhering to a prescribed fueling regimen difficult. Consuming any sports foods on the course may also be impractical because participants want to avoid carrying bulky items that could get caught on obstacles or caked in mud. Intrarace fueling requires thought and planning. "For speed and obstacle proficiency, minimal gear is paramount, which means hydration and fueling options can get neglected" (Coffin, email, October 24, 2022).

Amy Culp, RDN, CSSD, (email, October 18, 2022) is a sports dietitian at the University of Texas who consults with OCRers, especially Spartan Race participants. She says that most Spartan Races have water stations every 2 to 3 miles (usually these offer only water and no additional supplementation, such as sports drink or gels). Some races loop the same route multiple times, and participants may have access to a drop bin in which they can store supplies. However, if an athlete wants food or electrolytes on the course, they must carry them. For Ultra Beast distances, participants are required to carry a personal hydration system. Postrace parties may be lacking in foods optimal for recovery and rehydration. Obstacle course racers need to expect the unexpected even more than when participating in traditional races. Fueling for these events is another part of the overall challenge and may give well-prepared athletes a distinct advantage.

BODY COMPOSITION

Because OCRs are a unique blend of endurance and strength, athletes are constantly trying to achieve the ideal strength-to-weight ratio (Culp, email, October 18, 2022). Some climbing obstacles may require participants to carry an additional 20 kg or more for females and 35 kg or more for males. Seebohar (email, October 7, 2022) also notes that, in his practice, the recreational athletes he sees are mostly focused on weight loss and body composition changes, whereas elite athletes want to maintain a lean and muscular physique. "The Paleo diet dominated this sport early on because many athletes were coming from CrossFit. Now, I would say [that] it is a blend of many different nutrition strategies from keto to high-carb/low-fat."

Culp (email, October 18, 2022) says that she constantly has to battle nutrition misinformation and has observed a trend of low-carbohydrate diets and a fear of sports drinks. She has seen some participants struggle with disordered eating and eating disorders (EDs). Coffin (email, October 24, 2022) agrees. "I think a lot of OCR athletes chase a perceived ideal aesthetic [that] they believe will set them up for greater performance. Unfortunately, this often results in an unnecessary (and unhealthy) preoccupation with body weight at the expense of performance. I also see the concept of 'clean' taking over in this space where individuals are overly fixated on eating nutrient-dense foods and wind up cutting out or avoiding certain foods and deeming them 'bad' yet failing to meet their required energy intake." Many racers are high-achieving perfectionists, which is a common phenotype of individuals with EDs.[23] RDNs working with this population should see that the energy needs of their clients are being met and be cognizant of symptoms of disordered eating patterns and body dysmorphia. For more detail, refer to Chapter 18.

Expert Nutrition Tips

Following are some tips for working with obstacle course race athletes:

- To gain an understanding of the physiological demands of OCRs and to better understand the associated nutritional requirements, Seebohar (email, October 7, 2022) recommends that RDNs who want to work with this population should at least train for an OCR. "They don't necessarily have to compete in one, but it does help to understand the logistics." He goes on to say that "an RDN definitely needs to understand the complexity of energy system contribution... [S]ome of these races are also done at altitude and [under] different environmental conditions, so understanding nutritional differences for those changes is beneficial."
- Participants need to do their homework and determine whether they will have access to a drop bin during the race and plan accordingly. They should always come to the race having eaten beforehand and prepared with their own postrace snacks; they should not assume that there will be anything available aside from what they bring for themselves.
- Depending on the race distance, participants may consider training with only water as a fluid replacement if it is known that no sports drinks or foods will be offered on the course.
- With the exception of the sprint distance, Culp (email, October 18, 2022) emphasizes calorie replacement every 45 minutes, as well as frequent hydration and electrolyte replacement. The easiest foods to carry and consume while racing are gels. If drop bins are available along the course, easily digestible carbohydrates, such as bananas, sports drinks, gels, and lower-fiber energy bars, are good choices. Practitioners may also recommend electrolytes, depending on the sweat rate of the athlete, the climate, and other available race foods and beverages. For longer race distances, such as Spartan Ultra Beasts, there should be an increased focus on energy-dense food options high in electrolytes (eg, peanut butter and jelly sandwiches, trail mix, chicken noodle soup, or egg-and-cheese biscuit sandwiches). Before any competition, participants should practice with the foods they plan on consuming during the race. For specific guidelines, refer to Chapter 22 (Nutrition for Endurance and Ultraendurance Athletes).

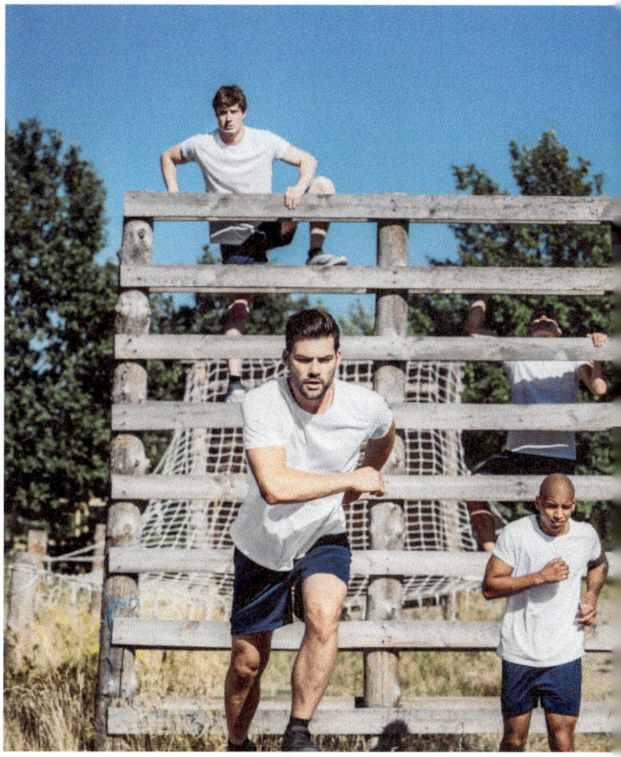

How to Get a Foot in the Door

With the sheer number of OCRs and participants, this is an arena for growth among sports RDNs. Begin by attending an OCR as a participant or observer to learn about the event and potentially make some client contacts (Seebohar, email, October 7, 2022; Culp, email, October 18, 2022; Coffin, email, October 24, 2022). Culp (email, October 18, 2022) points out that OCR is a unique sport, so simply applying the same principles one would with a marathon runner is not enough. Being well-versed in the types of obstacles; race lingo; and even the best types of clothes, shoes, and equipment is important for counseling and gaining credibility with clients. Also, given that many OCR athletes train in gym settings, Coffin (email, October 24, 2022) says that gyms are a good place to network. Finally, it is important for the RDN to know their audience and their "why" for doing OCR. Seebohar (email, October 7, 2022) says, "the beauty about OCR racing is that anyone can and will do them for different reasons." Whether it is to meet a performance goal, to lose weight, or to improve overall health, RDNs should keep the athlete's "why" in mind.

MOTORSPORTS

Description

Box 24.2 provides an overview of the main motorsport categories.[24,25]

BOX 24.2 Basic Motorsport Categories and Racing Circuits[24,25]

Open wheel	A vehicle in this class has wheels that are outside the car's main body. It also typically has a single-seat cockpit that encloses the driver's body, leaving the head exposed to the air (includes Formula 1 and Indy).
Formula 1	This class of open-wheel, closed-road course racing is the most glamorous and expensive class of motor racing, as well as the most popular motorsport outside the United States. Races are usually approximately 300 km and last less than 2 hours.
Indy racing	This class of open-wheel, oval-track racing in the United States is organized by IndyCar. The Indianapolis 500 is the signature race.
Enclosed wheel	A vehicle in this class has wheels that are inside the car's main body (includes stock cars, touring cars, and sports cars).
NASCAR (National Association for Stock Car Auto Racing)	Vehicles are raced on an oval speedway track. The NASCAR Cup Series is the sport's highest level of competition and involves 26 points races that count in the regular season standings, followed by a 10-race playoff among the 16 top point earners; races extend over 10 months, February through November. The longest races are 500 to 600 miles and can last several hours.
Touring car	These vehicles are modified street cars that race on closed-road courses or street circuits. The cars are usually based on family cars (eg, hatchbacks) but are very similar to sports cars.
Stock car	In the traditional sense, this is a car that has not been modified from its original factory configuration, although the vehicles are now based on a shared custom design, for example, NASCAR.
Sports car	This modified street car is raced on closed-road courses or street circuits. The cars are usually based on more powerful and expensive sports cars rather than touring cars.
Rally car racing	This form of racing takes place on roads (usually unpaved) with modified-production or specialty-built road-legal cars. Events can last several days and cover hundreds of miles. This is one of the most popular motorsports among amateurs. Unlike for most other motorsports, there is a codriver.
Motocross	This is a form of off-road motorcycle racing that is held on enclosed, off-road loops.

Basic Physiological Demands

Researchers have established that the physiological demands of race care driving based on oxygen consumption (VO_2) and heart are similar to those of other sports, such as basketball and soccer.[26,27] In a study with 7 professional, open-wheel drivers on both a roadway and an oval course, the average VO_2 and heart rate responses were approximately 79% and 82% of maximum, respectively. Experts believe, in part, that the elevated heart rate observed in this population is due to emotional stress in addition to physical effort. Drivers can reach speeds of 322 km/h for roughly 3 to 4 hours at potentially high temperatures (~50°C).[28,29] Even if the cockpit temperature can be cooled, the driver may still experience high levels of thermal strain.[29] In 1 study comparing 6 male and 6 female open and closed cockpit race cars, the only difference in physiological responses observed between sexes was higher breathing rates among females.[30] Females in the luteal phase of their menstrual cycle had a more elevated heart rate, breathing rate, skin temperature, core temperature, and physiological strain than those in the follicular phase.[30] It is also important to note that different styles of racing require different physical demands.[28] Open-wheel racing on a non–oval-shaped course is particularly difficult because the drivers are constantly reacting to turns of varying degrees and high gravitational forces, whereas oval racing is more consistent. Being in a closed cockpit elicited higher skin and core temperatures compared to an open cockpit.

PIT CREWS

Although motorsports are often considered individual events, they are, in many ways, team sports. A race car driver will not be successful without a strong pit crew. Some research has been conducted on the physical training of pit crews. During a pit stop, the crew must refuel the vehicle, change the tires, and make adjustments, all within approximately 15 seconds. In a sport where every second counts, the physical fitness of the pit crew is crucial to the team's success. In some cases, elite teams recruit former professional and collegiate athletes to be pit crew members. They train as high-intensity power athletes who must optimize strength and speed. No known studies have been published on the nutritional habits of this population, although descriptive data indicate that they tend to lose lean body mass in the offseason.[31] Pairing a strength program with nutritional strategies to optimize the development and maintenance of lean body tissue could have a significant impact on the success of the team.

Nutrition Issues

HYDRATION AND THERMOREGULATION

Although all athletes should be concerned about proper hydration, this is especially true for those operating a machine traveling at extremely high speeds—mental acuity is crucial. In 1 study of 9 male stock car drivers during a NASCAR race, the average body-weight loss was 0.77%, and the mean sweat rate was 0.63 L/h.[32] Motorsport athletes may compete for several hours without a break, which makes it difficult to consume foods and fluids during competition. Depending on the type of car and race, some drivers may be able to drink water and sports drinks through hydration systems installed in their cars. Small amounts of solid foods may be consumed during a pit stop, which averages about 15 seconds, or if there is a red flag (eg, a race delay for a crash).[24,33] Such situations, however, are few and far between, so making sure that the driver is adequately fueled and hydrated before racing is crucial.

Not only is it very difficult for drivers to safely ingest fluids and food during the race, but the fire-protective clothing they must wear can also significantly impede heat loss.[26,28] This cloth is capable of resisting temperatures up to 700 °C, but it blocks ventilation to the surface of the skin. As the driver sweats, the clothing becomes soaked, and the transference of environmental heat to the driver's skin is increased, which exacerbates the problem.[34] Other environmental exposures are also of concern. In a study of 8 elite motorsport athletes driving a simulator, the combined effect of carbon monoxide and heat exposure resulted in greater sweat loss and increased core temperature compared with exposure to heat alone.[35] The specific mechanism for this effect is unknown.

ENERGY AVAILABILITY AND BODY COMPOSITION

In a sport focused on speed, any extra weight is dead weight. This is especially true with the ultralight sports cars used in Formula 1 racing.[36] Motorsport drivers want to optimize their strength, especially the upper body, while minimizing their overall weight. Achieving a low body fat percentage is a common goal among this population. Although some drivers may see the role that optimal fitness can play in improving their finishes, many have the eating habits and overall fitness of the general population. Jennifer Brunelli, MS, RDN, LDN, (email, November 8, 2022) works in private practice and has consulted with NASCAR teams. Many of the athletes with whom she works are involved in other outdoor sports and entertainment and therefore care about how their bodies look. She says, "underfueling, additional training outside of their team's gym, and heavy muscle building supplements are often used." The length of the season and frequent travel can make it difficult for drivers and their teams to develop consistent habits. "They are on the road or at the facility more often than they are home. They need to understand how to order and shop when on the road or they will not be successful." It is important to work not only with the individual driver to develop a realistic eating plan but also with the crew managers who may coordinate the food choices available, although many teams may not be set up to individualize food options on race days.

Expert Nutrition Tips

Following are some tips for working with motosports athletes:

- Danielle LaFata, MA, RDN, CSSD, (email, October 5, 2015) has worked in the past with many professional athletes, including those involved in motorsports, and notes that what separates a good driver from a great driver is their ability to focus for a full race. Racing involves significant physical and mental stress. LaFata frames her nutrition recommendations in the context that optimal fuel will help decrease the negative effects experienced before and after racing: fatigue, decreased stamina and focus, impaired reaction time, and poor recovery. Drivers often feel fatigued for days after a race, so nutrition strategies that aid in recovery should be a primary focus for them.
- Over the years that Brunneli (email, November 8, 2022) has worked with NASCAR teams, she has noticed that they have become more educated about the importance of nutrition and are demanding a higher level of care, including sweat testing and blood-work analysis.
- LaFata (email, October 5, 2015) notes that, in her experience, drivers may lose 1.4 to 2.7 kg in only a few hours. Dehydration is a certain route to fatiguing their muscles and brains and doing so quickly. A hydrated driver is a more mentally aware driver.

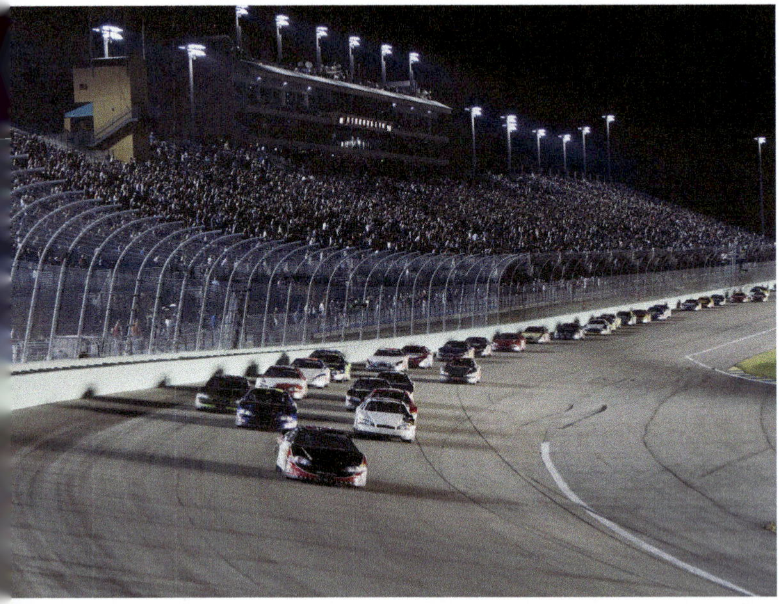

How to Get a Foot in the Door

Racing teams that work with an RDN often do so under the umbrella of other exercise professionals, such as certified strength and conditioning specialists, athletic trainers, and personal trainers. Having a background in these areas or building a network of professionals in exercise training can be a huge help. RDNs who want to break into this profession have to do their homework on the specific motorsport and be able to sell their services to a potentially skeptical audience. Partnering with other exercise professionals is an easier way to gain buy-in. Brunelli (email, November 8, 2022) started in motorsports through a connection that she had with strength coaches in NASCAR and then grew opportunities through word of mouth after showing her value to the team. She says that the opportunities are expanding. "Budgets are beginning to be approved to use for food and supplementation purchasing for the team as whole, so RDNs are becoming more and more valuable in these environments. There are also significant opportunities to support the corporate side of the team as well." Motorsport RDNs should be self-starters who are confident in their abilities and are authoritative and firm in their recommendations. Working with motorsport athletes is not for the timid. RDNs also need to be flexible. "This role is not 9 to 5. There are needs that often need to be addressed on a weekend and their schedules change if a race is delayed due to weather, pit crew members can change frequently in season due to performance or injury, and a much bigger focus on team collaboration with strength and condition and ATCs [certified athletic trainers] is necessary."

ARTISTIC PERFORMERS

The category of artistic performers is so vast and diverse that it could warrant its own book! Although dance may be the first sport that comes to mind, this category also includes cheerleading, figure skating, acrobatics, aerial arts, marching arts, music, theater, and more. Some of these overlap with other sports such as gymnastics (eg, cheerleading) or have their own dedicated sections in this text already (eg, figure skating). Athletes and the Arts,[37] a coalition of sports medicine, performing arts, and wellness organizations, provides many helpful resources and tools for this population. Dancers, marching artists, and musicians and actors are discussed in the following sections.

DANCE

Basic Physiological Demands

Ballet, jazz, modern, tap, hip-hop, ballroom, folk—the types of dance are as varied as the individuals who participate in them. Similar to gymnastics and figure skating, dance involves intermittent bursts of moderate-to-intense activity and predominantly uses the anaerobic system, although longer performances may have high aerobic demands as well.[38,39] Maximal oxygen consumption (VO_2 max) across many styles of dance, genders, and levels of technical ability has been estimated to range from 37 to 57 mL/kg/min.[39] Among female professional dancers, dance intensity can reach greater than 11 metabolic equivalents (METs), although most of a dancer's day is spent at about 3 METs.[40] Dancers are unusual among athletes in that even with a full day of rehearsal, they may burn only a few hundred calories per hour because of the stop-and-go nature of the activity. Their nutritional needs exceed those of the less-active, general population; however, their body-type expectations and potential societal pressures may create barriers to meeting these needs (Rachel Fine, MS, RDN, CSSD, email, September 11, 2022). Refer to Chapter 21 for specific recommendations on nutrition for intermittent, high-intensity sports.

Nutrition Issues

ENERGY AVAILABILITY AND BODY COMPOSITION

A majority of the research literature on dance has focused on female ballet dancers, particularly because of concerns about low energy intake and body composition. Among the different types of dance, ballet dancers tend to be the leanest and may have very low body fat percentages, resulting in higher rates of amenorrhea among female dancers.[38,41] Contributing to this situation is the fact that dancers tend to have low energy intakes (70%–80% of recommended) and are therefore at high risk of relative energy deficiency in sport (REDs) and EDs such as anorexia nervosa and bulimia nervosa. Energy intake among dancers has been reported as lower than that among matched controls.[41] In a study comparing 15 professional ballet dancers to nondancing control subjects matched by age, BMI, and fat-free mass (FFM), the energy intake of the dancers was significantly less (1,577 ± 89 kcal/d vs 2,075 ± 163 kcal/d). In addition, they had significantly lower resting metabolic rates (RMRs) and bone mineral densities (BMDs). These results support work by Kaufman et al,[42] who observed a significant positive correlation between the FFM-adjusted RMR and the BMD in the arms and spines of dancers compared with those of control subjects. The lower FFM-adjusted RMRs were predicted by dancers having a history of amenorrhea.

In a descriptive study of 26 female student dancers in South Africa, 24% of the dancers were assessed as having low energy availability (LEA) (<30 kcal per kilogram of FFM per day) compared to 8% of age-matched controls.[43] About 81% of the dancers were found to be in negative energy balance, with an average energy balance of −931 kcal/d. Keay et al[44] developed a Dance-Specific Energy Availability Questionnaire (DEAQ) to assess LEA in an international sample of mostly female dancers (n = 225; mean age = 20.5 years) along with some male dancers (n = 22; mean age = 22.5 years) training at the amateur and professional levels. LEA was reported by 57% of the female dancers and 29% of the male dancers. Of the females not taking hormonal contraception (n = 184), 33% experienced primary or secondary amenorrhea and 17% experienced oligomenorrhea in the previous year; 19% reported starting their periods at the age of 15 years or later.

Several studies have been published on the prevalence of EDs in this population. In a meta-analysis of 33 international studies published from 1966 to 2013, the prevalence of EDs among dancers in general was found to be 12% (range: 13.1%–20.5%), with that among ballet dancers reaching 16.4% (range: 1.9%–26.6%).[45] Compared with nondancer control subjects, dancers had a 3-fold higher risk of having an ED, particularly anorexia nervosa and other specified feeding or eating disorders. All included studies were of female dancers, and a majority of the study participants were dance students rather than professionals. Although it was not statistically assessed in this analysis, a higher number of cases of EDs occurred among students not attending elite ballet schools. Whether students in preprofessional programs are less likely to develop EDs or those with EDs are less likely to make it to the elite levels is unknown. In an assessment of ED risk using the Eating Disorder Inventory-3 (EDI-3), 69% of student dancers (18 of 26) were identified as at-risk compared to 39% of controls (10 of 26; $\chi^2 = 4.95$, $P = .025$).[43]

Wyon et al[46] assessed BMI and nutrition knowledge in student and professional ballet dancers and found that those dancers with disordered eating behaviors had lower levels of nutrition knowledge. In addition, the student dancers had lower BMIs (possibly because they had less muscle mass) and higher scores (which indicate higher concern) on the Eating Attitude Test-26 (EAT-26) screener. These results raise red flags, particularly among dance students, who, along with preprofessional and professional dancers, should be monitored closely. In studies of professional American ballet dancers, participants still had significantly higher EAT-26 scores than matched controls.[41,42] In 1 systematic review of disordered eating behaviors in dancers, the lifetime prevalence of EDs in professional dancers was 50%.[47] In a small (N = 15) group of professional ballet dancers, 40% met the criteria for the female athlete triad.[41] Among 31 collegiate modern dancers, the incidence of EDs was 12.9%.[48] Even if the more conservative estimates by Arcelus et al[45] are used, the rates of EDs in this population warrant vigilance among those who work with these athletes. Among professional dance companies, awareness of this issue has certainly increased, as have efforts to address EDs and healthy eating. The Dance/USA Taskforce on Dancer Health provides guidelines for screening dancers for health concerns, including nutrition, and they provide informational papers to guide health education amongst dance companies.[49] Nutrition knowledge may be improved through nutrition education interventions, but whether this translates into lasting behavior change and improved health overall is uncertain.[50]

Shannon Sterne, MS, MA, RDN, (email, July 29, 2015) is a dancer, choreographer, and former college instructor who runs her own Gyrotonic studio and has seen many types of disordered eating in the dance population, from fad diets to restrictive eating behaviors resulting in REDs. Among dance students in particular, Sterne has observed frequent meal skipping when they have back-to-back classes and rehearsals. Dancers usually do not like to have a full stomach before practices and performances because of tight clothing and demanding choreographies.[38] In addition, preperformance anxiety may have a negative impact on appetite, and performance days can be incredibly busy, with the venues often lacking ideal fueling options. It is therefore common for dancers to not eat within a couple of hours of a performance. Although performances themselves are relatively short, the demanding schedule could make maintaining adequate energy levels difficult.

Rachel Fine, MS, RDN, CSSD, (email, September 11, 2022) is a former professional dancer who is also a Certified Intuitive Eating Counselor and works with dancers of all levels. She sees a great deal of variation in what dancers may eat, but one commonality among many of them is an obsession with healthy eating and risk for disordered eating. She emphasizes the importance of first addressing a dancer's beliefs and emotions around food. "A dancer's relationship with food should be the first line of intervention, even prior to specific nutrition education."

Yasi Ansari, MS, RDN, CSSD, (email, October 19, 2022) is owner of Yasi Ansari Nutrition and a lifelong dancer who consults with dancers in ballet, tap, jazz, hip-hop, and lyrical dance, as well as performing artists in musical theater. She has observed an increase in "fear foods," such as carbohydrates, cow's milk, and animal products, among the dancers she counsels. She sees more of her clients following plant-based eating patterns and notes that "dancers are bombarded with food and diet messages from fellow dancers, parents, instructors, social media, etc, that can lead to unhealthy eating patterns." Situations that can be triggering for disordered eating include always facing the mirror while practicing their routines, being measured for costumes, long hours of training, and not wanting to "feel the food" as they get back on stage. Fine (email,

September 11, 2022) echoes Ansari's observations about the amount of nutrition misinformation from non-credible sources that dancers receive. "Many educators and coaches will intervene [on] a dancer's nutritional status and risk providing these dancers with triggering content that can lead to disordered eating behaviors." Fine has found that her clients have become more open to intuitive eating as this approach has gained visibility, and she uses it in her practice.

Deanna Busteed, MS, RDN, CSSD, (email, October 12, 2022) works at George Mason's Center for Sports Performance and also has a background in EDs. She has noticed an uptick in the number of EDs since the beginning of the COVID-19 pandemic among the dancers, cheerleaders, tumblers, and gymnasts with whom she works. "Many dancers experience REDs and are not menstruating." She highlights that "there is incredible pressure for dancers to remain thin while still being powerful and explosive," so she considers it important to focus on nutrient-dense foods. See Chapter 18 for more information on disordered eating and eating disorders.

INJURIES AND BONE HEALTH

Injuries have been studied more frequently among ballet dancers than other types of dancers. In an epidemiological review (5 studies) of injuries among preprofessional ballet dancers, injury rates per 1,000 training hours range from 0.8 to 2.9 injuries diagnosed by a medical professional, although the self-reported rates in 1 study were higher (4.7 times).[51] Most reported injuries appear to be related to overuse and to occur in the lower extremities, especially the feet, toes, and ankles. In 1 of the reviewed studies that assessed time lost from full participation because of injury, bone injuries resulted in the most time lost, with an average of 177 days lost for tibial stress fractures.[52] Along with LEA and menstrual disturbances among female dancers, ballet dancers experienced a prevalence of low BMD and osteopenia ranging from 10% to 46.5%.[47] Some researchers, however, have observed BMDs in dancers that were higher than or no different from those of nondancer controls.[53-55] There is evidence, however, that the BMDs of dancers are lower than those of athletes involved in other weight-bearing sports and that the non–weight-bearing sites are particularly at risk.[54,56] Compared to ballet dancers, those involved in other styles of dance (eg, modern dance and break dancing) may be more likely to experience traumatic injury and injury of the upper extremities.[57]

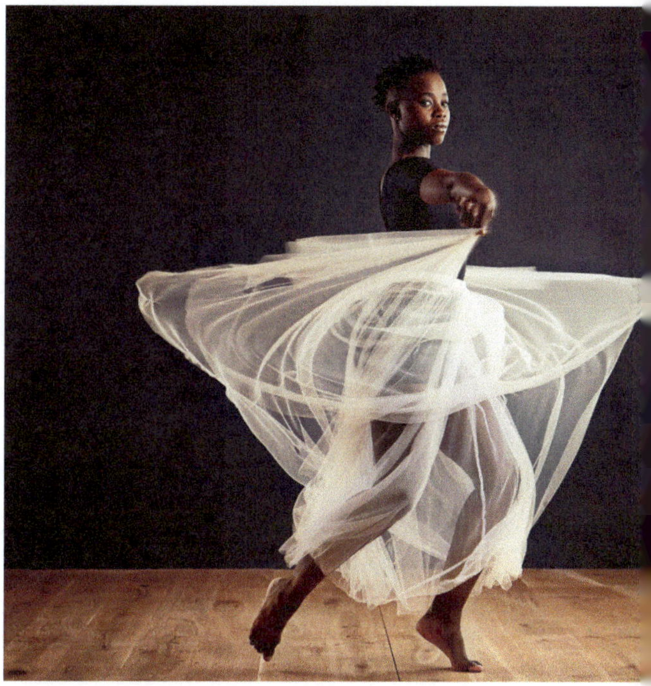

MICRONUTRIENT INTAKE

If dancers are not consuming adequate calories, they are at risk for various micronutrient deficiencies, with calcium, vitamin D, and iron being of particular concern. Adequate calcium intake is crucial for optimal bone health. In a study of 37 professional dance students, those who had the highest intakes of dietary calcium also had the highest BMD values.[53] Adolescents may be at particular risk for low dietary calcium. Khan et al[54] found that retired professional dancers self-reported inadequate calcium intake during their adolescence. In a study of 47 female adolescent ballet dancers in New Zealand, fewer than 40% met the daily recommendations for calcium, folate, magnesium, and selenium, and 28% were found to have suboptimal iron status.[58] In addition to poor dietary intake, the lack of sun exposure among dancers also puts them at risk for vitamin D deficiency.[59] Wolman et al[60] studied 19 professional ballet dancers in the winter and found that all were either insufficient or deficient in serum 25-hydroxyvitamin D. Although Doyle-Lucas et al[41] did not observe differences in macronutrient or micronutrient intakes between elite female dancers and lean controls (only energy intake was lower), the mean reported intakes for calcium (851 mg), vitamin D (5 mcg), and iron (13 mg) were still lower than recommended, even for nonathletes. A 4-month, randomized, double-blinded vitamin D intervention (120,000 IU over the course of 1 week) among 84 elite male and female adolescent ballet dancers resulted in a decrease in vitamin D deficiency and insufficiency and was negatively associated with the occurrence of traumatic injury.[46]

Expert Nutrition Tips

Following are some tips for working with dancers:

- Although both Sterne (email, July 29, 2015) and Fine (email, September 11, 2022) take a "food-first" approach, they frequently advise their clients to take a vitamin D or vitamin D plus calcium supplement because of the high risk of deficiency.[60] For those with more restrictive diets (eg, vegetarian, celiac), an iron-containing multivitamin–mineral supplement may also be warranted.
- Among high-level dancers who tour, finding appropriate foods is another major concern. Sterne (email, July 29, 2015) encourages her clients to pack meal-replacement bars for emergencies and to scout out dining options in advance. Busteed (email, October 12, 2022) advises that "[an] RDN needs to be compassionate, open-minded, and creative. Many times, dancers are training in studios for many consecutive hours and are in need of quick, easy, and creative ideas that they can easily implement."
- It is important for an RDN to understand not only the physical demands of the sport but the psychological aspects as well. This can vary greatly depending on the level of the dancer and the genre. Sterne (email, July 29, 2015) explains, "This art form is often very deeply intertwined with the dancer's ego and a drive for perfection. Sometimes, dancing is more important than their health." She encourages clients to view their bodies as instruments that need enough fuel to function at their peak. Ansari (email, October 19, 2022) finds satisfaction in "helping dancers tackle their fears around food and learning how to shift the focus from food and physical appearance to food and its impact on energy, strength building, and overall dance performance."
- Like most athletes, dancers can benefit from frequent reminders to take a break and eat. Ansari (email, October 19, 2022) says that "dancing is like another muscle and a part them, that some may forget how much energy it actually takes to dance, especially for long hours at a time."
- Fine (email, September 11, 2022) notes that RDNs who work with this population need to be both compassionate and realistic. They need compassion to understand the psychology behind aesthetic sports because it is very difficult to steer dancers away from the ideal body image goal, and they need to be realistic and frank about the importance of maintaining a healthy weight to prevent malnutrition and injury. Her goal for clients is that they achieve a happy, nonrestrictive, and realistic lifestyle in which dessert is an acceptable indulgence.

How to Get a Foot in the Door

Fine (email, September 11, 2022) says that it is crucial to have "familiarity with the dance world and the unique physical and emotional demands that go alongside it." Ansari (email, October 19, 2022) emphasizes that an understanding of the culture and history of dance and the perceived pressure to maintain a lean physique is crucial. "I think it is vital for the RDN to have experience with athletes who have struggled with an eating disorder and disordered eating." In Sterne's (email, July 29, 2015) experience, most professional companies either cannot afford to have an RDN on staff or do not prioritize it. She also notes that, since the COVID-19 pandemic, "dance company budgets are now tighter than ever." However, that does not mean that companies are not open to working with an RDN. In their 2011 report, Dance/USA recommended that professional dance companies have a nutrition specialist as part of the in-house team.[49] This person is encouraged to provide educational sessions to dancers and staff at least at the beginning of the season and to arrange periodic check-ins. Recommended seminar topics include self-awareness and body image (especially at a young age), EDs, cooking demonstrations and healthy food preparation, smoking cessation, stress management, and issues of special interest to females (eg, amenorrhea). An RDN with a broad range of experience in health-related topics would have a definite advantage. "Dance companies and studios are understanding the importance of nutrition education. In recent years, there has been a shift, and nutrition education is becoming part of a dancer's curriculum" (Ansari, email, October 19, 2022). Contacting a dance company and seeing how they are addressing these recommendations is a good place to start. In addition, many dance schools will offer a 1-hour nutrition class during their summer intensive program (Fine, email, September 11, 2022; Busteed, email, October 12, 2022; Ansari, email, October 19, 2022). Fine (email, September 11, 2022) suggests that RDNs who want to work with dancers individually should contact dance schools and offer to teach a group workshop for a given age group or topic. This is one way to generate interest in nutrition and establish rapport with the dancers and hopefully make them more willing to reach out for private counseling either in person or via telehealth. Finally, networking with other health care professionals such as sports medicine physicians, orthopedists, physical therapists, and mental health professionals specializing in eating disorders and disordered eating is a great way to attract future referrals and ensure a balanced treatment program for the client (Busteed, email, October 12, 2022; Ansari, email, November 27, 2022).

Box 24.3 highlights a form of dance known as aerial arts.[61-70]

BOX 24.3 Spotlight on Aerial Arts[61-70]

An *aerialist* includes anyone who "performs feats in the air or above the ground, especially on the trapeze."[61] Aerialists may incorporate yoga moves (yoga aerials) and dance (dance aerials) in their performances.[62,63] Aerial arts originated from circus arts and employs different apparatuses. Some of the most common apparatuses are silks, hammocks, hoops, and poles. Silks and hammocks can use the same material (a long piece of fabric), but the difference is in how it is hung. Silks have one end of the fabric attached to an overhead anchor (rigging), whereas hammocks make a folded loop out of the fabric and have both ends anchored at the same point above. Hoops, also called lyras, are circular apparatuses that are usually made of steel; they resemble hula hoops and can be suspended from the ceiling.[64] Poles are anchored to the ground, and athletes climb up, spin from, hang off, flip onto, jump off, and/or invert themselves on the poles.[65] Whereas aerial and circus arts are centuries old, their emergence as a sport for the masses likely came out of the Canadian acrobatic troupe Cirque du Soleil in the 1990s.[62] Since then, aerial arts have become mainstream at both the amateur and professional levels. The International Pole Sports Federation (IPSF) formed in 2009 and has held world championships since 2012, endeavoring to have pole and aerial sports included in the Olympic games.[66]

Research on the physical demands of aerial arts such as silks and poles is scant, with 1 published study on the physiological profile of recreational aerial athletes and a handful on pole dancing in individuals at various levels of training and experience.[67-70] Aerial arts are full-body activities that require, and can develop, flexibility, balance, strength, and cardiorespiratory fitness.[67] At present, there appears to be no published research on the nutritional habits or needs of aerial artists, and most recommendations have been based on those for gymnasts and dancers.

Lauren MacLeod, RDN, (email, October 7, 2022) is the lead dietitian for Outdoor Women's Wellness and is a writer and nutrition consult for outdoor and wellness brands. She started training in the aerial arts in 2017 as a creative outlet when injuries kept her from continuing her dance career and quickly fell in love with it. "I started by taking aerial classes, and when the other students found [out that] I was a sports dietitian, the questions flooded in." She quickly discovered, however, that aerialists struggled with many of the same nutrition difficulties as dancers. She has since worked with a range of aerialists from recreationalists to professionals who perform at festivals. She notes that "most aerialists haven't done this their whole life—they found aerial from another path. Many, like me, are former dancers looking for another way to move and flow. Others have never danced but come from a climbing background and want to use their strength in a creative way. It can be a frustrating art at times, but once an athlete falls in love with aerial, it becomes a lifelong journey."

Although aerials share many similarities with other sports, there are some unique challenges, particularly an aerialist's interaction with the air. MacLeod (email, October 7, 2022) stated that "Unlike other athletes, suddenly you're working in a three-dimensional space, including spinning, hanging upside down, and dropping. All this movement can

Continued on next page

BOX 24.3 *Spotlight on Aerial Arts*[61-70] (CONTINUED)

create complications when it comes to ensuring aerialists are eating enough without losing their lunch." Nutrition counseling typically involves helping the aerialist find easily digested foods and optimizing timing so that they are not eating too close to or too long before training. They also run the risk of getting dizzy and nauseous. "High-carb snacks like candied ginger are perfect for providing carbs and settling the stomach." MacLeod also acknowledges that, as with all artistic sports, body image is very important. "Especially in the professional sphere, there is an unhealthy obsession with appearing thin, plus the false belief that you have to be under a certain weight in order to be taken seriously as an aerialist. I process thoughts and feelings about body image with clients and encourage them to nourish for their training goals, not for the body they think they should have."

MacLeod (email, October 7, 2022) highly recommends working with this population if you have personal experience in dance, aerial arts, or circus; "it's just so niche." After she started taking classes and received questions from fellow students, she was able to use that flood of interest to express to her instructors the need for nutrition education. "They were happy to work with me because of my personal experience with aerial."

MARCHING ARTS

Description

Marching arts include any group of fine-arts–related activities that are closely associated with wind music.[71] This includes but is not necessarily limited to classifications such as marching band, drum corps, pep band, show band, color guard, winter guard, and indoor percussion. Historically, the first organized marching bands were military bands. This style is characterized by marching in straight formations and can include specific field units such as drum and bugle corps and pipe bands. It is commonly seen in parades. Corps-style bands differ from military bands in that the step sizes and formations are constantly changing, and the music style can vary from marches to contemporary rock music. Corps-style is probably the most intense and competitive category of marching band. Finally, show bands are focused on crowd entertainment, such as half-time shows at football games.[72] Whereas the corps band season runs from May to August, high school and collegiate military and show bands perform at least through the fall football season and usually march in spring parades. In addition to the instrumentalists, corps and show bands typically have a color guard and dancers. A college marching band may have upward of 300 participants of all shapes, sizes, and levels of fitness.

Basic Physiological Demands

Classifying the marching arts in terms of its physiological demands can be tricky. When considering 12-hour rehearsal days as well as parade marching, it is an endurance activity. Erdmann et al[73] estimated the exercise intensity of adolescent marching band members in a laboratory setting as 4.5 to 6 METs. This is similar to the intensity levels of recreational activities such as tennis, easy swimming, golfing, and mowing the lawn. Elite-level drum corps members, however, are likely on par with athletes in intermittent, high-intensity sports.[72] Drum corps programs are 10 to 12 minutes in duration, and a summer tour usually consists of 25 to 40 competitions.[74] It is worth noting that the energy cost of the participant will vary widely depending on the instrument (eg, bass drum vs flute) and role (instrumentalist vs flag bearer) played. Performance anxiety has also been shown to contribute to elevated heart rates before and during a performance.[75] Finally, as with other outdoor sports, performers will be exposed to all types of weather, from sweltering heat and humidity to wind, rain, and snow. Refer to Chapters 21 and 22 for more information on the energy demands for intermittent and endurance sports.

Nutrition Issues

BODY COMPOSITION AND CHRONIC DISEASE RISK

Marching artists vary considerably in their fitness levels and overall health. In a study by Sharma et al[76] on the association between diet and cardiovascular disease risk factors among 232 university marching band, dance team, and cheer squad members (n = 225 for band members), 45% were classified as overweight or obese (BMI ≥25), and 30% of women and 4.3% of men had high waist-to-hip ratios. In a 2022 national survey of college students, the prevalence of overweight and obesity was estimated to be approximately 40%, indicating that university marching band members are not necessarily in any better physical condition than the average college student.[77] The Sharma et al study[76] suggests that risk for cardiovascular disease and other chronic conditions among collegiate marching artists is also a concern because 7.8% of participants were found to have high blood glucose (>110 mg/dL), 10.3% had high total blood cholesterol (>200 mg/dL), and 14.7% had high systolic blood pressure (>140 mm Hg). These values are lower than those reported in a study by Morrell et al[78] published during a similar time frame on the general college population using the National Heart, Lung, and Blood Institute (NHLBI) guidelines for metabolic syndrome diagnosis. It is worth noting that the NHLBI guidelines are more stringent[79] than those used in the study by Sharma et al.[76] Depending on the criteria used, this could mean that the risk for cardiovascular or metabolic diseases among university marching band members may be underestimated.

Note, however, that drum and bugle corps members appear to have lower BMIs compared to members of other forms of marching band, which is likely due to their higher intensities of activity. In a longitudinal study of Drum Corps International (DCI) world-class performers (n = 501), 37% had BMIs that would classify them as overweight or obese.[74] By the end of the competitive season (3 months later), only 23% were classified as overweight or obese. After a 1-year follow-up, however, participants' BMIs had returned to their initial levels. In a more recent study comparing DCI members and nonelite drum corps members, the average BMIs were found to be 23.4 ± 3.7 and 25.0 ± 5.8, respectively.[80] It is worth noting that, among female study participants, 71% (76 of 107) of the female DCI members reported menstrual cycle changes during the season. This could have impacts on their energy availability and risk for REDs.

DIETARY PATTERNS AND HYDRATION

To date, only a few studies have been published on the dietary habits of marching band members.[76,80] Most recently, in a self-administered survey of 356 drum corps participants, the overall healthy eating index score was 58.8 ± 10.3, with only 1 participant falling within the "good" range with a score greater than 80.[80] The recommendations for fatty acid ratio, sodium limits, and limits on empty calories were met by only 8%, 2%, and 7% of participants, respectively. Participants were closest to meeting the recommendations by food group for protein foods (60%) and whole fruits (51%). Regarding meal-skipping behaviors, nonelite drum corps participants were more likely to skip meals than DCI members. In Sharma et al's[76] survey of 232 marching band, dance, and cheer participants, 85% consumed fewer than 5 servings of fruits and vegetables per day. Higher intakes of both grains (including non-whole grains) and alcohol were positively associated with higher BMI values. No data have been collected on the total energy intake of this population and how it aligns with total energy expenditure. Among high school programs, parents and booster clubs may provide meals during long competition days, or band members may have to rely on what is available at stadium concession stands. When meals are provided, choices may be limited and difficult for participants who have specialized dietary needs or requests (eg, gluten-free or vegetarian).

Marching artists are at a particular risk for fluid imbalance, especially during early-season training camps when they may spend all day outside.[72,76,81] Emerson et al[82] studied 19 collegiate marching band members at rehearsals and football games and observed that the maximum core body temperature at games was significantly higher than at that rehearsals (39.1 ± 1.1 °C vs 38.4 ± 0.7 °C, $P = .003$). This may be because the maximum game time was more than twice as long as the mean rehearsal time (260.5 ± 47.7 minutes vs 102.8 ± 19.8 minutes). The fluid consumption rates of the study participants were higher than their sweat rates, minimizing percent body mass loss; however, 63.6% of the time, the participants reported to games hypohydrated. It is also worth noting that maximal core temperature was significantly predicted by the wet-bulb globe temperature, the relative humidity, the ground surface, the use of mental health medications, and the number of hours of sleep. In a noncontrolled assessment of hydration management among high

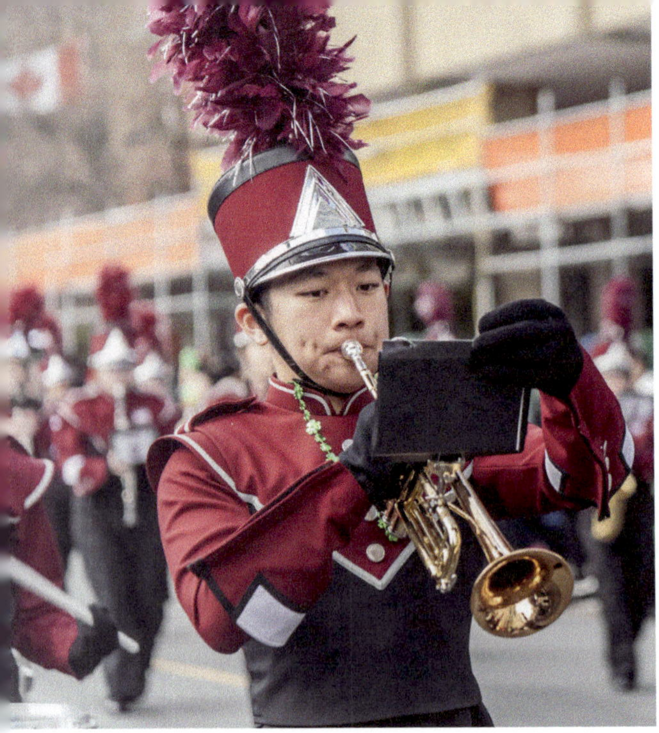

school marching band students, barriers to adequate fluid intake included the logistical difficulties of taking the time to break formation, participants not wanting to call attention to themselves if they were having a problem, and the lack of training in health-related issues of most music directors.[81]

Expert Nutrition Tips

Following are some tips for working with marching artists:

- Julie Brake, MS, RDN, (email, October 31, 2022) is an Atlanta-based dietitian who works in private practice in family nutrition, sports nutrition, and the prevention and treatment of disordered eating. She has had clients in the marching arts and helped develop a culinary nutrition guide for DCI. She says that getting a clear picture of the marching artist's activity is an important first step. "While it [marching arts] has not traditionally been considered a sport, the level of physical activity required can be very high. Asking questions and listening to the artist to determine the level of activity is crucial to adequately address nutrition needs and concerns."
- Brake (email, October 31, 2022) emphasizes the importance of hydration, often recommending sports drinks because of the large amounts of sweat loss in this population, particularly among those carrying heavy instruments. In a report on the fueling of high school marching band members, Vepraskas[81] found that providing them with fuel belts to hold their water bottles was an easy way to provide fluids without interrupting rehearsals. Subjective feedback from these students included improved mental acuity, more productive rehearsals, feeling better overall, and fewer episodes of heat-related stress.
- In addition to fluids, RDNs can provide convenient snack options for consumption before and during rehearsals that can withstand extreme temperatures (eg, trail mix, fruit cups, jerky, nut butter crackers, granola bars, fruit pouches or purees, pretzels, and dry cereal).[83] Brake (email, October 31, 2022) says that the timing of nutrition during intense rehearsal schedules is important. "Eating and drinking during rehearsals or band camps can be very difficult and limited to specific, sometimes narrow, time windows. This can lead to limited nutrition during activity and extreme hunger and thirst after activity."
- Education should not only take place with the marching artist, but it is also important to get directors, parents, and booster club members on board as potential allies. As with any large group, there will be a wide range of food preferences and special dietary needs. Some parents and boosters are less nutrition savvy than others, so there is a role for the RDN in educating and providing guidance to these supporters.

How to Get a Foot in the Door

The literature on the health of marching artists is sparse, but there is an increasing awareness on the importance of their overall health. The National Association of Schools of Music, which is the national accrediting agency for music and music-related disciplines, requires that music program policies, protocols, and operations reflect attention to health maintenance and injury prevention among musicians.[84] RDNs can use this accreditation requirement as a way to market their skill set. Although many marching directors are often receptive to nutritional guidance and resources, they may need to have its importance explained to them. This takes time and effort on the part of the RDN to work with directors, parents, and boosters. Brake (email, October 31, 2022) recommends connecting with local schools, particularly those with very competitive marching arts programs. Offering to give a short presentation at camp or a parent/booster meeting is a good place to start. Brake has also found her background in disordered eating to be very helpful given that the marching arts are highly appearance-driven. "I started working with marching artists because of my work with disordered eating and sports nutrition." She highlights that this can be a fun population to work with because they are typically "very motivated by wanting to improve performance . . . and have great input into how to accomplish nutrition and hydration goals."

MUSICIANS AND ACTORS

Physiological and Nutrition Issues

Actors, vocalists, and instrumental musicians are a relatively untapped group in the field of sports nutrition. They have diverse needs that can vary considerably because of the physicality of their craft (sitting vs whole-body movement), the length of time of a performance (minutes vs hours), and aesthetic expectations (eg, needing to look a certain way for a specific role). Among this population, it is important to note that there is a paucity of data in the research literature, so most of the information in this section is based on expert experience.

A limited number of studies on the physicality of performing artists have been performed. Playing a wind instrument while seated is estimated to expend approximately 1.8 METs, whereas drumming in a rock band is a high-intensity activity of about 8.1 METs, an estimated energy expenditure of 623 kcal/h, and a peak heart rate of 186 beats/min.[85,86] Libby Parker, MS, RDN, CEDRD, (oral communication, September 23, 2022) is a Manhattan-based dietitian who has personally been involved in musical theater and has work experience in private practice, corporate wellness, campus nutrition, and eating disorder treatment centers. She says that the schedules of theater performers are so packed that optimizing the timing of fueling, and options available, are critical. "They [performers] run through McDonald's, or they're not eating until 11 PM, and they've gone from breakfast to 11 PM without eating and then having work and rehearsal and dancing. . . . This is sports nutrition directly!"

Parker (oral communication, September 23, 2022) notes the importance for vocal performers of caring for the vocal cords and how timing and accessibility can be difficult. Some vocalists avoid dairy products because of concerns of excess mucous production; however, reports of this side effect of dairy appear to be mostly anecdotal. What is not debatable is the importance of hydration. Vocalists can use systemic means of hydration (eg, ingesting fluid) or superficial or surface methods (eg, humidifiers).[87] During rehearsals, "people tend to be pretty good about keeping their water bottle with them and drinking, but when they get to performances, it can be a little more hit or miss unless they've really locked it in." Parker has personally experienced heat stroke on stage, a situation exacerbated by the bright lights and limited access to fluids. In addition, there is also the rule of no eating once performers are in costume. "Unlike someone on the sidelines at a soccer game who can just pound something down, you step off stage, and you have a couple of scenes before you're back on. You still can't eat anything."

Kathy LaBella, RDN, CDN, CSSD, ACE-CMES/CPT, (oral communication, September 23, 2022) works in private practice consulting with a wide range of performers including professional musicians (vocal and instrumental) and radio announcers. She got her start as a sports dietitian at an athletic club and then became a certified medical exercise specialist. She agrees that feeding around performances is difficult and that "timing is everything." Even if the performer has time during the day before an evening performance to eat, nerves (even among seasoned performers) are common. "I was working with this one percussionist, a drummer, and he said, 'I get the jitters and an upset stomach, and I can't eat.' And it's true. I've talked to so many [performers], and so what they do is they starve themselves, and they get what's called drummer's fatigue. It is the same thing as a runner hitting the wall." Drummers aren't the only performers at risk for fatigue and/or overuse injuries, which can happen to almost any musician. Depending on the performer's schedule, they may have days without a break in performances. Most professional traveling musicians are still on their own for meal procurement (ie, no personal chef) and need education about how to eat on the road. Because most performances are in the evening, restaurants are usually closed by the time musicians are done, so planning ahead is important (LaBella, oral communication, September 23, 2022; Parker, oral communication, September 23, 2022).

Late nights, varied schedules, and long commutes are likely to cause many performers to resort to caffeine or other drugs to stay awake and alert. For vocal performers, caffeine has often been discouraged because of concerns that it may lead to dehydration. There is some limited evidence that moderate caffeine consumption (eg, 100-mg dose) does not appear to have an impact on vocal quality, although anecdotal reports indicate that many performers may be consuming much more than this.[88] Parker (oral communication, September 23, 2022) says that, among performers she knows, "caffeine is huge . . . whether it's coffee or energy drinks." LaBella (oral communication, September 23, 2022) adds that alcohol use can also be a concern, particularly among performers who get complimentary drinks and also because of the lack of venues open for food after performances.

Limited research has been published on disordered eating and body image among musical and theater performers compared to dancers. In a review of 10 studies on EDs in nondance performing artists by Kapsetaki and Easmon,[89] study heterogeneity and variable quality led to inconsistent results across studies, resulting in no clear picture on the prevalence of eating disorders among this population. In Parker's (oral communication, September 23, 2022) experience, she sees a lot of similarities between musical theater performers and dancers. "They are very much presenting their body type first, and they are getting cast based on what they look like as a part of their package. So, it's not strictly performance-based, even though it should be so." This can lead to performers falling into diet traps, skipping meals, and resorting to substance abuse, such as smoking, to push off hunger. More recently, since the COVID-19 pandemic, she has noticed that performers have been more vocal about what they need to do to take care of themselves. LaBella (oral communication, September 23, 2022) echoes this observation, reporting that she has had performing artists reach out to her wanting to become more in-tune with their bodies.

Expert Nutrition Tips

Following are some tips for working with musicians and actors:

- Timing is key. Both LaBella (oral communication, September 23, 2022) and Parker (oral communication, September 23, 2022) emphasize the importance of developing personalized hydration and fueling plans that provide consistent nutrition while offering flexibility amid chaotic schedules and late-night performances. If nerves are a problem, LaBella recommends consuming a larger carbohydrate meal the day before to top off carbohydrate stores, followed by smaller meals and plenty of fluid throughout the day. Performers should consider juice or slushies (low in dairy) if they struggle to get solid food down. It is also important to understand that performance days can be very different than rehearsal days—sometimes, they are less time-demanding, but fueling could be difficult because of nerves.
- Traveling performers need to plan ahead. If they are staying in a bus or hotel, they may have only a microwave available, if that. LaBella (oral communication, September 23, 2022) has her clients come up with a packed food list of simple snacks and meals that they prepare in advance and that require minimal equipment. If they are performing in a club and have access to food there, the RDN should provide suggestions for postperformance snacks or meals that provide a balanced mix of carbohydrates and proteins. If the performers live locally and are commuting home, the same principles apply. They should be prepared and make consuming a healthy meal or snack as convenient and easy as possible.

How to Get a Foot in the Door

If an RDN does not have a background in theater or music, LaBella (oral communication, September 23, 2022) emphasizes that having a passion for it is important. She encourages practitioners interested in working with this population to watch performances and get to know the performers. LaBella also recommends having a background or taking courses in exercise physiology and learning about body mechanics. This is a great population to work with through telehealth because of their variable schedules and potential travel. It is still important, however, to get out there and observe performances. Also, Parker (oral communication, September 23, 2022) emphasizes that many performing artists do not make much money. "They're always kind of hustling for the next thing. They're in a show, and they're auditioning for their next one, because they know their contract is ending. They can go without work for long periods of time, and that can be hard financially and can lead to lack of access to food or a variety of food and health care in general." Therefore, Parker says, it is crucial for the RDN to demonstrate their value by "showing that nutrition is a really important part of taking care of their instrument." An RDN's ability to share specific examples of how they have helped other clients is an important asset. Parker loves working with this population and sees this as a way to provide solid nutrition advice that is not just dieting. She says that it is crucial to know what the lifestyle is like and that the key to building a successful practice in this field is meeting performers and networking with the performing arts community.

ESPORTS

Description

What exactly is a "sport"? The Oxford English Dictionary defines *sport* as "an activity involving physical exertion and skill, especially one regulated by set rules or customs in which an individual or team competes against another or others."[90] The first video game competition took place in 1972 at Stanford University, and the question of whether video games should be classified as "sport" or not has been up for debate ever since.[91] What cannot be disputed, however, is the rapid growth and popularity of gaming and, more specifically, the electronic sports (or esports) industry—both are here to stay. *Esports* is a form of competition using video games that often take the form of organized, multiplayer competitions between individuals or between teams.[92] It is important to note that esports differ from playing video games as a recreational activity (general gaming) in that they are organized and highly competitive.[93] There are many different genres of games, but the most popular are multiplayer online battle arena games (eg, *League of Legends*, *Dota*), first-person shooter games (eg, *Valorant*), fighting games (eg, *Street Fighter*), real-time strategy games (eg, *Starcraft*), card games (eg, *Hearthstone*, *Magic: the Gathering*), and sports games like the *FIFA World Cup* (Casey Thomas, MS, RDN, oral communication, October 3, 2022).[92] See Box 24.4 for definitions used in esports.[94]

BOX 24.4 Common Gameplay Types in Esports[9]

Battle royale game	Form of first-person-shooter (FPS) game that blends last-person-standing gameplay with the survival, exploration, and scavenging elements of a survival game
Exergame	Game that is used as a form of fitness by tracking body movement or reaction time
Fighting game	Game that involves combat between 2 or more players, usually hand-to-hand combat and often some form of martial arts
FPS	Game centered on gun- and other weapon-based combat in a first-person perspective, with the player experiencing the action through the eyes of the protagonist
Multiplayer online battle arena (MOBA) game	Form of strategy game in which 2 teams of players compete against each other on a predefined battlefield and each player controls a single character with a set of distinctive abilities that can improve over the course of the game and contribute to the team's overall strategy
Real-time strategy (RTS)	Game that is ongoing in a defined level where a player is usually competing against 1 other opponent and both start out with equal amounts of resources; once the game starts, there are no breaks
Role-playing game (RPG)	Game in which the player controls 1 or more in-game characters in a defined world

Esports leagues exist at many levels from recreational to high school, collegiate, and professional, with most participants associated with a team.[92] No overarching regulatory body exists for all esports; instead, several associations of different professional teams have formed around the world (eg, International Esports Federation, World Esports Association, Korean e-Sports Association). Similarly, at the collegiate level, esports are not currently regulated by the National Collegiate Athletic Association, but instead are regulated by independent associations, with the largest in the United States being the National Association of Collegiate Esports (NACE). Its membership includes more than 260 colleges and universities, including a small number each from Canada and Puerto Rico.[95] The publisher of the game typically regulates the competition and dictates the rules, so there are no standardized regulations, and competition lengths (minutes to many hours) and formats (single- or double-elimination, group stages) can vary widely (Casey Thomas, MS, RDN, oral communication, October 3, 2022).[92] Generally, esports are played in tournament formats where individuals or teams participate in qualifying matches before entering a tournament. These can be virtual or physical events that are played on a local area network (LAN) in front of a live audience. A LAN is a computer network that interconnects computers within a limited area, resulting in less lag time and a higher-quality experience and decreasing the risk of cheating compared to an online game.

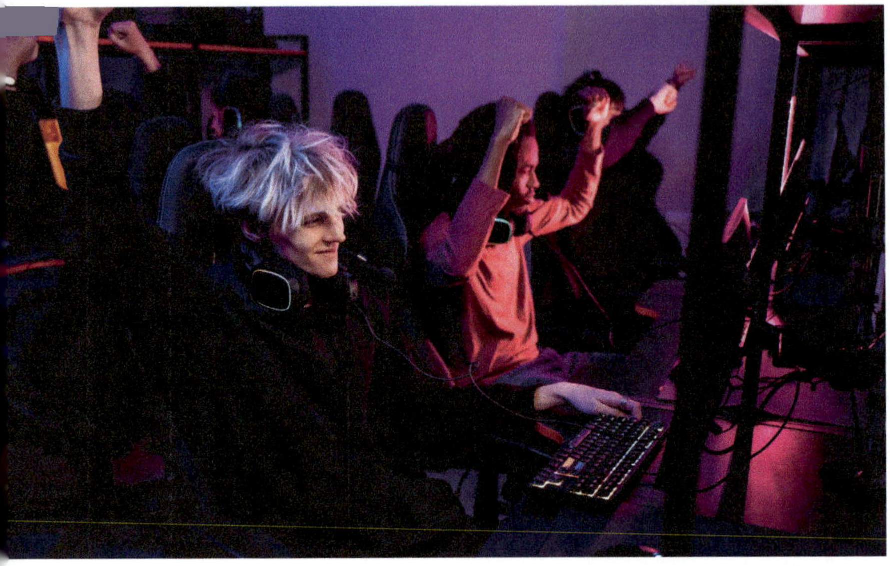

Although actual participation in esports has not been clearly measured, global viewership via online streaming media platforms in 2022 was estimated to be 432.1 million people, with about half of those being regular viewers (enthusiasts).[96] Viewership for the League of Legends World Championship Finals, for example, has rivaled that of the SuperBowl.[97] The largest single-game earnings by 1 individual in 2021 was almost $7 million.[98] Collegiate esport club teams started appearing in the United States in about 2009, with many schools now offering esports as a varsity sport including scholarship opportunities.[99]

Even though esports competitions are open to all genders, experts estimate that 35% of all participants are female but the professional ranks are heavily male-dominated (95% male).[100] Currently, longevity in the professional ranks is limited, with many players joining professional teams in their teens and retiring by their mid-20s (Thomas, oral communication, October 3, 2022).[101] Esports are popular worldwide, but they are most dominant and widely viewed in Asia.

Physiological Demands

Whereas most research in this area has been on video gaming in general and is not specific to competitive esports, a handful of studies have focused on the specific physiological demands of esports. Going back to the definition of *sport* as an activity involving physical exertion and skill, it can be argued that esports require both.[90] In a study of 14 males participating in a live, collegiate tournament, their mean heart rate (HR) during competition was 131 bpm, and their average peak HR during competition reached 188 bpm.[102] These values are higher than in a study that did not take place during an actual competition in which the peak HR was found to be 120 bpm, indicating that the environment or type of game may make a difference in HR response.[103] In a case report of a male playing a 30-minute video game compared to riding for 30 minutes on a cycle ergometer at a matched heart rate (where the matching is achieved by adjusting the cycling intensity), the peak heart rate while the participant was playing the game was 137 bpm even though his VO_2 max and energy expenditure did not change from rest and were 3 times lower than the values observed when he was cycling.[104] One would expect that exergaming, a less common competition within esports, would increase energy expenditure because of the active movement required. Most research on this topic, however, is on video gaming in children rather than on organized competition.[105] The cognitive requirements of esports share commonalities with those of nondigital sports in that they involve strong motor skills, mental agility, and quick reaction times (Thomas, oral communication, October 3, 2022).[93,105]

Some experts have raised concerns that participation in esports encourages young people to be less physically active and could contribute to health problems later in life. In a survey of 65 collegiate varsity esports players, researchers found that the players practiced between 3 and 10 hours per day.[106] In a scoping review of 33 studies evaluating the associations between esports and health, the percentage of esports players who said that they exercised regularly ranged from 65.0% to 88.7%, which is higher than the average rate among the general population. However, the percentage of players reporting that they did not do any type of physical activity ranged from 11.3% to 40.0%.[93] The authors of this scoping review concluded that esports players, particularly at higher levels, showed "satisfactory lifestyle habits" that did not appear to be worse than those of non-esports players. Overuse injuries among esports players do appear to be common, with the most frequent complaints being eye fatigue followed by pain in the neck, back, wrist, and hands. Sitting in the same position in front of a screen for hours, sometimes including during the night, may have a negative impact on sleep hygiene.[105]

Nutrition Issues

DIET QUALITY

Casey Thomas, MS, RDN, (oral communication, October 3, 2022) is a sports dietitian who has experience working with collegiate and professional athletes of many different sports and now specializes as a private consultant to professional and collegiate esports athletes. He highlights many challenges but also areas for improvement in this population. Among the professional teams with whom he works, players are usually in their teens or early 20s, come from all over the world, and are living with teammates or on their own. "Understanding who they are is really important. You get a lot of international kids, and they just miss their home-cooked foods." This can be difficult if a team has a private chef and everyone has different food preferences. Middle-tier teams may have a manager who orders all the food and may not have any concerns about nutritional quality. Lower-tier teams may provide food stipends and leave athletes to purchase food on their own.

Thomas (oral communication, October 3, 2022) also says that, compared to other athletes in traditional sports, "the amount of picky eaters in esports is significantly higher. It stems from a lack of nutrition knowledge as well as a lack of being in an established system since they were a kid. . . . They're living with their parents, and then, all of a sudden, a team says, 'We want to sign you for $2 million. Do you want to come?' They're young, with limited experience taking care of themselves, but agree anyway. They'll start ordering in all their food because it's easy." Some of the professional esports athletes that with whom Thomas has worked may sign a contract and then move into a place without a kitchen and nothing more than a refrigerator. "So, some of them are going to Google, 'good meal prep,' and they'll look at the first link, and it's gonna require all the sheet pans and that kind of stuff . . . So then they just say, 'I'm just gonna go order from Doordash.'"

Thomas (oral communication, October 3, 2022) also sees a lack of understanding among players about the link between nutrition and their performance, let alone health overall. He emphasizes that, even though esports are largely cognitive, he has seen many professionals retiring in their 20s because of health issues such as musculoskeletal injuries and type 2 diabetes. Some teams are starting to take notice. "They [team owners] are recognizing that physical health is important, especially if you want longevity with these players. . . . So, you are seeing things like personal trainers and strength coaches who come in. From there, it's easy to tack on nutritional considerations to whatever the physical stuff is that they're doing."

One of Thomas' (oral communication, October 3, 2022) main goals is to optimize players' cognitive performance, and he identifies 3 main arms for this: (1) remove the negative, (2) improve the hardware of the brain, and (3) improve the software of the brain. To begin, he evaluates anything that the players are doing that may acutely impair their performance, health, or recovery, such as excessive alcohol intake. Thomas defines the "hardware" as the raw materials of the brain, such as fluid, omega-3 fats (particularly docosahexaenoic acid), and micronutrients for efficient metabolic functioning. Because the brain is composed mostly of water, maintaining adequate hydration is crucial. Long competitions with few or no opportunities for fluid intake increase the risk of dehydration. In addition, water may not always be the go-to choice, particularly if events are sponsored by beverage companies. Finally, Thomas defines the "software" as all of the metabolic reactions occurring in the brain. He says that the main way to address this is by "ensuring good vascular health, and specifically methods to increase brain perfusion. . . . There's significant decreases in brain blood flow that occur across a day of sedentary behaviors." This can be improved by increased movement, as well as nutrients important for brain health such as essential fats and high-nitrate foods.

CAFFEINE AND NOOTROPICS

Caffeine-containing products, especially energy drinks, are very popular among this population, and the companies that make these products are major industry sponsors.[107] Thomas (oral communication, October 3, 2022) says that "the quick-fix mindset is real," and this population is very prone to reach for caffeine (eg, 5–6 drinks per day) or other supplements. He even conducted a randomized, double-blind, placebo-controlled crossover trial investigating the effects of energy drink consumption vs placebo on performance in 9 elite esports players.[108] No differences in cognitive measures and performance were observed between groups.

Thomas also highlights the growing field of nootropics, also known as "smart drugs" or "cognitive enhancers." Most research in this field has focused on elderly individuals and people with dementia or Alzheimer disease, so little is known about the effectiveness of these types of supplements among younger, healthier populations. Aside from caffeine, there is growing attention on various nootropic compounds such as l-theanine, polyphenols (eg, cocoa flavanols), creatine, and probiotics as possibly improving cognitive function in healthy young adults; however, these substances need to be studied more closely in this population before any conclusions can be drawn.[109]

Expert Nutrition Tips

Following are some tips for working with esports players:

- Focus on the development of basic cooking skills and food options that require minimal equipment and are fast and convenient (Thomas, oral communication, October 3, 2022).
- To improve blood perfusion to the brain, esports players should get up and move regularly. Thomas (oral communication, October 3, 2022) recommends getting up for at least 2 minutes of every 30 minutes of sitting. Nutritionally, he advocates eating foods that are high in nitrates, such as beets and arugula, as well as berries, which may also improve cerebral blood flow. Depending on food preference, a high-quality supplement, such as L-citrulline, may be warranted.
- Education on supplements, particularly caffeine, should be a part of any esports nutrition education program (Thomas, oral communication, October 3, 2022). Because esports is an indoor activity, a vitamin D supplement is likely warranted.
- Although esports players may not have had any nutrition education, Thomas (oral communication, October 3, 2022) says that they can be more savvy than other athletes in that they are more likely to question things and ask "why?" Thomas recommends that the RDN use this to their advantage and be ready to provide evidence (ie, research) to back up their claims.

How to Get a Foot in the Door

Thomas (oral communication, October 3, 2022) says that esports are decades behind traditional sports in that most teams may have 1 health staff member, if that. He emphasized the importance of understanding gamer culture and being able to talk the language. Start by being in the places where gamers hang out (eg, live streaming platforms, social media). Thomas started with pro bono work and was able to expand his practice from there. He said that "colleges are dying for free help," and starting with that could lead to paying positions. He also noted that high schools are also starting to offer support programs. Thomas acknowledges that "you have to understand that walking in is going to be very challenging and people aren't going to appreciate you or see the value in what you're doing, but hopefully you can get support from someone." That is why it is important for the RDN to focus on the value that they can bring to the team by making the manager's life easier, reducing the risk of injury, and improving a player's energy. RDNs wanting to work in this space need to be ready to back up their recommendations with sound, clear, data-driven evidence. Finally, because the esports science community is still quite small, Thomas encourages RDNs to reach out to others in the field so that research expands and evidence-based guidelines for professional practice develop.

TRANSGENDER AND GENDER-NONCONFORMING ATHLETES

Description

It is estimated that more than 1.6 million adults (aged 18 years and older) and youth (aged 13–17 years) identify as transgender or gender-nonconforming (TGNC) in the United States (0.6% of those aged 13 years and older). The percentage of youth who identify as TGNC is higher than the percentage of adults (1.4% vs 0.5%).[110] Regardless of how the legal landscape impacts the participation of TGNC individuals in competitive sports, there currently are and will continue to be TGNC athletes in need of nutritional guidance. This section reviews the current knowledge base and best practices for providing evidence-based, compassionate care, recognizing that there is much that health care practitioners still do not know and still have to learn about this understudied population.

To begin, words matter. It is important to understand the key terms listed in Box 24.5,[111] which are currently considered to be the most inclusive. The RDN can honor and affirm an athlete's gender identity by using their preferred name and pronouns. It is also worth noting that, although transgender is represented by the "T" in LGBTQ+ (lesbian, gay, bisexual, transgender, queer or questioning, and additional identities), it does not refer to a person's sexual orientation as the other letters do.

BOX 24.5 Sex and Gender Terminology[111]

Transgender	An adjective that is an umbrella term used to describe the full range of people whose gender identity and/or gender role do not conform to what is typically associated with their sex assigned at birth. Although the term *transgender* is commonly accepted, not all transgender or gender-nonconforming (TGNC) people self-identify as transgender.
Cisgender	An adjective used to describe a person whose gender identity and gender expression align with their sex assigned at birth; a person who is not TGNC.
Female-to-male (FTM)	Individuals who were assigned female sex at birth and who have changed, are changing, or wish to change their body and/or gender identity to a more masculine body or gender identity. FTM persons are also often referred to as *transgender men*, *transmen*, or *trans men*.
Male-to-female (MTF)	Individuals who were assigned male sex at birth and who have changed, are changing, or wish to change their body and/or gender identity to a more feminized body or gender identity. MTF persons are also often referred to as *transgender women*, *transwomen*, or *trans women*.
Gender identity	A person's deeply felt, inherent sense of being a boy, a man, or male; a girl, a woman, or female; or an alternative gender (eg, genderqueer, gender-nonconforming, gender neutral) that may or may not correspond to this person's sex assigned at birth or to this person's primary or secondary sex characteristics.
Gender expression	The presentation of an individual, including physical appearance, clothing choice and accessories, and behaviors that express aspects of gender identity or role. Gender expression may or may not conform to a person's gender identity.

Continued on next page

BOX 24.5 Sex and Gender Terminology[111] (CONTINUED)

Gender-nonconforming (GNC)	An adjective used as an umbrella term to describe people whose gender expression or gender identity differs from gender norms associated with their assigned birth sex.
Genderqueer	A term to describe a person whose gender identity does not align with a binary understanding of gender (ie, a person who does not identify fully as either a man or a woman). People who identify as genderqueer may redefine gender or decline to define themselves as gendered altogether.
Gender dysphoria	Discomfort or distress related to incongruence between a person's gender identity, sex assigned at birth, and/or primary and secondary sex characteristics.
Hormone therapy (gender-affirming hormone therapy, hormone replacement therapy)	The use of hormones to masculinize or feminize a person's body to better align that person's physical characteristics with their gender identity. People wishing to masculinize their body receive testosterone; those wishing to feminize their body receive antiandrogens and/or estrogens. Hormone therapy may be an important part of medically necessary treatment to alleviate gender dysphoria.
Trans	Common shorthand for the terms transgender, transsexual, and/or gender-nonconforming. Although the term trans is commonly accepted, not all transsexual or gender-nonconforming people identify as trans.
Transsexual	A term to describe TGNC people who have changed or are changing their bodies through medical interventions (eg, hormones, surgery) to better align their bodies with a gender identity that is different than their sex assigned at birth. Not all people who identify as transsexual consider themselves to be TGNC. For example, some transsexual individuals identify as female or male, without identifying as TGNC.
Sexual orientation	A component of identity that includes a person's sexual and emotional attraction to another person and the behavior and/or social affiliation that may result from this attraction. A person may be attracted to men, women, both, or neither, or they may be attracted to people who are genderqueer, androgynous, or have other gender identities. Individuals may identify as lesbian, gay, heterosexual, bisexual, queer, pansexual, or asexual, among others.

Nutrition and Health Considerations

The nutrition considerations for TGNC individuals are both clinical and psychosocial. If a person is undergoing a medical transition and receiving hormone therapy, this can lead to weight gain, body composition changes, altered lipid profiles, and changes in bone composition and other metabolic factors.[112] For example, an individual undergoing female-to-male transition on testosterone therapy will likely exhibit weight gain, increased lean body mass, decreased fat mass, changes in lipoproteins (increased low-density lipoprotein and decreased high-density lipoprotein), delayed prothrombin time, increased hemoglobin and hematocrit, and increased creatinine levels. An individual undergoing male-to-female transition on estrogen therapy will likely have changes in lipoprotein levels and blood pressure (increased or decreased), increased bone density, and decreased creatinine. Spironolactone, a potassium-sparking diuretic that blocks testosterone synthesis, can create electrolyte imbalances and increase the risk of hyperkalemia.[113] Pubertal blockers, such as gonadotropin-releasing hormone analogues, may put individuals at greater risk for impaired bone mineral density and skeletal stress injuries.

Psychosocial concerns in both the adult and youth TGNC populations include higher rates of disordered eating, body dysmorphia, and food insecurity compared with cisgender populations.[112,114] Julie Brake, MS, RDN, LD, (email, October 31, 2022) is a sports dietitian also specializing in eating disorders who has worked with some TGNC clients in her private practice. She says that "there is a high risk of disordered eating due to a high rate of body dissatisfaction in this [the TGNC] population. Sometimes the body dissatisfaction and body image distortion is related to trauma. . . . For these athletes, there is a lot of motivation to eat well but often a struggle due to mentally disconnecting from the physical body. This makes discerning hunger and fullness cues challenging."

Whitney Linsenmeyer, PhD, RDN, LD, (email, November 2, 2022) is an Assistant Professor at Saint Louis University whose research and clinical practice center on gender-affirming nutrition care for the TGNC population. She notes that TGNC youth are less likely to engage in physical activity and compete in school sports than cisgender youth and that TGNC adults are also less physically active than cisgender adults.[115,116] She says that reported barriers to physical activity and sport participation include "fear of being 'outed' as transgender, 'passing' as male or female, fear of body exposure, lack of safety in bathrooms and locker rooms, body dissatisfaction, and transphobic verbal and physical abuse." Despite the potential challenges and barriers to physical activity and sports participation among TGNC individuals, Linsenmeyer highlights the transformative power sports can have by providing "increased body satisfaction, improved gender congruence, improved self-esteem and well-being, and increased school belonging and social connectivity."[117]

Many aspects of nutrition assessment are binary and require RDNs to choose between male and female biological sex. For example, predictive energy equations use sex as a variable, and some Dietary Reference Intakes and acceptable laboratory values are sex-specific. Linsenmeyer et al[114] published a comprehensive practice paper that provides a detailed overview of sex-specific aspects of the Nutrition Care Process with consideration of the implications for TGNC individuals. Their recommendations for working with TGNC clients can be summarized as follows:

- Use reference values consistent with sex assigned at birth for clients who have not medically transitioned. It is estimated that 62% of TGNC adults in the United States have medically transitioned with hormone therapy (HT) and that 23% plan to do so in the future. A much smaller number have had gender-affirming surgeries (4%–43% depending on surgery type). Therefore, the RDN cannot assume that a client has medically transitioned and should gather this information as part of the client's medical history.
- Individualize nutrition assessment to align with the client's medical transition. The timing and scale of physical changes that occur with HT vary among individuals; however, the general timelines provided by the World Professional Association for Transgender Health can be used.
  - Masculinizing HT may increase muscle mass and strength starting at 6 to 12 months with an expected maximum effect at 2 to 5 years.
  - Feminizing HT may decrease muscle mass and strength starting at 3 to 6 months with an expected maximum effect at 1 to 2 years.[114,118]
- Express data as a range between the female and male reference values, especially in cases where ranges are routinely used (eg, estimating energy and protein needs).[114] This may be appropriate for clients on short-term HT (<6 months) or who are on low to moderate HT regimens.

Expert Nutrition Tips

Following are some tips for working with transgender and gender-nonconforming athletes:

- Make sure that all educational and other materials are gender-affirming. Linsenmeyer (email, November 2, 2022) says that "it's a first and crucial step to ensure [that] patients know they are respected. Skills include using a patient's preferred name and pronouns, apologizing for a mistake, and getting comfortable with gender-neutral terms. The National LGBTQIA+ Health Education Center (wwwlgbtqiahealtheducation.org) has excellent resources on communication."

» Because HT can alter a person's ability to sense hunger and fullness, it is particularly important to focus on the timing of nutrition and on foods that meet the athlete's needs whether they have an appetite or not (Brake, email, October 31, 2022).

» The discourse on the exclusion of TGNC individuals from organized sports has permeated many layers of society. Although it can be difficult to keep track of the constantly shifting legislative landscape, Linsenmeyer emphasizes that, to best support and understand the needs of their clients, RDNs need to be attuned to these political realities (Linsenmeyer, email, November 2, 2022).

» The unique histories and stages of therapy require a highly individualized nutrition approach. Brake (email, October 31, 2022) notes that it is crucial to stay up to date on all aspects and perspectives on care for this population and to consider current best practices when providing evidence-based recommendations grounded in science. She starts with sex at birth for all calculations and then monitors progress toward nutrition goals, making adjustments to recommendations as needed. "There is no cookie-cutter approach to helping individuals in this population. The most important thing to remember is that these are athletes and should be treated with care just like all of our athletes."

How to Get a Foot in the Door

Brake (email, October 31, 2022) says that she started working with TGNC athletes because they walked through her office door. "There is a segment of the general population that identifies as LGBTQ so there will be a segment of the population, including the athlete population, that identifies as LGBTQ as well. . . . Because I specialize in disordered eating care and sports nutrition, I had clients who were LGBTQ athletes." It was the lack of research and professional resources among the TGNC population that led Linsenmeyer (email, November 2, 2022) along her current professional path. She recommends becoming an ally and partner with community-based organizations by and for the TGNC community. "Since I am cisgender, it's especially important for me to center transgender individuals in my work." Both Brake and Lisenmeyer highlight the strong need for competent and compassionate RDNs working with the TGNC population.

KEY TAKEAWAYS

The traditional sports that practitioners most often associate with sports nutrition comprise a small percentage of the opportunities available. This chapter has not covered all of the opportunities that exist.

Any individual or group involved in regular, organized physical activity could benefit from the expertise of a sports dietitian.

Although RDNs clearly see the impact that they can make with these groups, it will take some convincing of these athletes, coaches, and organizing bodies, as well as collaborations with other health and fitness practitioners who are already established in each field. The research literature on these emerging sports, as it relates to nutrition, is often sparse. To make a case for working with any of these emerging populations, RDNs should begin to collect data and ensure that the guidelines they provide are evidence-based.

Self-motivated, curious, and entrepreneurial RDNs have much to offer and gain from working with these emerging sports.

The nutrition considerations for TGNC individuals are both clinical and psychosocial, and the unique histories and stages of therapy require a highly individualized nutrition approach. Sports RDNs should be aware of the best practices for providing evidence-based, compassionate care to transgender and gender-nonconforming athletes.

REFERENCES

1. The original crossfit box: then and now. Morning Chalk Up website. October 2016. Accessed October 15, 2022. https://morningchalkup.com/newsletters/original-crossfit-box-now
2. Glassman G. Understanding CrossFit. *CrossFit J.* 2007;56:1-2. Accessed October 14, 2024. https://library.crossfit.com/free/pdf/CFJ_56-07_Understanding.pdf
3. Feito Y, Heinrich KM, Butcher SJ, Poston WSC. High-intensity functional training (HIFT): definition and research implications for improved fitness. *Sports (Basel).* 2018;6(3):76. doi:10.3390/sports6030076
4. About the Games. CrossFit Games website. Accessed October 15, 2022. https://games.crossfit.com/about-the-games
5. CrossFit Kids Certificate Course. CrossFit website. Accessed October 15, 2022. wwwcrossfit.com/certificate-courses/online-kids
6. The Ultimate Guide to CrossFit Lingo: 100 Terms You Need to Know. WODHopper website. Accessed October 15, 2022. wwwwodhopper.com/crossfitlingo
7. Brisebois M, Kramer S, Lindsay KG, Wu C-T, Kamla J. Dietary practices and supplement use among CrossFit participants. *J Int Soc Sports Nutr.* 2022;19(1):316-335. doi:10.1080/15502783.2022.2086016
8. de Souza RAS, da Silva AG, de Souza MF, et al. A systematic review of CrossFit workouts and dietary and supplementation interventions to guide nutritional strategies and future research in CrossFit. *Int J Sport Nutr Exerc Metab.* 2021;31(2):187-205. doi:10.1123/ijsnem.2020-0223
9. Nutrition FAQ. CrossFit website. Accessed October 15, 2022. wwwcrossfit.com/faq/nutrition
10. The Complete CrossFit Macros Guide. WODReview website. Accessed October 15, 2022. https://wodreview.com/nutrition/crossfit-macros-guide
11. The Zone Diet. Zone Living website. Accessed July 28, 2015. https://zonediet.com/the-zone-diet
12. Cheuvront S. The Zone Diet and athletic performance. *Sports Med.* 1999;27(4):213-228. doi:10.2165/00007256-199927040-00002
13. Dos Santos Quaresma MVL, Guazzelli Marques C, Nakamoto FP. Effects of diet interventions, dietary supplements, and performance-enhancing substances on the performance of CrossFit-trained individuals: A systematic review of clinical studies. *Nutrition.* 2021;82:110994. doi:10.1016/j.nut.2020.110994
14. Obstacle Sports :A Brief History. World Obstacle website. Accessed October 28, 2022. wwwworldobstacle.org/history
15. Schuckies E. The rise of obstacle course races. Active.com website. 2022. Accessed October 28, 2022. wwwactive.com/running/articles/the-rise-of-obstacle-course-races
16. 2014 state of the sport—Part I: non-traditional running events. Running USA website. Published April 27, 2014. Accessed July 28, 2015. wwwrunningusa.org/non-traditional-running-events-special-report
17. Obstacle Racing. World Obstacle website. Accessed October 28, 2022. wwwworldobstacle.org/sub-sports-obstacle-racing
18. Kallet B. Spartan Race Types: The Full Guide to Finding the Right Race for You. Spartan website. Accessed October 28, 2022. wwwspartan.com/blogs/unbreakable-race-stories/different-spartan-race-types
19. Tough Mudder USA website. Accessed October 28, 2022. https://toughmudder.com
20. Frequently asked questions. Tough Mudder USA website. Accessed October 28, 2022. https://toughmudder.com/frequently-asked-questions
21. Spartan World Championships. Spartan website. Accessed October 28, 2022. https://race.spartan.com/en/race/championships
22. Thomas DT, Erdman KA, Burke LM. American College of Sports Medicine joint position statement. Nutrition and athletic performance. *Med Sci Sports Exerc.* 2016;48(3):543-568. doi:10.1249/MSS.0000000000000852
23. Halmi K, Sunday S, Kaye W, et al. Perfectionism in anorexia nervosa: variation by clinical subtype, obsessionality, and pathological eating behavior. *Am J Psychiatry.* 2000;157(11):1799-1805. doi:10.1176/appi.ajp.157.11.1799
24. Gifford C. *Racing: The Ultimate Motorsport Encyclopedia.* Kingfisher Publications; 2006.
25. What is rally? Rally America website. Accessed November 4, 2022. wwwrally-america.com/what_is_rally
26. Reid MB, Lightfoot JT. The physiology of auto racing. *Med Sci Sports Exerc.* 2019;51(12):2548-2562. doi:10.1249/MSS.0000000000002070
27. Jacobs P, Olvey S, Johnson B, Cohn K. Physiological responses to high-speed, open-wheel racecar driving. *Med Sci Sports Exerc.* 2002;34(12):2085-2090. doi:10.1097/00005768-200212000-00033
28. Carlson L, Ferguson D, Kenefick R. Physiological strain of stock car drivers during competitive racing. *J Thermal Biol.* 2014;44:20-26. doi:10.1016/j.jtherbio.2014.06.001
29. Barthel SC, Ferguson DP. Cockpit temperature as an indicator of thermal strain in sports car competition. *Med Sci Sports Exerc.* 2021;53(2):360-366. doi:10.1249/MSS.0000000000002483
30. Ferguson DP, Barthel SC, Pruett ML, Buckingham TM, Waaso PR. Physiological responses of male and female race car drivers during competition. *Med Sci Sports Exerc.* 2019;51(12):2570-2577. doi:10.1249/MSS.0000000000001997
31. Ferguson D, Davis A, Lightfoot J. Optimizing the physical conditioning of the NASCAR Sprint Cup pit crew athlete. *J Strength Cond Res.* 2015;29(3):567-577. doi:10.1519/JSC.0000000000000659
32. Carlson LA, Lawrence MA, Kenefick RW. Hydration status and thermoregulatory responses in drivers during competitive racing. *J Strength Cond Res.* 2018;32(7):2061-2065. doi:10.1519/JSC.0000000000002268

33. Ganguli T. Race car drivers eating during a race gives new meaning to fast food. *Orlando Sentinel.* May 22, 2009. Accessed August 27, 2015. http://articles.orlandosentinel.com/2009-05-22/sports/ractic_1_race-eat-snack
34. Rodrigues L, Magalhaes F. Car racing: in the heat of competition. *Rev Bras Med Esporte*. 2004;10(3):212-215. doi:10.1590/S1517-86922004000300011
35. Walker SM, Ackland TR, Dawson B. The combined effect of heat and carbon monoxide on the performance of motorsport athletes. *Comp Biochem Physiol A Mol Integr Physiol.* 2001;128(4):709-718. doi:10.1016/s1095-6433(01)00277-x
36. Rimmer L. How much does an F1 car weigh in 2022 and what's included in the limit? Autosport website. April 26, 2022. Accessed August 29, 2015. wwwautosport.com/f1/news/how-much-does-an-f1-car-weigh/10246442
37. Athletes and the Arts website. Accessed October 28, 2022. http://athletesandthearts.com
38. Sousa M, Carvalho P, Moreira P, Teixeira V. Nutrition and nutritional issues for dancers. *Med Probl Perform Art*. 2013;28(3):119-123.
39. Rodrigues-Krause J, Krause M, Reischak-Oliveira Á. Cardiorespiratory considerations in dance: from classes to performances. *J Dance Med Sci.* 2015;19(3):91-102. doi:10.12678/1089-313X.19.3.91
40. Twitchett E, Angioi M, Koutedakis Y, Wyon M. The demands of a working day among female professional ballet dancers. *J Dance Med Sci.* 2010;14(4):127-132.
41. Doyle-Lucas A, Akers J, Davy B. Energetic efficiency, menstrual irregularity, and bone mineral density in elite professional female ballet dancers. *J Dance Med Sci.* 2010;14(4):146-154.
42. Kaufman B, Warren M, Dominguez J, Wang J, Heymsfield S, Pierson R. Bone density and amenorrhea in ballet dancers are related to a decreased resting metabolic rate and lower leptin levels. *J Clin Endocrinal Metab.* 2002;87(6):2777-2783. doi:10.1210/jcem.87.6.8565
43. Robbeson JG, Kruger HS, Wright HH. Disordered eating behavior, body image, and energy status of female student dancers. *Int J Sport Nutr Exerc Metab.* 2015;25(4):344-352. doi:10.1123/ijsnem.2013-0161
44. Keay N, AusDancers Overseas, Francis G. Indicators and correlates of low energy availability in male and female dancers. *BMJ Open Sport Exerc Med.* 2020;6(1):e000906. doi:10.1136/bmjsem-2020-000906
45. Arcelus J, Witcomb G, Mitchell A. Prevalence of eating disorders amongst dancers: a systemic review and meta-analysis. *Eur Eat Disorder Rev.* 2014;22(2):92-101. doi:10.1002/erv.2271
46. Wyon M, Hutchings K, Wells A, Nevill A. Body mass index, nutritional knowledge, and eating behaviors in elite student and professional ballet dancers. *Clin J Sport Med.* 2014;24(5):390-396. doi:10.1097/JSM.0000000000000054
47. Hincapié C, Cassidy J. Disordered eating, menstrual disturbances, and low bone mineral density in dancers: a systematic review. *Arch Phys Med Rehabil.* 2010;91(11):1777-1789.e1. doi:10.1016/j.apmr.2010.07.230
48. Friesen K, Rozenek R, Clippinger K, Gunter K, Russo A, Sklar S. Bone mineral density and body composition of collegiate modern dancers. *J Dance Med Sci.* 2011;15(1):31-36.
49. 4Dancers. The dance/USA taskforce for dancer health – an introduction. 4Dancers.org website. April 7, 2019. Accessed October 19, 2024. https://4dancers.org/2019/04/the-danceusa-taskforce-for-dancer-health-an-introduction
50. Mathisen TF, Sundgot-Borgen C, Anstensrud B, Sundgot-Borgen J. Intervention in professional dance students to increase mental health- and nutrition literacy: A controlled trial with follow up. *Front Sports Act Living.* 2022;4:727048. doi:10.3389/fspor.2022.727048
51. Caine D, Goodwin BJ, Caine CG, Bergeron G. Epidemiological review of injury in pre-professional ballet dancers. *J Dance Med Sci.* 2015;19(4):140-148. doi:10.12678/1089-313X.19.4.140
52. Ekegren C, Quested R, Brodrick A. Injuries in pre-professional ballet dancers: incidence, characteristics and consequences. *J Sci Med Sport.* 2014;17(3):271-275. doi:10.1016/j.jsams.2013.07.013
53. Yannakoulia M, Keramopoulos A, Matalas A. Bone mineral density in young active females: the case of dancers. *Int J Sport Nutr Exerc Metab.* 2004;14(3):285-297. doi:10.1123/ijsnem.14.3.285
54. Khan K, Green R, Wark J, et al. Retired elite female ballet dancers and nonathletic controls have similar bone mineral density at weightbearing sites. *J Bone Miner Res.* 1996;11(10):1566-1574. doi:10.1002/jbmr.5650111025
55. Karlsson M, Johnell O, Obrant K. Bone mineral density in professional ballet dancers. *Bone Miner.* 1993;21(3):163-169. doi:10.1016/s0169-6009(08)80227-9
56. Quintas M, Ortega R, López-Sobaler A, Garrido G, Requejo A. Influence of dietetic and anthropometric factors and of the type of sport practiced on bone density in different groups of women. *Eur J Clin Nutr.* 2003;57(suppl 1):S58-S62. doi:10.1038/sj.ejcn.1601817
57. Vassallo AJ, Trevor BL, Mota L, Pappas E, Hiller CE. Injury rates and characteristics in recreational, elite student and professional dancers: a systematic review. *J Sports Sci.* 2019;37(10):1113-1122. doi:10.1080/02640414.2018.1544538
58. Beck KL, Mitchell S, Foskett A, Conlon CA, von Hurst PR. Dietary intake, anthropometric characteristics, and iron and vitamin D status of female adolescent ballet dancers living in New Zealand. *Int J Sport Nutr Exerc Metab.* 2015;25(4):335-343. doi:10.1123/ijsnem.2014-0089
59. Constantini N, Arieli R, Chodick G, Dubnov-Raz G. High prevalence of vitamin D insufficiency in athletes and dancers. *Clin J Sport Med.* 2010;20(5):368-371. doi:10.1097/JSM.0b013e3181f207f2
60. Wolman R, Wyon M, Koutedakis Y, Nevill A, Eastell R, Allen N. Vitamin D status in professional ballet dancers: winter vs. summer. *J Sci Med Sport.* 2013;16(5):388-391. doi:10.1016/j.jsams.2012.12.010
61. Aerialist. Merriam-Webster website. Accessed October 22, 2022. wwwmerriam-webster.com/dictionary/aerialist
62. AcroSchool. What is Acrobatics? August 20, 2020. Accessed January 15, 2025. wwwacroschool.com/acrobatics
63. Everything you need to know about aerial arts. Aerial Practice website. Accessed October 22, 2022. https://aerialpractice.com/articles/aerial-progress/what-is-aerial-arts

64. All about lyra hops – benefits, history, workouts, and rigging. Uplift Active. January 14, 2020. Accessed January 15, 2025. https://upliftactive.com/blogs/aerial-fitness/the-art-of-aerial-hoop
65. How to get started in pole fitness and dancing. SkyDancer Supply Co. July 30, 2021. Accessed January 15, 2025. https://skydancersupply.com/blogs/how-to-get-started/how-to-get-started-in-pole-fitness-and-dancing
66. International Pole Sports Federation website. Accessed October 22, 2022. wwwpolesports.org
67. Ruggieri RM, Costa PB. Contralateral Muscle Imbalances and Physiological Profile of Recreational Aerial Athletes. *J Funct Morphol Kinesiol.* 2019;4(3):49. doi:10.3390/jfmk4030049
68. Naczk M, Kowalewska A, Naczk A. The risk of injuries and physiological benefits of pole dancing. *J Sports Med Phys Fitness.* 2020;60(6):883-888. doi:10.23736/S0022-4707.20.10379-7
69. Nawrocka A, Mynarski A, Powerska A, Rozpara M, Garbaciak W. Effects of exercise training experience on hand grip strength, body composition and postural stability in fitness pole dancers. *J Sports Med Phys Fitness.* 2017;57(9):1098-1103. doi:10.23736/S0022-4707.16.06510-5
70. Gołuchowska AM, Humka MI. Types of the locomotor system injuries and frequency of occurrence in women pole dancers. *J Sports Med Phys Fitness.* 2022;62(5):661-666. doi:10.23736/S0022-4707.21.12239-X
71. Marching arts. Wikipedia website. Accessed October 31, 2022. https://en.wikipedia.org/wiki/Marching_arts
72. Pape L. More than just marching band: musical athletes redefine 'sport.' *Austin Fit Magazine.* October 1, 2014. Accessed September 3, 2015. wwwaustinfitmagazine.com/October-2014/More-Than-Just-Marching-Band
73. Erdmann LD, Graham RE, Radlo SJ, Knepler PL. Adolescents' energy cost in marching band. *Percept Mot Skills.* 2003;97(2):639-646. doi:10.2466/pms.2003.97.2.639
74. Levy J, Statham W, VanDoren L. BMI changes among marching artists: a longitudinal study. *Med Prol Perform Art.* 2013;28(4):236-241.
75. Jin Y, Obert M, Siivola C, LeBlanc A. Effect of audience on music performance anxiety. *J Res Music Ed.* 1997;45(3):480-496. doi:10.2307/3345541
76. Sharma S, Bush J, Bertman D, et al. Diet and cardiovascular risk in university marching band, dance team and cheer squad members: a cross-sectional study. *J Int Soc Sport Nutr.* 2008;5:9. doi:10.1186/1550-2783-5-9
77. American College Health Association. National College Health Assessment III: Spring 2022 Reference Group Executive Summary. 2022. Accessed October 31, 2022. wwwacha.org/wp-content/uploads/2024/07/NCHA-III_SPRING_2022_REFERENCE_GROUP_EXECUTIVE_SUMMARY.pdf
78. Morrell J, Lofgren I, Burke J, Reilly R. Metabolic syndrome, obesity, and related risk factors among college men and women. *J Am Coll Health.* 2012;60(1):82-89. doi:10.1080/07448481.2011.582208
79. Metabolic syndrome diagnosis. National Heart, Lung, and Blood Institute website. Last updated May 18, 2022. Accessed November 19, 2022. wwwnhlbi.nih.gov/health/metabolic-syndrome/diagnosis
80. McConnell C, McPherson A, Woolf K. Competition level not associated with diet quality in marching artists. *Int J Sport Nutr Exerc Metab.* 2018;28(1):66-74. doi:10.1123/ijsnem.2017-0096
81. Vepraskas C. Beat the heat: managing heat and hydration in marching band. *J Sch Nurs.* 2002;18(4):237-243. doi:10.1177/10598405020180042001
82. Emerson DM, Torres-McGehee TM, Yeargin SW, et al. Core body temperatures in collegiate marching band artists during rehearsals and performances. *J Athl Train.* 2021;56(3):302-310. doi:10.4085/1062-6050-0245.20
83. Burden M. Nutrition for marching arts: fueling athletes and the arts. Athletes and the Arts; 2020. Accessed October 31, 2022. http://athletesandthearts.com/dev/wp-content/uploads/SCAN-Factsheet-Nutrition-Marching-2020.pdf
84. National Association of Schools of Music Handbook 2023-24. Reston, VA: National Association of Schools of Music; January 11, 2024. https://nasm.arts-accredit.org/wp-content/uploads/sites/2/2024/01/M_2023-24_Handbook_Final_01-11-2024.pdf
85. Baadjou VA, van Eijsden-Besseling MD, Samama-Polak AL, Smeets RJ, Passos VL, Westerterp KR. Energy expenditure in brass and woodwind instrumentalists: the effect of body posture. *Med Probl Perform Art.* 2011;26(4):218-223.
86. De La Rue SE, Draper SB, Potter CR, Smith MS. Energy expenditure in rock/pop drumming. *Int J Sports Med.* 2013;34(10):868-872. doi:10.1055/s-0033-1337905
87. Sivasankar M, Leydon C. The role of hydration in vocal fold physiology. *Curr Opin Otolaryngol Head Neck Surg.* 2010;18(3):171-175. doi:10.1097/MOO.0b013e3283393784
88. Franca MC, Simpson KO, Schuette A. Effects of caffeine on vocal acoustic and aerodynamic measures of adult females. *CoDAS.* 2013;25(3):250-255. doi:10.1590/s2317-17822013000300010
89. Kapsetaki ME, Easmon C. Eating disorders in non-dance performing artists: a systematic literature review. *Med Probl Perform Art.* 2017;32(4):227-234. doi:10.21091/mppa.2017.4039
90. Sport. Oxford English Dictionary website. Accessed October 29, 2022. wwwoed.com/viewdictionaryentry/Entry/187476
91. Kane D, Spradley BD. Recognizing esports as a sport. *Sport J.* May 11, 2017. Accessed October 29, 2022. https://search.ebscohost.com/login.aspx?direct=true&db=s3h&AN=123066341&site=ehost-live
92. Leroux-Parra M. Esports Part 1: What are Esports? Harvard International Review April 24, 2020. Accessed January 15, 2025. https://hir.harvard.edu/esports-part-1-what-are-esports
93. Monteiro Pereira A, Costa JA, Verhagen E, Figueiredo P, Brito J. Associations between esports participation and health: a scoping review. *Sports Med.* 2022;52(9):2039-2060. doi:10.1007/s40279-022-01684-1
94. Gamer Lingo. Discover Esports website. Accessed October 31, 2022. https://discoveresports.com/gamer-lingo
95. National Association of Collegiate Esports website. Accessed October 29, 2022. https://nacesports.org

96. eSports audience size worldwide from 2020 to 2025, by type of viewers. Statistica website. Accessed October 24, 2024. wwwstatista.com/statistics/490480/global-esports-audience-size-viewer-type
97. Dunn, J. The rise of esports. Federal Reserve Bank of St. Louis website. August 24, 2022. Accessed October 29, 2022. wwwstlouisfed.org/open-vault/2022/aug/rise-of-esports-industry
98. Esports Earnings website. Accessed October 29, 2022. wwwesportsearnings.com
99. Cohen P. Video game becomes spectator sport. *New York Times*. April 12, 2009. wwwnytimes.com/2009/04/12/sports/othersports/12star.html
100. Rogstad ET. Gender in eSports research: a literature review. *Eur J Sport Soc.* 2021:19(3):195-213. doi:10.1080/16138171.2021.1930941
101. 75 Significant Esports Statistics: 2022 Market, Viewership & Investment Growth. Finances Online website. Accessed October 29, 2022. https://financesonline.com/esports-statistics
102. Andre TL, Walsh SM, ValladÃo S, Cox D. Physiological and perceptual response to a live collegiate esports tournament. *Int J Exerc Sci.* 2020;13(6):1418-1429.
103. ValladÃo SP, Middleton J, Andre TL. Esport: Fortnite acutely increases heart rate of young men. *Int J Exerc Sci.* 2020;13(6):1217-1227.
104. Haupt S, Wolf A, Heidenreich H, Schmidt W. Energy expenditure during eSports – a case report. *Dtsch Z Sportmed.* 2021;72(1):36-40. doi:10.5960/dzsm.2020.463
105. Yin K, Zi Y, Zhuang W, et al. Linking Esports to health risks and benefits: current knowledge and future research needs. *J Sport Health Sci.* 2020;9(6):485-488. doi:10.1016/j.jshs.2020.04.006
106. DiFrancisco-Donoghue J, Balentine J, Schmidt G, Zwibel H. Managing the health of the eSport athlete: an integrated health management model. *BMJ Open Sport Exerc Med.* 2019;5(1):e000467. doi:10.1136/bmjsem-2018-000467
107. A guide to: energy drinks in esports. Esportsinsider website. December 29, 2020. Accessed October 30, 2022. https://esportsinsider.com/2020/12/energy-drinks-esports-guide
108. Thomas CJ, Rothschild J, Earnest CP, Blaisdell A. The effects of energy drink consumption on cognitive and physical performance in elite league of legends players. *Sports (Basel).* 2019;7(9):196. doi:10.3390/sports7090196
109. Szot M, Karpęcka-Gałka E, Dróżdż R, Frączek B. Can nutrients and dietary supplements potentially improve cognitive performance also in esports? *Healthcare (Basel).* 2022;10(2):186. doi:10.3390/healthcare10020186
110. Herman JL, Flores AR, O'Neill KK. How many adults and youth identify as transgender in the United States? UCLA School of Law Williams Institute. June 2022. Accessed November 4, 2022. https://williamsinstitute.law.ucla.edu/publications/trans-adults-united-states
111. American Psychological Association. Guidelines for psychological practice with transgender and gender nonconforming people. *Am Psychol.* 2015;70(9):832-864. doi:10.1037/a0039906
112. Rahman R, Linsenmeyer WR. Caring for transgender patients and clients: nutrition-related clinical and psychosocial considerations. *J Acad Nutr Diet.* 2019;119(5):727-732. doi:10.1016/j.jand.2018.03.006
113. Marra J, Law AMY, Conlon E. Clinical considerations in caring for transgender athletes. *Am Fam Physician.* 2021;103(9):518-520.
114. Linsenmeyer W, Garwood S, Waters J. An examination of the sex-specific nature of nutrition assessment within the Nutrition Care Process: considerations for nutrition and dietetics practitioners working with transgender and gender diverse clients. *J Acad Nutr Diet.* 2022;122(6):1081-1086. doi:10.1016/j.jand.2022.02.014
115. Bishop A, Overcash F, McGuire J, Reicks M. Diet and physical activity behaviors among adolescent transgender students: school survey results. *J Adolesc Health.* 2020;66(4):484-490. doi:10.1016/j.jadohealth.2019.10.026
116. Jones BA, Haycraft E, Bouman WP, Arcelus J. The levels and predictors of physical activity engagement within the treatment-seeking transgender population: a matched control study. *J Phys Act Health.* 2018;15(2):99-107. doi:10.1123/jpah.2017-0298
117. Linsenmeyer W, Heiden-Rootes K, Drallmeier T, Thomure M, Nye E, Armstrong E. Nutrition and exercise as a 'source of empowerment': a narrative inquiry of transgender men. *SSM Qual Res Health.* 2022;2. doi:10.1016/j.ssmqr.2022.100128
118. Coleman E, Radix AE, Bouman WP, et al. Standards of care for the health of transgender and gender diverse people, version 8. *Int J Transgend Health.* 2022;23(suppl 1):S1-S259. doi:10.1080/26895269.2022.2100644

CHAPTER 25

Dietary Patterns and Athletes

Hope Barkoukis, PhD, RDN, LD, FAND

LEARNING OBJECTIVES

- Define the term *dietary pattern* and explain its role in health and disease.
- Characterize the core elements of the main "healthy" dietary pattern characterized in the *Dietary Guidelines for Americans*, 2020-2025.
- Differentiate the dietary characteristics representing the standard American diet from the healthy US dietary patterns discussed in the *Dietary Guidelines for Americans*, 2020-2025.
- Review popular dietary patterns embraced by athletes that are not included in the *Dietary Guidelines for Americans*, 2020-2025.
- Examine the challenges in determining dietary patterns in athletes.
- Identify the main dietary restrictions followed by athletes that have the greatest likelihood of impacting their overall dietary patterns.

INTRODUCTION

This chapter introduces the term *dietary pattern* and discuss its role in health promotion and sports performance, along with providing a general overview of the core elements of the main US dietary patterns identified as "healthy" in the *Dietary Guidelines for Americans, 2020–2025* (DGA).* The metabolic impact of each discussed dietary pattern as it relates to athletes is also described. Special attention is given to identifying the considerable gaps in knowledge regarding the prevalence of and adherence to the specific dietary patterns by athletes.

THE DIETARY GUIDELINES FOR AMERICANS AND HEALTHY DIETARY PATTERNS

The DGA is the cornerstone of evidence-based nutrition information for nutrition and health professionals. These guidelines are intended to assist all healthy individuals in meeting nutrition recommendations, promoting health, and reducing the risk of chronic disease through dietary advice. To do so, the DGA translates the quantitative requirements for nutrients and food components (eg, dietary fiber) established by the National Academies of Science, Engineering and Medicine into recommendations for foods and beverages that can help individuals meet their nutritional needs. The DGA serves as the foundation for all federally produced nutrition education materials for the public, in addition to providing the basis for the development, implementation, and evaluation of all federal food and nutrition programs.[1]

*The *Dietary Guidelines for Americans*, 2025-2030 is anticipated shortly after the publication of this book.

The fundamental principle guiding the DGA is the shift from recommending specific foods and beverages in isolation to focusing on how to create healthy dietary patterns throughout the life cycle. Extensive research has accumulated strong evidence to support the role of dietary patterns in impacting one's health significantly and positively, more so than specific choices of individual foods or beverages.[1]

Defining Dietary Patterns

A *dietary pattern* refers to the collective quantity, variety, proportion, and frequency of foods, beverages, and nutrients consumed by an individual over time.[1,2] Research has clearly established that regardless of what label is attributed to a particular dietary pattern, those reflecting nutrient-dense eating patterns are associated with a plethora of metabolic benefits, including a significant reduction in all-cause mortality.[3] The elements that are common to nutrient-dense or "healthy" dietary patterns are listed in Box 25.1.[3]

BOX 25.1 Elements Common to Healthy Dietary Patterns[3]

Include high intakes of	*Limit or omit*
Fruits	Processed meats or meat products
Vegetables	Refined grains
Nuts	High-fat dairy
Whole or unrefined grains	Added sugars
Legumes	Sugar-sweetened beverages
Fish and seafood	Excess sodium
Lean meat or poultry	Saturated and *trans* fats
Low-fat dairy	
Heart-healthy oils	

It is also important to note that a wide variety of food choices can be included to create a healthy dietary pattern.[3]

Healthy US-Style Dietary Pattern

The overarching recommended dietary pattern characterized by the DGA is called the Healthy US-Style Dietary Pattern or the US Department of Agriculture's primary Dietary Pattern. This pattern forms the framework for individuals of all ages, ethnicities, races, and sexes to consume a dietary pattern of nutrient-dense foods consistent with the appropriate quantity of daily calories.[1] Of note, the DGA does not specifically address the needs of athletes but instead focuses on life-cycle nutrient and energy recommendations. Quantities recommended for specific food groups differ based on appropriate energy needs, but the daily pattern consists of fruits; vegetables (including dark green, red, orange, and starchy ones); beans, peas, and lentils; whole grains; dairy and fortified soy foods; protein foods (meat, poultry, eggs, seafood, nuts, seeds, soy products); and oils.[1] This pattern meets nutrition and food component recommendations while remaining within the limitations set for saturated and *trans* fats, added sugars, and sodium.

It is also important to note that the dietary pattern recommendations from numerous expert organizations (eg, the National Heart, Lung, and Blood Institute; the National Cancer Institute; the American Heart Association; and the American Diabetes Association) do have minor differences, but all are in overall agreement with the healthy dietary pattern defined in the DGA.[4] The underpinning points of agreement include an abundant consumption of fruits, vegetables, whole grains, high-fiber choices, low-fat or no-fat dairy, lean meats, fish and seafood, and nuts, coupled with limited intake of processed foods, added sugars, *trans* fats, and saturated fats. The recommendations of these organizations do vary somewhat regarding the restriction of added sugars, snack foods, *trans* fats, and saturated fats, but they are essentially congruent. Additional recommendations for the consumption of fish (particularly oily fish) at least twice weekly are included by the American Heart Association.[5]

THE STANDARD AMERICAN DIET

The stereotypical dietary pattern consumed in the United States is known as the *Western diet* or the *standard American diet* (SAD), and includes less than 1 daily serving of fruit, less than 2 daily servings of vegetables, 15 to 22 tsp of added sugar, and the following defining characteristics[1,6]:

- 63% of daily total calories from refined and processed foods, such as soft drinks, potato chips, and packaged desserts;
- 25% of daily total calories from animal-based foods; and
- 12% of daily total calories from plant-based foods, with half of this amount being from French fries.

Refined and processed foods referenced in the SAD are considered a health concern and should not be confused with foods that are categorized as *minimally processed foods*. These minimally processed foods are exposed to various processing procedures that retain their nutritional properties and may extend their shelf life but do not add salt, sugar, fat, or oils. Some examples of these types of food-processing procedures include drying, crushing, grinding, roasting, boiling, vacuum sealing, pasteurization, and alcohol fermentation.[7] Accordingly, when a nutrition or other health care practitioner is counseling clients, they should take care to explain that not all forms of food processing are deleterious to health.

DIETARY PATTERNS INCLUDED IN THE DIETARY GUIDELINES FOR AMERICANS

Vegetarian Dietary Pattern

The Healthy US-Style Dietary Pattern can be individualized to meet personal preferences. One example currently practiced by approximately 5% to 6% of adults in the United States is the vegetarian dietary pattern, which excludes all animal meats, seafood, and poultry. The DGA includes a vegetarian dietary pattern for toddlers aged 12 through 23 months, as well as 12 different calorie levels for older individuals.[1] Emerging evidence shows an increasing interest in vegetarian or vegan diets among athletes, with reports of 8% of international athletes following a vegetarian diet and 1% following a fully vegan approach.[8,9] Note that the DGA discusses only the lacto-ovo form of vegetarianism (which includes dairy and eggs). Refer to Chapter 16 (where this pattern is referred to as ovolactovegetarianism) for a complete review of the various types of plant-based diets. It is important for the practitioner to acknowledge the wide variations in dietary practices and food choices among individuals who adhere to plant-based diets.

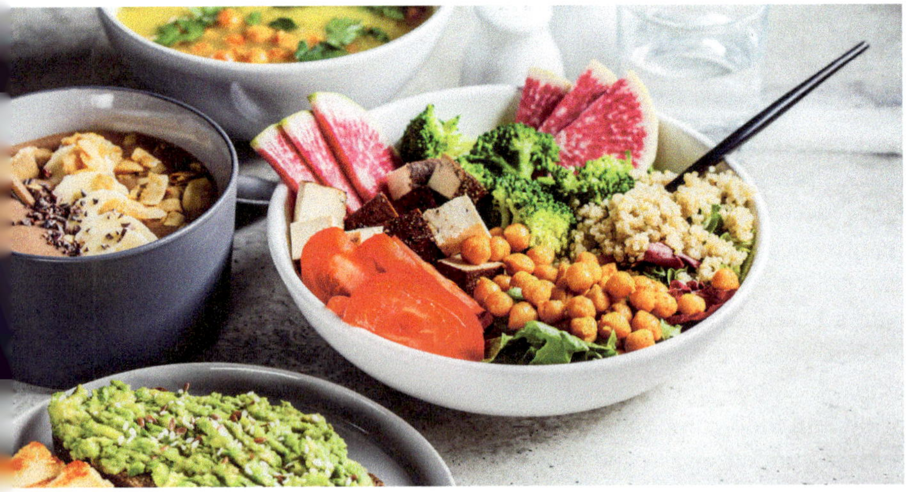

The plethora of data demonstrating the health benefits of vegetarian dietary patterns translates into wide acceptance by health care professionals. An increase in interest in vegetarianism among athletes in the United States has been noted, with data to support the observation that vegetarian athletes can meet their nutritional needs without compromising performance.[10,11] Data to date identify no clear pattern regarding a positive or negative impact of vegetarianism on strength, exercise capacity, and performance in endurance athletes.[12-14] Reported benefits include blunting oxidative stress and positively impacting the anti-inflammatory response.[15,16] However, other studies have not demonstrated differences between endurance athletes following vegetarian and omnivorous diets when assessing nitric oxide (a commonly used biomarker for inflammation) and exercise-induced malondialdehyde (an end product of lipid peroxidation that is used to assess oxidative stress).[17,18]

The key to providing sufficient nutritional support for athletes following a vegetarian diet lies in a well-planned dietary pattern that meets energy and nutrient demands.[11,19] Nutrients that warrant special consideration for the vegetarian athlete because of reduced absorption or bioavailability or limited presence in the diet include vitamin B12, vitamin D, calcium, iron, iodine, and zinc.[10] Protein adequacy can be achieved with attention to sufficiency of total energy intake and use of a variety of protein sources. However, optimal stimulation of muscle protein synthesis is dependent on protein quantity and quality.[19] Intake of an equivalent amount of plant-derived protein vs animal-derived protein has been found to result in decreased postprandial muscle protein synthesis. Therefore, special attention to leucine and the overall adequacy of essential amino acid intake should be noted, as leucine and essential amino acid levels are lower in plant-based diets.[19-22] What remains unknown at this time is the impact of vegetarian diets on the enhancement or blunting of molecular exercise adaptation in endurance and resistance exercise.[19] Refer to Chapter 16 for a full review of vegetarian diets in athletes.

Mediterranean Dietary Pattern

The Mediterranean-style diet is also included in the DGA as a healthy dietary pattern. The term *Mediterranean diet* technically reflects a range of dietary patterns. It is characterized by the use of olive oil as the primary fat source; daily inclusion of fruits, vegetables, legumes, nuts, seeds, and a variety of grains; infrequent consumption of animal meats; moderate amounts of dairy, eggs, and poultry; and exclusion of processed foods. Although not considered mandatory, one differentiating detail is the inclusion of moderate wine intake.[23] The Mediterranean dietary approach also incorporates foods reflecting an abundance of plant- and marine-based omega-3 fatty acids, monounsaturated fatty acids, and a reduced intake of saturated, omega-6, and *trans* fatty acids. This results in overall lower omega-6 levels and higher omega-3 levels (congruent with a favorable ratio of omega-6 to omega-3 essential fatty acids), a high intake of dietary fiber secondary to the heavy focus on plant-based foods, and liberal consumption of polyphenols and antioxidants.[5] Extensive research has demonstrated the wide array of metabolic benefits reaped from this type of dietary pattern, including increased longevity, reduced risk of cardiovascular and chronic diseases, a positive impact on the maintenance of cognitive functioning, reduced inflammation and insulin resistance, and an overall high dietary quality.[24-26] In addition to these noted health benefits, consideration for including this type of dietary pattern in sports nutrition is rationalized by its lack of rigid prescriptive approaches to the various food groups and its ability to be customized to the needs of the individual. The high inclusion of a wide variety of vegetables, fruits, and whole grains in the Mediterranean diet allows the athlete to put forward a "food-first" approach to achieving adequate intakes of vitamins, minerals, antioxidants, and potent anti-inflammatory dietary components.[23]

A 2022 review by Calella et al[27] noted that information regarding athlete adherence to a Mediterranean dietary pattern is "scarce, and available information does not permit clear conclusions." Their exhaustive systematic review of 16 studies of adolescent and adult athletes living in Mediterranean countries and participating in diverse sports noted that it was particularly challenging to assess adherence to this type of dietary pattern because of the 7 different Mediterranean diet assessment tools used among the different studies. The data revealed an average level of adherence to a Mediterranean dietary pattern across different sports, with higher levels of adherence than for the general population and inactive individuals.[28]

Considerably more research is needed to delineate the role of the Mediterranean diet in advancing a healthy dietary pattern for athletes, particularly for endurance performance. Baker et al[28] performed a randomized-sequence crossover study with 11 recreational athletes. A short-term Mediterranean diet (4 days) was given with a 16-day washout period, followed by 4 days of a typical Western dietary pattern. No significant differences were noted in any of the anerobic tests, whereas the 5-km treadmill time trial indicated a 6% improvement.

CHALLENGES IN DETERMINING DIETARY PATTERNS IN ATHLETES

Despite the millions of student and adult athletes in the United States, no comprehensive database exists to track the prevalence of specific dietary pattern habits for this important subgroup of the population. By contrast, the typical daily dietary patterns of Americans throughout the life cycle (beginning at 12 months of age) are well-described in the DGA.[1] The degree to which the dietary patterns of Americans compare to nutrient recommendations throughout the life cycle is also well-delineated.[1]

In addition, published research regarding the current state of adherence to specific dietary patterns in athletes of all ages is extremely limited. Yet, regardless of age, sex, or sport, optimal nutrition is universally considered imperative for athletic performance and effective recovery.[29] Several key organizations, including the Academy of Nutrition and Dietetics, Dietitians of Canada, the American College of Sports Medicine, and the International Society of Sports Nutrition have published recommendations on sports nutrition. The information presented in these documents predominantly focuses on energy, macronutrients, micronutrients, meal timing, fluids, performance and body composition goals, and correction needs related to biochemical or metabolic parameters. Numerous studies published on athletes have focused on protocol design and outcomes of specific nutrition interventions or observations of athlete nutrition habits, without including details regarding the overall dietary patterns.[30-32] Consider the following examples:

- A 2022 study employed a sophisticated statistical model to identify the frequency of intake of "pro-healthy" (ie, nutrient-dense) food groups, determining a resultant pro-healthy dietary index and noting the number of meals per day; however, no global dietary pattern assessments were included.[33]
- In 2021, the largest assessment of nutrition knowledge, dietary supplement use, fluid intake, and meal and snack frequency using a validated sports nutrition knowledge questionnaire was published using data from National Collegiate Athletic Association Division III student athletes.[34] The study added valuable knowledge on this population of student athletes, but it did not assess actual dietary intakes, making determinations of overall dietary patterns impossible.
- A 2017 comprehensive review focused on determinants of eating patterns and nutrient intake in competitive adolescent athletes.[35] This systematic review of 5,399 articles covering a 10-year period of time (2006–2016) resulted in data predominantly focused on nutrients with only a select few delineating eating patterns.[36-39]

Castillo et al[40] have specifically noted how critical it is to include future data on overall dietary patterns because "research on eating patterns and food sources is indispensable" and this knowledge gap represents an important future research opportunity. The combination of small study sample sizes and little attention to the overall dietary patterns of athletes unfortunately compromises the ability to gather a comprehensive appreciation of athletes' overall adherences to healthy dietary patterns.

POPULAR DIETARY PATTERNS NOT INCLUDED IN THE DIETARY GUIDELINES

As initially stated, the DGA represents the cornerstone of evidence-based information for nutrition and health professionals designed to guide all healthy individuals to meet nutrition recommendations, promote health, and reduce the risk of chronic disease through dietary advice.[1] However, several other dietary patterns are popular among Americans (including athletes), but they are not included in the DGA because they are not supported by the preponderance of evidence required to demonstrate overall health benefits for the public. The following sections discuss dietary patterns that are not included in the DGA but warrant consideration because of their popularity with athletes.

Low-Carbohydrate, High-Fat Diets

KETOGENIC DIETS

A widely accepted tenet of sports nutrition is the importance of high muscle glycogen stores, which necessitates high carbohydrate intake for optimal athletic performance.[41] Despite this, interest in lowering carbohydrate intake through a ketogenic diet (KD) has increased among athletes. In this context, a KD is defined as an intake of no more than 50 g of carbohydrate daily with moderate protein and high fat intake (≥75% of total energy intake from fat). The individual should also experience an elevation of free fatty acids and the presence of ketone bodies, as well as a β-hydroxybutyrate level of 0.5 to 3.0 mmol/L in circulation.[42]

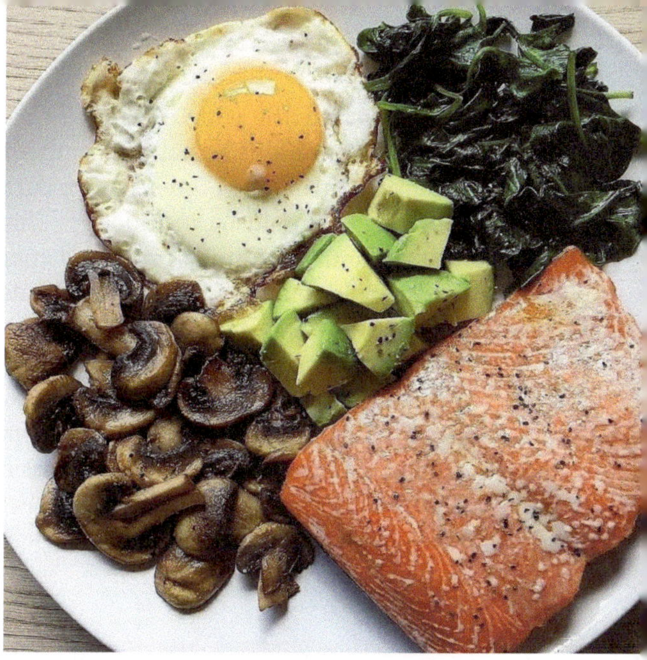

Exploring the plethora of reasons that athletes choose to follow a KD is beyond the scope of this chapter. However, endurance athletes have been known to use a KD because of their desire to avoid the need to replenish diminished glycogen stores during an event (as doing so potentially compromises digestive homeostasis and redirects fuel from muscle to the gut). Additionally, these athletes seek to embrace the molecular changes that enhance endurance adaptations, including increased fat oxidation during low-intensity exercise, spared carbohydrate oxidation, and the reduced postexercise lactate accumulation often observed on ketogenic diets.[42-45] The operational theory is that an endurance athlete who has adapted to a KD could potentially maintain sustained energy levels for a longer period of training, thus reducing the need for event refueling while at the same time maximizing their aerobic training benefits.[44-46] This keto-adaptation is discussed in more detail in Chapter 22.

Three systematic reviews on professionally trained and recreationally trained athletes following KDs for at least 3 weeks gave inconsistent results. Most of the reviewed studies demonstrated no clear performance benefit on maximal oxygen uptake (VO_2 max), time to exhaustion, maximum heart rate, or perceived exertion.[44,46,47] However, a KD was not necessarily a performance impediment for short-duration, high-intensity trials.[42,46,47] The respiratory exchange rate was significantly reduced secondary to adoption of a KD, demonstrating that increased fat oxidation was involved in supplying the energy used during exercise.[47,48] In addition, decreases in metabolic efficiency have been noted among trained athletes after a 3- to 4-week adaptation period when competitions were at the level of at least 70% of VO_2 max.[48,49] The wide heterogeneity of study design, the inclusion of predominantly male study participants, and the limited number of peer-reviewed published studies make it necessary to further engage in high-quality research trials to better understand the effects of KDs on performance, body composition, gut microbiota, and overall impact on health.

LOW-CARBOHYDRATE DIETS

Although standardized criteria are used to define KDs, this is not the case with low-carbohydrate diets. When an individual is following a low-carbohydrate diet, their intake of carbohydrates is reduced to an arbitrary threshold. The only available guidance to determine a defined and agreed-upon "low-carbohydrate" cut-off point is from the acceptable minimum distribution range established for macronutrients by the Dietary Reference Intakes.[50] The acceptable minimum distribution range for carbohydrate is established at 45% to 65% of total daily energy intake. Therefore, a low-carbohydrate diet should consist of carbohydrate intake less than 45% of total daily calories.

A dietary pattern embracing a low-carbohydrate, high-fat approach without increased plasma ketone levels can be observed in endurance athletes. Studies to date remain equivocal with regard to the efficacy of high-fat dietary patterns (that do not induce nutritional ketosis) in sparing muscle glycogen, positively affecting exercise performance and perceived fatigue, or impacting cognitive performance. The most promising work appears to be decreasing muscle damage biomarkers during the postrecovery period, but more research is needed.[41,45] Training under low-carbohydrate conditions is further discussed in Chapter 2. Burke[49] has provided a very detailed review of the available published studies on ketogenic and low-carbohydrate, high-fat diets, noting that "[t]he available literature suggests that keto-adaptation may impair muscle glycogen utilization." Chapter 4 provides an in-depth discussion of the molecular adaptations that occur in response to a low-carbohydrate, high-fat diet, the training responses to this type of dietary pattern, and factors that the sports dietitian should consider when discussing dietary fat intake with athletes.

Low-Carbohydrate, High-Protein Diets

One popular example of a low-carbohydrate, high-protein diet is the paleolithic dietary pattern (or Paleo diet). This dietary pattern focuses on the food options that would have been available to ancient hunter-gathers, resulting in a low to moderate carbohydrate intake.[51] Key challenges in defining the Paleo dietary pattern include the wide diversity of ancestral dietary patterns, the lack of current expertise as to what paleolithic hominins actually consumed, the reality that a considerable number of plant and animal foods consumed during the Stone Age are currently extinct, and a vigorous debate regarding which core dietary components should be included.[4,51] This dietary pattern typically excludes refined cereal grains, refined sugars, mammalian milk, processed energy-dense but low-nutrient-density choices, oils, and legumes. As such, the diet often includes pasture-raised animal meats, vegetables, fruits, fungi, roots, nuts, and seeds. A high quantity of branched-chain amino acids and creatine exists in the diet because of the increased inclusion of animal proteins. A wide range of macronutrient distributions has been reported by those following this dietary pattern, including 8% to 35% of calories from protein, 20% to 72% from fat, and 19% to 48% from carbohydrate. To date, no comprehensive study has been published assessing the impact of this dietary pattern on professional athletes or on the body compositions, exercise capacities, or overall health of competitive athletes. In addition, because of the wide range of macronutrient distributions within the Paleo diet, a standardized macronutrient range would be necessary to identify any potential benefits and risks to athletes.[51]

RESTRICTIONS THAT MAY AFFECT DIETARY PATTERNS

Gluten-Free Diets

A gluten-free diet is not a dietary pattern per se, but it warrants discussion here because of its prevalence among athletes and its potential to impact dietary patterns and intake. An athlete following a gluten-free diet may also be following a number of different dietary patterns.

Gluten ingestion can mediate several clinical manifestations in those diagnosed with celiac disease, wheat allergy, or nonceliac gluten sensitivity.[52,53] Gluten is a protein found in the alcohol-soluble fraction of gliadin and glutenins within wheat, barley, and rye.[54] It is also widely present within the US food supply in sauces (eg, soy sauce), malt vinegar, additives, fillers, and flour because of its ability to enhance processed foods, improve the baking process, and retain air within protein matrixes.[55,56]

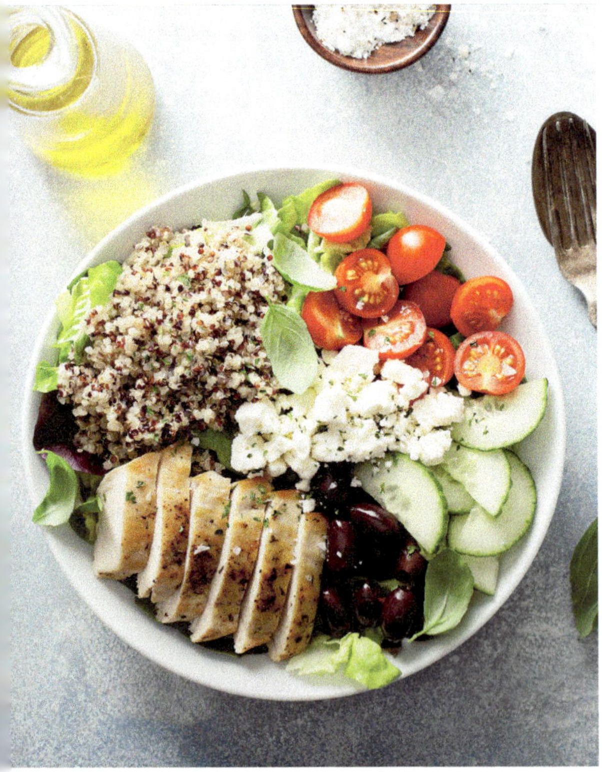

Recent data from Malsagova et al[29] indicated that a dietary pattern that excludes all identified sources of gluten is very popular among athletes. The authors noted that the percentage of athletes adhering to a gluten-free diet is 4 times greater than that within the general population. Lis et al[57] noted that, within their sample of 910 athletes (ranging from recreational athletes to Olympians), approximately 20% followed a gluten-free diet 90% to 100% of the time and approximately 70% of endurance athletes adhered to this style of eating approximately 50% of the time. Of the athletes following the gluten-free approach, less than 10% had a clinical diagnosis requiring a gluten-free diet.

The gluten-free diet may be popular among athletes because of the belief that gluten ingestion is universally associated with gastrointestinal inflammation and distress.[57] No data are currently available regarding the specific types of general dietary patterns followed by athletes who consume a gluten-free diet, but it is assumed that numerous carbohydrate choices would be eliminated.[58] Based on knowledge of the nutrient compositions of foods that are omitted, a gluten-free diet can put an athlete at risk for low intakes of protein as well as micronutrient deficiencies (ie, B vitamins, calcium, vitamin D, iron, and potassium).[57,59-62]

The Glycemic Index

In the 1980s, the term *glycemic index* (GI) was introduced. The GI serves to classify the total amount of glucose in the bloodstream, as measured by the area under the glucose curve, for 2 hours after the consumption of a

50-g portion of a carbohydrate test food. This is contrasted to the area under the glucose curve observed after consumption of the same quantity of a standard carbohydrate food, originally white bread and subsequently glucose. Carbohydrates were then indexed or classified according to their postprandial responses into the following categories[63]:

- high-GI food (GI ≥70)
- medium-GI food (GI = 56–70)
- low-GI food (GI ≤55)

Insufficient evidence exists to support the position that athletes should consider the GI of carbohydrates consumed in preexercise meals in order to enhance performance.[64] This is despite differences in a lower insulin stimulation between low- and high-GI carbohydrates and, thus, maintenance of a more stable blood glucose. More detailed information on the GIs of preexercise meals can be found in Chapter 2.

Short-term studies on athletes have predominantly failed to observe significant differences in fat oxidation following the consumption of low- vs high-GI carbohydrates.[65] Both enhanced performance[66] and no change in exercise performance have been observed in comparisons of low- vs high-GI foods.[67-71]

Although no parallel data exist for athletes, a 2021 exhaustive systematic review and meta-analysis of 43 cohorts from 34 publications involving more than 1.9 million adults observed no significant differences in BMI between the highest and lowest dietary GI groups. The authors concluded that there "is scant scientific evidence that low-GI diets are superior to high-GI diets for weight loss and obesity prevention."[72] It would therefore be an appropriate extrapolation to state that this observation would likely hold true for athletes as well.

GI characterizes the quality of a carbohydrate and does not define the total dietary quantity or percentage of carbohydrates in the athlete's diet. Determining the role of GI in helping healthy athletes maintain glucose control and the impact of GI on performance has been hampered by the wide heterogeneity of study methodologies, small sample sizes, and differing levels of total carbohydrates in the intervention diets.[65] More research is needed in this area.

Intermittent Fasting

Intermittent fasting (IF) is a dietary practice that consists of several different approaches. These may include[73]:

- time-restricted eating (which includes a feeding window of approximately 8–10 hours per day, with a restriction time of 14–16 hours)
- *fasting* (eating ad libitum for 1 day, followed by a day of total fasting or partial fasting, ingesting no more than 40% of one's recommended daily intake)
- 5:2 diet (eating ad libitum for 5 days per week, with 2 days per week of energy restriction)

The 2 most common approaches are time-restricted eating and alternate-day fasting. The total energy intake and the use of a specific dietary pattern are not factors considered in IF protocols.[73] The potential metabolic benefits to athletes who incorporate IF are theorized to include:

- decreased total energy intake, as well as reduced glucose and insulin plasma levels secondary to increased fat oxidation,[73-75] and
- decreased production of reactive oxygen species and, hence, a blunted inflammatory milieu.[75]

Keenan et al[74] published a comprehensive systematic review of 60 studies to assess the impact of IF and resistance training on body composition in recreationally active adults and nonelite adult athletes. These studies had a high heterogeneity in methodology, with half of participants using each of the 2 main types of IF (time-restricted eating and alternate-day fasting) for a period of 4 to 8 weeks. The only consistency in all protocols was the inclusion of a resistance training program. Total caloric intake was rarely reported, whereas the total protein intake ranged from 1.2 to 1.9 g per kilogram of body weight. The results indicated that lean body mass was maintained on all IF protocols, and the authors attributed this outcome to the inclusion of resistance training.[74]

Moro et al[75] published the results of an 8-week IF intervention involving adult athletes. This intervention randomized 38 male athletes into groups consuming a 16-hour time-restricted eating pattern or a standardized diet, with both arms of the trial tightly controlled for total caloric intake and macronutrient intake (carbohydrates, 53% ± 1.4%; protein, 22.1% ± 2.6%; fat, 24.7% ± 3.1%). The results showed that there were no differences in total caloric intake between groups and that both groups maintained strength and fat-free mass. However, individuals in the IF group showed decreased inflammation markers, baseline glucose, and plasma insulin levels. The authors noted that more work is necessary to clarify the total impact of IF dietary patterns on athletes. This is due to the many variations in study methodology among the investigations of IF diets performed to date, poorly defined dietary protocols, and the predominant use of male athletes; a definitive picture of the full impact on athletes' performance is not available.

Although the available data indicate that short-term studies of time-restricted eating in adult athletes do not show detriments to strength training adaptations, the long-term risks and benefits to athletes remain to be seen.[73-75] In addition, it must be noted that no comprehensive data exist to assess the types of additional dietary patterns being followed by those choosing to include an IF component. The extensive studies on athletes who fast during Ramadan have provided the most detailed information about this type of dietary pattern and potential health concerns. Specifically, fasting during Ramadan has been observed to put athletes at risk for dehydration; short-term studies using various IF protocols have not necessarily offered the opportunity to fully assess hydration.[73-75] This style of eating is not conducive to a frequent eating pattern that is beneficial to athletes, especially with regard to muscle protein synthesis, as discussed in Chapter 3. The authors note that the IF dietary approach is not optimal and, in fact, may be counterproductive to remodeling skeletal muscle protein.

SUMMARY

The nutrition and dietetics community has come to appreciate that dietary patterns are increasingly critical for their impact on overall health. One's dietary pattern, or the collective array of foods consumed on a habitual basis, broadly impacts metabolic well-being. These observations remain robust even after adjusting for a wide variety of specific factors such as the use of medications.[76] In addition, it is now widely accepted that the additive influence of the various nutrient and nonnutrient components within each food, or the "food matrix," influence one's metabolic milieu, as well as the synergistic interplay between foods within a dietary pattern.[77]

The sports dietitian must recognize that it is often challenging to balance focus on an athlete's overall dietary pattern while concurrently bringing necessary attention to very specific nutrient recommendations. A focused attention to specific food sources in sports nutrition is often warranted for many reasons, including manipulating plasma glucose levels, maximizing muscle protein synthesis, adjusting body composition, and responding to specific nutrient deficiencies. The skilled practitioner should recognize the importance of both addressing the overall dietary pattern and also highlighting specific nutrient considerations.

KEY TAKEAWAYS

A *dietary pattern* refers to the collective quantity, variety, proportion, and frequency of foods, beverages, and nutrients consumed over time.

Common elements of a healthy dietary pattern include intake of fruits, vegetables, whole grains, nuts, fish or seafood, lean meats and poultry, and low-fat dairy, as well as limited intake of processed foods, added sugars, *trans* fats, and specific saturated fats.

An extensive body of literature supports the position that one's overall dietary pattern, rather than intake of individual nutrients, is critical to optimal metabolic well-being and the reduction of disease risk.

A variety of dietary patterns can meet the nutritional and performance needs of athletes, regardless of the specific sport. Athletes should seek nutritional guidance from a sports dietitian before engaging in any new dietary pattern, particularly those that deviate from the ones described as "healthy" in the DGA.

REFERENCES

1. US Department of Agriculture and US Department of Health and Human Services. *Dietary Guidelines for Americans, 2020-2025*. 9th ed. December 2020.
2. US Department of Agriculture, Center for Nutrition Policy and Promotion, Nutrition Evidence Library, Dietary Patterns Technical Expert Collaborative. A series of systematic reviews on the relationship between dietary patterns and health outcomes. March 2014. Accessed May 12, 2020. https://nesr.usda.gov/sites/default/files / 2019-06/DietaryPatternsReport-FullFinal2.pdf5
3. English LK, Ard JD, Bailey RL, et al. Evaluation of dietary patterns and all-cause mortality: a systematic review. *JAMA Netw Open*. 2021;4(8):e2122277. doi:10.1001/jamanetworkopen.2021.22277
4. Katz DL, Meller S. Can we say what diet is best for health? *Annu Rev Public Health*. 2014;35:83-103. doi:10.1146/annurev-publhealth-032013-182351
5. Arnett DK, Blumenthal RS, Albert MA, et al. 2019 ACC/AHA guideline on the primary prevention of cardiovascular disease: executive summary: a report of the American College of Cardiology/ American Heart Association Task Force on Clinical Practice Guidelines. *Circulation*. 2019;140:e563-e595. doi:10.1161/CIR.0000000000000678
6. Grotto D, Ziel E. The Standard American Diet and its relationship to the health status of Americans. *Nutr Clin Pract*. 2010;25(6);603-612. doi:10.1177/08845336
7. dos Santos Leff P. Ultra-processed foods. In: Cheskin LJ, Franco M, Hoffman DJ, eds. *Encyclopedia of Human Nutrition*. 4th ed. Vol 4. Academic Press; 2023:653-662. doi:10.1016/B978-0-12-821848-8.00009-3
8. Meyer N, Reguant-Closa A. "Eat as if you could save the planet and win!" Sustainability integration into nutrition for exercise and sport. *Nutrients*. 2017;9(4):412. doi:10.3390/nu9040412
9. Melina V, Craig W, Levin S. Position of the Academy of Nutrition and Dietetics: vegetarian diets. *J Acad Nutr Diet*. 2016;116(12):1970-1980. doi:10.1016/j.jand.2016.09.025
10. Larson-Meyer DE. Vegetarian and vegan diets for athletic training and performance. *Sports Sci Exchange*. 2018;29(188):1-7.
11. Devrim-Lanpir A, Hill L, Knechtle B. Efficacy of popular diets applied by endurance athletes on sports performance: beneficial or detrimental? a narrative review. *Nutrients*. 2021;13(2):491. doi:10.3390/nu13020491
12. Shaw KA, Zello GA, Rodgers CD, Warkentin TD, Baerwald AR, Chilibeck PD. Benefits of a plant-based diet and considerations for the athlete. *Eur J Appl Physiol*. 2022;122(5):1163-1178. doi:10.1007/s00421-022-04902-w
13. Nebl J, Haufe S, Eigendorf J, Wasserfurth P, Tegtbur U, Hahn A. Exercise capacity of vegan, lacto-ovo-vegetarian and omnivorous recreational runners. *J Int Soc Sports Nutr*. 2019;16(1):23. doi:10.1186/s12970-019-0289-4
14. Leischik R, Spelsberg N. Vegan triple-ironman (raw vegetables/fruits). *Case Rep Cardiol*. 2014;2014:317246. doi:10.1155/2014/317246
15. Craddock JC, Probst YC, Peoples GE. Vegetarian and omnivorous nutrition—comparing physical performance. *Int J Sport Nutr Exerc Metab*. 2016;26(3):212-220. doi:10.1123/ijsnem.2015-0231
16. Kennedy DO. Phytochemicals for improving aspects of cognitive function and psychological state potentially relevant to sports performance. *Sports Med*. 2019;49(suppl 1):39-58. doi:10.1007/s40279-018-1007-0
17. Nebl J, Drabert K, Haufe S, et al. Exercise-induced oxidative stress, nitric oxide and plasma amino acid profile in recreational runners with vegetarian and non-vegetarian dietary patterns. *Nutrients*. 2019;11(8):1875. doi:10.3390/nu11081875
18. Potthast AB, Nebl J, Wasserfurth P, et al. Impact of nutrition on short-term exercise-induced sirtuin regulation: vegans differ from omnivores and lacto-ovo vegetarians. *Nutrients*. 2020;12(4):1004. doi:10.3390/nu12041004
19. Pohl A, Schünemann F, Bersiner K, Gehlert S. The impact of vegan and vegetarian diets on physical performance and molecular signaling in skeletal muscle. *Nutrients*. 2021;13(11):3884. doi:10.3390/nu13113884
20. Pinckaers PJM, Trommelen J, Snijders T, van Loon LJC. The anabolic response to plant-based protein ingestion. *Sports Med*. 2021;51(suppl 1):59-74. doi:10.1007/s40279-021-01540-8
21. Brennan JL, Keerati-U-Rai M, Yin H, et al. Differential responses of blood essential amino acid levels following ingestion of high-quality plant-based protein blends compared to whey protein—a double-blind randomized, cross-over, clinical trial. *Nutrients*. 2019;11(12):2987. doi:10.3390/nu11122987
22. Clarys P, Deliens T, Huybrechts I, et al. Comparison of nutritional quality of the vegan, vegetarian, semi-vegetarian, pesco-vegetarian and omnivorous diet. *Nutrients*. 2014;6(3):1318-1332. doi:10.3390/nu6031318
23. Cena H, Calder PC. Defining a healthy diet: evidence for the role of contemporary dietary patterns in health and disease. *Nutrients*. 2020;12(2):334. doi:10.3390/nu12020334
24. Ryan MC, Itsiopoulos C, Thodis T, et al. The Mediterranean diet improves hepatic steatosis and insulin sensitivity in individuals with non-alcoholic fatty liver disease. *J Hepatol*. 2013;59(1):138-143. doi:10.1016/j.jhep.2013.02.012
25. Sexton P, Black P, Metcalf P, et al. Influence of mediterranean diet on asthma symptoms, lung function, and systemic inflammation: a randomized controlled trial. *J Asthma*. 2013;50(1):75-81. doi:10.3109/02770903.2012.740120
26. Griffiths A, Matu J, Whyte E, et al. The Mediterranean dietary pattern for optimising health and performance in competitive athletes: a narrative review. *Br J Nutr*. 2022;128(7):1285-1298. doi:10.1017/S0007114521003202
27. Calella P, Gallè F, Di Onofrio V, Cerullo G, Liguori G, Valerio G. Adherence to Mediterranean diet in athletes: a narrative review. *Sport Sci Health*. 2022;18:1141-1148. doi:10.1007/s11332-022-00899-z

28. Baker ME, DeCesare KN, Johnson A, Kress KS, Inman CL, Weiss EP. Short-term Mediterranean diet improves endurance exercise performance: a randomized-sequence crossover trial. *J Am Coll Nutr.* 2019;38(7):597-605. doi:10.1080/07315724.2019.1568322
29. Malsagova KA, Kopylov AT, Sinitsyna AA, et al. Sports nutrition: diets, selection factors, recommendations. *Nutrients.* 2021;13(11):3771. doi:10.3390/nu13113771
30. Kerksick CM, Wilborn CD, Roberts MD, et al. ISSN exercise & sports nutrition review update: research & recommendations. *J Int Soc Sports Nutr.* 2018;15(1):38. doi:10.1186/s12970-018-0242-y
31. Thomas DT, Erdman KA, Burke LM. Position of the Academy of Nutrition and Dietetics, Dietitians of Canada, and the American College of Sports Medicine: nutrition and athletic performance. *J Acad Nutr Diet.* 2016;116(3):501-528. doi:10.1016/j.jand.2015.12.006
32. Burke LM, Castell LM, Casa DJ, et al. International Association of Athletics Federations Consensus Statement 2019: nutrition for athletics. *Int J Sport Nutr Exerc Metab.* 2019;29(2):73-84. doi:10.1123/ijsnem.2019-0065
33. Bykowska-Derda A, Zielińska-Dawidziak M, Czlapka-Matyasik M. Dietary-lifestyle patterns associated with bone turnover markers, and bone mineral density in adult male distance amateur runners—a cross-sectional study. *Nutrients.* 2022;14(10):2048. doi:10.3390/nu14102048
34. Klein DJ, Eck KM, Walker AJ, Pellegrino JK, Freidenreich DJ. Assessment of sport nutrition knowledge, dietary practices, and sources of nutrition information in NCAA Division III collegiate athletes. *Nutrients.* 2021;13(9):2962. doi:10.3390/nu13092962
35. Noll M, de Mendonça CR, de Souza Rosa LP, Silveira EA. Determinants of eating patterns and nutrient intake among adolescent athletes: a systematic review. *Nutr J.* 2017;16(1):46. doi:10.1186/s12937-017-0267-0
36. Diehl K, Yarmoliuk T, Mayer J, Zipfel S, Schnell, A. Eating patterns of elite adolescent athletes: results of a cross sectional study of 51 Olympic sports. *Dtsch Z Sportmed.* 2013;64(5):126-131. doi:10.5960/dzsm.2012.067
37. Iglesias-Gutiérrez E, García-Rovés PM, García A, Patterson AM. Food preferences do not influence adolescent high-level athletes' dietary intake. *Appetite.* 2008;50(2-3):536-543. doi:10.1016/j.appet.2007.11.003
38. Martínez S, Pasquarelli BN, Romaguera D, Arasa C, Tauler P, Aguiló A. Anthropometric characteristics and nutritional profile of young amateur swimmers. *J Strength Cond Res.* 2011;25(4):1126-1133. doi:10.1519/JSC.0b013e3181d4d3df
39. Aerenhouts D, Hebbelinck M, Poortmans JR, Clarys P. Nutritional habits of Flemish adolescent sprint athletes. *Int J Sport Nutr Exerc Metab.* 2008;18(5):509-523. doi:10.1123/ijsnem.18.5.509
40. Castillo M, Lozano-Casanova M, Sospedra I, Norte A, Gutiérrez-Hervás A, Martínez-Sanz JM. Energy and macronutrients intake in indoor sport team athletes: systematic review. *Nutrients.* 2022;14(22):4755. doi:10.3390/nu14224755
41. Burke LM, Ross ML, Garvican-Lewis LA, et al. Low carbohydrate, high fat diet impairs exercise economy and negates the performance benefit from intensified training in elite race walkers. *J Physiol.* 2017;595(9):2785-2807. doi:10.1113/JP273230
42. McSwiney FT, Wardrop B, Hyde PN, Lafountain RA, Volek JS, Doyle L. Keto-adaptation enhances exercise performance and body composition responses to training in endurance athletes. *Metabolism.* 2018;81:25-34. doi:10.1016/j.metabol.2017.10.010
43. Costa RJS, Hoffman MD, Stellingwerff T. Considerations for ultra-endurance activities: part 1- nutrition. *Res Sports Med.* 2019;27(2):166-181. doi:10.1080/15438627.2018.1502188
44. Hawley JA, Burke LM, Phillips SM, Spriet LL. Nutritional modulation of training-induced skeletal muscle adaptations. *J Appl Physiol (1985).* 2011;110(3):834-845. doi:10.1152/japplphysiol.00949.2010
45. Carr AJ, Sharma AP, Ross ML, Welvaert M, Slater GJ, Burke LM. Chronic ketogenic low carbohydrate high fat diet has minimal effects on acid-base status in elite athletes. *Nutrients.* 2018;10(2):236. doi:10.3390/nu10020236
46. Bailey CP, Hennessy E. A review of the ketogenic diet for endurance athletes: performance enhancer or placebo effect? *J Int Soc Sports Nutr.* 2020;17(1):33. doi:10.1186/s12970-020-00362-9
47. Cao J, Lei S, Wang X, Cheng S. The effect of a ketogenic low-carbohydrate, high-fat diet on aerobic capacity and exercise performance in endurance athletes: a systematic review and meta-analysis. *Nutrients.* 2021;13(8):2896. doi:10.3390/nu13082896
48. Shaw DM, Merien F, Braakhuis A, Maunder ED, Dulson DK. Effect of a ketogenic diet on submaximal exercise capacity and efficiency in runners. *Med Sci Sports Exerc.* 2019;51(10):2135-2146. doi:10.1249/MSS.0000000000002008
49. Burke LM. Ketogenic low-CHO, high-fat diet: the future of elite endurance sport? *J Physiol.* 2021;599(3):819-843. doi:10.1113/JP278928
50. Panel on Macronutrients; Panel on the Definition of Dietary Fiber; Subcommittee on Upper Reference Levels of Nutrients; Subcommittee on Interpretation and Uses of Dietary Reference Intakes; Standing Committee on the Scientific Evaluation of Dietary Reference Intakes; Food Nutrition Board, Institute of Medicine. *Dietary Reference Intakes for Energy, Carbohydrate, Fiber, Fat, Fatty Acids, Cholesterol, Protein, and Amino Acids.* National Academies Press; 2005. doi:10.17226/10490
51. Smith MM, Trexler ET, Sommer AJ, Starkoff BE, Devor ST. Unrestricted paleolithic diet is associated with unfavorable changes to blood lipids in healthy subjects. *Int J Exerc Sci.* 2014;7:128-139.
52. Catassi C, Bai JC, Bonaz B, et al. Non-celiac gluten sensitivity: the new frontier of gluten related disorders. *Nutrients.* 2013;5(10):3839-3853. doi:10.3390/nu5103839
53. Bascuñán KA, Roncoroni L, Branchi F, et al. The 5 Ws of a gluten challenge for gluten-related disorders. *Nutr Rev.* 2018;76(2):79-87. doi:10.1093/nutrit/nux068
54. Bascuñán KA, Elli L, Vecchi M, et al. Mediterranean gluten-free diet: is it a fair bet for the treatment of gluten-related disorders? *Front Nutr.* 2020;7:583981. doi:10.3389/fnut.2020.583981
55. Parada A, Araya M. History of gluten and its effects on celiac disease. Article in Spanish. *Rev Med Chil.* 2010;138:1319-1325. doi:10.4067/S0034-98872010001100018

56. Elli L, Ferretti F, Orlando S, et al. Management of celiac disease in daily clinical practice. *Eur J Intern Med.* 2019;61:15-24. doi:10.1016/j.ejim.2018.11.012
57. Lis D, Stellingwerff T, Kitic CM, Ahuja KD, Fell J. No effects of a short-term gluten-free diet on performance in nonceliac athletes. *Med Sci Sports Exerc.* 2015;47(12):2563-2570. doi:10.1249/MSS.0000000000000699
58. Black KE, Skidmore P, Brown RC. Case study: nutritional strategies of a cyclist with celiac disease during an ultraendurance race. *Int J Sport Nutr Exerc Metab.* 2012;22(4):304-310. doi:10.1123/ijsnem.22.4.304
59. Wu JH, Neal B, Trevena H, et al. Are gluten-free foods healthier than non-gluten-free foods? An evaluation of supermarket products in Australia. *Br J Nutr.* 2015;114(3):448-454. doi:10.1017/S0007114515002056
60. Kulai T, Rashid M. Assessment of nutritional adequacy of packaged gluten-free food products. *Can J Diet Pract Res.* 2014;75(4):186-190. doi:10.3148/cjdpr-2014-022
61. Missbach B, Schwingshackl L, Billmann A, et al. Gluten-free food database: the nutritional quality and cost of packaged gluten-free foods. *PeerJ.* 2015;3:e1337. doi:10.7717/peerj.1337
62. D'Angelo S, Cusano P. Gluten free diets in athletes. *J Phys Educ Sports.* 2020;20(suppl 4):2330-2336. doi:10.7752/jpes.2020.s4314
63. Jenkins DJ, Wolever TM, Taylor RH, et al. Glycemic index of foods: a physiological basis for carbohydrate exchange. *Am J Clin Nutr.* 1981;34(3):362-366. doi:10.1093/ajcn/34.3.362
64. Burdon CA, Spronk I, Cheng HL, O'Connor HT. Effect of glycemic index of a pre-exercise meal on endurance exercise performance: a systematic review and meta-analysis. *Sports Med.* 2017;47(6):1087-1101. doi:10.1007/s40279-016-0632-8
65. Dudar MD, Bode ED, Fishkin KR, et al. Pre-sleep low glycemic index modified starch does not improve next-morning fuel selection or running performance in male and female endurance athletes. *Nutrients.* 2020;12(9):2888. doi:10.3390/nu12092888
66. Wu CL, Williams C. A low glycemic index meal before exercise improves endurance running capacity in men. *Int J Sport Nutr Exerc Metab.* 2006;16(5):510-527. doi:10.1123/ijsnem.16.5.510
67. Moore LJ, Midgley AW, Thomas G, Thurlow S, McNaughton LR. The effects of low- and high-glycemic index meals on time trial performance. *Int J Sports Physiol Perform.* 2009;4(3):331-344. doi:10.1123/ijspp.4.3.331
68. Wong SH, Chan OW, Chen YJ, Hu HL, Lam CW, Chung PK. Effect of preexercise glycemic-index meal on running when CHO-electrolyte solution is consumed during exercise. *Int J Sport Nutr Exerc Metab.* 2009;19(3):222-242. doi:10.1123/ijsnem.19.3.222
69. Febbraio MA, Keenan J, Angus DJ, Campbell SE, Garnham AP. Preexercise carbohydrate ingestion, glucose kinetics, and muscle glycogen use: effect of the glycemic index. *J Appl Physiol (1985).* 2000;89(5):1845-1851. doi:10.1152/jappl.2000.89.5.1845
70. Jentjens RL, Jeukendrup AE. Effects of pre-exercise ingestion of trehalose, galactose and glucose on subsequent metabolism and cycling performance. *Eur J Appl Physiol.* 2003;88(4-5):459-465. doi:10.1007/s00421-002-0729-7
71. Kern M, Heslin CJ, Rezende RS. Metabolic and performance effects of raisins versus sports gel as pre-exercise feedings in cyclists. *J Strength Cond Res.* 2007;21(4):1204-1207. doi:10.1519/R-21226.1
72. Gaesser GA, Miller Jones J, Angadi SS. Perspective: Does glycemic index matter for weight loss and obesity prevention? examination of the evidence on "fast" compared with "slow" carbs. *Adv Nutr.* 2021;12(6):2076-2084. doi:10.1093/advances/nmab093
73. Correia JM, Santos I, Pezarat-Correia P, Minderico C, Mendonca GV. Effects of intermittent fasting on specific exercise performance outcomes: a systematic review including meta-analysis. *Nutrients.* 2020;12(5):1390. doi:10.3390/nu12051390
74. Keenan S, Cooke MB, Belski R. The effects of intermittent fasting combined with resistance training on lean body mass: a systematic review of human studies. *Nutrients.* 2020;12(8):2349. doi:10.3390/nu12082349
75. Moro T, Tinsley G, Bianco A, et al. Effects of eight weeks of time-restricted feeding (16/8) on basal metabolism, maximal strength, body composition, inflammation, and cardiovascular risk factors in resistance-trained males. *J Transl Med.* 2016;14(1):290. doi:10.1186/s12967-016-1044-0
76. Jacobs DR, Tapsell LC. Food synergy: the key to a healthy diet. *Proc Nutr Soc.* 2013;72(2):200-206. doi:10.1017/S0029665112003011
77. US Department of Agriculture. National Agriculture Library. Food matrix. December 22, 2015. Accessed December 22, 2023. https://agclass.nal.usda.gov/vocabularies/nalt/concept?uri=https://lod.nal.usda.gov/nalt/17238

CHAPTER 26

Nutrition Operations and Management

Matthew Frakes, PhD, RD, LDN, CSCS, ISAK-2, and Melissa L. Brown, PhD, RD, CSSD, LD

LEARNING OBJECTIVES

- Describe the role of the sports registered dietitian in nutrition operations and management.
- Apply foodservice concepts to the athletics field in the areas of menu development, safety, sanitation, purchasing, receiving, storage, inventory, distribution, and service.
- Compare and contrast the unique foodservice needs of an athletics department with traditional foodservice.
- Identify inputs, transformations, and outputs in the foodservice systems model as it pertains to athletics.
- Understand the contributing factors to the design and layout of foodservice facilities.
- Apply management and leadership concepts to sports nutrition operations including resource management, staffing, and finances.

INTRODUCTION

The information presented in the previous chapters of this book collectively underscores the vital importance of performance nutrition for health and athletic performance. The preferred provider of performance nutrition services is the registered dietitian nutritionist (RDN) with advanced training in sports nutrition, often with the added credential of Board-Certified Specialist in Sports Dietetics (CSSD). The role of the sports RDN has expanded tremendously over the years to truly maximize the training and education that is part of the pathway to becoming an RDN. The *Standards of Practice and Standards of Professional Performance for Registered Dietitian Nutritionists (Competent, Proficient, and Expert) in Sports and Human Performance Nutrition*[1] describes in detail what constitutes competent, proficient, and expert levels of practice for sports RDNs. After reviewing the indicators for each standard, one can clearly see the growth and expansion of the role of the sports RDN that goes well beyond the provision of medical nutrition therapy. Sports RDNs are tasked with providing behavioral and educational counseling, gaining knowledge and understanding of exercise physiology and sports science, running culinary nutrition programs and nutrition operations, and overseeing foodservice management and administration. A 2022 publication by Lambert et al[2] further describes the unique qualifications of the sports RDN.

Sports RDNs are responsible for providing the highest quality of care to athletes within the collegiate, professional, and Olympic athletic settings or within tactical and law enforcement settings. Moreover, "sports RDNs are both uniquely qualified to supply a broad scope of sports nutrition services that adheres to current evidence-based practices and uniquely positioned to assist athletic departments in administering, evolving, and optimizing all aspects of a program's sports nutrition service model."[2] Current objectives listed in job descriptions include oversight of the nutrition department and community initiatives; development of nutrition education; administrative responsibilities including staff management, preceptorship, and professional development; policy and procedure development for nutrition interventions in clinical services; and management of all foodservice operations.

This chapter is not intended to serve as a comprehensive resource on nutrition operations and management, but rather it is meant to provide a general overview with specific application to athletics and sports nutrition. The minimum standards for integrated services established in the Lambert et al[2] publication can be found in Box 26.1 and underscore the variety of roles the sports RDN serves. Note that the minimum standards were established specifically with respect to collegiate athletics, but they are still highly relevant to other areas of athletics. This chapter is divided into 2 sections, with the first section focusing on nutrition operations and the second focusing on management and administration, with some necessary overlap between the 2 sections.

BOX 26.1 Minimum Standards for Integrated Services[2]

Foodservice management services

Collaborate with dining services professionals on the planning, selection, and delivery of meals

Establish the food supply chain and select quality vendors in partnership with dining services

Set guidelines for menu planning and establish menu cycles to be implemented by the dining services department

Ensure that student-athletes with food allergies; religious, cultural, or cuisine preferences; and clinical diagnoses that require prescription diets have access to appropriately modified meals

Set standards for and advise athletics operations staff on negotiating with foodservice providers for meal price and quality, particularly with respect to off-site meals

Negotiate cost-effective purchasing of National Collegiate Athletic Association (NCAA)-compliant products and supplements

Provide food safety education for athletes and staff, especially as it pertains to the storage and consumption of food and meals away from dining facilities as needed

Sports nutrition services and staffing

Leadership

Set mission, vision, and values statements for the sports nutrition program or department

Participate in organization-wide strategic planning

Collaborate on departmental initiatives

Serve on administrative committees and act as a liaison for campus collaboration

Personnel management

Recruit, hire, and mentor staff dietitians and train individuals for positions

Assign and delegate department responsibilities effectively

Serve as an expert in nutrition services

Budget management

Develop an operating budget for the department and multisport program

Organize billing and invoice procedures

Monitor departmental expenses

Clinic management

Supervise the provision of services and access to care

Develop appropriate documentation processes

Build secure, confidential Health Insurance Portability and Accountability (HIPAA)- and Family Educational Rights and Privacy Act (FERPA)-compliant services

Monitor and implement all federal and state regulatory requirements related to the practice of dietetics and foodservice

Contract and compliance management

Interact with fundraising and sponsorship personnel to support nutrition initiatives

Build a culture of supplement safety across the interdisciplinary departments and sports programs

Assess product selection and use for compliance with NCAA rules and regulations

Evaluate meal and snack provision for compliance with NCAA rules and regulations

NUTRITION OPERATIONS

Overview of the Foodservice Industry

The foodservice industry is an essential part of the US economy and in 2020 employed approximately 12.1 million individuals according to the Bureau of Labor and Statistics.[3] Prior to the COVID-19 pandemic, Americans were consuming more meals away from home than ever before. In 1970, Americans were consuming 26% of meals away from home, and in 2018, that had increased to 44%.[3] Food consumption patterns changed dramatically during the COVID-19 pandemic and led to the growth of online ordering and delivery platforms such as GrubHub (GrubHub Inc, Chicago, IL) and DoorDash (DoorDash Inc, San Francisco, CA), as well as an increase in online grocery shopping services such as PeaPod (PeaPod Digital Labs, formerly, PeaPod Online Grocer LLC, Chicago, IL) and Instacart (Maple Bear Inc, San Francisco, CA). Finally, according to *QSR* (an online magazine covering the quick-service foodservice industry), "virtual" or "ghost" kitchens that specialize in meal production followed by delivery or pickup also grew during the pandemic.[4] The use of similar online ordering and delivery services became an integral component of meal management within athletics as well.

The foodservice industry includes commercial foodservices and noncommercial foodservices, which includes the military. Commercial foodservices are profit-making and include all varieties of restaurants (limited service, fast-casual, pop-up, family, casual dining, fine dining, and hotel dining),[5,6] contracted onsite foodservices, foodservices for sporting activities, caterers, vending, and retail operations that have a section for meals such as those found in grocery stores.[5] Noncommercial foodservices include onsite foodservices that are run by the organization in which they are housed such as businesses, colleges/schools, and hospitals.[5] Box 26.2 on page 692 describes the different types of operations and services included in the foodservice industry.

Each foodservice has its own mission statement. A mission statement is a general statement describing what the foodservice does, why the foodservice exists, and what purpose it serves for its customers. For

BOX 26.2 Types of Foodservice Operations and Services

Type	Description
Conventional	Preparation and serving of the meals are performed in the same facility and often use menu items that are made from scratch; input of labor is high.
Assembly-serve	The majority of the meals are prepared from convenience foods in that the meals need only to be assembled and not made from scratch; input of labor is less than in conventional settings.
Ready-prepared	Most of the meal preparation is completed in advance, and foods are stored chilled or frozen for later use.
Commissary	Meals are prepared in one central location and then shipped out or delivered to external sites for serving.
Limited service	Customers order their food and pay before sitting down to eat or taking the food to go; also known as quick service and includes fast-food restaurants.

example, a restaurant's mission may be to provide "a relaxing and enjoyable dining experience with distinctive food, drinks, and service for our guests, as well as offer a cooperative, rewarding environment for our employees." A school's foodservice mission may be "to promote good nutrition by providing quality meals while maintaining the highest level of customer satisfaction."[5] In contrast, a foodservice mission within the athletics environment might be to "promote the highest level of overall health and athletic performance by providing quality performance-based meals while maintaining the highest level of customer satisfaction."

Most foodservice operations use a systems approach, in which the interrelated and interdependent parts are arranged in a manner that produces a unified whole.[5,6] *Operations* in the context of this chapter refers to how the products or services of a business are produced, and specifically in regard to foodservice operations, it examines the processes from planning menus to production and service to sanitation and cleanup. Foodservice operations consist of the following components:

- menu planning
- purchasing
- receiving and storage
- ingredient assembly
- production
- distribution and service
- sanitation and safety
- design and layout of facility services
- department budget and menu forecasting

Menu Development and Planning

Sports RDNs are often involved in menu development and should therefore be experienced in that area. When developing menus, it is important to consider cost, taste, ability to standardize the recipes, nutrient profiles, variety, balance, cultural and dietary needs, length of each menu cycle, availability and accessibility of equipment and facilities, and the hours and convenience of dining areas around the athletes' personal and/

or academic schedules. The ability to standardize recipes is critical to cost-containment efforts.

In an area unique to sports nutrition and athletics, the menu development process also needs to consider performance needs and nutrient periodization. This includes game preparation and recovery meals as well as enhanced, expanded, and more frequent meal offerings during training camps and periods when the athletes will be training multiple times per day. Time and effort will also need to go into planning travel meals.

When one is developing a menu, catering to the needs of a single individual is not typically possible, nor is it advised. If an athlete will only eat certain foods, this should be handled outside the menu development process. One individual should not dictate the menu development process. Menus should be revised often to purge unpopular or expensive items and to add newer or trendy items to minimize menu cycle fatigue.

Box 26.3 lists examples of the factors that impact menu development and planning. Box 26.4 on page 694 lists the sequential steps one should take when planning a menu.

BOX 26.3 Considerations That Impact Menu Development and Planning

How often will the cycle change?

How will the pricing work (eg, á la carte, complete meal)?

Is the menu intended for a single-use event (eg, a meal served at a banquet)?

How much choice will customers be given to select their meal? (The fewer the choices, the more cost-effective the menu will be; however, it will still be necessary to develop alternative options for preference, allergies, client routines, etc). Options include:

- selective menus (at least 2 choices per category)
- semiselective menus (1-2 choices per category)
- nonselective or preselected menus

Will a cycle menu be used?

- A cycle menu repeats over a specified period of time.
- A cycle menu adds variety to meals in foodservices that serve a constant clientele.
- A cycle menu makes food production more complicated than a static menu (usually a larger menu with multiple categories and infrequent changes).
- The cycle length depends on the ability to incorporate variety and maintain interest.
  - A 1-week menu cycle works well for training camps that may last up to 2 to 3 weeks.
  - A 5 to 10-day menu cycle works well for situations lasting longer than 1 month.
  - A 1 to 2-week menu cycle works well in hospitals where patient stays are less than 1 week.
  - A 3 to 4-week menu cycle is typical for high school students.
  - A 4 to 6-week menu cycle is designed for operations that serve customers for an extended period of time, such as long-term care facilities, academic dining centers that work in semesters, and businesses.

Will more than 1 type of menu be used (for example, for different populations within the same organization)?

- Patients may choose meals from a static or restaurant-style menu.
- Employees who eat in the cafeteria may choose meals from a 4- to 6-week cycle menu that is à la carte.
- The catering manager may employ single-use menus.

Continued on next page

BOX 26.3 Considerations That Impact Menu Development and Planning (CONTINUED)

Does the menu meet the following conditions?

- The menu is consistent with the concept and mission of the foodservice program, as well as the preferences and cultural backgrounds of the target customers.
- The menu offers visually appealing and flavorful foods with different colors, sizes, shapes, and textures that were prepared using various cooking methods.
- The menu consists of low-cost items that balance out the higher-cost items so that the overall menu is cost-effective in terms of food and labor costs.
- The menu includes ingredients that can be effectively purchased, produced, and served on a consistent basis.
- The menu meets appropriate government regulations.
- The menu includes environmentally responsible foods and items that reflect a focus on sustainability? (In athletics, these factors need to be considered with health and performance as the driving force and according to periodized nutrition strategies.)
- The menu considers sourcing from and cost of local vendors, local farms, seasonal produce, and surrounding restaurants for catering services and special meals.
- The menu considers the location of services and the need to work with various culinary teams during in-season team travel.

BOX 26.4 Sequential Steps in Planning a Menu for Athletics[a]

1. Survey team preferences, aversions, and allergens.
2. Decide on a meal pattern.
3. Plan meal components as follows:
   a. dinner entrées (plan these first, as they are typically the most expensive);
   b. lunch entrées;
   c. side dishes for lunch and dinner;
   d. appetizers;
   e. desserts for lunch and dinner;
   f. beverages, condiments, and breads; and
   g. breakfast, if served.
4. Plan portion sizes.
5. Modify dishes to meet prescribed diets.
6. Complete a nutrient analysis.
7. Design menu engineering concepts for situations in which it matters, such as placement of certain items to increase likelihood of selection, etc.

[a] In athletics, these decisions are all made with health and performance as the driving factors and according to periodized nutrition strategies.

COLLEGE DINING AND CONTRACT COMPANIES

College athletics is one of the largest sectors that employs sports RDNs and illustrates the breadth of services that sports RDNs can provide. (Refer to Chapter 13 for comprehensive coverage of collegiate athletics.) College dining can be commercial or noncommercial, and it can be self-operated or outsourced to a foodservice contract company such as Aramark Corporation (Philadelphia, PA), Chartwells Higher Ed (division of Compass, Rye Brook, NY), or Sodexo USA (Gaithersburg, MD). The sports RDN will need to be aware of such contracts and know their contents and provisions. For instance, some contracts may be exclusive-use contracts, which would prohibit the ordering of outside food. In addition, many of these foodservice companies have contract RDNs that work with the general student body but not necessarily with the student-athletes.

Dining halls on college campuses have changed dramatically over the years. Dining halls now offer many stations and concepts using innovative foodservice equipment such as brick or stone hearth pizza ovens, tandoori ovens, and display cooking woks. College menus have evolved to be dynamic, healthful, global, fresh, and sustainable and also to allow for student customization. In the past, students may have been provided with 2 to 3 choices per meal in the dining halls. Currently, the choices have expanded to include made-to-order entrées, salad bars, deli and pasta bars, grill stations, specialty areas for prescribed diets and allergy-free zones, fresh baked desserts and sundae bars, and smoothie stations. Food services at colleges and universities primarily serve current students but also feed faculty, staff, administrators, and visitors. Customers no longer have to eat all meals in 1 main dining hall. Options have expanded to offer retail dining such as microrestaurants, chain restaurants in the form of a kiosk such as Starbucks (Seattle, WA), and convenience stores that sell grab-and-go items. Many of the college dining operations now remain open in some capacity 24 hours per day and have apps that display the weekly menus. These can be an excellent tool for nutrition education and plate building.

Figure 26.1 on pages 696 through 698 provides an example of a 1-week cycle menu.

Safety and Sanitation

All foodservice operations need to place a high priority on safety and sanitation to protect employees and customers. Causes of food contamination may include chemical exposures such as spraying a cleaning solution too close to uncovered food; however, the most prevalent cause is biological.[5] Biological hazards can be categorized as bacteria, viruses, fungi, parasites, and toxins. A full discussion of biological hazards goes beyond the scope of this chapter, but in general, sports RDNs should be knowledgeable about the following resources:

- the US Food and Drug Administration's *Food Code*, which provides guidance on food safety and sanitation[7];
- the role of the US Department of Agriculture's Food Safety and Inspection Service (FSIS)[8];
- the role of the Centers for Disease Control and Prevention[9];
- ways of preventing foodborne illness;
- types of bacteria, viruses, and parasites that cause foodborne illness;
- minimum internal cooking temperatures to ensure food safety;
- proper food storage temperatures;
- the Hazard Analysis Critical Control Point (HAACP) system which is a prevention-based food safety system[10]; and
- ways to ensure an accident-free workplace and the role of Occupational Safety and Health Administration (OSHA).[11]

Organizations such as ServSafe (part of the National Restaurant Association Educational Foundation, Inc) provide training that includes safe food manager, safe food handling, safe alcohol, safe allergen, and safe workplace programs.

Purchasing, Receiving, Storage, Inventory, Distribution, and Service

Once the menus have been developed and the safety and sanitation protocols are in place, the remaining steps in the foodservice operation can be considered. When purchasing and storing ingredients and materials, the sports RDN should prepare as follows:

Breakfast							
Monday	Tuesday	Wednesday	Thursday	Friday	Saturday	Sunday	
6:00 AM–10:00 AM	6:00 AM–10:00 AM	6:00 AM–10:00 AM	6:00 AM–10:00 AM	6:00 AM–10:00 AM	6:00 AM–10:00 AM	6:00 AM–10:00 AM	
Bananas	Bananas	Bananas	Bananas	Bananas	Bananas	Bananas	Island 1
Strawberries	Strawberries	Strawberries	Strawberries	Strawberries	Strawberries	Strawberries	
Watermelon	Watermelon	Watermelon	Watermelon	Watermelon	Watermelon	Watermelon	
Cantaloupe	Cantaloupe	Cantaloupe	Cantaloupe	Cantaloupe	Cantaloupe	Cantaloupe	
Pineapple	Red grapes	Kiwi	Dragon fruit	Mango	Oranges	Pineapple	
Fresh blueberries	Fresh blueberries	Fresh blueberries	Fresh blueberries	Fresh blueberries	Fresh blueberries	Fresh blueberries	
Oatmeal/yogurt toppings:	Oatmeal/yogurt toppings:	Oatmeal/yogurt toppings:	Oatmeal/yogurt toppings:	Oatmeal/yogurt toppings:	Oatmeal/yogurt toppings:	Oatmeal/yogurt toppings:	Island 2
Walnuts, cranberries	Walnuts, cranberries	Walnuts, cranberries	Walnuts, cranberries	Walnuts, cranberries	Walnuts, cranberries	Walnuts, cranberries	
Shredded cheese, butter	Shredded cheese, butter	Shredded cheese, butter	Shredded cheese, butter	Shredded cheese, butter	Shredded cheese, butter	Shredded cheese, butter	
Brown sugar, cinnamon	Brown sugar, cinnamon	Brown sugar, cinnamon	Brown sugar, cinnamon	Brown sugar, cinnamon	Brown sugar, cinnamon	Brown sugar, cinnamon	
Granola, honey	Granola, honey	Granola, honey	Granola, honey	Granola, honey	Granola, honey	Granola, honey	
Greek yogurt	Greek yogurt	Greek yogurt	Greek yogurt	Greek yogurt	Greek yogurt	Greek yogurt	
Syrup	Syrup	Syrup	Syrup	Syrup	Syrup	Syrup	Soup
Oatmeal	Oatmeal	Oatmeal	Oatmeal	Oatmeal	Oatmeal	Oatmeal	
Scrambled eggs	Scrambled eggs	Scrambled eggs	Scrambled eggs	Scrambled eggs	Scrambled eggs	Scrambled eggs	Hot line
Bacon	Bacon	Bacon	Bacon	Bacon	Bacon	Bacon	
Turkey sausage patty	Chicken-and-apple sausage	Turkey sausage patty	Turkey sausage link	Turkey sausage patty	Chicken-and-apple sausage	Oven-fried chicken tenders	
Breakfast potatoes	Breakfast potatoes	Breakfast potatoes	Breakfast potatoes	Breakfast potatoes	Breakfast potatoes	Breakfast potatoes	
Build your own omelet	Build your own omelet	Build your own omelet	Build your own omelet	Build your own omelet	Build your own omelet	Build your own omelet	
Hot biscuits/jelly	Hot biscuits/jelly	Hot biscuits/jelly	Hot biscuits/jelly	Hot biscuits/jelly	Hot biscuits/jelly	Hot biscuits/jelly	Island 3
Pancakes	Waffles	French toast	Cinnamon rolls	Banana nut muffin	Pancakes	Waffles	
Country gravy	Country gravy	Country gravy	Country gravy	Country gravy	Country gravy	Country gravy	
Syrup, sugar-free syrup, honey	Syrup, sugar-free syrup, honey	Syrup, sugar-free syrup, honey	Syrup, sugar-free syrup, honey	Syrup, sugar-free syrup, honey	Syrup, sugar-free syrup, honey	Syrup, sugar-free syrup, honey	

FIGURE 26.1 **Example 1-week cycle menu**

Lunch							
Monday	Tuesday	Wednesday	Thursday	Friday	Saturday	Sunday	
12:00 PM–3:00 PM	12:00 PM–3:00 PM	12:00 PM–3:00 PM	12:00 PM–3:00 PM	12:00 PM–3:00 PM	12:00 PM–3:00 PM	12:00 PM–3:00 PM	
Burger/chicken sandwich	Burger/chicken sandwich	Burger/chicken sandwich	Burger/chicken sandwich	Burger/chicken sandwich	Burger/chicken sandwich	Burger/chicken sandwich	BYO Burger station
Flatbread pizza	Flatbread pizza	Flatbread pizza	Flatbread pizza	Flatbread pizza	Flatbread pizza	Flatbread pizza	Stone hearth pizza oven
Mediterranean chicken breast	Honey-lime chicken breast	Kung pao beef	Grilled beef	Garlic parmesan chicken breast	Red wine beef	Blackened chicken	Hot line
Rosemary beef	Spaghetti and meatballs	Sweet-and-sour pork loin	Sausage and peppers	Strip loin steak	BBQ pork loin	Bacon	
Lemon-garlic tilapia	Fried catfish	Shrimp stir fry	Lemon-butter Swai fish	Glazed salmon	Shrimp kabobs	Shrimp and grits	
Herbed orzo	Fresh pasta	Fried rice	Steamed rice	Roasted sweet potatoes	Scallion rice	Rice and gravy	Hot line
Rice pilaf	Roasted red potatoes	Lo mein	Red beans	Brown rice and peas	Olive oil smashed potatoes	Beef lasagna	
Roasted cauliflower	Baked broccoli	Sautéed green beans	Mustard greens	Roasted carrots	Balsamic green beans	Fried okra	
Stewed chickpeas	Squash and zucchini	Miso soup	Vegetable medley	Grilled corn	Stir-fried root vegetables	Carrot souffle	Vegetarian
Artichoke and shallots	Sweet peas and onions	Sautéed sugar snaps	Sautéed spinach	Steamed asparagus	Stir-fried mushrooms and peppers	Roasted Brussels sprouts	
Corn and peppers	Chili roasted Brussels sprouts	Roasted okra	Braised cabbage	Sautéed bok choy	Roasted broccoli	Roasted sweet potatoes	
Chef's special	Chef's special	Chef's special	Chef's special	Chef's special	Chef's special	Chef's special	
Fruit bar	Fruit bar	Fruit bar	Fruit bar	Fruit bar	Fruit bar	Fruit bar	

Continued on next page

Dinner							
Monday	Tuesday	Wednesday	Thursday	Friday	Saturday	Sunday	
5:00 PM–8:00 PM	5:00 PM–8:00 PM	5:00 PM–8:00 PM	5:00 PM–8:00 PM	5:00 PM–8:00 PM	5:00 PM–8:00 PM	5:00 PM–8:00 PM	
Carved leg of lamb	Boudin/sausage links	Prime rib	Whole duck	Marinated pork tenderloin	Carved local beef	BBQ chicken	Carving
Chef's special	Chef's special	Chef's special	Chef's special	Chef's special	Chef's special	Chef's special	
Pizza bar	Pizza bar	Pizza bar	Pizza bar	Pizza bar	Pizza bar	Pizza bar	
Pasta bar	Pasta bar	Pasta bar	Pasta bar	Pasta bar	Pasta bar	Pasta bar	
Fried catfish	Shrimp and grits	Korean beef	Honey-garlic cod	Beef tips	Shrimp-and-peppers pasta	Chicken piccata	Hot line
Shrimp alfredo	BBQ brisket	Meatballs and marinara	Hamburger steak	Oven-roasted chicken quarters	Beef lasagna	Honey baked ham	
Chipotle chicken breast	Chicken thighs carnitas	Blackened salmon	General Tso's chicken	Panéed redfish	Chicken cordon bleu	Pepper steak	
Brown rice	Grilled corn	Herbed pasta	Mashed potatoes	Steamed rice	Pasta	Wild rice pilaf	Hot line
Grilled corn	Cilantro rice	Roasted fingerlings	Scallion rice	Sweet potato hash	Roasted red potatoes	Sautéed potatoes	
Roasted broccoli	Mixed vegetable	Zucchini and squash	Roasted carrots	Grilled asparagus	Squash and peppers	Broccoli and mushrooms	
Eggplant parmesan	Black beans	Sautéed bok choy	Braised greens	Lima beans	Tomato soup	Garlic green beans	Vegetarian
Mushroom and peppers	Roasted cauliflower	Vegetable stir fry	Fried okra	California vegetable medley	Sautéed spinach	Sautéed edamame	
Sautéed cabbage	Glazed carrots	Roasted chickpeas	Green peppers and onions	Roasted whole okra	Stir-fried carrots	Mixed greens	
Garlic toast	Corn muffins	Biscuits	Corn muffins	Garlic toast	Cornbread	Biscuits	Bread
Hawaiian rolls	Dinner rolls	Breadsticks	Hawaiian rolls	Cheddar biscuits	Bacon	Breadsticks	
Fruit bar	Fruit bar	Fruit bar	Fruit bar	Fruit bar	Fruit bar	Fruit bar	

FIGURE 26.1 **Example 1-week cycle menu (continued)**

- Be knowledgeable about and adhere to all local, state, and federal laws and undergo inspections on the schedules outlined in those laws.
- Plan and organize storage space, cooling, refrigeration, and freezing for products planned for purchasing.
- Use reputable preapproved vendors.
- Use training and education in sports nutrition and exercise physiology to assess and purchase food products and supplements that are supportive of the vision of the sports nutrition program and team or individual athlete outcomes.
- Use the menu to dictate what ingredients are needed for purchase, their quantities, and the estimated cost using the standardized recipes.
- Once the purchase needs have been determined, request and evaluate quotes before deciding from whom to purchase.
- Negotiate the price prior to securing an order or contract.
- Always inspect products upon delivery to make sure that they meet quality standards and match the purchase order prior to processing and paying invoices.
- Follow policies for food safety and storage.

A more expanded discussion of distribution and service is presented later in this chapter, including specifics on training tables, fueling stations, catering, travel, and meal management.

Trends and Concepts

The foodservice industry is constantly evolving and developing innovative concepts to enhance operations, increase customer and employee satisfaction, and improve financial outcomes. New trends are emerging in menu design, cooking methods, and foodservice equipment. In addition, modern technology has dramatically changed the foodservice industry through the advent of the internet, smartphones, and foodservice-related and meal-management-related apps. There are even new concepts that involve meal delivery though the use of drones, as well as robotic devices that produce food. Those working in foodservice operations, including sports RDNs, should stay apprised of these trends to keep their operations relevant. This is especially true in the sports nutrition field because of the plethora of new scientific findings directly impacting the care provided for athletes, as well as their health and performance needs. Modern athletes want increased options that enhance their health and performance with a focus on authentic ethnic dishes, taste, and sustainability. Modern athletes also place convenience in high demand, with the ability to make their meal management simple, easy, and quick. Specific meal-management apps and automated logistics tailored toward their daily schedules can help with this convenience.

The following list provides examples of drivers of foodservice trends:

- economic and business environment (increased competition or rising labor costs can affect menu prices)
- societal trends (increased awareness of the environment has encouraged farm-to-table and farm-to-counter eating)
- customer demographics (younger generations prefer fresh ingredients and freshly prepared menu items)
- customer demands (more consumers want healthy foods and/or convenient meals that will enhance athletic performance)
- technology and big data (online options for ordering food have rapidly expanded)

Foodservice involves more than just the food itself; foodservice also includes concepts such as the environment in which food is served and the time when it is served. For instance, what meals during what parts of the day (breakfast, lunch, dinner, snack) will be served? What is the décor of the dining area, along with the table settings, tone, and atmosphere? What are the demographics of the people being served, and does the menu cater to them appropriately? Where is the dining area located? Is it in close proximity to target customers and visible with plenty of signage to identify it? For example, if the foodservice operation has a fueling station, is that fueling station located in close proximity to where the athletes typically eat, and do they know it is there?

Finally, foodservice operations are important when it comes to attracting athletes and can impact their decision on where to play. Athletes often have a choice on where to play, and the more "perks" an organization can offer to them, the more attractive it will be to them. Athletes like to know that they will be taken care of in all aspects, and not just through on-the-field coaching.

Facilities and Design Layout

One of the less common responsibilities that may fall to the sports RDN is participating in facilities and design layout. Often, the sports RDN will be hired to work in an existing facility, but there are situations in which a brand new facility is being built or an existing facility is being renovated that require input from the RDN. In these situations, the sports RDN can provide guidance on selecting the new location, designing the overall concept, and creating the dining environment. These opportunities add to the value and vision of services the sports RDN provides. Sports RDNs should have input into what foodservice equipment is needed; the workflow within the kitchen, satellite facilities, and storage areas; and even how the dining areas will be organized (table and chair layout; placement of walls, ovens, and dishwashing stations; etc). This requires serving on the design team that interacts with the administration, donors, architects, and contractors.

Factors for sports RDNs to consider when building or renovating a new space include:

- efficient use of space
- bottlenecks and poor traffic patterns
- athlete pathways from sports practice and weight training to the fueling station and dining facility
- distance to storage areas and employee/staff footprint
- adequate amounts and types of cooking equipment
- maintenance of appropriate sanitation standards
- minimal risk of injury
- energy efficiency
- comfortable work environment, including appropriate temperature and humidity, clean air, adequate lighting, and noise control
- ample and adequate storage, receiving area, and parking for vendors
- logistic proximity to the customer base
- compliance with all regulations
- estimated cost of equipment and construction of space and communication with project donors
- completing the project within budget
- possible closure of existing facilities during renovations, with potential loss of income during that time

MANAGEMENT AND ADMINISTRATION OF SERVICES

Introduction to Management

Management occurs when the "work activities of others are overseen and coordinated so that jobs are completed according to standards and in an efficient way."[5] Someone who manages is responsible for overseeing and coordinating all operations under their purview. High-efficiency managers are able to maximize the output of goods and/or services while using the least amount of inputs. In foodservice, *outputs* include customer and employee satisfaction and quality meals; *inputs* include materials, facilities, and people, as well as money, time, equipment, technology, and information. Required managerial skills can be categorized as technical, human, interpersonal, and conceptual. Functions performed include planning, organizing, controlling, and leading. In addition, the roles can vary between interpersonal (figurehead, leader, liaison), informational (monitor, disseminator, spokesperson), and decisional (entrepreneur, disturbance handler, resource, allocator, negotiator).[5,6]

A full comprehensive discussion of the various approaches to management and theory goes beyond the scope of this chapter. In brief, common approaches to management include classical, behavioral, quantitative, and contemporary. A classical management approach is based on scientific management with the intent to increase worker efficiency. A behavioral management approach places the focus on the people involved in the organization and how they behave and act in that setting; it can include components of Theory X and Theory Y managers, as well as the Hawthorne studies. A quantitative management approach relies on statistics and computer modeling to dictate managerial actions. Finally, a contemporary management approach is based mainly on systems theory and contingency theory.[5,6]

Sports RDNs involved in management should know who the key stakeholders are within the organization, as well as the proper chain of command or reporting tree. The management of daily foodservice and nutrition operations requires teamwork and active relationships and partnerships with athletics administrators, sport coaches, operations managers, sports medicine practitioners, strength and conditioning coaches, sports psychologists, and foodservice and academic professionals (high school or collegiate setting). There is a delicate balance between being an efficient manager and not devaluing the role of the sports RDN, which is further discussed throughout this chapter. In brief, sports RDNs should be performing higher-level tasks equal to their level of education, experience, and skill, not just making recovery smoothies. (Job descriptions are further covered in the appendixes to this chapter.)

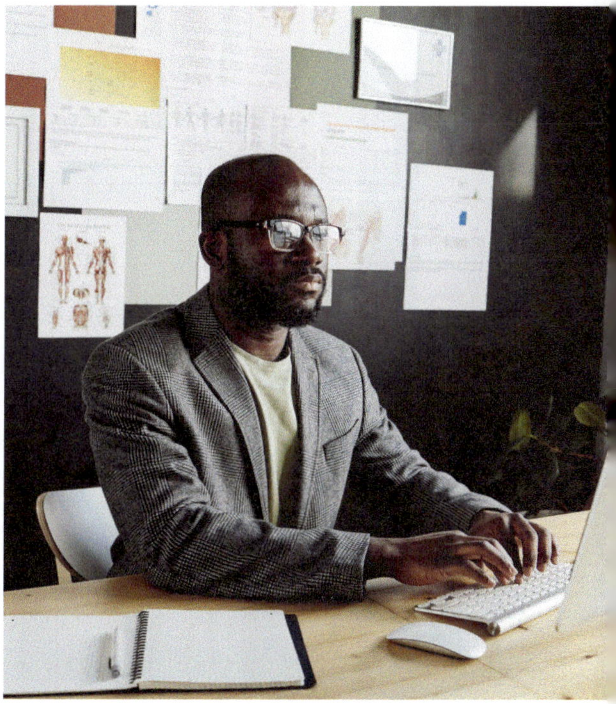

Sports RDNs are expected to add value to organizations by establishing and delivering high-quality, effective nutrition services in a cost-effective manner. One of the strongest indicators of successful athletics programs is player availability. Anything a sports RDN can do to help keep players healthy and available to play when coaches need them will be viewed favorably. A strong emphasis is also placed on tracking outcomes from the nutrition services provided to show the effectiveness of the sports RDN and the sports nutrition program as a whole. An important component of effective nutrition operations and management is to ensure that the standards of professional practice are being met. In 2021, the Academy of Nutrition and Dietetics published *Standards of Practice and Standards of Professional Performance for Registered Dietitian Nutritionists (Competent, Proficient, and Expert) in Sports and Human Performance Nutrition.*[1] This updated version should be used as a guide when assessing nutrition operations and management services. The standards of professional performance indicators that encompass (1) quality in practice, (2) competence and accountability, (3) provision of services, (4) application of research, (5) communication and application of knowledge, and (6) use and management of resources are the most relevant to nutrition operations and management.

Planning, Organizing, and Educating

STRATEGIC PLANNING

Sports RDNs should be experienced in designing strategies not just for individual athletes but for teams and groups of athletes. The strategic planning logic model illustrates the interconnected factors involved in the creation of a new sports nutrition program, as well as the ongoing operation of an existing program. Logic models are common tools for strategic planning and start with a needs assessment. The results of the needs assessment then drive the goals and objectives of the program in conjunction with the overall organizational mission. From there, the logic model illustrates how the inputs, outputs, and outcomes are all interrelated, with impacts from assumptions and external factors.[12] Figure 26.2 on page 702 provides an example of a strategic planning logic model.

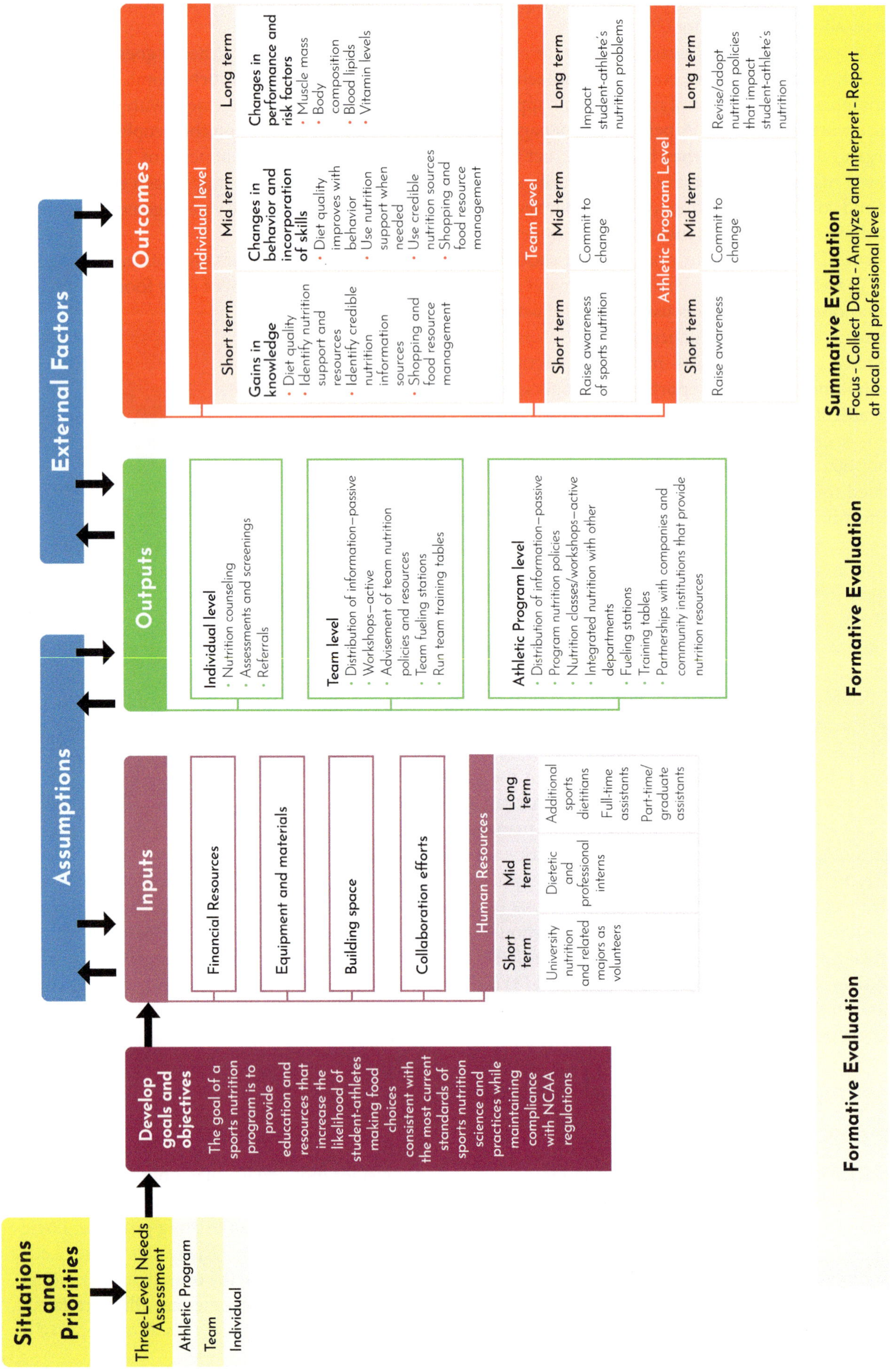

FIGURE 26.2 Example of a sports nutrition strategic planning logic model

DESIGNING QUALITY-IMPROVEMENT PROGRAMS, POLICIES, AND PROCEDURES

One of the most critical components of a successful program is the willingness and ability of the RDN to perform quality-improvement evaluations. As mentioned earlier, sports RDNs need to demonstrate their value to organizations, and one way to do that is by tracking outcomes, which is a form of evaluation.

The sports RDN is also responsible for designing standard operating procedures and policies dictating nutrition screening (eg, screening for eating disorders and return-to-play policies and dietary supplement screening and use policies); the various steps in the Nutrition Care Process, including how data will be collected (eg, HIPAA-compliant electronic health records); and the policies and procedures regarding billing for services. Each sports nutrition program will need to determine whether the athlete's medical insurance will be billed, if athletes are required to pay out of pocket, or if the athletics organization will cover the costs and provide the services free of charge to the athletes. In addition, the sports RDN may serve a role in securing contracts with local laboratory services to process discounted orders for the organization.

EDUCATIONAL OPPORTUNITIES, INCLUDING TRAINING TABLES AND FUELING STATIONS

The deregulation of feeding by the National Collegiate Athletic Association (NCAA) was pivotal in changing the way collegiate athletics programs could meet the nutritional needs of their athletes.[13] This subject is covered further in Chapter 13, but a few key concepts that have evolved from this decision are relevant to the discussion here. Comprehensive fueling stations and training tables have become integral components of sports nutrition programs, and both can serve to not only feed the athletes but educate them at the same time. Training tables provide nutrition primarily through meals, and fueling stations help supplement the nutrition available through meals by providing snacks before and after training and competition. Sports RDNs can use various visual cues and signage at the stations and tables to educate the student-athletes on the nutrient content and purpose of certain foods. Sideline provision of fueling and hydration also helps to keep the athletes performing optimally during training and competition. Boxes 26.5 and 26.6 on pages 704 and 705 provide points for the sports RDN to consider when planning and managing training tables and fueling stations, respectively.[14]

In addition to training tables and fueling stations, sports RDNs can incorporate many other nutrition education strategies into their services. These include team talks and presentations, as well as grocery store tours and dining hall tours. As a component of the dining hall tours, the sports RDN can perform what is known as "plate coaching." Plate coaching helps the athlete build their performance plate on the basis of the nutritional information and education provided. Arrangements can also be made with local grocery stores to use their facilities for tours and educational opportunities for the athletes who need to learn about selecting and purchasing healthy food.

The use of social media and "pop-ins" are also useful ways to provide nutrition education. Social media can be highly efficient when one needs to reach large numbers of athletes. In addition, it is important for sports RDNs to make themselves visible to the athletes and get to know the athletes in order to guide the education needed. An effective, informal way to accomplish this is to "pop in" to team practices and training sessions to observe how the players are performing; this also shows support for the athletes.[14] Such pop-ins can provide the sports RDN with quite a bit of information as they get to know the normal habits and performance levels of the athletes. This will also allow the sports RDN to be able to recognize when athletes are not having a normal training session based on their history. If the athlete seems like they are struggling more than usual and seems tired compared to their norm, the RDN can intervene if necessary. Pop-ins also serve as an excellent way to prompt athletes to approach with questions. Athletes often have a number of nutrition questions that they would like to ask, but they may be reluctant to schedule a formal appointment with the sports RDN for a variety of reasons.

Travel Meals and Catering

TRAVEL MEALS

Sports RDNs are often responsible for ensuring that their athletes receive appropriate meals and snacks when traveling domestically or internationally. They advocate for their athletes' nutritional needs while being mindful of budgetary and time constraints. To excel in this meal management task, sports RDNs need to

BOX 26.5 Considerations for Training Tables

Training tables are defined as meals provided specifically to athletes in a designated location that are not offered to nonathletes.

Training tables are used not just at the collegiate level but also at other levels of athletics such as the professional level, although a different term may be used.

The majority of restrictions and regulations on training tables apply mainly in the collegiate setting. However, even at the professional level, the budget is often not unlimited, so the issue of cost should always be taken into consideration.

Training tables can take the form of an entire dining hall designated for athletes, a section of the general dining hall, or catering provided in a private room or locker room setting.

In the collegiate setting, the number of meals provided by the organization varies based on the budget and/or the interpretation of meal compliance policies between universities, conferences, and intercollegiate division settings. Therefore, the sports registered dietitian nutritionist (RDN) will need to be part of the decision-making process to strategically select which meals and snacks will be provided.

The timing of meals varies and is decided based on needs assessments and the times that are most impactful. For instance, if a team has a game at 7:00 PM, should the organization provide breakfast, lunch, and/or dinner and, if so, at what times? The answer will depend on knowing the players on that particular team as well as their habits. Do the players tend to skip breakfast? Do they prefer not to have a big meal close to game time?

Training table meals will need to account for any special dietary needs of the athletes, protect any athletes with food allergies, and provide for any cultural preferences of the athletes.

If a team meal is going to be on the road, the sports RDN should serve a role in selecting the restaurant and should do so based on which one can provide the type of performance meal needed within the allowed budget. If a certain dollar amount is allocated for each athlete, what type of meal falls within this budget that also meets performance nutrition guidelines? Fast food? Sit-down steak house? Buffet-style restaurant? Italian restaurant or pizza? The decision should be based on the specific preferences of the team. Typically, an Italian- or American-style restaurant with a wide variety of selections works best and can be purchased within the budget allowed. If there is a time limitation, someone should call ahead to make arrangements for the meals to be ready when the team arrives; otherwise, a great deal of time will be spent looking at the menu and ordering. A preferred option may be to preorder a family-style meal to be prepared based on the pregame meal specifications set such as grilled chicken, pasta with red sauce, choice of vegetable, salad and dressing, and bread on the side.

Catering is often preferred for providing team meals, especially during travel. The sports RDN will need to take into account the budget, which catering company will allow specification of the types of food desired and how they will be prepared, and which company can provide the meals at the times and locations needed.

It is also important to consider the provision of meals to athletes during vacation periods, especially in collegiate athletics when the campus dining halls may be closed. This is particularly true for athletes participating in winter sports when their season extends over the winter break between semesters. Finding budget-friendly ways to adequately fuel athletes during these times becomes crucial.

Sports RDNs will need to be aware of any exclusive foodservice contracts with the university or organization and whether there are any restrictions on where the athletes' food can be purchased. Some campus foodservice providers demand an exclusive contract even for catered meals, so the sports RDN may be required to use them rather than order from an outside caterer.

Adapted with permission from reference 14: Brown M, Gomez-Hixson K. *Study Guide for the CSSD Board Exam*. 2nd ed. Pro-Style Nutrition Consulting; 2021. Accessed January 16, 2023. wwwpro-stylenutritionconsulting.com/

BOX 26.6 Considerations for Fueling Stations

Fueling stations can be mobile, permanent, or "pop-up" (ie, for temporary use based on a particular event or situation).

Fueling stations should be conveniently located in places where athletes are frequently present such as on the athletic fields (mobile), in the strength and conditioning rooms/weight rooms, in locker rooms, and in the common areas of the athletic facilities.

Fueling stations should provide allergy-free options with the possibility of 1 designated allergy-free fueling station to protect any athlete with an airborne food allergy; other fueling stations should at least have a designated section for allergy-free products.

Sports registered dietitian nutritionists (RDNs) should take advantage of the captive audience when athletes come to the fueling stations and display educational messaging in prominent view.

Sports RDNs should develop a method for athletes to grab "fuel packs" for away games and events using items from the fueling stations. Prepacked fuel packs that the athletes can grab before they hop on the bus or plane are ideal.

Sports RDNs will need to develop an inventory tracking system, so that expired items are discarded immediately to ensure food safety.

RDNs will also need to train the staff, schedule the hours of operation, and decide whether the fueling stations will use self-serve options or whether staff will be needed to manage the stations and be available to answer questions and to help athletes make appropriate selections.

Sports RDNs will need to decide what food and beverage items will be offered as grab-and-go only, nonperishables, perishables, or smoothies. These decisions will determine space allocation and storage space; the need for electricity and/or plumbing; and the need for refrigeration units, high-capacity durable blenders, and dishwashing capabilities. Also note that, in some states, the Department of Public Health may consider fueling stations under their regulation as a food service entity, in which case the sports RDN will need to consult with them to obtain approval and certification. It is best to check on this possibility well in advance during the planning stages.

RDNs will need develop a marketing strategy for the fueling stations. Do the athletes know who the sports RDN is and where to find them? What is offered at the fueling stations? What are the locations and hours of operation?

Adapted with permission from reference 14: Brown M, Gomez-Hixson K. *Study Guide for the CSSD Board Exam*. 2nd ed. Pro-Style Nutrition Consulting; 2021. Accessed January 16, 2023. wwwpro-stylenutritionconsulting.com/

become comfortable contacting various food providers and arranging meals. For example, if a sports RDN encounters a situation in which the food items they are looking for are not available on the standard menu, they will need to communicate directly with the chef to see if obtaining the necessary items is possible. It is often in the chef's best interest to accommodate these requests given the volume of business that comes with feeding a professional or collegiate athletic team. It is important to ensure that, if any special accommodations are needed, they are requested with ample lead time and not at the last minute. It is also important to notify the food provider if the athletes will be eating on a tight schedule. In fact, most establishments prefer to be called 2 to 3 weeks ahead of time to confirm that the team will be arriving at the establishment, along with the expected arrival time; that tables should be ready; and that the team should be seated right away whenever possible.

Having a preordered meal list or standardized menu for each mealtime is most efficient under time constraints, as allowing each athlete to peruse the menu and order what they would like typically takes much more time. In addition, the normal hours of operation for some food providers may not coincide with the team travel schedule. Again, this is when it is beneficial for the sports RDN to have a high comfort level with relaying the needs of the team to the chef or manager. The sports RDN can inquire about the possibility of opening the establishment to meet the travel needs of the athletes, which may or may not be possible. It is highly likely that the establishment will benefit from these special accommodations. They will be guaranteed revenue from the high-volume food order and the event will establish a standing relationship with the RDN and the team, which often leads to more referrals for them.[14] Also important to note is that not all sports RDNs will be required to travel with the team, in which case they may need to rely on other staff members for meal management. For example, if the sports RDN does not travel with a professional sports team, there is usually a trusted member from the operations division (eg, the director of operations, coordinator of operations, or team administrator) who is responsible for implementing the nutrition plans. The sports RDN should communicate frequently with this individual and provide clear and concise instructions to be carried out during the travel period.

CATERING

Catering can take on many different forms in athletics. Catering may be needed for meals provided on a quick overnight trip for an away game or an extensive trip lasting a week or more, or it could be in the form of meal provision for a major sporting event such as the International Olympics. For short-term trips, it is typical to use hotel catering services because of the relative ease of meal management and logistics. In this situation, the sports RDN should arrange for the meals well in advance and work with the hotel catering staff and chef to ensure that the athletes receive appropriate performance-based meals and snacks. When budget and finances prohibit the use of hotel catering (which can be expensive), the sports RDN will be responsible for securing a budget-friendly food source. For example, this could be accomplished by having meals delivered to the venue locker room. The sports RDN can either arrange for the menu in its totality to provide the same options to all athletes or use a meal management app with preapproved choices for athletes to select from.[14]

Major international sporting events can be the biggest logistical challenge for sports RDNs. Sports RDNs traveling with their athletes will be at the mercy of the venue's contracted caterer. Therefore, whenever possible, the sports RDN should investigate the planned options ahead of time and determine what additional items might be needed based on the needs of the athletes they are representing. For example, if the sports RDN knows in advance that precompetition and postcompetition snacks will not be readily available at the venue, they should task their staff with either providing these snacks through local sourcing, transporting the snacks with the team or athletes, or shipping the snacks in advance.

The catering for major international events is an enormous undertaking for the contracted foodservice provider. As athletes become more nutritionally savvy, foodservice providers can no longer focus solely on taste and ignore important factors such as the nutritional quality of the food, food allergies, sustainability, and the availability of culturally appropriate menu items. The planning for these events begins years in advance. As soon as the caterer is selected, they should consult with nutrition experts. Expert review of the menu in advance by qualified sports nutrition practitioners can lead to improvement in the food supply. When planning for major events, the sports RDN should have input into the menus and timing of the meals and snacks, and they should also provide the athletes with relevant education on selecting appropriate amounts and types of performance-specific foods to meet their individual needs. Burkhart and Pelly[15] performed a dietary intake study at the Delhi 2010 Commonwealth Games and found that the athletes consumed suboptimal levels of fruits, vegetables, iron, zinc, calcium, vitamin C, and vitamin A. Use of point-of-choice nutrition labeling and visuals illustrating periodized nutrition concepts can aid athletes in selecting appropriate items to meet their own individual needs and help prevent suboptimal intake levels.[16,17]

Although it is common to evaluate foodservice operations using foodservice systems models in general, these models are less often used to evaluate the catering at major sporting events. In a first of its kind study, Pelly and Tweedie[18] used the foodservice systems model and the program logic model to evaluate the integration of nutrition into the catering operation of a major sporting event. They found that nutrition expertise should be included early in the planning process to help prevent barriers to the provision of nutritionally adequate, culturally appropriate, and safe food. In a different study, Pelly et al[19] evaluated food provision and nutrition support at the 2012 London Summer Olympics. Sports nutrition experts who participated in the study were asked to provide feedback on menu quality, food safety, sustainability, nutrition labeling, cultural food offerings, and special diets. The results indicated that the participants ranked the overall food provision fairly high; they also ranked the freshness, presentation, variety, temperature, accessibility, cultural offerings, and postcompetition foods average to good. However, participants found the selection of recovery-focused foods and beverages, the availability of food at satellite venues, and the suitability of takeout snacks to be below average.

Barter System

Not all athletics organizations have a substantial budget that covers all meals and snacks without concern for the costs. In the professional sports world, some organizations may have a very limited budget and need to be creative in how they can provide performance meals and snacks to their athletes. This has led to the creation of the "barter system," which is a practice with which sports RDNs should be familiar when preparing to work with professional teams. The barter system is essentially the provision of goods or services in exchange for an agreed-upon value. For example, a catering company could agree to provide a certain amount of meals for the team each week throughout the season in exchange for promotional deals and marketing of their business by the team. This promotion and marketing would be the "value" provided to the caterer in exchange for the meals. The caterer may be recognized during broadcasts of the games and with signage placed in the stadium, as well as in social media posts from the team. Some barter contracts may even establish a particular food provider as the "official caterer" of the team.

Managing Resources, Staffing, and Finances

The sports nutrition staffing model helps programs identify the level of nutrition services that will best meet the needs of the organization. The sports nutrition model selected should be based on the size of the athletic program and the resources available. Lambert et al[2] described 4 different sports nutrition models, as listed in Box 26.7. The box also includes recommendations for staffing based on full-time equivalents (FTEs). FTEs are a common unit used in management to assist in staffing decisions. One FTE is equivalent to a 40-hour work week. Finally, Box 26.7 provides suggestions for staff reporting structure. Examples of these structures include:

- the medical model reporting structure, in which sports nutrition is a component of the comprehensive sports medicine organizational structure alongside the physician, athletic trainers, and strength and conditioning personnel, without any direct report to the athletics department;
- the head of athletic medicine structure, in which sports nutrition reports to the head athletic trainer or director, who subsequently reports to the athletic director; and
- the high-performance team structure, in which sports nutrition reports directly to the director of performance alongside other members of the sports medicine team.

Chapter 13 provides a more comprehensive discussion of the different reporting structures set forth in the publication by Lambert et al,[2] which were designed for collegiate athletes but have relevance to other areas, including professional sports.

BOX 26.7 Staffing Models in Sports Nutrition[2]

Job title Full-time equivalent (FTE)/ hours per week	Suggested reporting structure	Scope of service
Part-time model		
Consultant or part-time hire 0.25 to 0.75 FTE	Reports to the Athletic Director (AD), head of sports medicine, head athletic trainer (AT), or director of performance	Clinical sports nutrition Limited performance nutrition Limited nutrition education Supplement safety

Continued on next page

BOX 26.7 *Staffing Models in Sports Nutrition*[2] **(CONTINUED)**

Job title Full-time equivalent (FTE)/hours per week	Suggested reporting structure	Scope of service
Full-time model		
Staff sports registered dietitian nutritionist (RDN) 1 FTE	Reports to the director of sports nutrition (DSN) or, in the absence of a DSN, to the AD, head AT, or head of performance	Clinical sports nutrition Limited performance nutrition Selected nutrition education Supplement safety Foodservice operations advising Policy advising Regulatory compliance
Program model		
DSN 1 FTE	Reports to the AD	Clinical sports nutrition Performance nutrition Nutrition education Supplement safety Limited foodservice operations Budget and finance Set policies and procedures Regulatory compliance Selected staff development and training
Football staff RDN 1 FTE	Reports to the DSN or, in the absence of a DSN, to the AD, head AT, or head of performance	
Olympic sports staff RDN 1 FTE	Reports to the DSN or, in the absence of a DSN, to the AD, head AT, or head of performance	
Sports nutrition intern 1 FTE	Reports to the sports RDN	
Student workers 75 to 80 h/wk	Reports to the sports RDN	
Department model		
DSN 1 FTE	Reports to the AD	Clinical sports nutrition Performance nutrition Nutrition education Supplement safety Selected foodservice operations Budget and finance
Assistant DSN 1 FTE	Reports to the AD	

Football staff RDN 1 FTE	Reports to DSN or in the absence of a DSN, reports to AD, head AT, or head of performance	Set policies and procedures Regulatory compliance Selected recruiting activities Staff development and training
Olympic sports staff RDN 1 FTE	Reports to DSN or in the absence of a DSN, reports to AD, head AT, or head of performance	
Nutrition operations specialist/culinary RDN 1 FTE	Reports to DSN or foodservice director	
Sports RDN fellow 1 FTE	Reports to sports RDN	
Sports nutrition graduate assistant 1 FTE	Reports to sports RDN	
Student workers 150 h/wk	Reports to sports RDN	

In addition, sports RDNs are often tasked with creating job descriptions and training new hires in their positions. Three appendixes to Chapter 26 provide examples of job descriptions for the following position titles:

- Director of performance/sports nutrition (Appendix 26A)
- Sports dietitian (Appendix 26B)
- Sports nutrition intern (Appendix 26C)

Effective Leadership

Leaders can either be formally appointed or become informal leaders. A formal leader may be the designated "boss," but that does not ensure that others will follow their lead. An informal leader is an individual whom others naturally follow but who has not been designated a formal role in the organization. Effective leaders should be both of these: hired to lead and followed voluntarily by others in the organization. Effective leaders can motivate their employees and use their own skills to guide and influence the actions of those employees. This process of leading is done with a critical focus on accomplishing the organizational mission, goals, and objectives. A thorough discussion of the many leadership theories and styles is beyond the scope of this chapter. In brief, leadership theories can revolve around a singular focus such as traits, behaviors, delegation, or negotiation. Modern leadership theories have shifted away from focusing solely on traits and now focus more on what effective leaders actually do in a behavioral approach. Examples of behavioral leadership theories include authoritarian, democratic, and laissez-faire approaches.[20] Authoritarian leaders prefer to make all or most of the decisions. Democratic leaders prefer to use guidance and coaching when leading and invite employees to be part of the decision-making process. Laissez-faire leaders rarely provide guidance or feedback and allow employees to carry out their tasks without any input.

The most appropriate type of leader depends on the organization, the mission, and the internal and external factors impacting the organization at any one time. A manager may have one main leadership style but should also remain dynamic and exhibit the ability to change when needed. For instance, in the early stages of the COVID-19 pandemic, a normally democratic leader might have had to quickly switch to an authoritarian style given the emergent nature of the external force impacting the organization. Under those conditions, decisions needed to be made quickly and urgently. However, as the pandemic continued, the manager could transition back to being a democratic leader and could once again enlist the employees in the decision-making process. This example illustrates how managers should be strategic thinkers and account for the unknown impact of internal or external factors through disaster planning and managing change.

SUMMARY

This chapter is intended not as a comprehensive resource on nutrition operations and management but rather as a general overview with specific application to athletics and sports nutrition. Currently, the available resources specific to nutrition operations and management in athletics and sports nutrition are scarce, and the training and education that sports RDNs typically receive is a "learn as you go" or "on the job" approach. The inclusion of this chapter will help to fill that gap in knowledge and provide some level of preparation to avoid the need for sports RDNs to fully learn on the job.

KEY TAKEAWAYS

Sports RDNs are responsible for the care of their athletes, including the oversight of nutrition departments and community initiatives; the development of nutrition education; administrative responsibilities with staff management, preceptorship, and professional development; the development of policies and procedures for nutrition interventions in clinical services and compliance management; and the management of all foodservice operations.

Foodservice within athletics may have a blend of operations and service types depending on the conference level in which the institution or professional sports organization participates and the revenue generated to support foodservice expenses.

Components within foodservice operations include menu planning, purchasing, receiving and storage, ingredient assembly, production, distribution and service, sanitation and safety, design and layout of facility service, and department budget and menu forecasting.

Several points should be considered when developing menus: cost, taste, the availability and accessibility of equipment and facilities, the ability to standardize the recipes, nutrient profiles, variety, balance, cultural and dietary needs, the length of each menu cycle, and the hours and convenience of dining areas with respect to the athletes' personal and/or academic schedules.

Contracts with outsourced foodservice companies should be negotiated and reviewed carefully and consistently.

Food safety and sanitation take a high priority in foodservice operations, to protect against the variety of causes of contamination and different types of biological hazards.

Trends that drive foodservice include economic and business environments, societal trends, customer demographics, customer demands, and technology and big data.

Sports RDNs should have knowledge of and be willing to participate in facilities and design layout. The sports RDN can provide guidance on the location, overall concept, dining environment, vision of services, determination of foodservice equipment needed, workflow within the kitchen, satellite facilities, storage areas, and organization of dining areas.

It is beneficial for the sports RDN to know the key stakeholders within the organization or athletics department and the proper chain of command. Sports RDNs should have technical, human, interpersonal, and conceptual managerial skills. Functions performed using these skills include planning, organizing, controlling, and leading.

Sports RDNs should be experienced in designing standard operating procedures, policies for nutrition screening and the Nutrition Care Process, and strategies for both individual athletes and specialized groups of athletes and teams.

The deregulation of feeding by the NCAA changed the way collegiate athletic departments can support the nutritional needs of their athletes. Sports RDNs must work closely with their financial departments to build and service training tables, catering and travel meals, and barter systems to ensure that athletes receive appropriate meals and snacks for their health and performance goals.

Structural models for sports nutrition departments include the medical model reporting structure, the head of athletic medicine structure, and the high-performance team structure.

High-efficiency managers are able to maximize the output of goods and/or services while using the least amount of inputs. In foodservice, outputs are considered customer and employee satisfaction and quality meals. Inputs are considered to be materials, facilities, and people, as well as money, time, equipment, technology, and information.

Effective leaders are able to motivate their employees and use their own skills to guide and influence the actions of those employees.

REFERENCES

1. Daigle K, Subach R, Valliant M. Academy of Nutrition and Dietetics: Revised 2021 Standards of Practice and Standards of Professional Performance for Registered Dietitian Nutritionists (Competent, Proficient, and Expert) in Sports and Human Performance Nutrition. *J Acad Nutr Diet.* 2021;121(9):1813-1830.e55. doi:10.1016/j.jand.2021.04.018
2. Lambert V, Carbuhn A, Culp A, Ketterly J, Twombley B, White D. Interassociation consensus statement on sports nutrition models for the provision of nutrition services from registered dietitian nutritionists in collegiate athletics. *J Athl Train.* 2022;57(8):717-732. doi:10.4085/1062-6050-0157.22
3. US Bureau of Labor Statistics. Accessed January 16, 2023. https://data.bls.gov/timeseries/CES7072200001?amp%253bdata_tool=XGtable&output_view=data&include_graphs=true
4. Adams C. Will the 'ghost kitchen' trend continue during and after COVID-19? *QSR Magazine.* May 1, 2020. Accessed November 18, 2022. wwwqsrmagazine.com/outside-insights/will-ghost-kitchen-trend-continue-during-and-after-covid-19
5. Drummond KE, Cooley M, Cooley TJ. *Foodservice Operations and Management: Concepts and Applications.* Jones and Bartlett Learning; 2022.
6. Gregoire M. *Foodservice Organizations: A Managerial and Systems Approach.* 9th ed. Pearson Education. 2017.
7. 2022 Food Code. US Food & Drug Administration website. Accessed January 16, 2023. wwwfda.gov/food/retail-food-protection/fda-food-code
8. About FSIS. US Department of Agriculture, Food Safety and Inspection Service website. Accessed January 16, 2023. wwwfsis.usda.gov/about-fsis
9. Centers for Disease Control and Prevention website. Accessed January 16, 2023. wwwcdc.gov
10. Hazard Analysis Critical Control Point (HACCP). US Food and Drug Administration website. Accessed January 16, 2023. wwwfda.gov/food/guidance-regulation-food-and-dietary-supplements/hazard-analysis-critical-control-point-haccp
11. US Department of Labor, Occupational Safety and Health Administration (OSHA) website. Accessed January 16, 2023. wwwosha.gov
12. Paradis A. *Elevating Sports Nutrition: Nutrition Program Building Guide for Dietitians, Athletic Trainers, and Strength Coaches.* 2022. Accessed January 16, 2023. wwwelevatehumanperformance.com/free-book
13. Collegiate and Professional Sports Dietitians Association. Deregulation of Feeding. Accessed January 16, 2023. https://sportsrd.org/ncaa-deregulation-of-feeding
14. Brown M, Gomez-Hixson K. *Study Guide for the CSSD Board Exam.* 2nd ed. Pro-Style Nutrition Consulting; 2021. Accessed January 16, 2023. wwwpro-stylenutritionconsulting.com
15. Burkhart SJ, Pelly FE. Dietary intake of athletes seeking nutrition advice at a major international competition. *Nutrients.* 2016;8(10):638. doi:10.3390/nu8100638
16. Burkhart SJ, Pelly FE. Athlete use and opinion of point of choice nutrition labels at a major international competition. *Appetite.* 2013;70:6-13. doi:10.1016/j.appet.2013.06.080
17. Pelly F, Parker Simmons S. Food provision at the Rio 2016 Olympic Games: expert review and future recommendations. *Int J Sport Nutr Exerc Metab.* 2019;29(4):382-387. doi:10.1123/ijsnem.2018-0175
18. Pelly FE, Tweedie J. Inclusion of nutrition expertise in catering operations at a major global sporting event: a qualitative case study using a foodservice systems approach. *J Acad Nutr Diet.* 2021;121(1):121-133.e1. doi:10.1016/j.jand.2020.06.260
19. Pelly F, Meyer NL, Pearce J, Burkhart SJ, Burke LM. Evaluation of food provision and nutrition support at the London 2012 Olympic Games: the opinion of sports nutrition experts. *Int J Sport Nutr Exerc Metab.* 2014;24(6):674-683. doi:10.1123/ijsnem.2013-0218
20. Lewin K, Lippitt R, White RK. Patterns of aggressive behavior in experimentally created social climates. *J Soc Psychol.* 1939;10:2:271-299. doi:10.1080/00224545.1939.9713366

Appendix 26A

Position Description

DIRECTOR OF PERFORMANCE NUTRITION

POSITION DETAILS

Position number: xxxxxxxxx

Working title: Director of Performance Nutrition

Job classification: Director

Position type: Full-time/standard

Salary: $XXX,XXX

Work schedule: Standard, 40 h/wk (exempt)

College/unit: Athletics

Department name: Performance Nutrition

ORGANIZATIONAL STRUCTURE

Reports to position: xxxxxxxxx

Supervises positions: xxxxxxxxx

JOB SUMMARY

The Director of Performance Nutrition (DPN) serves in a leadership and supervisory role, overseeing the administrative and clinical work of *number of full-time registered dietitians* as well as paid student workers and a robust dietetic student internship program. The DPN is expected to provide nutrition assessments and support, meet the performance nutrition needs of elite student-athletes, and bolster day-to-day operations of the performance nutrition program. With direction over *number of type of sports (Olympic or football)*, the DPN assists their staff in providing expert sports nutrition resources, education, and consulting services and assists in the coordination of team meals. The DPN is engaged in a multidisciplinary team approach, working collaboratively with administration, team physicians, athletic training staff, strength and conditioning coaches, sports psychology and counseling professionals, sport coaches, and the performance chef to support each team and individual student-athlete. The DPN assists with research efforts, as well as the thoughtful creation of policies and procedures to enhance the overall health and well-being of student-athletes.

JOB RESPONSIBILITIES/PERCENTAGE OF TIME SPENT

1. MANAGEMENT OF NUTRITION EDUCATION AND CLINICAL COUNSELING DEVELOPMENT AND INITIATIVES — 30%

- Facilitates nutrition education and counseling resources for *name of sport oversight* teams and oversight of all *number of Division I/II/III teams and* creates meaningful education on a wide range of topics related to performance nutrition and general health.
- Meets regularly with support staff to discuss and implement proper preseason, in-season, and postseason nutrition for *name of sport oversight* athletes. Works with support staff to effectively disseminate this information to coaching staff. Serves as a nutrition resource for coaches, sports medical staff, academic services staff, and others within the department as appropriate. Provides consistent communication to coaching staff, strength and conditioning staff, athletic trainers, team physicians, mental health staff, and administration regarding sports nutrition and sports performance-related issues.
- Coordinates grocery tours and meal demonstrations for student-athletes to enhance their overall understanding of food and its relationship to performance and health.

Continued on next page

JOB RESPONSIBILITIES/PERCENTAGE OF TIME SPENT

- Meets with prospective student-athletes as part of the recruiting process, as requested. Provides recruiting services as requested by *name of sport oversight* during official and unofficial recruiting tours. Addresses concerns that parents and prospective athletes may have regarding specific dietary needs.
- Researches and analyzes scientific and lay reports related to nutrition and athletic performance, evaluates nutritional supplements and diets purported to enhance performance, and translates the findings into recommendations for coaches, athletic trainers, and student-athletes.
- Conducts 1-on-1 nutritional consultations as requested or referred by athletic trainers, coaches, mental health counselors, or physicians or by athlete request.
- Attends practices and competitions periodically to increase awareness and visibility to student-athletes and coaches; travels with teams when needed.
- Uses social media proficiently for the delivery of communication related to nutrition for teams on multiple health platforms.

2. ADMINISTRATIVE RESPONSIBILITIES AND PROFESSIONAL DEVELOPMENT

25%

- Supports the implementation of the vision, mission, and elite standards for *name of department*. Directs the day-to-day operation of the sports nutrition program, nutritional counseling, and education services provided to student-athletes.
- Provides supervision of *job position(s)*, including evaluations and planning sessions.
- Supervises all *name of sport* performance nutrition fellows, student workers, and dietetic interns.
- Effectively collaborates with the Assistant Athletic Director of Performance Nutrition in all aspects of management and oversight of the Performance Nutrition Department.
- Participates in necessary administrative meetings to advocate for and support the advancement of nutrition resources.
- Networks with other sports nutrition professionals and develops, implements, and maintains a monitoring system to evaluate Performance Nutrition Department outcomes.
- Manages yearly educational safety trainings that are required by the university and Athletics Department.
- Maintains professional competency and skills required for professional practice, including but not limited to current food, nutrition, and health issues, as well as research related to sports nutrition.
- Facilitates the process of cross-disciplinary collaboration and coordinates the exchange of pertinent information within the performance team.

3. POLICY AND PROCEDURE DEVELOPMENT

25%

- Works closely with mental health professionals and team physicians in the development of policies and procedures meant to ensure the general health and safety of the student-athlete.
- Provides assessment and counseling recommendations and supervises all other sport-specific and gender-specific recommendations regarding optimal body composition and weight for good health and optimal athletic performance.
- Develops and implements plans that align with meeting individual health and sport-specific physiological needs.
- Coordinates care and collaborates with health care professionals and other performance team members as appropriate.
- Addresses nutritional challenges to performance with special preference to food allergies, bone disturbances, gastrointestinal disturbances, iron depletion/anemia, vitamin deficiencies, food intolerances, and other medical nutrition therapies.
- Completes training and certification in the use of dual-energy x-ray absorptiometry (DXA) *(and/or other body composition assessment tool[s] available at institution)* to provide body

composition testing; disseminates clinical data to those deemed part of the student-athletes' care team in accordance with department policy.

- Reviews and assigns incoming athlete eating disorder screenings that are conducted biannually during preparticipation physical examinations.
- Provides assessment of and counseling to student-athletes regarding appropriate and legal use of dietary supplements as well as restricted substances in compliance with sport governing bodies, eg, National Collegiate Athletic Association (NCAA), US Anti-Doping Agency (USADA), World Anti-Doping Agency (WADA), and *name of institution* athletics policies; educates teams on topics such as appropriate use of nutritional supplementation, misuse of performance-enhancing drugs found in nutritional supplements, use of reliable resources to evaluate nutritional supplements, and proper supplementation regimens and protocols for correcting nutritional deficiencies in conjunction with the athletic trainer and team physicians.
- Collaborates with relevant health care providers within the Sports Medicine Department's existing health care network by making referrals when appropriate.
- Designs, assesses, and analyzes sports dietetics and clinical wellness practices.
- Oversees the evaluation, recommendation, purchasing, receiving, and distribution of dietary supplements for legality, safety, quality, and efficacy consistent with NCAA regulations and Athletics Department policies and procedures.

4. DIVERSITY, EQUITY, AND COMMUNITY INITIATIVES

10%

- Advances and supports *name of institution's* and the Athletics Department's diversity, inclusion, and community advancement initiatives through personal participation in educational and developmental opportunities, as well as participation in the creation of an inclusive culture consistent with the values of *name of institution* and its Athletics Department.

5. FOOD-RELATED OPERATIONS MANAGEMENT

10%

- Assumes responsibility for the coordination, staffing, and management of *number of fueling stations* located around athletic facilities, as well as oversight of inventory and stocking of individual team facility satellites.
- Works collaboratively with dining staff, including a foodservice dietitian and performance chef, on menu design and quality options provided in the athletic dining hall as well as all snacks provided in fueling stations.
- Assists Director of Operations for *assigned sports* with menu planning for precompetition and postcompetition meals.
- Ensures adherence to all requirements of the US Food & Drug Administration (FDA) Food Code, as well as all Occupational Safety and Health Administration (OSHA) employee safety regulations, in areas where food is prepared and distributed.
- Works with accounting office to ensure that appropriate spending and payment practices are maintained according to state law. Follows a system of checks and balances with separate individuals involved in the ordering of supplies and receiving of supplies.
- Forecasts, manages, and audits department budget, delivering fiscal responsibility while meeting the needs of the student-athletes' health and wellness goals.

REQUIRED QUALIFICATIONS

- Master's degree in nutrition science, kinesiology, exercise physiology, or the equivalent, along with a minimum of 3 years of experience working in a college or professional athletic environment.
- Registered dietitian with active registration by the Commission on Dietetic Registration; licensure and/or certification by the state of *name of state* (or the ability to immediately apply for certification upon hire).

REQUIRED SKILLS/TRAITS

- Ability to work collaboratively with a team of sports performance experts.
- Demonstrated ability to connect with and inspire a diverse student and staff population (race/ethnicity, sexual orientation, gender identity, disability, etc) and to help foster a culture of respect and accountability to enhance the student-athlete experience and maximize potential.
- Expertise in nutrition counseling and life skill development for athletes and coaches.
- Broad understanding of and/or background of research in the physiological, nutritional, motor movement, and training principles that influence athletic performance.
- Highly developed creative and organizational skills. Ability to multitask and manage several projects simultaneously.
- Excellent organizational, analytical, and communication skills with the ability to design and implement a sports nutrition program through empirically supported interventions.
- Attention to detail, strong organizational skills and planning, timeliness in the turnaround of projects, prioritization skills, and a strong work ethic.
- Ability to work within the framework of federal (Family Educational Rights and Privacy Act [FERPA], Health Insurance Portability and Accountability Act [HIPAA]) and *name of state* laws and regulations regarding privacy and confidentiality.
- Understanding of and alignment with the core values of *name of organization*.

PREFERRED QUALIFICATIONS

- Board Certified Specialist in Sports Dietetics (CSSD)

Appendix 26B

Position Description

PERFORMANCE DIETITIAN

POSITION DETAILS

Position number: xxxxxxxxx

Working title: Performance Dietitian

Job classification: XXXXXXXX

Position type: Full-time/standard

Salary: $XX,XXX

Work schedule: Standard, 40 h/wk (exempt)

College/unit: Athletics

Department name: Performance Nutrition

ORGANIZATIONAL STRUCTURE

Reports to position: xxxxxxxxx

Supervises positions: xxxxxxxxx

JOB SUMMARY

The Performance Dietitian for *football or Olympic sports* provides scientifically based counseling to student-athletes to optimize health and performance. Responsibilities include, but are not limited to, performing individual consults, conducting team talks, providing visual and verbal education, screening supplements, conducting and analyzing body composition scans, and developing menus for *names of assigned teams.* The position coordinates student-athlete care with athletic training, strength and conditioning, sports science, sports psychology and counseling, and coaching staff.

JOB RESPONSIBILITIES/PERCENTAGE OF TIME SPENT

1. **PROVISION OF SCIENTIFICALLY BASED COUNSELING TO STUDENT-ATHLETES TO OPTIMIZE HEALTH AND PERFORMANCE** — **50%**
   - Performs individual consults, develops meal plans tailored toward performance and recovery goals, conducts team talks, provides visual and verbal education, screens supplements, conducts and analyzes anthropometric scans, and develops menus for assigned teams.
   - Coordinates student-athlete care with athletic training, strength and conditioning, sports science, performance innovation, sports psychology and counseling, and coaching staffs.
   - Coordinates care with mental health staff in the disordered eating/eating disorder task force.

2. **OVERSIGHT OF FUELING STATIONS AND PRE- AND POSTEXERCISE FUELING INITIATIVES** — **25%**
   - Screens all supplements that may be provided to *name of sport* players or that student-athletes may express interest in purchasing.
   - Oversees the *assigned teams* fueling station and players' lounge and manages the undergraduate interns and fellows who work the stations to include, but not limited to, ordering products, inventory, researching new products, and scheduling students.

Continued on next page

JOB RESPONSIBILITIES/PERCENTAGE OF TIME SPENT

3. DIVERSITY, EQUITY, AND COMMUNITY INITIATIVES

10%

- Advances and supports *name of institution* and Athletics Department diversity, inclusion, and community advancement initiatives through personal participation in educational and developmental opportunities, as well as participation in the creation of an inclusive culture consistent with the values of *name of institution* and its Athletics Department.

4. OTHER DUTIES AS ASSIGNED

15%

- Assists in recruiting by meeting with prospective student-athletes.
- Assists in the organization of nutrition needs during summer camps with Director of Football Operations.
- Works closely with the chef and performance dining hall staff to develop menus.
- Aids operation staff in planning meals and logistics for home and away competitions.
- Supports advanced travel during away games (if applicable).
- Makes grocery trips to buy additional food product if needed.

REQUIRED QUALIFICATIONS

- Bachelor's degree in dietetics or a related field with 1 year of experience as a graduate assistant, intern, or full-time dietitian in a collegiate or other athletics setting.
- Registered dietitian with active registration by the Commission on Dietetic Registration; licensure or certification by the state of *name of state* (or the ability to immediately apply for certification upon hire).

REQUIRED SKILLS/TRAITS

- Ability to work collaboratively with a team of sport performance experts
- Demonstrated ability to connect with and inspire a diverse student and staff population (race/ethnicity, sexual orientation, gender identity, disability, etc) and to help foster a culture of respect and accountability to enhance student-athlete experience and maximize potential
- Ability to multitask and manage several projects simultaneously.
- Excellent organizational, analytical, and communication skills
- Ability to work within the framework of federal (Family Educational Rights and Privacy Act [FERPA], Health Insurance Portability and Accountability Act [HIPAA]) and *name of state* state laws and regulations regarding privacy and confidentiality.
- Understanding of and alignment with the core values of *name of organization*.

PREFERRED QUALIFICATIONS

- Master's degree in nutrition science, kinesiology, exercise physiology, or the equivalent
- Board Certified Specialist in Sports Dietetics (CSSD)

Appendix 26C

Position Description

PERFORMANCE NUTRITION INTERN

POSITION DETAILS

Position number: xxxxxxxxx
Working title: Performance Nutrition Intern
Job classification: 1- to 2-year intern
Position Type: Full-time/standard
Salary: $XX,XXX
Work schedule: Standard, 40 h/wk
College/unit: Athletics
Department name: Performance Nutrition

ORGANIZATIONAL STRUCTURE

Reports to position: xxxxxxxxx
Supervises positions: xxxxxxxxx (student workers)

JOB SUMMARY

The performance nutrition intern is a full-time professional position that works with *Division I/II/III* athletic teams. The intern provides assistance in individual and team nutrition counseling and education to enhance the health and performance of elite student-athletes and learn techniques for conducting body composition testing such as bioelectrical impedance analysis (BIA) and dual-energy x-ray absorptiometry (DXA). This position is limited to a 2-year appointment period.

JOB RESPONSIBILITIES/PERCENTAGE OF TIME SPENT

1. **KNOWLEDGE DEVELOPMENT AND ASSISTANCE WITH PROVIDING DAILY NUTRITION EDUCATION AND RESOURCES TO ASSIGNED SPORTS TEAMS** — **80%**
   - Assists teams with meals, menu planning, and game-time fueling for competition. Assists with planning and providing preseason fueling for practices and snacks for teams.
   - Learns appropriate procedures for conducting team talks, including team nutrition guides and supplemental education programs on topics such as ergogenic aids and banned substances and maintaining accurate records of nutritional needs for individuals.
   - Maintains direct communication with mentors, coaches, and student-athletes of assigned sports.
   - Gains an understanding of day-to-day performance nutrition services that are needed for intercollegiate athletics.
   - Learns the essential requirements of proper body composition testing in accordance with department policy, using BIA and DXA in conjunction with the Kinesiology Department. Assists with and learns essential requirements for facilitating annual eating disorder screening and medical documentation.

2. **MANAGEMENT OF FUELING STATIONS AND PRE- AND POSTEXERCISE FUELING INITIATIVES** — **10%**
   - Oversees and manages student workers assigned to the fueling station and players' lounge of assigned teams.

Continued on next page

JOB RESPONSIBILITIES/PERCENTAGE OF TIME SPENT

3. **DEVELOPS AN UNDERSTANDING OF DIVERSITY, EQUITY, AND COMMUNITY INITIATIVES** **5%**
   - Supports the initiatives of *name of institution* and Athletics Department's diversity, inclusion, and community advancement through personal participation in educational and developmental opportunities, as well as participation in the creation of an inclusive culture consistent with the values of *name of institution* and its Athletics Department.

4. **OTHER DUTIES AS ASSIGNED BY PERFORMANCE NUTRITION DEPARTMENT** **5%**

REQUIRED QUALIFICATIONS

» Bachelors' degree in dietetics or a related field

PREFERRED QUALIFICATIONS

» Registered dietitian with active registration by the Commission on Dietetic Registration; licensure or certification by the state of *name of state* (or the ability to immediately apply for certification upon hire)

» Master's degree in nutrition science, kinesiology, sports science, or a related field

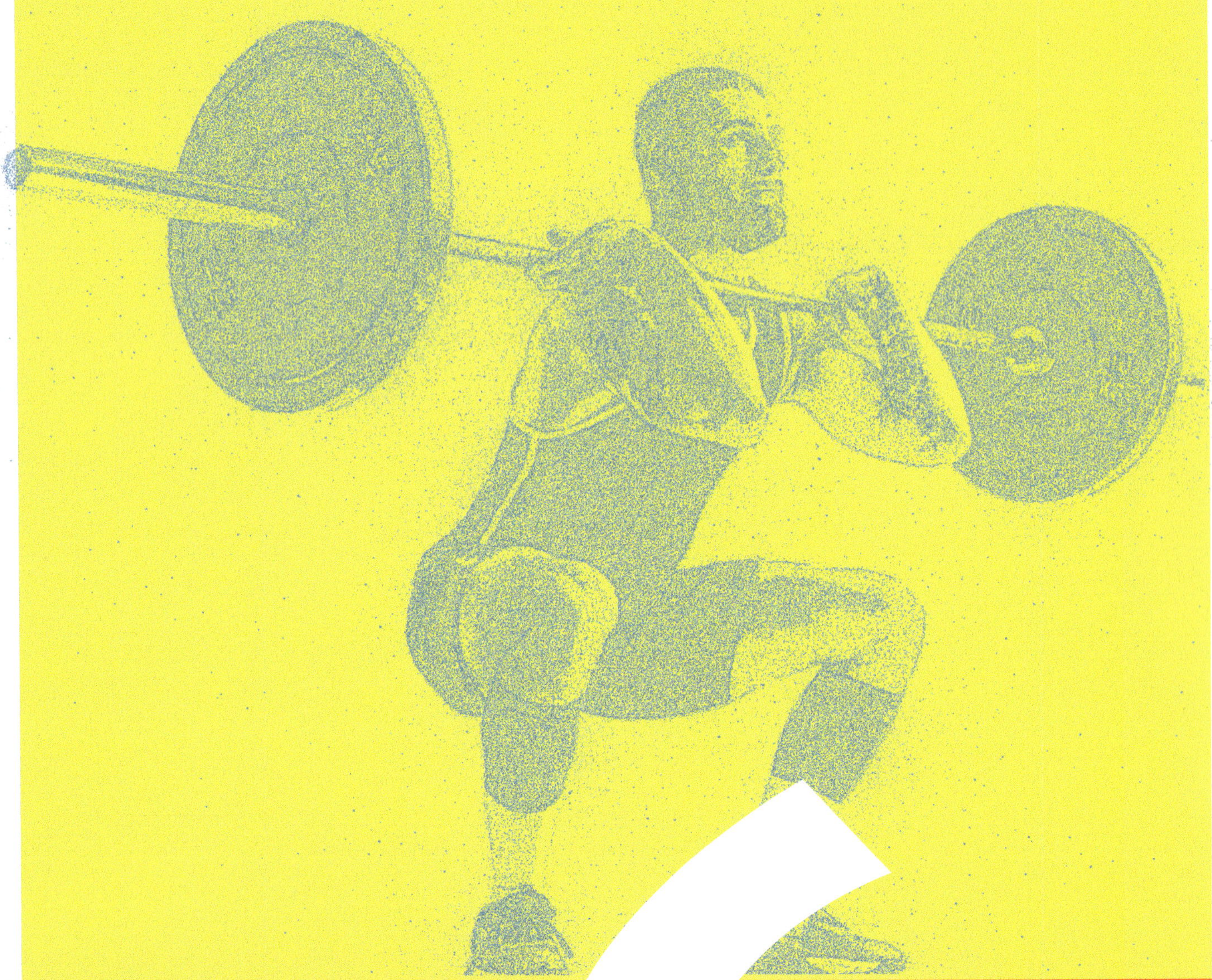

SECTION 6

AT A GLANCE

This At a Glance section features summaries for 24 sports. These summaries provide brief descriptions of the sports, along with the URLs for websites where more information is available. General nutrition guidelines are included and can serve as a basis for individualized nutrition plans. Common nutritional concerns are highlighted and briefly explained. These summaries may be helpful to the sports dietitian in the preparation of sports nutrition presentations for teams or as a topical guideline for an individual counseling session with an athlete.

AT A GLANCE

Alpine Skiing

Alpine ski racing is an individual winter snow sport that mixes speed, agility, balance, coordination, and stamina for various distances in the outdoor elements of the mountains. The sport originates from the winter recreational activity of downhill skiing and consists of 4 primary events, namely, downhill, super G, giant slalom, and slalom, as well as the combined or super combined event, which merges downhill and slalom in 1 event. All ages and sexes may compete in these events, and training consists of weightlifting, dry-land endurance conditioning, and on-snow gate training for up to 3-hour blocks of time. Competitions range from recreational leagues, age-group club teams, and high school teams to college, World Cup, and Olympic levels.

Alpine skiing events result in very high– or high-intensity exercise, depending on the length of training and the course. Other important factors to consider when an athlete is fueling for alpine skiing include weather, outdoor temperature, altitude, and distance from both shelter and the base of the mountain; these factors can affect an athlete's ability to hydrate and fuel properly. Hydration is fundamentally difficult for many skiers, as cold temperatures and altitude can decrease thirst. In addition, speed suits may limit an athlete's desire to undress for bathroom breaks (if nearby facilities are even available), especially for females. Access to high-density, compact carbohydrate-rich fuel that will not freeze is essential, along with warm liquids in insulated containers. Learn more about this sport at the US Ski & Snowboard website (www.usskiandsnowboard.org).

Common Nutritional Concerns

ELEVATION/ALTITUDE

Understanding nutrition guidelines for altitude is a key consideration for alpine skiing. Altitudes between 8,000 and 14,000 ft are considered high altitudes. Altitudes between 5,000 and 8,000 ft are considered moderately high altitudes. Guidelines for fueling at altitude include increasing hydration and carbohydrates and avoiding high-altitude anorexia by eating small frequent meals.

HYDRATION

Skiers have increased hydration needs as a result of elevation and exposure to the elements (sun, wind, cold) and rarely consume enough fluid while on the mountain. Encouraging intake, having fluids available, and timing fluids for appropriate bathroom breaks are all essential to meeting daily needs. Even at moderate altitudes (<5,000 ft), skiers can lose up to an additional 1 to 1.5 L/d through respiration alone.

FUEL AVAILABILITY AND TIMING

Ski racing and training often begin before most food establishments in ski areas are open. Athletes and coaches should plan for nutritious options on the road or at the mountain, bringing fuel with them whenever traveling. Skiers should also carry fuel and hydration with them to the training or racing venue, which can be a significant distance from any base or shelter.

INJURY PREVENTION

With the long alpine skiing season, intense strain on ligaments, joints, and the spine can cause weakness from repeated stress. The inclusion of adequate amounts of protein for muscle retention and repair, timed collagen supplementation, and micronutrient supplementation can help to maintain late-season strength. In addition, foods with a high omega-3 content or omega-3 supplementation should be considered for the prevention of severe concussion symptoms.

TRAVEL

Elite skiers train all year, many times traveling to foreign countries for training camps in areas where natural snow is available during opposite seasons. If unprepared, an athlete may experience jet lag, altitude sickness, and unfamiliar menu options all at once. Athletes should consider traveling with familiar and well-tolerated fuel sources to help prevent and alleviate symptoms. Working with customs authorities, researching local supermarkets, and understanding the culture of destination locations can optimize nutrition and performance.

GENERAL NUTRITION GUIDELINES

Energy

Recommended intake should be individualized, and expenditure varies based on the training cycle. Ski racing is considered a high-intensity sport, requiring the availability of glycogen for short bursts during a race, but energy expenditure during training can be much higher, especially for endurance conditioning and long training blocks at elevation.

Carbohydrate

Recommended intake is between 5 and 7 g per kilogram of body weight per day.

Protein

Recommended intake is between 1.2 and 2.0 g per kilogram of body weight per day.

Fat

Recommended intake is approximately 1.0 g per kilogram of body weight per day, or the remainder of kilocalories should be consumed as fat, with an emphasis on heart-healthy fats.

Acknowledgment

Thanks are due to Michelle Mix, MS, RD, LDN (Registered Dietitian, The Nutrition Mix), for authoring this section, cross-checking it with current recommendations, and assuring that the organizational information is current.

Resources

Aerenhouts D, Chapelle L, Clarys P, Zinzen E. Hydration status in adolescent alpine skiers during a training camp. *J Hum Kinet*. 2021;79:55-63. doi:10.2478/hukin-2021-0062

Ladd E, Shea KM, Bagley P, et al. Hydration status as a predictor of high-altitude mountaineering performance. *Cureus*. 2016;8(12):e918. doi:10.7759/cureus.918

Viscor G, Corominas J, Carceller A. Nutrition and hydration for high-altitude alpinism: a narrative review. *Int J Environ Res Public Health*. 2023;20(4):3186. doi:10.3390/ijerph20043186

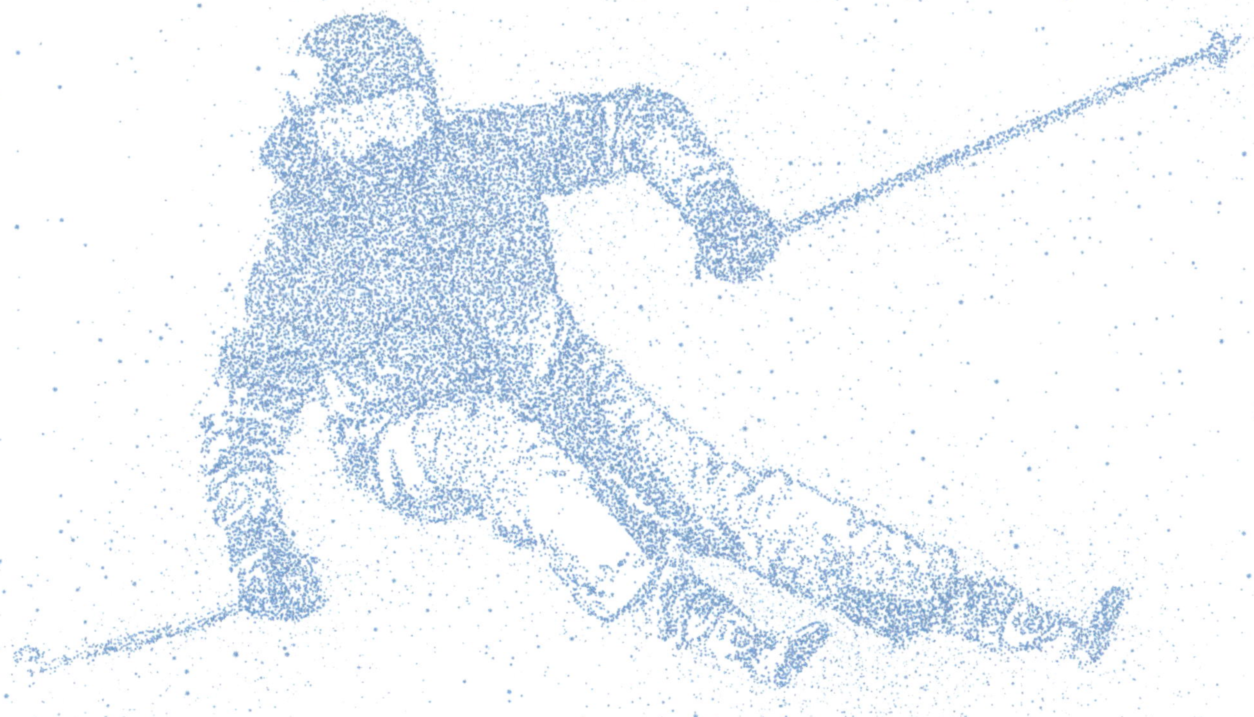

AT A GLANCE

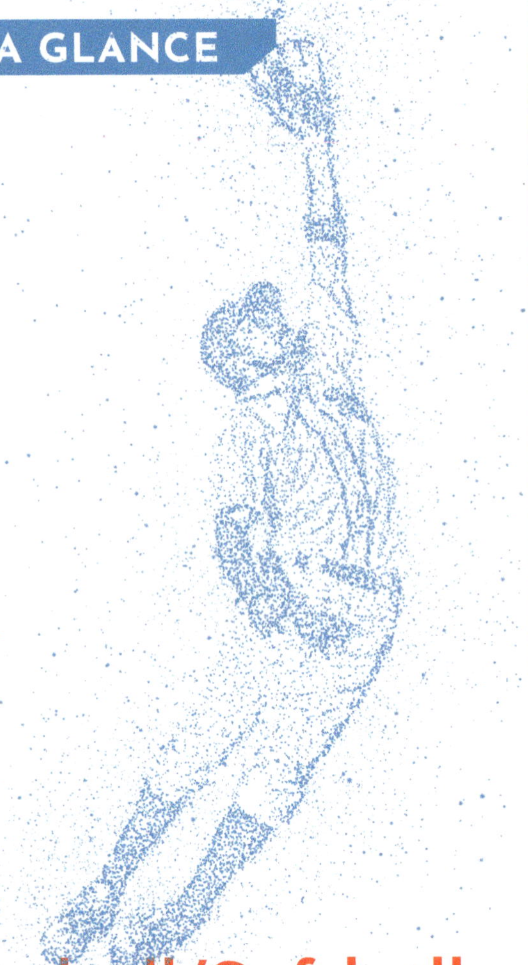

Baseball/Softball

Baseball and softball are skill sports requiring fine-motor control, superb coordination, and quick reaction time, as well as anaerobic power and general fitness conditioning. Baseball and softball are not sports with high energy demands because they do not involve continuous activity. Professional baseball players begin spring training in February, whereas professional softball begins in May. The regular season of professional baseball extends from April through September and is followed by postseason play in October. The professional softball season runs from late May through late August. Collegiate and youth baseball and softball are spring sports in school (generally running from February or March to June), and some players continue throughout the summer in recreational leagues. Learn more about baseball at the Major League Baseball website (www.mlb.com), and find out more about softball at the websites of USA Softball (www.usasoftball.com) and Women's Professional Fastpitch (www.wprofastpitch.com).

GENERAL NUTRITION GUIDELINES

Energy
Baseball and softball are relatively low-energy-expenditure sports.

Carbohydrate
Recommended intake is between 5 and 7 g per kilogram of body weight per day.

Protein
Recommended intake is between 1.2 and 1.7 g per kilogram of body weight per day.

Fat
Recommended intake is approximately 1.0 g per kilogram of body weight per day.

Common Nutritional Concerns

WEIGHT GAIN

Professional players may skip meals and then overeat, consume excess alcohol, and eat high-calorie snacks such as sunflower seeds during the game, all habits that can contribute to weight gain. Many overeat and reduce activity during the offseason.

FLUID INTAKE

Baseball and softball are often played under hot, humid conditions and are some of the only sports without a time limit. Dehydration is a daily concern, and players are encouraged to consume fluids during the half-inning when their team is not on the field.

PREGAME MEALS

Players often arrive for games without having eaten and must eat food that is accessible at the game site, which is often high in calories, fat, sugar, and salt. Minor league players have a limited budget and may seek out inexpensive food, which is often low in nutritional quality.

POSTGAME MEALS

Late-night eating, large postgame meals, and alcohol intake often result in weight gain. Minor league and collegiate players typically eat fast food to break up long bus rides.

FREQUENT TRAVEL

Frequent travel makes it difficult for players to maintain a routine and increases exposure to high-calorie foods that are low in nutritional quality.

AT A GLANCE

Basketball

Basketball is an intermittent, high-intensity sport requiring strength, power, cardiovascular fitness, agility, and skill. It is usually played in 4 quarters with a break at halftime, although overtime periods are necessary if the game is tied at the end of regulation play. All of the body's energy systems are used to fuel the sport: the adenosine triphosphate-phosphocreatine system to jump and pass, the lactic acid system for multiple sprints, and the aerobic system to support several hours of play. The game may be played casually or with great intensity and duration and in a variety of venues, from the playground to the professional arena. Learn more about the sport at the National Basketball Association (NBA) website (www.nba.com) and the Women's National Basketball Association (WNBA) website (www.wnba.com).

GENERAL NUTRITION GUIDELINES

Energy
Energy needs of basketball players differ, depending on body size, intensity of training, cross-training, and playing time, but in general, basketball is a high-energy-expenditure sport.

Carbohydrate
Recommended intake is more than 5 g per kilogram of body weight per day. This recommendation increases to between 7 and 12 g per kilogram of body weight per day during heavy training or competition.

Protein
Recommended intake is between 1.4 and 1.7 g per kilogram of body weight per day.

Fat
The remainder of kilocalories should be consumed as fat, with an emphasis on heart-healthy fats.

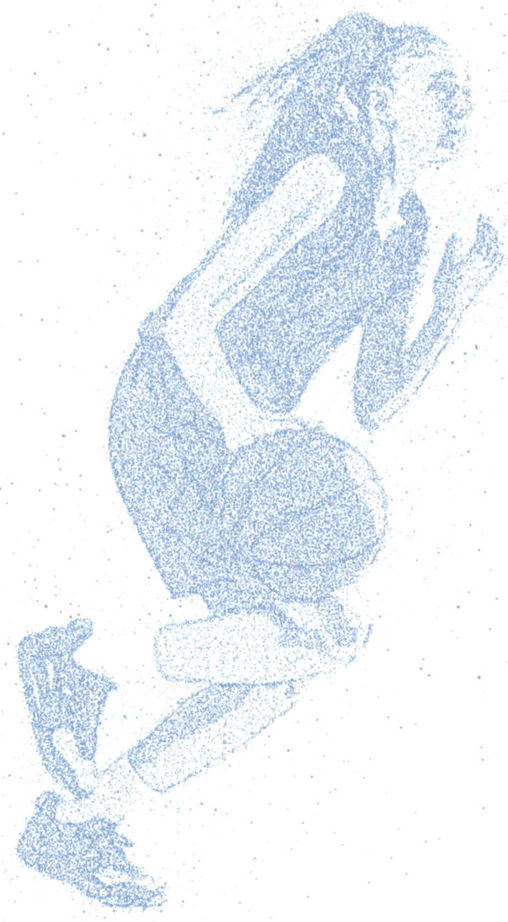

Common Nutritional Concerns

ENERGY INTAKE

Male professional basketball players may need up to 6,000 to 7,000 kcal/d, whereas other players, such as high school or recreational players, need considerably less. Low energy and nutrient intakes over the course of the long basketball season may contribute to fatigue, especially during playoffs, and to weight loss.

CARBOHYDRATE INTAKE

Basketball players need a large amount of carbohydrate daily to replenish glycogen used during demanding training sessions and games.

FLUID INTAKE

Training and games are often held in hot environments. Dehydration can lead to early fatigue and heat illness. Fluid intake should balance fluid losses.

RESTORATION OF GLYCOGEN, FLUIDS, AND ELECTROLYTES

Basketball seasons are long and intense. A good nutrition plan can prevent the staleness that many athletes report as the season wears on. Demanding practices, games, and training sessions deplete glycogen, fluids, and electrolytes. Glycogen stores and fluid and electrolyte losses must be replenished beginning immediately after competition or training. Some postexercise protein consumption is also encouraged. Appetite may be depressed, so liquid meal replacements may become an important option.

AT A GLANCE

Bodybuilding

Bodybuilding is a subjectively judged sport based on muscular development and body presentation. Males and females participate in contests at the amateur and professional levels. Bodybuilders are a variety of weights and sizes, and training and nutrient intakes change as bodybuilders prepare for contests. Competitive bodybuilders spend about 1½ hours in the gym each day during the offseason and 2 to 3 hours per day during precompetition. Training and nutrition must be well-matched and will vary depending on the demands of the training period—maintaining muscle mass, building muscle mass, tapering (precontest dieting), or cutting weight immediately before competition. The muscle-building phase begins after rest from the previous competitive season. The tapering phase is started approximately 12 weeks before competition with the goal of decreasing body fat and defining muscle mass, and the cutting phase is used if the tapering phase did not meet all of the goals for body composition. A maintenance phase should be used during the offseason.

Success in the sport requires discipline, consistency, and a long-term commitment to both training and dietary goals. Recovery, sleep, and supplementation may also play key roles in performance and physique outcomes. Learn more about the sport at the International Federation of Bodybuilding and Fitness website (www.ifbb.com).

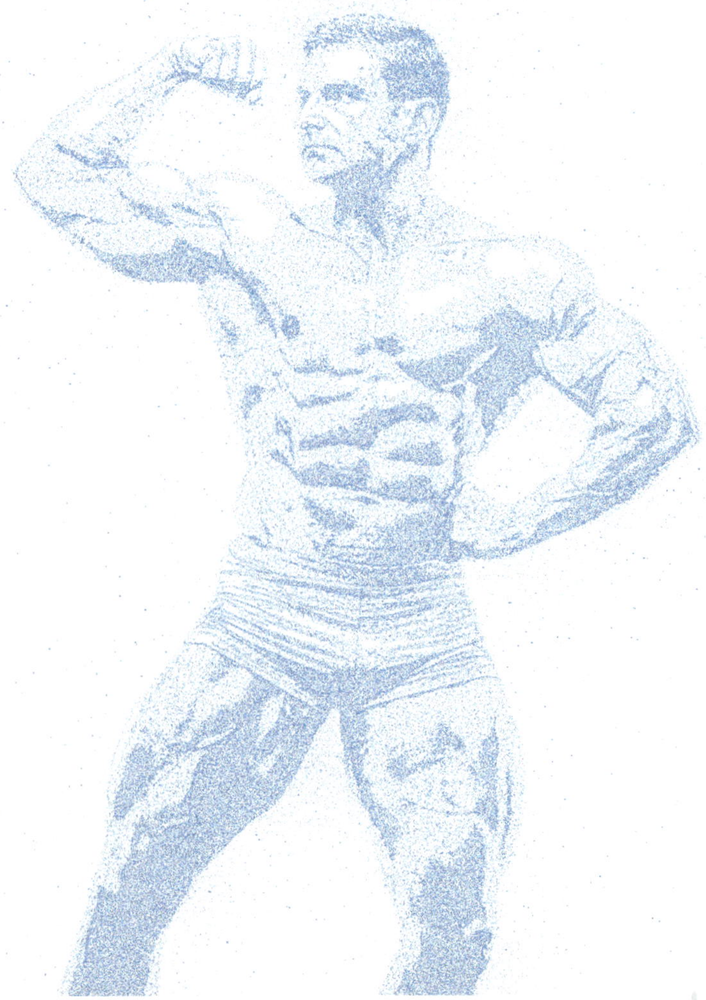

Common Nutritional Concerns

ENERGY INTAKE

Baseline energy intake varies tremendously, and energy needs change as contests approach. Bodybuilders need personalized meal plans that reflect various energy (kilocalorie) levels.

OTHER MACRONUTRIENTS

Excessive intake of any 1 macronutrient may result in low intake of another. The focus must be on macronutrient balance (not just protein intake), with the understanding that the demands of training and competition change the relative balance. Sufficient carbohydrate is needed to meet the demands of training. Protein intakes generally increase during the muscle-building, tapering, and cutting periods. As energy and protein intakes change, the relative contributions of carbohydrates and fats change. These general guidelines must be highly individualized.

FLUID INTAKE

Fluid loss must be balanced with fluid intake. Voluntary dehydration is one method that is used for cutting weight before competition and may be dangerous or life-threatening.

LACK OF VARIETY

Diets tend to be repetitive and to lack variety. Meal plans or suggestions for foods that contain similar energy and nutrient profiles are helpful.

BODY IMAGE AND DISORDERED EATING

Because of the nature of the sport, there is a risk for distorted body image and disordered eating.

GENERAL NUTRITION GUIDELINES

Energy
Energy intake and expenditure must be individually determined and will vary with the phase and amount of training. Estimated energy needs are as low as 30 kcal per kilogram of body weight per day for females trying to lose fat weight and maintain muscle mass and as high as 60 kcal per kilogram of body weight per day for males trying to build muscle mass.

Carbohydrate
Recommended intake is between 5 and 7 g per kilogram of body weight per day.

Protein
Recommended intake is between 1.4 and 1.7 g per kilogram of body weight per day. (Low overall energy intakes or individual preferences may result in higher intakes, reaching 2 g per kilogram of body weight per day during periods of the lowest energy intake.)

Fat
The remainder of kilocalories should be consumed as fat, with an emphasis on heart-healthy fats.

AT A GLANCE

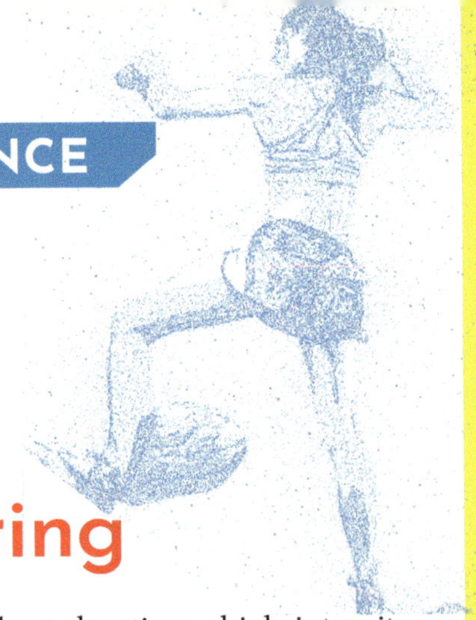

Bouldering

Bouldering is a short-duration, high-intensity sport that can be performed indoors or outdoors. Nutritional needs when bouldering outdoors may be greater than those when bouldering indoors because of the need for the participant to hike to the climbing area while carrying gear. Although energy production for bouldering is primarily anaerobic in nature, reliance on aerobic energy production may increase if training is to last for many hours. Learn more about the sport at the USA Climbing website (https://usaclimbing.org/climb/bouldering).

GENERAL NUTRITION GUIDELINES

Energy
Individual needs should be calculated based on the demands of training.

Carbohydrate
Recommended intake is approximately 5 g per kilogram of body weight per day.

Protein
Recommended intake is between 1.4 and 2.0 g per kilogram of body weight per day depending on individual goals.

Fat
The remainder of kilocalories should be consumed as fat, with an emphasis on heart-healthy fats.

Common Nutritional Concerns

ENERGY AND CARBOHYDRATE INTAKE

Climbers are generally noted to be at risk for chronically low energy and carbohydrate intake, which can be detrimental to health and performance. Practitioners should give special consideration to educating boulderers on the necessity of carbohydrates for performance. Meals eaten approximately 1 hour before climbing with a carbohydrate content of 1 g per kilogram of body weight should be adequate to support activity. Overall energy intake should be assessed individually to ensure that daily needs are met.

BODY COMPOSITION

Boulderers can have a variety of body types, but a lean physique is considered advantageous because a high power-to-weight ratio can make the activity easier. As a result, some athletes may choose to focus on fat loss in combination with the development of sport-specific strength. If fat loss is desired, practitioners should emphasize maintaining adequate carbohydrate and protein intakes to support training and the maintenance of muscle mass.

FLUID INTAKE

Hydration may be of particular concern when an individual is bouldering outdoors. Depending on the geographic location and time of year, higher temperatures and humidity may require greater replenishment of fluid and electrolytes. Reluctance to add additional weight to a backpack may lead to inadequate preparedness for hydration needs. Sports drinks may be a good option to satisfy both hydration and carbohydrate intake needs. When an individual is bouldering indoors, activity is generally not continuous, and fluid loss is not excessive.

MACRONUTRIENT INTAKE DURING EXERCISE

Carbohydrate intake during exercise is of particular concern during long training sessions and during outdoor bouldering that occurs in combination with hiking. Practitioners should consider identifying carbohydrate-predominant snacks that are lightweight and packable. On day-long hiking/climbing trips, packable meals containing fat and protein will need to be prepared as well.

Acknowledgment

Thanks are due to Tara Hites, RDN (Graduate Assistant, College of Health & Human Services, Bowling Green State University), for authoring this section, cross-checking it with current recommendations, and assuring that the organizational information is current.

Resources

Smith EJ, Storey R, Ranchordas MK. Nutritional considerations for bouldering. *Int J Sport Nutr Exerc Metab.* 2017;27(4):314-324. doi:10.1123/ijsnem.2017-0043

AT A GLANCE

Cycling

Cycling is a sport of various intensities and durations involving participants ranging from sprinters, whose races last only seconds, to endurance cyclists, such as Tour de France riders who traverse more than 2,000 miles (much of it over mountainous terrain). Energy and nutrient needs vary according to the type of cycling (eg, track, road racing, mountain biking, and bicycle motocross [BMX]), the demands of training, and the intensity and duration of the race. Learn more about the sport at the USA Cycling website (www.usacycling.org).

Common Nutritional Concerns

ENERGY AND CARBOHYDRATE INTAKES

Nutrient needs are often high, and a well-balanced diet is important. Distance cyclists need carbohydrate during the ride and must learn to consume food on the bike. Carbohydrate-electrolyte drinks, energy bars, gels, and bananas are some foods that work well for cyclists, but individual preferences and tolerances must be determined by trial and error.

FLUID INTAKE

Meeting fluid needs is challenging, as road cyclists can carry only 2 water bottles and can get additional fluids only at special feed zones along the course. Moreover, in road cycling and mountain biking, taking 1 hand off the bike to drink can lead to crashes.

Dehydration is a daily concern. Sweat rates should be calculated, and an individualized hydration plan should be developed. Cyclists should take precautions to prevent hyponatremia, especially in hot, humid environments.

RESTORATION OF GLYCOGEN, FLUIDS, AND ELECTROLYTES

Glycogen stores and fluid and electrolyte losses must be replenished beginning immediately after competition or training. Some postexercise protein consumption is also encouraged. Appetite may be depressed, so liquid meal replacements may become an important option.

GENERAL NUTRITION GUIDELINES

Endurance cycling guidelines can be found under Endurance and Ultraendurance Sports in this At a Glance section. Sprint cycling is a short-duration, very high-intensity sport, and the general guidelines for such sports include the following.

Energy
Individual needs should be calculated based on the demands of training.

Carbohydrate
Recommended intake is between 7 and 12 g per kilogram of body weight per day.

Protein
Recommended intake is between 1.2 and 1.7 g per kilogram of body weight per day.

Fat
The remainder of kilocalories should be consumed as fat, with an emphasis on heart-healthy fats.

Many cyclists are between the 2 extremes of sprinting and endurance, and energy and macronutrient requirements must be adjusted accordingly to reflect the demands of training and competition.

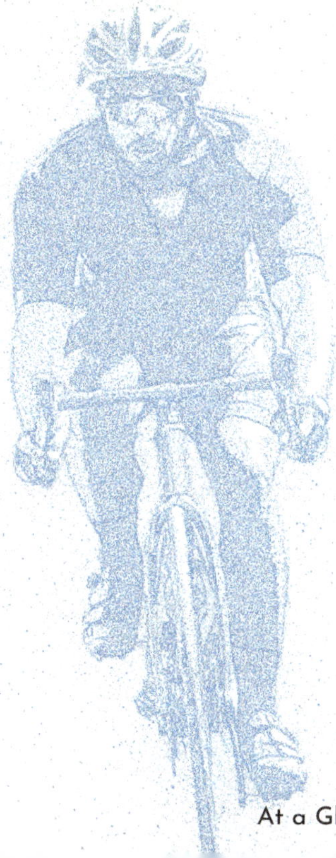

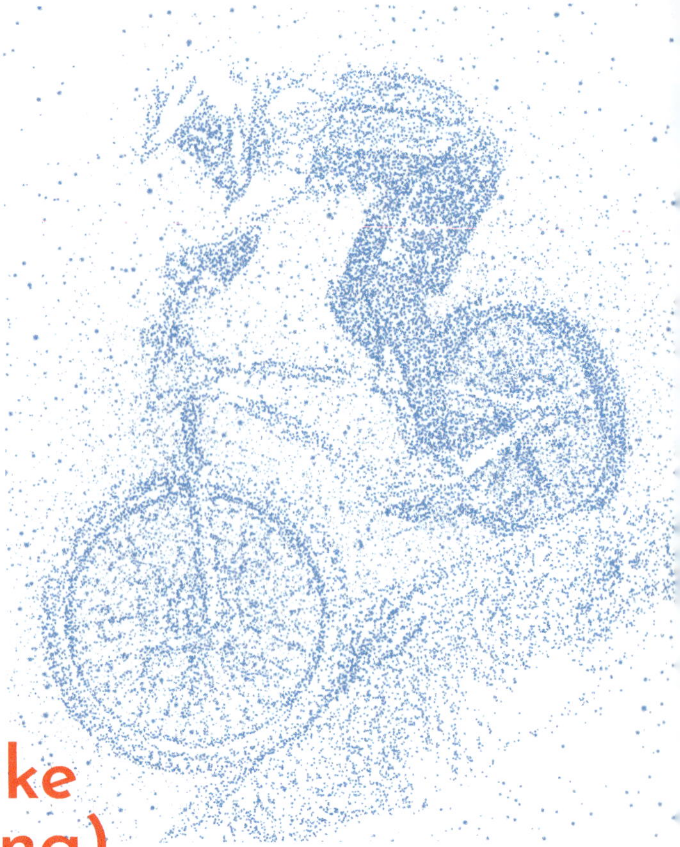

Downhill Mountain Bike Racing (Gravity Cycling)

Downhill mountain biking or gravity cycling is an extreme sport in which athletes race mountain bikes at high speeds on a timed course through steep, densely wooded terrain, often over rocks, cliffs, and drops. Bikes weigh, on average, 40 lb, and racing requires intense concentration, precision, agility, strength, balance, coordination, and stamina. Downhill mountain bike is therefore categorized as a very high– or high-intensity sport, depending on the length of training and the intensity of the course.

The downhill mountain biking season is held from early spring through late fall in remote mountain locations, but races can be held all year depending on the location. Outdoor conditions vary widely, and events may take place in extreme heat during the summer or freezing temperatures in late fall. Courses vary in length and difficulty, averaging 2 to 5 minutes of maximal effort per run. Each race lasts from 2 to 3 days and includes course walks (hiking down the mountain to view the course), training blocks on the course, and timed training runs before the final competition. Each training day is lengthy, beginning early in the morning and lasting 6 to 8 hours, with riders sometimes completing 8 to 12 runs per day.

Injuries occur daily, as the sport is inherently dangerous, and airlift evacuation from the venues is not uncommon; it is not unusual for many athletes to be competing while recovering from minor injuries, such as lacerations, heavy bruising, scrapes, strains, sprains, or even smaller broken bones. Prevention, recovery, and repair with appropriate nutrition are vital. Athletes range in age from elementary school-age through adulthood, and competition levels begin with local and regional race series, culminating with national and elite World Cup racing. Collegiate downhill mountain biking competitions occur at the club level, and events are not sanctioned unless they are registered with USA Cycling or Union Cycliste Internationale (UCI). Learn more about this sport at the USA cycling website (https://usacycling.org) and the UCI website (www.uci.org).

Common Nutritional Concerns

AVAILABILITY OF RESOURCES

Many races take place in remote mountain locations during the skiing offseason. As a result, ski resorts and seasonal businesses may not be open. Therefore, racers are advised to plan menus and shop for meals before traveling and to research the availability of area supermarkets and sources of fresh water (not always available at the venue). Another option is for teams to establish an accessible fuel station for athletes near the bottom of the racecourse.

HYDRATION

USA Cycling and UCI World Cup regulations require racers to wear protective body pads under long sleeves, long heavy pants, and a full-face helmet. Athletes can easily become overheated, especially in warmer climates. Racers should focus on hydration before the event to improve reaction time and performance, as well as prevent dehydration, heat exhaustion, and heat stroke. Weight loss through sweat is also common and should be measured to calculate individual fluid needs.

RECOVERY FUEL OR MEALS

Maintaining muscle and promoting recovery, especially from injury, is a priority; therefore, posttraining or race-day meals should contain higher protein contents, complex carbohydrates, and vitamin C to promote healing. Athletes should aim to include healthy fats for additional energy needs and for healing and physical body protection.

CONCUSSION RECOVERY

Concussion is common in downhill mountain biking; thus, all athletes should have impact testing done prior to participation and should supplement daily with omega-3 fatty acids. Athletes recovering from a concussion should follow available reputable nutrition concussion guidelines (as outlined on the Nutritional Support for Injury Recovery and Return-to-Play fact sheet provided on the website of the American Sports and Performance Dietitians Association [formerly, Collegiate and Professional Sports Dietitians Association (CPSDA)] at www.sportsrd.org/wp-content/uploads/2018/11/Nutrition-Support-for-Inury-Recovery-Return-to-Play.pdf).

GENERAL NUTRITION GUIDELINES

Energy
Recommended intake should be individualized and varies based on the training cycle. Downhill mountain bike racing is considered a high-intensity sport, requiring an adequate availability of glycogen during a race, but energy expenditure can be much higher during training days.

Carbohydrate
Recommended intake is between 5 and 7 g per kilogram of body weight per day.

Protein
Recommended intake is between 1.8 and 2.0 g per kilogram of body weight per day.

Fat
Recommended intake is approximately 1.0 g per kilogram of body weight per day, or the remainder of kilocalories should be consumed as fat, with an emphasis on heart-healthy fats.

Acknowledgment

Thanks are due to Michelle Mix, MS, RD, LDN (Registered Dietitian, The Nutrition Mix), for authoring this section, cross-checking it with current recommendations, and assuring that the organizational information is current.

Resources

Heileson JL, Anzalone AJ, Carbuhn AF, et al. The effect of omega-3 fatty acids on a biomarker of head trauma in NCAA football athletes: a multi-site, non-randomized study. *J Int Soc Sports Nutr*. 2021;18(1):65. doi:10.1186/s12970-021-00461-1

AT A GLANCE

Endurance and Ultraendurance Sports (Distance Running, Cycling, Swimming, Triathlons, and Cross-Country Skiing)

Endurance and ultraendurance sports include marathons, distance cycling, distance swimming, triathlons, and cross-country skiing. All require year-round training and nutrition support. Training and nutrition must be well-matched with the current activity level and will vary depending on the training period—preparation, prerace, race, or active recovery. Reducing body fat or weight should be attempted only during active recovery or early in the preparation period so that high-volume training and competition are not compromised. Learn more about these sports at the websites of the following organizations:

- USA Track & Field (www.usatf.org)
- World Ultra Cycling Association (www.ultracycling.com)
- US Masters Swimming: Long-Distance Swimming (www.usms.org/longdist)
- USA Triathlon (www.usatriathlon.org)
- US Ski & Snowboard: Cross Country (https://usskiandsnowboard.org/teams/cross-country)

Common Nutritional Concerns

ENERGY AND MACRONUTRIENT INTAKE

Energy and macronutrient needs are high in endurance and ultraendurance sports, and proper food intake must be an integral part of training. A structured eating plan must be developed to support training and competition throughout the year.

WEIGHT GAIN

After the racing season is over, energy intake must be adjusted to reflect the decreased volume and intensity of training to prevent unwanted weight gain.

BODY COMPOSITION

Leanness and low body weight are advantageous in sports in which the body must be moved. Excess body fat can be detrimental because, unlike muscle, it is non–force-producing mass. However, rapid weight or fat loss can be detrimental to training and performance, so changes to body composition must be slow. Small reductions in daily energy intake and some increase in activities of daily living will promote slow weight loss. Weight loss is best attempted during the recovery period or early in the preparation period.

FLUID AND SODIUM INTAKES

To an endurance athlete, fluids are like coolant to a car's radiator—without it, both will overheat and exhibit signs of breakdown. Fluid intake must be balanced with fluid losses to avoid dehydration and prevent hyponatremia. Sodium needs must be individually established. The inclusion of sodium in products consumed during training and racing is recommended.

LACK OF VARIETY

Variety and balance can be difficult to maintain day after day. However, athletes must avoid getting in a rut, so they should focus on whole foods, especially on off days.

FOOD INTOLERANCES

Some foods are not tolerated well during competition. Athletes should practice using various race foods and beverages during training to prevent problems during competition.

GENERAL NUTRITION GUIDELINES

Energy
This category of sport is associated with high energy expenditure.

Carbohydrate
Recommended intake is between 5 and 7 g per kilogram of body weight per day when training is reduced and as high as 10 to 12 g per kilogram of body weight per day during heavy training and the racing season. Carbohydrate loading (glycogen supercompensation) for competition is common.

Protein
Recommended intake is between 1.2 and 1.7 g per kilogram of body weight per day, with higher levels consumed during the prerace and racing seasons.

Fat
Recommended intake is between 0.8 and 2.0 g per kilogram of body weight per day to match energy expenditure, with an emphasis on heart-healthy fats.

AT A GLANCE

Field Events

Indoor field events include high jump, pole vault, long jump, triple jump, and shot put. Outdoor field events also include discus, hammer, and javelin throws. Both males and females compete in these events. The necessary athletic skills and body composition differ between jumpers and throwers. Jumpers tend to be leaner because they must move their body through space, whereas throwers depend on their strength and body mass to propel an object through space. Jumpers consume less energy than throwers. Learn more about the sports at the USA Track & Field website (www.usatf.org).

GENERAL NUTRITION GUIDELINES

Energy
Recommended intake varies depending on the individual and the event.

Carbohydrate
Recommended intake is between 5 and 7 g per kilogram of body weight per day.

Protein
Recommended intake is between 1.2 and 1.7 g per kilogram of body weight per day.

Fat
The remainder of kilocalories should be consumed as fat, with an emphasis on heart-healthy fats.

Common Nutritional Concerns

BODY COMPOSITION AND WEIGHT LOSS

Jumpers are encouraged to have a low percentage of body fat. There is a performance disadvantage to having excess body fat because fat is non–force-producing mass. However, if an athlete aims to lose weight, they should follow a weight-loss plan that allows for sufficient carbohydrate and protein intakes to support training as well as weight (fat) loss.

HIGH-FAT DIETS

Throwers have a tendency to consume high-fat diets. Such diets may also be high in saturated fat. All athletes should be aware of the advantages of consuming heart-healthy fats and should be encouraged to substitute such fats for saturated fats. If weight loss is desired, reducing dietary fat would be appropriate.

FLUID INTAKE

Several factors unique to track and field contribute to dehydration, including workouts that are unsupervised (thus placing the responsibility for hydration on the athletes), limited availability of fluids at the training facility, frequent travel from cool environments to hot climates with little time to acclimate to the change in temperature, increased fluid loss during air travel due to the low humidity in an airplane cabin, and the competitive nature of the sport, which might push an athlete to exercise even when dehydrated. Fluid loss must be balanced with fluid intake.

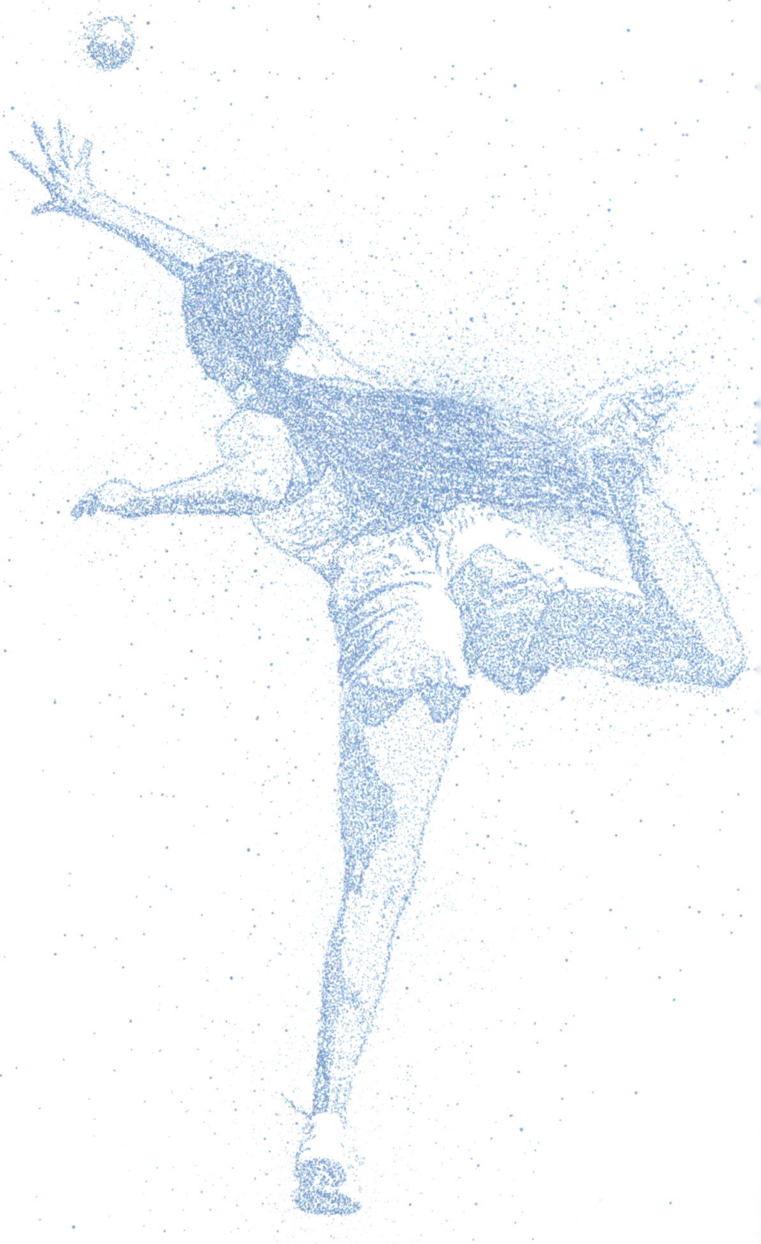

AT A GLANCE

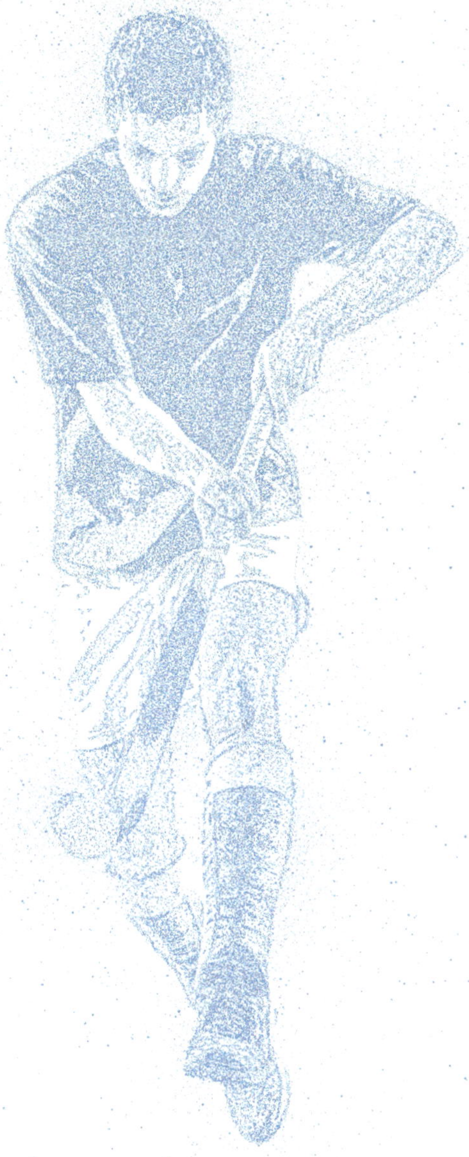

Field Hockey

Field hockey requires anaerobic power, aerobic conditioning, strength, agility, and speed. Similarly to other intermittent, high-intensity sports, field hockey involves constant changes in speed and direction. A game generally consists of four 15-minute quarters (youth games may be divided into just 2 halves of 25 minutes each) with a 2-minute break between quarters and a 15-minute break at halftime. Frequent player substitutions reduce playing time to about half of the overall game time. Learn more about the sport at the website for USA Field Hockey (www.usafieldhockey.com).

GENERAL NUTRITION GUIDELINES

Energy
Recommended intake should be individualized and varies based on the level of training, but field hockey is generally considered a high-energy-expenditure sport.

Carbohydrate
Recommended intake is between 5 and 10 g per kilogram of body weight per day during training and competition to ensure adequate glycogen.

Protein
Recommended intake is between 1.4 and 1.7 g per kilogram of body weight per day.

Fat
The remainder of kilocalories should be consumed as fat, with an emphasis on heart-healthy fats.

Common Nutritional Concerns

CARBOHYDRATE AND PROTEIN INTAKES

Field hockey players need a large amount of carbohydrate daily to replenish glycogen used during demanding training sessions and games. In addition, protein is important to repair the wear and tear on muscles that occurs in field hockey.

HYDRATION DURING EXERCISE

Hydration during training and competition is similar to that recommended for other high-intensity sports that do not require the wearing of protective padding. Sipping on fluids between shifts can help prevent dehydration and improve performance.

RESTORATION OF GLYCOGEN, FLUIDS, AND ELECTROLYTES

Demanding practices, games, and training sessions deplete glycogen, fluids, and electrolytes. Glycogen stores and fluid and electrolyte losses must be replenished beginning immediately after competition or training. Some postexercise protein consumption is also encouraged. Appetite may be depressed, so liquid meal replacements may become an important option.

AT A GLANCE

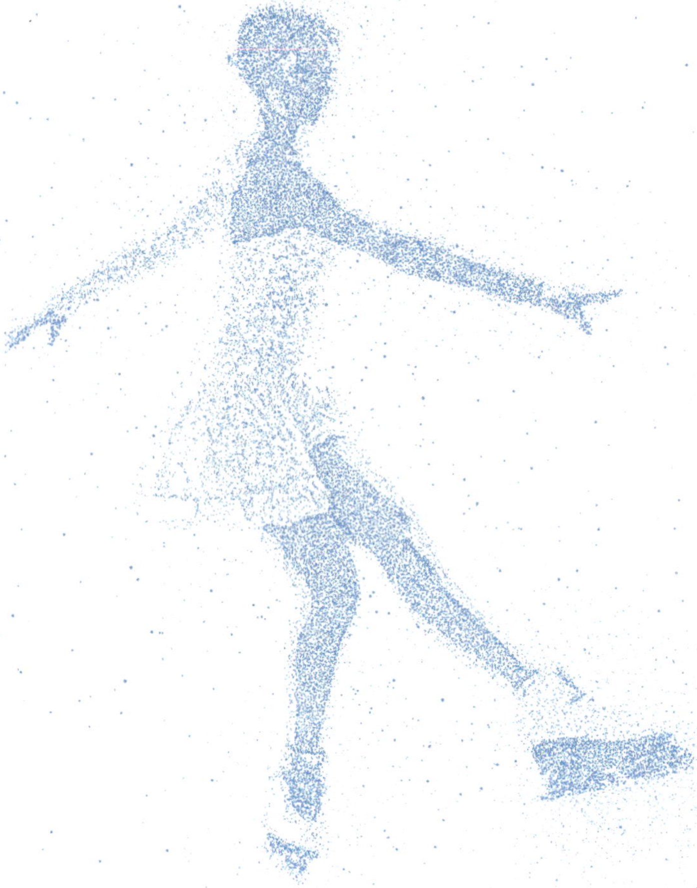

Figure Skating

Figure skating requires strength, power, and endurance. Individual competitions are held for males and females. Couples compete in pairs and ice dancing events, and team skating competitions are also held. Training starts very early, sometimes at the age of 3 years, and many world champions are in their teens. Technique and speed are important, and the degree of skating difficulty increases as skaters reach the elite level. An elite figure skater's training includes learning new skills, such as jumping and spinning, and repeatedly practicing those skills. High-intensity work coupled with lower-intensity skating and training 6 days per week in 2 sessions per day is a typical routine. Artistry plays a critical role, and many subjective elements are considered in scoring. Competitions at the elite level include a short program that lasts for 2 minutes and 40 seconds and a long program that lasts for 4 minutes (females) or 4.5 minutes (males and pairs). Learn more about the sport at the US Figure Skating website (www.usfigureskating.org).

GENERAL NUTRITION GUIDELINES

Energy
Recommended intake should be individualized based on body composition goals.

Carbohydrate
Recommended intake is between 3 and 7 g per kilogram of body weight per day.

Protein
Recommended intake is between 1.2 and 1.7 g per kilogram of body weight per day.

Fat
The remainder of kilocalories should be consumed as fat, with an emphasis on heart-healthy fats.

Common Nutritional Concerns

ENERGY RESTRICTION

Despite the high energy demands of training, many female figure skaters limit energy intake in an effort to attain or maintain a low percentage of body fat. Weight loss must be slow, with small restrictions of energy so that muscle mass can be protected and training is not negatively impacted.

BODY COMPOSITION

A low percentage of body fat, particularly for females, is considered necessary for success because of the physical demands of the sport as well as the importance of appearance, which is part of the subjective scoring system. The potential for disordered eating or eating disorders is high, and early intervention is imperative.

NUTRIENT INTAKE

The consumption of nutrient-dense foods is important, especially if overall energy intake is restricted. Many figure skaters are children and adolescents and need adequate nutrition to support growth and development.

AT A GLANCE

Football

American football is played by 2 teams of 11 players each. Each play involves some short-duration, high-intensity activity, and there is a short rest between plays. Professional football games have four 15-minute quarters with a halftime break, but the clock is frequently stopped during the course of gameplay, so each game takes about 4 hours to complete. Body composition varies by position, with receivers being lean and fast, whereas linemen depend on their strength and body mass to block. College football players usually have a smaller body mass than professional players and must increase size if they move into the professional ranks. Learn more about the sport at the National Football League website (www.nfl.com).

Common Nutritional Concerns

ENERGY INTAKE

Energy intake goals vary among athletes but can be more than 5,000 kcal/d. Many football players wish to change their body composition by increasing muscle mass (which may require a higher energy intake) or decreasing body fat.

OFFSEASON WEIGHT GAIN

Players need to match their offseason energy intake and balance it with energy expenditure. Some football players arrive at training camp or spring football practice overweight and out of shape. When this is the case, they often look for quick weight-loss methods. Some of these methods may be dangerous, such as voluntary dehydration, use of drugs thought to reduce body fat, and severe restriction of food intake. A nutrition and training plan implemented during the offseason can help athletes prevent unwanted weight gain.

HIGH FAT INTAKE

Some football players eat at restaurants frequently and consume a diet that is high in fat and high in saturated fat.

FLUID AND ELECTROLYTE INTAKE

Football players may play under hot, humid conditions, often early in the season before they are acclimated to the heat. Dehydration is a serious and potentially life-threatening problem. Sweating rates can be as high as 10 L/d, and a football player can lose as much as 12 lb of sweat in a practice session.

Hydration can be challenging because the weight of the uniform and pads presents an additional burden when players are exercising in the heat. If heat illness occurs, it is most likely to happen on the first day or 2 of preseason practice when players are not used to the heat. Fluid and electrolyte intakes must be balanced with losses. Approximately 10% of players may be cramp-prone because of substantial losses of sodium in sweat. As a result, they may need additional sodium in addition to fluids to prevent heat cramps.

GENERAL NUTRITION GUIDELINES

Energy
Energy expenditure varies depending on the level of the sport (professional, college, high school, or youth), level of training, amount of muscle mass, growth, and other factors and must be individually determined.

Carbohydrate
Recommended intake is more than 5 g per kilogram of body weight per day, and between 7 and 12 g per kilogram of body weight per day may be needed during rigorous training.

Protein
Recommended intake is between 1.4 and 1.7 g per kilogram of body weight per day.

Fat
The remainder of kilocalories should be consumed as fat, with an emphasis on heart-healthy fats.

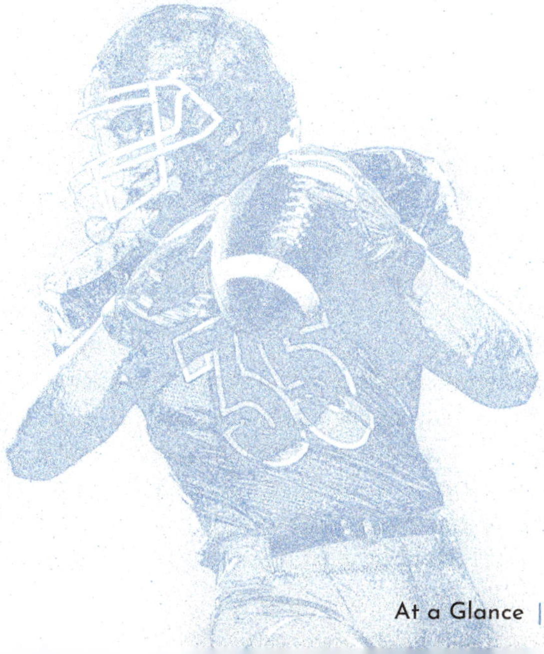

AT A GLANCE

Golf

Golf is a low-endurance, precision-skill sport. It requires fine-motor control and coordination. Swinging a club requires power, and walking the course requires general fitness, especially if the golfer is carrying clubs. Golf courses vary in length, but championship courses are approximately 6,000 to 7,000 yards, and an 18-hole course takes several hours to play. Females play shorter distances because of the location of the tees. Professional tournaments include 4 rounds (72 holes over 4 days), with additional holes played on the last day in the case of ties. Learn more about the sport at the websites of the Professional Golf Association (PGA) of America (www.pga.com) and the Ladies Professional Golf Association (www.lpga.com).

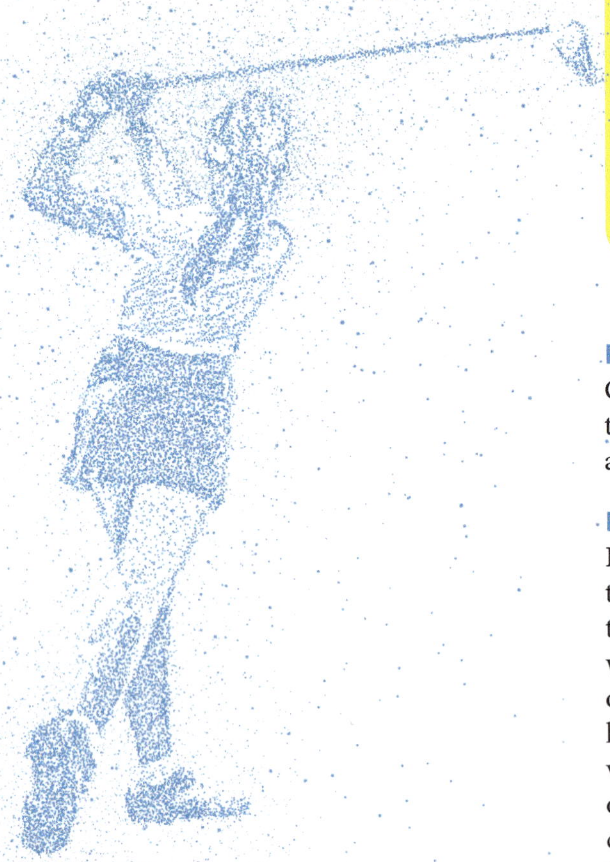

GENERAL NUTRITION GUIDELINES

Golfers do not have significantly increased demands for energy or nutrients; thus, general nutrient guidelines should be used and adjusted on an individual basis.

Energy
Golf is considered a relatively low-energy-expenditure sport.

Carbohydrate
Recommended intake is between 3 and 5 g per kilogram of body weight per day.

Protein
Recommended intake is between 1.2 and 1.7 g per kilogram of body weight per day (often closer to the lower end of this range).

Fat
Recommended intake is approximately 1.0 g per kilogram of body weight per day, or the remainder of kilocalories should be consumed as fat, with an emphasis on heart-healthy fats.

Common Nutritional Concerns

ENERGY INTAKE

The focus for golfers is typically on energy balance, although some players may wish to reduce energy intake to lose body fat. Slow weight loss should not affect performance, but severe restriction could lead to inadequate total energy intake and/or low blood glucose, which could negatively affect performance.

FLUID INTAKE

Golf often takes place under hot, humid conditions. Dehydration is a daily concern, and golfers are encouraged to consume fluids between holes.

PRECOMPETITION MEAL

Players need to eat a meal prior to play because they will be on the course for many hours. Start times vary and may be changed as a result of weather delays. Breakfast is vital because golfers often start early in the morning. Golfers should have a plan for a pregame meal that considers volume, macronutrient composition, and timing of intake that can be adjusted if the start time changes. In addition, they should avoid the high-fat and high-sugar foods at the halfway house or in the clubhouse. Golfers usually carry snacks, such as energy bars or sports drinks, to prevent hunger while on the course.

FREQUENT TRAVEL

Frequent travel makes it difficult to maintain a routine and increases exposure to high-calorie, low-nutrient-density foods.

AT A GLANCE

Gymnastics

Gymnastics involves activities that are typically characterized as short-duration and high-intensity to very high–intensity. In competition, athletes perform and then rest before beginning a new event. Gymnastics requires strength, power, and flexibility. Training is demanding, often involving many repetitions of individual skills or routines, but athletes can rest when it is not their turn to perform. Female gymnasts tend to be shorter and lighter than most other athletes and other females their age. A high percentage of lean body mass and a low percentage of body fat are desirable, not only because these body characteristics support the strength and power needed to excel at gymnastics skills but also because such bodies are considered aesthetically appealing. It is biologically easier for males to attain the currently held "ideal" body type than it is for females to do so. Learn more about the sport at the USA Gymnastics website (https://usagym.org).

Common Nutritional Concerns

ENERGY RESTRICTION

Despite the high energy demands of training, surveys suggest that many female gymnasts limit their energy intake. If loss of body fat is an appropriate goal, it must be slow, with small restrictions of energy, so that muscle mass can be protected and training will not be negatively affected.

BODY COMPOSITION

A low percentage of body fat, which may be difficult for females to attain or maintain, is considered necessary for success because of appearance and the physical demands of the sport. Amenorrhea may be present and is a warning sign associated with excessive energy restriction or anorexia. The potential for disordered eating and eating disorders is high, and early intervention is imperative.

NUTRIENT INTAKE

The consumption of nutrient-dense foods is important, especially if overall energy intake is restricted. Many gymnasts are children and adolescents and need adequate nutrition to support growth and development.

GENERAL NUTRITION GUIDELINES

Energy
Intake should be individualized based on body composition goals.

Carbohydrate
Recommended intake is between 3 and 7 g per kilogram of body weight per day.

Protein
Recommended intake is between 1.2 and 1.7 g per kilogram of body weight per day.

Fat
The remainder of kilocalories should be consumed as fat, with an emphasis on heart-healthy fats.

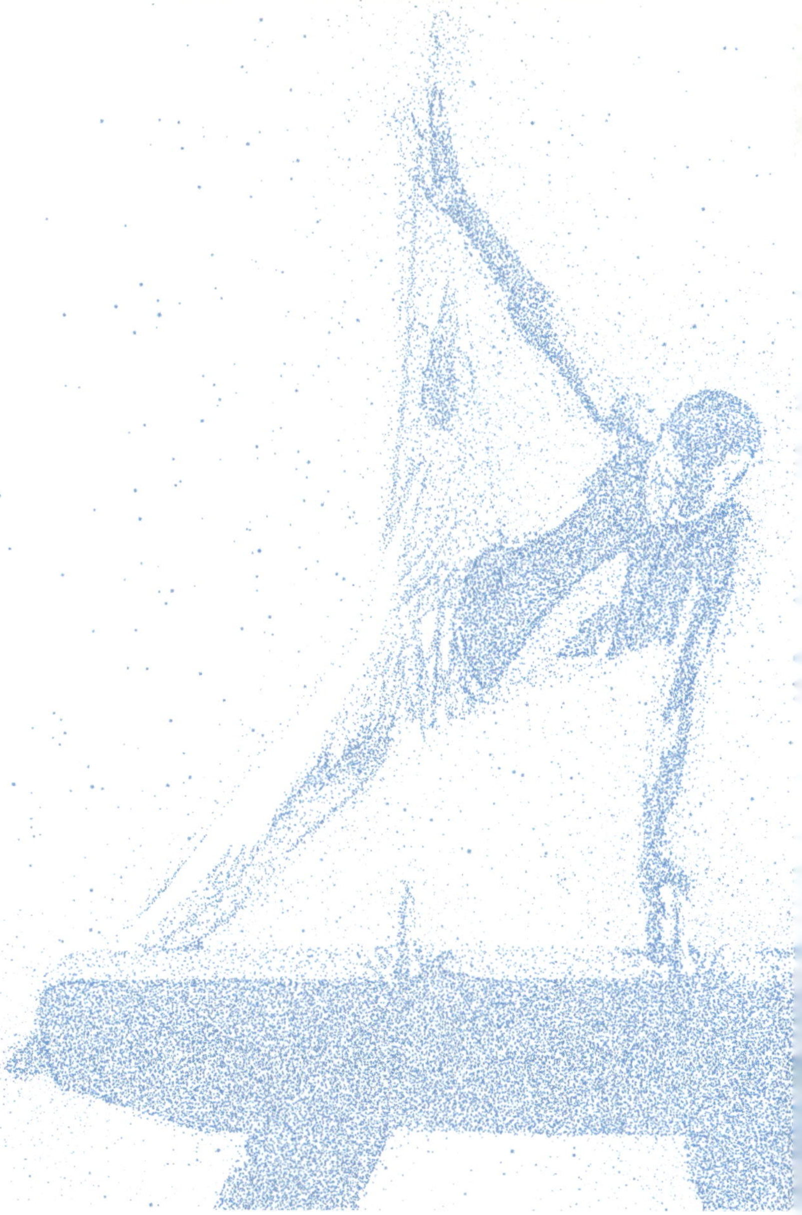

AT A GLANCE

Ice Hockey

Ice hockey requires anaerobic power, aerobic conditioning, strength, agility, and speed. Similarly to other intermittent, high-intensity sports, ice hockey involves constant changes in speed and direction, but ice hockey differs from soccer and basketball in that it also involves full body contact. A game consists of three 16-minute periods, but frequent player substitutions reduce playing time to about half of the overall game time. Learn more about the sport at the websites for the National Hockey League (www.nhl.com), USA Hockey (www.usahockey.com), and the Professional Women's Hockey League (www.thepwhl.com).

Common Nutritional Concerns

CARBOHYDRATE AND PROTEIN INTAKE

Hockey players need a large amount of carbohydrate daily to replenish glycogen used during demanding training sessions and games. Protein is also important to repair the wear and tear on muscles that occurs in hockey. Constant body-checking can take its toll on muscles, bones, tendons, and teeth.

HYDRATION DURING EXERCISE

Hydration during training and competition is important because players can sweat profusely under their gear even though they are on ice. Many hockey players spit out fluids instead of swallowing them. Sipping on fluids between shifts can help prevent dehydration and improve performance.

RESTORATION OF GLYCOGEN, FLUIDS, AND ELECTROLYTES

Demanding practices, games, and training sessions deplete glycogen, fluids, and electrolytes. Glycogen stores and fluid and electrolyte losses must be replenished beginning immediately after competition or training. Some postexercise protein consumption is also encouraged. Appetite may be depressed, so liquid meal replacements may become an important option.

GENERAL NUTRITION GUIDELINES

Energy
Recommended intake should be individualized and varies based on the level of training, but ice hockey is generally considered a high-energy-expenditure sport.

Carbohydrate
Recommended intake is more than 5 g per kilogram of body weight per day and should increase to between 8 and 10 g per kilogram of body weight per day during training and competition to ensure adequate glycogen in the quadriceps.

Protein
Recommended intake is between 1.4 and 1.7 g per kilogram of body weight per day.

Fat
The remainder of kilocalories should be consumed as fat, with an emphasis on heart-healthy fats.

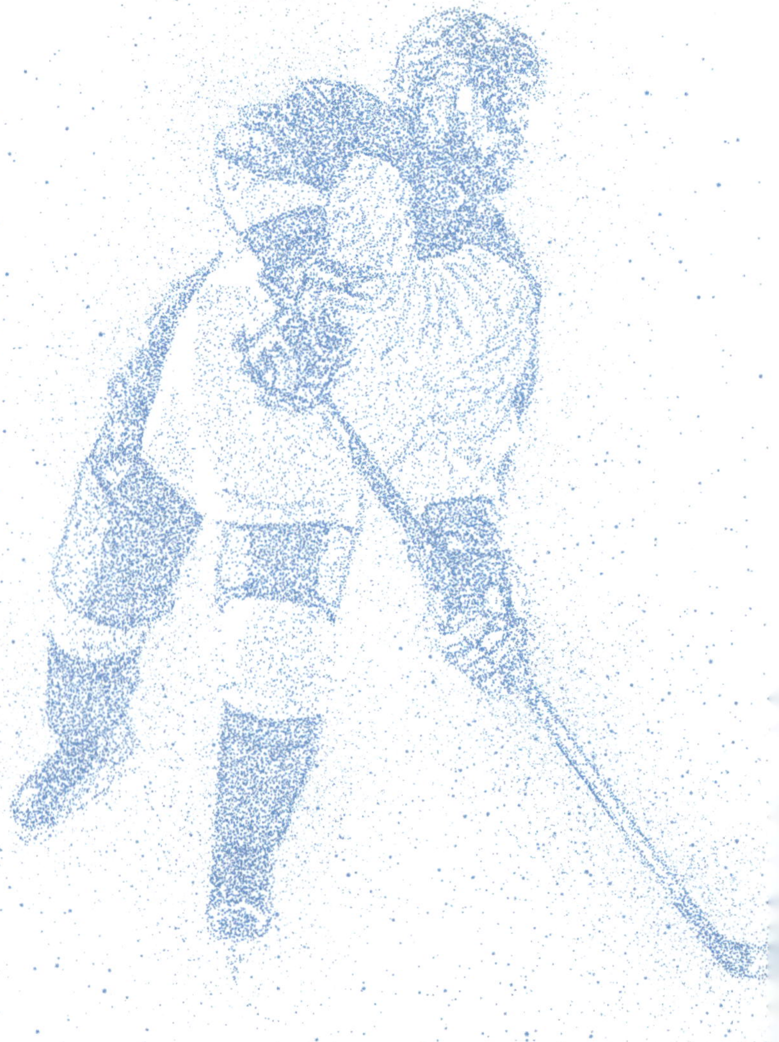

AT A GLANCE

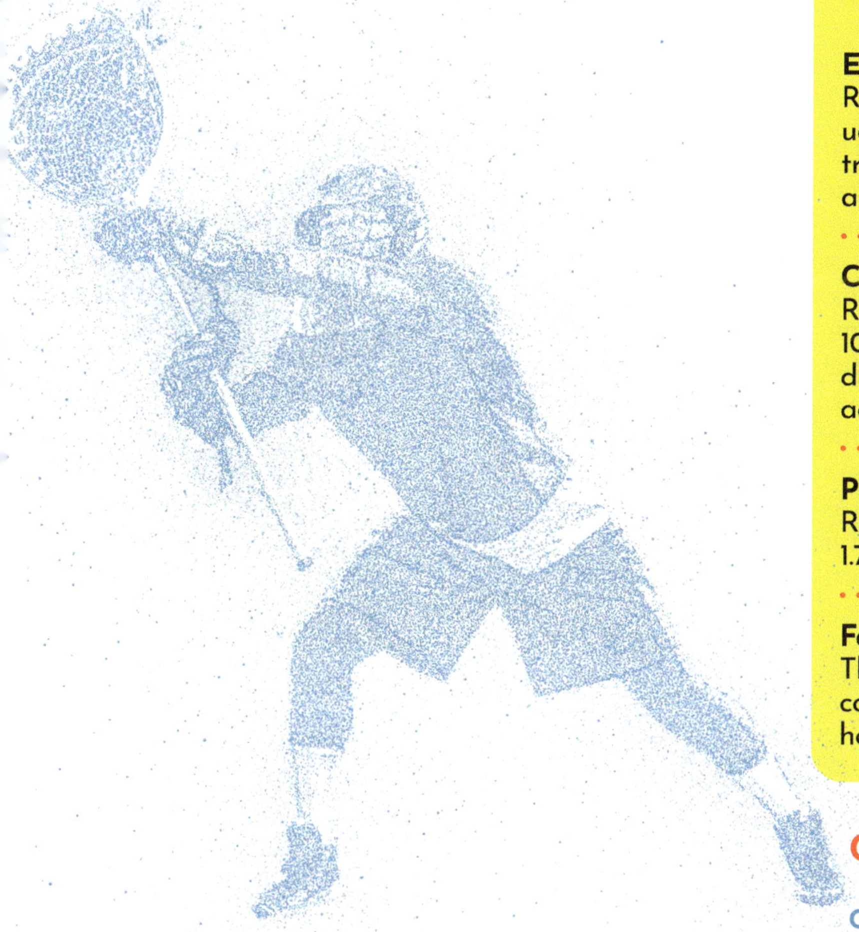

Lacrosse

Lacrosse requires anaerobic power, aerobic conditioning, strength, agility, and speed. Similarly to other intermittent, high-intensity sports, lacrosse involves constant changes in speed and direction, but lacrosse differs from soccer and basketball in that increased body contact occurs for male players (whereas women's lacrosse is considered a noncontact sport). A game generally consists of four 15-minute quarters (less for youth games) with a 2-minute break between quarters and a 10-minute break at halftime. Frequent player substitutions reduce playing time to about half of the overall game time. Learn more about the sport at the website of USA Lacrosse (www.usalacrosse.com).

GENERAL NUTRITION GUIDELINES

Energy
Recommended intake should be individualized and varies based on the level of training, but lacrosse is generally considered a high-energy-expenditure sport.

Carbohydrate
Recommended intake is between 5 and 10 g per kilogram of body weight per day during training and competition to ensure adequate glycogen.

Protein
Recommended intake is between 1.4 and 1.7 g per kilogram of body weight per day.

Fat
The remainder of kilocalories should be consumed as fat, with an emphasis on heart-healthy fats.

Common Nutritional Concerns

CARBOHYDRATE AND PROTEIN INTAKE

Lacrosse players need a large amount of carbohydrate daily to replenish glycogen used during demanding training sessions and games. Protein is also important to repair the wear and tear on muscles that occurs in lacrosse. In addition, the increased level of contact between male players can take a toll on muscles, bones, tendons, and teeth.

HYDRATION DURING EXERCISE

Hydration during training and competition is important because players can sweat profusely under their protective gear. Sipping on fluids between shifts can help prevent dehydration and improve performance.

RESTORATION OF GLYCOGEN, FLUIDS, AND ELECTROLYTES

Demanding practices, games, and training sessions deplete glycogen, fluids, and electrolytes. Glycogen stores and fluid and electrolyte losses must be replenished beginning immediately after competition or training. Some postexercise protein consumption is also encouraged. Appetite may be depressed, so liquid meal replacements may become an important option.

AT A GLANCE

Martial Arts

Martial arts is a broad term that describes several combat sports; boxing, fencing, judo, and tae kwon do may be the best known because they are Olympic sports, but there are hundreds of types of martial arts. Each martial art is different, but most involve strength, flexibility, and agility, and some also include explosive movements. Each martial art requires a strong level of mental and physical fitness. Many have weight classes, and some martial artists use a variety of methods to make weight. Participants in some competitions, such as judo and tae kwon do, compete several times over the course of a day. Learn more about these sports at the USA Dojo website (www.usadojo.com).

GENERAL NUTRITION GUIDELINES

Energy
Intake should be individualized based on body composition and weight goals.

Carbohydrate
Recommended intake is between 5 and 7 g per kilogram of body weight per day.

Protein
Recommended intake is between 1.2 and 1.7 g per kilogram of body weight per day.

Fat
The remainder of kilocalories should be consumed as fat, with an emphasis on heart-healthy fats.

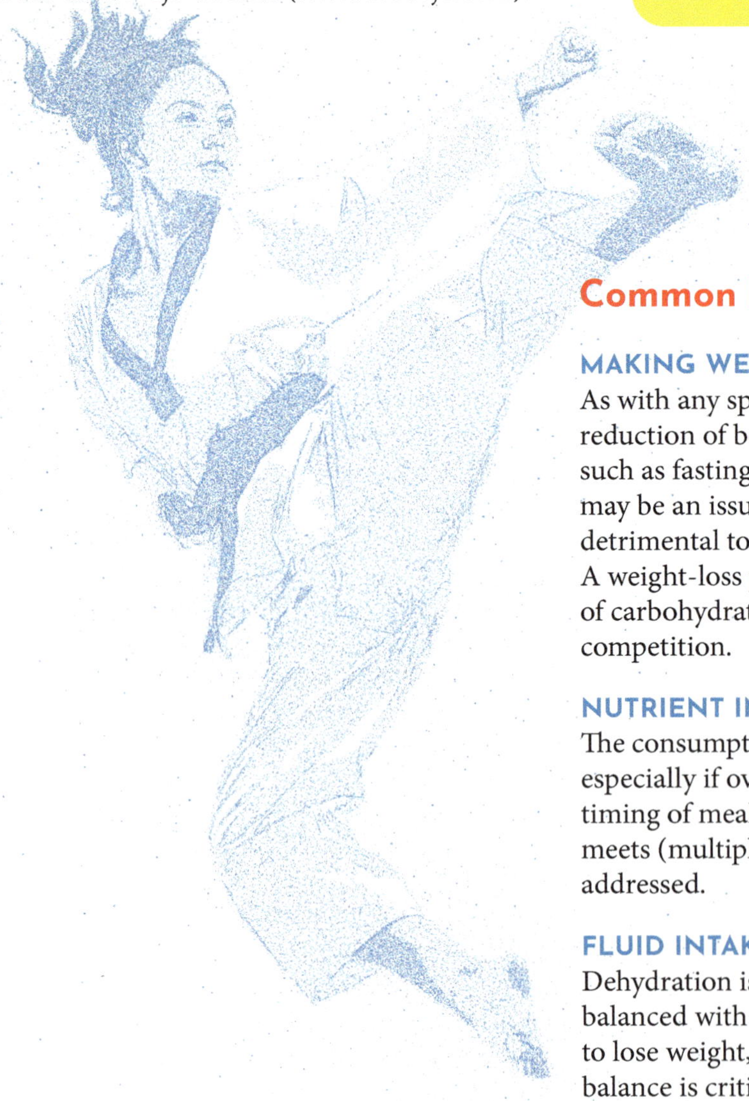

Common Nutritional Concerns

MAKING WEIGHT

As with any sport that has weight categories, rapid reduction of body weight, including extreme methods such as fasting, fluid restriction, and semistarvation, may be an issue. Rapid weight loss is more likely to be detrimental to performance than gradual weight loss. A weight-loss plan must allow for sufficient intakes of carbohydrate and protein to support training and competition.

NUTRIENT INTAKE

The consumption of nutrient-dense foods is important, especially if overall energy intake is restricted. The timing of meals and the adequacy of intake during meets (multiple bouts during 1 day) should be addressed.

FLUID INTAKE

Dehydration is a daily concern. Fluid losses should be balanced with fluid intake. If an athlete uses dehydration to lose weight, restoration of their fluid and electrolyte balance is critical.

AT A GLANCE

Rowing (Crew)

A typical crew race is 2,000 meters long; lasts for about 5.5 to 8 minutes; and requires strength, power, and endurance. The crew season begins in the fall with preseason training. Winter is a time of intense training and muscle building, and the spring racing season is known for its long daily practices leading up to a rest day and weekend competition. Summer is the offseason. The racing weight categories are lightweight and open (also called heavyweight). Learn more about the sport at the US Rowing website (www.usrowing.org).

GENERAL NUTRITION GUIDELINES

Energy
Rowing is considered a relatively high-energy-expenditure sport.

Carbohydrate
Recommended intake is between 5 and 7 g per kilogram of body weight per day.

Protein
Recommended intake is between 1.2 and 1.7 g per kilogram of body weight per day.

Fat
Recommended intake is approximately 1.0 g per kilogram of body weight per day.
Fat intake, in the form of heart-healthy fats, may be increased to meet high energy needs during training and should be decreased during the offseason.

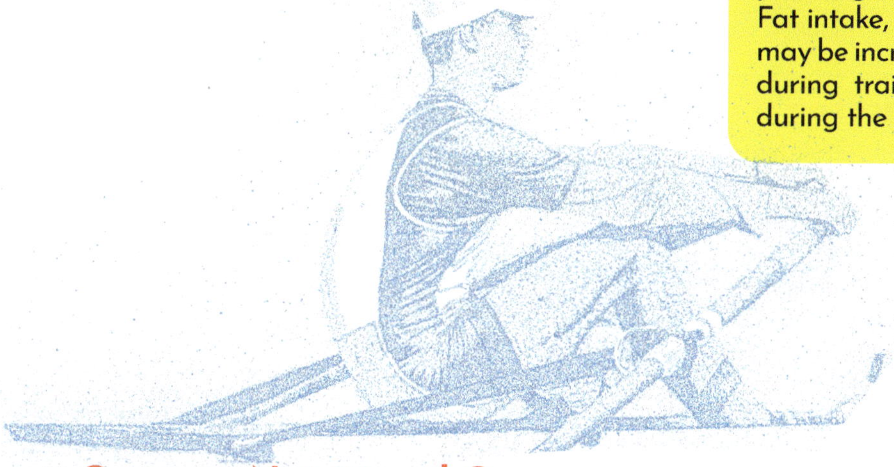

Common Nutritional Concerns

ENERGY INTAKE

Fatigue and lack of appetite may result in the involuntary underconsumption of energy. Lightweight rowers may voluntarily restrict energy intake to make weight.

MAKING WEIGHT

Lightweight rowers who are genetically lean and biologically small can comfortably meet the requirements for lightweight rowing. Problems with disordered eating and eating disorders occur when extraordinary efforts must be made to attain and maintain a low body weight. Voluntary dehydration may also be an issue. Learning to manage weight in the off-season is preferred to cutting weight during the season. Dangerous weight-cutting practices and disordered eating can be found in both male and female rowers.

CONSUMPTION OF FOODS WITH LOW NUTRIENT DENSITY

Rowers have high energy needs, and both male and female heavyweight rowers quickly discover that they must eat a lot of food to maintain their energy balance. High-fat, high-sugar snack foods and beverages can provide the energy needed but not the nutrients.

BALANCING FLUID INTAKE WITH FLUID LOSSES

Dehydration is a daily concern. Rowers have water bottles in the boat during training, but they do not have access to their water bottles during long training pieces (approximately 30–45 minutes each). It is unlikely that rowers can maintain fluid balance during training. Therefore, they should pay special attention to consuming sufficient fluids before and after training.

AT A GLANCE

Soccer

Soccer involves short, intense bursts of activity combined with moderately intense exercise and occasional rest periods. When soccer is played outdoors, the field is larger than a football field, and the average soccer player will cover between 8 and 12 km (between 5 and 7 miles) during a match. Each game consists of two 45-minute halves with a 15-minute halftime and may go into overtime, although the game is shorter for younger players. Learn more about the sport at the websites of US Soccer (www.ussoccer.com) and FIFA (Fédération Internationale de Football Association), the governing body of international soccer (www.fifa.com).

Common Nutritional Concerns

ENERGY INTAKE

Energy expenditure is high during training and games. A 75-kg male soccer player may expend more than 1,500 kcal during a game. Many players, both male and female, do not consume adequate energy, which can lead to the early onset of fatigue and poor nutrient intake.

FLUID INTAKE

Players should consume fluid early and at regular intervals during a game. Needs are especially high under hot, humid conditions. Consuming carbohydrate-electrolyte solutions during games is beneficial. Special attention should be paid to youth soccer players because they do not sweat as much as adults, so youths are at a higher risk for dehydration and heat illness. Youth players should consume fluid at least every 15 to 20 minutes during practice and frequently during games.

RESTORATION OF GLYCOGEN, FLUIDS, AND ELECTROLYTES

Glycogen stores and fluid and electrolyte losses must be replenished beginning immediately after competition or training. Soccer games are often scheduled close to each other with little time between games to replace muscle glycogen. Recovery nutrition helps soccer players make it through the season without fatigue. Some postexercise protein consumption is also encouraged. Appetite may be depressed, so liquid meal replacements may become an important option.

GENERAL NUTRITION GUIDELINES

Energy
Recommended intake should be individualized and varies based on the level of training, but soccer is considered a relatively high-energy-expenditure sport.

Carbohydrate
Recommended intake is approximately 5 g per kilogram of body weight per day and increases to between 7 and 12 g per kilogram of body weight per day during training and competition.

Protein
Recommended intake is between 1.4 and 1.7 g per kilogram of body weight per day

Fat
The remainder of kilocalories should be consumed as fat, with an emphasis on heart-healthy fats.

FREQUENT TRAVEL

Frequent travel makes it difficult to maintain a routine and increases exposure to foods that are high in calories but low in nutrient density.

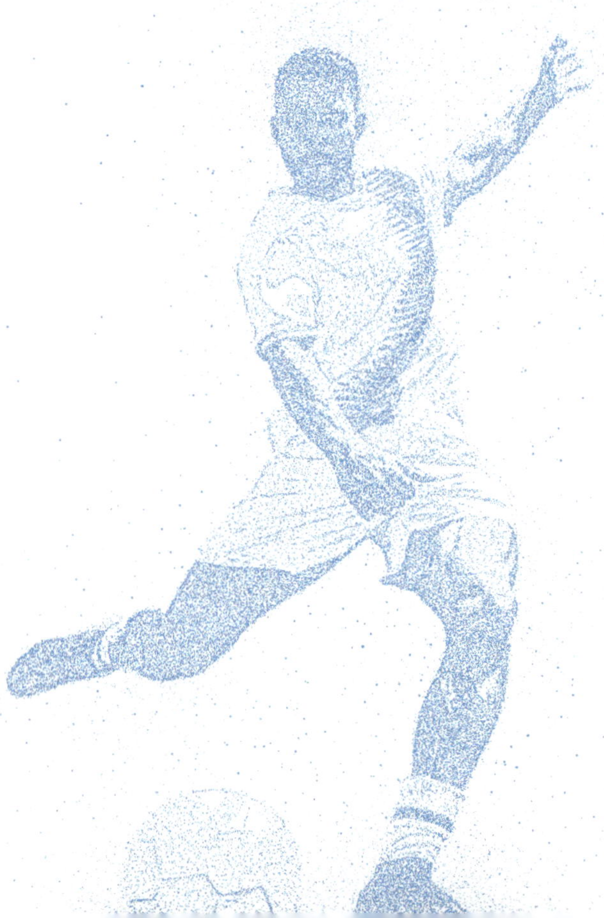

AT A GLANCE

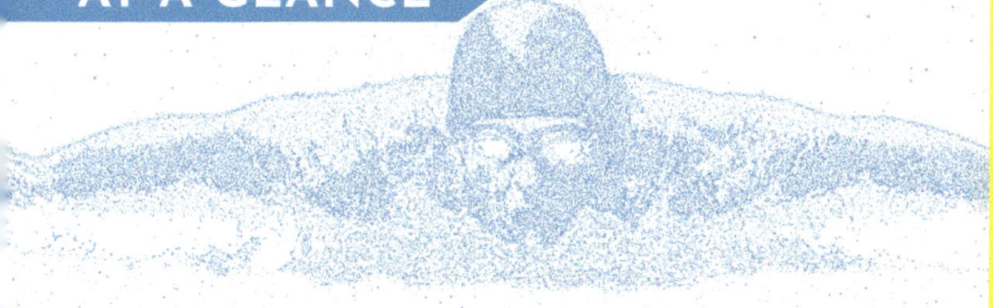

Swimming

Swimming is a sport of various intensities and durations. Swimming events include race lengths of 50 and 100 meters (sprints), 200 and 400 meters (middle distances), and 800 and 1,500 meters (distance). Long-distance swimming encompasses the swim portion of the full triathlon (2.4 miles) and ultraendurance events, such as swimming the English Channel (~24 miles). All swimmers have demanding training, so adequate daily energy and nutrient intakes are important. Learn more about the sport at the USA Swimming website (www.usaswimming.org).

Common Nutritional Concerns

ENERGY AND CARBOHYDRATE INTAKE

Energy and nutrient needs are high, and a well-balanced diet is important. Chronic undereating can be a problem. Swimmers often complain of chronic fatigue; hard training coupled with poor nutrition leads to fatigue. Athletes should aim for a minimum of 500 g of carbohydrate each day during the competitive season. Frequent meals and/or snacks are important.

FLUID INTAKE

Dehydration is a daily concern and can occur within 30 minutes of swimming. Many swimmers ignore fluid intake because they are surrounded by water, but the environmental conditions of swimming (warm pool water, warm air temperatures, and high humidity) can lead to dehydration.

RESTORATION OF GLYCOGEN, FLUIDS, AND ELECTROLYTES

Glycogen stores and fluid and electrolyte losses must be replenished beginning immediately after competition or training. Some postexercise protein consumption is also encouraged. Two-a-day swim practices are often conducted, and rapid replenishment of glycogen and fluid balance between practice sessions is critical.

GENERAL NUTRITION GUIDELINES

Recommendations must be tailored to the individual based on the level of training and the distance. Guidelines for long-distance swimming can be found under Endurance and Ultraendurance Sports in this At a Glance section. For swimming events ranging from 50 to 1,500 meters, the general guidelines include the following.

Energy
Intake should be individualized based on the demands of training.

Carbohydrate
Recommended intake is between 7 and 12 g per kilogram of body weight per day.

Protein
Recommended intake is between 1.2 and 1.7 g per kilogram of body weight per day.

Fat
Recommended intake is approximately 1.0 g per kilogram of body weight per day, or the remainder of kilocalories should be consumed as fat, with an emphasis on heart-healthy fats.

BODY COMPOSITION

A swimmer's appropriate percentage of body fat varies depending on the distance. Reducing body fat should be a slow process because too great of a reduction in energy, carbohydrate, and protein intakes can negatively affect training and performance.

RISK FOR DISORDERED EATING AND EATING DISORDERS

Swimmers are at risk for developing disordered eating and eating disorders. Refer the athlete to qualified health professionals when necessary.

AT A GLANCE

Tennis

Tennis requires anaerobic power, aerobic conditioning, strength, and agility. The game may be played casually or with great intensity and duration; thus, training and nutrient requirements vary tremendously. During a tennis match, 1 (singles) or 2 (doubles) players are on each side of the court. Male professional singles players must win 3 of 5 sets, and their singles matches typically last 2 to 4 hours. Females play the best of 3 sets, and their singles matches last, on average, between 1.5 and 3 hours. Most singles players hit from the baseline, and long rallies require excellent fitness. Most tournaments span 1 week, but major tournaments last 2 weeks. Most points in tennis take less than 10 seconds, but there are only 25 seconds of rest between points and 90 seconds between games, so endurance is needed for long matches. Tennis requires about 300 to 500 bursts of energy over the course of a match, so maintaining energy levels and hydration is critical for success. Recreational players play at a variety of intensities, and depending on the level of play, some do not have significantly increased demands for energy or nutrients. Learn more about the sport at the US Tennis Association website (www.usta.com).

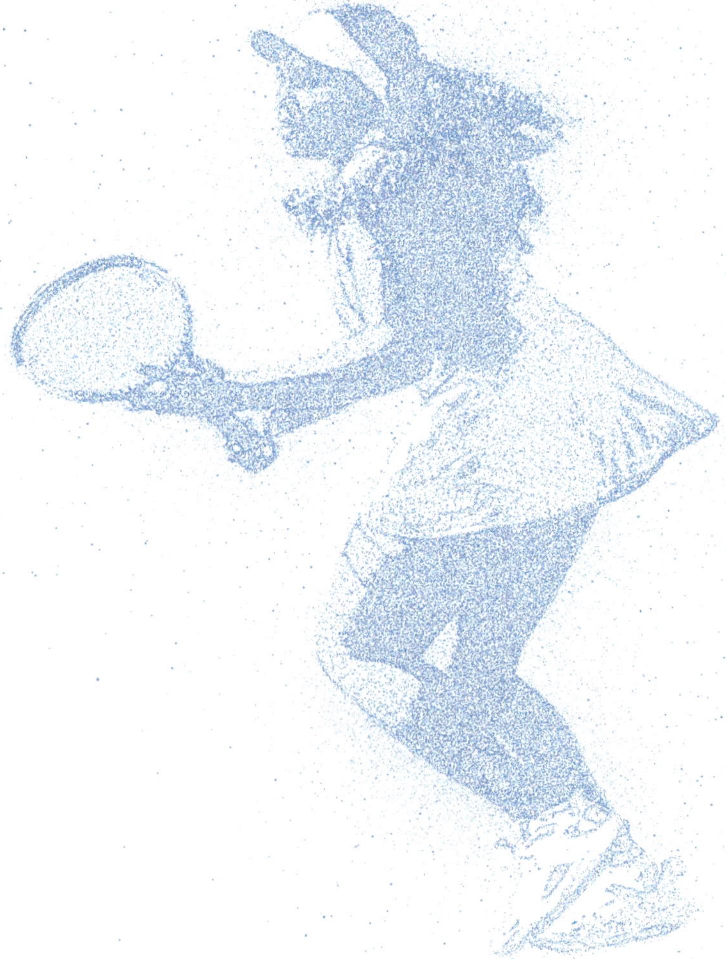

Common Nutritional Concerns

FLUID AND ELECTROLYTE INTAKE

Practice and play typically take place under hot and humid conditions. Dehydration is a daily concern. Some players may be cramp-prone as a result of large losses of sodium in sweat. These players may need additional sodium in addition to fluids to prevent heat cramps. Tennis players who are prone to cramps can try adding ½ teaspoon of table salt to 32 oz of sports drink, or they can choose an endurance formula sports drink, which will contain more sodium than a regular sports drink.

RESTORATION OF GLYCOGEN, FLUIDS, AND ELECTROLYTES

Demanding practices, training sessions, and match play deplete glycogen, fluids, and electrolytes. Glycogen stores and fluid and electrolyte losses must be replenished beginning immediately after competition or training. Some postexercise protein consumption is also encouraged. Near the end of a tournament, replenishment is especially important for peak performance.

GENERAL NUTRITION GUIDELINES

Energy
Recommendations vary depending on the level of training and the intensity and duration of play. Professional and collegiate players have high energy expenditures.

Carbohydrate
Recommended intake is between 7 and 12 g per kilogram of body weight per day.

Protein
Recommended intake is between 1.2 and 1.7 g per kilogram of body weight per day.

Fat
Recommended intake is approximately 1.0 g per kilogram of body weight per day, or the remainder of kilocalories should be consumed as fat, with an emphasis on heart-healthy fats.

PREMATCH MEAL

Tennis players, especially males, will be on the court for many hours, and they need to eat a meal before play. The start time may not be known (because of the length of other matches), and play may be stopped and restarted with short notice because of rain. Tennis players should have a plan for a prematch meal that considers volume, macronutrient composition, and timing of intake. The meal can be adjusted based on the actual start time.

MULTIPLE MATCHES IN 1 DAY

Tennis players may play more than 1 match in a day. This is especially true for younger athletes who compete in tournaments. Minimeals or snacks may be needed because sports drinks alone may not be substantial enough.

FREQUENT TRAVEL

Frequent travel makes it difficult to maintain a routine and increases exposure to foods are high in calories but low in nutrient density.

AT A GLANCE

Track Events

Track events range from the very fast 100-meter race to the much longer 10,000-meter run and 20,000-meter walking events. Nutrition recommendations must consider the distance involved. Daily workouts for track athletes are intense. Athletes may compete several times a day. For most short-duration, very high–intensity events, diet has less of an impact than other factors such as genetics and training. Compared with long-distance runners, middle-distance runners have more moderate carbohydrate needs. Learn more about the various track events and the demands of training at the USA Track & Field website (www.usatf.org).

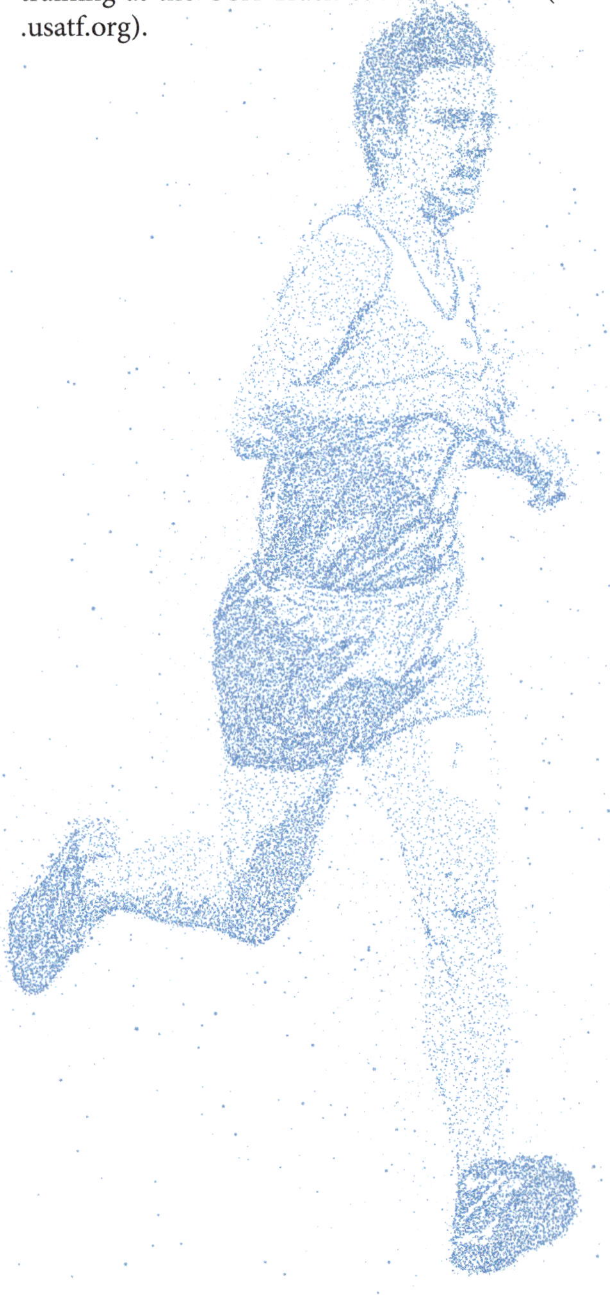

GENERAL NUTRITION GUIDELINES

Energy
Recommendations should be individualized based on body composition goals.

Carbohydrate
Experts recommend intake between 5 and 7 g per kilogram of body weight per day for very short-duration, very high-intensity events (100–400 m), recommended. For short-duration, high-intensity events (800–10,000 m), recommended intake is between 5 and 7 g per kilogram of body weight per day.

Protein
Recommended intake is between 1.2 and 1.7 g per kilogram of body weight per day.

Fat
Recommended intake is approximately 1.0 g per kilogram of body weight per day, or the remainder of kilocalories should be consumed as fat, with an emphasis on heart-healthy fats.

Common Nutritional Concerns

ENERGY INTAKE

In general, daily energy expenditure is high because of the demands of training. Reported daily intakes of track athletes are often less than estimated needs.

WEIGHT LOSS

High muscularity is valued, so many track athletes attempt to lose body fat. However, rapid weight loss is more likely to be detrimental to performance than gradual weight loss. A weight-loss plan must allow for the intake of sufficient carbohydrate and protein to support training.

POTENTIAL FOR DISORDERED EATING OR EATING DISORDERS

Pressure to attain or maintain a low percentage of body fat and an undue focus on body appearance increase the risk for athletes, particularly female middle-distance runners, to develop disordered eating or eating disorders.

AT A GLANCE

GENERAL NUTRITION GUIDELINES

Energy
Energy needs of volleyball players differ, depending on body size, the intensity of training, cross-training, and playing time, but in general, volleyball is a high-energy-expenditure sport.

Carbohydrate
Recommended intake is between 5 and 10 g per kilogram of body weight per day

Protein
Recommended intake is between 1.2 and 1.7 g per kilogram of body weight per day.

Fat
The remainder of kilocalories should be consumed as fat, with an emphasis on heart-healthy fats.

Volleyball

Volleyball is an intermittent, high-intensity sport requiring strength, power, cardiovascular fitness, agility, and skill. It is usually played as 3 or 5 sets of 25 points per set, but with the final set played to 15 points. With each set lasting approximately 25 to 30 minutes, an entire match can last from 75 to 150 minutes. Teams are allowed brief breaks between sets and may call timeouts during sets, which provide ample time to rest, refuel, and rehydrate. All of the body's energy systems are used to fuel the sport. Learn more about the sport at the website for USA Volleyball (https://usavolleyball.org).

Common Nutritional Concerns

CARBOHYDRATE AND PROTEIN INTAKE

Volleyball players need a large amount of carbohydrate daily to replenish glycogen used during demanding training sessions and games. Protein is also important to repair the wear and tear on muscles that occurs in volleyball.

FLUID INTAKE

Training and games are often held indoors in hot environments. Dehydration can lead to early fatigue and heat illness, so fluid intake should balance fluid losses.

RESTORATION OF GLYCOGEN, FLUIDS, AND ELECTROLYTES

Demanding practices, games, and training sessions deplete glycogen, fluids, and electrolytes. Glycogen stores and fluid and electrolyte losses must be replenished beginning immediately after competition or training. Some postexercise protein consumption is also encouraged. Appetite may be depressed, so liquid meal replacements may become an important option.

AT A GLANCE

Wrestling

Wrestling involves hand-to-hand combat and requires strength and stamina. A high power-to-weight ratio is desirable. Competitions are organized based on weight divisions, and some wrestlers make weight using drastic measures. Deaths have resulted from the combined use of a variety of techniques, including voluntary dehydration and starvation. Rule changes have been instituted to reduce excessive weight loss, including assessing body fat at the beginning of the season, determining a minimum competitive weight for each athlete, and holding weigh-ins close to the start of competition. No longer just a men's sport, women's wrestling became an Olympic sport in 2004, and the number of female wrestlers at the high school and collegiate levels is expected to grow. Learn more about the sport at the websites of USA Wrestling (https://themat.com), the National Collegiate Athletic Association (www.ncaa.com/sports/wrestling), and the National Federation of State High School Associations (www.nfhs.org/activities-sports/wrestling).

Common Nutritional Concerns

ENERGY INTAKE

Appropriate energy intake must be individually determined. A focus on performance and health, not just weight, can help wrestlers view energy intake from a positive perspective.

CUTTING WEIGHT OR MAKING WEIGHT

Weight-cutting practices can be severe and life-threatening, although new rules have been instituted to encourage less extreme weight-cutting behaviors than in the past. Collegiate wrestlers tend to use more extreme methods than high school wrestlers. Wrestlers in lower weight classes have relatively larger weight changes than those in heavier weight classes. Fasting, fluid restriction, and semistarvation are popular methods to make weight at all levels. Saunas, sweat suits (although banned), and diuretics may also be used. Nutrition counseling throughout the season is important to develop individualized plans, discuss weight loss methods, and monitor weight changes.

NUTRIENT INTAKE

The consumption of nutrient-dense foods is important, especially if overall energy intake is restricted. Wrestlers have demanding training programs, and sufficient macronutrient and micronutrient intakes are important to support training, performance, and health. Many wrestlers are adolescents and need adequate nutrition to support growth and development.

FLUID INTAKE

Dehydration is a daily concern. Fluid losses should be balanced with fluid intake. If dehydration is used as a weight-loss method, restoration of the athlete's fluid and electrolyte balance is critical. Some wrestlers believe that they can lose weight for the weigh-in and then rehydrate before a match. This is a false belief because it takes up to 6 hours for a body to reach normal hydration.

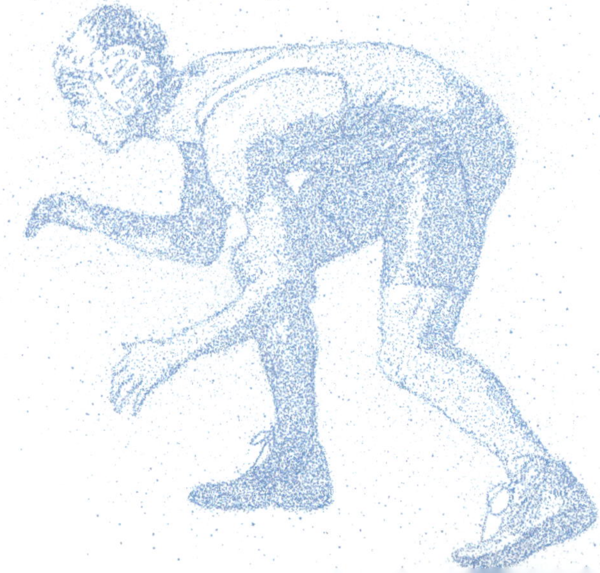

GENERAL NUTRITION GUIDELINES

Energy
Recommendations should be individualized based on body composition and weight goals.

Carbohydrate
Recommended intake is between 5 and 7 g per kilogram of body weight per day.

Protein
Recommended intake is between 1.2 and 1.7 g per kilogram of body weight per day. Protein requirements may increase to 2 g per kilogram of body weight per day during periods of lowest overall energy intake planned to achieve weight loss.

Fat
The remainder of kilocalories should be consumed as fat, with an emphasis on heart-healthy fats.

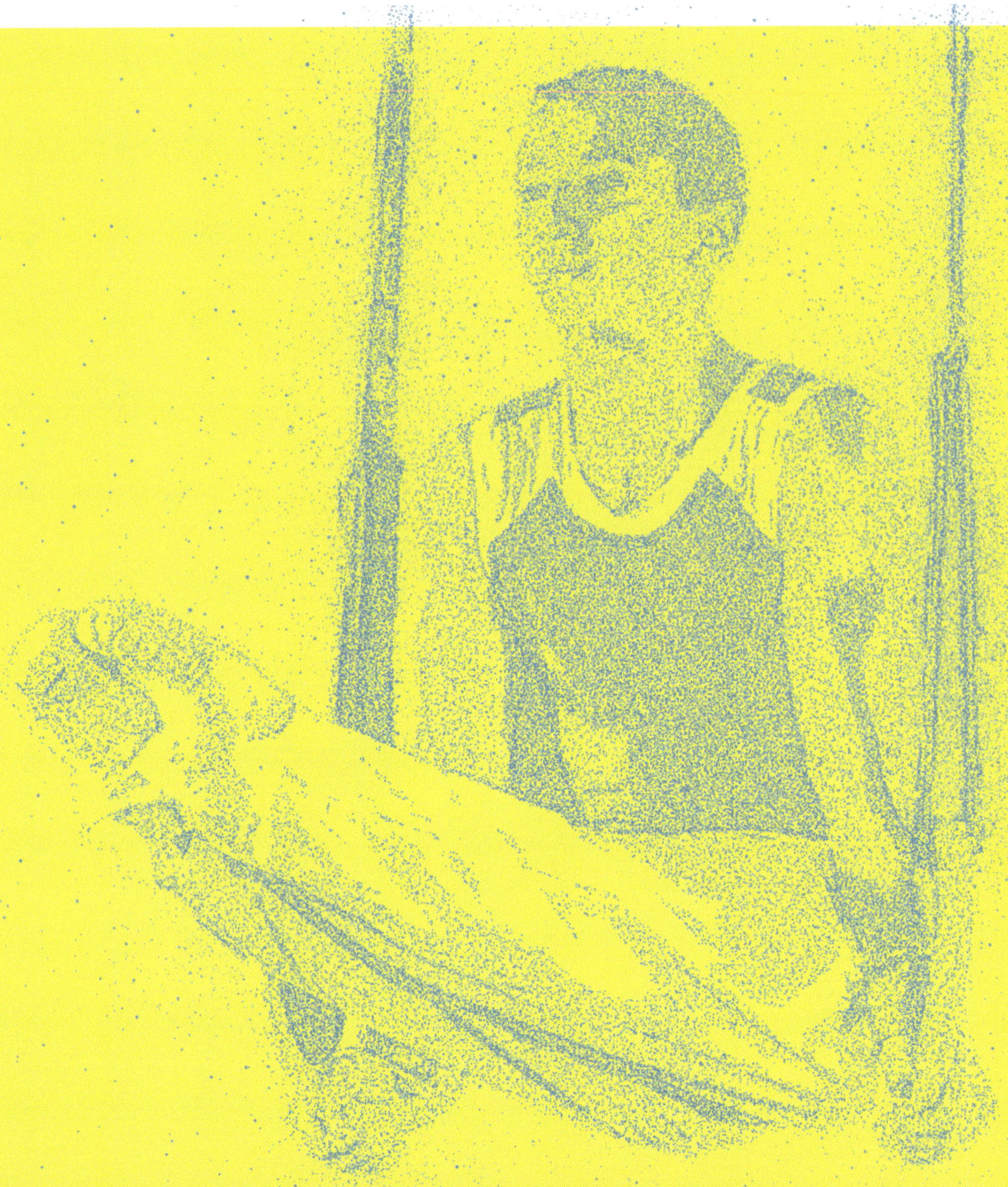

APPENDIXES

This section includes 2 helpful appendixes designed to support and expand on the core material presented in this textbook. Appendix A provides a selection of position statements, position stands, and consensus statements from leading organizations in sports nutrition. These documents reflect current expert recommendations and serve as authoritative resources for evidence-based practice. Appendix B offers a list of reputable websites related to sports nutrition, including professional organizations, research institutions, and educational platforms, to facilitate continued learning and access to up-to-date information.

Appendix A

SELECTED SPORTS NUTRITION-RELATED POSITION STATEMENTS, POSITION STANDS, AND CONSENSUS STATEMENTS

ACADEMY OF NUTRITION AND DIETETICS POSITION PAPERS

The Academy of Nutrition and Dietetics posts a number of position papers on www.eatrightpro.org. These papers are constantly evaluated and, if expired, archived via the *Journal of the Academy of Nutrition and Dietetics.* Visit www.eatrightpro.org/practice/guidelines-and-positions/academy-positions for current position papers.

AMERICAN COLLEGE OF SPORTS MEDICINE POSITION STANDS

The following position stands are available from www.acsm.org:

- Nutrition and Athletic Performance (Joint Position Statement of the Academy of Nutrition and Dietetics, Dietitians of Canada, and the American College of Sports Medicine)
- Exercise and Type 2 Diabetes (Joint Position Statement with the American Diabetes Association)
- Exercise and Physical Activity for Older Adults
- Appropriate Physical Activity Intervention Strategies for Weight Loss and Prevention of Weight Regain for Adults
- The Female Athlete Triad
- Exertional Heat Illness during Training and Competition
- Prevention of Cold Injuries During Exercise
- Exercise for Patients With Coronary Artery Disease
- Exercise and Fluid Replacement
- Physical Activity and Bone Health
- Exercise and Hypertension
- Weight Loss in Wrestlers

NATIONAL ATHLETIC TRAINERS' ASSOCIATION POSITION STATEMENTS

The following position statements are available from www.nata.org:

- Fluid Replacement for the Physically Active
- Exertional Heat Illnesses
- Evaluation of Dietary Supplments for Performance Nutrition
- Safe Weight Loss and Maintenance Practices in Sport and Exercise
- Preventing, Detecting, and Managing Disordered Eating in Athletes
- Management of the Athlete With Type I Diabetes Mellitus

INTERNATIONAL OLYMPIC COMMITTEE CONSENSUS STATEMENTS

The following consensus statements are available from the *Journal of the International Society of Sports Nutrition* at www.tandfonline.com/journals/rssn20/collections/issn-position-stands:

- Relative Energy Deficiency in Sport (REDs)
- Dietary Supplements and the High-Performance Athlete
- Recommendations and Regulations for Sport Events in the Heat

INTERNATIONAL SOCIETY OF SPORTS NUTRITION POSITION STANDS

The following position stands are available from www.sportsnutritionsociety.org:

- Diets and Body Composition
- Probiotics

SPORTS DIETITIANS AUSTRALIA POSITION STATEMENTS

The following position statements are available from www.sportsdietitians.com.au:

- Nutrition for Exercise in Hot Environments
- Sports Nutrition for the Adolescent Athlete
- Disordered Eating in High Performance Sport (Joint Position Statement of the Australian Institute of Sport and National Eating Disorders Collaboration)

These are not exhaustive lists. At the time of publication, all URLs were correct.

Appendix B

SPORTS NUTRITION-RELATED WEBSITES

This appendix lists websites that may be valuable to sports dietitians and other health professionals. The inclusion of a website does not constitute an endorsement of that site.

- Academy of Nutrition and Dietetics: www.eatright.org and www.eatrightpro.org
  - Sports and Human Performance Nutrition Dietetic Practice Group: www.shpndpg.org
- Amateur Athletic Union: www.aausports.org
- American College of Sports Medicine: www.acsm.org
- American Council on Exercise: www.acefitness.org
- American Diabetes Association: www.diabetes.org
- American Medical Society for Sports Medicine: www.amssm.org
- Athletics and Fitness Association of America: www.afaa.com
- Australian Sports Commission's Australian Institute of Sport: www.ausport.gov.au
- Body Positive: www.bodypositive.com
- American Sports and Performance Dietitians Association: www.sportsrd.org
- Dietitians of Canada: www.dietitians.ca
- Endurance Nation: www.endurancenation.us
- Gatorade Sports Science Institute: www.gssiweb.org/en
- IDEA Health & Fitness Association: www.ideafit.com
- Korey Stringer Institute at University of Connecticut: https://koreystringer.institute.uconn.edu
- National Athletic Trainers' Association: www.nata.org
- National Collegiate Athletic Association: www.ncaa.com
- National Eating Disorders Association: www.nationaleatingdisorders.org
- National Recreation and Park Association: www.nrpa.org
- Nicholas Institute of Sports Medicine and Athletic Trauma: www.nismat.org
- Olympic Games: www.olympics.com
- Physical Activity Guidelines for Americans: https://odphp.health.gov/our-work/nutrition-physical-activity/physical-activity-guideliness
- Runner's World: www.runnersworld.com
- SHAPE America Society of Health and Physical Education-Society of Health and Physical Educators: www.shapeamerica.org
- ShapeUpUS.org: https://shapeupus.org
- Special Olympics: www.specialolympics.org
- Sports Dietitians Australia: www.sportsdietitians.com.au
- SportsOracle: www.sportsoracle.com

- **Sports Science Insights:** www.sportsscienceinsights.com
- **The Vegetarian Resource Group:** www.vrg.org
- **US Anti-Doping Agency:** www.usada.org
- **World Anti-Doping Agency:** www.wada-ama.org/en
- **World Ultra Cycling Association** (formerly UltraMarathon Cycling Association): ultracycling.com

At the time of publication, all URLs were correct.

Continuing Professional Education and Additional Notes

Sports Nutrition: A Handbook for Professionals, 7th edition, offers readers Continuing Professional Education (CPE) credit. Please check the expiration date and the number of hours offered at the link below, on the product page at www.eatrightSTORE.org, or at the QR code below. Readers may earn credit by completing the interactive online quiz at:

https://publications.webauthor.com/SN_7e

The Academy of Nutrition and Dietetics Product Strategy & Revenue Operations team can be reached by email at publications@eatright.org. Additional notes, errata, related products, and information on licensing and permissions can be found on the product page at www.eatrightSTORE.org or at the QR code below.

Index

B

C

D

E

F

G

H

I

O

P

Q

R

S

T

U

V

W

Y

Z